Integrative Medicine in Veterinary Practice

Integrative Medicine in Veterinary Practice

Lisa P. McFaddin *DVM, GDCVHM, CVSMT, CVMRT, FCoAC, CVA, CVFT*

Caring Hands Animal Hospital,
Bristow, USA

WILEY Blackwell

Library of Congress Cataloging-in-Publication Data
Names: McFaddin, Lisa P. (Lisa Pinn), author.
Title: Integrative medicine in veterinary practice / Lisa P. McFaddin.
Description: First edition. | Hoboken, New Jersey : Wiley-Blackwell, [2024]
  | Includes bibliographical references and index.
Identifiers: LCCN 2024000369 (print) | LCCN 2024000370 (ebook) |
  ISBN 9781119879541 (hardback) | ISBN 9781119879572 (adobe pdf) |
  ISBN 9781119879565 (epub)
Subjects: MESH: Animal Diseases | Integrative Medicine | Complementary
  Therapies–veterinary
Classification: LCC SF745.5 (print) | LCC SF745.5 (ebook) | NLM SF 745.5
  | DDC 636.089/55–dc23/eng/20240124
LC record available at https://lccn.loc.gov/2024000369
LC ebook record available at https://lccn.loc.gov/2024000370

Cover Images: Courtesy of Lisa P. McFaddin
Cover Design: Wiley

Set in 9.5/12.5pt STIXTwoText by Straive, Chennai, India

SKY10070156_032024

To my parents who have always supported me and my harebrained endeavors. See dad, it's a good thing I never worked at Blockbuster.

To my key and my husband. Thank you for harmonizing, encouraging, and loving me.
To my son, who will be so glad his mom does not spend every spare minute in her office typing, thank you for not letting me take myself too seriously.

Contents

Preface

My Story

Most of my childhood memories center around being eight years old. During this time my dad said "Lisa, you seem to like animals a lot: you should be a veterinarian." As your classic goal-oriented type-A personality when presented with a challenge, I saddled up, buckled down and committed until the job was done. You often hear veterinarians describe a calling to help those who cannot help themselves, to care for the innocent, or an innate preference for non-human company. While I agree with these sentiments and love animals, at its core I became a veterinarian because the proposition seemed like an exciting and difficult pursuit.

I then spent the better part of my adolescence and young adult life with one mission: *Get into vet school*. I studied like crazy in high school. I attended a liberal arts college for my undergraduate studies, in large part to appear cultured on my application. I worked summers as a kennel and veterinary assistant at multiple animal hospitals trying to sponge up as much information and experience as possible.

Thankfully I was accepted on my first attempt. I was technically wait-listed, and in a non-dramatic fashion decided I would give up vet med and move to a remote island and open a craft store. That was until I was accepted and suddenly my island lifestyle seemed impractical.

With all the effort to get into vet school, I never gave much thought to what I would do afterward. While in high school I volunteered at a local animal shelter for two years. As this was my first veterinary "job" there was a huge learning curve. It was here I learned how to properly restrain animals, to interpret animal behavior, to clean lots and lots of poop, to cherish the moment when a cat or dog found their forever home, and the sadness associated with mass euthanasia due to overcrowding. During this time, I became the lead euthanasia assistant. One of my primary jobs was to inventory the shelter at least once a month, noting which cats and dogs had been there the longest, were ill, or had behavioral issues. This "kill list" was given to the shelter veterinarian. The doctor would euthanize the pet while I held. Some days we would have to cull over 15 animals. As you can imagine this is a lot for anyone to handle, especially someone whose frontal cortex had not yet fully formed. I only worked in this position for a couple of months. Eventually the stress and grief became too taxing, and I took reprieve in a summer job working at a greenhouse. The thought of being the doctor performing those mass euthansias was too much, and I decided shelter work was not for me.

Academia had and has always interested me. I love that light bulb moment when a student, intern, or team member understands a new concept or solves a puzzle. There is nothing more rewarding than contributing to another human being's "aha" moment. While I find the time in the lecture hall and clinics thrilling, I have trepidations regarding research. I have never considered myself a talented science writer, mostly because the necessity for brevity eludes me. To top it all off the dog-eat-dog nature of research funding seems too exhausting, so academia was out.

I have always loved neurology; there is something about the logicality of the field that soothes my need for structure and order. I am not, however, a fan of surgery in any form, especially surgeries which require drills and dissecting microscopes. I am also impatient and find the waiting period from first cut to the appearance of the spinal cord or brain excruciating. As an aside when I was an intern, during my first neurosurgery I tried too hard to impress the clinician. I attempted to set up the surgical suite myself. I, of course, threw the wrong end of the drill cord off the surgery table which, as you can imagine, did not a happy neurologist make. I spent the remainder of that neurology rotation on pins and needles trying not to screw up any more procedures. I did master the ability to make the most perfectly tiny bone wax balls and the smallest slices of gel foam.

Like many vet students, without a clue as to what to do once I graduated, I decided to delay my adulting decisions and pursue an internship. My then boyfriend, now husband, and I packed up our two cats, brand new puppy, and two 5-gal buckets of saltwater fish and drove 14 hours from Blacksburg, Virginia to Northbrook, Illinois for my one year rotating surgical–medical internship. While my internship year was most comparable to a year-long poorly paid hazing event, I did learn an incredible amount about being a veterinarian, trusting myself, and developing a tougher exterior shell.

Unfortunately, I still had not figured out what I wanted to do when I grew up. Over the next seven years I worked as a general practitioner, relief emergency veterinarian, and eventually created my own relief business. During this time, I still felt lost, and slightly disenfranchised by veterinary medicine. I was not prepared for the financial reality of how veterinarians are paid and the gravity of paying back my student loans. I also began to find the routine of general practice mundane. Before I created my relief business, I decided to study veterinary acupuncture as a way to carve out my own niche within a veterinary practice and hopefully increase my production numbers.

When choosing an acupuncture school, I decided to go big or go home. I wanted to immerse myself in this new field of study and who better to learn from then Dr. Xie at Chi University. During my studies my dog fell ill with a fungal infection, Blastomycosis, and the treatment nearly fried his liver. I used all my Western tools, but his liver values worsened. I decided to incorporate acupuncture, and with the help of my instructors added in Chinese herbal medicine and Chinese food therapy. Amazingly, his liver values improved, he got better and even thrived. He had more energy, his coat was softer, and he seemed happier. I also started using my acupuncture training when working emergency and general practice. I noticed a pattern. My patients improved faster with the incorporation of acupuncture. One of the beauties of working with animals is the general absence of placebo effect.

At that point I was hooked. Learning various aspects of integrative medicine was like eating potato chips: I could not have just one. After completing my acupuncture training over the next four years I studied Chinese food therapy (Chi University), Chinese herbal medicine (College of Integrative Veterinary Therapies), and veterinary spinal manipulation therapy (Healing Oasis). And most recently I completed my veterinary massage and rehabilitation therapy training (Healing Oasis). I would joke that while some people collected shoes, I was collecting initials. This alphabet soup of initials resulted in one client dubbing me Dr. LOL (Lots of Letters).

My diagnostic and treatment abilities improved greatly because of my integrative training. Figure 1 depicts me hard at work with one of my favorite bulldogs. My physical examinations seemed more thorough. My patients seemed healthier and happier. My clients

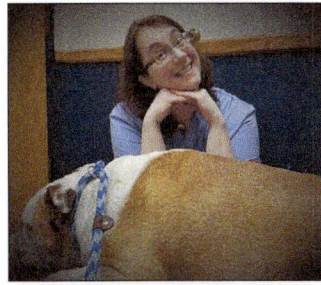

Figure 1 Myself working tirelessly with one of my integrative patients, Seamus. Source: Lisa P. McFaddin.

seemed more engaged and satisfied. Don't get me wrong, it has not been all puppies and daisies. I still have setbacks, frustrations, stubborn never-resolving cases. But I love that I have more options for treating my patients. I am grateful for the knowledge I have gained about veterinary medicine, my patients, and myself. I will never stop learning and trying to improve. Besides there are still a few initials I would like to add to my collection.

My Pet Tales

Scientific evidence, highlighting the benefits of each modality, is referenced throughout the book. Before we delve into the nitty-gritty, I thought an old-fashioned Top 10 list describing the ways in which my own pets have benefited

from integrative medicine would be appropriate. And yes, I know testimonials are not a form of evidence-based medicine. I would, however, argue there is still benefit in hearing the owner's stories and experiences.

Top 10 Personal Pet Tales

1. **Lysine + ocular herpes**: Since adoption my first-born, a tuxedo kitty named Ringo (Figure 2) would have periodic ocular herpes outbreaks. I would come home to find him squinty- and puffy-eyed with thick goopy discharge. Within a month of starting daily lysine therapy, the outbreaks lessened in severity and duration, and eventually stopped. And yes, I am aware a systematic review of lysine supplementation by Bol and Bunnik (2015) found no evidence the amino acid has antiviral properties and could increase the frequency and severity of infection. Additionally, correlation does not equal causation and it is possible the outbreak would have self-resolved. But as this was my first experience as a veterinary student with animal supplements it left a lasting impression.

2. **Acupuncture + tail pain**: Winston, my then six-year-old beagle mix pictured in Figure 3, woke up one morning and could not lift or wag his tail. This was limber tail

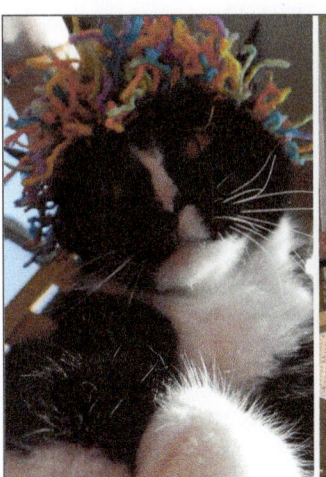
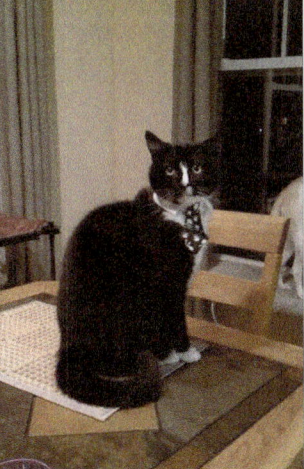

Figure 2 This was my tuxedo domestic shorthair "Ringo Rooney-Face." I adopted him my first year of vet school from an undergrad who could not handle an eight-week-old kitten. His favorite pastimes include hiding toys and trinkets in my shoes and listening to his own echo when he screams at the top of his lungs in the shower at 3 a.m. Sadly, Ringo passed two months shy of his 18th birthday. Source: Lisa P. McFaddin.

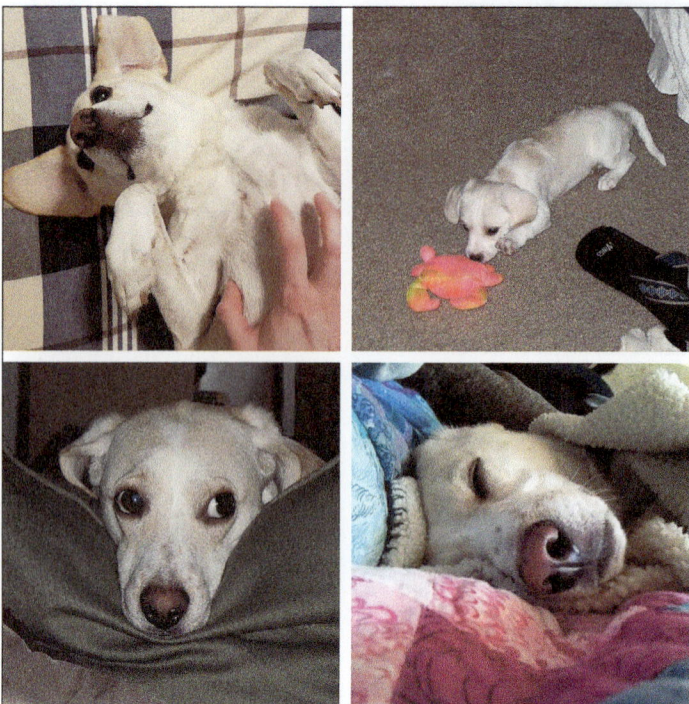

Figure 3 This was my beagle-mix "Sir Winston Poopy Pants." He was born in a research laboratory at my alma mater, Virginia Maryland College of Veterinary Medicine. He was part of a multidisciplinary study evaluating the effects of hypothyroidism on fertility. He was one of seven puppies in his litter who all turned seven weeks old the day the fourth years found out we had passed our boards. Nothing says "I need a puppy" like finding out you are going to be a veterinarian. Sadly, Winston passed shortly after his 15th birthday. Source: Lisa P. McFaddin.

gone crazy. He would banshee scream and beagle howl whenever he had to defecate. Radiographs were unremarkable, and no neurologic abnormalities were found, aside from pain. All traditional treatments failed: anti-inflammatories, opioids, steroids, gabapentin, amantadine, and methocarbamol. I was about halfway through my acupuncture training, so I only knew a few points. Within 24 hours of acupuncturing around the tail base he could poop without screaming. Within one week, after two additional treatments, he could raise his tail and wag like crazy without so much as a whimper.

3. **Chinese herbs + liver enzyme elevations**: While on oral antifungals for his second blastomycosis infection, Winston developed this insatiable thirst and a rotary sprinkler-like urinary habit. (In veterinary medicine we routinely call increased thirst polydipsia and increased urination polyuria. The combination of both issues is called PU/PD.) Recheck blood work showed his liver enzymes had spiked. Unfortunately, the PU/PD and liver values did not improve with the implementation of standard liver supplements. Knowing I could not stop the antifungals, for fear of a relapse, I felt lost. Amid my acupuncture training, and long before I started my Chinese veterinary herbal medicine training, I spoke with my acupuncture instructors who advised the use of a Chinese herbal formula. Within three weeks of starting the herbs his PU/PD normalized. Six weeks after starting the herbs his liver enzymes were almost half their original value. Within nine weeks his

liver values were normal and remained normal for the rest of the antifungal treatment, which lasted another three months.

4. **New food + food aversion**: Winston used to despise eating his kibble, especially if the pieces touched. I finally resorted to using a puzzle ball to feed him. He could bat it around and eat one kibble at a time. Every meal took a solid 20 minutes to ingest. During his second round of oral antifungal medications, he lost all interest in food. With the help of an integrative mentor, we developed a food plan with the goal of supporting his weakened immune and digestive systems. He started with a nutritionally balanced home-cooked diet then transitioned to a combination of home-cooked and dehydrated. For the first time in six years, he ate every meal with gusto. He also developed a very reliable internal meal timer, alerting all who would listen when it was time for breakfast and dinner.

5. **Acupuncture + food poisoning**: Returning home one morning, from a 14-hour overnight shift during my internship, my husband hugged me as we passed in the hallway of our apartment building. Walking away I heard him say "I think something's wrong with the dog." In my fog of sleep deprivation, I was unable to ask questions before he was out the door and on his way. Crossing the threshold, the unmistakable smell of vomit and diarrhea saturated my nasal cavities. Turned out my well-meaning husband had shared some questionably old turkey deli meat. As a beagle, my dog is a huge wimp when sick or injured. He becomes fly-paper clingy and snaps at the thought of pain which, unfortunately, makes him a less than ideal candidate for acupuncture. I sat with him on the floor while he belched and off gassed. When he was not looking, I placed acupuncture needles in his back and pelvic limbs. If he noticed and whipped his head around, I would pause

until he put his head back down. Ten minutes after needle placement he let out the loudest dog fart, which was impressive given his lack of butt cheeks. Fifteen minutes after needle placement he groaned, burped, and fell asleep. After 20 minutes I removed the needles. My exhaustion, coupled with the threat of another overnight shift in a few short hours, prevented movement. My dog and I slept on the floor together for at least four hours. When we awoke, he asked to go outside. He urinated but did not defecate. Happily, he did not have another bout of diarrhea or vomiting, and by dinner time he readily ate his bland diet.

6. **Chiropractic + lumbosacral spondylosis**: Prior to taking X-rays I thought Ringo's reluctance to jump was due to hip arthritis. But the orthogonal views did not lie. His hips looked great. His lumbosacral junction, however, was sad as he had significant bridging spondylosis. Spondylosis deformans is the formation of bony projections (bone spurs) from the edges of the vertebrae. The bone spurs represent degenerative changes and instability within a particular region. Bridging spondylosis involves connection of the bone spurs from the edge of the vertebrae and mineralization of the ventral longitudinal ligament. Bridging spondylosis, especially in the lumbosacral region, often reflects underlying arthritic changes and disk disease. The condition can cause pain and neurologic deficits, when severe. Ringo's chronic kidney disease prevented the use of anti-inflammatories. His complete distrust of all adulterated food items meant mixing supplements with his canned food was out. His Houdini-like ability to refuse pilling barred the use of all oral medications and supplements. While Ringo did not mind acupuncture, he would only allow the needles to stay in place for at most five minutes; then his skin would ripple, and the needles would shoot out.

He seemed less painful, and his jumping improved after three treatments. Before learning veterinary spinal manipulation therapy, I would repeat his acupuncture treatments monthly, and he seemed happy and comfortable. During my chiropractic training I figured "why not" and attempted to adjust him. The next day he was like a new cat: jumping, running, and getting into trouble. I had never been so happy to have him jump on the counter and bat around my pens and tchotchkes.

7. **Chinese herbs + hyperthyroidism**: The vomiting, skitzy nature, weight loss, poor haircoat, and the new heart murmur all screamed hyperthyroidism. A quick blood test confirmed Ringo was hyperthyroid. I started him on transdermal methimazole. Within five days his face looked like it had exploded, all swollen and scabbed. After stopping the drug for two weeks his face shrunk, I tried the oral medication just in case he was allergic to the carrier agents in the transdermal formulation. Unsurprisingly the same problem occurred this time after three days. The recent arrival of my newborn human prohibited pursuing radioiodine at the time. My absent desire to feed my two cats separately, and transition to meal-feeding, prevented the use of a prescription diet. Knowing how picky he was I was skeptical he would eat a powdered Chinese herbal formula mixed with the canned food. Much to my surprise he not only at it, he devoured it. Three weeks after starting the herb the vomiting stopped and his spastic demeanor improved. Six weeks after starting the herb his fur was once again soft and silky and his weight improved. Eight weeks after starting the herb both his T4 and free T4 by equilibrium dialysis fell well within the normal range.

8. **Manual therapy + chronic arthritis**: Poor Winston was diagnosed with arthritis in his neck, left hock and right shoulder over three years ago. Fortunately, I was able to maintain his comfort and activity level for 2.5 years with regular acupuncture and chiropractic adjustments. To be honest I did not initially notice him limping. What I noticed was he seemed to have more energy and was happier the day after I used him to practice my adjustments. One of the best things about my veterinary spinal manipulation training (which I lovingly called chiro-camp), I was able to start adjusting after the first session. And why do veterinarians have pets? So, we can practice on them. Afterall they must earn their keep somehow. I noticed Winston always seems happier and more comfortable a day after I practiced motion palpation and adjustments. Initially this improvement lasted a week or so. But the more I practiced, the better he felt, and the longer the beneficial effects lasted. During this time, I also re-started regular monthly acupuncture. I now try to maintain him on quarterly acupuncture and adjustments. If he does something silly and injures himself, I increase the frequency.

9. **Chinese herbs + protein-losing nephropathy**: I suspect Winston developed a protein-losing kidney disease (or nephropathy) due to antigen–antibody formation in the kidneys from his repeat blastomycosis infections, but genetics likely also played a role. His extensive workup did not reveal an obvious underlying cause. As an admirer of the International Renal Interest Society (IRIS) guidelines, I followed their protocol to a T, but after three months of treatment the protein loss did not improve. I did not start herbal therapy right away because I like to treat issues in a stepwise fashion. If you try all the treatments at once, you often have no idea what is and is not helping. After three months of an ACE inhibitor, fish oil, and a low protein diet his urine protein levels remained unchanged. I started him on two Chinese veterinary herbal formulations. Within eight weeks of starting the herbs his protein loss was a

third of the starting value. After 12 weeks of herbal therapy, I stopped his traditional medications. Recheck urine protein two months later showed continued improvement, and his classification changed to borderline urine protein loss.

10. **CBD oil + anxiety**: Winston became increasingly anxious after my child was born. The loud noises, drastic routine changes, and third-wheel status took an emotional toll. His kidneys and joints were doing so well, I was hesitant to make too many adjustments to his treatment regimen. Given the recent spotlight on CBD oil I decided to give it a try. I must say I saw a dramatic improvement. His anxiety, resource guarding, and dog aggression lessened. He also jumped less when the baby crawled toward him or made sudden jerky movements. When my son started eating solid food Winston became his best friend. I think Winston realized he now had a continual source of falling table scraps. After eight months I weaned him off the CBD oil and noticed his anxiety did not return.

My Lessons: Integrative Medicine Deep Thoughts

Training is expensive: You must factor in the financial cost of the course, books, certification, travel, lodging, and time, paid time off (PTO), and time away from family. I lovingly call my wall of certificates and degrees my "Wall o' Debt."

You need a plan for your return on investment (ROI). While learning for learning's sake is great, most of us are not in a financial position to spend money on education without expecting the training to advance our careers. A plan of attack is crucial. This includes surveying your surrounding clinics to determine if other practices offer the same services. If so, how much do they charge and how successful are they? How often can you realistically incorporate this new treatment modality? Jumping

into a training program without considering the financial windfall will generally result in further debt and frustration.

We can stop the stigma: There is significant stigma around the practice of integrative medicine. Many people (veterinarians and clients) fear what they do not know. Evidence-based medicine is the catchphrase vets like to throw around when dismissing integrative medicine. Many people are unaware of available scientific studies supporting nontraditional treatment options.

The desire for alternative pet therapies is out there, especially as millennials become the predominate pet–parent demographic. The 2021–2022 American Pet Products Association (APPA) National Pet Owners Survey Statistics on Pet Ownership and Annual Expenses found 69 million households in the United States own dogs and 45.3 million own cats (APPA 2022). The same study found millennials make up 32% of pet ownership in the United States, while baby boomers make up 27% and generation X 24% (APPA 2022). Millennials place a higher value on the human–animal bond and tend to focus on integrative therapy options (Tricarico 2019).

The 2018 American Veterinary Medical Association (AVMA) Pet Ownership and Demographics Sourcebook cites 57% of American households owned pets at the end of 2016, with 76.8 million dogs and 58.4 million cats (Burns 2018). The 2022 AVMA Pet Ownership and Demographics Sourcebook showed a moderate increase in the populations of owned cats (4% to a total of 29%) and dogs (7% to a total of 45%) with the number of households increasing, while the number of pets per household decreased slightly (Burns 2022; Nolen 2022). The estimate total number of owned dogs in 2022 was over 81.1 million with cats totaling over 60.7 million.

The Michelson Found Animals Foundation 2019 Pet Trends noted 68% of the 1000 companion animal owners surveyed used alternative treatments for their pets (MFAF 2018). These treatments included the use of supplements, especially CBD oil, acupuncture, chiropractic, massage, and physical therapy. Put another way, there are potentially 96 million patients (over 41.2 million cats and 55.1 million dogs) who could receive integrative therapies.

Even pet health insurance companies are catching on. By the end of 2017 over 2 million companion animals were insured in the United States and Canada, a 17% increase from the previous year (Carrns 2019). The 2021 North American Pet Health Insurance Association (NAPHIA) survey found 3.45 million pets in the United States had pet insurance, an over 57% increase in five years (NAPHIA 2023). The 2022 NAPHIA survey revealed the number increased another 27.7% to 4.41 million pets with the vast majority being dogs at 82% (NAPHIA 2023).

Many pet insurance plans include coverage for integrative therapies, especially acupuncture (Woodley 2018). The presence of this type of coverage re-emphasizes the mainstream incorporation of these treatment modalities, as well as reflecting client demand.

The bottom line is clients want these integrative options and veterinarians should have at least a basic understanding regarding the rationale for their use, safety, and efficacy. If veterinarians cannot answer client questions, flippantly disprove of these treatment modalities, or criticize clients for their line of thinking, they run the risk of alienating their client base. Nothing shuts down dialog like negativity and judgment.

Unfortunately, this animosity exists on the integrative medicine side as well. Many integrative practitioners are defensive and dismissive of their Western peers. Some strictly holistic veterinarians look down upon the integrative practitioners because integrative practitioners muddy the waters by using Western diagnostics and incorporating Western treatments. If we decided as a group to open our minds, drop our armor, shrink our egos, and combine forces we could help more patients and clients.

The AVMA is slowly evolving: Through educating veterinarian and client, and supporting continued scientific research, many veterinary integrative medicine (VIM) organizations and associations are becoming well known within the veterinary community. In particular, the American Holistic Veterinary Medical Association (AHVMA) has made great strides in promoting integrative medicine to other veterinarians and the public. This is accomplished through the regular publication of their scientific journal, *Journal of the American Holistic Veterinary Medical Association* (JAVHMA), and working closely with the AVMA as a member of the AVMA House of Delegates.

Currently, the AVMA has no specific position on VIM. In my opinion, this is due to a lack of knowledge and understanding regarding the practices of VIM and the availability of scientific research.

The AVMA recommends all branches of veterinary medicine, including integrative, be held to the same standards or care. These standards include:

- Always keep the health and welfare of the animal in mind.
- Evidence-based medicine should be used to diagnose and treat patients.
- Veterinarians should be appropriately trained before performing treatments on their patients.
- A valid veterinarian–client–patient relationship is mandatory.
- Documentation of owner consent for diagnostics and treatments is required.
- Treatment outcome should be noted in medical records.
- Veterinarians are responsible for understanding and adhering to local, state, and federal laws regarding the practice of veterinary medicine.

Know your state laws: All states have statutes defining and regulating the practice of veterinary medicine. Some states are stricter than others. For instance, some states allow non-veterinarians to practice acupuncture, spinal manipulation (chiropractic), and physical therapy. Other states consider the use of these modalities the practice of veterinary medicine, allowing only trained veterinarians to perform them. Still other states allow non-veterinarians to practice certain therapies under the direct supervision of a veterinarian with a pre-established veterinary–client–patient relationship. State licensing boards and state veterinary medical associations are excellent sources for understanding local legislation. As an aside some states limit or exclude the use of integrative medicine continuing education units (CEUs) toward the annual state CEU requirements.

Document, Document, Document: The medical record is considered a legal document, and as such should be as complete as possible. This is especially true when it comes to client communication and client consent. Basically, if it is not written down, then legally speaking it did not happen.

Because some aspects of integrative medicine are not yet considered mainstream medicine, it is very important clients understand the full array of services offered. I have a small consent form new clients review and sign when they first come to my practice. The form was adapted from examples available to members on the AHVMA website. An editable copy of the consent form is available on the website.

XXX

Consent for Integrative Medicine Treatment

In addition to traditional medical diagnostics and treatments, some of the veterinarians at xxx offer integrative medicine therapies. Services offered include acupuncture, chiropractic (veterinary spinal manipulation), Chinese herbal therapy, Western herbal therapy, homeopathy, nutritional supplementation, whole-food nutrition, and ozone therapy.

Veterinary integrative medicine, unlike traditional medications and treatments, frequently has beneficial effects on multiple body systems and conditions. While the integrative therapies offered are generally safe, some patients may experience transient discomfort or side effects, which can be the same or more severe than traditional options.

All xxx team members want to ensure our clients understand the integrative modalities available and, more importantly, how those treatments may benefit your pet. If you have questions regarding any of the services we offer please ask the veterinarian for more information.

To ensure we discuss integrative options with only interested pet parents please select one of the options below, as well as saign and date you understand the information provided.

I **am** interested in learning more about Integrative Veterinary Medicine and how it may help my pet.

☐

I **am not** interested in learning more about Integrative Veterinary Medicine and how it may help my pet.

☐

Date:_____   Signature:_____

I also ensure the following information is recorded in the medical record at every visit:

1. Complete patient history, including current preventatives, supplements, herbs, and medications.
2. Physical examination, including the findings of my traditional Chinese veterinary medical exam.
3. Traditional (Western) diagnoses.
4. Traditional Chinese veterinary medicine diagnoses, when applicable.
5. Diagnostic test options offered, approved, and declined by the client.
6. Treatments options offered, approved, and declined by the client.
7. Client communication regarding the length of treatment, recheck recommendations, and prognosis.

While this amount of record keeping may initially seem tedious, remember that you worked hard for your license. The last thing you want is there to be a legal question regarding your medical judgment and treatment. Having everything documented, including consent to discuss integrative medicine, is the best "CYA" you can have. Additionally, this "checklist" of documentation has made me a better practitioner and communicator with my clients. I have these concepts preloaded in my electronic medical record template, which I use as a reminder to cover all my bases during my appointments.

Everything is connected: Ever had clients mention something that seemed random and unrelated to the underlying problem during an appointment? Well, that obviously still happens to me, but a lot of times those "random" observations can be explained once you understand Chinese veterinary medicine, Western herbal medicine, functional medicine, and whole food therapy.

To me the cool thing about integrative medicine is that you really do look at the *whole* patient. I have always been one to hope for zebras, when I hear hoof beats. The "out of the box" thinking, the interconnectedness of the body systems, and connecting the dots are all embraced wholeheartedly in integrative medicine.

One example of this synergy is the circadian body clock discussed in traditional Chinese medicine (TCM), shown in Figure 4. TCM utilizes a 24-hour clock where each organ system has a two-hour period during which it is most active. For example, the large intestine is considered most active during 5–7 a.m., followed by the stomach at 7–9 a.m. Guess when you usually wake up to have your morning BM or eat breakfast?

Seizures and severe anxiety are often associated with liver dysfunction in TCM. The liver is most active during 1–3 a.m. Ever notice most pets' seizure in the middle of the night between 1 and 3 a.m.? Ever wake up in the middle of the night with a nagging worry or unending thought? I certainly do, and it is usually between 1 and 3 a.m.

Fewer cases make me moan in frustration: Overall, I dread treating certain chronic diseases less, including skin, pain, liver, kidney, anxiety, and cancer. Through the incorporation of acupuncture, Chinese herbs, spinal manipulation, nutraceuticals, and whole food therapy I have seen improvement in many patients. This is not to say I have "cured" them all, but I now can offer alternative therapies which improve quality and length of life.

I will preface this observation with the caveat that many people seek integrative therapy when all other options have failed. In these instances, it is crucial to set realistic expectations regarding the degree of expected improvement and length of treatment. Often, I see patients when the owners are on the verge of euthanasia. I used to view this as a negative and felt a lot of pressure to work miracles. I now see this as an opportunity. At the very least I can help the patient feel better, if only for a short period of time. And even if what I try does not work, at least I tried. No patient should die without the benefit of integrative medicine.

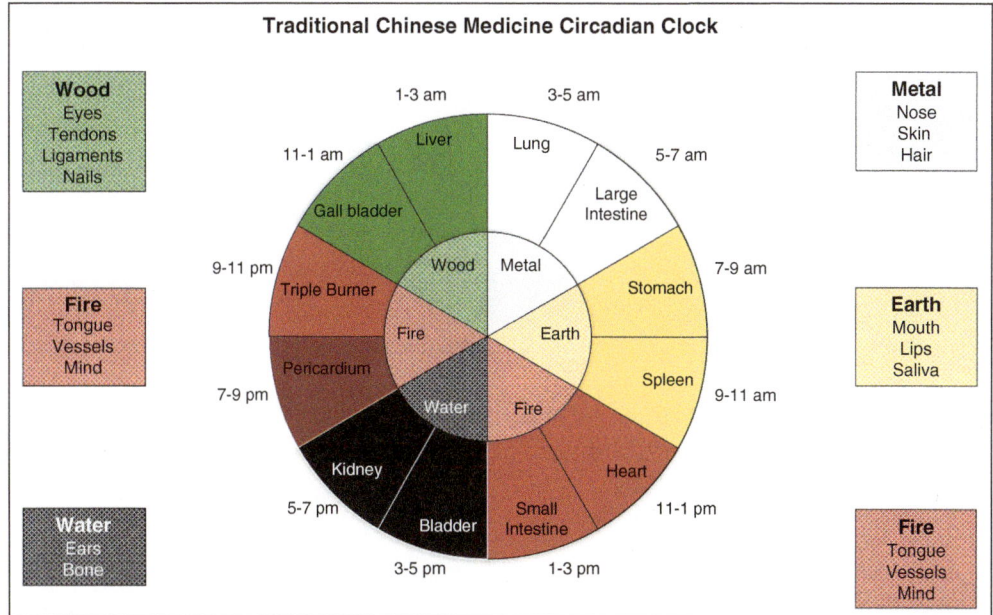

Figure 4 Schematic illustration of the body clock described in traditional Chinese medicine (TCM). There are 12 main body systems in TCM. All body systems are active throughout the day, but each organ has a two-hour period during which its effects on the body are the greatest. The outer portion of the clock illustrates when each organ is most active. TCM further divides all mater into five elemental systems: Wood, Fire, Earth, Metal and Water. The inner portion of the clock shows the division of each organ within the five element system. Source: Lisa P. McFaddin.

I still have ups and downs in my career: I am a firm believer that veterinary medicine works in three-week waves: You have three good weeks followed by one humbling week. Learning integrative medicine did not solve all my problems and magically make practicing veterinary medicine perfect. Adding these tools helped me become a better doctor, understand my role in the profession better, and provide me with a different way of viewing medicine. But I am still an imperfect human.

Acknowledgments

I want to thank the patients, clients, veterinary assistants, veterinary technicians, and veterinarians who served as mentors (both intentionally and inadvertently) over the years. I am honored and humbled to have been molded by your wisdom and experience. A special heartfelt thank you goes out to Dr. Pedro Rivera who helped open my eyes to the world of neurology and the musculoskeletal system.

I want to recognize the patience, grace, compassion, and humor gifted to me by my former team over the past years, especially Tama, Kathleen, Claudia, and Deh. Thank you for tolerating and supporting me while I toiled, grumbled, and struggled to write this book. We will all be happy to never hear me say "I have to go home to work on the book" again.

I want to thank the veterinarians who reviewed many of the chapters for content. You are all mentors in whom I hold the utmost respect. I have placed individualized acknowledgments at the end of those chapters.

Introduction

The Purpose

I want to empower all veterinarians with the knowledge that anyone can practice integrative medicine. I do not just mean anyone can learn the information, which they can. Integrative medicine has legitimate science behind it, proving its efficacy and legitimacy. We should all be proud to offer these treatment modalities to our clients and patients.

It is also important to know integrative medicine is not an all or nothing concept. There are many treatment modalities covered under the umbrella term integrative medicine. These modalities can be used individually or in combination, and they can be used with every case or select patients.

Integrative medicine can also be profitable. Veterinarians do not like to think about money. Sorry to burst your bubble, but *you have to think about money*. To thrive as a practice, to pay your staff, to grow your business, and to treat patients you have to make a profit. Remember knowledge for the sake of knowledge is great, but you cannot help anyone if your business is closed. There is a way to offer integrative treatments to your patients without sacrificing your bottom line.

By establishing integrative medicine as a scientifically accepted, readily accessible, easily incorporated, and profitable option, I hope to encourage more veterinarians to respect these treatments modalities. I want to inspire the profession as a whole to be more open-minded

and embrace non-Western scientifically proven treatments. Integrative medicine has a lot to offer our patients, as expressed by my cats in Figure 5, and our clients want to learn more about it. Would you prefer they learn the information from you or Dr. Google?

Ultimately, I would love all veterinarians to receive introductory information on integrative

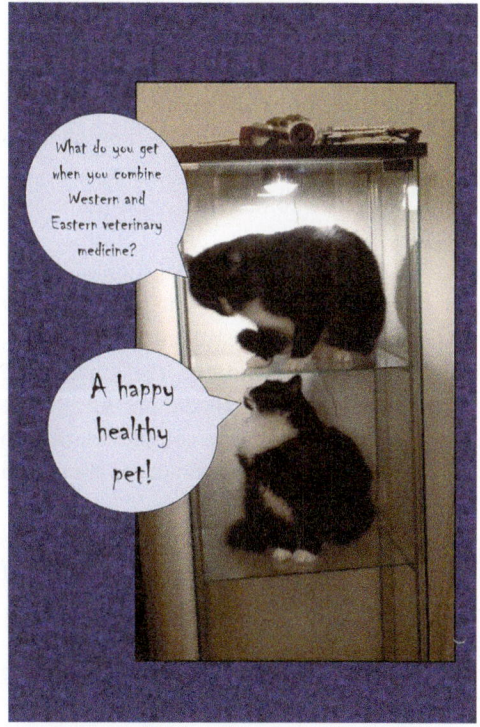

Figure 5 My cats, Ringo (above) and Samantha (below), discussing why they love veterinary integrative medicine. Source: Lisa P. McFaddin.

medicine in vet school. Memon et al. (2016) wrote an excellent introductory paper proposing the incorporation of integrative medicine within veterinary schools. I encourage anyone curious about the pros and cons, challenges and benefits of this curriculum to read the article.

The Terminology

Practically every medical organization has a unique and finely tuned definition of integrative medicine. My personal definition is as follows: veterinary integrative medicine (VIM) is a blended practice in which traditional (aka Western) and non-traditional (aka Eastern, holistic, and alternative) diagnostics and treatments are used to provide the best possible veterinary care to patients. Integrative medicine is the best of both worlds. As integrative practitioners we can pick and choose the best diagnostics and treatments traditional medicine has to offer admixed with the greatest non-traditional diagnostic and treatment options.

Complementary medicine is an analogous but outdated term. The phrase "complementary medicine" inadvertently supports the antiquated viewpoint that non-traditional therapies (i.e. acupuncture, Chinese and Western herbal therapy, spinal manipulation, prolotherapy, etc.) are non-scientific and cannot be used as a sole treatment. For example, acupuncture complements "real" medicine but is itself not "real" medicine. And while integrative treatments are complementary to traditional medicine, these practices are a form of "real" medicine.

Additionally, a simple spelling error, *complimentary*, can result in the assumption that your services are free of charge. A cautionary tale told to newbies is that some poor veterinarian opened a brand-new practice offering *complimentary* medicine. Within a few weeks she was bankrupt and forced to close. She had been sued multiple times by clients claiming she falsely advertised free services and then charged for them. A quick Google search

suggests this story is fabricated, but the lesson further supports the use of the phrase integrative medicine.

The terms "alternative" and "holistic" are used to describe the individual non-traditional modalities available. Veterinarians who practice strictly alternative or holistic medicine occasionally use traditional diagnostic methods but rarely incorporate Western medicine. The school adage "a square is a rectangle, but a rectangle is not a square" comes to mind. Thus, alternative and holistic therapies are contained within integrative medicine, but integrative medicine is not a part of alternative and holistic medicine.

Complementary and alternative veterinary medicine (CAVM) is another term thrown around by veterinarians. This loquacious term suggests non-traditional and alternative treatments are used to complement traditional medicine. Complementary and alternative medicine (CAM) was the term favored in human medicine for years until the adoption of the phrase integrative medicine. IM and VIM connote the feeling of fusion and harmony between the medical practices. Often the word "alternative" is associated with unscientific or unproven methods. It was for this reason the name of the National Institutes of Health (NIH) Center for Complementary and Alternative Medicine (NCCAM) was changed in 2014 to the National Center for Complementary and Integrative Health (NCCIH).

In summary, an integrative practitioner's foundation of medicine is reliant on traditional methods taught in veterinary school while incorporating non-traditional diagnostic techniques. Integrative practitioners then use both traditional and non-traditional treatments to correct imbalances, restore homeostasis, and prevent further disease.

The Science

A beloved idiom in veterinary medicine is evidence-based medicine (EBM). Unfortunately, like many trendy phrases, there is a lot of misconception regarding its meaning. While my then one-year-old son shown in Figure 6 believed he had discovered EBM, the concept has been around for centuries, but the actual phrase first appeared in human medicine in the early 1990s.

EBM developed out of necessity. Science and medicine were, and still are, advancing so quickly that concepts previously thought doctrine were becoming half-truths within a few years. Practitioners were concerned they were not treating their patients with the most up-to-date options available, while on the flip side feeling overwhelmed with the mountain of research articles available on each subject.

EBM was introduced to help human doctors rationally and systematically monitor the literature for new information, allowing easier incorporation in everyday practice. Masic et al. (2008) outlined a five-step approach for family medicine practitioners to readily utilize EBM in their daily practice:

1. Define the medical problem of interest.
2. Search available sources for information about the specific problem.

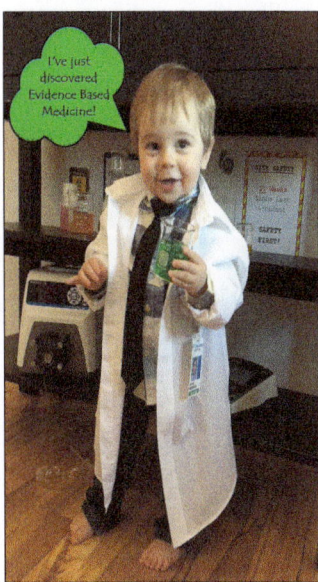

Figure 6 My almost one year-old budding scientist practicing evidence-based medicine. Source: Lisa P. McFaddin.

3. Critically review the available information.
4. Apply information to help the patient.
5. Determine if the application of the information improved the outcome for the patient.

EBM was created to help all practitioners, veterinary and human alike, improve patient care and quality of life. Somewhere along the line this conspiracy regarding EBM developed. Brennen McKenzie, a veterinarian and member of the Evidence-Based Veterinary Medicine Association, very clearly outlined the common myths associated with EBM in his 2013 lecture "Myths and Misconceptions About Evidence Based Medicine" at the American Board of Veterinary Practitioners.

Veterinarians tend to shy away from EBM because of three common misconceptions: there is a lack of scientific evidence in veterinary medicine; veterinarians promoting EBM believe only the results of randomized clinical trials are valid; and EBM cannot be used efficiently in daily practice (McKenzie 2013). Let's examine each of these myths a little more closely.

Lack of evidence: While there are less scientific studies in veterinary medicine compared to human medicine, a lot of valid articles and research studies still exist.

While randomized controlled trials (RCTs) are considered the gold standard for research studies, other information is still valuable. The beauty of EBM is that it utilizes the best available scientific evidence for a particular subject or problem. Depending on the problem an RCT may not be available or, if one is available, it may not pertain to the specific problem being evaluated.

When categorizing the type of available scientific information, the most common representation is a pyramid. This schematic, depicted in Figure 7, demonstrates the *quality* of information increases while the *quantity* of available resources decreases. The categories of information within the pyramid include meta-analysis, systematic review, RCTs, cohort

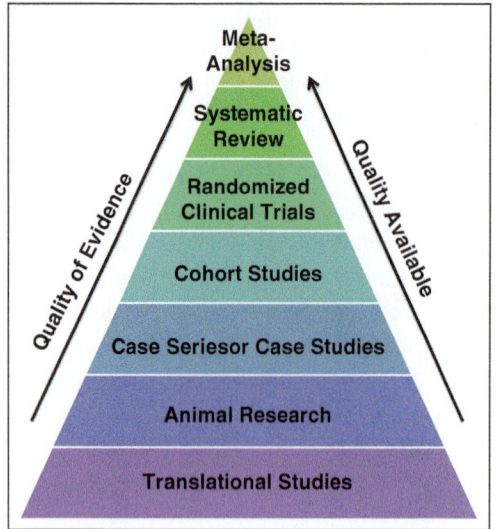

Figure 7 Schematic representation of available scientific information. The pyramid demonstrates that as the quality of the studies increase, the available research decreases. Source: Lisa P. McFaddin.

studies, case series/studies, animal research, and translation studies.

A **meta-analysis** is a statistical analysis of information from multiple studies generally addressing similar questions. A **systematic review** examines previous studies allowing for collection and extrapolation of information from multiple sources. **RCTs** utilize randomly assigned control and treatment groups which reduces researcher bias. **Cohort studies** investigate the risk factors for disease in a group of individuals. **Case series or studies** consist of individual or a group of case examples used to extrapolate information and apply it to the whole. **Animal research** are studies conducted in controlled settings in the laboratory using animal patients. **Translation studies** combine information from multiple scientific disciplines to apply those principles to medical treatment.

For some reason many veterinarians and human doctors latched onto the idea that only RCTs or meta-analyses could be used when revising medical decisions. The reality is EBM is not a pyramid. EBM is more appropriately

represented by three overlapping rings where each component is equally important and vital to improving patient health, as depicted in Figure 8. EBM emphasizes the incorporation and combination of information from valid scientific studies, individual clinical experience, and the needs of the patient.

Daily use of EBM is impractical: Most veterinarians barely have time to eat lunch let alone read dozens of articles daily or even weekly. Am I the only one who keeps stacks of journal articles as paper weights until the size of the pile causes twinges of guilt, and I recycle them, only to start all over?

Look, if we could spend hours reading and educating ourselves every day or even every week we would likely be in academia. It is just not practical to expect any full-time veterinarian, let alone someone with a life and family, to have that much time outside of clinics to devote to more work.

The good news is it does not actually take that much more time to use sound science to support your medicine. Ever searched VIN or other online veterinary sources for information about a particular case? Ever used PubMed or MedlinePlus to investigate recent journal articles and studies? Well, that right there is

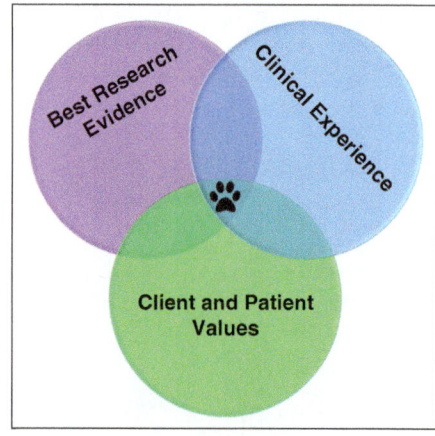

Figure 8 A visual representation of veterinary evidence-based medicine emphasizing the equal importance of scientific research, clinical experience, and patient needs. Source: Lisa P. McFaddin.

steps 1–3 of the five-step EBM plan. All you have left to do is apply the information and monitor the outcome, completing steps 4 and 5.

There is more to it than this, but not that much more. Learning to critically evaluate articles and studies is very important, and just like learning any new skill with a little practice it becomes second nature. The Evidence-Based Veterinary Medicine Association (EBVMA) has helpful resources and information about further training on their website, https://www.edvma.org.

Why bring this up in a book about VIM? As you have probably guessed I pride myself on offering the best medicine for my patients. I have found that incorporating VIM allows me to do just that. I strive to use EBM to guide my decisions as I forge ahead in my career, and the use of EBM within VIM helps legitimize the practice itself. Throughout the book I will emphasize the importance of EBM within VIM. Numerous articles, covering the entire pyramid, will be referenced for each treatment.

The Tool Box

VIM, much like feline lower urinary tract disease, is an umbrella term under which many disciplines fall. The most common therapies include the following (and also briefly described in Figure 9):

- Acupuncture
- Applied kinesiology*
- Aromatherapy*
- Chinese food therapy
- Chinese herbal medicine
- Cold laser therapy
- Homeopathy*
- Hyperbaric oxygen therapy*
- Nutraceuticals
- Ozone therapy
- Prolotherapy
- Regenerative medicine
- Rehabilitation and sports medicine*
- Reiki*

- Trigger point therapy
- Veterinary spinal manipulation therapy
- Western herbal medicine.

The treatments marked with an asterisk are not covered in this book. Applied kinesiology, aromatherapy, homeopathy, and Reiki each have their own value, but the general lack of scientific studies precludes their inclusion. While there are numerous well-performed studies involving hyperbaric oxygen therapy (HBOT), the start-up cost is often prohibitive unless practicing within a large tertiary referral practice. For this reason, HBOT was not included in this book.

Rehabilitation and sports medicine is proven to be effective in veterinary medicine, with extremely varied start-up costs dependent on the equipment utilized, e.g. underwater treadmill, therapeutic ultrasound. In a survey of VIM training in veterinary colleges accredited by the AVMA, Memon et al. (2021) discovered rehabilitation and acupuncture were the most common topics covered in the curriculum. Interestingly the authors found the number of VIM courses decreased over the past seven years, while the number of faculty trained in specific VIM modalities increased.

Despite its inclusion in this study, the classification of rehabilitation and sport medicine under the umbrella of VIM is a contentious topic. Many practitioners, especially those who are Diplomates of the American College of Veterinary Sports Medicine and Rehabilitation, consider this modality separate from VIM. As such it was not included in the book.

All these treatment modalities can be utilized individually or as a multimodal approach. When used together they build upon each other, opening new doors to understanding our patients and how best to help them. Integrative medicine in some ways offers a whole new world of possibilities and treatments for veterinary patients. Embracing and exploring this world can be exciting, rewarding, and profitable.

A is for **ACUPUNCUTRE** which **ACTIVATES** nerves, muscles, blood vessels, and lymphatics through **ACCURATE** needle placement just below the skin.

A is for **APPLIED** Kinesiology which uses muscle **ASSESSMENT** to evaluate nervous system function.

A is for **AROMATHERAPY** which **AWAKENS** the senses and soothe **ANXIOUS** minds through the inhalation and **APPLICATION** of essential oils.

C is for **CHINESE** Herbal Medicine which **CULTIVATES** homeostasis through the **CESSATION** of inflammation and pain, improving **COMMUNICATION** of **CELLULAR** signals, and allowing **CENTRALIZED** flow of energy, blood and lymphatics.

C is for **COLD** Laser which **CORRECTS** inflammation and blood flow using **CERTAIN** wavelengths of light.

F is for Chinese **FOOD** Therapy which embraces the idea that **FOOD** is medicine, **FORMULATING** diets to meet the exact nutritional needs of the pet based on signalment and concurrent illnesses.

H is for **HOMEOPATHY** which uses micro-titrated doses of single remedies to **HELP HARMONIZE** the body, restoring **HOMEOSTASIS.**

H is for **HYPERBARIC** Oxygen Therapy which uses **HIGHLY** pressurized oxygen in specialized chambers to reduce inflammation, stimulate angiogenesis, improve wound **HEALING**, and **HELP** control infections.

M is for Veterinary Spinal **MANIPULATION** Therapy which uses high-velocity low-amplitude thrust on one or more vertebral joints to improve areas of reduced **MOBILITY**, **MAXIMIZING** nervous system function and **MINIMIZING** pain.

N is for **NEUTRACEUTICALS** which **NOURISH, NURTURE,** and heal the body from various disease processes using dietary supplements.

O is for **OZONE** Therapy which relies on the powerful **OXIDATIVE** abilities of gas made of three **OXYGEN** atoms to reduce inflammation and control infection.

P is for **PROLOTHERAPY** which uses injections of natural irritants to **PROMOTE** healing in joints, ligaments and tendons.

R is for **REIKI** which promotes stress **REDUCTION, RELAXATION,** and physical healing through shared meditation.

R is for **REGENERATIVE MEDICINE** which uses injections of substances to **REPLACE** and promote **REGROWTH** of cells and tissues, in joints, ligaments and tendons.

R is for **REHABILITATION** and Sports Medicine which **RELIES** on manual therapies, therapeutic exercises, and specialized equipment to **REDUCE** pain and lameness and **RESTORE** normal musculoskeletal function.

T is for **TRIGGER** Point **THERAPY** which uses manual pressure or dry needling **TECHNIQUES** to reduce **TENSION** in a hyperirritable area of pathologically contracted skeletal muscle.

W is for **WESTERN** Herbal Medicine **WHICH** uses unprocessed plant material to treat dysfunction and imbalance **WITHIN** the body.

Figure 9 The alphabet of veterinary integrative medicine. Source: Lisa P. McFaddin.

Book Structure

This book is designed as a compendious overview of the cornucopia that is VIM, focusing on the successful integration of each modality within the practice. The next 11 chapters are dedicated to specific categories within the VIM umbrella. Each chapter will cover The What, The Why, and The How. Chapter 12, entitled "Multimodal Approach," ties it all together, demonstrating the benefit of using multiple VIM treatments at one time and providing real-world examples of each treatment in the form of case studies.

Verbal permission was obtained from all clients regarding the discussion of their pets and/ or use of their pets' images within the book. Every effort was made to obtain written permission as well. In the event written permission could not be obtained, the name of the patient was not used and/or the patient's face was not included in the image.

Introduction

A brief summary of the treatment modality and explanation of the chapter's contents is provided.

The What

An overview of the integrative therapy for the entire veterinary team broken down by word origin, definition, history (human and veterinary), background information, techniques, mechanisms of action, and safety. There is expanded information for veterinarians when applicable.

Word Origin: Whenever available the etymology of the therapy's name is provided.

Definition: A concise description of the VIM therapy is defined.

History: A summary of the evolution of each treatment in human and veterinary medicine.

Terminology: Each therapeutic modality comes with its own vocabulary. A basic understanding of these terms facilitates effective communication between professionals and clients. A summary of common terms is provided in this section.

Background Information: Typically contains multiple subdivisions describing necessary background information. Veterinarian-specific information may be provided, and is designated as such, which includes more in-depth information.

Techniques: Describes, when applicable, various techniques applicable to the modality. Veterinarian-specific information may be provided and is designated as such.

Mechanisms of Action: Summarizes the mechanism or mechanisms of action. Veterinarian-specific information may be provided and is designated as such.

Safety: Discusses safety, potential adverse effects, cautions, and contraindications. Veterinarian-specific information may be provided and is designated as such.

The Why

Justifies the use of the modality by discussing those disease processes and conditions which routinely benefit from the treatment in human and veterinary medicine, and examples of VIM research, when applicable.

Applications in Human Medicine: Summarizes the primary use of the modality in human medicine.

Applications in Veterinary Medicine: Summarizes the primary use of the modality in veterinary medicine.

Veterinary Research: Summaries of up to three scientific studies, when available, are provided. Additionally, when applicable, a table documenting the efficacy of each modality in the treatment of various conditions in veterinary medicine is provided, including author names and publication dates.

The How

The meat and potatoes of the book, outlining how each team member can effectively incorporate VIM into daily practice. After all, everyone has their own role in the success of the business. The subdivision into team members and veterinarians helps streamline the preparation process.

Team Members
Practice Managers

Let's start with the glue that holds the practice together, the practice manager (PM) also called the hospital manager or clinic manager. The PM has a difficult job, most of which is done behind the scenes. When asked to describe the most important detail(s) to consider when introducing a new service into a practice, two successful practice managers had similar answers.

Claudia Amaya (Figure 10) has functioned as both a customer service representative (CSR) and now a PM. Having worn multiple hats, she can provide unique insight by answering the same question from two viewpoints. As a PM she stated

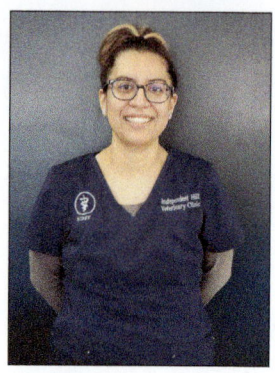

Figure 10 Claudia Amaya has worked in the veterinary field for over nine years. She spent 7.5 years as a customer service representative and is now a practice manager. Source: Lisa P. McFaddin.

The most important thing to think about when introducing a new service is marketing. You want to make sure clients are aware of the service you are providing and the benefits that it provides.

Another PM, Jennifer Ackerman (Figure 11) had this to say:

Although from an operations standpoint return on investment (pricing) must be considered, it becomes secondary when considering what the customer/community is asking for

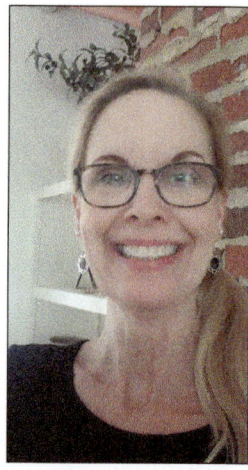

Figure 11 Jennifer Ackerman has worked both as a regional manager and practice manager for over five years. Source: Lisa P. McFaddin.

(demand). What do the doctors see as a need for their patients (standard of care)? Care and need for the patients is always paramount.

When introducing a new service into the hospital the PM needs to know a few details right off the bat: What is the new service? What is the return on investment? How to train the support staff most effectively? How to promote the service to the public?

The What and The Why sections define the purpose and methods of each therapy.

Return on Investment

Return on investment (ROI) is a term borrowed from the economic literature. When applied to veterinary medicine, ROI basically asks the question "Is the investment or change going to be profitable for the clinic?" Many people working in the veterinary field are uncomfortable discussing the financial aspects of veterinary medicine. Veterinary medicine is a business. Our goal is to help our patients thrive. To accomplish this goal, we need a healthy practice. A healthy practice is a profitable practice. We cannot effectively treat our patients if we cannot keep the doors open or pay our employees.

Anytime a hospital wants to introduce a new service, purchase new equipment, or improve the facility the question at the front of the PM's mind should be "What is the return on investment?" If the change or improvement are not profitable the hospital should not pursue it.

Imhoff (2001) outlines in detail how to analyze ROI in human healthcare. These recommendations are applicable to veterinary medicine. Imhoff specifies two ways to approach ROI: increase the hospital's revenue or reduce the cost of producing products/services. Revenue can be increased by increasing the market share and/or improving the quality of services offered (Imhoff 2001). Reducing production costs can be achieved by reducing resource consumption, increasing the number of procedures performed (without increasing the consumption of resources), and/or reducing complications from performed procedures (Imhoff 2001). VIM ROI should focus on increasing hospital revenue through the introduction of a novel service, improving the quality and breadth of medical care available to the patients.

The expectation is that VIM will increase hospital revenue by expanding the variety of services offered to the patients, as well as increasing the number of clients/patients seen at the hospital. The next variables to consider include client interest, veterinarian demand, hospital costs, regularity of use, scheduling, and pricing.

Client Interest

The Michelson Found Animals Foundation 2019 Pet Trends found 68% of the 1000 companion animal owners surveyed used alternative treatments for their pets (MFAF 2018). If there are specific studies documenting client interest or opinion regarding a specific modality it will be discussed in this section.

Veterinarian Demand

There is a need for more integrative practitioners as the number of pet owners interested in integrative therapy steadily increases, coupled with a shortage of veterinarians. The current and projected number of practicing veterinarians does not meet the ever-expanding volume of companion animals.

Ouedraogo et al.'s (2019) veterinarian census stated the number of veterinarians approaching retirement age outweighs the number of graduating veterinarians; 36% (40 800 individuals) of practicing veterinarians fall within the Baby Boomer and Silent generations and are approaching retirement, while only 3750 United States citizens graduate from US-based and foreign veterinary schools annually (Ouedraogo et al. 2019). The mean age of graduating veterinarians has continued to rise, 25 years of age in 1975 to 28 years of age in 2018, potentially reducing the average career length (Ouedraogo et al. 2019).

VIM is still in its infancy, and the number of veterinarians offering VIM is growing.

The market is far from saturated with integrative veterinarians. I practice in Manassas, Virginia, a suburb 45 minutes away from Washington DC. There are over 100 veterinary practices within a 20-mile radius of my practice. As of 2021, there were less than 12 practices offering veterinary acupuncture, and only one additional practice offering small animal spinal manipulation, within that same 20-mile radius.

Hospital Costs

Depends on the specific treatment. Each chapter will discuss the start-up costs for that modality. Start-up costs include more than just the cost of the classes and equipment. The cost of veterinarian training, staff training, supplies and equipment, staffing, facilities, and advertising must be considered.

Veterinarian Training

Include course cost, textbooks, travel expenses, and time off. The hospital management team must decide if they will cover any or all expenses. Travel costs are applicable to on-site courses only and typically include the flight, lodging, car rental, and meals.

With respect to time-off, most hospitals expect online courses be completed on the veterinarian's own time. Time-off required for on-site courses is a little trickier. Clinics offer an average of 4.1 paid continuing education (CE) days per year (AAHA 2019). The hospital must decide if the veterinarian can use CE PTO for the course. If more than four days are needed, the hospital must decide if the veterinarian will be required to use their contractual PTO days or if additional PTO days will be provided. If the clinic agrees to pay the veterinarian for some or all of the CE days, there is an added expense to the hospital.

Staff Training

Team training expenses are highly variable and dependent on the answers to the following questions. Will the training consist of an all-staff mandatory meeting in which the hospital is closed for appointments? Are team members responsible for independent learning between appointments? Does the hospital already have regular all-staff meetings, or would a special day and time need to be designated?

While considering staff training the management team must also examine negligible and tangible costs. There are two scenarios in which training costs would be extremely low: preexisting staff meetings and self-study. If the hospital has regular all-staff meetings, the time and staff schedule are already set; the only item that changes is the content. Training can be completed during one to two meetings (depending on meeting length) without requiring the reservation of additional non-appointment times. Initial training will take approximately 1–1.5 hours. With self-study, the employees are responsible for learning the material on their own without blocking appointments. This is not the preferred or recommended method of training.

If the hospital does not have regular meetings and elects to hold an all-staff meeting the costs would include ink and paper for printed materials, all-staff lunch, loss of revenue from blocked appointment times, and overhead cost for the length of training.

Supplies

Depend on the modality being introduced and includes equipment and hospital renovation/redecoration costs.

Staffing

The use of support staff beyond their normal duties. The American Animal Hospital Association (AAHA) recommendations a veterinary assistant or licensed technician always restrain patients for physical examinations and procedures. If a support staff member is required for a longer period than that of a typical appointment, additional staffing costs should be considered.

Facilities

This includes the costs needed to keep the doors open (aka overhead). Overhead includes rent or mortgage, utilities, administrative costs, and employee costs divided by the minutes the practice is open (Stevenson 2016). The price per minute equals the amount of revenue needed just to break even. Overhead is extremely hospital specific. The range tends to be $2–5/minute.

Advertising

The money spent promoting the service to the public. Much of the advertisement can be done with little to no additional expenditures. According to the AVMA 2019 Economic State of the Veterinary Profession, companion animal practices spend an average of 0.7% of their revenue on promotion and advertisement, with mean revenue of $1 207 938. It is unlikely the promotion of any integrative service would significantly affect this percentage.

Applicability

One of the amazing things about VIM is the variety of cases which can be helped with alternative therapies. Each chapter will discuss in more detail how that modality can be utilized on a daily basis.

Appointment Scheduling

The four factors to consider when planning VIM appointment protocols are appointment length, support staff availability, exam room availability, and follow-up appointment scheduling.

At my practice the initial integrative appointments are 60 minutes. Follow-up appointments are 30, 40, 50, or 60 minutes depending on the case. In the beginning, while the clinician is building his or her skillset and confidence, it may be a good idea to make all follow-up appointments at least 40 minutes long.

Our doctor to veterinary assistant (VA)/licensed technician (LT) ratio is 1 : 1.5 ensuring there is a VA/LT available to assist with patient restraint. There are three exam rooms with one to two doctors seeing appointments at a time. The exam rooms are different sizes: one small room (primarily used for cats), one medium room (used for cats and small to medium dogs), and one large room (used for large dogs and multi-pet appointments). The VA/LTs are instructed to check the schedule throughout the day to plan for integrative appointments. The goal is to ensure the right room is available at the right time, and that use of any given exam room does not negatively affect productivity for either doctor

When entering charges, a separate line item is created indicating when the patient should recheck: one, two four weeks, etc. On the same line item in parentheses the desired appointment length is entered: 30, 40, 50 minutes, etc. Having the information on the invoice helps communicate the doctor's goals for the next appointment with the CSR and client. This also prompts the CSR to forward book the appointment, with the appropriate appointment length, at the time of checkout. If the client cannot book the appointment at checkout the information is stored for easy access when the client calls back, ensuring the doctor has adequate time for the treatment.

As a rule, I do not incorporate VIM treatments with wellness examinations. In my opinion the wellness examination should focus on the overall health and husbandry of the patient. There is generally not enough time to cover all the wellness protocols while also performing adjustments, acupuncture, other manual therapies, and discussing changes to herbal formulas and/or diet. The administration of vaccinations at the same time as manual therapies (spinal manipulation, trigger point, and acupuncture) is a controversial and hotly debated topic amongst integrative practitioners.

Scheduling integrative appointments presents a unique opportunity not afforded by traditional Western appointments. Most appointments in veterinary medicine are scheduled linearly: 8 a.m., 8:30 a.m., 9 a.m., etc. For many VIM appointments the veterinarians are really only in the exam room for the initial history, examination, and treatment. If a hospital has enough exam rooms and personnel, integrative appointments could be staggered very easily. This would in essence double the DVM revenue per half hour to hour. Staggered appointments should be considered once the veterinarian amasses enough demand. This tactic does require double the exam room capacity, support staff, and requires careful planning when scheduling appointments.

Pricing

Service cost is a surprisingly complicated topic. When designing a pricing system, the following factors should be considered: facility costs; support staff time requirements; desired average client transaction; desired average number of daily doctor appointments; desired doctor revenue per hour; materials and equipment costs; and amortization of education/certification costs (if applicable).

Pricing, another hot-button issue in veterinary medicine, has as many approaches as there are opinions about pricing. Multiple components must be considered when discussing VIM pricing in the veterinary hospital: overhead, supply costs, amortization of veterinarian training, desired average transaction per client (ATC), desired veterinarian revenue per hour, and opportunity cost.

An in-depth discussion of these variables is beyond the scope of this book. There are numerous sources covering everything a practice would and should know about veterinarian fees, financial and productivity benchmarks, and compensation and benefits. Listed below are supplementary reference materials which discuss hospital pricing in further detail.

1. Business Management for an Integrative Veterinary Practice: A 19-hour online continuing education course offered through the Chi Institute of Traditional Chinese Veterinary Medicine (https://www.tcvm.com/Home.aspx).
2. *The Veterinary Fee Reference*, 10th edition: A statistical reference book created by AAHA establishing evidence-based fee structures and guidance.
3. *Financial and Productivity Pulsepoints*, 10th edition: An AAHA statistical reference book defining current financial benchmarks in veterinary medicine.
4. *Compensation and Benefits*, 9th edition: An AAHA statistical reference book outlining current veterinary compensation and benefit packages.

As an aside, opportunity cost is something we do not consider nor discuss much in veterinary medicine. Opportunity cost represents the amount of potential lost revenue. For example, if the average ATC for a hospital is $150 and a 30-minute acupuncture session is $100, then the opportunity cost is −$50. Opportunity cost provides another guideline when considering the pricing structure for acupuncture appointments.

For the sake of brevity each chapter will focus its attention on two aspects of VIM pricing: current market fees (when available) and hospital cost-based pricing. Hospital cost-based pricing uses the following formula:

> **Hospital Cost-Based Pricing = Hospital Cost per Patient × Percentage Markup**

Hospital costs, as outlined earlier, include veterinarian training assumptions, overhead, and supply assumptions. Both the veterinarian training assumptions, and occasionally supply assumptions, are calculated as amortized startup costs. Amortization is calculated using the expected number of daily VIM appointments and the desired time allotted to recoup expenses. The percent markup typically falls between 40 and 100%.

Using my current appointment prices, assuming a $3.5/minute overhead, my VIM appointments have an 80–85% markup. When developing a pricing system my PM and I evaluated market demand, hospital costs, average client transaction, and doctor revenue per hour.

To determine market demand, we called the clinics within a 20-mile radius offering acupuncture (and other integrative therapies) and requested service quotes. Hospital costs were calculated using the amount needed to break even for a 30- and 60-minute VIM appointment as our starting point. Finally, we used both the ATC and the goal veterinarian revenue per hour to define the desired service fee. The resulting fee schedule has been both successful and lucrative.

Most service charges in veterinary medicine are calculated arbitrarily. Understanding both the current market value and awareness of hospital costs are crucial to strategically designing a profitable pricing scheme. Remember, profit is not a dirty word. Profit not only keeps the lights on, pays employees, but also allows for hospital improvements, and the purchase of new equipment.

Veterinarians frequently feel guilty charging appropriately for their time. Veterinarians practicing integrative medicine spend a lot of time and money studying these therapies. They have a skillset not possessed by all veterinarians. Their training allows them to approach cases from a different, and often more inclusive, perspective. This special training provides valuable services to the patients. This value must be embraced by the practitioner, the entire staff, and then conveyed to the client.

Team Training

Alright, the veterinarian has received their training and is eager to start helping their patients the integrative way. What's next? The rest of the staff needs to know their new roles and what is expected of them. Enter training phase training.

Phase training is my go-to method of training for all support staff new hires. I call them "training checklists." These checklists outline very clearly the expected tasks all new hires are required to complete. The checklists are broken down into levels of difficulty, two to three depending on the position, with specific time requirements for completion. Most tasks require demonstration of competency on two separate occasions. The team member observing completion of the task dates and initials the checklist. Once all the required tasks are complete the team member is considered trained in that level or phase.

Accompanying these checklists are the compendium standard operating procedures, or SOPs, which explain, in detail, how to perform the required tasks. All team members who have completed the checklists are permitted to train new hires or those progressing through the higher levels of phase training. This design ensures everyone is familiar with the hospital protocols and preferred procedures, as well as encouraging staff member participation and ownership in the acclimation and training of new hires.

The concept of phase training can be used when introducing VIM to the hospital team. The phases can be broken down as follows:

- Phase 1: Background information about the VIM treatment.
- Phase 2: Demonstrate knowledge proficiency.
- Phase 3: Outline expectations for each team member.
- Phase 4: Demonstrate proficiency in client education.

A multi-media approach will assist training for each VIM service. This book, and compendium online materials, aim to provide a one-stop-shopping experience when it comes to successfully training the entire support team.

Teaching and Learning Styles Learning is an adaptive behavior that increases the likelihood of survival. If we see or hear a bear, we either freeze or run, and we avoid being eaten. We smell rotten food, do not eat it, and avoid food poisoning. We feel heat from a hot stove, hopefully do not touch it, and we avoid burning our skin.

As we age the role of learning becomes less about survival and more about self-development. Education helps advance our careers and enrich our daily lives. Most people consider themselves either visual or auditory learners. The truth is we learn using all our senses: vision, sound, smell, and touch.

The VIM team training relies primarily on visual and auditory cues. A large portion of our brain is devoted to recognizing and interpreting visual and auditory stimuli. The actual process through which our brains analyze and respond to these stimuli is extremely complex and not completely understood (Dosher and Lu 2017).

The brain learns by making new connections and pathways between the nerve cells, or neurons, in a process called neuroplasticity. The goal of any educator is to ensure neuroplasticity (aka memory) about the subject of interest. Ensuring neuroplasticity involves a two-part approach: repeat exposure to the desired information and keep the information short and to the point.

- **Repeat exposure**: Perceptual learning refers to the process of improving sensory information through experience, i.e. practice makes perfect. A study by Zhang et al. (2016) demonstrated perceptual learning requires the development of neuroplasticity between the cognitive and sensory portions of the brain. The sensory portions take in the information, the cognitive centers interpret the information, and the connections established between these regions aids in utilization and retention of the information (Zhang et al. 2016). Zhang et al. (2016) also showed that repeat exposure to the same stimulus is necessary to stimulate these connections and establish memory.
- **KISS (Keep it simple silly)**: Many learning models reference a signal-to-noise ratio. The signal is the information to be learned, while the noise is any other stimulus the brain is exposed to at any given moment in time. The goal is to increase the likelihood of the brain receiving the desired signal while reducing the noise (Dosher and Lu 2017).

Phase training hits both requirements for neuroplasticity: repetition and high signal intensity. The handouts and videos ensure both the auditory and visual centers are stimulated. The phases or levels ensure repetition of pertinent information throughout the learning process. And, unlike this section of the book, brevity within the phase training is crucial. Time is money in veterinary medicine. Time spent training is time not spent seeing patients. Any training program must be designed to ensure the maximum amount of information is retained in the most efficient means possible.

The PM's Role in Training

The PM's role is like the conductor of an orchestra where all of the musicians have been replaced with cats. All too often it falls on the shoulders of the PM to ensure the team is successfully trained.

To conquer this task the PM needs his or her own checklist which includes scheduling time for team training; ensure all information pertaining to the new service is reviewed with the staff; confirming all team members have completed the training; certifying all team members understand the information and can successfully educate clients; and ensuring staff buy-in.

The phase training, with accompanying handouts and PowerPoints, greatly reduces the PM's workload, assuring comprehensive employee education in a timely fashion. The quizzes solidify employee understanding of the materials. Finally, the client information provides a foundation for open client communication and education.

I highly recommend setting aside a specific day(s) and time(s) for all-team training to ensure everyone can concentrate and absorb the new material. These meetings should focus on training only, increasing signal intensity while eliminating the noise of non-VIM-related items. Ultimately scheduling team training is up to each PM, as you are the most familiar with the ebb and flow of the clinic.

Staff buy-in is perhaps the most elusive and important component of any service offered at a veterinary hospital. If your team does not believe in a product or service, it is very difficult to promote and utilize said item. With regards to staff buy-in, I thought I would turn to an expert in the field of veterinary leadership, Randy Hall. Randy is the cofounder and CEO of VetLead, an online leadership and management resource for veterinary professionals.

I was able to sit down with Randy Hall and discuss in detail the idea of employee engagement. Below are excerpts from the interview. The key points are summarized in Figures 12 and 13. The full interview, entitled "The Five Elements of Employee Engagement," is available for download on my veterinary podcast, Vetsplaining.

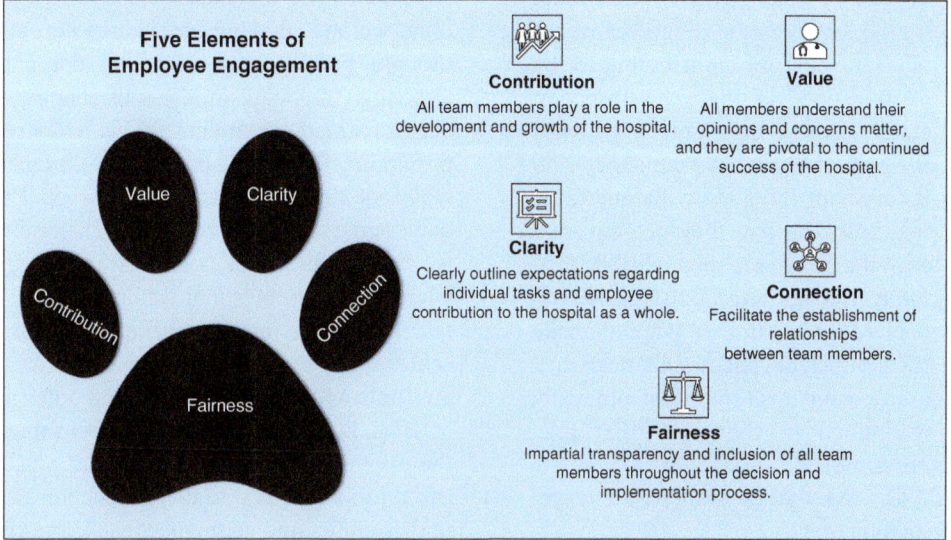

Figure 12 Summary of the five elements of employee engagement as outlined by Randy Hall. Source: Lisa P. McFaddin.

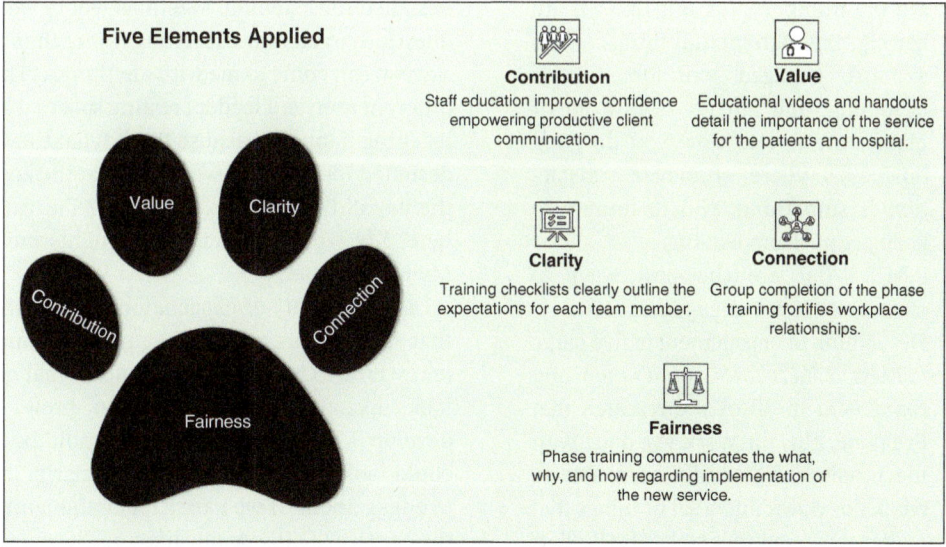

Figure 13 The application of the five elements of employee engagement utilizing the phase training described in the previous section. Source: Lisa P. McFaddin.

An Interview with Randy Hall

L.P.M. Could you define employee engagement versus employee satisfaction?

R.H. Employee engagement is really about people bringing discretionary effort to their job. . .They show up because of what they get to contribute to the organization not because of what they get for contributing to the organization. . .Employee satisfaction simply means they are happy with their job. You can have somebody who is very happy to go to work and satisfied with the pay they get, satisfied with the hours, satisfied with the flexibility, but not engaged. That is relatively easy to find. . .We can make them satisfied. That doesn't mean they are showing up at their best and really committed to the work that they are doing.

L.P.M. Why does employee engagement matter?

R.H. 21% greater profitability in highly engaged workforces. 41% reduction in absenteeism. 59% less turnover. They are big numbers. It's not like we are getting tiny incremental things out of a more engaged workforce. It is becoming, and already is in a lot of places, the key to how you do good business. Where employee satisfaction is something, you do purely to keep people from leaving.

L.P.M. What are the best ways to ensure employee engagement?

R.H. I think of engagement in five parts: *fairness, value, clarity, contribution*, and *connection*. In all of the research that I've done, plus the work I've done with the hospitals, I've really been able to break this down into a set of things that matter most and that cover the kind of organization [which] if you build it, you will have engaged people.

Fairness: I start with that because it's probably one of the tougher ones because fairness is kind of in the eye of the beholder. It relies on other peoples' beliefs on what is fair and is not. . .What we do to increase fairness in the organization is increase transparency. . .[We cannot] assume equal equals because it doesn't. . .The transparency is important. Here's why we are making decisions; here's how we are making decisions; here's the thought process that went into doing this. Showing your work in terms of changes and decisions made in the hospital is really really important. Because if people can understand what's behind it, it feels more fair, even if they don't agree with the decision. . .The reality is we have parts of our brain that get triggered when we find things that we don't believe are fair. They are actually the same as the disgust center in our brain. . .And the reason is parts of our brain are built to filter and find unfairness.

Value: By value I mean people feel valued in the organization. . .And things that practices can do to in general to drive value are things like listening, and getting feedback, and creating time for listening, not just saying I listen if you bring something to me. But specifically building spaces where we listen, that are designed for listening. Meetings where we ask questions to facilitate listening rather than just say you can come to me with anything. . .That's different then as a leader creating spaces where listening happens because that's what they are designed for...When I went home at the end of the day did I matter to that place? I'm valued here. My words matter. My thoughts matter. My ideas matter.

Clarity: Clarity of expectations is something that really does create engagement. Meaning I know how to be great here. I know what good looks like. I know how to learn, grow, and develop. I know what my future could be and could look like here. That level of clarity leads to engagement. If we have a lot of ambiguity in the system. . .it's really hard to be engaged because I don't have a path. . .Ambiguity kills engagement.

Contribution: Contribution means I get to show up and contribute to the future. . . I get to play a role in how we make decisions. I get to be involved in what the next quarter, month, year looks like. I get to make a difference. Not just people believe I matter, but I get to see a difference made because of my inputs. And that's where contribution really matters. . .In veterinary medicine we are kind of lucky because what we do matters.

Connection: I'm doing this with people I like being around. That I enjoy connecting with. That I have bonds with. That I communicate well with.

L.P.M. How do you apply those five factors when introducing a new service?

R.H. So, you can actually go right around those five components and think about it. How do I introduce this in a way that seems fair?. . .The transparency is where we get fairness. . .The value piece, I want your ideas about how we do this well to be incorporated. I want to listen to you. Clarity let's decide what good looks like in terms of how we role this out. Let's decide what are our expectations for how many people should use this or how often we should talk about it. Let's do that so we know what good looks like really well. Contribution, allowing people to contribute to the success of this. And this, if anywhere, is where the practice comes in because now, I'm also developing the ability to have conversations that the clients value more. So, I get to contribute in that way to the process. And then the connections, having a team go away and say alright I want you guys to think about this as a group. Figure out how you are going to get great at it. Figure out how I can help. But we get to have teams working on things that they feel are making a difference. . .That's a team building exercise.

Randy Hall, Cofounder and CEO of VetLead (www.vetlead.com).

Promotion

There are six common avenues of promotion for a VIM service: hospital website, social media, email blasts, mailers, in-hospital promotions, and client education. Specific recommendations for each category are in the treatment chapters of the book. Multiple categories can, and should, be used to ensure effective promotion of the service.

Hospital Website: Utilize the hospital website to advertise the VIM treatment under the "Services" section. Include a description of the specialized training and professional initials, if applicable, on the veterinarian's biography page. Create a VIM blog page discussing patient success stories.

Social Media: Utilize Facebook and Instagram to post fun and intriguing facts about VIM, photos of patients receiving VIM treatments, VIM-specific hashtags, and patient success stories.

Email Blasts: Send fun mass emails to your clients introducing the new service. Consider monthly case presentations illustrating how the service has benefited patients. Almost everyone has at least one email address these days. Customer service representatives (CSRs) should be amassing client emails at the same rate as phone numbers.

Mailers: I personally do not recommend mailers. In this digital age it is best to communicate hospital changes with clients electronically or in person. Most people throw away junk mail without ever reading it. Why waste your money on future trash? At least if your email blasts end up in the trash folder all it cost was the time spent creating the email. There are ideas for mailers within each chapter and on the website for those who cannot help but spend money on stamps.

In-Hospital Promotions: Capture your client's attention while in the clinic with their pet.

Each chapter offers in-hospital advertisement suggestions such as small signs, teasers on the invoice, and wearable buttons for the staff.

Client Education: Education is crucial to understanding the purpose and importance of any given treatment. The client handouts and videos solidify the pet owner's knowledge base, reducing concerns and conveying value. Downloadable and editable handouts and PowerPoint presentations can be found online. The handouts were reviewed by two amazing team members, Deh Tarchie-Singletary (CSR) and Melissa Duffy (veterinary assistant). The PowerPoint presentations were reviewed by the entire team at my clinic.

Integration

Ultimately the veterinarian decides which patients will benefit from and receive VIM therapies. The PM needs to support the veterinarian's regular use of the treatment. This is best accomplished through proper appointment and support staff scheduling.

Appointment times must be long enough to allow performance of the procedure but not too long to negatively affect the number of patients seen. Adequate support staff scheduling is crucial for services requiring additional patient restraint or treatments. Appropriate scheduling of team members also helps keep the doctor running on time while preventing escalating staff costs. Suggested appointment lengths and support staff specifics are discussed in the subsequent chapters.

Customer Service Representative

The first line of defense within any veterinary hospital. These amazing men and women are often the first persons with whom a client speaks, either on the phone or in person. As such our CSRs are one of the best advertisers for the hospital, especially when introducing a new treatment. The following attributes are necessary to ensure these hospital influencers are successful: a general understanding of the new VIM treatment; an appreciation of how

the treatment can help patients; and proficiency and confidence when speaking with clients about the new modality.

While the veterinarian and PM are frequently the ones designing the digital and print materials, the CSR must be aware of the available client information to answer client questions and/or refer clients to the appropriate information.

As the gatekeepers of the appointment schedule, CSRs are critical to VIM integration by ensuring appointments are scheduled appropriately. Appointment times should be long enough to allow performance of the procedure but not too long so as to negatively affect the number of patients seen. CSRs must be aware of specific patient recommendations for the appointments, i.e. fasting is needed for sedated trigger point procedures. Appointment length suggestions, as well as specific pre-appointment client reminders, are discussed in each chapter.

According to two of the best darn CSRs I have had the pleasure to work with, the most important detail to consider when introducing a new service into a practice is a knowledgeable staff. As Deh Tarchie-Singletary (Figure 14) put it "knowledge of the recommended services and treatment plan are important so we are able to educate the client, assuring they

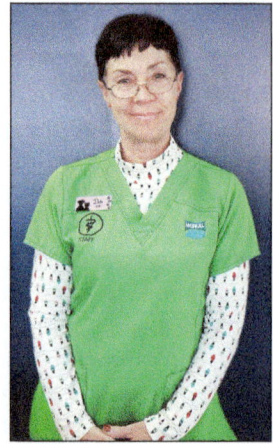

Figure 14   Deh Tarchie-Singletary has been working as a veterinary customer service representative for over 21 years. Source: Lisa P. McFaddin.

fully understand what is involved and why this is our recommendation."

Claudia Amaya seconded the sentiment stating

> As a CSR it is important to be knowledgeable and well educated on a new service before introducing it to a client. The most important information to give a client is how a service will benefit and improve the health of their pet. After all what good is a new service if it doesn't help the pet?

Veterinary Assistant and Licensed Technicians

The heart and soul of patient care within a veterinary hospital. These men and women frequently have more hands-on time with the patients than the veterinarian. VAs and LTs often develop strong emotional bonds with the patients and clients. Compassion and trust reinforce this VA/LT–client–patient bond. What this boils down to is VA and LT buy-in is extremely important. VAs and LTs regularly answer questions the clients are too embarrassed to ask the doctor or forgot to ask the doctor while he or she was in the exam room. VA and LT endorsements are essential to encourage client perusal of a new treatment avenue. The VAs and LTs should utilize their VIM training, client–patient bond, and available promotion information to educate clients and promote the VIM services.

For the purposes of this book VAs are defined as all non-licensed technicians. LTs are those who underwent schooling, passed the national boards, and obtained certification as a veterinary technician. Different states use different initials, including licensed veterinary technician (LVT), certified veterinary technician (CVT), and registered veterinary technician (RVT). To avoid confusion and favoritism, licensed technicians will be referred to as LTs in this book.

VAs and LTs help integrate VIM treatments by assisting veterinarians with appointments and providing reliable client education. Specific recommendations for appointments will be discussed within each chapter. The client education information can be found in the Training and Promotion sections.

My LTs did not disappoint when asked their opinion regarding the most important detail to consider when introducing a new service. Tama Allison (Figure 15) said "I need to know why the doctor thinks the new service is important and how it will help my patients. If I understand why the doctor thinks it's cool and useful, I can more easily promote and educate both staff and clients."

Kathleen Brooks (Figure 16) stated "Assisting with integrative appointments, much like all

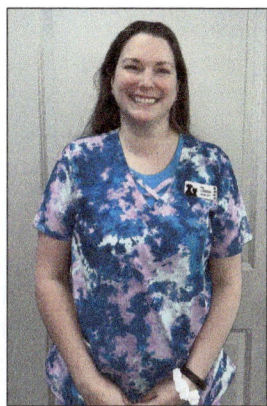

Figure 15 Tama Allison has been working in the veterinary field as a licensed technician for over 22 years. Source: Lisa P. McFaddin.

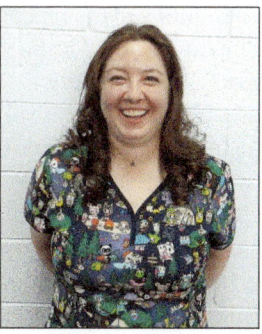

Figure 16 Kathleen Brooks has been working in the veterinary field for over 10 years and has spent the last five years as a licensed veterinary technician. Source: Lisa P. McFaddin.

aspects of veterinary medicine, boils down to three key principles: practice patience; less is more when it comes to restraint; and the perfect treat is *key*."

Veterinarians

Veterinarians, as the ones performing the treatments, are pivotal to the introduction of VIM within a practice. Veterinarians frequently have many non-medical questions regarding VIM. These questions can be broken down into six categories: state requirements and restrictions, return on investment, course availability, supplies and equipment, veterinary organizations, and reference books.

State Requirements and Restrictions

Factors to consider include a state's definition of what constiutes the "practice of veterinary medicine," integrative continuing education hours, and liability insurance.

The Practice of Veterinary Medicine: Each state has its own veterinary provisions outlining what is and is not considered the practice of veterinary medicine. Many states include provisions allowing non-veterinarians certified in certain integrative therapies, such as acupuncture and spinal manipulation, to practice under the direct supervision of a veterinarian. These rules can change, and careful review of your specific state requirements and restrictions is recommended. Links to each state's veterinary board and their rules and regulations pertaining to the practice of veterinary medicine can be found online.

Integrative Continuing Education Hours: Some states limit the use of integrative medicine continuing education (CE) hours toward the annual CE requirement for license renewal. Review your specific state's requirements for further details.

Liability Insurance: Professional liability insurance policies cover the veterinarian when accused of medical malpractice or negligence. This protection generally covers all allegations pertaining to veterinary-related activities. In most negligence and malpractice complaints the issue boils down to "standard of care," namely was the standard of care met. This can be tricky with respect to integrative medicine. Given the gray-zone that is liability protection and integrative medicine, veterinarians are encouraged to speak with their insurance companies directly to determine if a specific integrative service is covered.

Return on Investment

Specifics are discussed in the Team Members section of each chapter.

Training Course Availability

Let's take a moment to review a few key terms often applied incorrectly and interchangeably when discussing postgraduate veterinarian training: accreditation, credentials, licenses, certification, and post-nominal initials.

Accreditation is a voluntary process used to determine if an educational program or institution meets certain standards of quality as determined by an outside non-governmental agency (AVMA 2020). The Council for Higher Education Accreditation (CHEA) states "accreditation is a major way that students, families, government officials, and the press know that an institution or program provides a quality education" (CHEA 2020).

Colleges and universities in the United States are accredited by at least one of the 19 recognized institutional accrediting organizations. There are approximately 60 recognized accrediting organizations responsible for accrediting programs in the United States. These accrediting organizations are reviewed by the CHEA or the United States Department of Education. The accrediting organizations or "accreditors are private, non-governmental organizations created for the specific purpose of reviewing higher education institutions and programs for quality" (CHEA 2020).

The AVMA Council on Education™ (COE) accredits veterinary educational programs in the United States and Canada. The AVMA COE guarantees the "minimum standards in veterinary medical education are met by all

AVMA-accredited colleges of veterinary medicine" (AVMA COE 2020). Some veterinary schools offer courses on various VIM topics. There are, however, no AVMA COE accredited non-veterinary school VIM programs or courses currently available.

There are two accredited post-secondary organizations offering training courses in VIM: Chi University and the Healing Oasis Wellness Center. As of February 2023, all other post-graduate programs in VIM are offered by member organizations, associations, or businesses.

Chi University is accredited by the Distance Education Accrediting Commission (DEAC) which is recognized by the CHEA and US Department of Education. The Master's degree program in traditional Chinese veterinary medicine (TCVM) is licensed by the Florida Commission for Independent Education.

The Healing Oasis Wellness Center (HOWC) is accredited by the Accrediting Council for Continuing Education and Training (ACCET) which is recognized by the CHEA and US Department of Education. All programs offered are approved by the Wisconsin Department of Safety and Professional Service Educational Approval Program (DSPS-EAP) and the College of Animal Chiropractors (CoAC). The veterinary massage and rehabilitation training (VMRT) and veterinary spinal manipulation therapy (VSMT) courses are approved for the GI Bill® by the Wisconsin State Approving Agency for Veteran's Education Benefits. HOWC is also partnered with National University of Health Sciences.

Credentials: The National Environmental Health Association (NEHA) defines credentials as "issued by a third party with authoritative power and is proof of an individual's qualification or competence in a given subject." There are degree and non-degree credentials.

Degree credentials are those received upon completion or graduation from a secondary school such as a college or university. For example, upon graduation from Virginia Maryland College of Veterinary Medicine I received a Doctor of Veterinary Medicine (DVM).

Non-degree credentials are those not associated with graduation from a college or university and include certificates, industry certifications, licenses, and apprenticeships. Individuals with or without a college or postgraduate degree can receive non-degree credentials (NCES 2018; Zanville 2019). For the purposes of this book, non-degree credentials refer to those credentials received following the successful completion of specific VIM training programs.

Credentialing, for both degree and non-degree credentials, is the process required to meet the specific professional and/or technical skills required to perform a task and achieve recognition (NEHA 2020). In the case of VIM this process usually involves successful completion of a course or courses, demonstration of knowledge proficiency (through written examinations), and demonstration of technical proficiency (through practical examinations, case studies, and/or internship requirements). Table 1 lists and describes my personal post-nominal initials.

License: The Interagency Working Group on Expanded Measures of Enrollment and Attainment (GEMEnA) defines a license as "a credential awarded by a government agency that constitutes legal authority to do a specific job. Licenses are based on some combination of degree or certificate attainment, certifications, assessments, or work experience; are time-limited; and must be renewed periodically" (NCES 2020).

State licensure to practice veterinary medicine is a prime example. State licensure requirements vary greatly, with some requiring the practitioner pass a state-specific veterinary examination. At the heart of it, all states require documentation proving successful graduation from an accredited school of veterinary medicine, passing the North American Veterinary Licensing Examination (NAVLE), annual CE requirements, and an annual or biennial renewal fee. Currently, there are no VIM licenses.

Certification: The GEMEnA defines certification as "a credential awarded by a certification body based on an individual demonstrating

Table 1 A breakdown of my post-nominal initials.

Lisa P. McFaddin, DVM, GDCVHM, CVSMT, FCoAC, CVA, CVFT		
DVM	Initials explained	Doctor of Veterinary Medicine
	Credential type	Degree
	Organization	Virginia-Maryland College of Veterinary Medicine (VMCVM)
	Accreditation	American Veterinary Medical Association's (AVMA) Council on Education (COE)
GDCVHM	Initials explained	Graduate Diploma Veterinary Chinese Herbal Medicine
	Credential type	Degree
	Organization	College of Integrative Veterinary Therapies (CIVT)
	Accreditation	Registered Training Organization Nationally Recognized Training
CVSMT	Initials explained	Certificate of Competency Veterinary Spinal Manipulation Therapy
	Credential type	Non-degree
	Organization	Healing Oasis Wellness Center
	Accreditation	US Department of Education
CVMRT	Initials explained	Certificate of Competency Veterinary Massage and Rehabilitation Therapy
	Credential type	Non-degree
	Organization	Healing Oasis Wellness Center
	Accreditation	US Department of Education
FCoAC	Initials explained	Fellow of the College of Animal Chiropractors
	Credential type	Non-degree
	Organization	College of Animal Chiropractors
	Accreditation	n/a
CVA	Initials explained	Certified Veterinary Acupuncturist
	Credential type	Non-degree
	Organization	Chi University
	Accreditation	n/a
CVFT	Initials explained	Certified Veterinary Food Therapist
	Credential type	Non-degree
	Organization	Chi University
	Accreditation	n/a

Source: Lisa P. McFaddin.

through an examination process that he or she has acquired the designated knowledge, skills, and abilities to perform a specific job (NCES 2020). The examination can be either written, oral, or performance-based."

As an example, Chi University offers a certification program for veterinary acupuncture. Upon completion of the course, passing three online quizzes, passing a final written examination, passing a clinical acupoint examination, submission and approval of one case report, and completion of 30 hours of advanced training or an internship with a certified veterinary acupuncturist, students are eligible for the Certified Veterinary Acupuncturist certification. This certification is endorsed by the Chi University and the World Association of Traditional Chinese Veterinary Medicine (WATCVM). The certified veterinary acupuncturist certification has the post-nominal initials CVA.

Post-Nominal Initials: Wikipedia (2020) defines post-nominal initials, also known as post-nominal letters, post-nominal titles, and designator letters, as "letters placed after a person's name to indicate that the individual holds a position, academic degree, accreditation, office, military decoration, or honor, or is a member of a religious institute or fraternity." The standard listing hierarchy in the US is as follows: religious institutions, theological degrees, military decorations, academic degrees, honorary degrees, honors, decorations, professional licenses, certifications and affiliations, and retired uniformed service (Wikipedia 2020).

Not all non-degree credentials come with post-nominal initials. In the world of VIM post-nominal initials are very common, often creating an alphabet soup after one's name. As an example, let's look at my initials.

With all this information in mind, there are multiple questions to ask yourself when considering which VIM course to take.

- Is formal training necessary to practice the VIM therapy?
- What organizations and programs are available?
- Is the organization or school accredited?
- Is the offered training considered a certification program?
- Are there post-nominal initials associated with the certification?
- How long does it take to complete the training?
- What are the veterinarian's time requirements to complete the training?
- What is the cost of the training, including the course, books, and travel?
- Is travel required for the training?
- Does the training utilize hands-on experience, remote learning, or a combination?
- What are the faculty credentials?
- What is the student to teacher ratio?
- What are the requirements for certification, if applicable?
- When can the veterinarian start utilizing the VIM service?

Each chapter provides the following information regarding veterinarian training:

1. Organizations or companies offering courses.
2. Course name.
3. Course description, including approved American Association of Veterinary State Boards Registry of Approved Continuing Education (AAVSB RACE) hours if applicable.
4. Training location.
5. Training length.
6. Price.
7. Certification process, if applicable.

Supplies and Equipment

The veterinarian, and hospital manager, should determine what supplies and equipment are needed, where to purchase said supplies, is additional space within the hospital required to perform the treatment, and will hospital remodeling or redecoration be required.

Veterinary Organizations

There are numerous veterinary organizations with a focus on integrative medicine. This section describes the organizations focusing on that modality. When available the approximate annual or biennial membership fee is provided.

Currently no states require additional CE hours for any modality within VIM. Some veterinary organizations require annual CE hours to maintain active memberships. Additionally, some veterinary organizations provide veterinary CE in the form of annual conferences, courses, and lectures (in-person and webinar).

All veterinarians interested in any aspect of integrative medicine are encouraged to join the American Holistic Veterinary Medical Association (AHVMA). The AHVMA was founded in 1982 at the Western States Veterinary Conference. This organization represents all veterinarians practicing all forms of integrative medicine. Current membership numbers are close to 1800 veterinarians. The AHVMA helps advance integrative medicine through the AHVMA's seat on the AVMA House of Delegates. As a member of the AHVMA you have a direct voice to the AVMA. The AHVMA also supports integrative research and promotes veterinary student awareness of integrative medicine through the student chapters and scholarships.

American Holistic Veterinary Medical Association (AHVMA)

PO Box 630, Abingdon, MD 21009
(410) 569-0795
office@ahvma.org

Reference Books

Lest we forget our trusted reference books. If you are like me, you have amassed quite a few books which look beautiful on the bookshelf in the hospital library, with their shiny covers and un-cracked spines. But how many of those books have you read? The sheer number of books can be overwhelming. A list and description of recommended books for the veterinarian's professional library are also provided.

Promotion

The PM and veterinarian are responsible for designing and implementing the new service to existing and new clients. Refer to the Team Members section of the chapter for further information.

Integration

Successful integration is ultimately reliant upon the veterinarian. Promotion and client education will not amount to much if the veterinarian does not recommend or perform the treatment. The following items are addressed to ensure regular use of the VIM service: team training; appointment scheduling; support staff scheduling; and when to use VIM.

Team Training: The veterinarian must be an active participant in team training. Veterinarian involvement solidifies team buy-in by highlighting the benefits of the new treatment and proving their solidarity for the success of the hospital. The veterinarian can also confirm the entire team understands the new information and can effectively communicate and educate clients.

Veterinarians are also encouraged to treat employee pets. First-hand experience with VIM therapies helps the team really understand the benefits of the service and greatly improves their ability to promote and educate clients.

Appointment Scheduling: Appointment times should be long enough to allow performance of the procedure but not too long to negatively affect the number of patients seen. Veterinarians must communicate their needs with the entire team. The rationale for the length of the appointments should be discussed with all team members. Specific pre-appointment client reminders should also be discussed, such as encouraging owners to physically bring all their supplements and medications to the appointment.

Support Staff Scheduling: The veterinarian must understand and plan for effective use of their support staff and be aware of the number of people necessary to perform the VIM treatments.

When to Use the VIM Modality: This information is obtained through introductory and advanced courses, as well as with hands-on experience.

Conclusion

A summary of the key points discussed in the chapter.

Acknowledgments

A word of thanks is provided acknowledging the veterinarian expert who reviewed the chapter.

References

References cited in each chapter are provided in alphabetical order.

References

AAHA (American Animal Hospital Association) (2019). *Compensation and Benefits*, 9e. Denver, CO: AAHA Press.

APPA (American Pet Products Association) (2022). *Pet industry market size and ownership statistics*. https://www.americanpetproducts .org/press_industrytrends.asp (accessed 23 February 2023).

AVMA (American Veterinary Medical Association) (2020). *AVMA center for veterinary education accreditation*. https:// www.avma.org/education/center-for-veterinary-accreditation (accessed 21 December 2020).

AVMA COE (American Veterinary Medical Association Council on Education) (2020). *AVMA Council on Education*. https://www .avma.org/education/accreditation-veterinary-colleges (accessed 21 December 2020).

Bol, S. and Bunnik, E. (2015). Lysine supplementation is not effective for the prevention or treatment of feline herpesvirus 1 infection in cats: a systematic review. *BMC Veterinary Research* 11: 284.

Burns, K. (2018). *Pet ownership stable, veterinary care variable*. https://www.avma.org/ javma-news/2019-01-15/pet-ownership-stable-veterinary-care-variable (accessed 11 August 2021).

Burns, K. (2022). *New report takes a deep dive into pet ownership*. https://www.avma.org/ news/new-report-takes-deep-dive-pet-ownership (accessed 6 November 2022).

Carrns, A. (2019). More pet insurance policies are being sold. But are they worth the cost? *The New York Times* (4 January).

CHEA (Council for Higher Education Accreditation) (2020). *Accreditation and Recognition*. https://www.chea.org/about-accreditation (accessed 21 December 2020).

Dosher, B. and Lu, Z.-L. (2017). Visual perceptual learning and modules. *Annual Reviews of Visual Science* 15 (3): 343–363.

Imhoff, M. (2001). How to measure return on investment. https://citeseerx.ist.psu.edu/docu ment?repid=rep1&type=pdf&doi=22d012541 ea392ed0ce0bbe532a2ea14a3d7f83b (accessed 26 July 2021).

Masic, I., Miokovic, M., and Muhamedagic, B. (2008). Evidence based medicine: new approaches and challenges. *Acta Informatica Medica* 16 (4): 219–225. https://doi .org/10.5455/aim.2008.16.219-225.

McKenzie, B. (2013). *Myths and misconceptions about evidence-based medicine*. https://www. vin.com/members/cms/project/defaultadv1 .aspx?pid=11393&catId=&id=5959806&said= &meta=&authorid=&preview=

Memon, M., Shmalberg, J., Adair, H.S. et al. (2016). Integrative veterinary medical education and consensus guidelines for an integrative medicine curriculum within veterinary colleges. *Open Veterinary Journal* 6 (1): 44–56.

Memon, M.A., Shmalberg, J.W., and Xie, H. (2021). Survey of integrative veterinary medicine training in AVMA-accredited veterinary colleges. *Journal of Veterinary Medical Education* 48 (3): 289–294. https://doi .org/10.3138/jvme.2019-0067.

MFAF (Michelson Found Animals Foundation) (2018). *Furred lines: Pet trends.* https://www .prnewswire.com/news-releases/furred-lines-pet-trends-2019-300741947.html (accessed 26 July 2021).

NAPHIA (North American Pet Health Insurance Association) (2023). *Industry Data.* https:// naphia.org/industry-data/#my-menu (accessed 18 February 2023).

NCES (National Center for Education Statistics) (2018). *Nondegree work credentials and work experience programs.* https://nces.ed.gov/ programs/coe/indicator/sae/nondegree-work-credentials (accessed 27 December 2020).

NCES (National Center for Education Statistics) (2020). *Working definitions of non-degree credentials.* https://nces.ed.gov/surveys/ gemena/definitions.asp (accessed 27 December 2020).

NEHA (National Environmental Health Association) (2020). *Difference between credentials and certifications.* https://www .neha.org/Credentials-Certifications (accessed 21 December 2020).

Nolen, R.S. (2022). *Pet ownership rate stabilizes as spending increases.* https://www.avma.org/ news/pet-ownership-rate-stabilizes-spending-increases (accessed 22 February 2023).

Ouedraogo, F., Bain, B., Hansen, C., and Salois, M. (2019). A census of veterinarians in the United States. *Journal of the American Veterinary Medical Association* 255 (2): 183–191.

Stevenson, P. (2016). *How to set practice service fees.* https://cliniciansbrief.com/article/ how-set-practice-service-fees (accessed 21 December 2020).

Tricarico, E. (2019). *Build the bond to reach millennial pet owners.* https://www.dvm360 .com/view/build-bond-reach-millennial-pet-owners (accessed 26 July 2021).

Wikipedia (2020). *Post-nominal letters.* https:// en.wikipedia.org/wiki/Post-nominal_letters (accessed 27 December 2020).

Woodley, K. (2018). *Pet insurance for holistic and integrative practice.* https://ivcjournal.com/ pet-insurance-integrative-practices (accessed 11 August 2021).

Zanville, H. (2019). *Inside the big confusing credentialing tent: a new mission to understand non-degree credentials.* https://evolllution .com/programming/credentials/inside-the-big-confusing-credentialing-tent-a-new-mission-to-understand-non-degree-credentials (accessed 27 December 2020).

Zhang, Y.-X., Moore, D.R., Guiraud, J. et al. (2016). Auditory discrimination learning: role of working memory. *PLoS One* 11 (1): e0147320.

About the Companion Website

This book is accompanied by a companion website.

www.wiley.com/go/mcfaddin/integrativemedicine

This website includes:

1. Client Education Handouts
2. Script - Question and Answers
3. Training Worksheets
4. Quizzes
5. Training Guides
6. Training Worksheets
7. Training Handouts
8. Figures
9. Audio
10. Power Points

1

Acupuncture

Introduction

Acupuncture has been used in veterinary medicine for almost 3000 years and is defined as the insertion of a needle, or other object, into the skin on a specific area of the body which causes a beneficial response. The stimulation of acupuncture points can cause positive local and systemic effects. Veterinary acupuncture is commonly used to help with the management of anxiety, gastrointestinal disorders, generalized and chronic pain, immune system support and disorders, musculoskeletal disorders, neurologic disorders, reproductive disorders, and respiratory arrest.

The introduction of acupuncture into a veterinary practice can be beneficial for both the patient and the health of the practice. The successful incorporation and utilization of veterinary acupuncture does not end with the veterinaria's training. Support staff training and client education are crucial. This chapter discusses the what, why, and how for effective integration of veterinary acupuncture within your practice.

The What

Word Origin

Acupuncture is derived from the Latin words *acus*, meaning needle, and *pungare*, meaning pierce.

Definition

In its most elemental form, acupuncture is the insertion of a needle, or other object, into the skin on a specific area of the body causing a beneficial response.

Human History

The first recorded use of human acupuncture was in the Neolithic period in China around

Integrative Medicine in Veterinary Practice, First Edition. Lisa P. McFaddin.
© 2024 John Wiley & Sons, Inc. Published 2024 by John Wiley & Sons, Inc.
Companion website: www.wiley.com/go/mcfaddin/integrativemedicine

8000 years ago and involved 2-inch-long flat stone needles (called *ban-shie*). The first acupuncture book was inscribed on the inside of tortoise shells during the Xia-Shang Dynasty (2100–1046 BCE) (Xie 2011a,b). The introduction of metal during the Shang Dynasty (1600–1100 BCE) led to the creation of nine types of metal needles used for acupressure, acupuncture, and surgery (Xie 2011a). The study and practice of acupuncture has continued to develop and mature with time.

Acupuncture is considered one of the five branches of medicine within traditional Chinese medicine (TCM): acupuncture, Chinese herbs, Tui-na (massage), Qi-gong, and Chinese dietary therapy. These five branches are used together to restore and maintain a person's health and balance within nature.

The use of acupressure outside China is suspected to have developed independently over 5000 years ago. The best-known example is Ötzi, the Similaun Man. A group of German tourists found an entombed Iceman while hiking off-trail through the Alps in 1991. Little did they know that Ötzi was the oldest naturally preserved human mummy in Europe, who lived between 3400 and 3100 BCE. Ötzi was found with well-preserved clothes, small tools, and weapons. Over three decades of research have been conducted on Ötzi and his belongings. He is believed to have died from trauma and blood loss shortly after being shot with an arrow that shattered his left shoulder blade and punctured his lung (Wikipedia 2018). Figure 1.1 depicts a life-size reconstruction of Ötzi in his Neolithic clothing, with his belongings uncovered near him.

Even more interesting than his preservation and death was the discovery that his body was covered with 61 linear carbon tattoo markings. The use of radiography, computed tomography, and endoscopy revealed the tattoos were located over areas of underlying musculoskeletal abnormalities, such as arthritis and referred nerve (radicular) pain (Kean et al. 2013).

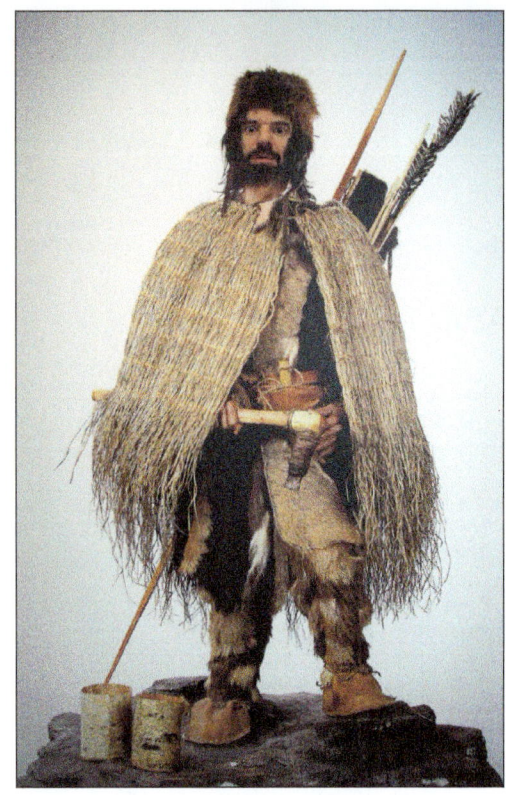

Figure 1.1 Meet Otzi, the over 5000-year-old iceman, whose medicinal tattoos mark regions of local and referred pain. Scientists believe acupressure was used on the carbon tattoos to provide temporary relief. Source: Melotzi/ Wikimedia Commons/CC BY-SA 4.0.

Kean et al. (2013) theorized that the markings were a form of "medicinal tattoos," mapping areas of chronic pain on his body. These authors speculated the tattoos were used as landmarks for acupuncture and acupressure treatment to relieve pain. In essence these were ancient "push here when injured" buttons covering his body. The markings would have allowed Ötzi to effectively communicate to other humans where to press, massage, or rub when experiencing pain. Ötzi's medicinal tattoos prove that the beneficial effects of manual therapy and acupuncture were developed and implemented by different cultures independently of each other.

Veterinary History

The development of veterinary acupuncture arose out of necessity to keep working horses healthy. The first recorded use of veterinary acupuncture was performed by Zhao Fu during the Zhou-mu-gong period (947–928 BCE) (Xie 2011a,b). Zhao Fu treated horse diseases through removal of blood (hemoacupuncture) in specific areas on horses' necks (Xie 2011a,b). The first veterinary acupuncture book, *Bole's Canon of Veterinary Acupuncture*, was written by Bo Le during the Qing-mu-gong period (659–621 BCE) (Xie 2011a,b). A more detailed account of the history of veterinary acupuncture can be found in Dr. Xie's book *Chinese Veterinary Herbology* (2011a,b).

The modern use and acceptance of veterinary acupuncture in the United States is largely due to the active efforts and scientific research spearheaded by the veterinarians working with Chi University and the International Veterinary Acupuncture Society (IVAS).

Terminology

The world of traditional Chinese veterinary medicine (TCVM) and acupuncture comes with its own vocabulary. A basic understanding of these terms facilitates effective communication between professionals and clients. A summary of common terms is provided below.

Acupoint: Also known as an acupuncture point. Anatomically, acupoints comprise free nerve endings, small vessels (arteries and veins), and lymphatics (this includes immune cells and channels carrying immune cells) (Clemmons 2007). Most are found along the 14 major meridians, and each channel has its own specific number of points. There are additional acupoints, called classical points, found elsewhere on the body.

Acupressure: The application of fingers and hands to specific acupoints or regions of multiple acupoints.

Acupuncture: The insertion of a sterile needle, or other object, into the skin on a specific area of the body causing a beneficial response.

Aquapuncture: The injection of sterile fluid into acupuncture points.

Bian Zheng: The utilization of one or more of the diagnostic systems to discern a TCVM diagnosis or pattern (Xie and Preast 2007a). The diagnostic systems include Five Element Theory, Yin–Yang Theory, Interior Versus Exterior Patterns, Cold Versus Hot Patterns, Deficiency Versus Excess Patterns, Five Treasures, and Zang-Fu Physiology.

Body Fluid: Fluid found within the body including tears, nasal discharge, sweat, urine, saliva, digestive juices, and joint fluid (Xie and Preast 2007d).

Damp: Used to describe environments and disease conditions. One of the six evils or conditions in TCVM. Represents conditions with excessive moisture, infection, heaviness, and often pain (Xie and Preast 2007b).

Deficiency Pattern: A condition in which the patient is lacking, often due to overwork, blood loss, or chronic illness. A patient can be deficient in one or more of the following: Qi, Blood, Yin, and Yang. Patients are often dry, thin, weak, lethargic, and have a pale tongue and weak pulse (Xie and Preast 2007a).

Drain: To remove from an area. Typically applied to Damp conditions.

Eight Principle Theory: A diagnostic system dividing the natural world into two categories (Yin or Yang) and three pairs (Interior vs. Exterior; Cold vs. Heat; and Deficiency vs. Excess) (Xie and Preast 2007a).

Electroacupuncture: An electric current is applied to pre-placed acupuncture needles using small leads.

The frequency and intensity of the current is controlled by the electroacupuncture unit. Electric stimulation mimics and exceeds repeat manual manipulation of the acupuncture needle (Shmalberg et al. 2014).

Excess Pattern: A condition in which the patient has too much of something. The condition is most often due to an exogenous (outside) pathogen (Wind, Cold, Dampness, Summer Heat, Dryness, and Fire) or secondary to another issue (overeating, blood stagnation, phlegm) (Xie and Preast 2007b). Patients often are excitable, breathe rapidly, and have a fever, distended abdomen, a red tongue with a coating, and surging pulse (Xie and Preast 2007a).

Exogenous pathogens: Also known as the 6 Exogenous Xie Qi or 6 Excessive Qi or 6 Evils. There are six weather changes that normally do not cause disease, but which under the right circumstances (i.e. extreme weather changes and/or preexisting disease) can invade the body causing illness: Wind, Cold, Summer Heat, Damp, Dryness, and Fire (Xie and Preast 2007b).

Exterior Patterns: Issues, typically chronic in nature, associated with organ systems (Xie and Preast 2007a).

Five Element Theory: Everything in the natural world can be broken down into five elements (Wood, Fire, Earth, Metal, and Water) which promote, restrain, and regulate each other, maintaining order (Xie and Preast 2007c).

Five Treasures: The organization of life into five substances: Qi, Shen, Jing, Blood, and Body Fluid (Xie and Preast 2007d).

Fu organs: Yang organs located within the interior of the body. These organs are hollow or tube-like and function to transport or excrete. Examples include the large intestine, stomach, small intestine, triple heater, gallbladder, and urinary bladder (Xie and Preast 2007g).

Interior Patterns: Issues, often acute in nature, affecting the inside of the body (Xie and Preast 2007a).

Jing (aka Essence): There are two forms of Jing: Prenatal and Postnatal Jing. You are born with Prenatal Jing, also known as Kidney Jing or Congenital Jing (Xie and Preast 2007d). Postnatal Jing (aka Zang-Fu jing or Acquired Jing) is acquired through the ingestion of food and stored in each Zang-Fu organ (Xie and Preast 2007d).

Jing Luo: A system of interconnected channels covering the outer surface of the body. The channels function as a conduit through which Qi (energy) and Blood circulate throughout the entire body (Xie and Preast 2007e).

Meridians: A set of 12 paired and two unpaired pathways or channels on the outer surface of the body through which blood and energy (Qi) flow to the main organ systems (Zang-Fu organs), joints, muscles, bone, and brain (Xie and Preast 2007e).

Meridian clock: Also known as the TCM circadian clock. Qi flows through the 12 Zang-Fu organ channels in a specific order: lung → large intestine → stomach → spleen → heart → small intestine → bladder → kidney → pericardium → triple burner → gallbladder → liver. There is a two-hour period during which the passage of qi through each meridian and corresponding organ is greatest (Xie and Preast 2007e).

Phlegm: An abnormal form of body fluid which can accumulate within the body (Xie and Preast 2007d). Often any "strange" condition or illness is due to phlegm.

Qi (Energy): There are eight primary forms of Qi: Yuan Qi, Zong Qi, Gu Qi, Ying Qi, Wei Qi, Zang-Fu Qi, Jing Luo Qi, and Zheng Qi (Xie and Preast 2007d).

Shen (aka Spirit or Affect): An outward expression of an individual's mental state (Xie and Preast 2007d).

TCVM: A Chinese medicine system used to treat animals and comprising four branches: acupuncture, Chinese herbal medicine or therapy, Tui-na, and food therapy.

TCVM therapeutic actions: A beneficial effect associated with a specific TCVM therapy.

Tonify: To increase energy (Qi), blood flow, Yin, Yang, or organ function in an area. A substance which tonifies is often referred to as a "tonic."

Wind: Used to describe environments and disease conditions. One of the six evils or conditions in TCVM. Often considered the primary cause of disease. Wind can invade the body from the outside world (Exogenous Wind) or originate within the body (Internal Wind) (Xie and Preast 2007b). The presence of Wind often allows other pathogens or conditions to develop concurrently.

Yang: Half of the Yin–Yang division. The descriptor can be applied to all manner of items both animate and inanimate. Characteristics considered Yang include day, brightness, summer, hot, fast, male, healthy, strength, birth, top or back, Qi, pungent or bitter, and Fu organs (Xie and Preast 2007f).

Yin: Half of the Yin–Yang division. The descriptor can be applied to all manner of items both animate and inanimate. Characteristics considered yin include night, darkness, winter, cold, slow, female, illness, weakness, death, bottom or belly, blood, salty and sweet, and Zang organs (Xie and Preast 2007f).

Yin–Yang Theory: Divides all things into two halves which oppose, complement, control, create, and transform into each other (Xie and Preast 2007f).

Zang-Fu physiology: The classification of the 12 organs as either Zang or Fu.

Zang organs: Yin organs located within the interior of the body, are solid in structure, and whose primary function is manufacturing and storage: lung, spleen, heart, pericardium, liver, and kidney (Xie and Preast 2007g).

Acupuncture and TCVM

An understanding of TCM and TCVM is crucial to understanding traditional acupuncture techniques. An in-depth discussion of TCVM is beyond the scope of this book, but a very brief introduction to the TCVM theories most applicable to acupuncture is discussed. Additional TCVM concepts are covered in Chapters 2 and 3.

Yin–Yang Theory

A philosophical view dividing all things into two halves which oppose, complement, control, create, and transform into each other (Xie and Preast 2007f). The Tai Ji symbol is a visual representation of Yin–Yang theory. Characteristics of both Yin and Yang are shown in Figure 1.2.

Five Element Theory

The Five Element Theory breaks down everything in the natural world into five elements: Wood, Fire, Earth, Metal, and Water. The five elements promote, restrain, and regulate each other, keeping the natural world in perfect working order and establishing homeostasis (Xie and Preast 2007c). Table 1.1 outlines the characteristics defining each element.

Zang-Fu Physiology

The classification of the 12 organ systems as either solid structures used for storage (Zang) or

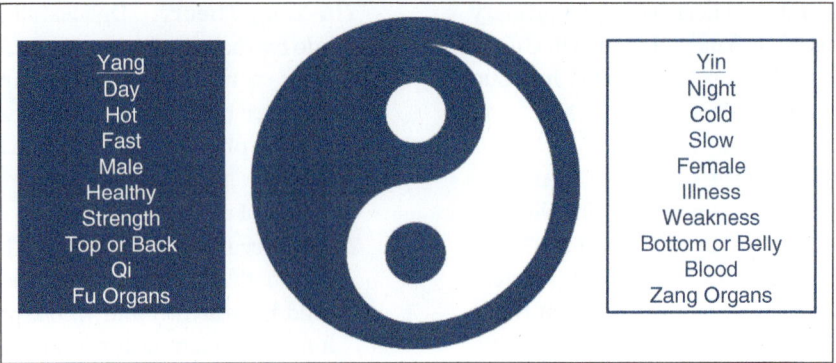

Figure 1.2 The Yin and Yang philosophy and archetypal Tai Ji symbol (Xie and Preast 2007f). Source: Lisa P. McFaddin.

hollow tube-like structures used to transmit and excrete (Fu). Zang organs include lung, spleen, heart, pericardium, liver, and kidney. Fu organs include large intestine, stomach, small intestine, triple heater, gallbladder, and urinary bladder.

The Zang-Fu systems are further divided into Yin and Yang organs. Zang or Yin organs are defined as those located within the interior of the body, are solid in structure, and whose primary function is to manufacture and store (Xie and Preast 2007g). Fu or Yang organs are hollow or tube-like and function to transport or excrete (Xie and Preast 2007g). Just as Yin and Yang complement each other, creating two halves of a whole, Zang and Fu are grouped together as wives and husbands. Each pair of Zang-Fu organs are further classified by their relationship to the five elements of the world: Wood, Fire, Earth, Metal, and Water.

Meridians

The Jing Luo is an intricate system of interconnected channels covering the outer surface of the body. The channels function as a conduit through which Qi (energy) and Blood circulate throughout the entire body. There are 14 major meridians which circle the body in specific patterns. The 12 meridians supply blood and energy to the 12 main organ systems, called Zang-Fu organs, as well as joints, muscles, bone, and brain. The Du, or

Governing Vessel, is located on the dorsal midline and the Ren, or Conception Vessel, is located on the ventral midline (Xie and Preast 2007e).

The Yin or Zang organ meridians are located more toward the center or inside of the body and limbs; while the Yang or Fu organ meridians are located on the outside of the body and limbs (Xie and Preast 2007). The 12 paired meridians are the most used channels due to their direct communication with the internal organ systems.

Meridians for Veterinarians

The Jing Luo comprises main highways, called Jing Mai, and smaller roads, called Luo Mai (Xie and Preast 2007e). The Jing Mai can be further broken down into 12 paired Regular Channels or meridians and eight unpaired Extraordinary Channels (Xie and Preast 2007e).

The eight extraordinary channels do not pair with internal organs, and many have branches which connect to the 12 regular channels. The Luo Mai are divided into the Branch Collaterals and 12 Muscle and Cutaneous Regions (Xie and Preast 2007e). The Luo Mai are additional subdivisions off the 12 Zang-Fu channels. See Figure 1.3 for a diagram of the Jing Luo.

Qi

Qi continuously runs throughout the body. Once Qi stops flowing the animal dies. Qi flows through the 12 Zang-Fu organ channels in a

Table 1.1 The Five Element Theory breaks down everything in the natural world into five elements: Wood, Fire, Earth, Metal, and Water. The Five Elements promote, restrain, and regulate each other keeping the natural world in perfect working order, establishing homeostasis (Xie and Preast 2007c). An incomplete list of characteristics commonly defining each element is provided.

	Wood	Fire	Earth	Metal	Water
Season	Spring	Summer	Late summer	Fall	Winter
Color	Green	Red	Yellow	White	Black
Orifice	Eyes	Tongue	Mouth	Nose	Ears
Sense	Vision	Speech	Taste	Smell	Hearing
Tissue	Tendons and ligaments	Blood vessels	Muscles	Skin and hair	Bones
Function	Purifying	Circulating	Digesting	Breathing	Excretion
Secretion	Tears	Sweat	Saliva	Nasal fluid	Urine
Zang organ	Liver	Heart and pericardium	Spleen	Lung	Kidney
Fu organ	Gallbladder	Small intestine and triple heater	Stomach	Large intestine	Bladder

Source: Lisa P. McFaddin.

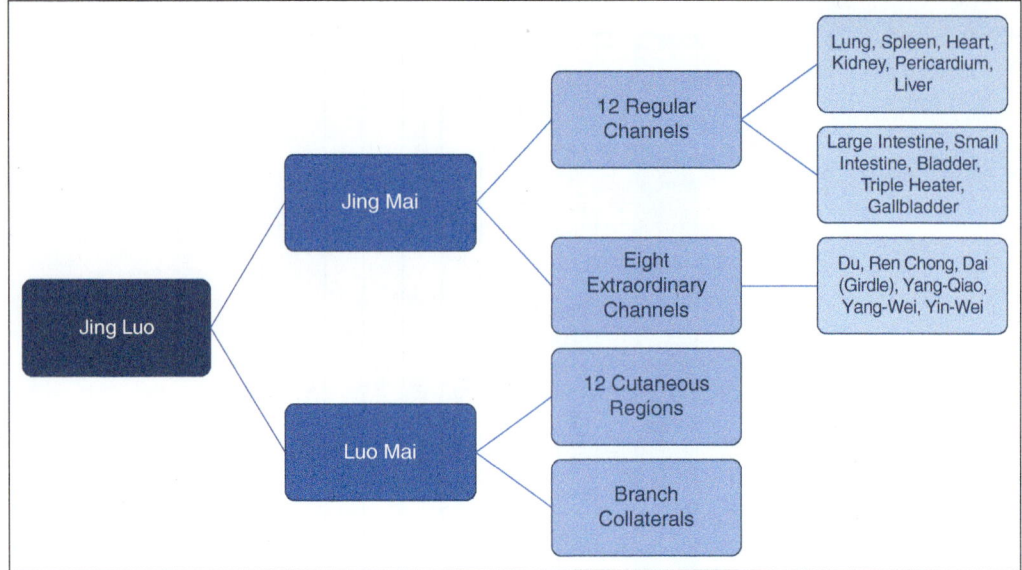

Figure 1.3 A schematic representation of the subdivisions of the Jing Luo (Xie and Preast 2007e). Source: Lisa P. McFaddin.

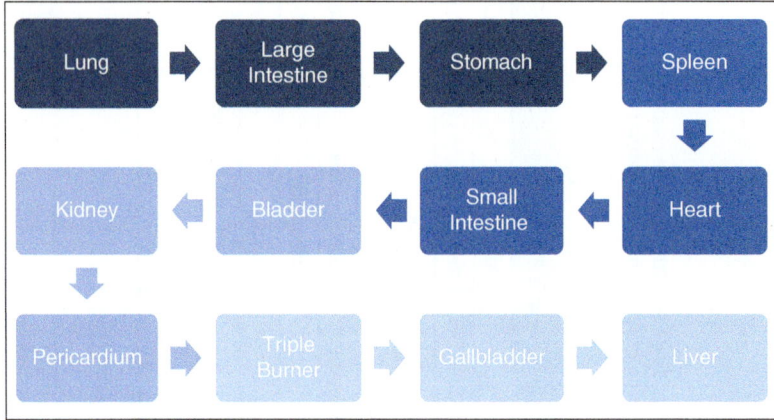

Figure 1.4 The order through which Qi flows through the 12 major meridians. Source: Lisa P. McFaddin.

specific order as depicted in Figure 1.4. There is a two-hour time period during which the passage of Qi through each meridian and corresponding organ is greatest. This is known as the TCM circadian clock, depicted in Figure 1.5.

Acupoints

Most acupuncture points, or acupoints, are found along the 14 major meridians. Each channel has its own specific number of

acupoints. Table 1.2 breaks down the acupoints on the 14 major meridians, while Figure 1.6 illustrates the approximate location of each meridian on the dog.

There are additional acupoints, known as Classical Points, not found on the common meridians. Acupoints found on the 14 major meridians are named using the initials of the channel and the number of the acupoint, for example LU-1 is the first acupoint on the lung channel. The total number of acupoints varies

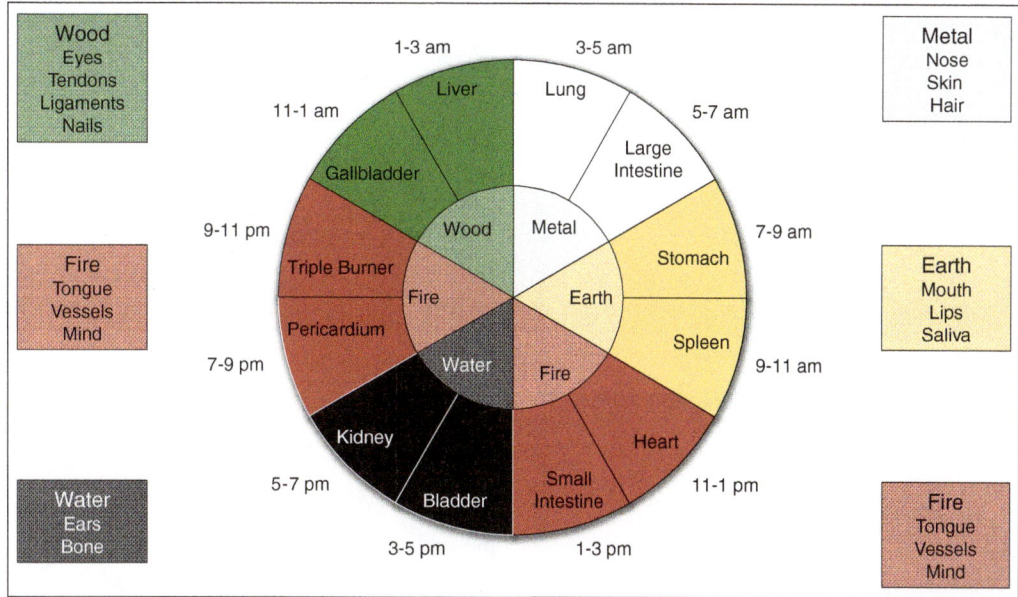

Figure 1.5 A visual representation of the order in which Qi or energy flows throughout the 12 Zang-Fu meridians throughout the day. Source: Lisa P. McFaddin.

Table 1.2 The primary location, origin, termination region, and number of acupoints on the 14 main meridians of the dog (Xie and Preast 2007e).

Channel	Primary location	Starting location	Ending location	Acupoints
Lung (LU)	Thoracic limb	Chest	First digit nail bed	11
Large intestine (LI)	Thoracic limb	Second digit nail bed	Outside of the nostril	20
Stomach (ST)	Pelvic limb	Below the pupil on the orbit	Second digit nail bed	45
Spleen (SP)	Pelvic limb	First or second digit nail bed	Outside of the chest	21
Heart (HT)	Thoracic limb	Center of the armpit	Fifth digit nail bed	9
Small intestine (SI)	Thoracic limb	Fifth digit	Tragus of the ear	19
Bladder (BL)	Pelvic limb	Inside corner of the eye	Fifth digit nail bed	67
Kidney (KID)	Pelvic limb	Behind the pad	Chest	27
Pericardium (PC)	Thoracic limb	Chest	Behind the pad	9
Triple heater (TH)	Thoracic limb	Fourth digit nail bed	Outside of the eyebrow	23
Gallbladder (GB)	Pelvic limb	Outside corner of the eye	Fourth digit nail bed	44
Liver (LIV)	Pelvic limb	First digit nail bed	Chest	14
Governing vessel (GV)	Dorsal midline	Just above the anus	Inside the upper gum	28
Conception vessel (CV)	Ventral midline	Between the anus and genitals	Chin	24

Source: Lisa P. McFaddin.

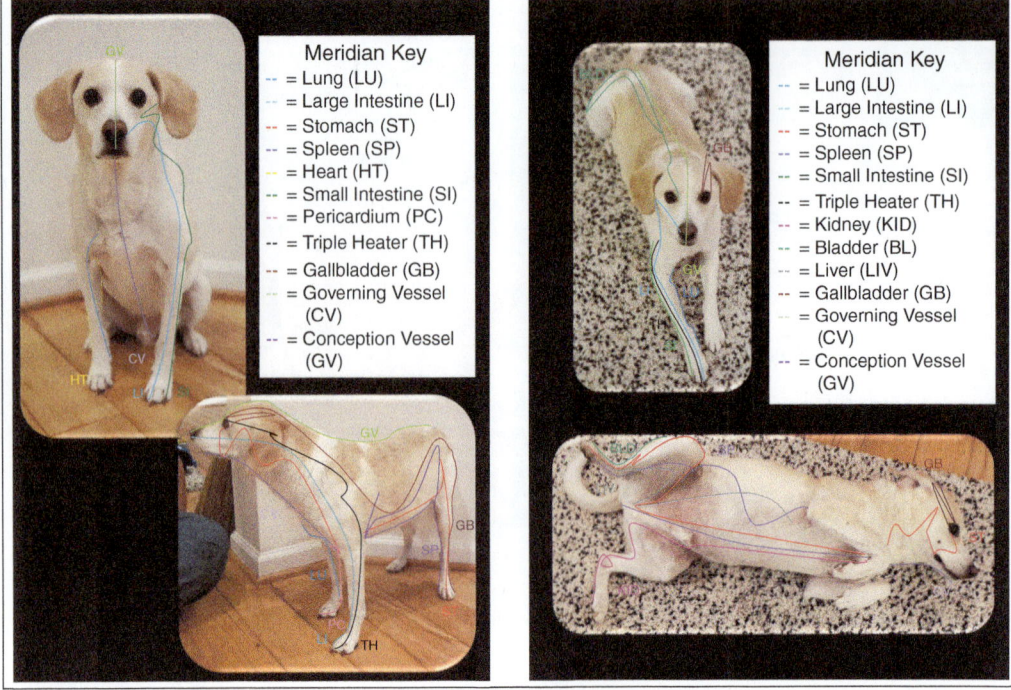

Figure 1.6 Winston modeling the approximate location of the 14 major meridians of the dog. Source: Lisa P. McFaddin.

by species. Depending on the acupuncture technique, humans have between 360 and 2000 acupoints, while dogs and cats have approximately 400 acupoints.

From a TCVM perspective the stimulation of acupoints directly affects the flow of Qi, and subsequently Blood, at the acupoint itself and throughout the meridian. The stimulation of distant body regions and internal organs is explained through the interconnectedness of the meridians.

Techniques

There are multiple forms or techniques used in veterinary acupuncture. Traditional acupuncture is also called dry needling. Other techniques include acupressure, electroacupuncture, aquapuncture, hemoacupuncture, pneumoacupuncture, moxibustion, and laser acupuncture.

Acupressure

The application of fingers and hands to specific acupoints or regions of multiple acupoints. Owners can be taught to perform acupressure at home. Acupressure can be used for most conditions treated with dry needle acupuncture, but it is most commonly implemented for relaxation and the treatment of conditions causing mild pain (Kober et al. 2003; Trentini III et al. 2005; Monson et al. 2019).

Aquapuncture

The injection of sterile fluid into acupuncture points. The most commonly used injectables include saline, vitamin B12, homeopathic remedies, the patient's blood (whole), or local anesthetic. Necessary materials may include 1- or 3-ml syringes, 27g or 25g needles, and sterile injectables. Figure 1.7 depicts materials commonly used during aquapuncture. If using

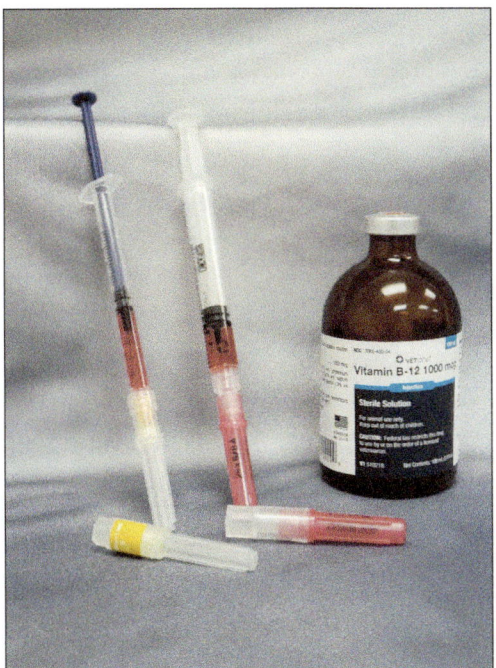

Figure 1.7 Vitamin B12 aquapuncture materials including multidose sterile bottle of vitamin B12, sterile single-use syringes (1 and 3 ml), and small needles (27g) used for injection. Source: Lisa P. McFaddin.

a multiple-dose syringe the needle should be changed every one to two acupoints.

Aquapuncture is used to lengthen and intensify the effects of traditional acupuncture by causing physical changes within the acupoint and stimulating the nervous system (Chen et al. 2014). This technique is also frequently used in patients who will not tolerate needle placement.

Dry Needle

Also known as traditional needle stimulation, this is the most common technique. A variety of sterile single-use filiform needles are used to puncture the skin at specific acupoints on the body. Needle manufacturer, gauge, and length are based on practitioner preference, patient size, disease condition, and desired treatment effects. Acupoint selection is based on patient presentation. Method of needle insertion (perpendicular, diagonal, or horizontal) is based on

acupoint location. The length of time needles remain in place is dependent on patient temperament and disease condition. The frequency of treatment is determined by the practitioner and is generally based on patient condition.

Acupuncture needles must be filiform, sterile, and single use. A variety of gauges (28, 30, 32, 34, 36, 38, and 40) and lengths (¼, ½, 1, 1.5, and 2 inch) are available (Figure 1.8). Dry needle acupuncture can aid in the treatment of numerous conditions including anxiety, cardiopulmonary disorders, cognitive disorders, dermatologic disorders, digestive disorders, hormone disorders, immune support, kidney disorders, liver disorders, metabolic disorders, neurologic disorders, ocular disorders, organ prolapse, pain, performance animals, reproductive disorders, and wound healing (see Table 1.7 for references).

Electroacupuncture

Electric current is applied to pre-placed acupuncture needles using small leads. The frequency and intensity of the current is controlled by the practitioner through the adjustment of the electroacupuncture unit. Electric stimulation mimics and exceeds repeat manual manipulation of the acupuncture needle. Necessary materials include acupuncture needles and an electroacupuncture unit (see Figure 1.9 for examples of two types of electroacupuncture units).

Electroacupuncture is primarily used to treat pain (especially nerve pain), neurologic weakness, and muscle spasms (Cassu et al. 2008; Ren et al. 2012; Shmalberg et al. 2014, 2019; Lewis, et al. 2020). Lower frequencies (5–20 Hz) stimulate local nerves, while higher frequencies (80–120 Hz) reduce muscle spasms and release endorphins prolonging the pain control.

Gold Bead Implantation

Very small 24-karat gold beads, approximately the size of the tip of a ballpoint pen, are inserted into specific acupuncture points. Gold

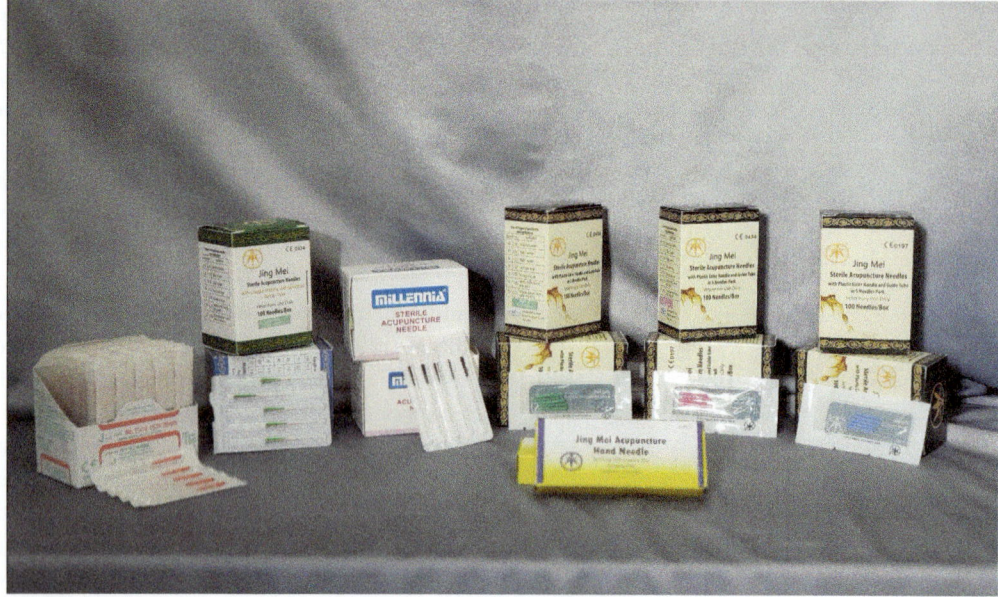

Figure 1.8 Acupuncture needles of various gauges (sizes) and lengths. All acupuncture needles are sterile, single-use, and filiform in shape with metal or plastic needle handles. Source: Lisa P. McFaddin.

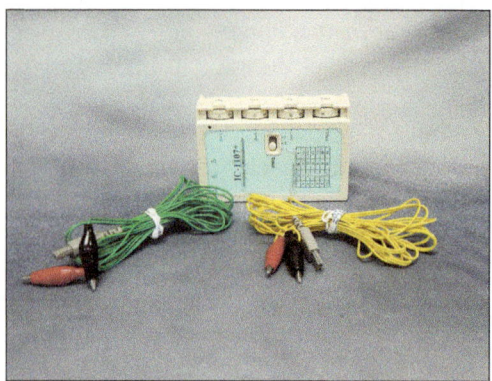

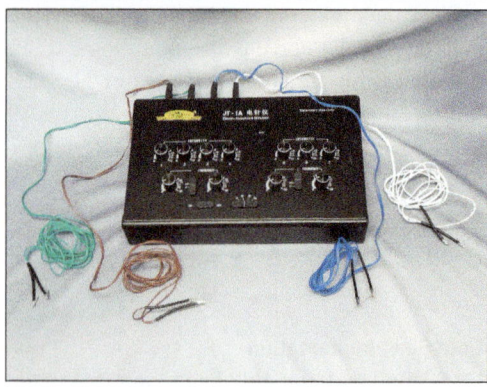

Figure 1.9 Electroacupuncture units and associated leads. Source: Lisa P. McFaddin.

bead implantation (GBI) provides long-term stimulation of acupuncture points. The technique was introduced to the veterinary field by a founding member of the IVAS, Dr. Grady Young, in the 1970s (Ben-Yakir 2009). The technique was later perfected by Dr. Terry Dukes in 1975.

Necessary materials include sterile 24-karat gold beads, sterile gloves, clippers, surgical scrub, alcohol, sterile syringes, and sterile needles for bead insertion.

GBI is primarily used to manage chronic musculoskeletal and neurologic conditions including degenerative joint disease, osteoarthritis, osteochondritis dessicans, vertebral spondylosis, hip dysplasia, urinary and fecal incontinence, lick granulomas, non-healing fractures, traumatic nerve injury, and seizures (Durkes 1992; Jaeger et al. 2006).

Hemoacupuncture

The intentional puncture of a blood vessel with a needle. The amount of blood removed is dependent on the size of the animal, generally only a few drops. Acupuncture needles, sterile single-use needles (27, 25, 23, or 22 g), and potentially sterile single-use 1-ml syringes are needed. This technique is most used in large animals. Primary indications include fever, infection, and chronic non-healing wounds (Faramarzi et al. 2017).

Laser Acupuncture

Low-power (5–30 mW) cold laser (generally 630–670 nm) applied to acupoints. Best suited for acupoints in areas of thin skin. A class III or IV therapeutic laser with a small head attachment is required. The technique is most often used to treat pain, anxiety, inflammation, and wound healing (Chon et al. 2019). This modality has the added benefit of minimal patient sensation and short duration of treatment, without the risk of infection, trauma or bleeding. Figure 1.10 shows one type of class IV veterinary therapeutic laser with laser acupuncture capabilities. Refer to Chapter 6 for more information on veterinary laser therapy (aka photobiomodulation).

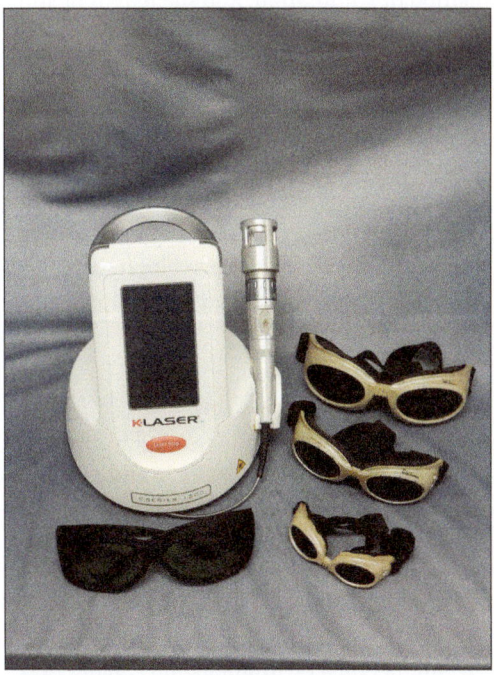

Figure 1.10 A class IV veterinary therapeutic laser with human and animal personal protective eyewear. Source: Lisa P. McFaddin.

Moxibustion

Moxa can be performed directly or indirectly. During direct moxa, uncommonly used in veterinary medicine, the moxa is placed and burned directly on the skin. During indirect moxa the herb is burned without direct skin contact.

For the indirect technique, moxa can be rolled into small balls, attached to the end of the acupuncture needles pre-placed in the skin, and burned. Moxa can also be burned as a pre-rolled stick above the skin over acupoints (Figure 1.11).

Depending on the technique used, moxa (*Artemisia vulgaris*), acupuncture needles, and a lighter are needed. Moxa is used for its warming properties, its ability to eliminate toxins, and its ability to improve peripheral blood flow (Deng and Shen 2013).

Pneumoacupuncture

Injection of air into specific acupoints or larger areas of subcutaneous tissue. Various sizes of sterile syringes and needles and air are required to perform this technique. Pneumoacupuncture is primarily used in large animals to tonify conditions causing weakness, especially focal nerve paralysis (Mittleman and Gaynor 2000; Ferguson 2007).

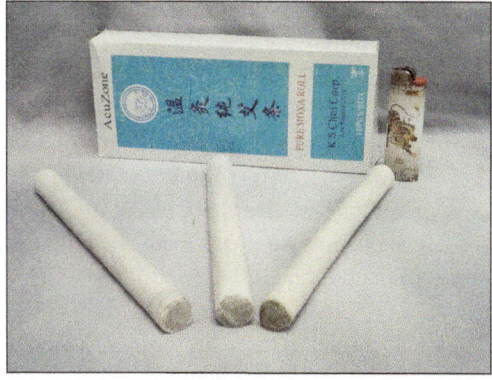

Figure 1.11 A brand of pre-rolled moxa (*Artemisia vulgaris*) used for moxibustion. Source: Lisa P. McFaddin.

Mechanisms of Action

From a Western medicine perspective, acupuncture results in nerve, blood vessel, lymphatic (immune system), and cellular stimulation that causes an immediate local effect which then spreads systemically (Clemmons 2007; Zhou and Benharash 2014). Unbeknownst to the first acupuncturists, most of the major meridians lay overtop nerve pathways. Before the invention of the microscope and magnetic resonance imaging (MRI), the beneficial effects of acupuncture were described using terms like Qi. With the advent of advanced imaging we can view Qi, at least in part, as the electrical activity transmitted from nerve cell to nerve cell.

Anatomically, acupoints comprise free nerve endings, small vessels (arteries and veins), and lymphatics (this includes immune cells and channels carrying immune cells). Placement of the acupuncture needle punctures the skin causing counter-irritation within the epidermis, dermis and subcutaneous tissues, leading to microtrauma (Clemmons 2007). This tissue disruption directly affects local nerves, blood vessels, and immune cells improving blood flow, immune response, and relaxation of tissues and muscles. Signals carried by the nerve cells spread from the point of impact to the spinal cord and eventually the brain, propagating the beneficial effects of acupuncture throughout the body (Chiu et al. 2001). This expanded description of the mechanism of action brings us back to the original definition of acupuncture: the insertion of a needle into a specific area of the skin causes a beneficial response.

Here we delve deeper into the complexity surrounding acupuncture's mechanisms of action, which is a well-studied and confusing topic in human and veterinary medicine. There are many moving parts occurring instantaneously and simultaneously, making it difficult to concisely break down what is happening and when. As such, there are numerous theories outlining the effect acupuncture has on various body systems. When combined the theories create a cohesive and complex pathophysiology through which acupuncture exerts its effect.

When discussing the science behind acupuncture there are two key questions. What differentiates acupuncture points from "normal" skin? How does placement of a tiny needle through the skin, subcutaneous tissue, and muscle benefit the patient?

Normal Skin Versus Acupoint

From a "western" medicine perspective most acupoints have several common physical characteristics. Acupoints often have a palpably different texture and temperature compared to the surrounding skin. Most acupoints are depressions within the skin, but the points can be turgid swellings.

Needle–Skin Interactions

The local, regional, and systemic effects generated by acupuncture are dependent on several variables: the acupuncture points selected, the method of stimulation, and the length of stimulation (Karavis 1997). Needle placement through the skin causes counter-irritation within the epidermis, dermis, and subcutaneous tissues, leading to microtrauma. This stimulation causes a combination of three potential, and often simultaneously occurring, reactions at the acupoint: nerve stimulation (neuronal reactions), physical changes (biophysical reactions), and chemical changes (biochemical reactions) (Zhu 2014).

Mechanisms for Veterinarians

This section examines the acupoint, neuronal reactions, biophysical reactions, and biochemical reactions in more detail.

Acupoint

Acupuncture points are in areas of the skin with low electrical resistance and high electrical conductance (Mittleman and Gaynor 2000; Longhurst 2010). Small changes in the energy dynamics of the tissue quickly and easily initiate and then propagate electrical changes to the surrounding tissues.

Acupoints usually contain neurovascular bundles: free nerve endings, small vessels (arterioles and venules), a robust lymphatic supply, and often mast cells (Longhurst 2010). Table 1.3 outlines the common nervous system components found in and around acupuncture points. Figure 1.12 illustrates the approximate location of each receptor within the skin layers. Acupoints can be categorized based on the type of nerves supplying the area (Garcia and Chiang 2007; Ferguson 2011). Table 1.4 summarizes the characteristics of each acupuncture category in more detail.

Meridians follow the peripheral nervous system. For example, the lung and pericardium meridians are found along the musculocutaneous and median nerves, respectively (Clemmons 2007; Longhurst 2010).

Neuronal Reactions

The initial sensation felt by the placement of an acupuncture needle is known as "De Qi" or "arrival of Qi." Acupuncture is the physical stimulus triggering the nervous system response. The intensity of needle placement, duration of stimulation (i.e. how long the needles remain in place), and the speed with which the needles are placed affect the afferent nerves and thus the sensory response (Karavis 1997; Zhao 2008). Given the complex series of events that occur following needle placement, De Qi can be thought of as the sensory results of multiple neuronal reactions.

In general, the acupuncture needle stimulates nociceptors and mechanoreceptors within free nerve endings in the skin, subcutaneous tissue, and muscles. Afferent pain signals are initially transmitted by thin, slow, unmyelinated C fibers (Group IV fibers) and

Table 1.3 The common neuronal receptors found within acupuncture points (Mittleman and Gaynor 2000; Purves et al. 2012b; Zhu 2014).

Receptor type	Location	Function
Free sensory nerve endings	Epidermis Dermis	Nociceptors: respond to damaging stimuli and their activation results in pain Thermoreceptors: respond to temperature changes both hot and cold
Follicular nerve endings	Root hair plexus	Mechanoreceptors: respond to deformation of surrounding tissue including pressure and stretch
Merkel's complexes	Bottom epidermis	Mechanoreceptors: slow adapting and respond to sustained pressure
Meissner's corpuscles	Top dermis	Mechanoreceptors: rapidly adapting and sensitive to fine or light texture and pressure
Ruffini corpuscles	Middle dermis	Mechanoreceptors: slow adapting and responsive to shearing stress and drag
Pacinian corpuscles	Deep dermis or subcutaneous	Mechanoreceptors: rapidly adapting and sensitive to strong pressure, jarring movements, and vibration
Muscle spindle cells	Skeletal muscle	Mechanoreceptors: stretch receptors within muscles assessing muscle length
Golgi tendon organs	Musculotendinous junction	Mechanoreceptors: measure muscle tension at the origin and insertion during concentric contraction

Source: Lisa P. McFaddin.

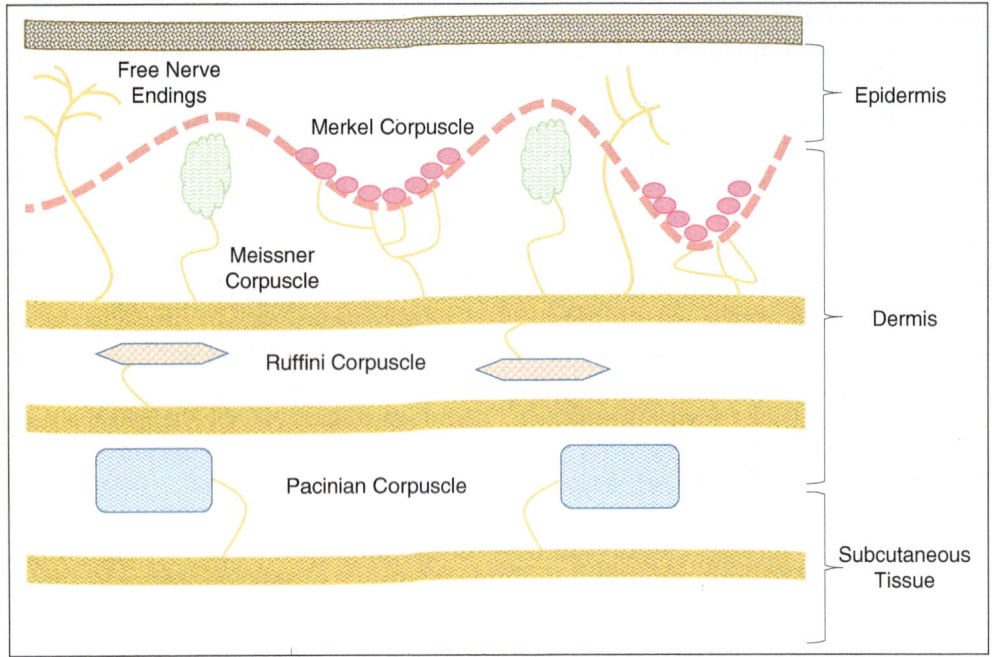

Figure 1.12 Schematic representation of common receptors found within the skin. Source: adapted from Purves et al. (2012b).

Table 1.4 The four types of acupuncture points designated by their neural relationship (Mittleman and Gaynor 2000; Garcia and Chiang 2007).

Name	Classification	Example acupoint
Type I (motor points)	• Found where nerves enter muscle • Minimal stimulation of the nerve causes maximum muscle contraction • Most common acupoint (67%)	LI-4 (dorsal metacarpus at the midpoint between the second and third metacarpal bones)
Type II	• Superficial nerves located along the dorsal and ventral midline	Bai-Hui (dorsal midline between L7 and S1)
Type III	• Associated with high concentrations of superficial nerves and nerve plexi	PC-6 (medial distal antebrachium in the groove between the flexor carpi radialis and superficial digital flexor)
Type IV	• Found on musculotendinous junctions (MCJ), more specifically associated with Golgi tendon organs (GTOs) • GTOs are spindle-shaped receptors located at the MCJ which measure muscle tension at the origin and insertion during concentric contraction	BL-57 (pelvic limb caudal to the tibia halfway between the popliteal crease and calcaneal tuber)

Source: Lisa P. McFaddin.

thin, faster, myelinated Aδ fibers; afferent mechanical signals are primarily transmitted through Aδ fibers (Zhu 2014). The involvement of Aδ and C fibers in the propagation of acupuncture analgesia, by selectively blocking conduction of the afferent fibers, was proven using the application of capsaicin bilaterally to the sciatic nerves (Okada et al. 1996).

Human experiments discovered the analgesic effects of acupuncture are due to afferent nerve signals from local muscles (Chiang et al. 1973). Specifically, Chiang et al. (1973) demonstrated the analgesic effects induced by the stimulation of LI-4 (located in the fleshy tissue between the thumb and index finger) were not inhibited by vascular occlusion of the forearm or cutaneous procaine injections. However, injections of procaine into the ulnar and median nerves eliminated the analgesic effects of LI-4 stimulation.

The principle of spinal segmental innervation explains the path through which afferent sensory information moves from the point of needle placement to the spinal cord. Groups of afferent sensory nerves in the skin (dermatomes) and muscle (myotomes) transmit information to specific segments of the spinal cord (neurotomes) (Karavis 1997). Once stimulated, the Aδ and C fibers transmit sensory information from their corresponding dermatomes and myotomes to the dorsal horn of the spinal cord, specifically the substantia gelatinosa (Yam et al. 2018).

C fiber first-order neurons terminate in laminae I (marginal zone) and II (substantia gelatinosa) of the dorsal horn of the spinal cord (Yam et al. 2018). Aδ first-order neurons from the periphery enter the spinal cord through Lissauer's tract, travel cranially or caudally for three to four spinal segments and then enter laminae II (substantia gelatinous) connecting to a second-order neuron (Purves et al. 2012a).

Once in the substantia gelatinosa a portion of the sensory information crosses midline below the central canal entering the spinothalamic tract, a set of sensory tracts located in the ventral funiculus of the spinal cord white matter (Purves et al. 2012a,b). Within the substantia gelatinosa inhibitory interneurons are also stimulated, blocking the transmission of nociceptive information to the higher centers of the brain (Mittleman and Gaynor 2000; Purves et al. 2012a,b). This local inhibition of pain is known as Melzack and Wall's gate theory.

Most of the sensory information then travels to the ipsilateral thalamus. The thalamus is a gate through which all sensory information, except olfactory, travels. The spinothalamic tract terminates at a third-order neuron where most information travels to the somatosensory region of the ipsilateral cortex, specifically the parietal lobe (Clemmons 2007; Purves et al. 2012a,b). On the way to the thalamus branches are sent to several connections in the midbrain, especially the periaqueductal gray matter (PAG) and rostral ventral medulla (RVM) (Yam et al. 2018).

The PAG helps regulate the response to nociceptive input by integrating information from the higher brain centers, including the cortex, and the dorsal horn of the spinal cord. The RVM downregulates excitatory information from the dorsal horn of the spinal cord. Both the PAG and RVM express a variety of neurotransmitters (endogenous opioids and cannabinoids, 5-hydroxytryptamine or 5-HT, and norepinephrine or NE) that are heavily involved in the regulation and recognition of pain (Yam et al. 2018). The importance of endogenous opioids in perpetuating the effects of acupuncture is emphasized by the fact that administration of drugs known to inhibit opioid biosynthesis (cycloheximide) or block opioid action (naloxone) reduce the analgesic effects of acupuncture (Mittleman and Gaynor 2000).

The acupuncture–brain connection was confirmed by Chiu et al. (2001). Using manganese-enhanced functional MRI on anesthetized rabbits, the group established that electroacupuncture stimulation of two acupoints, ST-36 and GB-34, resulted in neural activation of specific regions of the brain. Chiu et al. (2001) further discovered the location of this neural activation was dependent on the acupoint being stimulated. Hippocampal activation was seen with the stimulation of ST-36, while stimulation of GB-34 caused activation in the hypothalamus, insula, and motor cortex. The specificity of neural activation was found to be time dependent, with specific brain centers triggered after

5 minutes of electroacupuncture and a more generalized stimulation after 20 minutes.

Numerous studies have confirmed the link between the specific acupoint stimulation and the type of neural activation within the brain. Zhang et al. (2015) demonstrated that acupuncture stimulation of Taichong and Taixi increased neuronal activity in areas relating to vision, emotions, and cognition (cerebral occipital lobe, middle occipital gyrus, inferior occipital gyrus and cuneus) while inhibiting areas related to emotion, attention, phonological and semantic processing, and memory (gyrus rectus of the frontal lobe, inferior frontal gyrus, and center of the posterior lobe of the cerebellum). Alternatively, activation of non-acupoints, or sham points, did not result in specific brain stimulation as demonstrated by Wu et al. (2002) and Zhu et al. (2015). Huang et al. (2012) provided a systematic review and meta-analysis of 34 studies using functional MRI to assess brain response to acupuncture. The study also mentioned the absence of neural response following stimulation of sham acupoints.

Internal organ response following acupuncture needle placement is often the result of afferent sensory information from cutaneous nerves producing patterns of reflex activity in segmentally related visceral structures (Karavis 1997). This cutaneo-visceral reflex occurs without the involvement of higher brain centers. A similar viscero-visceral reflex functions to propagate internal organ response to acupuncture. Figure 1.13 summarizes this information in an algorithmic depiction of the neurophysiology of acupuncture.

Biophysical Reactions

Needle insertion and subsequent adjustment of the needle (twisting, seating, and flicking) causes mechanical pressure and distortion within the connective tissue and muscle (Zhao 2008). Langevin et al. (2007) repeatedly demonstrated that unidirectional and bidirectional acupuncture needle rotation in mouse

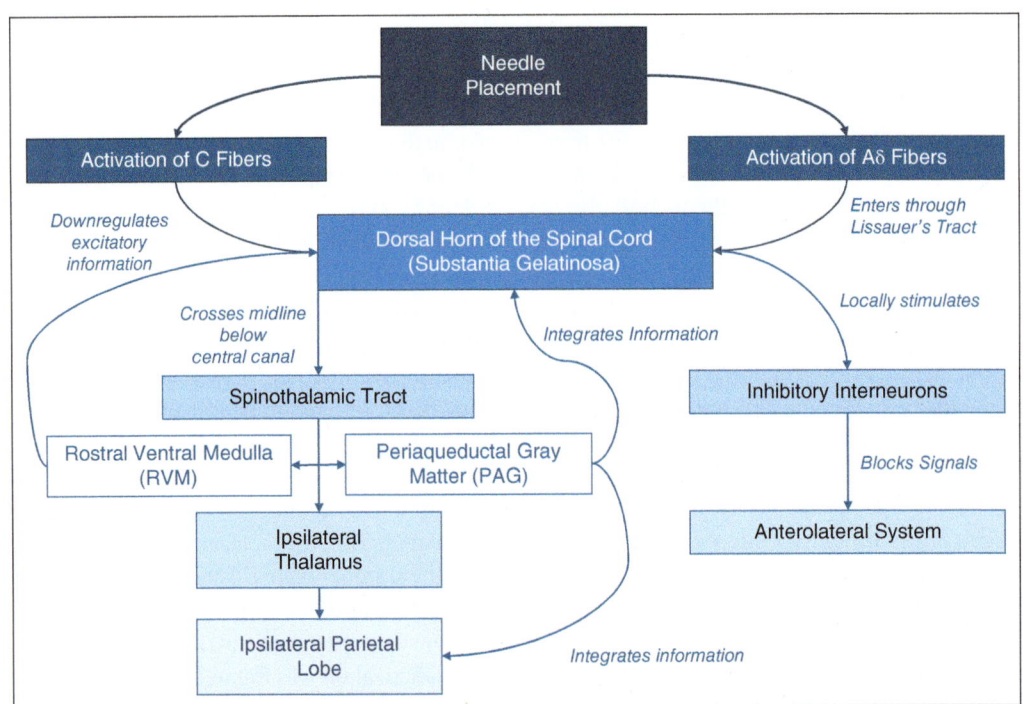

Figure 1.13 Flow diagram of the neurophysiology of acupuncture. Source: Lisa P. McFaddin.

subcutaneous tissue resulted in collagen winding around the needle, activating local connective tissue fibroblasts.

Needle placement and manipulation triggers mechanoreceptors at the level of the skin, muscle, and tendons. The role of skin mechanoreceptors and nociceptors in acupuncture is discussed in the preceding section. The primary mechanoreceptors within striated muscles are muscle spindle cells (MSC) and Golgi tendon organs (GTO).

Two afferent sensory nerves innervate MSC, Group Ia and II, which assess muscle length and, over time, the speed with which muscle moves or contracts. MSC run parallel to muscle fibers and are comprise four to eight specialized intrafusal muscle fibers encased in connective tissue. Activation of Group Ia and II can stimulate both alpha and gamma motor neurons innervating the affected MSC, inhibit MSC in contralateral homologous and antagonistic muscles, and inhibit pain through the spinothalamic tract (Purves et al. 2012a,b).

GTO are collagen bundles with spindle-shaped receptors surrounded by a thin capsule located in the musculotendinous junction. Group Ib afferent sensory nerves within the GTO are responsible for measuring muscle tension at the origin and insertion. Activation of Group Ib nerves inhibits alpha and gamma motor neurons innervating the muscle, as well inhibiting pain through stimulation of interneurons within the dorsal horn of the spinal cord (Purves et al. 2012a,b).

Shear force- and stress-induced tissue displacement, caused by the acupuncture needle, stimulates local MSC and GTO. MSC and GTO activation initially causes muscle contraction around the needle followed by relaxation of the muscle and connective tissue. Continued activation of local MSC and GTO results in propagation of the mechanical signals through the surrounding connective tissue and muscle. Zhang et al. (2012) describe this expanding effect of MSC and GTO stimulation as a vase-like pattern. Figure 1.14 illustrates the location

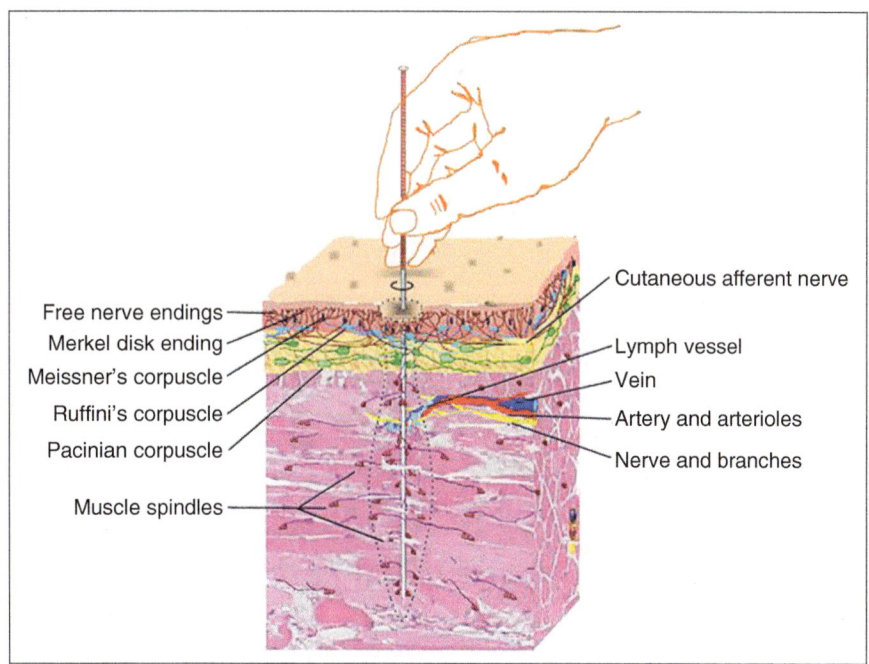

Figure 1.14 The components of the skin, subcutaneous tissue, and muscle layers affected by placement of an acupuncture needle, as well as the vase-like activation of muscle spindle cells caused by twisting and manipulation of the needle (Zhang et al. 2012). Source: Zhang, et al., 2011/Public Domain CC BY 3.0.

and anatomy affected by acupuncture needle placement as well as the proposed vase-like distribution of MSC activation caused by twisting and manipulation of the acupuncture needle (Zhang et al. 2012).

Biochemical Reactions

Needle placement causes local tissue injury and, more importantly, initiates tissue healing. Needle stimulation causes the release of a whole host of neural and nonneuronal bioactive factors (Zhu 2014). These biochemical substances contribute to the local and systemic beneficial effects of acupuncture primarily through regulation of blood and lymphatic flow, as well as stimulation of afferent signals to the central nervous system (Clemmons 2007). Figure 1.15 depicts the most common biochemical reactions and resultant mediators involved in acupuncture.

Opioid peptides, β-endorphins, enkephalins, dynorphins, serotonin, noradrenaline and gamma-aminobutyric acid (GABA) are also released and produced within the central nervous system as a direct result of acupuncture, particularly electroacupuncture (Zhao 2008). The primary function of these biochemical modulators and neurotransmitters is the central inhibition of pain. Table 1.5 outlines the source and primary function of the most common biochemical mediators involved in acupuncture.

Safety

Acupuncture is a very safe and well-tolerated medicinal practice. Like all therapies, there are conditions under which acupuncture should not be used or used with caution, as well as a few mild potential adverse effects. Table 1.6 outlines these cautions, contraindications, and potential adverse effects.

The Why

Applications in Human Medicine

The National Institutes of Health (NIH) issued a consensus statement on the beneficial effects of acupuncture in 1998. The NIH outlined the conditions and diseases for which acupuncture had demonstrated scientifically advantageous effects, including adult postoperative pain, postoperative dental pain, chemotherapy nausea, vomiting, addiction, stroke rehabilitation, headache, menstrual cramps, tennis elbow, fibromyalgia, myofascial pain, osteoarthritis, and asthma (NIH 1998).

Since that time vast research has been completed on the efficacy of acupuncture in human medicine. The NIH National Center for Complementary and Integrative Medicine (NCCIH) website (https://nccih.nih.gov) is an excellent resource to learn more about the effectiveness and usefulness of acupuncture in people.

Applications in Veterinary Medicine

Pain control is the most common reason for which acupuncture is used in veterinary medicine. The American Animal Hospital Association (AAHA) referenced the use of acupuncture for pain control in the 2015 and 2022 Pain Management Guidelines for Dogs and Cats (Epstein et al. 2015; Gruen et al. 2022). Veterinary acupuncture is also commonly used to aid in the treatment of arthritis, degenerative joint disease, gastrointestinal issues (vomiting, diarrhea, and inappetence), hip dysplasia, immune system support (chronic infections, cancer, autoimmune diseases), intervertebral disk disease (IVDD), muscle and tendon injury, oncology, reproductive disorders, and respiratory arrest (Chan et al. 2001; Lana et al. 2006; Xie and Ortiz-Umpierre 2006; Gülanber 2008; Chrisman 2011).

> "Acupuncture offers a compelling and safe method for pain management in veterinary patients and should be strongly considered as part of multimodal pain management plan" (Epstein et al. 2015).

Veterinary Research

Veterinary acupuncture is a well-studied treatment modality (Miscioscia and Repac 2022).

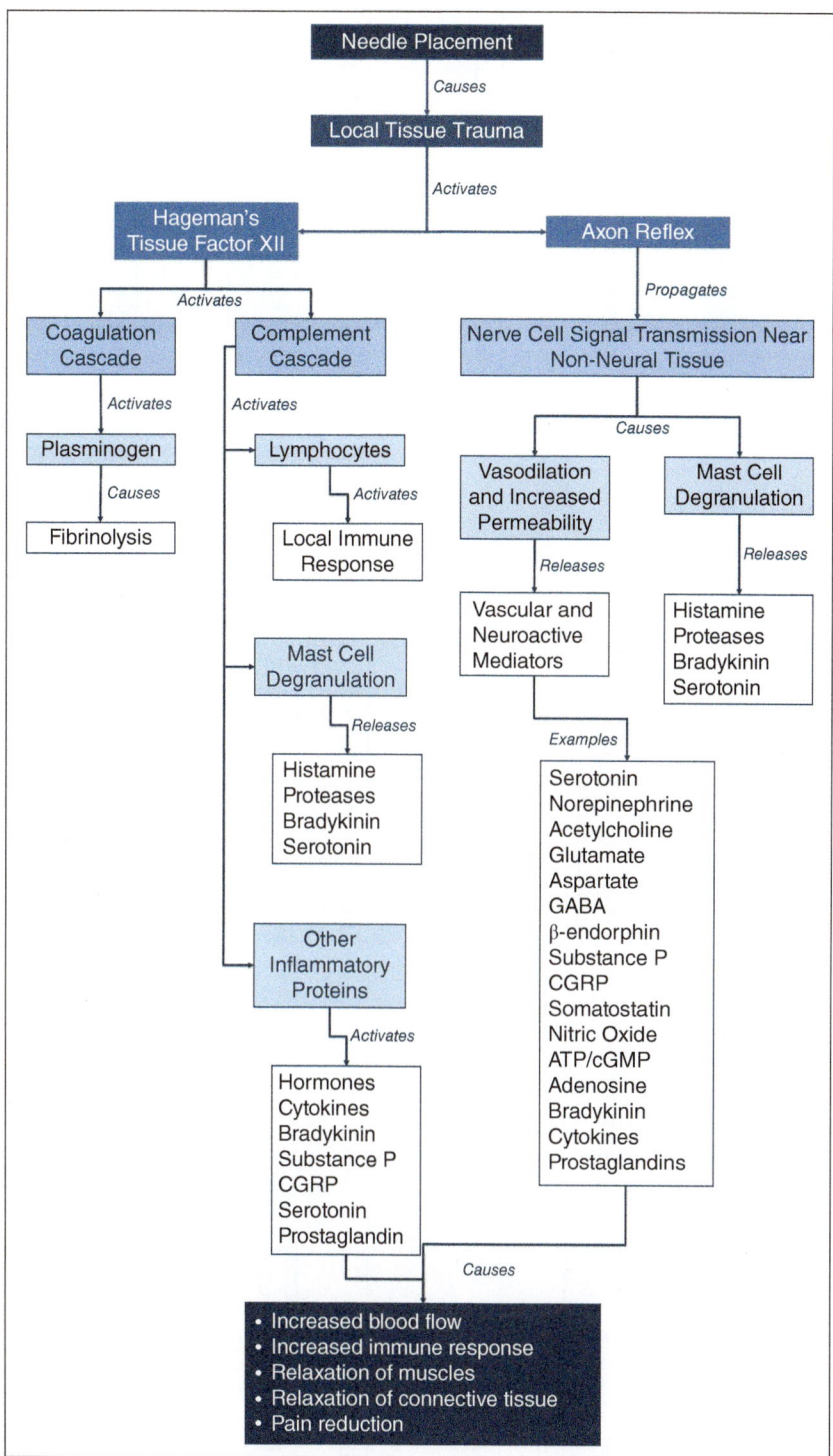

Figure 1.15 Flow chart of the most common biochemical reactions and mediators caused by acupuncture (Clemmons 2007; Zhang et al. 2012; Zhu 2014). ATP, adenosine triphosphate; cGMP, cyclic guanosine monophosphate; CGRP, calcium gene-related peptide. Source: Lisa P. McFaddin.

Table 1.5 The source and primary function of the most common biochemical mediators involved in acupuncture.

Mediator	Source	Function
Acetylcholine	Keratinocytes Injured efferent nerves	Induces muscle contractions and modulates pain
Adenosine	Breakdown product of ATP	Reduces pain through activation of Ia receptors on ascending afferent nerves from muscle spindle cells (Goldman et al. 2010)
ATP and cGMP	Damaged epidermal cells and peripheral nerve tissue	Sensitizes sensory afferent nerves reducing pain sensation (Ren et al. 2012)
β-Endorphin	Keratinocytes Melanocytes Dermal fibroblasts Leukocytes	Opioid peptide reducing pain through stimulation of μ-opiate receptors (Zhang et al. 2012)
Bradykinin	Mast cells Blood vessels	Inflammatory mediator of cardiovascular homeostasis, inflammation, and nociception through activation of bradykinin 1 and 2 receptors (Zhang et al. 2012)
Calcitonin gene-related peptide (CGRP)	Epithelial cells Immune cells	Neuropeptide modulating pain sensation through interaction with an autoreceptor (Zhang et al. 2012)
Cytokines	Epithelial cells Local tissue and cells	Inflammatory proteins which augment afferent sensory nerve response reducing pain sensation and reducing production of additional inflammatory mediators from afferent terminals (Zhang et al. 2012)
GABA	Macrophages Lymphocytes	Inhibitory neurotransmitter affecting autoreceptors within the CNS modulating the pain response (Zhao 2008)

Mediator	Source	Function
Glutamate Aspartate	Epithelial cells Macrophages	Excitatory amino acid modulating pain information peripherally and centrally through stimulation of autoreceptors, including N-methyl-D-aspartate (NMDA) receptors (Zhao 2008)
Histamine	Mast cells	Stimulation of H_1 receptors causes increased vascular permeability, relaxation of vascular smooth muscle, reduction in pain sensation, and increased concentration of β-endorphin in the cerebrospinal fluid (Huang et al. 2018)
Nitric oxide	Local tissues	Enhances acetylcholine and β-endorphin release while inhibiting release of substance P from primary afferent nerves (Zhang et al. 2012)
Norepinephrine	Sympathetic nerves	Norepinephrine modulates neuropathic pain through spinal α_2 receptors (Zhao 2008)
Plasminogen	Local tissues	Precursor to plasmin involved in fibrinolysis
Prostaglandins	Local tissues	Proinflammatory factor affecting afferent sensory nerve excitability (Zhang et al. 2012)
Protease	Mast cells	Enzyme involved in proteolysis and functions as a proinflammatory mediator
Serotonin (5-hydroxytryptamine)	Platelets Mast cells	Neurotransmitter involved in modulation of nociception through interactions with 5-HT_1 and 5-HT_3 receptors (Zhang et al. 2012)
Somatostatin	Merkel cells Keratinocytes	Endogenous nonopioid neuropeptide which modulates nociception (Zhao 2008)
Substance P	Mast cells Fibroblasts Platelets Keratinocytes Macrophages	Tachykinin neuropeptide involved in peripheral and spinal nociception (Zhao 2008)

Source: Lisa P. McFaddin.

Table 1.6 The conditions under which acupuncture should not be used or should be used with caution. Acupuncture is very safe with minimal and infrequent adverse effects.

Cautions	Contraindications	Adverse effects
• Extra caution should be used when placing needles around the eye • Shorter needles should be used at specific points over the chest • Fewer needles should be used in severely debilitated and geriatric patients • Avoid certain points around the lower back and abdomen during pregnancy • Avoid electroacupuncture on animals with seizures and pacemakers	• Do not needle through skin infections • Do not needle through open wounds • Do not needle through tumors • Avoid moxibustion in the summer • Avoid hemoacupuncture in weak or geriatric patients • Do not needle CV-8	• Bleeding • Bruising • Local irritation • Bent needle • Difficult to remove needle • Needle ingestions

Source: Adapted from Xie and Ortiz-Umpierre (2006).

Randomized Cross-Over Clinical Study Evaluating the Effect of Acupuncture on Blood Pressure, Blood Glucose, and Hematological Parameters in Healthy Dogs

Author: Erol Güçlü Gülanber, DVM, PhD
Journal: *American Journal of Traditional Chinese Veterinary Medicine*
Date: 2018
Study design: Randomized clinical trial
Study hypothesis: Acupuncture of specific known acupuncture points will reduce blood pressure, reduce blood glucose, increase white blood cells, and increase red blood cells in normal canines. Placement of needles in non-acupuncture (sham) points will not have the same effects.
Sample size: 100 companion canines of varying breeds, ages, and sex.
Materials and methods: A normal physical examination and fasted blood work was required to qualify the subjects as normal canines. Dogs were randomly divided into two groups: acupuncture (Group A) versus sham acupuncture (Group B). A fasted blood sample and blood pressure was obtained on the day of the experiment before needle placement. Group A dogs had needles placed by a certified veterinary acupuncturist in four acupuncture points (LI-4, ST-36, GB-34, and SP-6). Needles remained in place for 20 minutes. Blood pressure and blood draw were performed immediately following needle removal, one hour later, and one week later. After the final measurement needles were placed in sham locations for 20 minutes with measurements obtained immediately following needle removal, one hour later, and one week later. Group B underwent the same experimentation with placement of the needles at sham points first, followed by the four acupuncture points. Data was evaluated using one-way analysis of variance (ANOVA).

Results

1. A reduction in blood pressure 20 and 60 minutes after acupuncture was statistically significant in both groups compared to the pre-acupuncture measurement. Blood pressure was slightly higher at 60 minutes compared to 20 minutes but still significantly lower than the pre-acupuncture level.

2. A reduction in blood glucose 20 and 60 minutes after acupuncture was statistically significant in both groups compared to the pre-acupuncture measurement. Blood glucose was slightly higher at 60 minutes compared to 20 minutes but still significantly lower than the pre-acupuncture level.
3. A statistically significant increase in the white blood cell count was noted 20 and 60 minutes after acupuncture compared to pre-acupuncture levels.
4. There was no statistically significant difference in the red blood cell count following acupuncture.
5. No statistically significant difference was noted in blood pressure, blood glucose, white blood cell count, and red blood cell count in the patients receiving sham acupuncture.

Study conclusions

1. Acupuncture effectively reduced blood pressure and blood glucose in normal canines.
2. Acupuncture effectively increased white blood cell counts in normal canines.
3. Acupuncture did not affect red blood cell counts in normal canines.

Study limitations

1. There was no true control group.
2. There was no statistical analysis comparing the acupuncture and sham-acupuncture variable measurements directly.

L.P.M. conclusions

1. Acupuncture reduced blood pressure and blood glucose in normal dogs for up to one hour post needle removal. The true duration of effect is unknown. Acupuncture may be a useful adjunct in the management of canine diabetes mellitus and hypertension, but additional studies are needed.
2. Acupuncture increased the white blood cell count of normal dogs for up to one hour post needle removal. The true duration of effect is unknown. Acupuncture may be a useful adjunct for patients needing immune system support, but additional studies are needed.
3. Acupuncture did not positively or negatively affect the red blood cell count of normal dogs.

Gülanber (2018)

Comparison of Decompressive Surgery, Electroacupuncture, and Decompressive Surgery Followed by Electroacupuncture for the Treatment of Dogs with Intervertebral Disk Disease with Long-Standing Severe Neurologic Deficits

Author(s): Jean G. Joaquim, DVM, PhD; Stelio P. L. Luna, DVM, PhD; Juliana T. Brondani, DVM, PhD; Sandra R. Torelli, DVM, PhD; Shelia C. Rahal, DVM, PhD; and Fernando de Paula Freitas, DVM
Journal: *Journal of the American Veterinary Medical Association*
Date: 2010

Study design: Clinical trial
Study hypothesis: The use of electroacupuncture (EAP) in dogs with severe neurologic deficits, lasting >48 hours after onset of thoracolumbar disk herniation, would result in better clinical improvement compared to those undergoing decompressive surgery (DSX).

(Continued)

Comparison of Decompressive Surgery, Electroacupuncture, and Decompressive Surgery   (Continued)

Sample size: 40 companion dogs between 3 and 6 years of age weighing 10–20 kg with a >48-hour history of severe neurologic deficits due to thoracolumbar IVDD.

Materials and methods: There were three experimental groups:

1. The DSX-only group consisted of 10 dogs retroactively selected from those seen and treated at the teaching hospital from 2003 to 2006.
2. 10 dogs received DSX and EAP between 2006 and 2008.
3. 19 dogs received EAP only between 2006 and 2008.

Dogs were placed in the DSX+EAP and EAP-only groups based on owner preference. IVDD was confirmed using myelography, MRI or CT. EAP was performed at BL-18 to BL-23 (bilaterally) and ST-36 to GB-34 (bilaterally) for 20 minutes at 2 and 15 Hz. Patients received EAP once a week for one to six months. Myelopathy scoring was performed prior to treatment and six months following treatment. Statistical analysis was performed using the Goodman test.

Results

1. The improvement rate in dogs receiving EAP was significantly higher compared to the DSX group.

2. There was no significant difference in improvement between dogs in the EAP group vs. those in the DSX+EAP group.

Study conclusions: EAP is a viable option for dogs experiencing severe neurologic deficits for >48 hours after onset due to thoracolumbar IVDD.

Study limitations

1. There was no control group.
2. Division of patients within the experimental groups was not random nor even.
3. The number of EAP sessions was not standardized.
4. Advancement in IVDD surgery between 2003 and 2008 may have affected patient outcome in the DSX and DSX+EAP groups.

L.P.M. conclusions: Patients with long-standing severe neurologic deficits, especially deep pain negative, historically have a poor outcome. The use of EAP, with or without DSX, appears an effective treatment option, especially when euthanasia is the most common alternative.

Joaquim et al. (2010)

Analgesic Efficacy of Laser Acupuncture and Electroacupuncture in Cats Undergoing Ovariohysterectomy

Authors: Felipe Nascimento, Virginia Marques, Giulianne Crociolli, Gabriel Nicácio, Isabela Nicácio, and Renata Cassu

Journal: *Journal of Veterinary Medical Science*

Date: 2019

Study design: Randomized blinded clinical trial

Study hypothesis: The use of laser acupuncture (LA) and electroacupuncture (EAP) would decrease postoperative pain and the need for rescue analgesics in cats undergoing elective ovariohysterectomy (OHE).

Sample size: 30 companion intact female cats aged six months to five years.

Materials and methods: Cats arrived 36 hours prior to the procedure to acclimate to the environment. Cats were divided randomly and evenly into three groups: control, LA, and EAP. Patients in the LA and EAP group were sedated with ketamine, midazolam, and tramadol. Two acupuncture points (bilaterally) were stimulated in both the EAP and LA groups: ST-36 and SP-6. Acupuncture points were stimulated for 20 minutes with EAP and 9 seconds each with LA. All OHEs were performed by the same surgeon using the same drug protocols. Pain was assessed using the Interactive Visual Analogue Scale and UNESP-Botucatu Multidimensional Composite Pain Scale (MCPS) by a blinded observer two hours prior to surgery and 0.5, 1, 2, 4, 6, 8, 12, 18, and 24 hours after extubation. Patients exhibiting pain received a rescue dose of tramadol followed by a single dose of meloxicam 30 minutes later, if needed. Statistical analysis of the results relied on Kruskal–Wallis test, Friedman test, and Dunn's post hoc test.

Results

1. The number of cats requiring rescue analgesia was not significantly different between the three groups.

2. The number of rescue doses needed was significantly higher in the control group compared to the EAP and LA groups, but not statistically different between the two treatment groups.

Study conclusions: Preoperative EAP and LA reduced postoperative pain lessening the need for rescue analgesia following routine OHE in cats.

Study limitations

1. Relatively small sample size within each group.
2. Opioids and ketamine can interfere with the effectiveness of acupuncture which may have dampened the effects.

L.P.M. Conclusions: EAP and LA reduced postoperative pain in normal feline patients undergoing routine OHE. Pretreatment with EAP and/or LA may be beneficial in reducing postoperative pain for other common surgical procedures.

Nascimento et al. (2019)

As of July 2021 a quick search on PubMed yielded 522 articles for "veterinary acupuncture," 301 articles for "acupuncture canine," and 267 for "acupuncture feline."

Not all studies of veterinary acupuncture present the therapy in a favorable light. Habacher et al. (2006) performed a systematic review of the available research on veterinary acupuncture up to 2004. The group concluded that while many patients benefited from acupuncture, sufficient evidence to support the use of acupuncture for the treatment of various veterinary ailments was lacking. The researchers admitted the existing studies should be repeated, and the lack of evidence of efficacy did not mean acupuncture was not effective (Habacher et al. 2006). More studies were needed to definitively prove acupuncture helped veterinary patients.

Numerous studies supporting the use of veterinary acupuncture have been conducted since 2004. Selmer and Shiau (2019) performed a meta-analysis of 16 human and eight veterinary clinical trials comparing the effectiveness of conventional therapies with those integrating TCM, including acupuncture. The systematic review and meta-analysis demonstrated a statistically significant improvement in patient outcome when both conventional and traditional Chinese medicine was utilized

(Selmer and Shiau 2019). Presented below are the summaries of three veterinary acupuncture studies.

Table 1.7 specifies many of the diseases and conditions for which veterinary acupuncture has shown a scientifically beneficial effect. This list is not all inclusive, as new studies documenting the beneficial effects of acupuncture in veterinary medicine are continually published.

The How

Team Members

This section reviews the potential return on investment (ROI), how to effectively train the entire team, how to promote, and how to integrate the integrative therapy.

Return on Investment

ROI can be determined by evaluating client interest, veterinarian demand, hospital costs, applicability of the service, appointment scheduling, and pricing.

Client Interest

Currently there are no studies documenting client interest or the popularity of acupuncture. By evaluating trends in client opinion and pet health insurance, interest in acupuncture can be inferred.

- *Client opinion*: Table 1.8 summarizes the pet owner demographics and statistics mentioned in the My Lessons section at the beginning of this book. Even if half of those owners are open to acupuncture, that is still 53.1 million potential patients.
- *Pet health insurance*: Many pet insurance plans include coverage for integrative therapies, especially acupuncture (Woodley 2018). The presence of this type of coverage re-emphasizes the mainstream incorporation of these treatment modalities, as well as reflecting client demand.

Veterinarian Demand

The number of certified veterinary acupuncturists (CVAs) has grown exponentially over the past 40 years. The IVAS and Chin University are two of the most recognized organizations in veterinary acupuncture. The IVAS was founded in 1974, with 80 members by 1975. As of January 2021, IVAS has over 1800 members (https://www.ivas.org/about-ivas). Chi University has trained and certified over 7500 veterinarians since 1988 (https://www.chivm.edu). Keep in mind that IVAS members and Chi University graduates are international and these totals reflect veterinarians worldwide.

While the number of CVAs has increased over the time, the upsurge of owned pets, especially those whose owners are interested in integrative therapy, coupled with the shortage of veterinarians (as defined by the veterinary census of Ouedraogo et al. and the 2023 economic report by the American Veterinary Medical Association (AMVA), indicates that there is a need for more integrative practitioners (Ouedraogo et al. 2019; AMVA 2023). The current and projected number of practicing veterinarians does not meet the ever-expanding volume of companion animals (see the Book Structure section at the beginning of this book for further information on the current veterinarian shortage).

While acupuncture certification is highly recommended, it is not required to practice veterinary acupuncture. This makes calculating the exact number of veterinarians currently practicing acupuncture difficult. If we use the IVAS members plus Chi University graduates, round up, and ignore duplicates, there are 6000 veterinarians currently practicing acupuncture in the United States. That represents a little over 5% of the total veterinarian population (AVMA 2018). Using the estimated 45.9 million potential integrative patients that is 7650 patients per veterinary acupuncturist. With these numbers, I would say there is room for more practitioners.

Another way to examine the need in your area is to compare the number of general

Table 1.7 Examples of studies demonstrating the efficacy of veterinary acupuncture in the treatment of multiple diseases and conditions as of 2023.

System category	Disease conditions studied	Studies
Anesthesia	Anxiolytic and sedative	Kim and Nam (2006), Fong and Xie (2019)
	Postoperative recovery and pain management	Lin et al. (2010), Laim et al. (2009), Gakiya et al. (2011), Groppetti et al. (2011), Luna et al. (2015), Marques et al. (2015), Ribeiro et al. (2017), Turner-Knarr (2018), Nascimento et al. (2019), Ferro et al. (2022)
Behavior	Anxiolytic and sedative	Kim and Nam (2006), Mier (2021)
Cardiovascular	Hypertension	Lin et al. (2010), Shengfeng et al. (2018), Gülanber (2018)
Dermatologic	Otitis	Sánchez-Araujo and Puchi (2011)
Endocrine	Cortisol reduction	Koh et al. (2017)
	Glucose reduction	Gülanber (2018)
Gastrointestinal	Enteritis	Gülanber (2008)
	Megaesophagus	Gülanber (2008)
	Vomiting	Koh et al. (2014), Scallan and Simon (2016), Yue et al. (2021)
Immune system	Increase white blood cells	Gülanber (2018)
	Wound healing	Pettermann (2015)
	Neoplasia	Lana et al. (2006), Xie et al. (2017)
	Vaccination	Perdrizet et al. (2019)
Musculoskeletal	Chronic pain	Lane and Hill (2016), Teixeira et al. (2016), Silva et al. (2017)
	Cruciate ligament disease	Shmalberg et al. (2014), Lee (2019)
	Hip dysplasia	Gülanber (2018), Teixeira et al. (2016)
	Myositis	Gülanber (2008)
	Osteoarthritis	Um et al. (2005), Gülanber (2018), Chomsiriwat and Ma (2019)
	Patellar luxations	Fuda et al. (2008)

(Continued)

Table 1.7 (Continued)

System category	Disease conditions studied	Studies
Neurologic	Cervical vertebral instability	Rovnard et al. (2018), Liu et al. (2015), Chen et al. (2019)
	Chronic pain	Silva et al. (2017)
	Congenital abnormalities	Fuda et al. (2008), Liu et al. (2016)
	Horner's syndrome	Cho and Kim (2008)
	Intervertebral disk disease	Hayashi et al. (2007), Gülanber (2018), Han et al. (2010), Chien (2011), Rovnard et al. (2018), Zuo et al. (2019), Dragomir et al. (2021), Sawamura et al. (2022)
	Neck and back pain	Liu et al. (2016), Collins (2021))
	Paresis and paralysis	Liu et al. (2016)
	Seizures	Tangjitjaroen and Mahatnirunkul (2017)
	Viral infections	Tangjitjaroen and Mahatnirunkul (2017)
Ophthalmic	Intraocular pressure reduction	Kim et al. (2005)
Respiratory	Resuscitation (respiratory arrest)	Gülanber (2018)

Source: Lisa P. McFaddin.

Table 1.8 Summary of the 2022 pet ownership and pet health insurance demographics in the United States discussed in the Introduction of the book (Burns 2018; MFAF 2018; Burns 2022; NAPHIA 2023; Nolen 2022; APPA 2022).

• 83% of pets are owned by millennials (32%), generation X (24%), and baby boomers (27%)
• 69 million households owned dogs
• 45.3 million households owned cats
• Estimated over 81.1 million owned dogs
• Estimated over 60.7 million owned cats
• 68% of owners are interested in alternative treatment modalities for their pets
• 4.41 million pets have pet health insurance
• 82% of insurance pets are dogs

Source: Lisa P. McFaddin.

practitioners within a 5-, 10-, or 20-mile radius to the number of advertised veterinary acupuncturists. The search radius is dependent on your hospital's demographics. Most comparisons tend to follow the 5% trend, meaning at least 5% of the surrounding hospitals are currently offering acupuncture. Ensuring your area is not saturated with veterinary acupuncturists prevents introduction of a redundant service.

Hospital Costs

Let's start by reviewing the potential costs associated with introducing and offering acupuncture: veterinarian training, staff training, supplies and equipment, staffing, facilities, and advertising. Tables 1.10 and 1.11 demonstrate varying start-up costs, dependent on the hospital's contribution toward the veterinarian's training and prior utilization of regular all-staff meetings. For more information on potential hospital costs, refer to the Introduction.

Veterinarian Training

Course Costs   There are five main training programs in the United States. Each program contains online and on-site training, with an average of three on-site sessions. On-site sessions generally last three to five days. Typical completion time, with certification, is six months. Additional information can be found in the Veterinarian section of this chapter (cost range, $6995–9750).

Textbooks   Textbooks may not be required for the certification courses but are often recommended. The price range for one to two books is $200–400 (average cost, $300).

Travel Expenses   Travel costs include airfare, lodging, car rental, and meals. The estimated pricing is based on three on-site sessions with four full days of training.

1. *Airfare*: Due to the global effects of the pandemic, the average roundtrip domestic flight within the United States was less expensive in 2021 compared to 2019, $293 versus $359 (Weir 2019; Damodaran 2021). Airfare rose precipitously in June 2022 to an average of $398 for a roundtrip domestic flight and has continued to rise by at least 3.4% in the last eight months to approximately $412 (US Bureau of Labor Statistics 2023; Trcek 2023). The $412 value was used when calculating the cost of airfare for three round-trip flights (total cost, $1236).
2. *Lodging*: As of February 2023 the federal per diem rate for lodging on business trips is $98 per night (FederalPay.org 2023). The federal per diem rate was used for calculations, with four nights of lodging over three sessions (total cost, $1176).

3. *Car rental*: Unfortunately the price of car rentals skyrocketed following the pandemic. First, rental car companies sold most of their inventory at the end of 2020 due to the drop in travel (Fields 2021). Secondly, the demand for car rentals spiked sooner than expected once travel resumed in 2021 (Fields 2021). Finally, there has been a microchip manufacturing shortage, slowing car production. As of January 2023, the average weekly car rental price is $551 (French and Kemmis 2023). Rideshare and cabbing are extremely popular, but the variability in travel distances makes calculating an average cost impractical. It is suspected this cost would be comparable, if not lower, than that of a rental car. The total was calculated using five-day car rentals for three sessions (total cost, $1653).

4. *Meals*: The federal per diem rate for business trip meals from October 2022 through September 2023 is $59 a day (FederalPay. org 2023). Most training programs provide at least one meal, as well as snacks. Meal expenditure is estimated to be $40 per day for a total of 15 days (total cost, $600).

5. *Time off*: Veterinarian paid time-off (PTO) for on-site courses only factors in as an added expense if additional PTO is provided outside of the veterinarian's contractual annual PTO. Clinics offer an average of 4.1 paid continuing education (CE) days per year according to the last AAHA Compensation and Benefits Guide (AAHA 2020). If the total number of CE days exceeds the allotted CE days per year, the hospital can either require the veterinarian use PTO or pay the veterinarian for some or all the remaining CE days. Requiring the use of PTO would not "cost" the hospital anything additional. The clinic accrues an added expense if they agree to pay for the additional CE days. The price range provided represents a clinic offering 5–12 days of additional paid CE leave. The median pay for a full-time veterinarian, calculated by the United States Bureau of Labor Statistics in 2022, was $100 370 or $48.26/hour (BLS 2022a). Each paid CE day was counted as eight hours. The total does not include potential lost revenue due to the veterinarian's absence, nor does it include relief veterinarian expenses. The average number of additional paid CE days was estimated to be 8.5 days (total cost, $3282).

Staff Training Team training expenses are highly variable and dependent on the preexistence staff meetings and use of a staff meeting for training (compared to self-study). Refer to the Introduction of this book for a breakdown of these variables (cost range, $230–1295).

Supplies The quantity and brand of supplies kept on-hand is dependent on practitioner preference and the hospital's goal for consumables on-hand. Given this variability, the expected expenditure for acupuncture supplies is based on the cost per patient. All pricing is current as of February 2023.

- *Acupuncture needles*: The range assumes a cost of $12 for a box of 100 needles with 10–30 needles used per patient (total per patient, $2.50).
- *Moxa:* The average cost of a box of 10 moxa sticks is around $15. Each stick can be used for at least three treatments (total per patient, $0.52).
- *Electroacupuncture*: An electroacupuncture unit, with leads, is not required but very helpful. The average cost is $400 per unit. The price range per patient is based on the frequency of use and the assumptions and calculations presented by a 2015 paper discussing the profitability of veterinary acupuncture (Marks and Shmalberg 2015) (total per patient, $0.76–$4.02).
- *Vitamin B12*: A 100-ml multidose bottle of vitamin B12 costs $8. On average a patient receives 1 ml of vitamin B12 divided into multiple acupoints. The price per bottle is based

on the average price across all major veterinary distributors (total per patient, $0.08).

- *Syringes:* A box of 100 syringes (1 ml with 25g or 3 ml with 22g) costs on average $15 per box. If a separate syringe is used for each 0.1 ml injection of vitamin B12 at most 10 syringes would be used for the aquapuncture session. Generally, a 1-ml syringe is used, unless larger quantities of vitamin B12 are injected, and the needle is changed every one to two injections. The price is based on using 10 syringes per patient (total per patient, $1.50).
- *Needles*: A box of 100 needles (27 or 25g) costs around $8. The presented cost assumes 10 needles are used per patient (total per patient, $0.80).

Staffing Acupuncture appointments range from 30 to 60 minutes depending on the condition(s) being treated. Following the American Animal Hospital Association (AAHA) recommendations a veterinary assistant or licensed technician (VA/LT) should restrain patients for physical examinations and procedures. A VA/LT may be utilized for the length of the entire appointment or only until the needles are placed.

Some practitioners prefer the VA/LT remain in the room following needle placement, ensuring the pet remains calm, is not walking around, and does not attempt to remove the needles. Other practitioners prefer the VA/LT leave the room.

If the VA/LT is only needed for the examination and needle placement there is no difference in staffing cost for an acupuncture appointment compared to a traditional appointment. If the VA/LT is required to stay in the exam room until the needles are removed the staff cost for the additional 15–45 minutes should be considered: $4.43–13.29 per patient. The provided expenses are based on a national average wage of $17.72 an hour for veterinary technologists and technicians as of September 2022 (BLS 2022b).

Facilities Facility expenses represent the costs needed to keep the doors open (aka overhead). Overhead includes rent or mortgage, utilities, administrative costs, and often employee costs divided by the minutes the practice is open (Stevenson 2016). The price per minute equals the amount of revenue needed just to break even. Overhead is extremely hospital specific, but the range tends to be $2–5/minute. The low end of the range in Table 1.9 represents the cost for a 30-minute appointment at a clinic with a $2/minute overhead, while the high end represents the cost for a 60-minute appointment at a clinic with a $5/minute overhead.

Designating a specific room for acupuncture minimizes the chances other associates will need the room for their appointments. However, there is then an added expense for designing the room and potential lost revenue if the room is not used regularly. The absence of a designated room theoretically reduces redecoration costs, but this can be disruptive for appointment flow if the treatment takes longer than the allotted time.

Advertising There are numerous ways to advertise a new service. On average, veterinary hospitals spend 0.7% of revenue on promotion and advertisement (AVMA 2019). Most of the advertisement can be done with little to no additional expenditure. The Promotion section discusses advertising ideas in further detail. The national median gross revenue for companion animal practices was $1.2 million in 2022 (AVMA 2023). Advertising costs are calculated assuming no more than 5% of the current advertising budget would be used for promotion of the new service (estimated maximal cost, $420).

Start-Up Costs Table 1.9 summarizes projected start-up costs for acupuncture. Table 1.10 calculates potential start-up costs based on the degree of hospital contribution toward veterinarian and staff training. Different scenarios are presented in which the hospital covers all, some, or none of the expenses.

Table 1.9 Total potential hospital start-up costs and per-pateint expenses for acupuncture as of 2023.

Category	Subcategories	Projected cost		
Veterinarian training	Course costs	$6995–9750		Average $8373
	Textbooks	$200–400		Average $300
	Travel expenses	$4199		
	Time-off	$1909–4581		Average $3245
Staff training	Variable	$230–1295		
Supplies	Acupuncture needles	$12 per box		$2.50 per patient
	Moxa	$15 per box		$0.52 per patient
	Electroacupuncture unit	$400 per unit		$0.76–4.02 per patient
	Vitamin B12	$8 per bottle		$0.08 per patient
	Syringes (1 and 3 ml)	$15 per box		$1.50 per patient
	Needles (27g and 25g)	$8 per box		$0.80 per patient
Staffing	Variable	≥$0		
Facilities	Overhead	$2–5 per minute for 30–60 minute appointment		$60–300 per patient
Advertising	Variable	≤$420		

Source: Lisa P. McFaddin.

Applicability

As stated earlier, acupuncture is extremely versatile and beneficial for numerous conditions and ailments. Acupuncture is used primarily for painful conditions (musculoskeletal and neurologic). As the clinician becomes more comfortable and confident in their acupuncture skills the variety of cases for which acupuncture is recommended typically increases.

Appointment Scheduling

There are four main factors to consider when planning acupuncture appointment protocols: appointment length, support staff availability, exam room availability, and follow-up appointment scheduling.

There are other issues to consider when scheduling acupuncture appointments. For example, will acupuncture appointments be scheduled separately from traditional Western appointments or will the appointment length be increased to allow time for needle placement? Will vaccinations be given during the acupuncture appointment? Some practitioners prefer to perform vaccines at the time of acupuncture; whiles others prefer to separate vaccine administration from acupuncture sessions by at least 24 hours.

The initial integrative appointment is longer, 60 minutes, compared to follow-up appointments. Follow-up appointments should be scheduled for 30–50 minutes depending on the patient and if additional treatments are performed.

Keep the appointment positive: you want the pet to enjoy the experience. A relaxed pet is more easily treated. Avoid ancillary procedures which may cause stress: nail trims, anal gland expression, sanitary trims, anything with the ears, etc. Additional information on appointment scheduling can be found in the Introduction at the beginning of this book.

Pricing

An in-depth look into appointment pricing can be found in the Introduction. Here I discuss two pricing methods: current market fees and hospital cost-based pricing.

Table 1.10 Projected acupuncture start-up costs for eight hospital scenarios, with varying hospital contributions toward veterinary certification and staff training as of February 2023. The cost of veterinarian training is based on the averages presented in Table 1.9. Staff training costs assume a 1.5-hour long all-staff meeting, using national averages for employee numbers: eight non-DVMs and two DVMs (AVMA 2019, 2023). The cost of office supplies and lunch as estimated based on 10 employees attending the meeting. The overhead is based on an average of $3.5/minute. Missed revenue is calculated using the 2022 national mean revenue per hour for companion animal practices ($567/hour) (AVMA 2023). Advertising includes printed materials, digital advertisement, and community engagement.

Category	Projected expenses	Ex. 1	Ex. 2	Ex. 3	Ex. 4	Ex. 5	Ex. 6	Ex. 7	Ex. 8
Veterinarian training	Average course cost	$8378	$8378	$8378	n/a	$8378	$8378	$8378	n/a
	Average textbooks	$300	n/a	n/a	n/a	$300	n/a	n/a	n/a
	Travel expenses	$4665	n/a	n/a	n/a	$4665	n/a	n/a	n/a
	Average time-off	$3283	$3283	n/a	n/a	$3283	$3283	n/a	n/a
Staff training	Office supplies	$30	$30	$30	$30	$30	$30	$30	$30
	Lunch	$200	$200	$200	$200	$200	$200	$200	$200
	Overhead	$315	$315	$315	$315	n/a	n/a	n/a	n/a
	Missed revenue	$851	$851	$851	$851	n/a	n/a	n/a	n/a
Supplies	Five boxes acupuncture needles	$50	$50	$50	$50	$50	$50	$50	$50
	Electroacupuncture unit	$400	$400	$400	$400	$400	$400	$400	$400
	One box of moxa	$15	$15	$15	$15	$15	$15	$15	$15
	One bottle vitamin B12	$6	$6	$6	$6	$6	$6	$6	$6
	One box 1-ml syringes	$12	$12	$12	$12	$12	$12	$12	$12
	One box 27g needles	$6	$6	$6	$6	$6	$6	$6	$6
Advertising		$420	$420	$420	$420	$420	$420	$420	$420
Total		$18931	$13966	$10683	$2305	$17765	$12800	$9517	$1139

Source: Lisa P. McFaddin.

Current Market Fees A study of five general practices within Central Florida found the price of acupuncture appointments ranged from $45–150 with a mean of $95.80 (Shmalberg 2016; Marks and Shmalberg 2015). The average length of these appointments was 47 minutes. According to the Nationwide® Purdue 2019 Veterinary Price Index, veterinary pricing increased by 21.1% between the end of 2014 and the end of 2018 (Purdue University 2019). Presuming services continued to increase by at least 5% annually, a 50-minute session would translate to $130 by January 2023.

Thervo (2019) lists veterinary acupuncture appointments costs at $65–85 a session but do not specify the length of the appointment. Speaking with other certified veterinary acupuncturists the current price range for a 30–60-minute acupuncture appointment is $85–200.

Hospital Cost-Based Pricing Table 1.11 outlines the hospital cost per patient for 30- and 60-minute acupuncture appointments. The

veterinarian training amortization per patient was calculated using the following assumptions:

1. The average companion animal practice employees 2.1 full-time veterinarians (AVMA 2023).
2. The average companion animal practice is open for appointments 5.6 days/week (AVMA 2023).
3. The average companion animal veterinarian sees two patients/hour (AVMA 2023).
4. The average companion animal veterinarian works 45 hours a week (AVMA 2023).
5. The average companion animal veterinarian spends 78% of their work week seeing appointments (AVMA 2023).
6. The average companion animal veterinarian receives 21 paid days of vacation and holiday pay annually (iVet360 2023).
7. The average companion animal veterinarian receives 4.1 paid days off for CE per year (AAHA 2019).
8. Acupuncture appointments account for 14% of a veterinarian's appointments (Marks and Shmalberg 2015).

Table 1.11 Estimated hospital costs per patient for 30- and 60-minute acupuncture appointments as of February 2023. Start-up costs are taken from the totals in Table 1.10. Amortization is per patient and is based on the veterinarian seeing 952 acupuncture patients in two years. Overhead is calculated using $3.5/minute in a practice with two veterinarians. Multiple examples are provided with the variance determined by the total cost within each category. The total is rounded to the nearest whole number.

	Ex. 1	Ex. 2	Ex. 3	Ex. 4	Ex. 5	Ex. 6	Ex. 7	Ex. 8
30-Minute appointments								
Table 1.9 totals	$18 931	$13 966	$10 683	$2305	$17 765	$12 800	$9517	$1 139
Amortization	$19.80	$14.61	$11.17	$2.41	$18.58	$13.39	$9.96	$1.19
Overhead	$52.50	$52.50	$52.50	$52.50	$52.50	$52.50	$52.50	$52.50
Total	**$72**	**$67**	**$64**	**$55**	**$71**	**$66**	**$62**	**$54**
60-Minute appointments								
Table 1.9 totals	$18 931	$13 966	$10 683	$2305	$17 765	$12 800	$9517	$1 139
Amortization	$19.80	$14.61	$11.17	$2.41	$18.58	$13.39	$9.96	$1.19
Overhead	$105	$105	$105	$105	$105	$105	$105	$105
Total	**$125**	**$120**	**$116**	**$107**	**$124**	**$118**	**$115**	**$106**

Source: Lisa P. McFaddin.

9. The amortization is calculated over a two-year period.

Using the above information, the typical companion animal veterinarian sees 3398 patients a year (70 patients a week, working 48.4 weeks a year). At least 476 of these patients would receive acupuncture, for a total of 952 patients in two years.

Supply assumptions were based on the average cost per patient for each supply listed in Table 1.9. Appointments with dry needling only would cost the hospital $5.29 less per patient.

Overhead includes rent or mortgage, utilities, administrative costs, and often employee costs divided by the minutes the practice is open (Stevenson 2016). A $3.5/minute overhead was used. The national average of two DVMs per hospital was used, rounded down from 2.1 (AAHA 2019; AVMA 2023).

The formula to determine service fees is quite simple: service fee = hospital cost + profit. The big question becomes how much profit? Table 1.12 illustrates the potential fee for 30- and 60-minute acupuncture appointments, based on hospital cost and variable markup percentages. It becomes readily apparent that the lower the hospital contribution, the higher the comparative profit.

Additional Considerations

Most of my patients receive other treatments or diagnostics when they come in for their treatments. We often adjust current medication regimens, run diagnostics (blood work, urinalysis, radiographs, etc.), discuss dietary and environmental modifications, and discuss nutrition and nutraceuticals, all of which increase revenue, average transaction charge (ATC), and DVM revenue per hour.

Offering acupuncture also helps improve current client retention and drive new client acquisition. Marks and Shmalberg (2015) found 29% of new acupuncture patients returned for wellness and other services. Improving client retention and new client acquisition helps drive revenue.

Scheduling acupuncture appointments presents a unique opportunity not afforded by traditional Western appointments. Most appointments in veterinary medicine are scheduled linearly: 8 a.m., 8:30 a.m., 9 a.m., etc. With acupuncture appointments the veterinarians may only be in the exam room for the initial history, examination, needle placement and again at the time of needle removal. In a hospital with enough exam rooms and personnel, acupuncture appointments could be staggered very easily. This would in essence double the DVM revenue per half hour to hour. This tactic requires double the exam room capacity, support staff, and requires careful planning when scheduling appointments.

As an additional resource several organizations offer online courses discussing the integration of acupuncture and TCVM into the veterinary practice. The IVAS offers a three-hour online prerecorded webinar series presented by Nell Ostermeier, DVM, CVA, FAAVA called Integrating Acupuncture into Practice. Chi University has a 19-hour online course on discussing TCVM Business Management.

Team Training

The concept of phase training is used when introducing acupuncture to the hospital team. A multimedia approach is used to assist with the training program and is outlined in Table 1.13.

In order for the practice manager to fulfill his or her role in training, they need their own checklist:

- Schedule a date and time for the team training.
- Ensure all information pertaining to the new service is reviewed with the staff.
- Confirm all team members have completed the training.
- Certify all team members understand the information and can successfully educate clients.

Table 1.12 Potential 30- and 60-minute acupuncture appointment prices using hospital costs from Table 1.11 at varying percentage markups as of February 2023.

		Ex. 1	Ex. 2	Ex. 3	Ex. 4	Ex. 5	Ex. 6	Ex. 7	Ex. 8
30-Minute appointments									
Total hospital cost		$72	$67	$64	$55	$71	$66	$62	$54
Potential appointment price	40% Markup	$101	$94	$90	$77	$99	$92	$87	$76
	50% Markup	$108	$101	$96	$83	$107	$99	$93	$81
	60% Markup	$115	$112	$107	$94	$118	$111	$105	$93
	70% Markup	$122	$114	$109	$94	$121	$112	$105	$92
	80% Markup	$130	$121	$115	$99	$128	$119	$112	$97
	90% Markup	$137	$127	$122	$105	$135	$125	$118	$103
	100% Markup	$144	$134	$128	$110	$142	$132	$124	$108
60-Minute appointments									
Total hospital cost		$125	$120	$116	$107	$124	$118	$115	$106
Potential appointment price	40% Markup	$175	$168	$162	$150	$174	$165	$161	$148
	50% Markup	$188	$180	$174	$161	$186	$177	$173	$159
	60% Markup	$200	$112	$107	$94	$118	$111	$105	$93
	70% Markup	$213	$204	$197	$182	$211	$201	$196	$180
	80% Markup	$225	$216	$209	$193	$223	$212	$207	$191
	90% Markup	$238	$228	$220	$203	$236	$224	$219	$201
	100% Markup	$250	$240	$232	$214	$248	$236	$230	$212

Source: Lisa P. McFaddin.

Table 1.13 The breakdown of veterinary acupuncture phase training steps and resources for the entire hospital team.

Phase 1: Background information	
Team training guide	• The handout walks the practice manager and/or veterinarian through Phase 1 of the training • A downloadable and editable copy of the handout is located on the companion website
Training presentation	• The video covers background information on the modality • PowerPoints can be downloaded, edited, and personalized from the companion website • The document can be used as a PowerPoint or saved as an mp4 creating a personalized movie
Team training handout	• The handout provides additional background information for the CSRs, VAs, and LTs to complement the knowledge gained from watching the training presentation • A downloadable and editable copy of the handout is located on the companion website
Phase 2: Knowledge proficiency	
Quiz	• A short quiz to ensure all team members have a good understanding of the service being offered • A downloadable and editable copy of the handout is located on the companion website • A key is provided
Phase 3: Expectations	
Training worksheets	• A training checklist is provided for CSRs and VA/LTs with role-specific expectations and tasks for each staff member • A recommended completion time is provided • A downloadable and editable copy of the handout is located on the companion website
Phase 4: Client education	
Client scripts	• Bullet point information and scripted examples used when discussing acupuncture with clients • A downloadable and editable copy of the handout is located on the companion website
Client education presentation	• A short (five to seven minute) client educational video about the therapeutic modality • PowerPoints can be downloaded, edited, and personalized from the companion website • The document can be used as a PowerPoint or saved as an mp4 creating a personalized movie
Client education handout	• An informational handout about the therapeutic modality written specifically for clients • A downloadable and editable copy of the handout is located on the companion website

CSR, customer service representative; VA, veterinary assistant; LT, licensed technician.
Source: Lisa P. McFaddin.

Promotion

There are six common avenues of promotion for a veterinary integrative medicine (VIM) service: hospital website, social media, email blasts, mailers, in-hospital promotions, and client education.

Hospital Website

Advertise "Acupuncture" in several locations on the website main page, services, veterinarian's biography, and blog page. On the main page create a button or banner stating "Now offering veterinary acupuncture" with a link to success stories or client testimonials. Utilize the hospital website to advertise the VIM treatment under the "Services" section. On the veterinarian's biograph section include a description of the specialized training and professional initials. Create an Acupuncture blog page discussing patient success stories.

Social Media

Utilize Facebook, Instagram, and/or Twitter to post facts, photographs, hashtags, and patient success stories. Include fun and intriguing facts about veterinary acupuncture. Clients love patient photographs, especially when receiving veterinary acupuncture treatments. Create or utilize veterinary acupuncture specific hashtags.

Email Blasts

Send fun mass emails to your clients introducing veterinary acupuncture. Consider monthly case presentations illustrating how the service has benefited patients. Almost everyone has at least one email address these days. Customer service representative should be amassing client emails at the same rate as phone numbers.

Mailers

Mailers can be expensive and are largely unnecessary in this digital age. Mailers can be used to announce the introduction of acupuncture to existing clients. The mailer should include the name of the new service, a brief description of how veterinary acupuncture can help pet patients, the name of the doctor performing the acupuncture, and maybe a brief description of the training the doctor received and a photograph of a pet receiving acupuncture.

In-Hospital Promotions

Advertise veterinary acupuncture within the hospital using small promotional signs, informational signs, invoice teasers, and staff buttons. Small promotional signs can be placed in the waiting room and exam rooms. Include photographs of pets receiving acupuncture. Consider catchphrases such as "Got Acupuncture" or "Veterinary Acupuncture Has a Point."

Informational signs should include a brief description of how veterinary acupuncture can help pet patients, photographs of pets receiving acupuncture, name of the doctor performing acupuncture, and a brief description of the training the doctor received.

Invoice teasers should consist of short phrases reminding and enticing owners regarding a new service offered at the practice. Examples include "Now offering Veterinary Acupuncture," "Curious if acupuncture can help your pet?," "Introducing Veterinary Acupuncture," and "Would your pet benefit from Veterinary Acupuncture?"

Buttons can be made for the staff to wear with kitchy phrases reminding owners, in a fun way, of the new VIM service. Examples include "Got Acupuncture" and "Want to learn more about Veterinary Acupuncture?".

Client Education

Education is crucial to understanding the purpose and importance of any given treatment. The client handouts and videos solidify pet owner knowledge base, reducing concerns and conveying value.

Integration

The key components for proper integration include availability of the service to the right patients, appropriate patient scheduling, appropriate support staff scheduling, and staff buy-in (understanding the benefits of the offered service).

Veterinarians

There are several factors to contemplate when veterinarians are considering, and preparing to incorporate, a VIM in their clinical repertoire: state requirements and restrictions, ROI, course availability, supplies and equipment, veterinary organizations, and continuing education.

State Requirements and Restrictions

Is Acupuncture Considered the Practice of Veterinary Medicine?

Table 1.14 details which states define acupuncture as the practice of veterinary medicine. Some states permit non-veterinarians certified in acupuncture to practice, usually under the supervision of a veterinarian. Table 1.14 also addresses which states allow human acupuncturists to practice on animals. These rules and regulations can change. Check your local state board for further information. Links to each state's veterinary board can be found online.

Does Acupuncture CE Count Toward Licensure CE Requirements?

Currently no states require specific CE hours for veterinary acupuncture. Some states limit the use of integrative medicine CE hours toward the annual CE requirement for license renewal. Most states permit the use of acupuncture CE if the lectures or webinars are performed by an approved provider. Review your specific state's requirements for further details. Table 1.14 outlines those states which permit the use of acupuncture CE toward the annual CE requirement.

Utilizing AVMA (2019) and each state's Board of Veterinary Medicine website, Table 1.14 addresses the following questions: Does the state define acupuncture as the practice of veterinary medicine? Are licensed human acupuncturists certified in animal acupuncture allowed to practice? Are they required to practice under the direct supervision of a veterinarian? Are acupuncture CE hours applicable to the annual or biennial CE requirement? Links to each state veterinary board are provided on the companion website.

Are Your Assets Covered?

Check with your liability insurance to determine if you are covered when practicing veterinary acupuncture. Refer to the Introduction at the beginning of this book for additional information.

Return on Investment

Specifics are discussed in the Team Members section of this chapter.

Course Availability

While certification is not strictly required, formal acupuncture training should be considered a requirement. Training and certification provide the foundation for understanding how acupuncture can best help your veterinary patients. Completion of formal training also helps legitimize the modality. Most training programs involve multiple online and on-site courses. Veterinarians can usually start practicing acupuncture after the first on-site training session. The following initial certification course offerings and pricing are current as of February 2023.

Many of the organizations offering the initial acupuncture certification offer advanced training as well. Board certification in acupuncture is possible through the American Board of Animal Acupuncture (ABAA). ABAA is a non-profit certification agency dedicated to establishing and promoting standards of care in veterinary acupuncture and Western medicine. Additionally, Chi University offers a Master of Science in Integrative Veterinary Medicine, a Master of Science in Traditional Chinese Veterinary Medicine, and a Graduate Certificate in Veterinary Acupuncture.

Veterinarians who are on the fence about committing to a full training course are encouraged to attend introductory lectures first. Familiarizing yourself with the information is a great way to determine if pursuing this

Table 1.14 The legality of veterinary acupuncture (VA) and applicability of continuing education (CE) hours by state as of 2023. A link to each state's veterinary board can be found on the companion website.

State	PVM	LA	LAE	ACE	References
Alabama	Yes	No	No	Yes	ASBVME (2021)
Alaska	No	No	No	Yes	ADCBPL (2023)
Arizona	Yes	Yes	No	Yes	ASVMEB (2022)
Arkansas	Yes	No	No	≤5 hours/year	ADAVMEB (2008, 2019)
California	No	Yes	No	Yes	CDCAVMB (2022)
Colorado	No	Yes	No	Yes	CDRASBVM (2019)
Connecticut	No	NS	NS	Yes	CBVM (2023)
Delaware	No	NS	NS	Yes	DBVM (2023)
District of Columbia	No	NS	No	Yes	DCVM (2023)
Florida	Yes	No	No	≤5 hours/year	FBVM (2022), eLaws.us (2020)
Georgia	Yes	NS	No	Yes	GSBVM (2022, 2023)
Hawaii	No	Yes	No	Yes	HDCCAPVLDBVM (2010)
Idaho	No	Yes	No	Yes	IBVM (2020)
Illinois	Yes	Yes	No	Yes	IGA (2004)
Indiana	Yes	Yes	No	Yes	IVMB (2019)
Iowa	No	NS	No	Yes	IBVM (2017)
Kansas	Yes	NS	No	Yes	KBVE (2020)
Kentucky	Yes	No	No	Yes	KYBVE (2020)
Louisiana	No	Yes	No	Yes	LBVM (2022)
Maine	Yes	No	No	Yes	MSBVM (2022)
Maryland	No	Yes	No	Yes	MBVME (2019)
Massachusetts	Yes	Yes	No	Yes	MBRVM (2022)
Michigan	Yes	NS	No	Yes	MBVM (2023)
Minnesota	No	NS	No	Yes	MNBVM (2022)
Mississippi	Yes	NS	Yes	Yes	MSBVM (2008)
Missouri	Yes	NS	No	Yes	MOVMB (2022)
Montana	Yes	NS	Yes	Yes	MCA (2021)
Nebraska	No	Yes	No	Yes	NLU (2019)
Nevada	Yes	No	No	Yes	NBVME (2023)
New Hampshire	Yes	No	No	Yes	NHBVM (2020, 2022)
New Jersey	Yes	Yes	No	Yes	NJSBVME (2021)
New Mexico	No	Yes	No	≤7 hours/year	NMBVM (2018), CaseText (2023)
New York	No	Yes	No	Yes	NYSLPV (2023)
North Carolina	No	No	No	Yes	NCVMB (2014)
North Dakota	Yes	NS	No	Yes	NDVBME (2007)

State	PVM	LA	LAE	ACE	References
Ohio	Yes	NS	No	Yes	ORC (2006)
Oklahoma	Yes	Yes	No	Yes	OVB (2022)
Oregon	No	Yes	No	Yes	OL (2021)
Pennsylvania	No	Yes	No	Yes	CP (2022)
Rhode Island	No	NS	No	Yes	RIDH (2006)
South Carolina	Yes	Yes	No	Yes	SCCL (2016)
South Dakota	No	NS	No	Yes	SDL (2023)
Tennessee	Yes	No	No	Yes	TBVME (2014)
Texas	Yes	Yes	No	Yes	TAC (2012)
Utah	No	Yes	No	Yes	UC (2020)
Vermont	No	NS	No	Yes	VGA (2023)
Virginia	Yes	No	No	Yes	DHP (2007)
Washington	No	NS	No	Yes	WSL (2023)
West Virginia	No	NS	No	Yes	WVBVM (2023)
Wisconsin	No	Yes	No	Yes	WVEB (2022)
Wyoming	No	NS	No	Yes	WBVM (2018)

PVM (Practice of Veterinary Medicine): the state board considers VA to be the PVM. 2023
LA (Licensed Acupuncturist): an LA may perform VA under the direct supervision of a veterinarian with an active veterinary–client–patient relationship.
LAE (Licensed Acupuncturist Exemption): an LA is not required to practice under direct veterinary supervision.
ACE (Applicable CE): VA CE is applicable to the state's mandated CE hours assuming approval by the American Association of Veterinary State Boards (AAVSB) Registry of Approved Continuing Education (RACE).
NS, information not specified.
Source: Lisa P. McFaddin.

modality is right for you and your practice. State and national veterinary conferences, as well as many online veterinary educational platforms, for example Veterinary Information Network (VIN), Vetfolio, DVM360 Flex, Vet Girl on the Run, and College of Integrative Veterinary Therapies (CIVT), frequently offer American Association of Veterinary State Boards (AAVSB) Registry of Approved Continuing Education (RACE)-approved lectures on various integrative topics.

Canine Rehabilitation Institute

- **Course name**: Certified Veterinary Acupuncture Therapist Program
- **Prerequisites**: License, in good standing, to practice veterinary medicine or third or fourth year veterinary student.
- **Description**

- 120-hour AAVSB RACE-approved certification course in small animal veterinary acupuncture, both dry needle and electroacupuncture.
- The course is accredited by the Association of Veterinary Anesthetists.
- The course is recognized by the American Academy of Veterinary Acupuncture (AAVA), an affiliate of the IVAS.
- The course focuses on the neurophysiology of acupuncture (medical acupuncture). TCVM is not discussed.
- Course comprises three modules: two required and one elective.
- Certification requirements:
  o Pass all written and practical examinations (score ≥70% required)
  o No internship required
  o No case studies required.

- **Online training**: Three 16-hour online modules (available for 60 days before the on-site portion).
- **On-site training**: Three (three-day) on-site modules in Wheat Ridge, CO. Limited on-site class size of 20 students with five faculty members.
- **Completion time**: Approximately six months.
- **Cost**: $7875.
  - Includes digital copy of the notes.
  - Program is recognized by the AAVA.

- **Contact information**
  - Address: 2137 S. Eastgate Avenue, Springfield, MO 65809
  - Website: www.caninerehabinstitute.com
  - Email: info@caninerehabinstitute.com

Chi University

- **Course name**: Veterinary Small Animal Acupuncture Certification Track
- **Prerequisites**: License, in good standing, to practice veterinary medicine or third or fourth year veterinary student.
- **Description**
  - 142-hour certification course in small animal veterinary acupuncture.
  - 138 hours are AAVSB RACE-approved.
  - The course focuses on:
    - The fundamentals of TCVM as a means of diagnosing and treating patients.
    - Emphasis is placed on the Western understanding of acupuncture's mechanisms of action.
    - Learned acupuncture techniques: dry needle, electroacupuncture, aquapuncture, and moxibustion.
    - The incorporation of acupuncture into daily practice.
  - Students are eligible for the Certified Veterinary Acupuncturist certification endorsed by Chi University and the World Association of Traditional Chinese Veterinary Medicine (WATCVM). Certification requirements include:
    - Successful completion of the program.

  - Pass three online quizzes (score >75% required).
  - Pass the final written on-site exam (score >75% required).
  - Pass the on-site clinical acupoint exam (score >75% required).
  - Submit one case report.
  - Complete 30 hours of advanced TCVM training or internship/observation with a certified veterinary acupuncturist.
  - Chi University is accredited by the Distance Education Accrediting Commission (DEAC).

- **Online training**: Three online sessions
- **On-site training**: Two (four-day) on-site sessions in Reddick, FL. There are live lectures on specific conditions and hands-on small laboratory groups working with live animals. There is now an option to take the program through University of California Davis Veterinary Medicine in which the on-site sessions ae held in Davis, CA.
- **Completion time**: The course takes approximately 6–10 months to complete. Variance in the completion time is due to the time needed for the internship or advanced TCVM training, as well as completion of the case report.
- **Cost**: $7580
  - Canine acupoint chart.
  - 32-hour evidence-based veterinary acupuncture course.
  - One-year membership with the WATCVM.
  - Lifetime case consultation with Chi faculty.
  - Digital class handouts and notes provided.
  - Lunch and snacks provided.
  - Printed binders available for an additional cost.
- **Contact information**
  - Address: 9650 W Hwy 318, Reddick, FL 32686, USA
  - Phone: (800) 860-1543
  - Website: www.chiu.edu
  - Email: register@chiu.edu

College of Integrative Veterinary Therapies

- **Course name**: Certification in Veterinary Acupuncture
- **Prerequisites**: License, in good standing, to practice veterinary medicine or third or fourth year veterinary student.
- **Description**
  - 93-hour RACE interactive distance online only, small animal acupuncture certification course. Quizzes are provided for RACE hours.
  - The course focuses on:
    - The fundamentals of TCVM as a means of diagnosing and treating patients.
    - Emphasis is also placed on the Western understanding of acupuncture's mechanisms of action.
    - Learned acupuncture techniques include dry needle, electroacupuncture, aquapuncture, and moxibustion.
    - The incorporation of acupuncture into daily practice.
  - Requirements for certification include:
    - Completion of all modules.
    - Completion of all module assessments.
    - Case log book with at least 10 cases.
  - Successful completion of the certification is a prerequisite for obtaining a Graduate Diploma of Veterinary Acupuncture, which is nationally accredited under the Australian Qualifications Framework at the postgraduate level.
  - **Online training**: Four online modules taking approximately three months each to complete.
  - **On-site training**: Not applicable.
  - **Completion time:** 12 months.
- **Cost**: $7020
  - Digital copy of the notes.
  - Case support from tutors.
  - Live case forums.
  - One-on-one practical sessions.
  - Virtual assessments using Skype.

- **Contact information:**
  - Address: PO Box 352, Yeppoon, 4703 QLD, Australia
  - Phone: (304) 930-5684
  - Website: www.civtedu.org
  - Email: admin1@civtedu.org

CuraCore

- **Course name**: Medical Acupuncture for Veterinarians (MAV)
- **Prerequisites**: License, in good standing, to practice veterinary medicine or third or fourth year veterinary student.
- **Description**
  - Up to 166 hours of AAVSB RACE-approved small animal acupuncture certification course.
  - The course focuses on medical acupuncture, both dry needle and electroacupuncture, with an emphasis on myofascial palpation. TCVM is not discussed.
  - Requirements for certification include:
    - Completion of all modules.
    - Completion of online interactive sessions.
    - Passing all assessments (score of ≥70% required).
    - Completion of interactive testing.
    - Submission of a case report.
  - Graduates are eligible for the MAV master class, a monthly program of 12 90-minute sessions available online.

- **Online training**: One (five-day) on-site session if the hybrid option is chosen. Hands-on portion takes place at the CuraCore Academy in Fort Collins, CO.
- **On-site training**: 10 online modules. There is an online-only option.
- **Completion time:** One year.
- **Cost**: $9750
  - Interactive group and individual sessions.
  - Technical skills tutorial.
  - Access to MAV private Facebook group.
  - Graduate listing on website.
  - CuraCore MAV acupuncture kit.

- **Contact information**:
  - Address: 4007 Automation Way, Fort Collins, CO 80525, USA
  - Phone: (970) 818-0851
  - Website: www.curacore.org
  - Email: info@curacore.org

International Veterinary Acupuncture Society

- **Course name**: US Certification Course in Veterinary Acupuncture
- **Prerequisites**: License, in good standing, to practice veterinary medicine or third or fourth year veterinary student.
- **Description**
  - 160-hour veterinary acupuncture certification course with the option to focus on small animal, equine, or both.
  - The course focuses on:
    - The fundamentals of TCVM as a means of diagnosing and treating patients.
    - Emphasis is also placed on the Western understanding of acupuncture's mechanisms of action.
    - Learned acupuncture techniques include dry needle, electroacupuncture, aquapuncture, and moxibustion.
    - The incorporation of acupuncture into daily practice.
  - Requirements for certification include:
    - Attendance and completion of all sessions.
    - 16 hour mentored internship.
    - Pass all written and practical examinations (score of $\geq 70\%$ required).
    - Case log book with at least 10 cases.
    - Submission of a peer-reviewed case report.

- **Online training**: One online session
- **On-site training**: Four (four to five day) on-site sessions whose location changes annually.
- **Completion time**: The course takes approximately six to nine months to complete. Completion time variance is due to the time needed to complete the care report.

- **Cost**: $6995
  - Digital class notes provided.
  - An additional 16 hours of mentored internship provided.
- **Contact information**
  - Address: PO Box 1283, Portland, TX 78374
  - Phone: (970) 266-0666
  - Website: www.ivas.org
  - Email: office@ivas.org

Supplies and Equipment

Recommended starting veterinary acupuncture supplies and suppliers are provided in Tables 1.15 and 1.16. Hospital remodeling and/or redecorating is generally not required when offering veterinary acupuncture. Most traditional exam rooms can be utilized for acupuncture sessions. Some practitioners prefer to have a dedicated acupuncture room while others use existing spaces. Having comfy places for the patient to lie down is highly recommended. This can be accomplished with yoga mats or puzzle floor mats and towels or blankets. Creating a relaxing environment with soft music and diffusors (lavender or pheromones) is also beneficial.

Veterinary Organizations

A description of the most common veterinary organizations with a special interest in acupuncture are provided below. Table 1.17 summarizes the organizations' names, contact information, and membership dues as of February 2023.

American Academy of Veterinary Acupuncture

- **Description**: The AAVA was founded in 1998 and is affiliated with IVAS. The goals of the AAVA are to promote the education, understanding, and professional development of veterinarians practicing veterinary acupuncture, TCVM, and other Eastern medicine practices. There is no annual CE requirement to maintain membership.

Table 1.15 Common veterinary acupuncture starting supplies with approximate costs as of February 2023.

Supplies	Price	Suggested starting quantity
Acupuncture needles	$12 per 100 needles	32g (0.5 and 1 inch) for large dogs = 1 box each 34g (0.5 and 1 inch) for medium dogs = 1 box each 36g (0.5 inch) for small dogs and cats = 1–2 boxes 38g (0.5 inch) for small dogs and cats = 1 box Korean hand needles for small dogs and cats = 1 box
Electroacupuncture unit	$400	One electroacupuncture unit with multiple leads ±carrying case
Moxa	$15	Regular sticks = 1 box Smokeless sticks = ±1 box Mini-sticks = ±1 box
Aquapuncture	$31	Vitamin B12 (100-ml multidose bottle) = 1 bottle 1-ml syringes = 1 box 3-ml syringes = ±1 box 27g needles = 1 box 25g needles = ±1 box

Source: Lisa P. McFaddin.

Table 1.16 The most used veterinary acupuncture suppliers.

Jing Tang Herbal	A Time to Heal	Lhasa Oms
9700 West Hwy 318, Reddick FL 32686	140 Webster Road, Shelburne, VT 05482	230 Libbey Parkway, Weymouth, MA 02189
(352) 591-2141 (800) 891-1986	(802) 497-2375	(800) 722-8775
https://store.tcvmherbal.com	https://atimetohealherbs.com	https://www.lhasaoms.com

Source: Lisa P. McFaddin.

- **Membership benefits**
  - Free subscription to the *American Journal of Traditional Chinese Veterinary Medicine*, a peer-reviewed journal.
  - Searchable member directory.
  - Help advance integrative medicine through the AAVA's seat on the AVMA House of Delegates.
  - Access to the career center with open positions and potential candidates.
  - Option to advance the veterinarian's acupuncture development through completion of the Fellows of American Academy of Veterinary Acupuncturists (FAAVA) certification process.
  - The AAVA hosts an annual CE.

American Holistic Veterinary Medical Association

- **Description**: The American Holistic Veterinary Medical Association (AHVMA) was founded in 1982 at the Western States Veterinary Conference with the goal of advancing integrative medicine through the education of integrative and non-integrative veterinarians, the introduction of integrative medicine to

Table 1.17 Veterinary associations and organizations with a special interest in acupuncture as of February 2023.

Organization	Contact information	Membership dues
American Academy of Veterinary Acupuncture (AAVA)	PO Box 803, Fayetteville, TN 37334 (931) 438-0238 office@aava.org	$150/year
American Holistic Veterinary Medical Association (AHVMA)	PO Box 630, Abingdon, MD 21009 (410) 569-0795 office@ahvma.org	$300/year
College of Integrative Veterinary Therapies (CIVT)	PO Box 352, Yeppoon, 4703 QLD, Australia (303) 800-5460 membership@civtedu.org	$185/year
International Veterinary Academy of Pain Management (IVAPM)	PO Box 1868, Mt Juliet, TN 371211 info@ivapm.org	$150/year
International Veterinary Acupuncture Society (IVAS)	PO Box 1283, Portland, TX 78374 (970) 266-0666 office@ivas.org	$110/year
World Association of Traditional Chinese Veterinary Medicine (WATCVM)	WATCVM and AATCVM PO Box 141324, Gainesville, FL 32614 (844) 422-8286 support@aatcvm.org	$85/year

Source: Lisa P. McFaddin.

veterinary students, the promotion of research, and representation in the AVMA House of Delegates. There is no annual CE requirement to maintain membership.

- **Membership benefits**
  - Free subscription to the *AHVMA Journal*, a peer-reviewed journal.
  - Online resources for client education.
  - Searchable member directory.
  - Discounted vaccination titers through Kansas State University (KSU) Diagnostic Lab.
  - Free access to the Natural Medicines Database, an online resource for supplements, natural medicines, and integrative therapies.
  - Reduced cost for the AHVMA annual conference.

College of Integrative Veterinary Therapies
- **Description**: An online organization open to all licensed animal health providers

interested in integrative medicine. There are two membership options: full membership for veterinarians and associate membership for registered animal health professionals. CIVT strives to promote all aspects of evidence-based integrative medicine through online education and discussion forums. CIVT provides financial support to veterinary students interested in studying integrative medicine. CIVT also helps fund integrative medicine research. There is no annual CE requirement to maintain membership.

- **Membership benefits**
  - Access to the online electronic library.
  - Access to the electronic *Journal of Integrative Veterinary Therapies*.
  - Three free CE webinars annually.
  - 20% discount on all webinars.
  - Discounts on specific CIVT courses.
  - Searchable member directory.

– Access to the Natural Medicines Databases and the American Botanical Council Library.

International Veterinary Academy of Pain Management

- **Description**: Originally known as the Companion Animal Pain Management Consortium, then the Academy of Pain Management Interest Group, and finally the International Veterinary Academy of Pain Management (IVAPM). Founded in 2001 to provide pain management education and certification programs. The organization's goal is to provide acute and chronic pain relief for veterinary patients. Both traditional and alternative therapies are embraced, including acupuncture and rehabilitation and physical therapy.
- **Membership benefits**
  - Members can become Certified Veterinary Pain Practitioners (CVPP).
  - Access to member's only Facebook group offering case consultations and questions.
  - Reduced subscription rate for IVAPM's journal *Veterinary Anaesthesia and Analgesia*.
  - Reduced registration fee for the International Veterinary Emergency and Critical Care conference.
  - Reduced registration for all IVAPM CE events (online and on-site).
  - Complimentary World Small Animal Veterinary Association membership.

International Veterinary Acupuncture Society

- **Description**: IVAS was founded in 1974 to promote and educate veterinarians and non-veterinarians on the subject of veterinary acupuncture. IVAS held the first veterinary acupuncture course in 1974 in Cincinnati, Ohio. Current membership numbers are over 1800 veterinarians. IVAS helps promote, educate, and set the global standards for veterinary acupuncture. Certified Veterinary Acupuncturists (CVA)

are required to have 10 hours of acupuncture CE every two years.
- **Membership benefits**
  - Searchable member directory.
  - Access to IVAS member-only publications: *The Point* published quarterly and *The Flashpoint* published monthly.
  - Discounted IVAS events and seminars.
  - Online access to IVAS Congress Proceedings.
  - Free digital subscription to the *American Journal of Traditional Chinese Veterinary Medicine*, a peer-reviewed journal.
  - Access to the in-print and online IVAS classifieds.
  - Access to online forums with other IVAS members.
  - Access to veterinary acupuncture templates for in-hospital promotion.
  - Access to veterinary acupuncture educational materials.
  - IVAS has multiple CE events annually.

World Association of Traditional Chinese Veterinary Medicine

- **Description**: The WATCVM promotes the education, research, and practice of TCVM throughout the world. The WATCVM provides financial support to veterinary students interested in studying TCVM as well as establishing student organizations within veterinary schools. The WATCVM funds TCVM research programs. There is no annual CE requirement to maintain membership.
- **Membership benefits**
  - Access to online case discussion forums.
  - Free subscription to the *American Journal of Traditional Chinese Veterinary Medicine*, a peer-reviewed journal.
  - Access to the quarterly online TCVM newsletter.
  - Access to the online TCVM library.
  - Discounted TCVM conferences.
  - Access to the online classified ads.
  - Assistance with scientific writing as well as research design of grant proposals.

– Dual membership in WATCVM and American Association of TCVM (AATCVM).
– The WATCVM and AATCVM offer an annual International Conference on TCVM.

Reference Books

The following is a list of my recommended TCVM and veterinary acupuncture books as of February 2023. A summary of each book is provided.

Acu-Cat: A Guide to Feline Acupressure
- Authors: Nancy Zidonis and Amy Snow
- Summary: An introduction to TCVM theory, the location of feline acupuncture points (acupoints), practical tips for performing acupressure, and suggested acupressure acupoints by disease condition. This book can be utilized by veterinarians, non-veterinarians working in the animal health field, and owners.

Acu-Dog: A Guide to Canine Acupressure
- Authors: Amy Snow and Nancy Zidonis
- Summary: A introduction to TCVM theory, the location of canine acupoints, practical tips for performing acupressure, and suggested acupressure acupoints by disease condition. This book can be utilized by veterinarians, non-veterinarians working in the animal health field, and owners.

Acupuncture for Dogs and Cats: A Pocket Atlas
- Author: Christina Matern, DVM
- Summary: A quick reference pocket guide introducing the basic concepts of TCVM and veterinary acupuncture. A brief outline of the location, indication, systemic effect, and technique for each canine acupoint is discussed.

Application of Traditional Chinese Veterinary Medicine in Exotic Animals
- Authors: Zhiqiang Yang and Huisheng Xie, DVM, MS, PhD
- Summary: Proceedings from the 13th Annual International TCVM Conference discussing the introduction and implementation of TCVM therapies for exotic animals.

Clinical Application of Different TCM Schools and Thoughts in Veterinary Practice
- Authors: Huisheng Xie, DVM, MS, PhD and Aituan Ma, DVM, PhD, MS
- Summary: Proceedings from the 18th Annual International TCVM Conference discussing the different TCVM schools and theories and TCVM therapy for infectious and inflammatory diseases, behavioral disorders, and other conditions.

Clinician's Guide to Canine Acupuncture
- Authors: Curtis Wells Dewey, DVM, MS, DACVIM (Neurology), DACVS and Huisheng Xie, DVM, MS, PhD
- Summary: An in-depth discussion of canine acupuncture focusing on the anatomic location of acupoints. A summary of the Western and Eastern indications for each acupoint is provided.

Essentials of Western Veterinary Acupuncture
- Authors: Samantha Lindley, BVSc, MRCVS and Mike Cummings, DVM
- Summary: A discussion of the history, mechanisms of action, safety, and practical uses of veterinary acupuncture from a Western medicine perspective.

Four Paws Five Directions: A Guide to Chinese Medicine for Cats and Dogs
- Author: Cheryl Schwartz, DVM
- Summary: An introduction to TCVM in veterinary medicine focusing on TCVM theory and acupuncture. Additional therapies are briefly covered: food therapy, herbal supplements, nutritional supplements, environmental modifications. The disease processes are organized by body system and the Five Element Theory.

Integrating Complementary Medicine into Veterinary Practice
- Authors: Robert S. Goldstein, VMD, Paula Jo Broadfoot, DVM, Richard E. Plamquist, DVM, Karen Johnstons, DVM, Jiu Jia Wen,

DVM, Barbara Fougère, BSc, BVMS (Hons), BHSc (comp Med), MODT, MHSc (Herb Med), CVA (IVAs), CVBM, CVCP, and Margo Roman, DVM
- Summary: A comprehensive review of multiple integrative therapies including Chinese herbal medicine, acupuncture, homotoxicology, nano-pharmacology, and therapeutic nutrition. The book aims to educate veterinary practitioners on the validity, effectiveness, and incorporation of each modality within daily practice.

Interactive Medical Acupuncture Anatomy
- Author: Narda G. Robinson, DO, DVM, MS, FAAMA
- Summary: A combination book and CD set providing detailed anatomic locations for human acupoints.

Manual of Natural Veterinary Medicine: Science and Tradition
- Authors: Susan G. Wynn, DVM and Steve Marsden, DVM, ND, MSOM, Lac, Dipl. CH., RH(AHG)
- Summary: A quick reference book discussing the integrative therapy options for numerous diseases in veterinary medicine. The book is organized by Western conditions. For each category the potential TCVM diagnoses and treatment options are reviewed in succinct detail. A must have for all integrative veterinarians.

Practical Guide to Traditional Chinese Veterinary Medicine: Emergencies and Five Element Syndromes
- Authors: Huisheng Xie, DVM, MS, PhD, Lindsey Wedemeyer, MA, VetMB, MRCVS, and Cheryl L Chrisman, DVM, MS, EdS, DACVIM (Neurology)
- Summary: The first of a four-volume series discussing the practical use of TCVM in veterinary medicine. The book breaks down the TCVM pattern diagnosis and treatment options (acupuncture, Chinese herbal formulas, Tui-na, food therapy, and environmental changes) for common small animal emergencies. The book is organized using the Five Element Theory of disease as it relates to emergent disorders.

Practical Guide to Traditional Chinese Veterinary Medicine: Exotic, Zoo, and Farm Animals
- Authors: Huisheng Xie, DVM, MS, PhD and Harvey E Ramirez
- Summary: The final book of a four-volume series discussing the practical use of TCVM in veterinary medicine. The book breaks down the TCVM pattern diagnosis and treatment options (acupuncture, Chinese herbal formulas, Tui-na, food therapy, and environmental changes) for exotic, zoo, and farm animals.

Practical Guide to Traditional Chinese Veterinary Medicine: Small Animal Practice
- Authors: Huisheng Xie, DVM, MS, PhD, Lindsey Wedemeyer, MA, VetMB, MRCVS, Cheryl L Chrisman, DVM, MS, EdS, DACVIM (Neurology), and Lisa Trevisanellow, DrMEDVET
- Summary: The second of a four-volume series discussing the practical use of TCVM in veterinary medicine. The book breaks down the TCVM pattern diagnosis and treatment options (acupuncture, Chinese herbal formulas, Tui-na, food therapy, and environmental changes) for common small animal diseases. The book is organized by Western medical diagnoses and then further divided into the possible TCVM diagnoses for each disease process.

Spark in the Machine: How the Science of Acupuncture Explains the Mysteries of Western Medicine
- Author: Daniel Keown
- Summary: A discussion of how Western medicine can be used to validate Chinese medicine theories.

Traditional Chinese Veterinary Medicine Approach to Gastrointestinal and Hepatobiliary Diseases
- Authors: Liting Cao, DVM, PhD and Huisheng Xie, DVM, PhD

- Summary: Proceedings from the 22nd Annual International TCVM Conference discussing the use of TCVM for the treatment of gastrointestinal and hepatobiliary diseases.

Traditional Chinese Veterinary Medicine Approach to Veterinary Dermatological and Immune-Mediated Diseases
- Authors: Aituan Ma, DVM, PhD, MS, Cui Liu, DVM, PhD, Chang Yu, DVM, MS, and Huisheng Xie, DVM, MS, PhD
- Summary: Proceedings from the 21st Annual International TCVM Conference discussing the use of TCVM for the treatment of dermatologic and immune-mediated diseases.

Traditional Chinese Veterinary Medicine Empirical Technique to Scientific Validation
- Authors: Zhiqiang Yang and Huisheng Xie, DVM, MS, PhD
- Summary: Proceedings from the 1st Annual International TCVM Conference discussing the scientific study of TCVM including basic scientific research, small animal specific studies, exotic animal specific studies, large animal specific studies, and pediatric and geriatric medicine.

Traditional Chinese Veterinary Medicine for the Diagnosis and Treatment of Kidney and Water Element Disorders
- Authors: Aituan Ma, DVM, PhD, MS and Huisheng Xie, DVM, MS, PhD
- Summary: Proceedings from the 23rd Annual International TCVM Conference discussing the use of TCVM for the treatment of kidney and water element disorders.

Traditional Chinese Veterinary Medicine for Geriatric Medicine and Palliative Care
- Authors: Huisheng Xie, DVM, MS, PhD and Aituan Ma, DVM, PhD, MS
- Summary: Proceedings from the 19th Annual International TCVM Conference discussing the use of TCVM for geriatric medicine and palliative care.

Traditional Chinese Veterinary Medicine for Neurologic Diseases
- Authors: Huisheng Xie, DVM, MS, PhD, Cheryl L Chrisman, DVM, MS, EdS, DACVIM (Neurology), and Lisa Trevisanellow, DrMEDVET
- Summary: Proceedings from the 13th Annual International TCVM Conference discussing the use of TCVM for a variety of neurologic conditions.

Traditional Chinese Veterinary Medicine from Dragon Legend to Modern Practice
- Authors: Xiuhuii Zhong, Aituan Ma, DVM, PhD, MS, Lisa Trevisanellow, DrMEDVET, and Qingbo Wang
- Summary: Proceedings of the 14th Annual International TCVM Conference discussing the use of TCVM for the treatment of liver, gastrointestinal, equine specific, and exotic animal specific diseases. A variety of other topics are also covered including the longitudinal muscle system, platelet-rich plasma in aquapuncture, and the adverse effects of Chinese herbal medicine and acupuncture.

Traditional Chinese Veterinary Medicine: Fundamental Principles
- Authors: Huisheng Xie, DVM, MS, PhD and Vanessa Preast, DVM, CVA
- Summary: The quintessential introduction to TCVM theory with self-study quizzes, case examples, and practical application of TCVM therapies for small animal and equine patients.

Traditional Chinese Veterinary Medicine for Pain, Lameness, Neurological and Endocrine Disorders
- Authors: Huisheng Xie, DVM, MS, PhD and Aituan Ma, DVM, PhD, MS
- Summary: Proceedings from the 20th Annual International TCVM Conference discussing the use of TCVM for the treatment of pain, lameness, neurologic disorders, endocrine disorders, infertility, and other conditions.

Veterinary Acupuncture
- Author: Allen M. Schoen, DVM, MS
- Summary: A detailed discussion of the history, anatomy, neurophysiologic mechanisms of action, scientific research, techniques, and practical application of veterinary acupuncture for small and large animals.

Promotion

Information regarding the hospital's promotion of acupuncture can be found in the Team Members section.

Integration

Key components for proper integration include availability, scheduling, and staff buy-in. Availability means offering the service to the right patient. Scheduling refers to appropriate patient and support staff scheduling. Staff buy-in ensures all team members understand the benefits of the offered service.

Conclusion

Veterinary acupuncture is a well-studied and broadly accepted therapeutic modality.

References

Acupuncture offers a multitude of beneficial effects for veterinary patients. This chapter and online resources describe in detail how veterinary acupuncture can be successfully introduced into daily practice, as well as provide practical tools for implementation.

Acknowledgments

I would like to thank Dr. Nell Ostermeier for the reviewing this chapter for content. Nell Ostermeier, DVM, CVA, FAAVA is a certified veterinary acupuncturist and fellow of the American Academy of Veterinary Acupuncture. Dr. Ostermeier wears many hats. She is an integrative veterinarian practicing at Lombard Animal Hospital in Portland, Oregon; an educator for the IVAS; a well-known lecturer within the United States and internationally; and founder of People + Pet Integrative Therapies providing consultation and education to veterinarians and owners on different aspects of integrative medicine.

AAHA (American Animal Hospital Association) (2020). *Compensation and Benefits*, 9e. Denver, CO: AAHA Press.

ADAVMEB (Arkansas Veterinary Medical Examining Board) (2008). 092.00.1-1 Rules and Regulations. https://arvetboard. statesolutions.us/wp-content/uploads/2019/ 01/Practice-Act-Rules-and-Regulations-2019. pdf (accessed 19 February 2023).

ADAVMEB (Arkansas Veterinary Medical Examining Board) (2019). Arkansas Veterinary Medical Practice Act. https:// arvetboard.statesolutions.us/wp-content/ uploads/2020/07/Practice-Act-2019.pdf (accessed 19 February 2023).

ADCBPL (Alaska Division of Corporations, Business and Professional Licensing) (2023). Veterinary Statutes and Regulations. https:// www.commerce.alaska.gov/web/portals/5/ pub/VeterinaryStatutes.pdf (accessed 19 February 2023).

APPA (American Pet Products Association) (2022). Pet industry market size and ownership statistics. https://www. americanpetproducts.org/research-insights/ industry-trends-and-stats (accessed 23 February 2023).

ASBVME (Alabama State Board of Veterinary Medical Examiners) (2021). Alabama Veterinary Practice Act. https://asbvme.

alabama.gov/wp-content/uploads/2021/07/
Alabama_Practice_Act_and_Administrative_
Code_Updated_Working_Copy_2018_3_5_
2019.pdf (accessed 19 February 2023).

ASVMEB (Arizona State Veterinary Medical
Examining Board) (2022). AZ Revised Statues
(Veterinary Practice Act). https://vetboard.
az.gov/sites/default/files/AZ%20Revised%20
Statutes%20Amended%20September%20
2022%20as%20of%209.24.22s.pdf (accessed
19 February 2023).

AVMA (American Veterinary Medical
Association) (2018). 2017–2018 Edition AVMA
Pet Ownership and Demographics
Sourcebook. https://www.avma.org/sites/
default/files/resources/AVMA-Pet-
Demographics-Executive-Summary.pdf
(accessed 8 September 2021).

AVMA (American Veterinary Medical
Association) (2019). Economic state of the
veterinary profession. https://www.avma.org/
news/press-release/AVMA-2019-Economic-
State-of-the-Veterinary-Profession-Report-
now-available (accessed 26 July 2021).

AVMA (American Veterinary Medical
Association) (2023). *2023 AVMA Report on the
Economic State of the Veterinary Profession*.
Schaumburg, IL: AVMA.

Ben-Yakir, S. (2009). Gold beads implantation:
the scientific basis. https://www.med-
vetacupuncture.org/english/articles/goldbead.
html (accessed 9 December 2023).

BLS (Bureau of Labor Statistics) (2022a).
Occupational outlook handbook:
veterinarians 2022 median pay. https://www.
bls.gov/ooh/healthcare/veterinarians.htm
(accessed 18 February 2023).

BLS (Bureau of Labor Statistics) (2022b).
Occupational outlook handbooks: veterinary
technologists and technicians median pay
2020. https://www.bls.gov/ooh/healthcare/
veterinary-technologists-and-technicians.htm
(accessed 18 February 2023).

BLS (Bureau of Labor Statistics) (2023). News
Release: Consumer Price Index January 2023.
https://www.bls.gov/news.release/pdf/cpi.pdf
(accessed 18 February 2023).

Burns, K. (2018). Pet ownership stable,
veterinary care variable. https://www.avma.
org/javma-news/2019-01-15/pet-ownership-
stable-veterinary-care-variable (accessed
11 August 2021).

Burns, K. (2022). New report takes a deep dive
into pet ownership. https://www.avma.org/
news/new-report-takes-a-deep-dive-pet-
ownership (accessed 6 November 2022).

CaseText (2023). N.M. Code R. 16.25.4.8, Register
Volume 34, No. 3. https://casetext.com/
regulation/new-mexico-administrative-
code/title-16-occupational-and-professional-
licensing/chapter-25-veterinary-medicine-
practitioners/part-4-continued-education-
requirements-veterinarians/section-162548-
general-requirements#:~:text= (accessed
19 February 2023).

Cassu, R., Luna, S., Clark, R., and Kronka,
S. (2008). Electroacupuncture analgesia in
dogs: is there a difference between uni- and
bi-lateral stimulation? *Veterinary Anaesthesia
and Analgesia* 35 (1): 52–61.

CBVM (Connecticut Board of Veterinary
Medicine) (2023). Chapter 384: Veterinary
Medicine. https://www.cga.ct.gov/
current/pub/chap_384.htm (accessed
19 February 2023).

CDCAVMB (California Veterinary Medical
Board) (2022). California Veterinary Medicine
Practice Act. www.vmb.ca.gov/laws_regs/
vmb_act.pdf (accessed 19 February 2023).

CDRASBVM (Colorado State Board of
Veterinary Medicine) (2019). Title 12: Division
of Professions and Occupations, Articles 315:
Veterinarians and Veterinary Technicians.
https://drive.google.com/file/d/0B-
K5DhxXxJZbTFdrR3FPZ0g0czg/
view?resourcekey=0-Ub47Cye48cDfikST
taciMg (accessed 19 February 2023).

Chan, W.-W., Chen, K.Y., Liu, H. et al. (2001).
Acupuncture for general veterinary practice.
Journal of Veterinary Medical Science 61 (10):
1057–1062.

Chen, C.-Y., Lin, C.-N., Chern, R.-S. et al. (2014).
Neuronal activity stimulated by liquid
substrates injection at Zusanli (ST36)

aqupoint: the possible mechanism of aquapuncture. *Evidence Based Complementary and Alternative Medicine* 2014: 627342.

Chen, B., Zhang, C., Zhang, R.-P. et al. (2019). Acupotomy versus acupuncture for cervical spondylotic radiculopathy: protocol of a systematic review and meta-analysis. *British Medical Journal Open* 9 (8): e029052.

Chiang, C., Chang, C., Chu, H., and Yang, L. (1973). Peripheral afferent pathway for acupuncture analgesia. *Scientia Sinica* B (16): 210–217.

Chien, C.H. (2011). Canine intervertebral disk disease treated with aquapuncture and Chinese herbal and western medicine. In: *Traditional Chinese Veterinary Medicine for Neurological Disease* (ed. H. Xie, C. Chrisman, and L. Trevisanello), 311. Reddick, FL: Jing Tang Publishing.

Chiu, J.-H., Cheng, H.C., Tai, C.H. et al. (2001). Electroacupuncture-induced neural activation detected by use of manganese-enhanced functional magnetic resonance imaging in rabbits. *American Journal of Veterinary Research* 62 (2): 178–184.

Cho, S.-J. and Kim, O. (2008). Acupuncture treatment for idiopathic Horner's syndrome in a dog. *Journal of Veterinary Science* 9 (1): 117–119.

Chomsiriwat, P. and Ma, A. (2019). Comparison of the effects of electro-acupuncture and laser acupuncture on pain relief and joint range of motion in dogs with coxofemoral degenerative joint disease. *American Journal of Traditional Chinese Veterinary Medicine* 14 (1): 11–20.

Chon, T., Mallory, M.J., Yang, J. et al. (2019). Laser acupuncture: a concise review. *Medical Acupuncture* 31 (3): 164–168.

Chrisman, C.L. (2011). Spinal cord disorders. In: *Traditional Chinese Veterinary Medicine for Neurological Diseases* (ed. H. Xie, C. Chrisman, and L. Trevisanello), 225–330. Reddick, FL: Jing Tang Publishing.

Clemmons, R.M. (2007). Functional neuroanatomical physiology of acupuncture. In: *Xie's Veterinary Acupuncture* (ed. H. Xie

and V. Preast), 341–347. Ames, IA: Blackwell Publishing.

Collins, P.J. (2021). A randomized, blinded and controlled study using digital thermal imaging to measure temperature change associated with acupuncture in dogs with back pain. *American Journal of Traditional Chinese Veterinary Medicine* 16 (2): 1–10.

CP (Commonwealth of Pennsylvania) (2022). Chapter 31: State Board of Veterinary Medicine. http://www.pacodeandbulletin.gov/Display/pacode?file=/secure/pacode/data/049/chapter31/chap31toc.html&d=reduce (accessed 19 February 2023).

Damodaran, A. (2021). Consumer airfare index report, May 2021. https://media.hopper.com/research/consumer-airfare-quarterly-index-report (accessed 8 August 2021).

DBVM (Delaware Board of Veterinary Medicine) (2023). Title 24: Progressions and Occupations, Chapter 33. Veterinarians, Subchapter I: General Terms. https://delcode.delaware.gov/title24/c033/sc01/index.html#:~:text=(9)%20%E2%80%9CVeterinary%20medicine%E2%80%9D,%2C%20%C2%A7%203302%3B%2057%20Del. (accessed 19 February 2023).

DCVM (District of Columbia Board of Veterinary Medicine) (2023). District of Columbia Municipal Regulations for Veterinarians. https://doh.dc.gov/sites/default/files/dc/sites/doh/publication/attachments/Veterinarian_DC_Municipal_Regulations_For_Veterinarians.pdf (accessed 19 February 2023).

Deng, H. and Shen, X. (2013). The mechanism of moxibustion: ancient theory and modern research. *Evidence Based Complementary and Alternative Medicine* 2013: 379291.

DHP (Department of Health Professions) 2007. Chapter 38 of Title 54.1 of the Code of Virginia Veterinary Medicine. https://www.dhp.virginia.gov/media/dhpweb/docs/vet/leg/Chapter38_VetMed.pdf (accessed 19 February 2023).

Dragomir, M., Pestean, C.P., Melega, I. et al. (2021). Current aspects regarding the clinical relevance of electroacupuncture in dogs with spinal cord injury: a literature review. *Animals* 11 (1): 219.

Durkes, T. (1992). Gold bead implants. *Problems in Veterinary Medicine* 4 (1): 207–211.

eLaws.us (2020). 61G18-16.002. Continuing Education Requirements for Active Status License Renewal. http://flrules.elaws.us/fac/61g18-16.002 (accessed 19 February 2023).

Epstein, M., Rodan, I., Griffenhagen, G. et al. (2015). 2015 AAHA/AAFP pain management guidelines for dogs and cats. *Journal of the American Animal Hospital Association* 51 (2): 67–84.

Faramarzi, B., Lee, D., May, K., and Dong, F. (2017). Response to acupuncture treatment in horses with chronic laminitis. *Canadian Veterinary Journal* 58 (8): 823–827.

FBVM (Florida Board of Veterinary Medicine) (2022). The 2022 Florida Statues, Chapter 474, Veterinary Medical Practice. http://www.leg.state.fl.us/statutes/index.cfm?App_mode=Display_Statute&URL=0400-0499/0474/0474.html (accessed 19 February 2023).

FederalPay.org (2023). FY 2023 Federal Per Diem Rates October 2022–September 2023. https://www.federalpay.org/perdiem/2023 (accessed 18 February 2023).

Ferguson, B. (2007). Techniques of veterinary acupuncture and moxibustion. In: *Xie's Veterinary Acupuncture* (ed. H. Xie and V. Preast), 329–339. Ames, IA: Blackwell Publishing.

Ferguson, B. (2011). An effective and simple protocol to treat intervertebral disk disease associated with a Qi-deficiency/stagnation pattern. In: *Traditional Chinese Veterinary Medicine for Neurological Diseases* (ed. H. Xie, C. Chrisman, and L. Trevisanello), 333–334. Reddick, FL: Jing Tang Publishing.

Ferro, A.C.Z.B., Cannolas, C., Reginato, J.C., and Luna, S.P.L. (2022). Postoperative acupuncture is as effective as preoperative acupuncture or meloxicam in dogs undergoing ovariohysterectomy: a blind randomized

study. *Journal of Acupuncture and Meridian Studies* 15 (3): 181–188.

Fields, S. (2021). Plannng to rent a car? It's going to cost you. https://www.marketplace.org/2021/05/27/planning-to-rent-a-car-its-going-to-cost-you. (accessed 8 August 2021).

Fong, P. and Xie, H. (2019). Comparison of the sedation effect of dry needle acupuncture of an-shen versus intramuscular butorphanol in 24 companion dogs. *American Journal of Traditional Chinese Veterinary Medicine* 14 (1): 5–10.

French, S. and Kemmis, S. (2023). Rental Car Pricing Statistics:2023. https://www.nerdwallet.com/article/travel/car-rental-pricing-statistics#:~:text=The%20average%20weekly%20rental%20price,in%20advance%2C%20it%20was%20%2420513. (accessed 18 February 2023).

Fuda, K., Bannai, Y., Kozai, N., and Abe, Y. (2008). Management of a dog with atlantoaxial instability and lateral patellar luxations using a combination of electroacupuncture and Chinese herbal therapy. *American Journal of Traditional Chinese Veterinary* 3 (1): 60–62.

Gakiya, H., Silva, D.A., Gomes, J. et al. (2011). Electroacupuncture versus morphine for the postoperative control pain in dogs. *Acta Cirúrgica Brasileira* 26 (5): 346–351.

Garcia, K. and Chiang, J. (2007). Acupuncture. In: *Pain Management* (ed. S. Waldam), 1093–1105. Phildelphia, PA: Elsevier.

Goldman, N., Chen, M., Fujita, T. et al. (2010). Adenosine A1 receptors mediate local anti-nociceptive effects of acupuncture. *Nature Neuroscience* 13 (7): 883–888.

Groppetti, D., Pecile, A.M., Sacerdote, P. et al. (2011). Effectiveness of electroacupuncture analgesia compared with opioid administration in a dog model: a pilot study. *British Journal of Anaesthesia* 107 (4): 612–618.

Gruen, M.E., Lascelles, B.D.X., Colleran, E. et al. (2022). 2022 AAHA pain management guidelines for dogs and cats. *Journal of the American Animal Hospital Association* 58 (2): 55–76.

GSBVM (Georgia State Board of Veterinary Medicine) (2022). Georgia Veterinary Practice Act. https://sos.ga.gov/sites/default/files/2022-02/veterinary_minutes_20180116_vparc_subcommittee.pdf (accessed 19 February 2023).

GSBVM (Georgia State Board of Veterinary Medicine) (2023). Department 700. Rules of Georgia State Board of Veterinary Medicine. https://rules.sos.ga.gov/gac/700 (accessed 19 February 2023).

Gülanber, E.G. (2008). The clinical effectiveness and application of veterinary acupuncture. *American Journal of Traditional Chinese Veterinary Medicine* 3 (1): 9–22.

Gülanber, E.G. (2018). A randomized cross-over clinical study evaluating the effect of acupuncture on blood pressure, blood glucose, and hematologic parameters in healthy dogs. *American Journal of Traditional Chinese Veterinary Medicine* 13 (1): 25–33.

Habacher, G., Pittler, M., and Ernst, E. (2006). Effectiveness of acupuncture in veterinary medicine: systematic review. *Journal of Veterinary Internal Medicine* 20 (3): 480–488.

Han, H.-J., Yoon, H.-Y., Kim, J.-Y. et al. (2010). Clinical effect of additional electroacupuncture on thoracolumbar intervertebral disc herniation in 80 paraplegic dogs. *American Journal of Chinese Medicine* 38 (6): 1015–1025.

Hayashi, A.M., Matera, J.M., Soares da Silva, T. et al. (2007). Electro-acupuncture and Chinese herbs for treatment of cervical intervertebral disk disease in a dog. *Journal of Veterinary Science* 8 (1): 95–98.

HDCCAPVLDBVM (Hawaii Department of Commerce and Consumer Affairs, Professional and Vocational Licensing Division, Board of Veterinary Medicine) (2010). Chapter 471: Veterinary Medicine. https://files.hawaii.gov/dcca/pvl/pvl/hrs/hrs_pvl_471.pdf (accessed 19 February 2023).

Huang, W., Pach, D., Napadow, V. et al. (2012). Characterizing acupuncture stimuli using brain imaging with FMRI: a systematic review and meta-analysis of the literature. *PLoS One* 7 (4): e32960.

Huang, M., Wang, X., Xing, B. et al. (2018). Critical roles of TRPV2 channels, histamine H1 and adenosine A1 receptors in the initiation of acupoint signals for acupuncture analgesia. *Scientific Reports* 8 (1): 6523.

IBVM (Idaho Board of Veterinary Medicine) (2020). Veterinary Practice Act State of Idaho. https://elitepublic.bovm.idaho.gov/IBVMPortal/IBVM/VPA/Idaho%20Veterinary%20Practice%20Act.pdf (accessed 19 February 2023).

IBVM (Iowa Board of Veterinary Medicine) (2017). Chapter 169: Veterinary Practice. https://www.legis.iowa.gov/docs/ico/chapter/169.pdf (accessed 19 February 2023).

IGA (Illinois General Assembly) (2004). Professions, occupations, and business operations: (225 ILCS 115/) Veterinary Medicine and Surgery Practice Act of 2004. https://www.ilga.gov/legislation/ilcs/ilcs3.asp?ActID=1326&ChapterID=24#:~:text=The%20practice%20of%20veterinary%20medicine,control%20in%20the%20public%20interest. (accessed 19 February 2023).

iVet360 (2023). Benefits Matter. : https://ivet360.com/recruiting-tool-kit/wages-benefits/benefits-matter/#:~:text=Most%20companies%20provide%20a%20minimum,and%20holidays%2C%20plus%20sick%20time (accessed 23 February 2023].

IVMB (Indiana Veterinary Medical Board) (2019). Title 25: Professions and Occupations, Article 38.1 Veterinarians. https://iga.in.gov/legislative/laws/2022/ic/titles/025/#25-38.1 (accessed 19 February 2023).

Jaeger, G., Larsen, S., Søli, N., and Moe, L. (2006). Double-blind, placebo-controlled trial of the pain-relieving effects of the implantation of gold beads into dogs with hip dysplasia. *Veterinary Record* 158 (21): 722–726.

Joaquim, J.G.F., Luna, S.P.L., Brondani, J.T. et al. (2010). Comparison of decompressive surgery, electroacupuncture, and decompressive surgery followed by electroacupuncture for the treatment of dogs with intervertebral disk disease with long-standing severe neurologic deficits. *Journal of the American Veterinary Medical Association* 236 (11): 1225–1229.

Karavis, M. (1997). The neurophysiology of acupuncture: a viewpoint. *Acupuncture in Medicine* 15 (1): 33–42.

KBVE (Kansas Board of Veterinary Examiners) (2020). State Board of Veterinary Examiners Statutes. https://kbve.kansas.gov/wp-content/uploads/2021/01/kbve-statutes-amp-regs-new-fees.pdf (accessed 19 February 2023).

Kean, W.F., Tocchio, S., Kean, M., and Rainsford, K. (2013). The musculoskeletal abnormalities of the Similaun Iceman ("Ötzi"): clues to chronic pain and possible treatments. *Inflammopharmacology* 21 (1): 11–20.

Kim, M.-S. and Nam, T.-C. (2006). Electroencephalography (EEG) spectral edge frequency for assessing the sedative effect of acupuncture in dogs. *Journal of Veterinary Medical Science* 68 (4): 409–411.

Kim, M.-S., Seo, K.-M., and Nam, T.-C. (2005). Effect of acupuncture on intraocular pressure in normal dogs. *Journal of Veterinary Medical Science* 67 (12): 1281–1282.

Kober, A., Scheck, T., Schubert, B. et al. (2003). Auricular acupressure as a treatment for anxiety in prehospital transport settings. *Anesthesiology* 98 (6): 1328–1332.

Koh, R., Isaza, N., Xie, H. et al. (2014). Effects of maropitant, acepromazine, and electroacupuncture on vomiting associated with administration of morphine in dogs. *Journal of the American Veterinary Medical Association* 244 (7): 820–829.

Koh, R., Xie, H., and Cuypers, M.-L. (2017). The therapeutic effect of acupuncture and Chinese herbal medicine in 12 dogs with hyperadrenocorticism. *American Journal of Traditional Chinese Veterinary Medicine* 12 (1): 55–68.

KYBVE (Kentucky Board of Veterinary Examiners) (2020). Kentucky Revised Statutes (KRS) Chapter 321. https://www.kybve.com/documents/laws-regulations-booklet.pdf (accessed 19 February 2023).

Laim, A., Jaggy, A., Forterre, F. et al. (2009). Effects of adjunct electroacupuncture on severity of postoperative pain in dogs undergoing hemilaminectomy because of acute thoracolumbar intervertebral disk disease. *Journal of the American Veterinary Medical Association* 234 (9): 1141–1146.

Lana, S., Kogan, L.R., Crump, K.A. et al. (2006). The use of complementary and alternative therapies in dogs and cats iwth cancer. *Journal of the American Animal Hospital Association* 42 (2): 361–365.

Lane, D. and Hill, S. (2016). Effectiveness of combined acupuncture and manual therapy relative to no treatment for canine musculoskeletal pain. *Canadian Veterinary Journal* 57: 407–414.

Langevin, H.M., Bouffard, N.A., Churchill, D.L., and Badger, G.J. (2007). Connective tissue fibroblast response to acupuncture: dose dependent effect of biodirectional needle rotation. *Journal of Alternative and Complementary Medicine* 13 (3): 355–360.

LBVM (Louisiana Board of Veterinary Medicine) (2022). Louisiana Veterinary Practice Act. https://lsbvm.org/wp-content/uploads/LA-Veterinary-Practice-Act-CURRENT.pdf (accessed 19 February 2023).

Lee, L. (2019). Non-surgical treatment for cranial cruciate ligament rupture in senior dogs: a retrospective case series. *American Journal of Traditional Chinese Veterinary Medicine* 14 (1): 49–64.

Lewis, M.J., Granger, N., Jeffery, N.D., and CANSORT-SCI (2020). Emerginc and adjunct therapies for spinal cord injury following acute canine intervertebral disc herniation. *Frontiers in Veterinary Science* 7: 579933.

Lin, J.-H., Shih, C.-H., Kaphle, K. et al. (2010). Acupuncture effects on cardiac functions measured by cardiac magnetic resonance imaging in a feline model. *Evidence Based Complementary and Alternative Medicine* 7 (2): 169–176.

Liu, C.M., Chang, F.C., and Lin, C.T. (2015). Retrospective study of the clinical effects of acupuncture on cervical neurological diseases in dogs. *Journal of Veterinary Science* 17 (3): 337–345.

Liu, C.M., Holyoak, G.R., and Lin, C.T. (2016). Acupuncture combined with Chinese herbs for the treatment in hemivertebral French bulldogs with emergent paraparesis. *Journal of Traditional and Complementary Medicine* 6 (4): 409–412.

Longhurst, J. (2010). Defining meridians: a modern basis of understanding. *Journal of Acupuncture and Meridian Studies* 3 (2): 67–74.

Luna, S.P.L., Di Martino, I., Rodolfo de Sá Lorena, S.E. et al. (2015). Acupuncture and pharmacopuncture are as effective as morphine or carprofen for postoperative analgesia in bitches undergoing ovariohysterectomy. *Acta Cirúrgica Brasileira* 30 (12): 831–837.

Marks, D. and Shmalberg, J. (2015). Profitability and financial benefits of acupuncture in small animal private practice. *American Journal of Traditional Chinese Veterinary Medicine* 10 (1): 43–48.

Marques, V.I., Cassu, R.N., Nascimento, F.F. et al. (2015). Laser acupuncture for postoperative pain management in cats. *Evidence Based Complementary and Alternative Medicine* 2015: 653270.

MBRVM (Massachusetts Board of Registration in Veterinary Medicine) (2022). Massachusetts law about veterinary practice. https://www.mass.gov/info-details/massachusetts-law-about-veterinary-practice (accessed 19 February 2023).

MBVM (Michigan Board of Veterinary Medicine) (2023). Public Health Code Act 368 of 1978, Article 15 Occupations, Part 161 General Provisions. http://www.legislature.mi.gov/(S(j2ynwbgd1j4kqisz4hw3osoq))/documents/mcl/pdf/mcl-368-1978-15.pdf (accessed 19 February 2023).

MBVME (Maryland Board of Veterinary Medical Examiners) (2019). Agriculture Article, Title 2, Subtitltes 3 and 17; Code of Maryland Regulations 15.01.11 and 15.4, Board of Veterinary Medical Examiners. https://mda.maryland.gov/vetboard/Documents/Laws-Regs/Veterinary-Practice-Act-COMAR.pdf (accessed 19 February 2023).

MCA (Montana Code Annotated) (2021). Title 37. Professions and Occupations, Chapter 18. Veterinary Medicine, Part 1. General - Veterinary Medicine Defined. https://leg.mt.gov/bills/mca/title_0370/chapter_0180/part_0010/section_0020/0370-0180-0010-0020.html (accessed 19 February 2023).

MFAF (Michelson Found Animals Foundation) (2018). Furred lines: Pet trends. https://www.prnewswire.com/news-releases/furred-lines-pet-trends-2019-300741947.html. (accessed 26 July 2021).

Mier, H. (2021). Effectiveness of aqua-acupuncture for reducing stress of canine patients in veterinary clinics. *American Journal of Traditional Chinese Veterinary Medicine* 16 (1): 41–50.

Miscioscia, E. and Repac, J. (2022). Evidence-based complementary and alternative canine orthopedic medicine. *Veterinary Clinics of North America Small Animal Practice* 52 (4): 925–938.

Mittleman, E. and Gaynor, J. (2000). A brief overview of the analgesic and immunologic effects of acupuncture in domestic animals. *Journal of the American Veterinary Medical Association* 217 (8): 1201–1205.

MNBVM (Minnesota Board of Veterinary Medicine) (2022). Minnesota Statutes 2022, Chapter 156: Veterinarian. www.revisor.mn.gov/statutes/cite/156/pdf (accessed 19 February 2023).

Monson, E., Arney, D., Benham, B. et al. (2019). Beyond pills: acupressure impact on self-rated pain and anxiety scores. *Journal of Alternative and Complementary Medicine* 25 (5): 517–521.

MOVMB (Missouri Veterinary Medical Board) (2022). Missouri Veterinary Medical Practice Act Chapter 340, RSMO Statutes. https://pr.mo.gov/boards/veterinary/RulesandRegulations.pdf (accessed 19 February 2023).

MSBVM (Maine State Board of Veterinary Medicine) (2022). Maine Veterinary Practice Act. https://www.mainelegislature.org/legis/statutes/32/title32sec4853.html (accessed 19 February 2023).

MSBVM (Mississippi Board of Veterinary Medicine) (2008). The Mississippi Board of Veterinary Medicine Rules. https://mississippivetboard.org/wp-content/uploads/2013/02/Rules-of-the-Board-of-Veterinary-Medicine.pdf (accessed 19 February 2023).

NAPHIA (North American Pet Health Insurance Association) (2023). Industry data. https://naphia.org/industry-data/#my-menu (accessed 18 February 2023).

Nascimento, F.F., Marques, V.I., Crociolli, G.C. et al. (2019). Analgesic efficacy of laser acupuncture and electroacupuncture in cats undergoing ovariohysterectomy. *Journal of Veterinary Medical Science* 81 (5): 764–770.

NBVME (Nevada Board of Veterinary Medical Examiners) (2023). Chapter 638 – Veterinary Medicine, Euthanasia Technicians. https://www.leg.state.nv.us/NRS/NRS-638.html#NRS638Sec001 (accessed 19 February 2023).

NCVMB (North Carolina Veterinary Medical Board) (2014). The North Carolina Veterinary Practice Act. https://www.ncvmb.org/content/laws/documents/PRACTICE_ACT_PF.pdf (accessed 19 February 2023).

NDVBME (North Dakota Board of Veterinary Medical Examiners) (2007). Chapter 43-29 Veterinarians. https://www.ndbvme.org/image/cache/North_Dakota_Practice_Act.pdf (accessed 19 February 2023).

NHBVM (New Hampshire Board of Veterinary Medicine) (2020). Chapter Vet 100 Organizational Rules. https://www.gencourt.state.nh.us/rules/state_agencies/vet100-700.html (accessed 19 February 2023].

NHBVM (New Hampshire Board of Veterinary Medicine) (2022). Chapter Vet 600 Practice of Veterinary Medicine. https://www.oplc.nh.gov/sites/g/files/ehbemt441/files/inline-documents/sonh/vet-600-adopted-text.pdf (accessed 19 February 2023).

NIH (National Institutes of Health) (1998). NIH consensus conference: acupuncture. *Journal of the American Medical Association* 280 (17): 1518–1524.

NJSBVME (New Jersey State Board of Veterinary Medical Examiners) (2021). New Jersey Administrative Coade Title 13, Law and Public Stafety, Chapter 44, State Board of Veterinary Medical Examiners. https://www.njconsumeraffairs.gov/regulations/Chapter-44-State-Board-of-Veterinary-Medical-Examiners.pdf (accessed 19 February 2023).

NLU (2019). Statutes relating to veterinary medicine and surgery practice act. https://dhhs.ne.gov/licensure/Documents/VeterinaryMedicineSurgery.pdf (accessed 19 February 2023).

NMBVM (New Mexico Board of Veterinary Medicine) (2018). 61–14-2 Definitions Veterinary Practice Act. https://www.nmbvm.org/wp-content/uploads/2021/07/Veterinary-Practice-Act-Turtle-image.pdf (accessed 19 February 2023).

Nolen, R.S. (2022). Pet owner ship rate stabilizes as spending increases. https://www.avma.org/news/pet-ownership-rate-stabilizes-spending-increases (accessed 22 February 2023).

NYSLPV (New York State Licensed Professions Veterinarian) (2023). Article 135, Veterinarian. https://www.op.nysed.gov/professions/veterinarian/laws-rules-regulations/article-135 (accessed 19 February 2023).

Okada, K., Oshima, M., and Kawakita, K. (1996). Examination of the afferent fiber responsible for the suppression of the jaw-opening reflex in heat, cold, and the manual acupuncture stimulation in rats. *Brain Research* 740 (1–2): 201–207.

OL (Oregon Legislature) (2021). Chapter 686 – Veterinarians; Veterinary Technicians. https://www.oregonlegislature.gov/bills_laws/ors/ors686.html (accessed 19 February 2023).

ORC (Ohio Revised Code) (2006). Section 4741.01 Veterinarian Definitions.

https://codes.ohio.gov/ohio-revised-code/section-4741.01 (accessed 19 February 2023).

Ouedraogo, F., Bain, B., Hansen, C., and Salois, M. (2019). A census of veterinarians in the United States. *Journal of the American Veterinary Medical Association* 255 (2): 183–191.

OVB (Oklahoma Veterinary Board) (2022). Oklahoma Veterinary Practice Act. https://www.okvetboard.com/practice-act/388-practice-act-effective-2022/viewdocument/388 (accessed 19 February 2023).

Perdrizet, J.A., Shiau, D.-S., and H.X. (2019). The serological response in dogs inoculated with canine distemper virus vaccine at the acupuncture point governing vessel-14: a randomized controlled trial. *Vaccine* 37 (13): 1889–1896.

Pettermann, U. (2015). Combination of laser acupuncture and low level laser therapy for treatment of non-healing and infected wounds. *American Journal of Traditional Chinese Veterinary Medicine* 10 (2): 33–42.

Purdue University (2019). Veterinary price index. https://assets.ctfassets.net/440y9b545yd9/5IsP0OgjAls6CbaXWvTDuS/81213899998ebb624d418b7521448a0a/FINAL_Nationwide-Purdue_2019-Veterinary-Price-Index.pdf (accessed 11 November 2023).

Purves, D., Augustine, G.J., Fitzpatrick, D. et al. (ed.) (2012a). Pain. In: *Neuroscience*, 5e, 209–228. Sunderland, MA: Sinauer.

Purves, D., Augustine, G.J., Fitzpatrick, D. et al. (2012b). The somatic sensory system: touch and proprioception. In: *Neuroscience*, 5e, 189–208. Sunderland, MA: Sinauer Associates.

Ren, W., Tu, W., Jiang, S. et al. (2012). Electroacupuncture improves neuropathic pain: adenosine, adenosine 5′-triphosphate disodium and their receptors perhaps change simultaneously. *Neural Regeneration Research* 7 (33): 2618–2623.

Ribeiro, M.R., de Carvalho, C.B., Pereira, R.H.Z. et al. (2017). Yamamoto new scalp acupuncture for postoperative pain management in cats undergoing ovariohysterectomy. *Veterinary Anesthesia and Analgesia* 44 (5): 1236–1244.

RIDH (Rhode Island Department of Health) (2006). Rules and Regulations for the Licensure of Veterinarians. https://risos-apa-production-public.s3.amazonaws.com/DOH/DOH_3841.pdf (accessed 19 February 2023).

Rovnard, P., Frank, L., Xie, H., and Fowler, M. (2018). Acupuncture for small animal neurologic disorders. *Veterinary Clinics of North America Small Animal Practice* 48 (1): 201–219.

Sánchez-Araujo, M. and Puchi, A. (2011). Acupuncture presents relapses of recurrent otitis in dogs: a 1-year follow-up of a randomized controlled trial. *Acupuncture in Medicine* 29 (1): 21–26.

Sawamura, M., Arai, T., and Kawasumi, K. (2022). Effect of acupuncture on the energy metabolism of dogs with intervertebral disk disease and cervical disk herniation: a pilot study. *Veterinary Research Communications* 47 (2): 879–884.

Scallan, E. and Simon, B. (2016). The effects of acupuncture point Pericardium 6 on hydromorphone-induced nausea and vomiting in healthy dogs. *Veterinary Anesthesia and Analgesia* 43 (5): 495–501.

SCCL (South Carolina Code of Laws) (2016). Title 40 – Professions and Occupations, Chapter 69 Veterinarians, Article 1, General Provisions. https://www.scstatehouse.gov/code/t40c069.php (accessed 19 February 2023).

SDL (South Dakota Legislature) (2023). Codified Laws Chapter 36-12 Veterinarians. https://sdlegislature.gov/Statutes/Codified_Laws/2060135 (accessed 19 February 2023).

Selmer, M. and Shiau, D.-S. (2019). Therapeutic results of integrative medicine treatments combining traditional Chinese with western medicine: a systematic review and meta-analysis. *American Journal of Traditional Chinese Veterinary Medicine* 14 (1): 41–47.

Shengfeng, L., Cao, X., Ohara, H. et al. (2018). Common parameters of acupuncture for the treatment of hypertension used in animal models. *Journal of Traditional Chinese Medicine* 35 (3): 343–348.

Shmalberg, J. (2016). Integrative medicine: the evidence, economics, and logistics of an emerging field. https://todaysveterinarypractice.com/practice-building-integrative-medicine-the-evidence-economics-logistics-of-an-emerging-field. (accessed 20 December 2020).

Shmalberg, J., Burgess, J., and Davies, W. (2014). A randomized controlled blinded clinical trial of electro-acupuncture administered one month after cranial cruciate ligament repair in dogs. *American Journal of Traditional Chinese Veterinary Medicine* 9 (2): 43–51.

Shmalberg, J., Xie, H., and Memon, M. (2019). Canine and feline patients referred exclusively for acupuncture and herbs: a two-year retrospective analysis. *Journal of Acupuncture and Meridian Studies* 12 (5): 145–150.

Silva, N.E.O.F., Luna, S.P.L., Joaquim, J.G.F. et al. (2017). Effect of acupuncture on pain and quality of life in canine neurological and musculoskeletal diseases. *Canadian Veterinary Journal* 58 (9): 941–951.

Stevenson, P.D. (2016). How to set practice service fees. https://cliniciansbrief.com/article/how-set-practice-service-fees. (accessed 10 June 2020).

TAC (Texas Admistrative Code) (2012). Title 22, Part 24 Texas Board of Veterinary Medical Examiners, Chapter 575 Practice and Procedure. https://texreg.sos.state.tx.us/public/readtac$ext.ViewTAC?tac_view=4&ti=22&pt=24&ch=575&rl=Y (accessed 19 February 2023).

Tangjitjaroen, W. and Mahatnirunkul, P. (2017). A retrospective study of the therapeutic effect of acupuncture in 9 dogs with neurologic deficits from suspected canine distemper virus infections. *American Journal of Traditional Chinese Veterinary Medicine* 12 (2): 77–83.

TBVME (Tennessee Board of Veterinary Medical Examiners) (2014). Chapter 1730-1 General Rules Governing Veterinarians. https://publications.tnsosfiles.com/rules/1730/1730-01.20140821.pdf (accessed 19 February 2023).

Teixeira, L.R., Luna, S.P.L., Matsubara, L.M. et al. (2016). Owner assessment of chronic pain intensity and results of gait analysis of dogs with hip dysplasia treated with acupuncture. *Journal of the American Veterinary Medical Association* 249 (9): 1031–1039.

Thervo (2019). How much does acupuncture cost. https://thervo.com/costs/acupuncture-cost#insurance. (accessed 12 January 2020).

Trcek, L. (2023). This is How Much Flight Prices Increase in 2023 (+FAQs). https://www.travelinglifestyle.net/this-is-how-much-flight-prices-increase-in-2023 (accessed 18 February 2023).

Trentini, J. III, Thompson, B., and Erlichman, J. (2005). The antinociceptive effect of acupressure in rats. *American Journal of Chinese Medicine* 33 (1): 143–150.

Turner-Knarr, K. (2018). Liver-3 acupoint effect on isoflurane anesthesia usage during canine orchiectomy: a controlled, randomized and blinded clinical study. *American Journal of Traditional Chinese Veterinary Medicine* 13 (1): 15–24.

UC (Utah Code) (2020). Chapter 28, Veterinary Practice Act, Part 1 General Provisions. https://le.utah.gov/xcode/Title58/Chapter28/C58-28_1800010118000101.pdf (accessed 19 February 2023).

Um, S.-W., Kim, M.-S., Lim, J.-H. et al. (2005). Thermographic evaluation for the efficacy of acupuncture on induced chronic arthritis in the dog. *Journal of Veterinary Medical Science* 67 (12): 1283–1284.

VGA (Vermont General Assembly) (2023). The Vermont Statutes Online, Title 26: Professions and Occupations, Chapter 44: Veterinary Medicine. https://legislature.vermont.gov/statutes/fullchapter/26/044 (accessed 19 February 2023).

WBVM (Wyoming Board of Veterinary Medicine) (2018). Veterinary Medicine Practice Act, Chapter 30 Veterinarians. https://vetboard.wyo.gov/rules (accessed 19 February 2023).

Weir, M. (2019). How much airfare in the US costs today compared to 10 years ago. https://www.businessinsider.com/fight-prices-airfare-average-cost-usa-2019-11 (accessed 10 December 2019).

Wikipedia (2018). Otzi. https://en.wikipedia.org/wiki/%C3%96tzi#cite_note-27 (accessed 26 July 2021).

Woodley, K. (2018). Pet insurance for holistic and integrative practice. https://ivcjournal.com/pet-insurance-integrative-practices (accessed 11 August 2021).

WSL (Washington State Legislature) (2023). Chapter 18.92 RCW Veterinary Medicine, Surgery, and Dentistry. https://app.leg.wa.gov/rcw/default.aspx?cite=18.92 (accessed 19 February 2023).

Wu, M.T., Sheen, J.M., Chuang, K.H. et al. (2002). Neuronal specificity of acupuncture response: a fMRI study with electroacupuncture. *Neuroimage* 16: 1028–1037.

WVBVM (West Virginia Board of Veterinary Medicine) (2023). Series 4 Standards of Practice. https://www.wvbvm.org/Home/Laws/Rules-/Series-4-Standards-of-Practice (accessed 19 February 2023).

WVEB (Wisconsin Veterinary Examining Board) (2022). Chapter VE1 Veterinarians. https://docs.legis.wisconsin.gov/code/admin_code/ve/1.pdf (accessed 19 February 2023).

Xie, H. (2011a). Chronicle of Chinese history and traditional Chinese veterinary medicine. In: *Xie's Chinese Veterinary Herbology* (ed. H. Xie and V. Preast), 558–591. Ames, IA: Wiley-Blackwell.

Xie, H. (2011b). *History of Veterinary Acupuncture*. Reddick, FL: Chi University.

Xie, H. and Ortiz-Umpierre, C. (2006). What acupuncture can and cannot treat. *Journal of the American Animal Hospital Association* 42: 244–248.

Xie, H. and Preast, V. (2007a). Diagnostic systems and pattern differentiation. In: *Traditional Chinese Veterinary Medicine: Fundamental Principles*, 305–468. Reddick, FL: Chi Institute Press.

Xie, H. and Preast, V. (2007b). Etiology and pathology. In: *Traditional Chinese Veterinary Medicine: Fundamental Principles*, 209–248. Reddick, FL: Chi Institute Press.

Xie, H. and Preast, V. (2007c). Five element theory. In: *Traditional Chinese Veterinary Medicine: Fundamental Principles*, 27–62. Reddick, FL: Chi Institute Press.

Xie, H. and Preast, V. (2007d). Qi, Shen, Jing, blood, and body fluid. In: *Traditional Chinese Veterinary Medicine: Fundamental Principles*, 69–100. Reddick, FL: Chi Institute Press.

Xie, H. and Preast, V. (2007e). The meridians. In: *Traditional Chinese Veterinary Medicine: Fundamental Principles*, 149–204. Reddick, FL: Chi Institute Press.

Xie, H. and Preast, V. (2007f). Yin and Yang. In: *Traditional Chinese Veterinary Medicine: Fundamental Principles*, 1–24. Reddick, FL: Chi Institute Press.

Xie, H. and Preast, V. (2007g). Zang-Fu Physiology. In: *Traditional Chinese Veterinary Medicine: Fundamental Principles*, 105–114. Reddick, FL: Chi Institute Press.

Xie, H., Hershey, B., and Ma, A. (2017). Review of evidence-based clinical and experimental research on the use of acupuncture and Chinese herbal medicine for the treatment or adjunct treatment of cancer. *American Journal of Traditional Chinese Veterinary Medicine* 12 (1): 69–77.

Yam, M.F., Loh, Y.C., Tan, C.S. et al. (2018). General pathways of pain sensation and the major neurotransmitters involved in pain regulation. *International Journal of Molecular Sciences* 19 (8): 1–23.

Yue, I., Shiau, D., Xie, H., and Ma, A. (2021). A randomized, blinded, controlled, clinical trial investigating the mitigation effect of acupuncture points PC-6, ST-36 and LI-4 on morphine induced nausea and vomiting in healthy dogs. *American Journal of Traditional Chinese Veterinary Medicine* 16 (1): 11–18.

Zhang, Z.-J., Wang, X.-M., and McAlonan, G.M. (2012). Neural acupuncture unit: a new concept for interpreting effects and mechanisms of acupuncture. *Evidence Based Complementary and Alternative Medicine* 429412.

Zhang, S.-Q., Wang, Y.-J., Zhang, J.-P. et al. (2015). Brain activation and inhibition after acupuncture at Taichong and Taixi: resting-state functional magnetic resonance imaging. *Neural Regeneration Research* 10 (2): 292–297.

Zhao, Z.-Q. (2008). Neural mechanism underlying acupuncture analgesia. *Progress in Neurobiology* 85 (4): 355–375.

Zhou, W. and Benharash, P. (2014). Effects and mechanisms of acupuncture based on the principle of meridians. *Journal of Acupuncture and Meridian Studies* 7 (4): 190–193.

Zhu, H. (2014). Acupoints initiate the healing process. *Medical Acupuncture* 26 (5): 264–270.

Zhu, B., Yang, Y., Zhang, G. et al. (2015). Acupuncture at KI3 in healthy volunteers induces specific cortical functional activity: an fMRI study. *BMC Complementary and Alternative Medicine* 15: 361.

Zuo, G., Gao, T.-C., Xue, B.-H. et al. (2019). Assessment of the efficacy of acupuncture and chiropractic on treating Cervical spondylosis radiculopathy. *Medicine* 98 (48): e17974.

2

Chinese Food Therapy

CHAPTER MENU

Introduction

Chinese food therapy (CFT) is one of the four branches within traditional Chinese veterinary medicine (TCVM): acupuncture, Chinese herbal medicine or therapy, Tui-na, and food therapy. CFT is a medicinal system utilizing food and herbs to aid in the prevention and treatment of diseases and disharmonies diagnosed using TCVM principles. CFT can be used as an adjunct to existing foods or to formulate complete diets in the short or long term.

The introduction of CFT into a veterinary practice can be beneficial for both the patient and the health of the practice. The successful incorporation and utilization of CFT does not end with the veterinarian's training. Support staff training and client education are crucial. This chapter discusses the what, why, and how for effective integration of CFT within your practice.

The What

Definition

CFT is one of the four branches of TCVM: acupuncture, Chinese herbal medicine or therapy, and food therapy. CFT is a medicinal system utilizing food and herbs to aid in the prevention and treatment of diseases and disharmonies diagnosed using TCVM principles.

Human History

Early books describing Chinese medicine, such as *Recipes for Fifty-Two Ailments* (200 BCE) and *Yellow Emperor's Inner Canon* (111 BCE), briefly mentioned food therapy to improve disease conditions and promote health (Wikipedia 2019). The first true CFT text was featured as a chapter in Sun Simiao's *Prescriptions Worth a Thousand Gold* (650 BCE). One of the first CFT books,

Integrative Medicine in Veterinary Practice, First Edition. Lisa P. McFaddin.
© 2024 John Wiley & Sons, Inc. Published 2024 by John Wiley & Sons, Inc.
Companion website: www.wiley.com/go/mcfaddin/integrativemedicine

Candid Views of a Nutritionist-Physician, was written in the mid-ninth century (Wikipedia 2019). The book described in detail the TCM properties of various foods and their application in the treatment and prevention of disease. Unfortunately the book is now lost. The concept of food therapy was even documented by the father of Western medicine, Hippocrates, as far back as 400 BCE (Xie 2015).

> "Let medicine be your food and food be your medicine."
>
> *Hippocrates*

Veterinary History

There are no historical texts discussing CFT in veterinary medicine. The evolution of CFT in TCVM is expected to follow the same trajectory as veterinary acupuncture. Like veterinary acupuncture and Chinese veterinary herbal medicine, veterinary CFT has gained traction as a useful therapeutic modality over the last 50 years (Shmalberg 2013).

Terminology

The world of TCVM and CFT comes with its own vocabulary. A basic understanding of these terms is crucial, allowing effective communication amongst professionals and with clients. A summary of common terms is provided below.

AAFCO (Association of American Feed Control Officials): Members are individuals from various governmental agencies throughout North America responsible for the regulation of animal feed. The US Food and Drug Administration (FDA) is a member. The individual members have the ability to regulate animal feed requirements within their jurisdiction, but AAFCO as a whole is not a regulatory body.

Bian Zheng: Utilization of one or more of the diagnostic systems to discern a TCVM diagnosis or pattern. The diagnostic systems include Five Element Theory, Yin–Yang Theory, Interior vs. Exterior Patterns, Cold versus Hot Patterns, Deficiency versus Excess Patterns, Five Treasures, and Zang-Fu Physiology (Xie and Preast 2007b).

Body fluid: Fluid found within the body including tears, nasal discharge, sweat, urine, saliva, digestive juices, and joint fluid (Xie and Preast 2007d).

Damp: Can be used to describe environments and disease conditions. One of the six evils or conditions in TCVM. Represents conditions with excessive moisture, infection, heaviness, and often pain (Xie and Preast 2007).

Deficiency Pattern: Condition in which the patient is lacking, often due to overwork, blood loss, or chronic illness. A patient can be deficient in one or more of the following: Qi, Blood, Yin, and Yang. Patients are often dry, thin, weak, and lethargic, and have a pale tongue and weak pulse (Xie and Preast 2007b).

Drain: Remove from an area. Generally applies to Damp conditions.

Eight Principles Theory: Diagnostic system dividing the natural world into two categories (Yin or Yang) and three pairs (Interior vs. Exterior; Cold vs. Heat; and Deficiency vs. Excess) (Xie and Preast 2007b).

Excess Pattern: Condition in which the patient has too much of something, often due to exogenous pathogens (Wind, Cold, Dampness, Summer Heat, Dryness, and Fire) or secondary to another issue (overeating, blood stagnation, phlegm). Patients often are excitable, breathe rapidly, and have a fever, distended abdomen, a red tongue with a coating, and surging pulse (Xie and Preast 2007b,c).

Exogenous pathogens (aka six Exogenous Xie Qi or six Excessive Qi or six Evils): There are six weather changes which normally do not cause disease, but under the right circumstances (i.e. extreme weather changes and/or preexisting disease) can invade the body causing illness: Wind, Cold, Summer Heat, Damp, Dryness, and Fire (Xie and Preast 2007c).

Exterior Patterns: Issues associated with organ systems. Generally chronic in nature.

Five Element Theory: Everything in the natural world can be broken down into five elements, Wood, Fire, Earth, Metal, and Water, which promote, restrain, and regulate each other, maintaining order (Xie and Preast 2007d).

Five Energies: Food can be divided by thermal properties into cold, cool, neutral, warm, and hot (Xie 2015).

Five Tastes: Food can be divided by taste into sour, bitter, sweet, pungent, and salty (Xie 2015).

Five Treasures: The organization of life into five substances: Qi, Shen, Jing, Blood, and Body Fluid (Xie and Preast 2007e).

Fu organs: Yang organs located within the interior of the body. They are hollow or tube-like and function to transport or excrete. Examples include the large intestine, stomach, small intestine, triple heater, gallbladder, and urinary bladder (Xie and Preast 2007h).

Interior Patterns: Issues affecting the outside of the body. Generally acute in nature.

Jing (aka Essence): There is Jing you are born with (Prenatal Jing, Kidney Jing, or Congenital Jing) and Jing you acquire through ingestion of food and stored in each Zang-Fu organ (Postnatal Jing, Zang-Fu Jing, or Acquired Jing) (Xie and Preast 2007e).

Meridians (aka regular meri**dians**): A set of 12 paired and two unpaired pathways or channels on the outer surface of the body through which blood and energy (Qi) flow to the main organ systems, called Zang-Fu organs, joints, muscles, bone, and brain (Xie and Preast 2007f).

Meridian clock (aka TCM circadian clock): Qi flows through the 12 Zang-Fu organ channels in a specific order: lung → large intestine → stomach → spleen → heart → small intestine → bladder → kidney → pericardium → triple burner → gallbladder → liver. There is a two-hour time period during which the passage of Qi through each meridian and corresponding organ is greatest (Xie and Preast 2007f).

Phlegm: An abnormal form of body fluid which can accumulate within the body. Often any "strange" condition or illness is due to phlegm (Xie and Preast 2007e).

Qi (Energy): There are eight primary forms of Qi: Yuan Qi, Zong Qi, Gu Qi, Ying Qi, Wei Qi, Zang-Fu Qi, Jing Luo Qi, and Zheng Qi (Xie and Preast 2007e).

Shen (Spirit or Affect): An outward expression of an individual's mental state (Xie and Preast 2007e).

TCVM: A Chinese medicine system used to treat animals and comprising four branches: acupuncture, Chinese herbal medicine or therapy, Tui-na, and food therapy.

TCVM therapeutic actions: Beneficial effect associated with a specific TCVM therapy.

Tonify (aka Tonic): Increases energy (Qi), blood flow, Yin, Yang, or organ function in an area.

Wind: Can be used to describe environments and disease conditions. One of the six evils or conditions in TCVM. Often considered the primary cause of disease. Wind can invade the body from the outside world (Exogenous Wind) or originate within the body (Internal Wind). Allows other pathogens or conditions to develop (Xie and Preast 2007c).

Yang: Half of the Yin–Yang division. The descriptor can be applied to all manner of items both animate and inanimate. Characteristics include day, brightness, summer, hot, fast, male, healthy, strength, birth, top or back, Qi, pungent or bitter, and Fu organs (Xie and Preast 2007g).

Yin: Half of the Yin–Yang division. The descriptor can be applied to all manner of items both animate and inanimate. Characteristics include night, darkness, winter, cold, slow, female, illness, weakness, death, bottom or belly, blood, salty, and sweet, and Zang organs (Xie and Preast 2007g).

Yin–Yang theory: Divides all things into two halves which oppose, complement, control, create, and transform into each other (Xie and Preast 2007g).

Zang-Fu physiology: Classification of the 12 organs as either Zang or Fu.

Zang organs: Yin organs located within the interior of the body, solid in structure, and whose primary function is manufacturing and storage: lung, spleen, heart, pericardium, liver, and kidney (Xie and Preast 2007h).

CFT and TCVM

TCVM Diagnosis

The safe and effective use of CFT begins with establishing a TCVM diagnosis. A fundamental understanding of the theories behind TCVM is necessary to properly diagnose patients. The factors used when making a TCVM diagnosis are outlined in Table 2.1.

Table 2.1 The key historical and physical components affecting a traditional Chinese veterinary medicine (TCVM) diagnosis (Xie and Preast 2007a).

Historical considerations	Examination considerations
• Chronicity of condition • Previous diseases • Environment • Diet • Current medications, supplements, or herbs • Habits • Dreaming • Attitude toward other dogs and people • Appetite • Thirst • Urinary habits • Stool consistency	• Complete traditional (Western) examination • Shen (affect or demeanor) • Personality • Areas of hot or cold • Smell (body and breath) • Active acupuncture points • Tongue • Pulse

Source: Lisa P. McFaddin.

TCVM Theories and Practices

The following is a review of the information provided in Chapter 1 with additional details demonstrating the interconnectedness of TCVM and CFT.

Yin–Yang Theory

A philosophical view dividing all things into two halves which oppose, complement, control, create, and transform into each other. There are five principles to Yin–Yang Theory. Everything in the world can be broken down into two components: Yin and Yang. These two facets can be further divided into smaller Yin–Yang components; Yin and Yang can control one another; Yin and Yang can help create one another; and Yin and Yang can transform into one another (Xie and Preast 2007g). The Tai Ji symbol is a visual representation of Yin–Yang Theory. Characteristics of both Yin and Yang are shown in Figure 2.1.

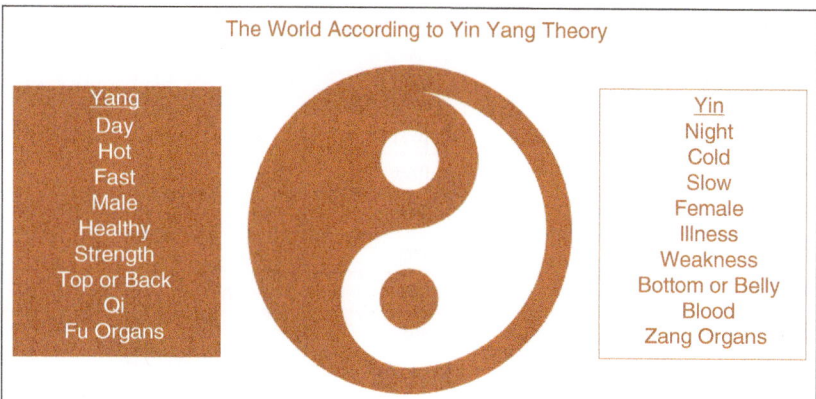

Figure 2.1 The Yin and Yang philosophy and archetypal Tai Ji symbol (Xie and Preast 2007g). Source: Lisa P. McFaddin.

Yin–Yang Theory is not binary but a continuum, just as the Tai Ji demonstrates there is a little bit of Yang (orange) within all Yin (yellow) and vice versa. Using the concept of day and night, the middle of the night is considered almost all Yin (complete darkness) followed by early morning which is mostly Yang with some residual Yin (early morning light but not full sun), while midday is considered almost all Yang (high-noon sun) followed by dusk which is mostly Yin with residual Yang (sunlight is fading but still present).

The Yin–Yang Theory can be applied to the categorization of diseases. Excess conditions involving heat, moisture, and/or infection (think hot spots) are characterized as Yang, while deficiency conditions involving weakness, cold, and often dryness (think hypothyroidism) are characterized as Yin.

The same principle can be applied to food. Yin (cooling) foods are used to treat Yang (hot) conditions. Table 2.2 outlines some common food items classified as either Yin or Yang tonics.

Five Element Theory

The Five Element Theory breaks down everything in the natural world into five elements: Wood, Fire, Earth, Metal, and Water. The Five Elements promote, restrain, and regulate each other, keeping the natural world in perfect working order, establishing homeostasis (Xie and Preast 2007d). Table 2.3 outlines the characteristics defining each element.

Our veterinary patients can be thought of in terms of the Five Element Theory as described in Table 2.4. These are generalizations and do not apply to every patient. Just as with Yin–Yang Theory, the Five Element Theory is fluid. Most patients are a combination of elements with one predominant element shining

Table 2.2 Common food items classified as either Yin or Yang tonics (Yifang and Yingzhi 2012; Pitchford 2002).

Yin tonics	Characterized as cooling and Tonifying Yin	Duck, rabbit, clams, egg whites, pork, tofu, cheese, whitefish, milk, black beans, kidney beans, wheat, barley, brown rice, string beans, asparagus, spinach, tomato, peas, celery, broccoli, apples, lemon, mango, pears, banana, pineapple, and honey
Yang tonics	Characterized as warming and Tonifying Yang	Venison, mutton, kidney, shrimp, lobster, goat, lamb, quinoa, buckwheat, chives, raspberry, walnuts, pistachios, chestnuts, garlic, cayenne, cinnamon, clove, nutmeg, dried ginger, dill seed, fennel seed, basil, rosemary, and thyme

Source: Lisa P. McFaddin.

Table 2.3 The characteristics of the five elements (Xie and Preast 2007d).

	Wood	Fire	Earth	Metal	Water
Season	Spring	Summer	Late summer	Fall	Winter
Color	Green	Red	Yellow	White	Black
Orifice	Eyes	Tongue	Mouth	Nose	Ears
Emotion	Anger	Joy	Worry	Grief	Fear
Flavor	Sour	Bitter	Sweet	Pungent	Salty
Sense	Vision	Speech	Taste	Smell	Hearing
Tissue	Tendons and ligaments	Blood vessels	Muscles	Skin and hair	Bones
Function	Purifying	Circulating	Digesting	Breathing	Excretion
Secretion	Tears	Sweat	Saliva	Nasal fluid	Urine
Zang organ	Liver	Heart and pericardium	Spleen	Lung	Kidney
Fu organ	Gallbladder	Small intestine and triple heater	Stomach	Large intestine	Bladder
Yin-Yang	Mostly Yang	Full Yang	Yin–Yang balance	Mostly Yin	Full Yin

Source: Lisa P. McFaddin.

through. The element(s) patient's most commonly associate with can also change with age. Winston, my beagle-mix, was a true Fire personality when younger, always hyper and easily excitable. After 10 years of age he started slowing down and has morphed into more of an Earth-Metal, calmer but definitely has boundaries.

The Five Element Theory is applied to food using each element's taste and internal organ association. An unbalanced diet often contains excessive or deficient components affecting the overall taste (Clemmons 2015). Disharmony within the diet can lead to disharmony within the patient. Conversely, the diet can be used to restore homeostasis, correct imbalances, and prevent disease within the body (Clemmons 2015). Table 2.5 lists the various foods associated with each of the Five Elements.

Five Element Theory for Veterinarians The Five Elements are depicted in a specific circular order: Wood → Fire → Earth → Metal →

Water. The elements can support and control one another through the Sheng and Ke Cycles, respectively (Xie and Preast 2007d). The Sheng (Inter-promoting) Cycle describes each element as both a parent (mother) and child (son) when compared to the other elements (Xie and Preast 2007d). The mother element serves to support and nourish the child element. The Ke (Inter-Restraining) Cycle defines each element as a grandparent (grandmother) and grandchild (grandson). The grandparent is responsible for controlling the grandchild. For example, Fire is the mother of Earth and the grandmother of Metal. The interactions of the Five Elements are illustrated in Figure 2.2.

Four pathologic cycles can affect the Five Elements (Xie and Preast 2007b–d). The mother element stifles, instead of supports, the son: Spleen (Earth) Deficiency leads to Lung (Metal) Deficiency. The son element shares its problem with the mother (reverse Sheng Cycle): Spleen (Earth) Deficiency leads to Heart (Fire) Deficiency. The grandmother

Table 2.4 The five element theory as it applies to veterinary patient personalities (Xie and Preast 2007d).

	Wood	Fire	Earth	Metal	Water
Breed	Rottweiler	Jack Russel Terrier	English Labrador	Most cats	Chihuahua
Personality traits	Dominant Aggressive Fast moving Impatient	Easily excited Loves attention Smart Fast	Loyal Sweet Laid back Slow	Aloof Likes routine Natural leader Good vision	Quiet Observer Fearful Consistent
Physical traits	Thin body Quick movements	Strong body Fast	Sturdy body Often overweight	Broad chest Luscious coat	Small Thin
Disease predilections	Cardiovascular behavioral	Cardiovascular behavioral	Gastrointestinal obesity	Respiratory issues Dermatologic	Urogenital issues Kidney issues

Source: Lisa P. McFaddin.

Table 2.5 Common food items classified by the five element theory (Clemmons 2015; Xie and Preast 2007d).

	Zang-Fu organs	Taste	Foods
Wood	Liver and gallbladder	Sour	Chicken, wheat, plums, lemon, peach, pineapple, tomato, and vinegar
Fire	Heart and small intestine	Bitter	Lamb, gallbladder, corn, asparagus, lettuce, celery, apricot, bitter melon, and rhubarb
Earth	Spleen and stomach	Sweet	Beef, egg, grains, corn, rice, yams, squash, pumpkin, carrot, and banana
Metal	Lung and large intestine	Pungent	Onion, ginger, garlic, cloves, fennel, nutmeg, mint, radish, and pepper
Water	Kidney and bladder	Salty	Pork, clam, crab, oyster, mussel, duck, beans, seaweed, and barley

Source: Lisa P. McFaddin.

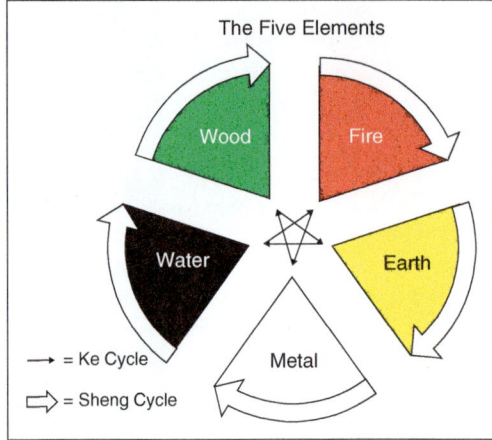

Figure 2.2 A visual representation of the Five Elements with the Sheng (inter-promoting) and Ke (inter-restraining) cycles (Xie and Preast 2007). Source: Lisa P. McFaddin.

excessively controls the grandson (Cheng Cycle): Spleen (Earth) Deficiency leads to Kidney (Water) Deficiency. The grandson insults the grandmother (Ru Cycle): Spleen (Earth) Deficiency leads to Liver (Wood) Deficiency.

The nourishing and pathologic cycles affecting the Five Elements can be used to treat imbalances (Clemmons 2015). Deficiencies can be corrected by tonifying or supporting the mother of the deficient element, while excess conditions can be controlled by supporting the grandmother. This concept, outlined in Table 2.6, is frequently used in CFT by focusing on the five tastes of food and their association with the Five Elements.

The Five Element Theory can also be used to prevent disease. Using an animal's constitution, foods can be chosen based on the five tastes which support and nourish the patient's personality (Clemmons 2015). For example an English Labrador with an Earth-type personality will flourish on a sweeter and slightly bitter diet, but during times of excess worry sour foods will help nourish the Spleen, preventing disease.

Eight Principles Theory

This diagnostic system contains three category pairs divided into Yin and Yang components (Xie and Preast 2007b,h). Think of this as a math problem: Yin–Yang + Three Root Pairs = Eight Principles.

	Yin	Yang
First pair	Interior	Exterior
Second pair	Cold	Heat
Third pair	Deficiency	Excess

Table 2.6 The five element theory as it applies to Chinese food therapy (Xie and Preast 2007d; Clemmons 2015; Xie 2015).

	Taste	Taste properties	Pathology due to excess	Imbalance correction
Wood	Sour	Astringent; aids digestion; bitter	Weakens the spleen; overproduction of saliva; muscle injury	Pungent foods
Fire	Bitter	Drying; strengthening	Dries the spleen; dries the skin; dry cough or asthma	Salty foods
Earth	Sweet	Harmonizing; moistening	Bone aches; kidney imbalance; phlegm formation; hair loss	Sour foods
Metal	Pungent	Aromatic; hot; dispersing	Muscle knots and spasms; damages the Shen; weak nails; exhausts Qi and blood	Bitter foods
Water	Salty	Softening; moistens	Weak muscles; weak skin; weak bones; depression	Sweet foods

Source: Lisa P. McFaddin.

Yin–Yang Refer to the previous section for specific information on Yin–Yang Theory. Yin–Yang Theory can be subdivided into three root pairs: Interior versus Exterior; Cold versus Heat; and Deficiency versus Excess. These four pairs create the Eight Principles Theory (Xie and Preast 2007g). Figure 2.3 outlines the multiple subcategories of potential conditions created by the Eight Principle Theory.

Interior and Exterior Patterns The first root pair refers to the location and extent of the disease or condition within the body. Exterior Patterns affect the outside of the body and are acute in nature, while Interior Patterns focus on internal organ systems and have a longer duration of effect (Xie and Preast 2007b).

CFT focuses on selecting foods which have attributes contrary to the presenting problem. Food therapy for an exterior condition, such as a virus causing fever, chills, and achy muscles, may include a reduction in the volume of food intake, foods which cause sweating (ginger, boneset leaves), and foods high in antioxidants (cabbage, green peppers) (Pitchford 2002). In contrast, an interior condition, such as chronic

vomiting, may benefit from foods which calm the digestive tract (sweet potato, rice) and support the immune system (mushrooms, probiotics) (Pitchford 2002).

Cold and Heat Patterns The second root pair reflect the thermal nature of a disease condition and can be subdivided by their location within the body (Xie and Preast 2007b). Cold Patterns include Exterior Cold, Interior Excess Cold, and Interior Deficient Cold (aka Yang Deficiency). Heat Patterns include Excess Heat, Interior Excess Heat, and Interior Deficient Heat (aka Yin Deficiency).

CFT also classifies food by their Five Energies using the concept of Cold and Heat Patterns: Hot, Warm, Neutral, Cool, and Cold (Xie 2015). Hot and Warm foods are also classified as Yang Tonics; while Cool and Cold foods are classified as Yin Tonics. Neutral foods contain equal parts Yin and Yang, neutralizing the thermal properties. Table 2.7 shows the division of food by their thermal properties.

Deficiency and Excess Patterns The third root pair reflect the body's ability to resist disease.

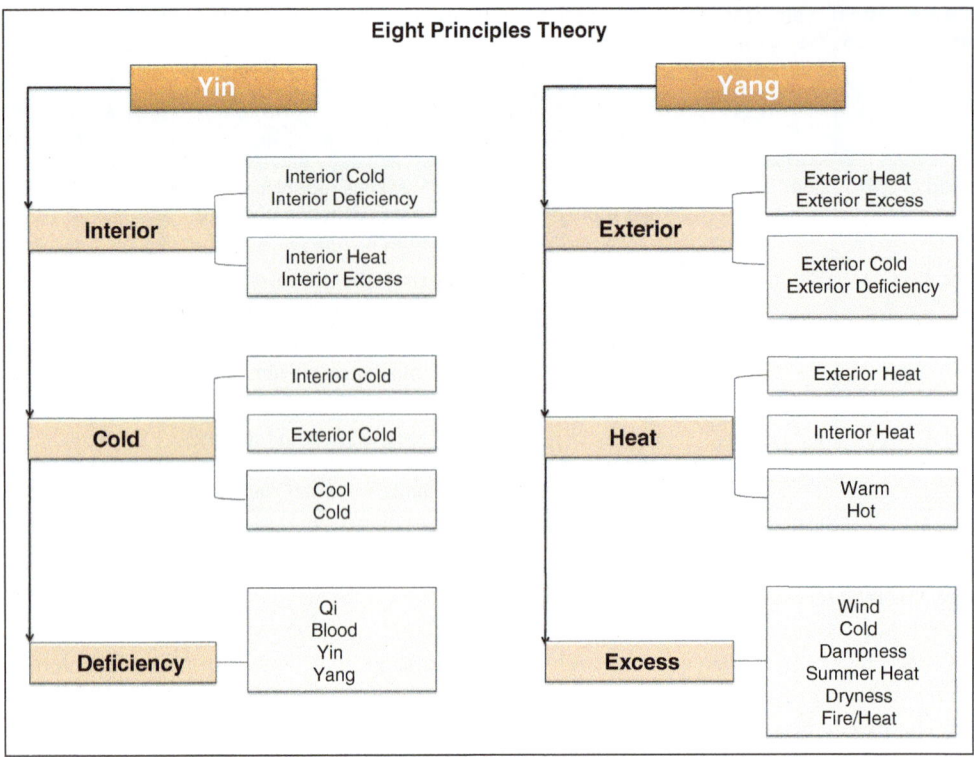

Figure 2.3 Pattern differentiation using the Eight Principles Theory (Xie and Preast 2007d). Source: Lisa P. McFaddin.

Table 2.7 The thermal spectrum of food (Pitchford 2002; Clemmons 2015; Xie 2015).

Cold	Asparagus, banana, bamboo, clam, crab, cucumber, eggplant, grapefruit, fritillaria, kelp, lemon, lettuce, millet, pear, sugar cane, and watermelon
Cool	Apple, barley, celery, egg, eggplant, grass, hay, honey, mung bean, mushroom, orange, pear, peppermint, radish, spinach, tofu, wheat, and wheat bran
Neutral	Abalone, apricot, beat pulp, beef, bran, cabbage, carrot, corn, egg yolk, grape, napa, oyster, peanuts, pineapple, pork, rice, white sugar, and yam
Warm	Brown sugar, cherry, chicken, garlic, ginger, ginseng, green onion, fennel, hawthorn, lychee, oat, onion, peach, pumpkin, shrimp, squash, raspberry, and walnut
Hot	Black pepper, cinnamon, ginger, green pepper, goat, lamb, red pepper, and soybean oil

Source: Lisa P. McFaddin.

There are four categories of Deficiency Patterns: Qi, Blood, Yin, and Yang (Xie and Preast 2007b). The Excess Patterns are defined by the type of pathogen (assaulting or infectious agent) that is present: Wind, Cold, Dampness, Summer Heat, Dryness, and Fire/Heat (Xie and Preast 2007b).

Once the specific pattern is identified CFT uses foods with the opposite characteristics to aid in the treatment of the condition and resolution of the clinical signs. Table 2.10 provides a detailed list of the foods divided by Deficiency and Excess Patterns.

Case Example

Case presentation: A 12-year-old male neutered beagle mix presenting with a chronic history of generalized weakness, increased thirst and urination, anxiety, weight loss, a red dry tongue, and a deep fast pulse.
TCVM diagnosis: Yin deficiency
TCVM treatment goals: Tonify Yin, Cool
Food therapy options: rabbit, brown rice, kidney beans, spinach, broccoli, apples

---

Eight Principles Theory for Veterinarians The complexity of the Eight Principle Theory is illustrated in Figure 2.3. The following paragraphs explain the three root pairs and their application in CFT in more detail.

Interior conditions typically involve internal organs. These issues generally occur later in the course of disease and/or with chronic conditions. With time, emotional distress (Shen disturbances) is common. Interior conditions can be subcategorized into Interior Excess Cold, Interior Deficient Cold, Interior Excess Heat, Interior Deficient Heat, Qi Deficiency, and Blood Deficiency (see Table 2.8) (Pitchford 2002; Xie and Preast 2007b).

Exterior conditions involve superficial surfaces including skin, hair, muscles, and meridians (energy channels located throughout the body). These disorders often start acutely or occur early within a disease process and resolve quickly (short duration) (Xie and Preast 2007b). Common clinical signs include fever, cold aversion, shaking or shivering, a thin coating on the tongue, and a superficial pulse. Exterior conditions are subcategorized into Exterior Cold, Exterior Heat, Exterior Excess, and Exterior Deficiency, as shown in Table 2.9.

By understanding the thermal nature of the patient's condition CFT can be used to correct imbalances. For example, a patient with a hot condition can be fed cooling foods to help alleviate symptoms. Awareness of the patient's constitution and propensity for hot or cold signs allows selection of foods which nourish and support the patient, preventing disharmony and disease.

Most foods fall into the cool, neutral, and warm categories. Fewer items are defined as

Table 2.8 The subcategories and clinical signs associated with interior conditions. These conditions affect internal organs, are noted in chronic conditions or later in the course of disease, often cause Shen (emotional) distress, the tongue may vary in color and often has a coating, and the pulse is deep (Pitchford 2002; Xie and Preast 2007c).

Subcategories	Clinical signs
Interior excess cold	Cold extremities; increased intestinal activity; tongue = purple, wet; pulse = deep, slow
Interior deficient cold	Cold extremities; lethargy; inappetance; diarrhea; tongue = pale purple, ± coating; pulse = deep, slow, weak; seen with **Yang deficiency**
Interior excess heat	Fever; hot extremities; tachypnea; dry stool; reduced urine production; tongue = red, dry, yellow coating; pulse = rapid, forceful
Interior deficient heat	Anxious; low-grade fever (chronic); small dry stool; reduced urine; tongue = red, dry, ± thin coating; pulse = rapid, thready; seen with **Yin deficiency**
Qi deficiency	Shortness of breath; cough; inappetance; diarrhea; organ prolapse; frequent urination or incontinence; tongue = pale, wet; pulse = weak
Blood deficiency	Anxious, scares easily; dull eyes; tendon weakness; tongue = pale, dry; pulse = deep, soft

Source: Lisa P. McFaddin.

Table 2.9 The subcategories and clinical signs associated with exterior conditions. These conditions affect superficial areas (skin, hair, muscles, and meridians), are acute or occur early in the course of disease, of short duration, often involve a fever, cold aversion, and shaking or shivering, the tongue typically has a thin coating, and the pulse is superficial (Pitchford 2002; Xie and Preast 2007b).

Subcategories	Clinical signs
Exterior cold	Serous nasal discharge; shivering; tongue = pale, thin coating; pulse = slow
Exterior heat	Mucoid nasal discharge; cough; tongue = red, thin coating; pulse = rapid
Exterior excess	Fever; tongue = red; pulse = forceful
Exterior deficiency	General weakness; tongue = pale; pulse = weak, soft

Source: Lisa P. McFaddin.

excessively hot or cold. When discussing the functions and indications for specific food items, hot and warm foods, as well as cold and cool foods, are often grouped together.

Cold and cool foods are characterized as quickly growing plants, raw food, refrigerated or frozen foods, and foods with blue, green, or purple coloring. The TCVM therapeutic actions may include Clears Heat, Drains or Purges Fire, Cools Blood, Clears Toxins, and Nourishes Yin. TCVM indications are Heat Patterns, Blood Heat, Blood Toxins, and Yin Deficiency (Xie 2015). Physiologic effects include anti-inflammatory properties, sedative effects, fever reduction, lowering blood pressure, calming, and soothing the nervous system (Clemmons 2015). A few example foods include apples, asparagus, bananas, barley, celery, citrus, cucumber, egg, eggplant, honey, lettuce, millet, mushrooms, pears, peppermint, radish, spinach, tofu, watermelon, and wheat (Pitchford 2002).

Hot and warm foods are characterized as slow-growing plants, more processed, cooked at a higher temperature and/or pressure, require extra mastication, and have a red, orange, or yellow color. The TCVM therapeutic actions may include Yang Tonics, Activating Channels, Tonify Yang Qi, and Warming. TCVM indications include Cold Extremities, Cold Bi Syndrome, and Yang Qi Deficiency (Xie 2015). These foods are known to promote circulation, warm the body, improving organ function, and strengthening the body. Some example foods are brown sugar, cherry, chicken, cinnamon, ginger, goat, green pepper, fennel, lamb, oat, peach, pumpkin, red pepper, squash, raspberry, and walnut (Pitchford 2002; Clemmons 2015).

Neutral foods are characterized as falling between the two extremes. From a TCVM perspective they are typically considered General Qi or Blood Tonics, maintenance foods, and help harmonize diets and herbs. TCVM indications include all conditions, Qi Deficiency, Yin Deficiency, and Blood Deficiency (Xie 2015). They are known to harmonize and be gentle on the body (Xie 2015). Example foods include apricots, beet pulp, beef, bran, cabbage, carrot, corn, egg yolk, peanuts, pineapple, pork, rice, and white sugar yam (Pitchford 2002; Clemmons 2015).

Patients can suffer from Yin, Yang, Qi, and Blood Deficiencies, as well as Zang-Fu organ deficiencies. Common foods used for deficiency patterns can be organized by the condition they support: Yin Tonics (egg whites, kidney beans, and apples), Yang Tonics (lamb, goat, and buckwheat), Qi Tonics (corn, chicken, and yams), and Blood Tonics (beef, aduki bean, and carrots) (Clemmons 2015; Xie 2015). Infections, Damp, Heat, and Wind are considered Excess conditions (Xie 2015). Common foods used for excess patterns include those which drain Damp (aduki bean, rice, and pumpkin) and clear Heat (turkey, cucumber, and celery) (Clemmons 2015).

Finally, foods can be categorized using the third root pair, deficiency/excess, as shown in Table 2.10.

Five Treasures

This is the categorization of life essence into five substances: Qi (Energy or Life), Shen (Spirit or Affect), Jing (Essence), Blood, and Body Fluid (all other excretions). Qi is the most important substance when discussing CFT. Of the seven common forms of Qi, described in Table 2.11, CFT focuses on Gu Qi. Gu Qi, also known as Food Qi or Food Essence, is formed from the processing of food by the Spleen (Xie and Preast 2007e). Gu Qi is the main source of the body's energy (or life) after birth. Good food creates good Gu Qi. Poor nutrition results in poor Gu Qi formation with excessive formation of unusable energy sources, such as dampness and phlegm (Marsden 2015).

Table 2.10 The categorization of food by its TCVM properties (Pitchford 2002; Clemmons 2015; Xie 2015). Some of the foods are characterized by more than one classification structure.

Deficiency patterns	
Yin tonic	Duck, rabbit, clam, mussel, eggs (white), goat milk, pork, sea cucumber, tofu, cheese, whitefish, milk, black bean, kidney beans, wheat, barley, brown rice, string beans, asparagus, spinach, tomato, peas, celery, broccoli, apples, lemon, mango, pears, banana, pineapple, honey, royal jelly, black sesame seed, coix, probiotics
Yang tonic	Venison, mutton, kidney, shrimp, lobster, prawn, goat, lamb, quinoa, buckwheat, chives, fenugreek seed, raspberry, walnut, pistachio, chestnut, garlic, cayenne, cinnamon, clove, nutmeg, dried ginger, dill seed, fennel seed, basil, rosemary, thyme
Qi tonic	Beef, chicken, rabbit, mutton, rumen, eel, eggs, goose, carp, trout, herring, mackerel, milk, tofu, ham, corn, oat, glutinous rice, brown rice, millet, lentil, potato, chickpea, soybean, pumpkin, squash, sweet potato, yam, shiitake, carrot, peppers, spinach, kale, lentil, microalgae, rutabaga, cherry, figs, lychee, coconut, grape, citrus, date, chestnut, peanut, lotus seed, tumeric, almond, hawthorn berry, fennel, coix, molasses
Blood tonic	Beef, bone marrow, organ meat, beef liver and heart, pork skin, hair tail fish, octopus, squid, sardines, eggs, liver, oyster, soy milk, kidney beans, aduki bean, tempeh, sweet rice, barley, black bean, corn, oats, carrot, chili peppers, beet, beetroot, seaweed/kelp, leafy greens, broccoli, parsley, chives, avocado, dark leafy greens, kelp, apricots, dates, lychee, cherry, fig, grape, vinegar, longan, black sesame, dandelion, dang gui, job's tears, longan, microalgae, molasses, mullberry, nettle, watercress
Excess patterns	
Resolve stagnation	Chicken, lamb, venison, shrimp, crab, carrot, radish, watercress, mustard greens, citrus peel, hawthorn berry, vinegar, ginger, garlic, turmeric, clove, dill, coriander, chestnut
Resolve phlegm	Beef, salmon, tuna, clam, oyster, millet, oats, rice, barley, rye, mung bean, soybean, sweet potato, pumpkin, winter squash, alfalfa, celery, radish, mushroom, mustard greens, seaweed, pepper, shiitake, watercress, apple, cherry, dates, lemon, pear, citrus and peel, plantain, jujube, ginger, garlic, thyme, horseradish, peppermint, almond, white pepper, black pepper, walnut, marjoram, licorice
Drain damp	Mackerel, quail, clam, duck, frog, sardine, anchovy, coix, buckwheat, aduki bean, rice, barley, kidney bean, rye, barley, kelp, water chestnut, celery, corn, plantain, squash, pepper, alfalfa, turnip, mushroom, pumpkin, rutabaga, alfalfa, turnip, pumpkin, plum, grapefruit, orange peel, pear, apple, black tea, coix, basil, ginger, horseradish, aloe, garlic, green tea, job's tears, parsley
Drain damp and clear heat	Turkey, white fish, gizzard, rabbit, sardines, salmon, oily fish, white meat chicken, barley, aduki beans, yuca, broccoli, bitter greens, leafy greens, orange vegetables, winter squash, radish, daikon, parsley, celery, kale, brussel sprouts, cabbage, cauliflower, cumin, cardamom, turmeric, coriander, fenugreek, thyme, raw cruciferous vegetables

Source: Lisa P. McFaddin.

Table 2.11 The seven primary forms of Qi (Xie and Preast 2007e).

	Also known as	Source	Primary function
Yuan Qi	Primary or source Qi	Kidney essence Gu Qi	Sustain normal growth and development
Zong Qi	Pectoral Qi Ancestral Qi	Gu Qi Cosmic Qi	Governs and controls the respiratory and circulatory systems
Gu Qi	Food Qi Food essence	Food processed by the spleen	Supplies and restores the Ying Qi, Wei Qi, Yuan Qi, and kidney essence
Ying Qi	Nutrient Qi	Gu Qi	Supplies and nourishes the blood and body
Wei Qi	Defensive Qi	Gu Qi	Protects the body from illness
Zang-Fu Qi	Named by organ	Yuan Qi	Function dependent on the organ involved
Jing Luo Qi	Meridian Qi	Yuan Qi	Allows communication between the meridians and the associated internal organ

Source: Lisa P. McFaddin.

Five Treasures for Veterinarians Qi can be thought of as energy. Without Qi there is no life. There are seven primary forms of Qi, each with their own properties and purposes: Yuan Qi, Zong Qi, Gu Qi, Ying Qi, Wei Qi, Zang-Fu Qi, and Jing Luo Qi. When Qi is weak (Qi Deficiency) or stuck (Qi Stagnation) disease can develop (Xie and Preast 2007e). The following box describes the forms of Qi.

Shen can be thought of as an animal's spirit, affect, or mental state. A healthy Shen is nourished by the Heart, Blood, and Yin, while a disturbance in Shen is usually due to Heart, Blood or Yin Deficiency or Excessive Heat (Xie and Preast 2007e).

Gu Qi and the Spleen

During the process of digestion, the Spleen extracts the clear (pure) from the impure (turbid). Only the turbid descends to the small intestine. The clear substance, called Gu Qi (Food Essence), ascends to the Lung, combining with Qing Qi (Universal Clean Air) to form Zong Qi (Pectoral Qi). Gu Qi also forms Ying Qi (Nutrient Blood) which circulates in the blood vessels and transforms into Blood (Xie and Preast 2007e).

The Spleen also extracts fluids from the food. The clear fluid ascends to the Heart where Blood is made under the influence of the Kidney (Xie and Preast 2007e). Any unusable or pathologic fluid, called Damp, extracted by the Spleen is stored in the body (Xie and Preast 2007e). The accumulation of Damp causes many diseases commonly seen in veterinary medicine. The less nutrient dense and more processed the diet, the more unusable fluid (Damp) is made.

If the diet is poor, then Gu Qi and clear fluid are poor and Blood is not made resulting in Blood Deficiency (Marsden 2015). Damp accumulation also impedes Qi flow. Qi propels Blood, and lack of Qi worsens Blood Deficiency (Xie and Preast 2007e).

Jing is the body's Essence, both what an individual is born with (Prenatal Jing) and what is acquired throughout life (Postnatal Jing). Prenatal Jing deficiency results in many congenital diseases. Postnatal Jing is generally depleted through chronic diseases, excessive behaviors, overworking, lack of sleep, and chronic dehydration (Xie and Preast 2007e).

The importance and function of blood in Chinese and Western medicine is similar. The difference lies in the philosophies behind the formation and pathologic effects of blood. In TCVM, blood is formed from Da Qi (air), Gu Qi, Ying Qi, and Jing (Xie and Preast 2007e). Diseases of the blood center around Blood Deficiency, defined by the organ involved, and blockage (Stagnation) of blood flow.

Jin Ye or Body Fluids are composed of the remaining bodily excretions: tears, urine, joint fluid, nasal discharge, saliva, gastrointestinal fluid, and sweat (Xie and Preast 2007e). Different organs are responsible for the formation and propagation of various body fluids. Jin Ye disease is dependent on the fluid involved but are generally a result of deficiencies.

Zang-Fu Physiology

The classification of the 12 organ systems as either solid structures used for storage (Zang) or hollow tube-like structures used to transmit and excrete (Fu). Zang organs include lung, spleen, heart, pericardium, liver, and kidney. Fu organs include large intestine, stomach, small intestine, triple heater, gallbladder, and urinary bladder.

Foods can be classified by the organ system(s) they support. The Five Element Theory divides foods by their taste properties, but keep in mind that each taste corresponds to that element's Zang-Fu organs as well (Table 2.5). Suggested foods for specific Zang-Fu pathologies can be found in Tables 2.17–2.20.

Zang-Fu Physiology for Veterinarians Each of the 12 organs communicates to the exterior of the body through a channel or meridian. Most acupuncture points are found along these 12 paired meridians (see Chapter 1 for a more detailed explanation of the meridians and acupuncture points).

Just as Yin and Yang complement each other, creating two halves of a whole, Zang and Fu are grouped together as wives and husbands. Each pair of Zang-Fu organs are further classified by their relationship to the Five Elements of the world as depicted in Table 2.5. Zang or Yin organs are defined as those located within the interior of the body, solid in structure, and whose primary functions are manufacturing and storage (Xie and Preast 2007h). Fu or Yang organs are hollow or tube-like and function to transport or excrete (Xie and Preast 2007h). The Fu organs help their associated Zang organs fulfill their roles.

Each organ has its own unique function and potential disease conditions as described in Tables 2.12–2.16. Most Zang-Fu diseases are classified as either excess (too much of

Table 2.12 The Zang-Fu physiology and pathology of the liver and gallbladder (Xie and Preast 2007; Xie and Preast 2007a,b,h; Chen and Chen 2012).

Liver	Functions	Stores blood; maintains the flow of Qi; ensures smooth digestion; maintains the body's vital activities; ensures smooth flow of water; controls the connective tissue; opens into the eyes
	Excess conditions	Liver Qi stagnation; liver fire; liver damp heat; liver Yang rising; liver cold
	Deficiency conditions	Liver blood deficiency; liver Yin deficiency; liver internal wind
Gallbladder	Functions	Descends Qi and bile to intestines
	Excess conditions	Gallbladder damp heat
	Deficiency conditions	No specific disease conditions

Source: Lisa P. McFaddin.

Table 2.13 The Zang-Fu physiology and pathology of the heart, small intestine, pericardium, and small intestine (Xie and Preast 2007a,b,h; Chen and Chen 2012).

Heart	Functions	Dominates the blood and vessels; houses the Shen; controls the sweat; opens in the tongue
	Excess conditions	Extreme heart heat; phlegm-fire disturbing heart; heart blood stagnation; phlegm obstructing the mind
	Deficiency conditions	Heart Qi deficiency; heart Yang deficiency; heart blood deficiency; heart Yin deficiency
Small intestine	Functions	Receive food from stomach and spleen; ensure nutrient absorption; separate nutrients from waste
	Excess conditions	Small intestine cold; small intestine heat
	Deficiency conditions	No specific disease conditions
Pericardium	Functions	Protect the heart
	Excess conditions	No specific disease conditions
	Deficiency conditions	
Triple burner	Functions	(aka San Jiao, triple heater, or triple warmer) Conduit for Qi to flow head to tail; divides the body upper, middle, and lower parts; connects to the pericardium
	Excess conditions	Triple burner obstruction
	Deficiency conditions	No specific disease conditions

Source: Lisa P. McFaddin.

Table 2.14 The Zang-Fu physiology and pathology of the spleen and stomach (Xie and Preast 2007a,b,h; Chen and Chen 2012).

Spleen	Functions	Governs digestion and absorption; transports and transforms Gu Qi; transports and transforms water; controls the blood; dominates the muscles and limbs; opens into the mouth
	Excess conditions	Spleen cold-damp; spleen damp-heat
	Deficiency conditions	Spleen Qi deficiency; spleen Qi sinking; spleen not controlling blood; spleen Yang deficiency
Stomach	Functions	Receive and digest food; prepares food for the spleen
	Excess conditions	Stomach cold; stomach heat; stomach food retention; Rebellious stomach Qi; stomach phlegm
	Deficiency conditions	Stomach Yin deficiency

Source: Lisa P. McFaddin.

something) or deficiency (weakness). Many of the excess disease conditions are due to the organs being attacked by pathogens which, ironically, is usually caused by a deficiency allowing the pathogen to invade. For example, Wei Qi (immune system) deficiency can allow outside pathogens (especially Wind Invasions) resulting in disease or infection. Additionally, deficiencies in the Spleen cause Damp accumulation. Both conditions, Wind Invasion and Dampness, are considered excess conditions but they occur because of an underlying deficiency.

Table 2.15 The Zang-Fu physiology and pathology of the lung and large intestine (Xie and Preast 2007a,b,h; Chen and Chen 2012).

Lung	Functions	Governs Qi; governs respiration; regulates water; controls the skin and hair; opens into the nose
	Excess conditions	Lung wind-cold; lung wind-heat; lung wind-dryness-heat; lung heat
	Deficiency conditions	Lung Qi deficiency; lung Yin deficiency; lung Yin and Qi deficiency; lung Qi and kidney Qi deficiency
Large intestine	Functions	Receives waste from the small intestine; reabsorbs available fluid; prepares feces for excretion
	Excess conditions	Large intestine food accumulation; large intestine damp heat; large intestine cold
	Deficiency conditions	No specific disease conditions

Source: Lisa P. McFaddin.

Table 2.16 The Zang-Fu physiology and pathology of the kidney and bladder (Xie and Preast 2007a,b,h; Chen and Chen 2012).

Kidney	Functions	Stores congenital and acquired Jing; governs water regulates cosmic Qi; dominates the bone; opens into the ears; controls the urogenital and anus
	Excess conditions	No specific disease conditions
	Deficiency conditions	Kidney Yang deficiency; kidney Qi not firm; kidney failing to receive Qi; kidney Yin deficiency; kidney Jing deficiency
Bladder	Functions	Receives waste from the kidneys
	Excess conditions	Bladder damp-heat
	Deficiency conditions	No specific disease conditions

Source: Lisa P. McFaddin.

All foods have an affinity for one or more Zang-Fu organ and/or their associated channels. The TCVM properties of each food can be used to aid in the resolution of clinical signs and disease conditions depending on the presenting Zang-Fu pathology. Example food therapy options for several common conditions affecting the heart, kidney, gastrointestinal System, and lungs, based on the desired TCVM treatment goals, are provided in Tables 2.17–2.20, respectively.

Bian Zheng

Bian Zheng refers to the utilization of one or more of the diagnostic systems for pattern differentiation. This is where all the theories are put together to generate a TCVM diagnosis.

Bian Zheng for Veterinarians There are seven primary classification systems used when obtaining a TCVM diagnosis: Eight Principles, Triple Heater Patterns, Meridian Patterns, Four Levels, Zang-Fu Physiology, Qi–Blood–Body Fluid Patterns, and Six Phases.

- *Eight Principles*: Diseases divided into four pattern pairs: Exterior versus Interior, Hot versus Cold, Excess versus Deficiency, and Yang versus Yin (Xie and Preast 2007b). This categorization is applicable to all disease conditions.
- *Triple Heater Patterns*: Diseases are categorized by their location within the three parts (Jiao) of the body: Upper Jiao (Heart and Spleen), Middle Jiao (Spleen and Stomach),

Table 2.17 Examples of Chinese food therapy defined by three TCVM heart pathologies (Pitchford 2002; Clemmons 2015; Xie 2015; DiNatale 2015; Rimar 2015).

	Heart Qi deficiency	Heart Yin deficiency	Heart blood deficiency
TCVM treatment goals	Qi tonic Drain damp	Avoid hot and bitter Avoid overeating	Warm or cool Avoid hot and very bitter
Meat protein	Beef, tripe, chicken liver, goose, ham, quail, and clam	Cuttlefish, duck, frog, oyster, pork, and tofu	Beef, bone marrow, eggs, liver, heart, and sardines
Grains, beans	Garbanzo, soybean, corn, oats, rye, and barley	Wheat, oats, rice, mung bean, kidney bean, and barley	Corn, oats, wheat, and adzuki beans
Vegetables	Shiitake, carrot, pumpkin, fennel, sweet potato, and asparagus	Endive, spinach, avocado, and tomato	Beet, carrot, kelp, and dark greens
Fruit	Apple, mullberry, and pear	Pineapple and cherry	Fig and date
Nuts, oils, spices	Coix and ginger	Coix	n/a

Source: Lisa P. McFaddin.

Table 2.18 Examples of Chinese food therapy defined by three TCVM kidney pathologies (Pitchford 2002; Clemmons 2015; Xie 2015; DiNatale 2015; Rimar 2015).

	Kidney Jing deficiency	Kidney Qi deficiency	Kidney Yin deficiency
TCVM treatment goals	Nourish essence Tonify kidney Qi Tonify Yin, and Yang Tonify spleen	Tonify kidney Qi and Yang	Nourish kidney Yin Clear false heat
Meat protein	Kidney, chicken, abalone, mussel, oyster, bone marrow, eggs	Raw milk, lamb, chicken, pheasant, venison, cheese, yogurt, duck	Pork, beef, quail, kidney, clams, mullet, eggs, cheese
Grains, beans	Quinoa, millet, wheat, black beans, kidney beans, amaranth, corn, oats	Quinoa, rice, rye, garbanzo, tempeh, barley, millet, lentil	Quinoa, spelt, rice, wheat germ, kidney bean, lima bean, mung bean, tofu
Vegetables	Microalgae, barley, wheat grass, beet, seaweed, reishi	Carrot, potato, pumpkin, yam, winter squash, alfalfa sprouts	Artichoke, asparagus, cabbage, carrots, sweet potato
Fruit	Mulberry, date, fig, raspberry, wolfberry, lycium	Grape, orange, tamarind, blueberry, apple	Avocado, mango, plum, pomegranate
Nuts, oils, spices	Almond, chestnut, walnut, aniseed, cinnamon, fennel seed	Nettle, chickweed, cinnamon, coconut milk, hemp	Ginseng, slippery elm, rose, sesame oil, honey, jasmine

Source: Lisa P. McFaddin.

Table 2.19 Examples of Chinese food therapy defined by three TCVM gastrointestinal disorders (Pitchford 2002; Clemmons 2015; Xie 2015; DiNatale 2015; Rimar 2015).

	Spleen Qi deficiency	Food and Qi stagnation	Megacolon
TCVM treatment goals	Tonify spleen Qi Drain damp	Promotes Qi movement Releases constraint	Moisten the intestines Drains heat Promotes Qi movement Unblocks the bowels
Meat protein	Chicken	Crab, chicken	Rabbit, beef, tofu
Grains, beans	Oats, rye, aduki bean	Wheat germ	n/a
Vegetables	Mushroom, rutabaga, yam, sweet potato, pumpkin	Carrot	Alfalfa sprouts, cabbage
Nuts, oils, spices	Coriander, cardamom, black pepper	Garlic	Honey, saffron

Source: Lisa P. McFaddin.

Table 2.20 Examples of Chinese food therapy defined by three TCVM lung disorders (Pitchford 2002; Clemmons 2015; Xie 2015; DiNatale 2015; Rimar 2015).

	Wind-heat	Lung Qi deficiency	Lung Yin deficiency
TCVM goals	Eliminate wind-heat Disperse lung and stop cough Cool Limit meat	Tonify lung Qi Disperse lung and stop cough	Nourish lung Yin Disperse lung and stops cough
Meat, grains, vegetables, fruit, and other	Turkey, barley, cucumber, celery, pear, honey, peppermint, honeysuckle flower, chrysanthemum	Mutton, beef lung, walnut	Duck, white fish, rabbit, eggplant, pear, honey, Yi Yi ren

Source: Lisa P. McFaddin.

and Lower Jiao (Kidney and Liver). Applicable to many water-metabolism and Damp-Heat conditions (Xie and Preast 2007b).

- *Meridian Patterns*: Pattern differentiation is based on the affected meridian or channel. Primarily used for musculoskeletal and infectious conditions (Xie and Preast 2007b,f).
- *Four Levels*: Divides the immune system into four levels: Wei Qi, Qi, Ying Qi, and Xue (Marsden 2015). Pattern differentiation is based on the level of the immune system affected. Wei Qi is the most superficial layer, basically the skin or outer barrier, and is generally attacked by Wind. Qi are the internal organs or systemic immune system (Marsden 2015). Attacks to the Qi level result in high fevers, thirst, sweating, and bounding pulses. Ying Qi is the plasma, while Xue is the Blood. Attacks reaching both levels cause serious illness such as that seen with septicemia, hemorrhage, immune-mediated thrombocytopenia, and autoimmune hemolytic anemia (Marsden 2015).

- *Zang-Fu pathology*: Diseases associated with a specific Zang-Fu organ and classified as Deficient or Excess. This classification is applicable to most disease conditions (see Tables 2.12–2.16 for examples).

- *Qi–Blood–Body Fluid Patterns*: Vital substances are needed to nourish and support the Zang-Fu organs. Disease patterns are based on the fluid being affected. These diagnoses are most applicable to chronic internal and endocrine diseases (Xie and Preast 2007b,e).
- *Six Phases*: Patterns are divided into Yin and Yang and subsequently divided into inner, middle, and outer levels: Tai Yang (Greater Yang), Shao Yang (Lesser Yang), Yang Ming (Bright Yang), Tai Yin (Greater Yin), Shao Yin (Lesser Yin), and Jue Yin (Terminal Yin) (Xie and Preast 2007b,g). These diagnoses are applicable to most diseases affecting the immune system, central nervous system, and many musculoskeletal disorders (Marsden 2015). The Six Phases correlate to the Zang-Fu organs, often allowing for a Zang-Fu diagnosis as well.

Tongue and Pulse Diagnosis

The importance of an accurate tongue and pulse diagnosis in aiding the Bian Zheng cannot be stressed enough. These two attributes are critical for the TCVM diagnosis and proper herb selection. Table 2.21 provides a brief look into the complexity and intricacies of tongue and pulse diagnosis.

Table 2.21 Examples of tongue and pulse characteristics with associated TCVM conditions (Scott 1994; Xie and Preast 2007a; Chen et al. 2012).

Tongue		Pulse	
Description	**TCVM conditions**	**Description**	**TCVM conditions**
Pale	Blood deficiency, Qi deficiency	**Taut**	LIV Qi stagnation, blood stasis
Lavender	LIV Qi stagnation, blood stasis	**Thin**	LIV blood deficiency, Yin deficiency, blood deficiency
Flabby	SP Qi deficiency, dampness	**Rapid, forceful**	Heat, damp heat
Wet	SP Qi deficiency, dampness	**Rapid**	Heat (excess or deficiency)
Dark red	Stasis type of heat	**Slow**	Cold
Purple	Qi or blood stasis, LIV Qi stagnation, cold	**Weak and thready**	Deficiency
Yellow	Heat	**Forceful**	Excess
Swollen	Dampness, Qi deficiency, Yang deficiency, SP Qi deficiency	**Wiry**	Stagnation, pain, liver disease, phlegm
Small and thin	Qi or blood deficiency, KID Jing deficiency	**Slippery**	Phlegm, dampness, food stagnation
Yellow and dull	SP Qi deficiency, damp	**Soft**	Qi deficiency, cold
Swollen and pale	KID Yang deficiency	**Choppy**	Blood deficiency, Qi deficiency, blood stagnation
Swollen and red	Heat	**Deep and wiry**	Qi contained
Cracked and red	Yin deficiency	**Deep**	Interior condition, Qi deficiency
White	LU Qi deficiency	**Middle to deep**	Interior but not severe
Dark	KID Yin deficiency	**Superficial**	Excess

LIV, Liver; SP, Spleen; KID, Kidney; LU, Liver.
Source: Lisa P. McFaddin.

In general terms the tongue is evaluated by its size, shape, color, and presence of a coating. Tongue diagnosis is actually very nuanced and complicated. For example, specific areas of the tongue correspond with certain Zang-Fu organs, making the diagnoses even more specific.

Typically, the femoral artery is used for pulse diagnosis in dogs and cats (Marsden 2015). The pulse is evaluated using the practitioner's fingertips. Special names are ascribed to the type of pulse based on the depth, intensity, tone, and rhythm, all of which are affected by things like vessel wall tone, vessel diameter, and heart rate. As with the tongue, pulse diagnosis is really complex. Unlike the tongue, unless the pet only has one pelvic limb, both femoral pulses should be palpated. Frequently the left and right pulses differ. In fact the left pulse is associated with Yin and Blood, while the right pulse is associated with Yang and Qi. Similar to the tongue, different areas of the femoral pulse also correspond to different Zang-Fu organs, again helping to home in on the diagnosis.

Five Tastes

The Five Tastes divide foods into well-defined categories, but the characteristics, properties, and indications of each taste are complex. Table 2.22 presents the Five Tastes in more detail. Each taste is broken down into its associated element, taste properties, what happens if too much of a specific taste is ingested (pathology due to excess), when to feed, and representative foods.

Classifications

Putting it all together, CFT classifies food using multiple characteristics simultaneously.

Table 2.22 The five tastes of food with their associated element, taste properties, pathology due to excess, indications for ingestion, and example foods (Clemmons 2015; Xie 2015).

Sour	Element	Wood
	Taste properties	Astringent; aids digestion; lowers intestinal acidity; stimulates peristalsis; and stimulates nutrient absorption
	Pathology due to excess	Weakens the spleen; overproduction of saliva; retains moisture; and muscle injury
	Indications	Excessive sweating; chronic diarrhea; and urinary incontinence
	Example foods	Chicken, wheat, plums, lemon, peach, pineapple, tomato, and vinegar
Bitter	Element	Fire
	Taste properties	Drying; strengthening; clears damp and heat; improves appetite; and stimulates digestion
	Pathology due to excess	Dries the spleen; dries the skin; and dry cough or asthma
	Indications	Excess heat; heat toxin; and damp
	Example foods	Lamb, gallbladder, corn, asparagus, lettuce, celery, apricot kernel, bitter melon, and rhubarb
Sweet	Element	Earth
	Taste properties	Harmonizing all other flavors; moistening; and rules taste
	Pathology due to excess	Bone aches; kidney imbalance; phlegm formation; and hair loss
	Indications	General weakness; deficiency patterns; Qi, blood, Yin, or Yang deficiency; pain reduction and relief
	Example foods	Beef, egg, grains, corn, rice, yams, squash, pumpkin, carrot, and banana

(Continued)

Table 2.22 (Continued)

Pungent	Element	Metal
	Taste properties	Aromatic, hot; disperses stagnation; improves blood/Qi circulation; and varying temperatures
	Pathology due to excess	Muscle knots and spasms; damages the Shen; weak nails; and exhausts Qi and blood
	Indications	Qi-blood stagnation; localized pain; edema; and tumors
	Example foods	Onion, ginger, garlic, cloves, fennel, nutmeg, mint, radish, and pepper
Salty	Element	Water
	Taste properties	Softening; moistens; and improves concentration
	Pathology due to excess	Weak muscles; weak skin; weak bones; and depression
	Indications	Lumps; nodules; masses; cysts; and constipation
	Example foods	Pork, clam, crab, oyster, mussel, duck, beans, seaweed, and barley

Source: Lisa P. McFaddin.

1) The Five Tastes: sour, bitter, sweet, pungent, and salty
2) The Five Energies: cold, cool, neutral, warm, and hot
3) The Eight Principles: yin, yang, interior, exterior, deficiency, excess, cold, and heat
4) Zang-Fu physiology: lung, spleen, heart, pericardium, liver, kidney. Fu organs include large intestine, stomach, small intestine, triple heater, gallbladder, and urinary bladder.
5) TCVM therapeutic actions

The CFT classification for five common foods (apple, carrot, chicken, rice, and sweet potato) are described below (Clemmons 2015; DiNatale 2015; Rimar 2015; Xie 2015; Pitchford 2002). Table 2.23 lists the Chinese food classification of common ingredients.

1) **Apple**
   a) Taste: sweet and sour
   b) Energy: cool
   c) Zang-Fu: spleen and stomach
   d) TCVM therapeutic actions: produce body fluids and reinforce the spleen
   e) Therapeutic indications: debility, indigestion, loss of appetite

2) **Carrot**
   a) Taste: sweet
   b) Energy: neutral
   c) Zang-Fu: spleen, liver, and lung
   d) TCVM therapeutic actions: reinforces and strengthens spleen; aids in digestion; reinforces liver energy; enhances vision; strengthens the lung; nourishes the skin; promotes Qi circulation; stops cough; and clears heat
   e) Detoxify
   f) Therapeutic indications: spleen Qi deficiency; weakness; emaciation; edema; increased urination; and chronic disease

3) **Chicken**
   a) Taste: sweet
   b) Energy: warm
   c) Zang-Fu: spleen and stomach
   d) TCVM therapeutic actions: nourish and tonify Qi and Blood; tonify Kidney Jing; tonifies spleen and stomach Qi; and promotes blood circulation
   e) Therapeutic indications: spleen Qi deficiency; weakness; emaciation; edema; increased urination; and chronic disease

Table 2.23 Chinese food therapy classification of common foods using taste and thermal properties, Zang-Fu organ affinity, TCVM therapeutic actions, and therapeutic indications (Pitchford 2002; Yifang and Yingzhi 2012; Clemmons 2015; DiNatale 2015; Rimar 2015; Xie 2015).

Food	Properties	Zang-Fu organ(s)	TCVM therapeutic actions	Therapeutic indications
Almond	Sweet Neutral	Lung Spleen Large intestine	Moistens the lungs and intestines; strengthens the spleen and stomach	Cough; difficulty breathing; constipation
Apple	Sweet Sour Cool	Spleen Stomach	Produces body fluids; reinforces the spleen	Debility; indigestion; loss of appetite
Apricot	Sweat Sour Neutral	Lung Stomach	Produces body fluids; moistens lungs; clears and warms wind-cold	Thirst; asthma; cough; constipation due to large intestinal dryness
Banana	Sweet Cold	Stomach Large intestine	Strengthens the stomach; promotes body fluids; moistens dryness; clear heat; detoxify; softens the intestines for constipation	Throat dryness; thirst; constipation
Barley	Sweet Cool	Spleen Stomach Bladder	Reinforces and strengthens the spleen; regulates the stomach; relieves thirst; induces urination; Yin tonic; dampening	Spleen and stomach; weakness; anorexia; diarrhea; thirst; difficult and painful urination
Beef	Sweet Warm or neutral	Spleen Stomach Large intestine	Reinforces and strengthens the spleen and stomach; enriches Qi and blood; nourishes Yin, Qi, and blood	Anorexia; diarrhea; edema; fatigue; diabetes; general weakness; underweight
Carrot	Sweet Neutral	Spleen Liver Lung	Reinforces and strengthens the spleen; aids in digestion; reinforces liver energy; enhances vision; strengthens the lung; nourishes the skin; promotes Qi circulation; stops cough; clears heat; detoxify	Indigestion; food stagnation; blurred vision; night blindness; lung heat cough; prevents colds; vitamin A deficiency
Celery	Pungent, sweet Cool	Liver Stomach Bladder	Clears heat; calms the liver; reinforces the stomach; eases urination	Fevers; liver heat; vomiting and anorexia from stomach heat; difficult urination from heat; hematuria; hypertension; dizziness; headache

(Continued)

Table 2.23 (Continued)

Food	Properties	Zang-Fu organ(s)	TCVM therapeutic actions	Therapeutic indications
Chicken	Sweet Warm	Spleen Stomach	Nourishes and enriches Qi and blood; tonifies kidney Jing; nourishes the spleen; tonifies the spleen and stomach Qi; improves blood circulation	Spleen Qi deficiency; weakness; emaciation; edema; frequent urination; weakness after surgery; chronic illness
Duck	Sweet, salty Neutral	Lung Spleen Kidney	Nourishes Yin; reinforces the stomach; removes damp	Yin deficiency; fever; cough. Removes edema; dry throat; edema
Egg	Sweet Neutral		Nourishes Yin and blood; Jing tonic	Blood deficiency; Yin deficiency
Eggplant	Sweet Cold	Stomach Large intestine	Clears heat; cools blood	Hemorrhoids; bloody stools
Garlic	Pungent, sweet Warm, hot	Spleen Stomach Lung	Warms middle burner; reinforces and strengthens the stomach; helps warm; aids digestion; kills parasites; food stagnation; resolves damp and phlegm; circulates Qi	Pain in upper abdomen; food poisoning; dysentery
Ginger	Pungent, spicy Warm	Lung Spleen Stomach	Warms the middle burner (spleen and stomach); stops vomiting; warms the lung; arrests cough; increases appetite; promotes bowel movements	Anorexia; weakness; cough; upper respiratory infection; vomiting; dysentery; dyspepsia
Goat	Sweet Hot	Spleen Kidney	Warms middle burner; enriches Qi and blood	Male impotence; cold intolerance; weakness in lower back; profuse clear urine; abdominal pain; cold limbs; fatigue
Honey	Sweet Neutral	Lung Stomach Large intestine	Moistens lung; stops cough; moistens bowel	Respiratory disease; cough
Honeysuckle flower	Sweet Cold	Lung Heart Stomach	Clears heat; detoxifies; antiviral effect	Fever; sore throat; boils and carbuncles
Kelp	Salty Cold	Liver Stomach Kidney	Dissolves phlegm; softens hard masses; relieves edema	Goiter; edema; hypertension; heart disease; carcinomas; hernia

Food	Properties	Zang-Fu organ(s)	TCVM therapeutic actions	Therapeutic indications
Lamb	Sweet Hot	Spleen Kidney	Warms middle burner; enriches Qi and blood; tonifies Yang	Male impotence; cold intolerance; weakness in lower back; profuse clear urine; abdominal pain; cold limbs; fatigue
Lemon	Sour Cold	Stomach Lung Liver	Produces body fluids; relieves heat	Cough; indigestion; diabetes
Lettuce	Bitter, sweet Cool	Stomach Large intestine	Promotes urination	Difficulty urinating; bloody urine
Millet	Sweet, salt Slightly cold	Spleen Stomach Kidney	Nourishes spleen and kidney; relieves thirst; induces urination; calms Shen; clears heat; Yin tonic but dampening	Vomiting; anorexia; thirst; difficult urination with fever; skin conditions; abnormal night behaviors
Mushroom (shiitake)	Sweet Neutral	Stomach	Resolves hard masses	Rickets; anemia; measles; cancers
Mussel	Salty Warm	Liver Kidney	Nourishes liver and kidney; tonifies blood and essence	Night sweats; lumbago; impotence; dizziness; headache
Napa	Sweet Neutral	Stomach Large intestine	Promotes urination	Constipation; ulcers
Oats	Sweet Warm	Spleen Kidney	Warms kidney Yang; tonifies Qi. Stops hemorrhage; use for Qi and Yang deficiency; strengthens spleen; dry damp	Decreases blood cholesterol and triglycerides; decreases blood pressure; hyperlipidemia; spleen Qi deficiency; Yin tonic but dampening
Orange	Sweet, sour Cool	Stomach Bladder	Produces body fluids; induces urination	Difficult urination; thirst
Pork	Sweet, salt Neutral	Lung Spleen Liver	Nourishes Yin; moistens dryness; enriches/tonifies blood	Dry cough; dry mouth; emaciation; fatigue; constipation
Potato	Sweet Neutral	Spleen Stomach Large intestine	Reinforces spleen and stomach; relieves spasm and pain	Indigestion; weak spleen and stomach; pain in the upper abdomen from spleen and stomach disharmony; GI ulcers
Pumpkin	Sweet Warm	Spleen Stomach	Reinforces middle burner; replenishes Qi; dissolves phlegm; promotes discharge of pus; expels roundworms; dries damp in gastrointestinal tract	Weak spleen, spleen Qi deficiency; coughing up thick sputum; gut parasites; malnutrition; chronic inflammatory bowel disease; diabetes

(Continued)

Table 2.23 (Continued)

Food	Properties	Zang-Fu organ(s)	TCVM therapeutic actions	Therapeutic indications
Quail	Sweet Neutral	Spleen Liver	Reinforces spleen Qi; removes damp	Removes edema; strengthens bones and tendons
Rabbit	Sweet Cool	Spleen Stomach Liver Large intestine	Reinforces spleen; enriches Qi; nourishes Qi and Yin	Anorexia; fatigue; thirst
Radish	Pungent Sweet Cool	Lung Stomach	Promotes digestion; eliminates phlegm	Respiratory infections; common cold
Rice (brown)	Sweet Cool	Spleen Stomach Kidney	Regulates spleen and stomach; clears heat; nourishes kidney	Yin tonic but dampening
Rice (white)	Sweet Warm or neutral	Spleen Stomach	Nourishes spleen; harmonizes stomach; relieves thirst; Yin tonic but dampening	Vomiting; anorexia; thirst and dry mouth; stomach Yin impairment and heat
Rye	Bitter Neutral	Spleen	Drains damp and water from spleen	Spleen Qi deficiency
Spinach	Sweet Cool	Large intestine Stomach Liver	Moistens dryness; eases bowel motions; promotes production of body fluids; quenches thirst; nurtures/nourishes liver; improves vision	Constipation; thirst; liver heat; liver Yin deficiency; dizziness; constipation from dryness in geriatric patients; thirst due to diabetes mellitus or stomach heart
Squash	Sweet Warm	Spleen Stomach	Heals inflammation; relieves pain; reinforces middle burner; replenishes and tonifies Qi; protects from cold; dissolves phlegm; promotes discharge of pus; expels roundworms	Bronchiectasis; pulmonary abscess; weak spleen; coughing up thick sputum; gut parasites; malnutrition; chronic inflammatory bowel disease; diabetes mellitus
Sweet potato	Sweet Neutral	Spleen stomach Large intestine	Reinforces spleen and stomach; assists with bowel movements; promotes production of body fluids; quenches thirst; tonifies spleen	Fatigue; constipation; thirst. General Qi deficiency; fatigue; inflammatory bowel disease; prevents diabetes mellitus
Tangerine	Sweet or sour Cool	Lung Stomach kidney	Promotes digestion; strengthens spleen	Chest congestion; vomiting; hiccups

Food	Properties	Zang-Fu organ(s)	TCVM therapeutic actions	Therapeutic indications
Tomato	Sweet or sour Cool	Stomach Liver	Clears heat and detoxifies; produces body fluids; nourishes Yin; cools blood and clears liver heat Often cooked	Dry throat; blurred vision; bleeding gums; nasal bleeding; hypertension; vitamin deficiency; cancer prevention
Tripe	Sweet Neutral	Spleen Stomach	Reinforces spleen and stomach	Anorexia; diarrhea
Vinegar	Sour, sweet warm or neutral	Liver Stomach	Food stagnation; anorexia	Hard abdominal masses; vomiting blood; bloody stools; nosebleed
Walnut	Sweet Warm	Kidney Lung Large intestine	Lubricates intestines; tonifies lung and kidney; helps kidney Yang	Asthma; cough; seminal emission; impotence; constipation; arthritis (worse in the winter)
Watermelon	Sweet Cold	Stomach Heart Bladder	Clears heat; induces urination; relieves thirst	Difficulty urinating; sore throat; mouth canker sores
Wheat	Sweet Cool	Heart Spleen Kidney	Nourishes heart; reinforces spleen; relieves thirst; induces urination; Yin tonic but dampening	Thirst; difficult urination with fever; hysteria; dry mouth; diarrhea
Yam	Sweet Neutral	Lung Spleen Kidney	Tonifies lung; tonifies spleen; tonifies kidney; spleen Qi deficiency	Diarrhea; cough; diabetes

Source: Lisa P. McFaddin.

4) **Rice**
   a) Taste: sweet
   b) Energy: warm or neutral
   c) Zang-Fu: spleen and stomach
   d) TCVM therapeutic actions: nourish spleen; harmonize stomach; relieve thirst; and Yin tonic but dampening
   e) Therapeutic indications: vomiting; anorexia; thirst and dry mouth; and stomach heat
5) **Sweet Potato**
   a) Taste: sweet
   b) Energy: neutral
   c) Zang-Fu: spleen, stomach, and large intestine
   d) TCVM therapeutic actions: reinforce spleen and stomach; assists with bowel movements; promote body fluid production; quench thirst; and tonify spleen
   e) Therapeutic indications: fatigue; constipation; thirst; general Qi deficiency; fatigue; inflammatory bowel disease; and prevents diabetes mellitus

Applying CFT

CFT is generally utilized through the application of at least one of the following approaches: guide commercial diet selection; supplement commercial diets; recreate an herbal formula;

temporary therapeutic diet; and/or maintenance diet.

Guide Commercial Diet Selection

The TCVM principles of food are used to select
commercially prepared diets based on the
requirements of a specific patient. For example, patients exhibiting heat signs will benefit
from a minimally processed diet with a cooling
protein, such as turkey. The more processed
the diet, the more energy required to break
down, absorb, and utilize the nutrients within
the food; thus, the hotter the food source
(Shmalberg 2013; Rimar 2015).

Just like individual food substances, prepared meals have their own thermal properties. The thermal energetics associated with a
meal is the result of the energy required to
digest, metabolize, and utilize the nutrients
within the food. This concept is known as Xing
(Rimar 2015).

The factors affecting Xing include food preparation, food animal age, food animal diet,
water content, and growth speed (Rimar 2015).
The more processed the food, the more heat is
released and the hotter the food becomes
(Rimar 2015). Figure 2.4 depicts the Xing associated with common food preparation techniques. Keep in mind the food preparation
method cannot overcome the underlying

thermal properties of the food. For example,
goat will always be hot whether cooked or raw.

The age at which the food animal is killed
affects its thermal properties. Younger animals
are generally warmer; while older animals are
typically cooler (Rimar 2015). The protein from
grain-fed food animals is warmer compared to
their free-range counterparts (Rimar 2015).
The administration of hormones and antibiotics also increases the temperature of food
animal protein.

Food sources with higher water contents
tend to be cooler (Rimar 2015). Plant sources
which grow faster (e.g. radishes) are cooler
compared to slower-growing plants (e.g. root
vegetables) (Rimar 2015).

Supplement Commercial Diets

Home-cooked protein, carbohydrates, vegetables, and/or fruits can be added to commercially prepared diets using TCVM treatment
principles. The category, type, and quantity of
food added is dependent on the individual
patient's needs as determined by the
veterinarian.

Recreate an Herbal Formula

Food can be used to recreate the therapeutic
properties of an herbal formula. A food
substitute matching the TCVM therapeutic

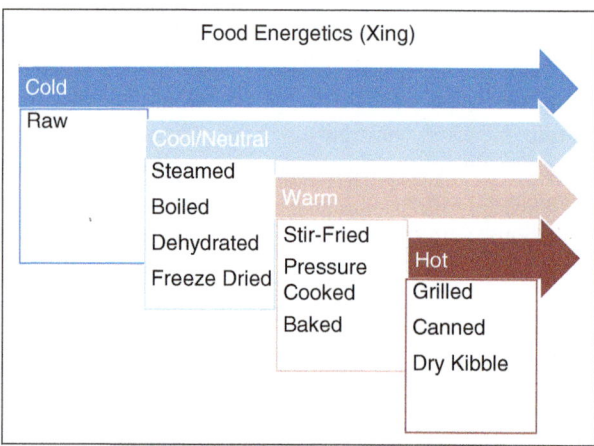

Figure 2.4 The energetics of common food preparations (Rimar 2015). Source: Lisa P. McFaddin.

properties of each individual herb within an herbal formula are chosen. The ratio of the foods within the diet is based on the ratio of herbs comprising the formula (Clemmons 2015). The total diet volume is based on the caloric requirement of the patient. The diet is then balanced using the addition of vitamins, minerals, fatty acids, and amino acids as needed. These diets are most often used short term but, if balanced, can be fed long term. Table 2.24 illustrates the formulation of a therapeutic diet meant to mimic the ingredients of a specific Chinese herbal formula: Bai Hu Tang (White Tiger Decoction).

Temporary Therapeutic Diet

Specific diets can be used short term to aid in the treatment of certain disease conditions. These diets are not often balanced and should only be used under the direction of a trained veterinarian. CFT teas can also be used as means to introduce specific herbal remedies in the diet, especially if the patient will not tolerate true herbal formulas.

There are thousands of ancient classical CFT recipes created to aid in human health. Many of these recipes can be adapted for cats and dogs. There are also newer recipes geared toward cats and dogs used to treat specific TCVM conditions. These therapeutic diets are

Table 2.24 A therapeutic diet created mimicking the Chinese herbal formula Bai Hu Tang. Formula percentage was calculated using a total weight of 51 g. Diet percentage was calculated using a total caloric count of 246 kcal; 300 mg of calcium supplementation is recommended per serving (Pitchford 2002; Chen and Chen 2012; Chen et al. 2012; Clemmons 2015).

Individual herb	TCVM properties	Formula percentage (%)	Food alternative	TCVM properties	Diet percentage (%)
Shi Gao (Gypsum)	Clears heat Drains fire	59	Crab	Promotes blood Nourishes Yin Clears heat	59
Zhi Mu (*Anemarrhena*)	Clears heat Enriches Yin	17.5	Millet	Nourishes spleen Nourishes kidney Calms Shen Clears heat Tonifies Yin	17.5
Zhi Gan Cao (Honey fried licorice)	Tonifies spleen Relieves pain Clears heat Harmonizing	6	Squash	Heals inflammation Relieves pain Reinforces middle burner Tonifies Qi Protects from cold	6
Geng Mi (nonglutinous rice)	Tonifies lung, spleen, and intestines	17.5	Coriander	Reinforces middle burner Protects from cold	17.5

Source: Lisa P. McFaddin.

meant for short-term use. Table 2.25 provides examples of traditional CFT recipes.

Maintenance Diet

If the diet based on the patient's current TCVM diagnosis, is balanced, the calorie content is appropriate for the patient, and the owner is able to routinely make the food, a CFT diet can

Table 2.25 Example of two therapeutic Chinese food therapy diets (Clemmons 2015; Xie 2015).

Classic recipe: Qi and blood tonic	Dog/cat recipe: Qi tonic
Chicken 200 g	Ground beef 4 oz
Astragalus 30 g	Beef liver 4 oz
Angelica 10 g	Spinach ¼ cup
Onion 20 g	String beans 3 oz
Ginger 20 g	Olive oil 1 tbsp
Salt 10 g	Calcium 1000 mg
Preparation: cook for 2 hours	Preparation: cook until well done
For dogs/cats: omit onion	Contains 704 kcal with 37% protein, 10% carbohydrate, and 53% fat

Source: Lisa P. McFaddin.

be fed long term. Maintenance diets must be appropriate for the age and health status of the patient. Different ratios of protein, carbohydrate, vegetable and fat are recommended for different disease conditions.

The inclusion of grains within the diet is based on the patient's nutritional needs and TCVM diagnosis. Given the current controversy surrounding grain-free diets the veterinarian must weigh the pros and cons of including or excluding grains. Open client communication is essential regarding the potential risks associated with a grain-free diet. A well-balanced diet is critical for patient health. Inclusion of vitamins and supplements, and consultation with a board-certified veterinary nutritionist may be warranted.

A majority of the diets discussed in CFT are home-cooked. The client is the person responsible for preparing the home-cooked diets. An open and frank discussion with the client regarding the time and cost requirements is critical, especially when used as a long-term feeding solution. A discussion of the pros and cons of raw diets is beyond the scope of this book.

A Bit About AAFCO

The Association of American Feed Control Officials (AAFCO) has been in existence since 1906. AAFCO members are individuals from various governmental agencies throughout North America responsible for the regulation of animal feed. The US FDA is a member of AAFCO. AAFCO exists as an animal-feed think tank in which members discuss potential rules and regulations pertaining to animal food. The ideas and models created by the AAFCO members are shared with the member's respective governmental agencies which then create laws.

The individuals comprising AAFCO have the ability to regulate animal feed requirements within their jurisdictions, but *AAFCO as a whole is not a regulatory body.*

Most states have adopted the AAFCO model for pet food regulations within their own laws, making the AAFCO model the default standard. The AAFCO model discusses recommendations for pet food labeling, i.e. what is written on the back of the bag of food. The model also covers the minimum recommended nutritional requirements and nutrient profiles for cats and dogs based on life stage.

The following statement is found on most cat and dog foods: "[Pet Food Product Name] is formulated to meet the nutritional levels established by the AAFCO Dog (or Cat) Food Nutrient Profiles for [pet life stage]."

Home-cooked diets do not carry the aforementioned label claim; however, the veterinarian's goal is to create a balanced maintenance diet. As a result, home-cooked diets often meet or exceed the nutrient profile recommendations established by AAFCO.

For additional information about AAFCO and its pet food recommendations visit https://www.aafco.org.

(AAFCO 2014)

Regardless of the treatment style chosen the goal is *balance*. The TCVM diagnosis is used to develop the TCVM treatment strategy, and the TCVM properties of the food are used to offset the TCVM diagnosis and fulfill the treatment goals. For example, a dog diagnosed with Damp Heat will be treated by clearing the heat and draining the damp. A diet consisting of duck, Adzuki bean, squash, and apple could be used.

Maintenance Diets for Veterinarians

There is no such thing as the perfect diet for a cat or dog, but diets can be formulated to meet the nutritional and metabolic needs of an individual pet. Any diet used for more than a week or two should be balanced. Most commercially available diets are created using the minimum nutrient profiles established by AAFCO.

These nutrient profiles contain minimum requirements for protein, fat, vitamins (fat and water soluble), and minerals based on the pet's species and life stage (AAFCO 2014). There is no minimum requirement listed for the carbohydrate content of cat and dog food. Review the AAFCO website (https://www.aafco.org) for specific pet food nutrient recommendations. Refer to Chapter 4 on nutraceuticals to learn more about the regulations of commercial animal food production and safety, as well as the AAFCO.

The diets discussed in CFT are typically cooked. The use of raw diets for companion cats and dogs, while controversial, has its place in veterinary medicine but is beyond the scope of this chapter. Reference material detailing raw food diets in veterinary medicine are provided in the Reference Materials section of this chapter and companion website.

Home-cooked diets offer many benefits for our veterinary patients including the use of minimally processed ingredients; the absence of preservatives and binding agents necessary for the long-term storage of commercially prepared foods; reduced numbers of advanced glycosylated end products (AGEs) and reactive oxygen species (ROS) which contribute to inflammation; diets tailor-made for each individual patient; improved digestibility, nutrient absorption, and assimilation; and improved palatability (Silver 2014; Rimar 2015). Potential negatives associated with home-cooked diets include owner time and cost constraints; lack of variety; over- or under-consumption of calories; unbalanced protein, fat, and carbohydrate levels; and vitamin and mineral deficiencies (Rimar 2015; Heinze 2016; Pedrinelli et al. 2017).

Owner Concerns   A frank discussion must be had with the owner regarding the potential time and cost commitment for home-cooked meals. These issues pertain to the purchasing, preparation, storage, and serving of homemade meals. Bulk purchasing and preparation, with freezing of meals, reduces the day-to-day time requirement. Bulk storage of prepared meals often requires the use of a large freezer.

The recipes must outline the exact ingredients and measurements for each food item. If the owner plans to prepare multiple meals at one time the veterinarian should discuss how best to prepare, divide, and store the meals. For example, plastic storage containers should be avoided (Silver 2014).

The best cooking methods (including temperatures and length of time) should be discussed with the owner. For example, the use of crockpots can be a huge time saver, and the appropriate temperature required to kill common bacteria, at least 140 °F (60 °C) but preferably 165 °F (74 °C), should be disclosed (Rimar 2015). Additionally, overcooking vegetables can denature enzymes reducing their nutrient density (Rimar 2015). Preparing a client handout detailing the ingredients list, preparation and storage instructions will greatly assist client compliance and reduce the risk of errors in the kitchen.

Dietary Variety Let's face it, most pets eat the same food day-in and day-out. The necessity for nutritional variety in companion animals is yet another contentious topic. Dietary variety can be helpful when dealing with picky eaters, ensuring adequate nutrient consumption without the routine use of multivitamins, and assisting with the management of certain disease conditions.

On the flip side, dietary variety can be detrimental to patients with food intolerances and allergies. Varying the diet may also adversely affect the owner's time and financial commitments depending on the ingredients needed and frequency of dietary changes. The pros and cons of feeding one versus multiple meals types should be discussed with the client.

Caloric Requirements To prevent over- and under-conditioning of our companion animal patients, the daily energy requirements for each pet must be calculated. The Oxford dictionary defines a *calorie* as the energy needed to increase the temperature of 1 g (or 1 ml) of water by 1 °C. In veterinary medicine we tend to use the term *kilocalories*, defined as the unit of energy of 1000 cal or 1 large calorie.

A cat or dog's daily energy requirements are calculated using maintenance energy requirement (MER). MER is the daily energy (kilocalorie) requirements needed to support an animal over time (Hand et al. 2010). Resting energy requirement (RER) is the energy needed to support an animal's metabolism just while existing: lying in a cage without exerting any additional energy aside from breathing, eating, drinking, voiding, and sleeping (Hand et al. 2010). MER uses RER as the baseline caloric need and then adjusts that need depending on their size and activity level. The MER is highly dependent on the species, age, sex, altered versus intact, activity level, gestation, and lactation (Wynn 2010).

There are numerous equations and online calculators available to calculate a pet's MER. I typically utilize the energy calculator on the Veterinary Information Network (VIN) and the formulas provided in the 5th edition of *Small Animal Clinical Nutrition* and in *Nutrient Requirements of Dogs and Cats*. Please refer to one of these sources for the MER and RER equations.

Ingredient Proportions The amount of protein, fat, and carbohydrates comprising the diet is dependent on the species, age, lifestyle, and health status. Based on the 2014 AAFCO nutrient profiles a healthy dog/cat should have a minimum of 18%/26% protein and 5.5%/9% fat on a dry matter basis (AAFCO 2014). AAFCO and the National Research Council (NRC) do not provide a recommended minimum carbohydrate amount for cat and dog food (NRC 2006; AAFCO 2014).

When designing a CFT recipe these proportions are broken down into protein, carbohydrate, and vegetable categories based on a percentage of the total calories not dry matter. Fruit generally encompass 0–5% of the vegetable portion of the diet. Additional oils may be added and the caloric requirements are often taken from the carbohydrate or protein portion of the diet. Table 2.26 provides example protein, grain, and vegetable ratios for potential home-cooked diets. Once the veterinarian has determined the ingredient proportions and ingredient list the MER is used to calculate the exact amounts of each food needed.

Table 2.26 Examples of potential ingredient proportions for a variety of home-cooked diets for cats and dogs (Feuer 2006a,b; Rimar 2015).

		Protein (%)	Carbohydrates (%)	Vegetables (%)
Canine	Allergies	20–50	0–60	20–50
	Cancer	50	20	30
	Diabetes	33	33	33
	Growth	25–33	25–33	25–33
	Healthy	50–75	15–25	10–15
	Liver disease	33	33	33
	Kidney disease	20–25	50–60	20–25
	Obesity	25–33	33–37.5	25–33
Feline	Allergies	90	0	10
	Cancer	90	0	10
	Diabetes	90	0	10
	Growth	90–100	0–5	0–5
	Healthy	75–80	10–15	3–5
	Liver disease	90	0	10
	Kidney disease	60	20	20
	Obesity	90	0	10

Source: Lisa P. McFaddin.

An Example of Recipe Portion Calculations

Signalment: Three-year-old male neutered mix breed dog
Weight: 22 lbs = 10 kg
Body condition score: Good (5/9)
MER: 630 kcal/day
Proposed ingredient proportions: 60% protein, 20% carbohydrates, and 20% vegetables
Ingredients chosen: Beef, brown rice, zucchini, broccoli

Ingredient quantities

- Beef (95% lean ground, cooked): 180 g = 308 kcal
- Brown rice (long grain, cooked): 85 g = 94 kcal
- Zucchini (cooked): 200 g = 32 kcal
- Broccoli (cooked): 200 g = 75 kcal
- Corn oil: 14 g = 120 kcal

Notes

- This would be the total amount of food per day and should be divided into at least two meals.
- This is not a balanced diet without the addition of supplements.
- http://CalorieKing.com was used to calculate the calories for each food item.

Balancing the Diet A balanced diet is imperative if fed for more than one to two weeks. A multitude of disease conditions can result from the chronic consumption of poor diets. Essential dietary nutrients, vitamins, and minerals include calcium, chlorine, choline, copper, essential amino acids, folic acid, iodine, iron, magnesium, manganese, niacin, pantothenic acid, potassium, riboflavin, selenium, sodium, vitamin A, vitamin B1, vitamin B6, vitamin B12, vitamin D, vitamin E, vitamin K, and zinc. The functions and diseases associated with deficiencies for three essential dietary nutrients are described in Table 2.27.

Table 2.27 The function and disease conditions, due to over- or under-consumption, associated with three essential dietary nutrients, vitamins, and minerals (Feuer 2006a,b; Hand et al. 2010).

Calcium	Functions	Bone and teeth health; coagulation; nerve signal transmission; muscle contraction; cell signaling
	Deficiency conditions	Nutritional secondary hyperparathyroidism; osteopenia; skeletal abnormalities
	Excess conditions	Skeletal abnormalities, especially in growing animals
Chlorine	Functions	Acid–base balance; cellular health and function
	Deficiency conditions	Poor weight gain and weakness in puppies and kittens
Choline	Functions	Component of phospholipid cell membranes
	Deficiency conditions	Weight loss; hepatic lipidosis
Copper	Functions	Connective tissue production; iron metabolism; red blood cell production; myelin production; protects against oxidative damage; melanin production
	Deficiency conditions	Loss of hair pigmentation in puppies and kittens; anemia
Essential fatty acids	Functions	Protein synthesis
		Amino acids dogs and cats cannot make: arginine, histidine, isoleucine, leucine, lysine, methionine, phanylalanine, threonine, tryptophan, valine, and taurine (cats only)
	Deficiency conditions	Inappetance; poor growth; weight loss; hair changes; compromised immune system; fertility problems; other signs dependent on the missing amino acid
		Taurine-specific problems: retinal degeneration; blindness; deafness; cardiomyopathy; heart failure; compromised immune system; fertility problems; congenital defects; poor neonatal growth
Folic acid	Functions	Metabolism of amino acids and nucleotides; synthesis of mitochondrial proteins
	Deficiency conditions	Weight loss; anemia due to reduced hemoglobin concentrations

Iodine	Functions	Thyroid hormone production; puppy and kitten growth and development; metabolism regulation
	Deficiency conditions	Goiter; poor hair coat; weight gain
	Excess conditions	Epiphora; ptyalism; nasal discharge; dandruff
Iron	Functions	Red blood cell production; energy metabolism
	Deficiency conditions	Poor growth; anemia; lethargy; weakness; diarrhea
	Excess conditions	Gastrointestinal signs; tissue damage
Magnesium	Functions	Enzyme; muscle and nerve cell integrity; endocrine system function; bone and teeth health
	Deficiency conditions	Poor weight gain; irritability; convulsions; carpal joint hyperextension; hindlimb paralysis
Manganese	Functions	Enzyme; bone health; neurologic health
	Deficiency conditions	None reported
Niacin	Functions	Enzyme
	Deficiency conditions	Anorexia; weight loss; facial inflammation; ptyalism; bloody stool
	Excess conditions	Bloody stools; convulsions
Pantothenic acid	Functions	Energy metabolism
	Deficiency conditions	Coma; tachypnea; tachycardia; convulsions; gastrointestinal distress; compromised immune system
Phosphorus	Functions	Skeletal structure; DNA and RNA structure; energy metabolism; motor control; acid–base balance
	Deficiency conditions	Poor weight gain; inappetance; distal limb skeletal malformations in puppies
Potassium	Functions	Acid–base balance; nerve signal transmission; enzyme function
	Deficiency conditions	Poor weight gain and growth in puppies and kittens; cervical muscle paralysis; hindlimb weakness
Riboflavin	Functions	Enzyme
	Deficiency conditions	Anorexia; weight loss; muscle weakness; dermatitis; eye lesions
Selenium	Functions	Protection from oxidative damage; immune system health
	Deficiency conditions	Anorexia; depression; difficulty breathing; coma; muscle loss
Sodium	Functions	Acid–base balance; blood pressure regulation; nerve health
	Deficiency conditions	Restlessness; tachycardia; polydipsia

(Continued)

Table 2.27 (Continued)

Vitamin A	Functions	Vision; growth; immune health; fetal development; cellular health
	Deficiency conditions	Anorexia; weight loss; ataxia; ocular disorders; skin lesions; respiratory disorders; compromised immune system
	Excess conditions	Bone and blood vessel changes; dehydration; neurologic changes; joint pain
Vitamin B1 (thiamin)	Functions	Responsible for energy and carbohydrate metabolism; activation of ion channels in neuronal tissue
	Deficiency conditions	Failure to grow; weight loss; neurologic deficiencies in puppies and kittens; nervous and cardiovascular system damage in adult dogs
Vitamin B6	Functions	Glucose production; red blood cell function; synthesis of niacin; supports the nervous, immune, and endocrine systems; gene expression
	Deficiency conditions	Anorexia; weight loss (especially in puppies and kittens); poor muscular control and weakness; anemia in adults
	Excess conditions	Poor motor control; weakness
Vitamin B12	Functions	Enzyme
	Deficiency conditions	Inappetance; compromised immune system; anemia; bone marrow changes
Vitamin D	Functions	Calcium and phosphorus balance
	Deficiency conditions	Rickets; lethargy; muscle loss; boney changes
	Excess conditions	Anorexia; weakness; gastrointestinal signs; soft tissue calcification; dehydration; bone density changes; hair changes; muscle loss
Vitamin E	Functions	Protects against oxidative damage
	Deficiency conditions	Loss of skeletal muscle; fertility issues; retinal degeneration
Vitamin K	Functions	Activated clotting factors and other proteins
	Deficiency conditions	None reported
Zinc	Functions	Enzyme functions; cell replication; protein and carbohydrate metabolism; skin health; wound healing
	Deficiency conditions	Poor weight gain; vomiting; skin lesions

Source: Lisa P. McFaddin.

We should also mention the current FDA investigation into a possible link between certain diets, predominantly those containing legumes and white potatoes, and an increased risk for the development of dilated cardiomyopathy (DCM) in non-predisposed canines (FDA 2019). Initially the concern centered on grain-free and pulse-rich diets (called non-traditional diets), but updated findings in June 2019 revealed that both commercial and home-made diets with and without grain have been implicated (FDA 2019). Pulses are a legume subgroup comprising peas, lentils, chickpeas, and dry beans that are harvested as a dry crop and contain low lipid levels (Marinangeli et al. 2017). Pulses have been used as ingredients in dog and cat food for over 20 years (Butterwick et al. 1994).

Clinicians and researchers within the veterinary community are still debating the cause for the increased incidence of DCM in non-predisposed breeds. Multiple papers have suggested taurine deficiency is responsible, due to poor absorption or increased excretion (Kaplan et al. 2018; Ontiveros et al. 2020). Additionally, some dogs diagnosed with DCM fed non-traditional diets demonstrated significant improvement in cardiac function once the diet was changed to a traditional feed (Freid et al. 2021). Other reviews and studies suggest taurine deficiency is not the cause (Mansilla et al. 2019; Donadelli et al. 2020; McCauley et al. 2020). Unfortunately, currently there appear to be more questions than answers.

The risk of developing dietary-related DCM should never be taken lightly. The risk still appears to be low when comparing the number of documented cases with the sheer number of companion dogs. The veterinarian should talk openly and honestly with the client about the potential risks associated with DCM development. Consultation with your local veterinary cardiologist, nutritionist, and state veterinary medical association may be advisable to ensure consistent, accurate, and timely information is provided to the owners.

Home-cooked meals often require supplementation with at least calcium and potentially a multivitamin. The type of supplement chosen is dependent on the patient's condition and practitioner's preference. The dosage is dependent on the diet chosen and patient's size. An in-depth discussion concerning available supplements is beyond the scope of this chapter but is discussed in more detail in Chapter 4.

There are numerous resources available to assist with recipe building and balancing.

Excellent reference texts include *Applied Veterinary Clinical Nutrition*, *Clinical Nutrition: Veterinary Clinics of North America Small Animal Practice*, *Nutrient Requirements of Dogs and Cats*, and *Small Animal Clinical Nutrition*, 5th edition. Suggested online sources include the American College of Veterinary Nutrition (ACVN), BalanceIT, NutriBase, and PetDiets.

The Why

Applications in Human Medicine

The National Institutes of Health Center for Complementary and Integrative Medicine does not specifically mention CFT as a treatment modality when discussing traditional Chinese medicine.

Studying food therapy is challenging in both human and veterinary medicine. Ensuring standardization of the recipes, food sourcing, and food preparation is difficult. Studies must also account for food intolerances and allergies, which may require substitutions. The concurrent use of pharmaceutical, nutraceuticals, or herbal products may affect food digestion and absorption. Conducting randomized controlled trials is difficult. Conducting blinded studies is extremely difficult, if not impossible. People tend to look at what they are eating, unless blindfolded, but even then they can taste different food substances.

There are limited studies in English pertaining to the use of CFT in human medicine. Kaminogawa and Nanno (2004) used literature reviews to outline the beneficial effects of food on the immune system. Shen et al. (2010) conducted a randomized controlled trial demonstrating the effectiveness of CFT in reducing blood pressure and treating Yin deficiency in 85 hypertensive patients. A subsequent literature review further supported the use of CFT in the management of hypertension (Zou 2016). Another literature review endorsed the use of CFT in the management of unregulated diabetes mellitus (Wong 2016).

Arjmandi et al. (2017) concluded the consumption of dried plum for one year by post-menopausal women improved their bone mineral density compared to a control group. The beneficial effects were maintained five years after completion of the study. A systematic literature review was also used to highlight the usefulness of CFT in the treatment of functional dyspepsia and irritable bowel syndrome in Sinosphere Asia (Chu et al. 2018).

Applications in Veterinary Medicine

Studies investigating the applications and benefits of CFT are extremely rare. Veterinary CFT recommendations are predominantly based on unpublished and published case studies, anecdotal evidence, and extrapolation from human medicine. CFT is commonly used in veterinary medicine to aid in the treatment of cancer, cardiovascular diseases, chronic inflammation, dermatologic disorders, endocrine dysfunction, gastrointestinal disorders, general health maintenance, geriatric patients, kidney disorders, and liver diseases (Clemmons 2015; DiNatale 2015; Rimar 2015; Xie 2015).

Veterinary Research

Currently, there are no veterinary-specific CFT studies in English. There are numerous studies in veterinary nutrition explaining the importance of species- and lifestyle-appropriate nutrition, but these articles focus on commercial diets and/or approaching nutrition from a Western medicine perspective. The lack of scientific evidence does not negate the therapeutic benefit of CFT but highlights the importance of appropriately studying this treatment modality in the future. Table 2.28 lists examples of current nutritional research in veterinary medicine.

The How

Team Members

This section reviews the potential return on investment (ROI), how to effectively train the entire team, how to promote CFT, and how to integrate the CFT.

Return on Investment

ROI can be determined by evaluating client interest, veterinarian demand, hospital costs, applicability of the service, appointment scheduling, and pricing.

Client Interest

As of February 2023, there are no studies documenting client interest or the popularity of TCVM, including CFT. We can infer veterinary client interested by looking at client opinion, demographic assessments, pet health insurance trends, and veterinary training program availability.

Client Opinion The sheer number of dietary options and plans available highlight how much people care about what they eat: gluten free, grain free, low carb, keto, South Beach diet, the Zone diet, the Blood Type diet, Atkins, raw diet, vegetarian, vegan, low histamine, FODMAP (fermentable oligosaccharides, disaccharides, monosaccharides, and polyols), anti-inflammatory diet, legume free, dairy free, and nut free to name a few. The sheer number of "specialized" diets showcases the interest humans have in modifying their diet to improve their own health. Whether people realize this or not, changing your diet to improve your physical and mental health is a form of food therapy.

The World Health Organization (WHO) included details about TCM for the first time in the 11th revision of their global compendium, the International Statistical Classification of Diseases and Related Health Problems (ICD), in August

Table 2.28 Examples of studies demonstrating the efficacy of veterinary food therapy in the management of health and disease conditions as of January 2023.

System category	Disease conditions studied	Studies
Cardiovascular	General support	Stoeckel et al. (2011)
	Taurine and cardiomyopathy	Kaplan et al. (2018), Donadelli et al. (2020), and Freid et al. (2021)
Dermatology	Atopic dermatitis	Stoeckel et al. (2011) and van Beeck et al. (2015)
Cancer	General support	Stoeckel et al. (2011) and Heinze et al. (2012)
Endocrinology	Glycemic control	Teixeira et al. (2018, 2019)
General health	Feline	Zoran and Buffington (2011), Allaway et al. (2018), and Donadelli and Aldrich (2019)
	Post-alteration	Spofford et al. (2014) and Vendramini et al. (2020)
	Puppy growth and development	Wang et al. (2017)
Hematology	Red blood cell stability	Stoeckel et al. (2011) and Anturaniemi et al. (2020)
Nephrology	Renal health	Geddes et al. (2016), Dobenecker et al. (2017), and Alexander et al. (2019)
Ophthalmology	Retinal health	Wang et al. (2016)
Urogenital	Urolithiasis	Dijcker et al. (2014)
	Feline idiopathic cystitis	Naarden and Corbee (2019)

Source: Lisa P. McFaddin.

2018 (WHO 2018). The purpose of the ICD is to influence the medical practices and standards for more than 100 countries (Cyranoski 2018). WHO's recognition of the viability of TCM reflects the public's growing interest in alternative and integrative therapies for their own health.

Demographic Assessments Millennials are now the predominant pet–parent demographic. Between 2007 and 2015 one in three US pet owners were classified as millennials, and their generation was responsible for 43% of the growth in the number of pet owners (Miller 2017). Millennials tend to be very health conscious with respect to themselves and their pets, helping drive the trend toward natural and organic pet food. The 2016 Packaged Facts' National Online Consumer Survey revealed 69% of millennial pet owners were more likely to purchase pet food advertising "natural" ingredients, and 75% of millennial dog owners believe pet food safety is paramount when considering which brands to purchase (Miller 2017).

This trend was further supported by a 2016 study which surveyed 3562 US and French pet owners with at least one dog or cat (Nielsen 2016). The owners were more likely to purchase a pet food if the product was labeled as non-genetically modified; the product was labeled as organic; the product was perceived to be "natural"; the product was perceived to be manufactured in a kitchen setting instead of a laboratory; the product was labeled as nutrient enhanced and/or the formulation was different (stew, freeze-dried, dehydrated, etc.); and the product contained unusual flavors or descriptors of common ingredients, for example "chicken tandoori" rather than "chicken" (Nielsen 2016).

A study conducted by Conway and Saker (2018) reinforced clients' desire to make informed decisions about their pet's food. Preexisting opinions could be changed with proper education (Conway and Saker 2018). Clients also showed a propensity for feeding their pets food obtained from sustainable and environmentally friendly sources (Conway and Saker 2018).

According to the 2021–2022 American Pet Products Association (APPA) National Pet Owners Survey, 63.4 million households in the United States own at least one dog while 42.7 million own at least one cat (APPA 2021). During the 2019 calendar year Americans spent \$38.4 billion on pet food and treats, including dogs, cats, exotic species, horses, and fish, and \$42 billion in 2020 (APPA 2021). The APPA estimates pet owners will spend \$44.1 billion on pet food and treats in 2021.

In 2020 the average dog and cat owner spent at least \$368 and \$326, respectively, on pet food and treats per companion animal (APPA 2021). In contrast the APPA estimated pet owners spent at least \$700 and \$379 annually on routine and surgical canine and feline veterinary visits, respectively.

Key Demographic Take Aways

- Millennials are the primary companion animal owners.
- Millennials are interested in providing the best nutrition possible for their pet.
- Pet owners want to be educated and involved in selecting their pet's diet.
- People are willing to spend money on their pet's food.

Pet Health Insurance The 2022 North American Pet Health Insurance Association (NAPHIA) survey found 4.41 million pets in the United States had pet insurance, a greater than 57% increase in five years (NAPHIA 2023).

Many pet insurance plans include coverage for integrative therapies, especially acupuncture (Woodley 2018). The presence of this type of coverage re-emphasizes the mainstream incorporation of these treatment modalities, as well as reflecting client demand.

Veterinarian Demand

The upsurge of pet owners interested in integrative therapy, coupled with the shortage of veterinarians, means there is definitely a need for more integrative practitioners (see the Introduction at the beginning of the book for further information on this topic).

The Chi University advertises 7500 graduates since 1998. If we assume 50% of those graduates undertook the CFT training, ignoring those who may not practice in the United States, that is roughly 3700 veterinarians training in CFT. This represents around 2% of the total veterinarian population.

The 2018 American Veterinary Medical Association (AVMA) Pet Ownership and Demographics Sourcebook states that 57% of American households owned pets at the end of 2016, with 76.8 million dogs and 58.4 million cats (AVMA 2018). Using the statistics from the Michelson Found Animals Foundation 2019 Pet Trends survey, if 68% of pet owners are interested in alternative treatments there are up to 52.2 million dogs and 39.7 million cats whose owners are willing to pursue integrative therapy (MFAF 2018). With these numbers I would say there is definitely room for more practitioners.

The Nutrition issue of *Veterinary Clinics of North America Small Animal Practice* had an entire chapter dedicated to advising veterinarians on how to assess the nutritional validity of alternative diets and how to properly discuss these dietary options with clients (Parr and Remillard 2014). The authors recommend veterinarians improve their nutritional knowledge base and offer client nutritional consultations to remain competitive as client involvement in their pet's dietary choices rise. These recommendations reinforce the need for trained veterinarians who can safely and effectively advise their clients regarding proper nutrition, whether that be commercial bought or home-cooked.

Another way to examine the need in your specific area is to compare the number of general practitioners within a 5-, 10-, or 20-mile radius to the number of veterinarians advertising CFT. The search radius is dependent on your hospital's demographics. Most comparisons tend to follow the 5% trend, meaning no more than 5% of the surrounding hospitals are currently offering CFT. Ensuring your area is not saturated prevents the introduction of a redundant service.

Hospital Costs

Let's start by reviewing all the potential costs associated with introducing and offering CFT: veterinarian training, staff training, supplies and equipment, staffing, facilities, and advertising. Table 2.29 through demonstrate Table 2.31 the different potential start-up costs, primarily dependent on the hospital's contribution toward the veterinarian's training and prior utilization of regular all-staff meetings. For more information on potential hospital costs refer to the Introduction chapter of this book.

Veterinarian Training

Course Cost Currently, there is only one organization in the United States offering a training program in CFT. The program can be completed online or as a hybrid online and on-site. The on-site portion lasts two days. Additional information can be found in the Veterinarians section of this chapter. The cost is $1500, as of February 2023.

Textbooks Textbooks may not be required for the course but are often highly recommended. The average cost ($250) is based on a two-book requirement as of February 2023.

Travel Expenses The value provided reflects the total travel expenses based on one on-site session with three full days of training. Here is a breakdown of the costs:

- *Airfare*: As of February 2023 the average roundtrip domestic flight within the United States is $412 (BLS 2023; Trcek 2023) (total cost, $412).
- *Lodging*: As of February 2023 the federal per diem rate for lodging on business trips is $98 per night (FederalPay.org 2023). The federal per diem rate was used for calculations, with

Table 2.29 Total potential hospital start-up costs for Chinese food therapy as of February 2023.

Category	Subcategories	Projected cost	
Veterinarian training	Course cost	$1500	
	Textbooks	$250	
	Travel expenses	$0–1377	
	Time-off	$0	
Staff training	Variable	$230–1295	
Supplies	None	$0	
Staffing	Variable	$230–1396	
Facilities	Overhead	$2–5/minute per 30–60-minute appointment	$60–300 per patient
Advertising	Variable	≤$538	

Source: Lisa P. McFaddin.

three nights of lodging for one session (total cost, $294).

- *Car rental*: Unfortunately the price of car rentals skyrocketed following the pandemic. As of January 2023, the average weekly car rental price is $551 (French and Kemmis 2023). Rideshare and cabbing are extremely popular, but the variability in travel distances makes calculating an average cost impractical. It is suspected this cost would be comparable, if not lower, than that of a rental car (total cost, $551).
- *Meals*: The federal per diem rate for business trip meals from October 2022 through September 2023 is $59 a day (FederalPay. org 2023). Most training programs provide at least one meal, as well as snacks. Meal expenditure is estimated to be $40/day for a total of three days (total cost, $120).
- *Time off*: Veterinarian paid time-off (PTO) for on-site courses only factors in as an added expense if additional PTO is provided outside of their contractual annual PTO. Clinics offer an average of 4.1 paid continuing education (CE) days per year (AAHA 2019). Allowing the veterinarian to use CE days for the on-site courses would not "cost" the hospital anything additional. There is also no additional cost if the hospital requires the veterinarian use their PTO for the on-site training.

Staff Training Team training expenses are highly variable and dependent on the preexistence of staff meetings and use of a staff meeting for training (compared to self-study). Refer to the Introduction at the beginning of the book for a breakdown of these variables (cost range, $230–1295).

Supplies No supplies are required.

Staffing Integrative appointments range from 30 to 60 minutes depending on the condition(s) being treated. Following the American Animal Hospital Association (AAHA) recommendations, a veterinary assistant or licensed technician (VA/LT) should always restrain patients for physical examinations and procedures. A VA/LT is usually required for 15–20 minutes. Support staff assistance is not required while discussing plans with the client, so there is no difference in staffing cost for CFT appointments compared to traditional appointments.

Facilities The costs needed to keep the doors open (aka overhead). This includes rent or mortgage, utilities, administrative costs, and often employee costs (aka staffing) divided by the minutes the practice is open (Stevenson 2016). The price per minute equals the amount of revenue needed just to break even. Overhead is extremely hospital specific, but the range tends to be $2–5/minute. The low end of the range provided in Table 2.29 represents the cost for a 30-minute appointment at a clinic with a $2/minute overhead, while the high end represents the cost for a 60-minute appointment at a clinic with a $5/minute overhead.

Designating a specific room, in a multi-exam room hospital, for integrative appointments minimizes the chances other associates will need the room for their appointments. However, there is then an added expense for designing the room and potential lost revenue if the room is not used regularly. The absence of a designated room theoretically reduces redecoration costs, but this can be disruptive for appointment flow if the appointment exceeds the scheduled time.

Advertising There are numerous ways to advertise a new service. On average veterinary hospitals spend 0.7% of revenue on promotion and advertisement (AVMA 2019). Most of the advertisement can be done with little to no additional expenditure. The national median gross revenue for companion animal practices was $1.2 million in 2022 (AVMA 2023). Advertising costs are calculated assuming no more than 5% of the current advertising budget

Table 2.30 Projected CFT start-up costs for six potential hospital scenarios, with varying hospital contributions toward veterinary certification and staff training, as of February 2023. The cost of veterinarian training is based on the averages presented Table 2.29. Staff training costs assume a 1.5-hour long all-staff meeting, using national averages for employee numbers: eight non-DVMs and two DVMs (AVMA 2019, 2023). The cost of office supplies and lunch as estimated based on 10 employees attending the meeting. The overhead is based on an average of $3.5/minute. Missed revenue is calculated using the 2022 national mean revenue per hour for companion animal practices ($567/hour) (AVMA 2023). Advertising includes printed materials, digital advertisement, and community engagement.

Category	Projected expenses	Ex. 1	Ex. 2	Ex. 3	Ex. 4	Ex. 5	Ex. 6
Veterinarian training	Average course cost	$1500	$1500	n/a	$1500	$1500	n/a
	Average textbooks	$250	n/a	n/a	$200	n/a	n/a
	Travel expenses	$1377	n/a	n/a	$945	n/a	n/a
Staff training	Office supplies	$30	$30	$30	$20	$20	$20
	Lunch	$200	$200	$200	$200	$200	$200
	Overhead	$315	$315	$315	n/a	n/a	n/a
	Missed revenue	$851	$851	$851	n/a	n/a	n/a
Supplies	None required	n/a	n/a	n/a	n/a	n/a	n/a
Advertising		$420	$420	$420	$420	$420	$420
Total		$4943.00	$3316.00	$1816.00	$3285.00	$2140.00	$640.00

Source: Lisa P. McFaddin.

Table 2.31 Hospital costs per patient for 30- and 60-minute CFT appointments as of February 2023. Factors affecting hospital cost are divided into veterinarian certification (start-up cost) and overhead costs. Amortization is based on the veterinarian seeing 952 integrative patients in two years. Overhead was calculated using $3.5/minute. Multiple examples are provided with the variance determined by the total cost within each category. The total is rounded to the nearest whole number.

Category	Projected expenses	Ex. 1	Ex. 2	Ex. 3	Ex. 4	Ex. 5	Ex. 6
Hospital costs	Table 2.30 totals	$4960	$3333	$1833	$3403	$2258	$758
	Amortization schedule per patient	$5.19	$3.48	$1.91	$3.45	$2.25	$0.67
Overhead	30-minute appointment	$52.50	$52.50	$52.50	n/a	n/a	n/a
	60-minute appointment	n/a	n/a	n/a	$105	$105	$105
Total		**$58**	**$56**	**$54**	**$108**	**$107**	**$106**

Source: adapted from Stevenson (2016).

would be used for promotion of the new service (estimated maximal cost, $420).

Start-Up Costs Table 2.29 summarizes projected start-up costs for CFT. Table 2.30 calculates potential start-up costs based on the degree of hospital contribution toward veterinarian and staff training. Different scenarios are presented in which the hospital covers all, some, or none of the expenses.

Applicability
As stated earlier, CFT is versatile and beneficial for numerous conditions and ailments. As the clinician becomes more comfortable and confident in their CFT skills the variety of cases for which CFT is recommended increases.

Appointment Scheduling
There are four main factors to consider when planning integrative appointment protocols: appointment length; support staff availability; exam room availability; and follow-up appointment scheduling.

The initial integrative appointment is longer compared to follow-up appointments, often 60 minutes. Follow-up appointments should be scheduled for 30–50 minutes depending on the patient and if additional treatments are performed.

Keep the appointment positive. You want to pet to enjoy the experience. A relaxed pet is more easily adjusted. Avoid ancillary procedures which may cause stress: nail trims, anal gland expression, sanitary trims, anything with the ears, etc.

Another issue to consider is whether the hospital will schedule CFT appointments separately from traditional Western appointments or increase the appointment length. Additional information on appointment scheduling can be found in the Introduction at tnhe beginning of this book.

Pricing
An in-depth look into appointment pricing can be found in the Introduction. Here we discuss two pricing methods: current market fees and hospital cost-based pricing.

Current Market Fees There are no studies examining the average cost of veterinary integrative appointments. In general clinicians practicing CFT also offer acupuncture and/or Chinese herbal medicine, so one could apply the average cost of acupuncture appointments to all integrative appointment costs.

A study of five general practices within central Florida found the price of acupuncture appointments ranged from $45 to $150, with a mean of $95.80 (Marks and Shmalberg 2015; Shmalberg 2016). The average length of these appointments was 47 minutes. According to the Nationwide® Purdue 2019 Veterinary Price Index, veterinary pricing increased by 21.1% between the end of 2014 and the end of 2018 (Purdue University 2019). Presuming services continued to increase by at least 5% annually, a 50-minute session would translate to $130 by January 2023.

Hospital Cost-Based Pricing   Table 2.31 outlines the hospital cost per patient for 30- and 60-minute integrative appointments. The veterinarian training amortization per patient was calculated using the assumptions listed in Chapter 1.

The formula for determining service fees is quite simple: Service Fee = Hospital Cost + Profit. The big question becomes how much profit? Table 2.32 illustrates the potential fee for integrative appointments based on hospital cost and variable markup percentages. It becomes readily apparent that the lower the hospital contribution, the higher the comparative profit.

Additional Considerations   Most of my patients receive other treatments or diagnostics when they come in for their treatments. Frequently we adjust current medication regimens, run diagnostics (blood work, urinalysis, radiographs, etc.), discuss dietary and environmental modifications, and discuss nutrition and nutraceuticals, all of which increases revenue, average transaction charge (ATC), and DVM revenue per hour.

Offering integrative medicine also helps improve current client retention and drives new client acquisition. Marks and Shmalberg (2015) found 29% of new acupuncture and integrative patients returned for wellness and other services. Improving client retention and new client acquisition helps drive revenue.

Team Training

The concept of phase training is used when introducing acupuncture to the hospital team. A multi-media approach is used to assist with the training program (see Table 2.33 for information).

Practice Manager's Role

To conquer this task the practice manager needs his or her own checklist which includes the following information:

- Schedule a date and time for the team training.

Table 2.32   Potential CFT appointment pricing using hospital cost at varying percentage markups as of February 2023. Examples 1–3 represent 30-minute appointments, while examples 4–6 represent 60-minute appointments.

Category	Projected expenses	Ex. 1	Ex. 2	Ex. 3	Ex. 4	Ex. 5	Ex. 6
Hospital cost per patient	(Nearest whole number)	$58	$536	$54	$108	$107	$106
Appointment price	40% Markup	$81	$750	$76	$151	$150	$148
	50% Markup	$87	$804	$81	$162	$161	$159
	60% Markup	$93	$112	$86	$173	$118	$111
	70% Markup	$99	$911	$92	$184	$182	$180
	80% Markup	$104	$965	$97	$194	$193	$191
	90% Markup	$110	$1018	$103	$205	$203	$201
	100% Markup	$116	$1072	$108	$216	$214	$212

Source: Lisa P. McFaddin.

Table 2.33 The breakdown of CFT phase training steps and resources for the entire hospital team.

Phase 1: Background information	
Team training guide	The handout walks the practice manager and/or veterinarian through Phase 1 of the training
	A downloadable and editable copy of the handout is located on the companion website
Training presentation	The video covers background information on the modality
	PowerPoints can be downloaded, edited, and personalized from the companion website
	The document can be used as a PowerPoint or saved as an mp4 creating a personalized movie
Team training handout	The handout provides additional background information for the CSRs, VAs, and LTs to complement the knowledge gained from watching the training presentation
	A downloadable and editable copy of the handout is located on the companion website
Phase 2: Knowledge proficiency	
Quiz	A short quiz to ensure all team members have a good understanding of the service being offered
	A downloadable and editable copy of the handout is located on the companion website
	A key is provided
Phase 3: Expectations	
Training worksheets	A training checklist is provided for CSRs and VA/LTs with role-specific expectations and tasks for each staff member
	A recommended completion time is provided
	A downloadable and editable copy of the handout is located on the companion website
Phase 4: Client education	
Client scripts	Bullet point information and scripted examples used when discussing the therapy with clients
	A downloadable and editable copy of the handout is located on the companion website
Client education presentation	A short (five to seven minute) client educational video about the therapeutic modality
	PowerPoints can be downloaded, edited, and personalized from the companion website
	The document can be used as a PowerPoint or saved as an mp4 creating a personalized movie
Client education handout	An informational handout about the therapeutic modality written specifically for clients
	A downloadable and editable copy of the handout is located on the companion website

CSR, customer service representative; VA, veterinary assistant; LT, licensed technician. Source: Lisa P. McFaddin.

- Ensure all information pertaining to the new service is reviewed with the staff.
- Confirm all team members have completed the training.
- Certify all team members understand the information and can successfully educate clients.

Promotion

There are six common avenues of promotion for a veterinary integrative medicine (VIM) service: hospital website, social media, email blasts, mailers, in-hospital promotions, and client education.

Hospital Website

Advertise "Veterinary Chinese Food Therapy" in several locations on the website. Check out AAHA's Publicity Toolbox, available free of charge to AAHA accredited hospitals, for client consent forms when discussing specific patients and using their photographs. On the made page insert "Now offering veterinary Chinese food therapy" with a link to success stories or client testimonials. Utilize the hospital website to advertise the VIM treatment under the "Services" section. Veterinarian biographs should include a description of the specialized training and professional initials. Create a veterinary CFT blog page discussing patient success stories.

Social Media

Utilize Facebook, Instagram, and/or Twitter to post facts, photographs, hashtags, and patient success stories. Include fun and intriguing facts about CFT. People love pictures of their pets and food, so combining the two is sure to increase views. Create or utilize CFT-specific hashtags.

Email Blasts

Send fun mass emails to your clients introducing veterinary CFT. Consider monthly case presentations illustrating how the service has benefited patients. Almost everyone has at least one email address these days. Customer service representatives should be amassing client emails at the same rate as phone numbers.

Mailers

Mailers can be expensive and are largely unnecessary in this digital age. Mailers can be used to announce the introduction of CFT to existing clients. The mailer should include the name of the new service, a brief description of how veterinary CFT can help pet patients, the name of the doctor, with their new initials, a brief description of the training the doctor received, and possibly a few photographs of home-made pet meals.

In-Hospital Promotions

Advertise veterinary CFT within the hospital using small promotional signs, informational signs, invoice teasers, and staff buttons. Small promotional signs can be placed in the waiting room and exam rooms. Include photographs of pets and their home-made meals. Consider catchphrases such as "Food is Medicine" or "You are what you eat."

Informational signs should also include a brief description of how CFT can help pet patients, name of the doctor certified in CFT, and a brief description of the training the doctor has received.

Invoice teasers should consist of short phrases reminding and enticing owners regarding a new service offered at the practice. Examples include "Now offering Veterinary Chinese Food Therapy"; "Curious if Chinese Food Therapy can help your pet?"; "Introducing Veterinary Chinese Food Therapy"; and "Would your pet benefit from veterinary Chinese Food Therapy?"

Buttons can be made for the staff to wear with kitchy phrases reminding owners, in a fun way, of the new VIM service. Examples include "Food is medicine" and "Want to learn more about veterinary Chinese Food Therapy?"

Client Education

Education is crucial to understanding the purpose and importance of any given treatment.

The client handouts and videos solidify pet owner knowledge base, reducing concerns and conveying value. A study by Oliveira et al. (2014) highlighted the importance of owner compliance when feeding home-made diets. Poor compliance can lead to malnutrition and vitamin/mineral deficiencies. In a survey of 46 owners feeding a home-made diet formulated by a veterinary nutritionist for at least six months, 30.4% of the owners modified the diets without the nutritionist's knowledge, 40% did not monitor the ingredient quantities, 73.9% did not use the recommended amount of soybean oil and salt, and 34.8% did not use the recommended vitamins and supplements correctly; 76.1% of the owners did report the recipes were easy to prepare. Over half (56.5%) of the owners stated their dogs would not eat the recommended diet.

Integration

The key components for proper integration include availability of the service to the right patients; appropriate patient scheduling; appropriate support staff scheduling; and staff buy-in (understanding the benefits of the offered service).

Veterinarians

There are several factors to consider when veterinarians prepare to incorporate CFT into their clinical repertoire: state requirements and restrictions, return on investment, course availability, veterinary organizations, and continuing education.

State Requirements and Restrictions
Is CFT Considered the Practice of Veterinary Medicine?
Each state has its own veterinary provisions outlining what is and is not considered the practice of veterinary medicine. Currently no state specifically defines CFT as the practice of veterinary medicine. Keep in mind that advice provided by a veterinarian regarding animal nutrition is typically considered the practice of

veterinary medicine. These rules can change, and careful review of your specific state requirements is recommended.

Does CFT Continuing Education Count toward Licensure Continuing Education Requirements?
Currently no states require specific CE hours for veterinarians offering CFT nor do they specifically reference CFT CE. Some states limit the use of integrative medicine CE hours toward the annual CE requirement for license renewal. Most states permit the use of integrative CE if the lectures or webinars are performed by an approved provider. Review your specific state's requirements for further details. Table 1.14 in Chapter 1 lists each state's CE requirements and provides links for their board of veterinary medicine on the companion website.

Are Your Assets Covered?
Check with your liability insurance to determine if you are covered when practicing CFT. Refer to the Introduction at the beginning of this book for additional information.

Return on Investment
Specifics are discussed in the Team Members section of this chapter.

Course Availability
Formal training and certification in veterinary CFT is not required but highly encouraged, given the complexity of TCVM and CFT and the risk of disease development if pets are fed poorly designed diets for prolonged periods of time.

Pedrinelli et al. (2017) evaluated the nutrient composition of 106 home-made Portuguese companion animal diets (80 dogs, 24 cats, and two diets intended for dogs and cats). The results were compared to the Nutritional Guidelines for Complete and Complementary Pet Food for Cats and Dogs. All diets had at least one nutrient below the recommended levels, with iron, vitamin E, zinc, calcium, copper, choline, riboflavin, thiamine, and vitamin

B12 being the most common deficiencies noted (Pedrinelli et al. 2017). This study emphasizes the importance of properly balancing homemade diets. Appropriate training and certification will reduce the risk of recommending an unbalanced diet to a patient.

Training (and ideally certification) in either veterinary acupuncture and/or Chinese herbal medicine is recommended before completing CFT training. This creates a foundation of TCVM knowledge. Chapters 1 and 3 discuss these treatment modalities in detail.

Currently there is only one program in the country offering CFT training through Chi University. Veterinarians can start utilizing CFT recipes while completing the training. Chi University also offers a Master of Science in Integrative Veterinary Medicine and a Master of Science in TCVM. Pricing is accurate as of February 2023.

Most of the Chinese herbal medicine certification programs briefly discuss CFT. The veterinary organizations listed in the following section offer CFT and other food therapy lectures, weekend courses, and webinars but do not offer certification courses.

Veterinarians who are on the fence about committing to a full training course are encouraged to attend introductory lectures first. Familiarizing yourself with the information is a great way to determine if pursuing this modality is right for you and your practice. State and national veterinary conferences, as well as many online veterinary educational platforms (VIN, Vetfolio, DVM360 Flex, Vet Girl on the Run, and College of Integrative Veterinary Therapies [CIVT]) frequently offer American Association of Veterinary State Boards (AAVSB) Registry of Approved Continuing Education (RACE)-approved lectures on various integrative topics.

Chi University
- **Course name**: Veterinary Food Therapy
- **Prerequisites**: Licensed veterinarians, in good standing, and third or fourth year veterinary students who have completed at least one session of veterinary acupuncture and completed the TCVM fundamental theories online lectures.
- **Description**
  - 41-hour RACE-approved veterinary food therapy course with 14 hours of lab and demonstrations:
    o Concepts in basic nutrition
    o TCVM food therapy principles
    o Food therapy for specific conditions
    o How to make the food.
  - Students who successfully complete the course are eligible for certification. Certified Veterinary Food Therapist certification is endorsed by the Chi University of Chinese Medicine. Certification requirements include:
    o Completion of all sessions
    o Pass the take-home exam
    o Submission of a case report.
- **Online training**: Students have the option of taking the entire course online with 10 hours of cooking demonstrations.
- **On-site training**: Students also have the option of taking a hybrid course of 27 hours online and two days on-site.
  - Includes four hours of TCVM diagnosis on live patients and the option to assist with food preparation and taste the final products.
- **Completion time**: Three to four months.
- **Cost**: $1500.00
  - Additional charges apply for:
    o TCVM Fundamental Theories course
    o CVFT certification
    o Printed notes.
- **Contact information**
  - Address: 9650 West Hwy 318, Reddick, FL 32686, USA
  - Phone: (800) 860-1543
  - Website: www.chiu.edu
  - Email: register@chiu.edu

College of Integrative Veterinary Therapies (CIVT)
- The CIVT started an online certification course in Veterinary Natural Nutrition in

October 2021. This course covers the principles of small animal nutrition from a variety of integrative medicine approaches.

- **Course name**: Certification in Small Animal Natural Nutrition
- **Prerequisites**: Licensed veterinarians or a Certificate Animal Health Sciences
- **Description**
  - Course covers:
    - o Concepts in basic nutrition
    - o Practical nutrition
    - o Commercial pet foods
    - o Alternative feeding practices
    - o Home-made diets
    - o Supplements and nutrigenomics
    - o Detoxification and fasting
    - o Weight control and obesity
    - o Naturopathic animal health care
    - o Therapeutic nutrition.
  - Students who successfully complete the course are eligible for certification endorsed by CIVT. Information regarding the requirements for certification, and post-nominal initials, were not available as of September 2021.
- **Online training**: Only option.
  - Students are granted access to the Animal Diet Formulator while enrolled in the course.
- **Completion time**: Two years
- **Cost**: $4680
  - CIVT also offers two other options
    - o Certification in Veterinary Natural Nutrition
    - • Veterinarians only
    - • Completion time is six months
    - • Contains 20 RACE-approved CE hours
    - • Online
    - • Cost: $1495
      - o Certification Veterinary Integrative Therapeutic Nutrition
    - • Must complete the Veterinary Natural Nutrition course first
    - • Completion time is 12 months
    - • Online
    - • Cost: $3495

- **Contact information**
  - Address: PO Box 352, Yeppoon, 4703 QLD, Australia
  - Phone: (304) 930-5684
  - Website: www.civtedu.org
  - Email: admin1@civtedu.org

Supplies

There are no specific supplies required when offering CFT. Hospital remodeling and/or redecorating is not required.

Veterinary Organizations

A description of the most common veterinary organizations with a special interest in TCVM and CFT is provided. Table 2.34 lists the contact names, contact information, and membership dues for these organizations.

American Holistic Veterinary Medical Association (AHVMA)

- **Description**: The AHVMA was founded in 1982 at the Western States Veterinary Conference with the goal of advancing integrative medicine through the education of integrative and non-integrative veterinarians, the introduction of integrative medicine to veterinary students, the promotion of research, and representation in the AVMA House of Delegates. There is no annual CE requirement to maintain membership.
- **Membership benefits**
  - Free subscription to the *AHVMA Journal*, a peer-reviewed journal.
  - Online resources for client education.
  - Searchable member directory.
  - Discounted vaccination titers through Kansas State University (KSU) Diagnostic Lab.
  - Free access to the Natural Medicines Database, an online resource for supplements, natural medicines, and integrative therapies.
  - Reduced cost for the AHVMA annual conference.

Table 2.34 Veterinary associations and organizations with a special interest in integrative medicine and/or CFT as of February 2023.

Organization	Contact information	Membership dues
American Holistic Veterinary Medical Association (AHVMA)	PO Box 630, Abingdon, MD 21009 (410) 569-0795 office@ahvma.org	$300/year
College of Integrative Veterinary Therapies (CIVT)	PO Box 352, Yeppoon, 4703 QLD, Australia (303) 800-5460 membership@civtedu.org	$185/year
Veterinary Botanical Medicine Association (VBMA)	6410 Highway 92, Acworth, GA 30102 office@vbma.org	$85/year
World Association of Traditional Chinese Veterinary Medicine (WATCVM)	WATCVM and AATCVM PO Box 141 324, Gainesville, FL 32614 (844) 422-8286 support@aatcvm.org	$85/year

Source: Lisa P. McFaddin.

College of Integrative Veterinary Therapies (CIVT)

- **Description**: An online organization open to all licensed animal health providers interested in integrative medicine. There are two membership options: full membership for veterinarians and associate membership for registered animal health professionals. CIVT strives to promote all aspects of evidence-based integrative medicine through online education and discussion forums. CIVT provides financial support to veterinary students interested in studying integrative medicine. CIVT also helps fund integrative medicine research. There is no annual CE requirement to maintain membership.
- **Membership benefits**
  - Access to the online electronic library.
  - Access to the electronic *Journal of Integrative Veterinary Therapies.*
  - Three free CE webinars annually.
  - 20% discount on all webinars.
  - Discounts on specific CIVT courses.
  - Searchable member directory.
  - Access to the Natural Medicines Databases and the American Botanical Council Library.

Veterinary Botanical Medicine Association (VBMA)

- **Description**: An online organization open to all veterinarians and herbalists interested in promoting the responsible application of herbal therapies on animals. The VBMA was founded by Susan Wynn, DVM, CVA, CVCH, AHG in 2002. No required annual CE to maintain membership.
- **Membership benefits**
  - Daily email discussion threads detailing real-life case questions and expert practical advice.
  - Weekly and monthly emails are also shared highlighting herbs commonly used in veterinary medicine.
  - Free subscription to the biannual online *Journal of Veterinary Botanical Medicine.*
  - Access to Herbal Wiki, an online herbal materia medica.

- Access to additional educational articles, websites, and videos.
- Discounted cost for telemedicine conferences and webinars.
- Searchable member directory.
- The VBMA offers an annual conference and multiple webinars.

World Association of Traditional Chinese Veterinary Medicine (WATCVM)
- **Description**: The WATCVM promotes the education, research, and practice of TCVM throughout the world. The WATCVM provides financial support to veterinary students interested in studying TCVM as well as establishing student organizations within veterinary schools. The WATCVM funds TCVM research programs. No required annual CE to maintain membership.
- **Membership benefits**
  - Access to online case discussion forums.
  - Free subscription to the *American Journal of Traditional Chinese Veterinary Medicine*, a peer-reviewed journal.
  - Access to the quarterly online TCVM newsletter.
  - Access to the online TCVM library.
  - Discounted TCVM conferences.
  - Access to the online classified ads.
  - Assistance with scientific writing as well as research design of grant proposals.
  - Dual membership in WATCVM and American Association of TCVM (AATCVM).
  - The WATCVM and AATCVM offer an annual International Conference on TCVM.

Reference Materials
This is my list of recommended TCVM, CFT, and veterinary nutrition books as of February 2023. A brief summary of each book is also provided.

Application of Traditional Chinese Veterinary Medicine in Exotic Animals
- Author: Zhiqiang Yang and Huisheng Xie, DVM, MS, PhD
- Summary: Proceedings from the 13th Annual International TCVM Conference discussing the introduction and implementation of TCVM therapies for exotic animals.

Applied Veterinary Clinical Nutrition
- Authors: Andrea Fascetti, VMD, PhD, DACVIM, DACVN and Sean Delaney, DVM, MS, DACVN
- Summary: Meant to be a quicker reference for the busy practitioner, allowing the practical application of canine and feline nutrition during daily practice. The book provides an overview of nutrition basics, pet food options, and dietary supplement information.

Bone Broth for Dogs and Cats: Supercharged Nutrition for Allergies, Stiffness, Skin Problems, Intestinal Issues, Inflammation, and the Immune System
- Author: Judy McFarlen, DVM
- Summary: An in-depth discussion of the beneficial effects of bone broth, as well as practical recipes.

Canine and Feline Nutrition: A Resource for Companion Animal Professionals
- Authors: Linda P. Case, MS, Leighann Daristotle, DVM, PhD, Michael G. Hayek, PhD and Melody Foess Rassch, DVM
- Summary: A point-of-reference guide for animal professionals regarding companion animal nutrition, as well as practical approaches to interpreting and understanding nutritional myths, pet food safety, pet food ingredient lists, pet food formulations, and dietary supplementation.

Canine Nutrigenomics: The New Science of Feeding Your Dog for Optimum Health
- Authors: Jean Dodds, DVM and Diana Laverdure
- Summary: An in-depth discussion into the study of how nutrition affects gene expression in canines.

Chinese Herbal Formulas for Veterinarians
- Authors: John Chen, PhD, Pharm D, OMD, Lac, Tina Chen, MS, Lac, Signe Beebe, DVM, and Michael Salewski, DVM
- Summary: Monograms of Chinese herbal formulas used in veterinary medicine

organized by their TCVM category. Each monogram discusses the nomenclature, formula composition, dosage, Chinese therapeutic actions, clinical manifestations, veterinary clinical applications, veterinary modifications, cautions and contraindications, pharmacological effects, human clinical studies and research, toxicology, suggested acupuncture therapies, and often additional author comments.

Chinese Medical Herbology and Pharmacology
- Authors: John Chen, PhD, Pharm D, OMD, Lac and Tina Chen, MS, Lac
- Summary: Monograms of Chinese herbs organized by their TCM category. Each monogram discusses the nomenclature, Chinese therapeutic actions, dosages, cautions and contraindications, chemical composition, pharmacological effects, clinical studies and research, herb-drug interactions, toxicology, and often additional author comments.

Chinese Veterinary Herbal Handbook: 216 Most Commonly Used Veterinary Herbal Formulas
- Author: Huisheng Xie, DVM, MS, PhD, Lauren Frank, DVM, CVA, Vanessa Preast, DVM, CVA and Lisa Trevisanello, DVM, CVA
- Summary: The third edition is an earlier version of the *Clinical Manual of Veterinary Herbal Medicine* functioning as a faster reference guide. Focuses on formulas carried by Jing Tang Herbal.

Clinical Application of Different TCM Schools and Thoughts in Veterinary Practice
- Author: Huisheng Xie, DVM, MS, PhD and Aituan Ma, DVM, PhD, MS
- Summary: Proceedings from the 18th Annual International TCVM Conference discussing the different TCVM schools and theories and TCVM therapy for infectious and inflammatory diseases, behavioral disorders, and other conditions.

Clinical Manual of Veterinary Herbal Medicine: 178 Commonly Used Veterinary Herbal Formulas
- Author: Huisheng Xie, DVM, MS, PhD and Aituan Ma, DVM, PhD, MS
- Summary: A quick reference book covering the safe use of Chinese herbal medicine in veterinary patients with an emphasis on practical information on commonly used Chinese herbal formulas as well as formula selection using TCVM and Western diagnoses. Scientific studies focusing on the referenced herbal formulas are provided. Focuses on formulas carried by Jing Tang Herbal.

Clinical Nutrition: Veterinary Clinics of North America Small Animal Practice
- Authors: Dottie Laflamme, DVM, PhD, DACVN and Debra Zoran, DVM, PhD, DACVIM
- Summary: A condensed summary covering the foundation of small animal nutrition, its practical applications to everyday life, and the nutritional management of common canine and feline diseases.

Dr. Becker's Real Food for Health Dogs and Cats: Simple Homemade Food
- Authors: Beth Taylor and Karen Becker, DVM
- Summary: An introduction to the theory and applications of raw food diets for dogs and cats, as well as multiple raw food diet recipes.

Dr. Pitcairn's Complete Guide to Natural Health for Dogs and Cats
- Authors: Richard Pitcairn, DVM, PhD and Susan Pitcairn
- Summary: An introduction into the applications of integrative pet care for owners.

Essential Guide to Chinese Herbal Formulas: Bridging Science and Tradition in Integrative Veterinary Medicine
- Author: Steve Marsden, DVM, ND, MSOM, Lac, Dipl.CH., RH(AHG)
- Summary: A quick reference book covering the safe use of Chinese herbal medicine in veterinary patients with an emphasis on

practical information on commonly used Chinese herbal formulas as well as formula selection using TCVM and Western diagnoses. Focuses on formulas carried by A Time to Heal Herbs.

Feeding Dogs: The Science Behind the Dry Versus Raw Debate
- Author: Conor Brady, BSC Hons, PhD
- Summary: A scientific review of the current commercial dog food, including its major pitfalls, and suggested canine diets going forward.

Four Paws Five Directions: A Guide to Chinese Medicine for Cats and Dogs
- Author: Cheryl Schwartz, DVM
- Summary: An introduction to TCVM in veterinary medicine focusing on TCVM theory and acupuncture. Additional therapies are briefly covered: food therapy, herbal supplements, nutritional supplements, environmental modifications. The disease processes are organized by body system and the Five Element Theory.

Healing with Whole Foods: Asian Traditions and Modern Nutrition
- Author: Paul Pitchford
- Summary: An in-depth look into the applications of CFT with traditional Chinese medicine descriptions of common food items and a multitude of recipes for various human diseases.

Home-Prepared Dog and Cat Diets
- Author: Patricia Schenck
- Summary: An introduction for owners into the basics of companion animal nutrition, the effect of diet on specific disease conditions, and home-cooked recipes.

Integrating Complementary Medicine into Veterinary Practice
- Authors: Robert S. Goldstein, VMD, Paula Jo Broadfoot, DVM, Richard E. Plamquist, DVM, Karen Johnstons, DVM, Jiu Jia Wen, DVM, Barbara Fougère, BSc, BVMs (Hons), BHSc (comp Med), MODT, MHSc (Herb Med), CVA (IVAs), CVBM, CVCP, and Margo Roman, DVM
- Summary: A comprehensive review of multiple integrative therapies including: Chinese herbal medicine, acupuncture, homotoxicology, nano-pharmacology, homotoxicology, and therapeutic nutrition. The book aims to educate veterinary practitioners on the validity, effectiveness, and incorporation of each modality within daily practice.

Integrative and Traditional Chinese Veterinary Medicine Food Therapy Small Animal and Equine
- Authors: Margaret Fowler, DVM and Huisheng Xie, DVM, MS, PhD
- Summary: A thorough explanation of Western and Eastern nutritional science with a TCVM foundation. Food therapy for specific disease conditions, based on TCVM pattern differentiation and traditional diagnoses, are discussed. The book includes information on specific dietary ingredients, as well as 300 AAFCO-compliant homemade small animal recipes and recipes for equine top-dressings.

Manual of Natural Veterinary Medicine: Science and Tradition
- Authors: Susan G. Wynn, DVM and Steve Marsden, DVM, ND, MSOM, Lac, Dipl. CH., RH(AHG)
- Summary: A quick reference book discussing the integrative therapy options for numerous diseases in veterinary medicine. The book is organized by Western conditions. For each category the potential TCVM diagnoses and treatment options are then discussed in succinct detail. A must-have for all integrative veterinarians.

Nutrient Requirements of Dogs and Cats
- Author: National Research Council
- Summary: A detailed description of the nutrient requirements for dogs and cats based on age and lifestyle, as well as nutrient metabolism and diseases related to nutritional deficiencies.

Pain, Lameness, Neurological and Endocrine Disorders
- Authors: Huisheng Xie, DVM, MS, PhD and Aituan Ma, DVM, PhD, MS
- Summary: Proceedings from the 20th Annual International TCVM Conference discussing the use of TCVM for the treatment of pain, lameness, neurologic disorders, endocrine disorders, infertility, and other conditions.

Practical Guide to Traditional Chinese Veterinary Medicine: Emergencies and Five Element Syndromes
- Authors: Huisheng Xie, DVM, MS, PhD, Lindsey Wedemeyer, MA, VetMB, MRCVS, and Cheryl L. Chrisman, DVM, MS, EdS, DACVIM (Neurology)
- Summary: The first of a four volume series discussing the practical use of TCVM in veterinary medicine. The book breaks down the TCVM pattern diagnosis and treatment options (acupuncture, Chinese herbal formulas, Tui-na, food therapy, and environmental changes) for common small animal emergencies. The book is organized using the Five Element Theory of disease as it relates to emergent disorders.

Practical Guide to Traditional Chinese Veterinary Medicine: Exotic, Zoo, and Farm Animals
- Authors: Huisheng Xie, DVM, MS, PhD and Harvey E. Ramirez
- Summary: The final book of a four-volume series discussing the practical use of TCVM in veterinary medicine. The book breaks down the TCVM pattern diagnosis and treatment options (acupuncture, Chinese herbal formulas, Tui-na, food therapy, and environmental changes) for exotic, zoo, and farm animals.

Practical Guide to Traditional Chinese Veterinary Medicine: Small Animal Practice
- Authors: Huisheng Xie, DVM, MS, PhD, Lindsey Wedemeyer, MA, VetMB, MRCVS, Cheryl L. Chrisman, DVM, MS, EdS,

DACVIM (Neurology), and Lisa Trevisanellow, DrMEDVET
- Summary: The second of a four-volume series discussing the practical use of TCVM in veterinary medicine. The book breaks down the TCVM pattern diagnosis and treatment options (acupuncture, Chinese herbal formulas, Tui-na, food therapy, and environmental changes) for common small animal diseases. The book is organized by Western medical diagnoses and then further divided into the possible TCVM diagnoses for each disease process.

Raw and Natural Nutrition for Dogs: The Definitive Guide to Homemade Diets
- Author: Lew Olson, PhD
- Summary: A reference guide for owners providing an introduction to canine nutrition, the benefits of a raw food diet, and practical raw food recipes.

Real Food for Dogs and Cats: A Practice Guide to Feeding Your Pet a Balanced, Natural Diet
- Author: Clare Middle, DVM
- Summary: A quick reference for pet owners regarding how to properly balance naturel diets.

See Spot Live Longer
- Authors: Steve Brown and Beth Taylor
- Summary: An introductory guide for pet owners to the complexity of canine nutritional science. The book includes background educational information, as well as practical tips for augmenting and designing companion canine diets.

Small Animal Clinical Nutrition, Fifth Edition
- Authors: Michael Hand, DVM, PhD, Craig Thatcher, DVM, MS, PhD, Rebecca Remillard, PhD, DVM, Philip Roudebush, DCM, and Bruce Novotny, DVM
- Summary: The gold-standard for small animal nutritional information covering dogs, cats, birds, reptiles, and small mammals with over 125 contributing authors. The book discusses the fundamental principles of small animal nutrition, commercial and

home-made pet foods, nutritional management of canine and feline diseases, and dietary husbandry information for many exotic species. There are now digital excerpts of the sixth edition available through Clinician's Brief.

Traditional Chinese Veterinary Medicine Approach to Gastrointestinal and Hepatobiliary Diseases
- Authors: Liting Cao, DVM, PhD and Huisheng Xie, DVM, PhD
- Summary: Proceedings from the 22nd Annual International TCVM Conference discussing the use of TCVM for the treatment of gastrointestinal and hepatobiliary diseases.

Traditional Chinese Veterinary Medicine Approach to Veterinary Dermatological and Immune-Mediated Diseases
- Authors: Aituan Ma, DVM, PhD, MS, Cui Liu, DVM, PhD, Chang Yu, DVM, MS, and Huisheng Xie, DVM, MS, PhD
- Summary: Proceedings from the 21st Annual International TCVM Conference discussing the use of TCVM for the treatment of dermatologic and immune-mediated diseases.

Traditional Chinese Veterinary Medicine: Empirical Technique to Scientific Validation
- Authors: Zhiqiang Yang and Huisheng Xie, DVM, MS, PhD
- Summary: Proceedings from the 1st Annual International TCVM Conference discussing the scientific study of TCVM including basic scientific research, small animal specific studies, exotic animal specific studies, large animal specific studies, and pediatric and geriatric medicine.

Traditional Chinese Veterinary Medicine for the Diagnosis and Treatment of Kidney and Water Element Disorders
- Authors: Aituan Ma, DVM, PhD, MS and Huisheng Xie, DVM, MS, PhD
- Summary: Proceedings from the 23rd Annual International TCVM Conference discussing the use of TCVM for the treatment of kidney and water element disorders.

Traditional Chinese Veterinary Medicine for Geriatric Medicine and Palliative Care
- Authors: Huisheng Xie, DVM, MS, PhD and Aituan Ma, DVM, PhD, MS
- Summary: Proceedings from the 19th Annual International TCVM Conference discussing the use of TCVM for geriatric medicine and palliative care.

Traditional Chinese Veterinary Medicine for Neurologic Diseases
- Authors: Huisheng Xie, DVM, MS, PhD, Cheryl L. Chrisman, DVM, MS, EdS, DACVIM (Neurology), and Lisa Trevisanellow, DrMEDVET
- Summary: Proceedings from the 13th Annual International TCVM Conference discussing the use of TCVM for a variety of neurologic conditions.

Traditional Chinese Veterinary Medicine from Dragon Legend to Modern Practice
- Authors: Xiuhuii Zhong, Aituan Ma, DVM, PhD, MS, Lisa Trevisanellow, DrMEDVET, and Qingbo Wang
- Summary: Proceedings of the 14th Annual International TCVM Conference discussing the use of TCVM for the treatment of liver, gastrointestinal, equine specific, and exotic animal specific diseases. A variety of other topics are also covered including, the longitudinal muscle system, platelet-rich plasma in aquapuncture, and the adverse effects of Chinese herbal medicine and acupuncture.

Traditional Chinese Veterinary Medicine: Fundamental Principles
- Authors: Huisheng Xie, DVM, MS, PhD and Vanessa Preast, DVM, CVA
- Summary: The quintessential introduction to TCVM theory with self-study quizzes, case examples, and practical application of TCVM therapies for small animal and equine patients.

Traditional Chinese Veterinary Medicine for Pain, Lameness, Neurological and Endocrine Disorders

- Authors: Huisheng Xie, DVM, MS, PhD and Aituan Ma, DVM, PhD, MS
- Summary: Proceedings from the 20th Annual International TCVM Conference discussing the use of TCVM for the treatment of pain, lameness, neurologic disorders, endocrine disorders, infertility, and other conditions.

Unlocking the Canine Ancestral Diet: Healthier Dog Food the ABC Way

- Author: Steve Brown
- Summary: A practical reference for dog owners on how to augment their dog's current diet to improve overall health. Recipes for complete dog foods are also included.

The Ultimate Pet Health Guide: Breakthrough Nutrition and Integrative Care for Dogs and Cats

- Author: Gary Richter, MS, DVM
- Summary: A practical reference for pet owners discussing integrative medicine and non-traditional (aka kibble) food options.

Xie's Chinese Veterinary Herbology

- Authors: Huisheng Xie, DVM, MS, PhD and Vanessa Preast, DVM, CVA
- Summary: A practical guide covering the theory and application of veterinary Chinese herbal medicine. The book is organized into three sections: herbal materia medica, herbal formulas, and clinical applications.

Yin and Yang Nutrition for Dogs: Maximizing Health with Whole Foods, Not Drugs

- Author: Judy Morgan, DVM
- Summary: Quick reference for pet owners discussing based concepts in Chinese veterinary medicine and dog food recipes.

Your Guide to Health with Foods and Herbs: Using the Wisdom of Traditional Chinese Medicine

- Authors: Zhang Yifang and Yao Yingzhi

- Summary: A quick-reference guide introducing the application of traditional Chinese medicine to common foods and herbs.

There are also multiple online reference materials available as of February 2023. A short description of each source is provided below, and links to the sites are provided on the companion website.

American College of Veterinary Nutrition

- Website: https://acvn.org
- Summary: Provides information pertaining to board certification in veterinary nutrition, links to useful articles and other websites for veterinarians and owners on all topics related to nutrition, and a directory for obtaining consultations with veterinary nutritionists.

Animal Diet Formulator

- Website: https://animaldietformulator.com
- Summary: A subscription-based online resource which formulates canine and feline diets using the United States Department of Agriculture (USDA) nutritional data. Diets are formulated to meet the AAFCO and the European Pet Food Industry Federation (FEDIAF) for various life stages. The formulator offers subscriptions for individuals, professionals, and commercial use. The software program was created by Steve Brown and presented by Royal Animal Health University.

BalanceIt

- Website: https://secure.balanceit.com/index.php
- Summary: This website is designed and run by board-certified veterinary nutritionists and provides tons of useful information and guidance for veterinarians and owners.

  – Videos discussing home-made food preparation, cooking demonstrations, and basic information explaining the application of nutrition in the management of many common canine diseases.
  – Free Autobalancer application allowing the creation of home-made food recipes

based on desired food type and weight. These recipes also include the dietary supplements necessary to balance the meals.

- The referenced supplements are developed and sold by veterinary nutritionists working for BalanceIt.
- Veterinary nutritionist consultations are available online for a fee.

NutriBase 18 Pro Edition Software
- Website: http://nutribase.org
- Summary: Paid software providing nutritional information on thousands of human food and restaurant items.

Veterinary Nutritional Consultations: PetDiets
- Website: https://www.petdiets.com
- Summary: Created by Rebecca Remillard, DVM, DACVN as an independent veterinary nutrition consultation service for owners and veterinarians online or over the phone. The website offers customized home-cooked recipes as well as articles discussing pertinent topics in veterinary nutrition.

Veterinary School Nutrition Services
There are multiple veterinary schools with board-certified veterinary nutritionists offering professional consultation services, including home-cooked diet development, for a fee.
- The Ohio State University Hummel and Trueman Hospital for Companion Animals: Nutrition Support Service
- Colorado State University Veterinary Teaching Hospital: Nutrition

- Cummings Veterinary Medical Center at Tufts University: Clinical Nutrition Service
- UC Davis Veterinary Medical Teaching Hospital: Nutrition Service

Zootrition
- Website: http://zootrition.org
- Summary: A free comprehensive database providing nutritional information and dietary calculators for zoo and wildlife managers.

Promotion
Information regarding the hospital's promotion of CFT can be found in the Team Members section.

Integration
The key components for proper integration include availability of the service to the right patients; appropriate patient scheduling; appropriate support staff scheduling; and staff buy-in (understanding the benefits of the offered service).

Conclusion

Veterinary CFT is an up-and-coming therapeutic modality. The potential effects and benefits of CFT are numerous for veterinary patients. This chapter and companion website describe in detail how CFT can be successfully introduced into daily practice, as well as provide practical tools for implementation.

References

AAFCO (Association of American Feed Control Officials) (2014). AAFCO Methods for Substantiating Nutritional Adequacy of Dog and Cat Foods. https://www.aafco.org/wp-content/uploads/2023/01/Pet_Food_Report_2013_Annual-Appendix_C.pdf (accessed 5 May 2020).

AAHA (American Animal Hospital Association) (2019). *Compensation and Benefits*, 9e. Denver, CO: AAHA Press.

Alexander, J., Stockman, J., Atwal, J. et al. (2019). Effects of the long-term feeding of diets enriched with inorganic phosphorus on the adult feline kidney and phosphorus metabolism. *British Journal of Nutrition* 121 (3): 249–269.

Allaway, D., de Alvaro, C.H., Hewson-Hughes, A. et al. (2018). Impact of dietary macronutrient profile on feline body weight is not consistent with protein leverage hypothesis. *British Journal of Nutrition* 11: 1310–1318.

Anturaniemi, J., Zaldívar-López, S., Moore, R. et al. (2020). The effect of raw vs dry diet on serum biochemical, hematologic, blood iron, B12, and folate levels in Staffordshire bull terriers. *Veterinary Clinical Pathology* 49: 258–269.

APPA (American Pet Products Association) (2021). Pet industry market size and ownership statistics. https://www .americanpetproducts.org/news/News-Public-Relations/pet-industry-market-size-trends-ownership-statistics#:~:text=2021%2D2022% 20APPA%20National%20Pet,U.S.%20 households%20owned%20a%20pet (accessed 8 September 2021).

Arjmandi, B., Johnson, S.A., Pourafshar, S. et al. (2017). Bone-protective effects of dried plum in postmenopausal women: efficacy and possible mechanisms. *Nutrients* 9 (5): 496.

AVMA (American Veterinary Medical Association) (2018). 2017–2018 Edition AVMA Pet Ownership and Demographics Sourcebook. https://www.avma.org/sites/ default/files/resources/AVMA-Pet-Demographics-Executive-Summary.pdf (accessed 8 September 2021).

AVMA (American Veterinary Medical Association) (2019). Economic state of the veterinary profession. https://www.avma.org/ news/press-release/AVMA-2019-Economic-State-of-the-Veterinary-Profession-Report-now-available (accessed 2021 26 July).

AVMA (American Veterinary Medical Association) (2023). *2023 AVMA Report on the Economic State of the Veterinary Profession*. Schaumburg, IL: AVMA.

van Beeck, F.L., Watson, A., Bos, M. et al. (2015). The effect of long-term feeding of skin barrier-fortified diets on the owner-assessed incidence of atopic dermatitis symptoms in Labrador Retrievers. *Journal of Nutritional Science* 4: e5.

BLS (Bureau of Labor Statistics) (2023). News Release: Consumer Price Index January 2023. https://www.bls.gov/news.release/pdf/cpi.pdf (accessed 18 February 2023).

Butterwick, R., Markwell, P., and Thorne, C. (1994). Effect of level and source of dietary fiber on food intake in the dog. *Journal of Nutrition* 124 (12 Suppl): 2695S–2700S.

Chen, J.K. and Chen, T.T. (2012). *Chinese Medical Herbology and Pharmacology*. City of Industry, CA: Art of Medicine Press.

Chen, J.K., Chen, T.T., Beebe, S., and Salewski, M. (2012). *Chinese Herbal Formulas for Veterinarians*. City of Industry, CA: Art of Medicine Press.

Chu, N., Yao, C., and Tan, V. (2018). Food therapy in Sinosphere Asia. *Gastroenterology* 52 (2): 105–113.

Clemmons, R. (2015). *Feeding According to TCM*. Reddick, FL: Jing Tang Publishing.

Conway, D. and Saker, K. (2018). Consumer attitude toward the environmental sustainability of grain-free pet foods. *Frontiers in Science* 5: 170.

Cyranoski, D. (2018). Why Chinese medicine is heading for clinics around the world. *Nature* 561: 448–450.

Dijcker, J., Hagen-Plantinga, E.A., Everts, H. et al. (2014). Factors contributing to the variation in feline urinary oxalate excretion rate. *Journal of Animal Science* 92 (3): 1029–1036.

DiNatale, C. (2015). *Dr. DiNatale's Lecture Notes*, 380–418. Reddick, FL: Jing Tang Publishing.

Dobenecker, B., Webel, A., Reese, S., and Kienzle, E. (2017). Effect of a high phosphorus diet on indicators of renal health in cats. *Journal of Feline Medicine and Surgery* 20 (4): 339–343.

Donadelli, R. and Aldrich, C. (2019). The effects of varying fiber sources on nutrient utilization, stool quality, and hairball managemetn in cats. *Journal of Animal Physiology and Animal Nutrition* 104 (2): 715–724.

Donadelli, R.A., Pezzali, J.G., Oba, P.M. et al. (2020). A commercial grain-free diet does not decrease plasma amino acids and taurine status but increases bile acid excretion when fed to Labrador Retrievers. *Translational Animal Science* 4 (3): txaa141.

FDA (Food and Drug Administration) (2019). FDA investigation into potential link between certain diets and canine dilated cardiomyopathy. https://www.fda.gov/animal-veterinary/outbreaks-and-advisories/fda-investigation-potential-link-between-certain-diets-and-canine-dilated-cardiomyopathy (accessed 3 January 2020).

FederalPay.org (2023). FY 2023 Federal Per Diem Rates October 2022-September 2023. https://www.federalpay.org/perdiem/2023 (accessed 18 February 2023).

Feuer, D. (2006a). *Your Cat's Nutritional Needs: A Science-Based Guide for Pet Owners*. Washington, DC: National Academies Press.

Feuer, D. (2006b). *Your Dog's Nutritional Needs: A Science-Based Guide for Pet Owners*. Washington, DC: National Academies Press.

Freid, K.J., Freeman, L.M., Rush, J.E. et al. (2021). Retrospective study of dilated cardiomyopathy in dogs. *Journal of Veterinary Internal Medicine* 35 (1): 58–67.

French, S. and Kemmis, S. (2023). Rental car pricing statistics:2023. https://www.nerdwallet.com/article/travel/car-rental-pricing-statistics#:~:text=The%20average%20weekly%20rental%20price,in%20advance%2C%20it%20was%20%24513. (accessed 18 February 2023).

Geddes, R., Biourge, V., Chang, Y. et al. (2016). The effect of moderate dietary protein and phosphate restriction on calcium–phosphate homeostasis in healthy older cats. *Journal of Veterinary Internal Medicine* 30 (5): 1690–1702.

Hand, M., Thatcher, C.D., and Remillard, R.L. (2010). *Small Animal Clinical Nutrition*, 5e (ed. P. Roudebush and B.J. Novotny). Topeka, KS: Mark Morris Institute.

Heinze, C. (2016). Should you make your own pet food at home? https://vetnutrition.tufts.edu/2016/07/should-you-make-your-own-pet-food-at-home.

Heinze, C., Gomez, F., and Freeman, L. (2012). Assessment of commercial diets and recipes for home-prepared diets recommended for dogs with cancer. *Journal of the American Veterinary Medical Association* 241 (11): 1453–1460.

Kaminogawa, S. and Nanno, M. (2004). Modulation of immune functions by food. *Evidence Based Complementary and Alternative Medicine* 1 (3): 241–250.

Kaplan, J.L., Stern, J.A., Fascetti, A.J. et al. (2018). Taurine deficiency and dilated cardiomyopathy in Golden Retrievers fed commercial diets. *PLoS One* 13 (12): e02909112.

Mansilla, W.D., Marinangeli, C.P., Ekenstedt, K.J. et al. (2019). Special topic: the association between pulse ingredients and canine dilated cardiomyopathy: addressing the knowledge gaps before establishing causation. *Journal of Animal Science* 97 (3): 983–997.

Marinangeli, C.P.F., Curran, J., Barr, S.I. et al. (2017). Enhancing nutrition with pulses: defining a recommended serving size for adults. *Nutrition Reviews* 75 (12): 990–1006.

Marks, D. and Shmalberg, J. (2015). Profitability and financial benefits of acupuncture in small animal private practice. *American Journal of Traditional Chinese Veterinary Medicine* 10 (1): 43–48.

Marsden, S. (2015). Lecture notes and videos: Nutritional strategies in Chinese herbal medicine: building on the success of herbs with diet change. Online, College of Integrative Veterinary Therapies, pp. 135–137.

McCauley, S.R., Clark, S.D., Quest, B.W. et al. (2020). Review of canine dilated cardiomyopathy in the wake of diet-associated concerns. *Journal of Animal Science* 98 (6): skaa155.

MFAF (Michelson Found Animals Foundation) (2018). Furred lines: Pet trends. https://www.prnewswire.com/news-releases/furred-lines-pet-trends-2019-300741947.html (accessed 26 July 2021).

Miller, N. (2017). 1 in 3 U.S. pet owners millennials: what it means for the pet food market. https://www.packagedfacts.com/Content/Blog/2017/02/07/1-in-3-US-Pet-Owners-Millennials-What-it-Means-for-the-Pet-Food-Market (accessed 2 December 2019).

Naarden, B. and Corbee, R. (2019). The effect of a therapeutic urinary stress diet on the short-term recurrence of feline idiopathic cystitis. *Veterinary Medicine and Science* 6 (1): 32–38.

NAPHIA (North American Pet Health Insurance Association) (2023). Industry Data. https://naphia.org/industry-data/#my-menu (accessed 18 February 2023).

Nielsen, T.N.C. (2016). The humanization of Pet Food. https://nap.nationalacademies.org/read/10668/chapter/2 (accessed 2 December 2020).

NRC (National Research Council) (2006). *Nutrient Requirements of Dogs and Cats.* Washington, DC: National Academies Press.

Oliveira, M., Brunetto, M.A., da Silva, F.L. et al. (2014). Evaluation of the owner's perception in the use of homemade diets for the nutritional management of dogs. *Journal of Nutritional Science* 3: e23.

Ontiveros, E.S., Whelchel, B.D., Yu, J. et al. (2020). Development of plasma and whole blood taurine reference ranges and identification of dietary features associated with taurine deficiency and dilated cardiomyopathy in Golden Retrievers: a prospective, observational study. *PLoS One* 15 (5): e0233206.

Parr, J. and Remillard, R. (2014). Handling alternative dietary requests from pet owners. *Veterinary Clinics of North America: Small Animal Practice* 44 (4): 667–688.

Pedrinelli, V., Gomes, M., de , O.S., and Carciofi, A.C. (2017). Analysis of recipes of home-prepared diets for dogs and cats published in Portuguese. *Journal of Nutritional Science* 6: e33.

Pitchford, P. (2002). *Healing with Whole Foods.* Berkley, CA: North Atlantic Books.

Purdue University (2019). Veterinary price index. https://assets.ctfassets.net/440y9b545yd9/5IsP0OgjAls6CbaXWvTDuS/81213899998ebb624d418b7521448a0a/FINAL_Nationwide-Purdue_2019-Veterinary-Price-Index.pdf (accessed 11 November 2023).

Rimar, T. (2015). *Dr. Rimar's Lecture Notes*, 177–269. Reddick, FL: Jing Tang Publishing.

Scott, J. (1994). An introduction to pulse diagnosis. *Journal of Chinese Medicine* 14: 1–20.

Shen, C., Pang, S., Kwong, E., and Cheng, Z. (2010). The effect of Chinese food therapy on community dwelling Chinese hypertensive patients with Yin-deficiency. *Journal of Clinical Nursing* 19 (7–8): 1008–1020.

Shmalberg, J. (2013). A comparison of the nutrient composition and Chinese food therapy energetics of common canine and feline dietary ingredients. *American Journal of Traditional Chinese Veterinary Medicine* 8 (1): 23–29.

Shmalberg, J. (2016). Integrative medicine: the evidence, economics, and logistics of an emerging field. https://todaysveterinarypractice.com/practice-building-integrative-medicine-the-evidence-economics-logistics-of-an-emerging-field/. (accessed 20 December 2020).

Silver, R. (2014). A veterinarian's approach to home prepared diets for dogs and cats. Rx Vitamins Technical Report.

Spofford, N., Mougeot, I., Elliott, D.A. et al. (2014). A moderate fat, low-energy dry expanded diet reduces gain in body condition score when fed as part of a post neutering weight-control regimen in growing fat cats. *Journal of Nutritional Science* 3: e40.

Stevenson, P. (2016). How to set practice service fees. https://cliniciansbrief.com/article/how-set-practice-service-fees (accessed 10 June 2020).

Stoeckel, K., Nielsen, L., Fuhrmann, H., and Bachmann, L. (2011). Fatty acid patterns of dog erythrocyte membranes after feeding of a fish-oil based DHA-rich supplement with a base diet low in n-3 fatty acids versus a diet containing added n-3 fatty acids. *Acta Veterinaria Scandinavica* 52: 57.

Teixeira, F.A., Machado, D.P., Jeremias, J.T. et al. (2018). Effects of pea with barley and less-pronounced maize on glycemic control in diabetic dogs. *British Journal of Nutrition* 120 (7): 777–786.

Teixeira, L., Pinto, C.F.D., Kessler, A.D.M., and Trevizan, L. (2019). Effect of partial substitution of rice with sorghum and inclusion of hydrolyzable tannins on digestibility and postprandial glycemia in adult dogs. *PLoS One* 14 (5): e0208869.

Trcek, L. (2023). This is how much flight prices increase in 2023 (+FAQs). https://www.travelinglifestyle.net/this-is-how-much-flight-prices-increase-in-2023/ (accessed 18 February 2023).

Vendramini, T., Amaral, A.R., Pedrinelli, V. et al. (2020). Neutering in dogs and cats: current scientific evidence and importance of adequate nutritional management. *Nutrition Research Reviews* 33 (1): 134–144.

Wang, W., Hernandez, J., Moore, C. et al. (2016). Antioxidant supplementation increases retinal responses and decreases refractive error changes in dogs. *Journal of Nutritional Science* 5: e18.

Wang, W., Brooks, M., Gardner, C., and Milgram, N. (2017). Effect of neuroactive nutritional supplementation on body weight and composition in growing puppies. *Journal of Nutritional Science* 6: e56.

WHO (World Health Organization) (2018). ICD-11 for Mortality and Mordbidity Statistics, 11th Global Compendium. https://icd.who.int/browse11/l-m/en (accessed 2 December 2019).

Wikipedia (2019). Chinese food therapy. https://en.wikipedia.org/wiki/Chinese_food_therapy. (accessed December 2019).

Wong, Y.C.P. (2016). Need of integrated dietary therapy for persons with diabetes mellitus and "unhealthy" body constitution presentations. *Journal of Integrative Medicine* 14 (4): 255–268.

Woodley, K. (2018). Pet insurance for holistic and integrative practice. https://ivcjournal.com/pet-insurance-integrative-practices/ (accessed 11 August 2021).

Wynn, S. (2010). Clinical aspects of energy metabolism. www.vin.com (accessed 9 Decmber 2023).

Xie, H. (2015). *Dr. Xie's Lecture Notes*, 1–176. Reddick, FL: Jing Tang Publishing.

Xie, H. and Preast, V. (2007a). Diagnostic methods. In: *Traditional Chinese Veterinary Medicine: Fundamental Principles*, 249–303. Reddick, FL: Chi Institute Press.

Xie, H. and Preast, V. (2007b). Diagnostic systems and pattern differentiation. In: *Traditional Chinese Veterinary Medicine: Fundamental Principles*, 305–468. Reddick, FL: Chi Institute Press.

Xie, H. and Preast, V. (2007c). Etiology and pathology. In: *Traditional Chinese Veterinary Medicine: Fundamental Principles*, 209–248. Reddick, FL: Chi Institute Press.

Xie, H. and Preast, V. (2007d). Five element theory. In: *Traditional Chinese Veterinary Medicine: Fundamental Principles*, 27–62. Reddick, FL: Chi Institute Press.

Xie, H. and Preast, V. (2007e). Qi, Shen, Jing, blood, and body fluid. In: *Traditional Chinese Veterinary Medicine: Fundamental Principles*, 69–100. Reddick, FL: Chi Institute Press.

Xie, H. and Preast, V. (2007f). The meridians. In: *Traditional Chinese Veterinary Medicine: Fundamental Principles*, 149–204. Reddick, FL: Chi Institute Press.

Xie, H. and Preast, V. (2007g). Yin and Yang. In: *Traditional Chinese Veterinary Medicine: Fundamental Principles*, 1–24. Reddick, FL: Chi Institute Press.

Xie, H. and Preast, V. (2007h). Zang-Fu physiology. In: *Traditional Chinese Veterinary Medicine: Fundamental Principles*, 105–114. Reddick, FL: Chi Institute Press.

Yifang, Z. and Yingzhi, Y. (2012). *Your Guide to Health with Food and Herbs*. New York: Better Link Press.

Zoran, D. and Buffington, T. (2011). Effects of nutrition choices and lifestyle changes on the well-being of cats, a carnivore that has moved indoors. *Journal of the American Veterinary Medical Association* 239 (5): 596–606.

Zou, P. (2016). Traditional Chinese medicine, food therapy, and hypertension control: a narrative review of Chinese literature. *American Journal of Chinese Medicine* 44 (8): 1579–1594.

3

Chinese Herbal Medicine

Introduction

Chinese herbal medicine (CHM) is one of the four branches within traditional Chinese veterinary medicine (TCVM): acupuncture, Chinese herbal medicine or therapy, Tui-na, and food therapy. CHM is a medicinal system which utilizes individual and combinations of herbs to prevent and aid in the treatment of disease. Proper veterinarian training, as well as utilizing and recommending herbal products from trusted sources, is vital. CHM can be used to aid in the treatment of almost all veterinary conditions. The introduction of CHM into a veterinary practice can be beneficial for both the patient and the health of the practice. The successful incorporation and utilization of CHM does not end with the veterinarian's training. Support staff training and client education are crucial. This chapter discusses the what, why, and how for effective integration of CHM within your practice.

The What

Definition

CHM is one of the four branches within TCVM: acupuncture, Chinese herbal medicine or therapy, Tui-na, and food therapy. CHM is a medicinal system which utilizes individual and combinations of herbs to aid in the diagnosis, prevention, and treatment of disease.

Human History

The first written documentation of CHM use dates to 1066–221 BCE (Chen and Chen 2012b). Included in these records was a list of botanical and animal substances used, case studies, and toxicity information. The first official book of CHM, *Shen Nong Ben Cao Jing* (*Divine Husbandman's Classic of the Materia Medica*), was written in the second century CE by several unknown authors (Chen and Chen 2012b).

Integrative Medicine in Veterinary Practice, First Edition. Lisa P. McFaddin.
© 2024 John Wiley & Sons, Inc. Published 2024 by John Wiley & Sons, Inc.
Companion website: www.wiley.com/go/mcfaddin/integrativemedicine

The book outlined the medicinal use of 365 herbs (Chen and Chen 2012b). A more detailed history of CHM can be found in *Chinese Medical Herbology and Pharmacology* by John K. and Tina T. Chen.

Veterinary History

The first organized utilization and records of CHM in veterinary patients, dated 770–476 BCE, were written by Sun Yang and Wang Liang, widely recognized as "the fathers of Chinese veterinary medicine" (Chen et al. 2012). The first published book on veterinary CHM, *Chi Ma Niu To Lu Ching* (*Various Treatises on the Treatment of Horses, Cattle, Camels, and Donkeys*), dates to 581–618 CE (Chen et al. 2012). A more detailed history of CHM in veterinary medicine can be found in *Chinese Medical Herbal Formulas for Veterinarians* (Chen et al. 2012).

Terminology

The world of TCVM and CHM comes with its own vocabulary. A basic understanding of these terms is crucial, allowing effective communication amongst professionals and with clients. A summary of common terms is provided below.

Bian Zheng: Utilization of one or more of the diagnostic systems to discern a TCVM diagnosis or pattern. The diagnostic systems include Five Element Theory, Yin–Yang Theory, Interior versus Exterior Patterns, Cold versus Hot Patterns, Deficiency versus Excess Patterns, Five Treasures, and Zang-Fu physiology (Xie and Preast 2007b).

Body fluid: Fluid found within the body including tears, nasal discharge, sweat, urine, saliva, digestive juices, and joint fluid (Xie and Preast 2007e).

Damp: Can be used to describe environments and disease conditions. One of the six evils or conditions in TCVM. Represents conditions with excessive moisture, infection, heaviness, and often pain (Xie and Preast 2007c).

Drain: Remove from an area. Generally applies to Damp conditions.

Eight Principles Theory: Diagnostic system dividing the natural world into two categories (Yin or Yang) and three pairs (Interior vs. Exterior; Cold vs. Heat; and Deficiency vs. Excess) (Xie and Preast 2007b).

Excess Pattern: Condition in which the patient has too much of something, often due to exogenous pathogens (Wind, Cold, Dampness, Summer Heat, Dryness, and Fire) or secondary to another issue (overeating, blood stagnation, phlegm). Patients often are excitable, breathe rapidly, and have a fever, distended abdomen, a red tongue with a coating, and surging pulse (Xie and Preast 2007b,c).

Exogenous Pathogens (aka **6** Exogenous Xie Qi or **6** Excessive Qi or **6** Evils): There are six weather changes which normally do not cause disease, but under the right circumstances (i.e. extreme weather changes and/or preexisting disease) can invade the body causing illness: Wind, Cold, Summer Heat, Damp, Dryness, and Fire (Xie and Preast 2007c).

Exterior Patterns: Issues associated with organ systems. Generally chronic in nature.

Five Element Theory: Everything in the natural world can be broken down into five elements, Wood, Fire, Earth, Metal, and Water, which promote, restrain, and regulate each other, maintaining order (Xie and Preast 2007d).

Five Energies: Food can be divided by thermal properties into cold, cool, neutral, warm, and hot (Xie 2015).

Five Tastes: Food can be divided by taste into sour, bitter, sweet, pungent, and salty (Xie 2015).

Fu Organs: Yang organs located within the interior of the body. They are hollow or tube-like and function to transport or excrete. Examples include large intestine, stomach, small intestine, triple heater, gall bladder, and urinary bladder (Xie and Preast 2007h).

Five Treasures: The organization of life into five substances: Qi, Shen, Jing, Blood, and Body Fluid (Xie and Preast 2007e).

Interior Patterns: Issues affecting the outside of the body. Generally acute in nature.

Jing (Essence): There is Jing you are born with (Prenatal Jing, Kidney Jing, or Congenital Jing) and Jing you acquire through ingestion of food and stored in each Zang-Fu organ (Postnatal Jing, Zang-Fu Jing, or Acquired Jing) (Xie and Preast 2007e).

Meridians (aka Regular Meri**dians**): A set of 12 paired and two unpaired pathways or channels on the outer surface of the body through which blood and energy (Qi) flow to the main organ systems, called Zang-Fu organs, joints, muscles, bone, and brain (Xie and Preast 2007f).

Meridian clock (aka TCM circadian clock): Qi flows through the 12 Zang-Fu organ channels in a specific order: lung → large intestine → stomach → spleen → heart → small intestine → bladder → kidney → pericardium → triple burner → gallbladder → liver. There is a two-hour time period during which the passage of Qi through each meridian and corresponding organ is greatest (Xie and Preast 2007f).

Phlegm: An abnormal form of body fluid which can accumulate within the body. Often any "strange" condition or illness is due to phlegm (Xie and Preast 2007b).

Qi (Energy): There are eight primary forms of Qi: Yuan Qi, Zong Qi, Gu Qi, Ying Qi, Wei Qi, Zang-Fu Qi, Jing Luo Qi, and Zheng Qi (Xie and Preast 2007e).

Shen (Spirit or Affect): An outward expression of an individual's mental state (Xie and Preast 2007e).

TCVM: A Chinese medicine system used to treat animals and comprising four branches: acupuncture, Chinese herbal medicine or therapy, Tui-na, and food therapy.

TCVM therapeutic actions: Beneficial effect associated with a specific TCVM therapy.

Tonify (aka Tonic): Increase energy (Qi), blood flow, Yin, Yang, or organ function in an area.

Wind: Can be used to describe environments and disease conditions. One of the six evils or conditions in TCVM. Often considered the primary cause of disease. Wind can invade the body from the outside world (Exogenous Wind) or originate within the body (Internal Wind). Allows other pathogens or conditions to develop (Xie and Preast 2007c).

Yin–Yang Theory: Divides all things into two halves which oppose, complement, control, create, and transform into each other (Xie and Preast 2007g).

Yang: Half of the Yin–Yang division. The descriptor can be applied to all manner of items both animate and inanimate. Characteristics include day, brightness, summer, hot, fast, male, healthy, strength, birth, top or back, Qi, pungent or bitter, and Fu organs (Xie and Preast 2007g).

Yin: Half of the Yin–Yang division. The descriptor can be applied to all manner of items both animate and inanimate. Characteristics include night, darkness, winter, cold, slow, female, illness, weakness, death, bottom or belly, blood, salty and sweet, and Zang organs (Xie and Preast 2007g).

Zang-Fu physiology: Classification of the 12 organs as either Zang or Fu.

Zang organs: Yin organs located within the interior of the body, solid in structure, and whose primary function is manufacturing and storage: lung, spleen, heart, pericardium, liver, and kidney (Xie and Preast 2007h).

CHM and TCVM

TCVM Diagnosis

The safe and effective use of CHM begins with establishing an accurate TCVM diagnosis. A fundamental understanding of the theories behind TCVM is necessary to properly diagnose patients. The factors used when making a TCVM diagnosis are outlined in Table 3.1.

TCVM Theories and Practices

Learning TCVM is literally and figuratively like learning another language. There is a ton of information which can be overwhelming. Years can, and should, be spent studying this field, and even then it is often only the tip of the iceberg with respect to the breadth and sophistication that is TCVM and CHM. I am still a student of TCVM, learning every day how to improve my practice and better help my patients. It would be impossible to teach any member of the veterinary team, especially those new to the field, everything about TCVM and CHM in a few pages. An introductory course in TCVM is a great start, but keep in mind I do mean start as there is always more to learn, really in all fields of medicine. An in-depth discussion of TCVM theory is beyond the scope of this book. To shed light on the complexity of TCVM diagnoses and CHM prescriptions, a brief overview of key TCVM

Table 3.1 The historical and physical components affecting a TCVM diagnosis (Xie and Preast 2007a).

Historical considerations	Historical considerations
• Chronicity of condition	• Complete traditional (Western) examination
• Previous diseases	• Shen (affect or demeanor)
• Environment	• Personality
• Diet	• Areas of hot or cold
• Current medications, supplements, or herbs	• Smell = body and breath
• Habits	• Active acupuncture points
• Dreaming	• Tongue
• Attitude toward other dogs and people	• Pulse
• Appetite	
• Thirst	
• Urinary habits	
• Stool consistency	

Source: Lisa P. McFaddin.

components are outlined. The suggested book list, in the Veterinarians section, references additional educational material pertaining to TCVM and CHM.

Yin–Yang Theory

A philosophical view dividing all things into two halves which oppose, complement, control, create, and transform into each other. There are five principles to the Yin–Yang Theory. Everything in the world can be broken down into two components: Yin and Yang. These two facets can be further divided into smaller Yin–Yang components; Yin and Yang can control one another; Yin and Yang can help create one another; and Yin and Yang can transform into one another (Xie and Preast 2007g). The Tai Ji symbol is a visual representation of Yin-Yang Theory. Characteristics of both Yin and Yang are shown in Figure 3.1.

Yin–Yang Theory is not binary but a continuum, just as the Tai Ji demonstrates there is a little bit of Yang (orange) within all Yin (yellow) and vice versa. Using the concept of day and night, the middle of the night is considered almost all Yin (complete darkness) followed by early morning which is mostly Yang with some residual Yin (early morning light but not full sun), whereas midday is considered almost all Yang (high-noon sun) followed by dusk which is mostly Yin with residual Yang (sunlight is fading but still present).

The Yin–Yang Theory can be applied to the categorization of diseases. Excess conditions involving heat, moisture, and/or infection (think hot spots) are characterized as Yang, while deficiency conditions involving weakness, cold, and often dryness (think hypothyroidism) are characterized as Yin.

Herbs can also be classified as having more Yin or Yang characteristics. For example, herbs which have a warming effect (Ginger, Cinnamon) are thought of as more Yang, while herbs with a cooling and/or drying effect (Salvia, Rhubarb) are considered more Yin. Table 3.2 characterizes common individual Chinese herbs as either Yin or Yang.

Yin–Yang Theory for Veterinarians Interestingly, Yin–Yang theory can be applied to the concept of redox reactions. Reduction–oxidation (redox) involves chemical reactions where atoms lose electrons (oxidation) or gain electrons (reduction). Antioxidants calm excessive oxidants just as Yin calms excessive Yang. Oxidants are known to cause inflammation, just as inflammation is associated with Yang. The relationship between Yin–Yang and redox reactions was illustrated concisely in the study by Ou et al. (2003). The authors measured the oxidative properties of 24 commonly used Chinese herbs using oxygen radical absorbance capacity (ORAC). Herbs with higher ORAC values (>433 μmol) were considered more potent free radical scavengers or antioxidants. Herbs with lower ORAC values (<243 μmol) had less antioxidant effects. Interestingly the herbs with the highest ORAC scores (aka antioxidants) were traditionally classified as Tonifying Yin (Yin Tonics), while the herbs with lower ORAC scores were classified at Tonifying Yang (Yang Tonics).

Yin–Yang and reduction–oxidation are opposite halves of a whole. They rely on control and transform into each other. Both strive to create and maintain an equilibrium. For Yin–Yang this homeostasis is seen within all organisms, and for redox this is seen at a molecular level. Imbalance in either system results in disease.

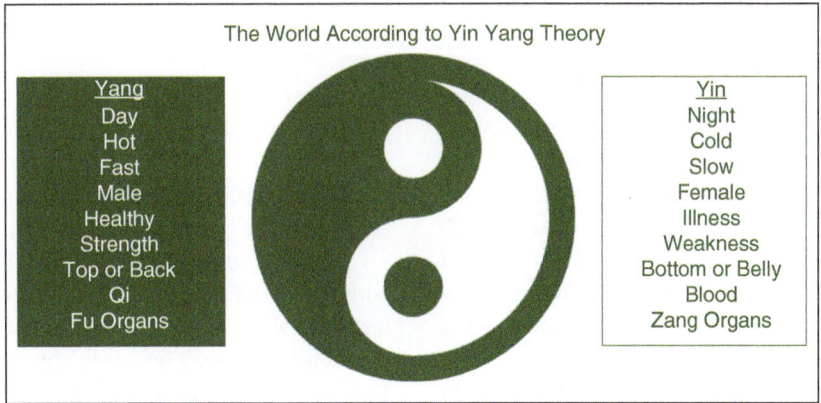

Figure 3.1 The Yin and Yang philosophy and archetypal Tai Ji symbol (Xie and Preast 2007g). Source: Lisa P. McFaddin.

Table 3.2 Common Chinese herbs classified as supporting, influencing, and/or tonifying Yin or Yang (Ou et al. 2003; Chen and Chen 2012a). Chinese and English names are shown; English names are broken down into the scientific and common name (in parentheses).

Yin tonics		Yang tonics	
Chinese name	**English names**	**Chinese name**	**English names**
Da Huang	*Rheum palmatum* (Rhubarb)	Bai Ji Tian	*Morinda officinalis* (Morinda)
Dan Pi	Cortex moutan (Moutan)	Bai Zhi	*Angelica dahurica* (Angelica)
Dan Shen	*Salvia miltorrhiza* (Salvia)	Dan Sheng	*Codonopsis pilosula* (Codonopsis)
Huang Bai	*Phellodendron amurense* (Amur Cork-Tree)	Fang Feng	*Ledebouriella divaricata* (Siler Root)
Huang Lian	Rhizoma Coptidis (Coptis)	Fu Zhi	*Aconitum carmichaelii* (Aconitum)
Huang Qin	*Scutellaria baicalensis* (Scullcap)	Gan Jiang	*Zingiber officinale* (Ginger)
Jin Yin Hua	*Lonicera japonica* (Japanese Honeysuckle)	Gui Zhi	*Cinnamomum cassia* (Cinnamon)
Lian Qiao	*Forsythia suspense* (Weeping Forsythia)	Rou Cong Rong	Herba Cistanches (Broomrape)
Long Dan Cao	*Gentiana scabra* (Chinese Gentian)	Tu Si Zi	*Cuscuta chinensis* (Cuscuta)
Mai Men Dong	*Ophiopogon japonicus* (Mondo Grass)	Xi Xin	Herba Asari (Wild Ginger)
Qing Hao	*Artemisiae annua* (Sweet Wormwood)	Yin Yang Huo	*Epimedium grandiflorum* (Epimedium)
Sheng Di Huang	*Rehmannia glutinosa* (Rehmannia Root)	Xu Duan	Radix Dipsaci (Teasel)
Zhi Mu	*Anemarrhena asphodeloides* (Anemarrhena)	Yi Zhi Ren	Fructus Alpiniae Oxyphylla (Sharpleaf Galangal)

Source: Lisa P. McFaddin.

Five Element Theory

The Five Element Theory breaks down everything in the natural world into five elements: Wood, Fire, Earth, Metal, and Water. The Five Elements promote, restrain, and regulate each other, keeping the natural world in perfect working order and establishing homeostasis (Xie and Preast 2007d). Table 3.3 outlines the characteristics defining each element.

TCVM is built upon interconnected layers of theory – everything is related. Within the Five Element Theory, Yin–Yang Theory still applies.

A nice example of this application is the transition between the seasons. Summer (Fire) is considered the most Yang season as it is the hottest followed by later summer/early fall (Earth) where the weather is more temperate. This time of year would have a fair balance of both Yin and Yang. Fall (Metal) is cooler with more Yin than Yang elements, followed by the cold winter (Water) which is almost full Yin. This then leads into spring (Wood) where the weather starts to warm and the Yang mixes more with the Yin.

Table 3.3 The characteristics of the Five Elements (Xie and Preast 2007d).

	Wood	Fire	Earth	Metal	Water
Season	Spring	Summer	Late Summer	Fall	Winter
Color	Green	Red	Yellow	White	Black
Orifice	Eyes	Tongue	Mouth	Nose	Ears
Emotion	Anger	Joy	Worry	Grief	Fear
Flavor	Sour	Bitter	Sweet	Pungent	Salty
Sense	Vision	Speech	Taste	Smell	Hearing
Tissue	Tendons and ligaments	Blood vessels	Muscles	Skin and hair	Bones
Function	Purifying	Circulating	Digesting	Breathing	Excretion
Secretion	Tears	Sweat	Saliva	Nasal Fluid	Urine
Zang organ	Liver	Heart and pericardium	Spleen	Lung	Kidney
Fu organ	Gallbladder	Small intestine and triple heater	Stomach	Large intestine	Bladder
Yin-Yang	Mostly Yang	Full Yang	Yin–Yang balance	Mostly Yin	Full Yin

Source: Lisa P. McFaddin.

Our veterinary patients can be thought of in terms of the Five Element Theory as described in Table 3.4. These are generalizations and do not apply to every patient. Just as with Yin–Yang Theory, the Five Element Theory is fluid. Most patients are a combination of elements with one predominant element shining through. The element(s) patient's most commonly associate with can also change with age. Winston, my beagle-mix, was a true Fire personality when younger, always hyper and easily excitable. After 10 years of age he started slowing down and has morphed into more of an Earth-Metal, calmer but definitely has boundaries.

Five Element Theory for Veterinarians The Five Elements are depicted in a specific circular order: Wood → Fire → Earth → Metal → Water. The elements can support and control one another through the Sheng and Ke Cycles, respectively (Xie and Preast 2007d). The Sheng (Inter-promoting) Cycle describes each element as both a parent (mother) and child (son) when compared to the other elements (Xie and Preast 2007d). The mother element serves to support and nourish the child element. The Ke (Inter-Restraining) Cycle defines each element as a grandparent (grandmother) and grandchild (grandson). The grandparent is responsible for controlling the grandchild. For example, Fire is the mother of Earth and the grandmother of Metal. The interactions of the Five Elements are illustrated in Figure 3.2.

Four pathologic cycles can affect the Five Elements (Xie and Preast 2007d). The mother element stifles, instead of supports, the son: Spleen (Earth) Deficiency leads to Lung (Metal) Deficiency. The son element shares its problem with the mother (reverse Sheng Cycle): Spleen (Earth) Deficiency leads to Heart (Fire) Deficiency. The grandmother excessively controls the grandson (Cheng Cycle): Spleen (Earth)

Table 3.4 The Five Element Theory as it applies to veterinary patient personalities (Xie and Preast 2007d).

	Wood	Fire	Earth	Metal	Water
Breed	Rottweiler	Jack Russel Terrier	English Labrador	Most cats	Chihuahua
Personality traits	Dominant Aggressive Fast moving Impatient	Easily excited Loves attention Smart Fast	Loyal Sweet Laid back Slow	Aloof Likes routine Natural leader Good vision	Quiet Observer Fearful Consistent
Physical Traits	Thin body Quick movements	Strong body Fast	Sturdy body Often overweight	Broad chest Luscious coat	Small Thin
Disease predilections	Cardiovascular Behavioral	Cardiovascular Behavioral	Gastrointestinal Obesity	Respiratory issues Dermatologic	Urogenital issues Kidney issues

Source: Lisa P. McFaddin.

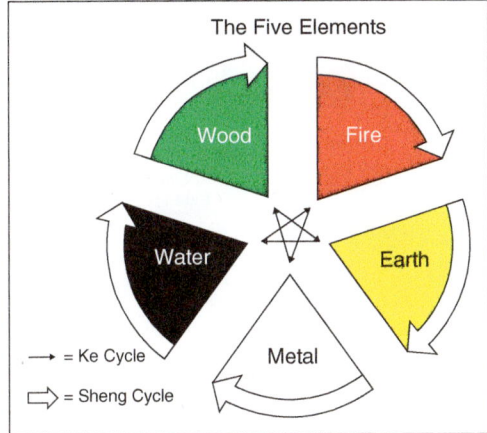

The Five Elements

Figure 3.2 A visual representation of the Five Elements with the Sheng (Inter-Promoting) and Ke (Inter-Restraining) Cycles (Xie and Preast 2007d). Source: Lisa P. McFaddin.

Deficiency leads to Kidney (Water) Deficiency. The grandson insults the grandmother (Ru Cycle): Spleen (Earth) Deficiency leads to Liver (Wood) Deficiency.

The nourishing and pathologic cycles affecting the Five Elements can be used to treat imbalances (Clemmons 2015). Deficiencies can be corrected by tonifying or supporting the mother of the deficient element, while excess conditions can be controlled by supporting the grandmother. The Five Element Theory can also be used to prevent disease.

Eight Principles Theory

This diagnostic system contains three category pairs divided into Yin and Yang components (Xie and Preast 2007g). Think of this as a math problem: Yin-Yang + Three Root Pairs = Eight Principles.

	Yin	Yang
First pair	Interior	Exterior
Second pair	Cold	Heat
Third pair	Deficiency	Excess

Yin–Yang   Refer to the previous section for specific information on Yin–Yang Theory. Yin–Yang Theory can be subdivided into three root pairs: Interior versus Exterior; Cold versus Heat; and Deficiency versus Excess. These four pairs create the Eight Principles Theory (Xie and Preast 2007g). Figure 3.3 outlines the multiple subcategories of potential conditions created by the Eight Principles Theory.

Interior and Exterior Patterns   The first root pair refers to the location and extent of the disease or condition within the body. Exterior Patterns affect the outside of the body and are acute in nature; while Interior Patterns focus on internal organ systems and have a longer duration of effect (Xie and Preast 2007b).

Cold and Heat Patterns   The second root pair reflect the thermal nature of a disease condition and can be subdivided by their location within the body (Xie and Preast 2007b). Cold Patterns include Exterior Cold, Interior Excess Cold, and Interior Deficient Cold (aka Yang Deficiency). Heat Patterns include Excess Heat, Interior Excess Heat, and Interior Deficient Heat (aka Yin Deficiency).

Deficiency and Excess Patterns   The third root pair reflect the body's ability to resist disease. There are four categories of Deficiency Patterns: Qi, Blood, Yin and Yang (Xie and Preast 2007b). The Excess Patterns are defined by the type of pathogen (assaulting or infectious agent) that is present: Wind, Cold, Dampness, Summer Heat, Dryness, and Fire/Heat (Xie and Preast 2007b).

Eight Principles Theory for Veterinarians   The complexity of the Eight Principles Theory is illustrated in Figure 3.3. Interior conditions typically involve internal organs. These issues generally occur later in the course of disease and/or with chronic conditions. With time, emotional distress (Shen disturbances) is

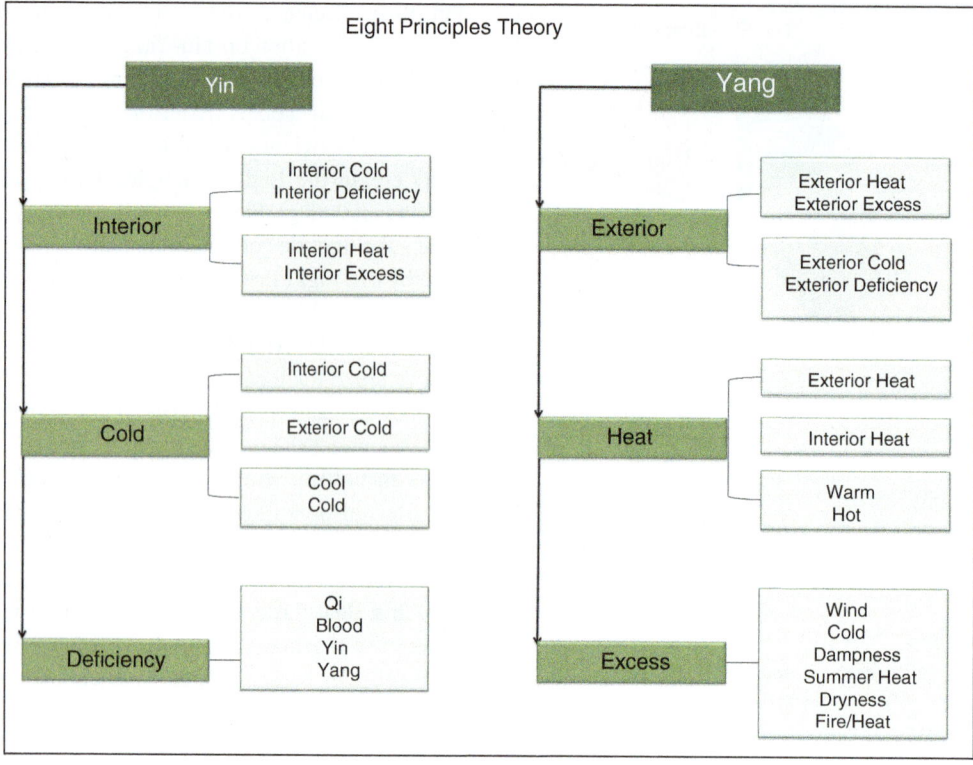

Figure 3.3 Pattern differentiation using the Eight Principles Theory (Xie and Preast 2007c). Source: Lisa P. McFaddin.

common. Interior conditions can be subcategorized into Interior Excess Cold, Interior Deficient Cold, Interior Excess Heat, Interior Deficient Heat, Qi Deficiency, and Blood Deficiency (see Table 3.5) (Xie and Preast 2007b).

Exterior conditions involve superficial surfaces including skin, hair, muscles, and meridians (energy channels located throughout the body). These disorders often start acutely or occur early within a disease process and resolve quickly (short duration) (Xie and Preast 2007b). Common clinical signs include fever, cold aversion, shaking or shivering, a thin coating on the tongue, and a superficial pulse. Exterior conditions are subcategorized into Exterior Cold, Exterior Heat, Exterior Excess, and Exterior Deficiency, as shown in Table 3.6 (Xie and Preast 2007b).

Zang-Fu Physiology

In TCVM the 12 internal organs are classified as either part of the Zang or Fu organ system. Each organ communicates to the exterior of the body through a channel or meridian. Most acupuncture points are found along these 12 paired meridians.

Just as Yin and Yang complement each other, creating two halves of a whole, Zang and Fu are grouped together as wives and husbands. Each pair of Zang-Fu organs is further classified by their relationship to the Five Elements of the world as depicted in Table 3.3. Zang or Yin organs are defined as those located within the interior of the body, are solid in structure, and whose primary functions are manufacturing and storage (Xie and Preast 2007h). Fu or Yang organs are hollow or tube-like and function to transport or excrete

Table 3.5 The subcategories and clinical signs associated with interior conditions. These conditions affect internal organs, are noted in chronic conditions or later in the course of the disease, often cause Shen (emotional) distress, the tongue may vary in color and often has a coating, and the pulse is deep (Xie and Preast 2007b).

Subcategories	Clinical signs
Interior excess cold	Cold extremities; increased intestinal activity; tongue = purple, wet; pulse = deep, slow
Interior deficient cold	Cold extremities; lethargy; inappetance; diarrhea; tongue = pale purple, ± coating; pulse = deep, slow, weak; seen with Yang Deficiency
Interior excess heat	Fever; hot extremities; tachypnea; dry stool; reduced urine production; tongue = red, dry, yellow coating; pulse = rapid, forceful
Interior deficient heat	Anxious; low-grade fever (chronic); small dry stool; reduced urine; tongue = red, dry, ± thin coating; pulse = rapid, thready; seen with Yin Deficiency
Qi deficiency	Shortness of breath; cough; inappetance; diarrhea; organ prolapse; frequent urination or incontinence; tongue = pale, wet; pulse = weak
Blood deficiency	Anxious, scares easily; dull eyes; tendon weakness; pulse = pale, dry; pulse = deep, soft

Source: Lisa P. McFaddin.

Table 3.6 The subcategories and clinical signs associated with exterior conditions. These conditions affect superficial areas (skin, hair, muscles, and meridians), are acute or occur early in the course of disease, of short duration, often involve a fever, cold aversion, and shaking or shivering, the tongue typically has a thin coating, and the pulse is superficial (Xie and Preast 2007b).

Subcategories	Clinical signs
Exterior cold	Serous nasal discharge; shivering; tongue = pale, thin coating; and pulse = slow
Exterior heat	Mucoid nasal discharge; cough; tongue = red, thin coating; pulse = rapid
Exterior excess	Fever; tongue = red; pulse = forceful
Exterior deficiency	General weakness; tongue = pale; pulse = weak, soft

Source: Lisa P. McFaddin.

(Xie and Preast 2007h). The Fu organs help their associated Zang organs fulfill their roles. Each organ has its own unique function and potential disease conditions as described in Tables 3.7–3.11.

All herbs have an affinity for one or more Zang-Fu organ and/or their associated channels. Herbs are said to enter specific organ channels as a means through which they exert their effect either directly or indirectly (Chen and Chen 2012a). Table 3.12 provides the Chinese name, scientific name, taste and thermal properties, associated Zang-Fu channels, and TCVM therapeutic actions for nine commonly used herbs.

Zang-Fu Physiology for Veterinarians Each Zang-Fu organ is susceptible to its own potential disease conditions. Most Zang-Fu diseases are classified as either excess (too much of something) or deficiency (weakness). Many of the excess disease conditions are due to the organs being attacked by pathogens which, ironically, is usually caused by a deficiency allowing the pathogen to invade. For example, Wei Qi (immune system) deficiency can allow outside pathogens (especially Wind Invasions) resulting in disease or infection. Additionally, deficiencies in the spleen can cause Dampness to accumulate. Both conditions, Wind Invasion

and Dampness, are considered excess conditions but they occur because of an underlying deficiency. Tables 3.7–3.11 discuss the functions and diseases associated with each Zang-Fu organ pair.

Five Treasures

The Five Treasures are the fundamental substances stored by each of the Zang-Fu organs. Life is controlled and supported by the Five

Table 3.7 The TCVM physiology and pathology of the liver and gallbladder (Xie and Preast 2007a,b,h; Chen and Chen 2012a).

Liver	Functions	Stores blood; maintains the flow of Qi; ensures smooth digestion; maintains the body's vital activities; ensures smooth flow of water; controls the connective tissue; opens into the eyes
	Excess conditions	Liver Qi stagnation; liver fire; liver damp heat; liver Yang rising; liver cold
	Deficiency conditions	Liver blood deficiency; liver Yin deficiency; liver internal wind
Gallbladder	Functions	Descends Qi and bile to intestines
	Excess conditions	Gallbladder damp heat
	Deficiency conditions	No specific disease conditions

Source: Lisa P. McFaddin.

Table 3.8 The TCVM physiology and pathology of the heart, small intestine, pericardium, and small intestine (Xie and Preast 2007a,b,h; Chen and Chen 2012a).

Heart	Functions	Dominates the blood and vessels; houses the Shen; controls the sweat; opens in the tongue
	Excess conditions	Extreme heart heat; phlegm-fire disturbing heart; heart blood stagnation; phlegm obstructing the mind
	Deficiency conditions	Heart Qi deficiency; heart Yang deficiency; heart blood deficiency; heart Yin deficiency
Small intestine	Functions	Receive food from stomach and spleen; ensure nutrient absorption; separate nutrients from waste
	Excess conditions	Small intestine cold; small intestine heat
	Deficiency conditions	No specific disease conditions
Pericardium	Functions	Protect the heart
	Excess conditions	No specific disease conditions
	Deficiency conditions	
Triple Burner (aka San Jiao, Triple Heater, or Triple Warmer)	Functions	Conduit for Qi to flow head to tail; divides the body upper, middle, and lower parts; connects to the pericardium
	Excess conditions	Triple burner obstruction
	Deficiency conditions	No specific disease conditions

Source: Lisa P. McFaddin.

Table 3.9 The TCVM physiology and pathology of the spleen and stomach (Xie and Preast 2007a,b,h; Chen and Chen 2012a).

Spleen	Functions	Governs digestion and absorption; transports and transforms Gu Qi; transports and transforms water; controls the blood; dominates the muscles and limbs; opens into the mouth
	Excess conditions	Spleen cold-damp; spleen damp-heat
	Deficiency conditions	Spleen Qi deficiency; spleen Qi sinking; spleen not controlling blood; spleen Yang deficiency
Stomach	Functions	Receive and digest food; prepares food for the spleen
	Excess conditions	Stomach cold; stomach heat; stomach food retention; rebellious stomach Qi; stomach phlegm
	Deficiency conditions	Stomach Yin deficiency

Source: Lisa P. McFaddin.

Table 3.10 The TCVM physiology and pathology of the lung and large intestine (Xie and Preast 2007a,b,h; Chen and Chen 2012a).

Lung	Functions	Governs Qi; governs respiration; regulates water; controls the skin and hair; opens into the nose
	Excess conditions	Lung wind-cold; lung wind-heat; lung wind-dryness-heat; lung heat
	Deficiency conditions	Lung Qi deficiency; lung Yin deficiency; lung Yin and Qi deficiency; lung Qi and kidney Qi deficiency
Large intestine	Functions	Receives waste from the small intestine; reabsorbs available fluid; prepares feces for excretion
	Excess conditions	Large intestine food accumulation; large intestine damp heat; large intestine cold
	Deficiency conditions	No specific disease conditions

Source: Lisa P. McFaddin.

Table 3.11 The TCVM physiology and pathology of the kidney and bladder (Xie and Preast 2007a,b,h; Chen and Chen 2012a).

Kidney	Functions	Stores congenital and acquired Jing; governs water; regulates cosmic Qi; dominates the bone; opens into the ears; controls the urogenital and anus
	Excess conditions	No specific disease conditions
	Deficiency conditions	Kidney Yang deficiency; kidney Qi not firm; kidney failing to receive Qi; kidney Yin deficiency; kidney Jing deficiency
Bladder	Functions	Receives waste from the kidneys
	Excess conditions	Bladder damp-heat
	Deficiency conditions	No specific disease conditions

Source: Lisa P. McFaddin.

Table 3.12 Nine commonly used individual Chinese herbs designated by their Chinese name (Pinyin), scientific name, common name, properties (taste and temperature), associated Zang-Fu organs, and their TCVM therapeutic effects (Chen and Chen 2012a).

Pinyin	Scientific name Common name	Properties	Zang-Fu	TCVM actions
Bai Zhi	*Angelica dahurica* Angelica root	Acrid Warm	Stomach Large intestine Lung	Exterior releasing: wind-cold
Bo He	*Mentha haplocalyx* and *M. arvensis* Mint herb	Acrid Cold	Lung Liver	Exterior releasing: wind-heat
Chen Pi	*Citrus reticulata* Blanco Citrus peel; orange peel; tangerine peel	Bitter Arid Warm	Lung Spleen	Qi regulating
Dang Gui	*Angelica sinensis* Angelica root	Sweet Acrid Warm	Heart Liver Spleen	Blood-tonifying
Fu Zhi (Fu Zi)	*Aconitum carmichaelii* Aconitum; monkshood; aconite root	Spicy Hot Toxic	Heart Kidney Spleen	Interior warming
Gan Cao	*Glycyrrhiza glabra* Licorice root	Sweet Neutral	Spleen Stomach Lung Heart	Qi-tonifying
Gan Jiang	*Zingiber officinale* Ginger root	Spicy Hot	Heart Lung Spleen Stomach	Interior warming
Huang Qi	*Astragalus membranaceus* Astragalus root	Sweet Slightly warm	Spleen Lung	Qi-tonifying
Ren Shen	*Panax ginseng* Ginseng	Sweet Slightly bitter Slightly warm	Lung Spleen	Qi-tonifying

Source: Lisa P. McFaddin.

Treasures: Qi, Shen, Jing, Blood, and Body Fluid. Qi can be thought of as energy. Without Qi there is no life. Shen can be thought of as an animal's spirit, affect, or mental state. Jing is the body's Essence, both what an individual is born with (Prenatal Jing) and what is acquired throughout life (Postnatal Jing). The importance and function of blood in Chinese and Western medicine is similar. The difference lies in the philosophies behind the formation and pathologic effects of blood. Jin Ye or Body Fluids comprise the remaining bodily excretions: tears, urine, joint fluid, nasal discharge, saliva, gastrointestinal fluid, and sweat (Xie and Preast 2007e).

Five Treasures for Veterinarians There are seven primary forms of Qi, each with their own properties and purposes, as described in Table 3.13: Yuan Qi, Zong Qi, Gu Qi, Ying Qi,

Table 3.13 The seven primary forms of Qi (Xie and Preast 2007e).

	AKA	Source	Primary function
Yuan Qi	Primary or source Qi	Kidney Essence Gu Qi	Sustains normal growth and development
Zong Qi	Pectoral Qi Ancestral Qi	Gu Qi Cosmic Qi	Governs and controls the respiratory and circulatory systems
Gu Qi	Food Qi Food Essence	Food processed by the spleen	Supplies and restores the Ying Qi, Wei Qi, Yuan Qi, and kidney Essence
Ying Qi	Nutrient Qi	Gu Qi	Supplies and nourishes the blood and body
Wei Qi	Defensive Qi	Gu Qi	Protects the body from illness
Zang-Fu Qi	Named by organ	Yuan Qi	Function dependent on the organ involved
Jing Luo Qi	Meridian Qi	Yuan Qi	Allows communication between the meridians and the associated internal organ

Source: Lisa P. McFaddin.

Wei Qi, Zang-Fu Qi, and Jing Luo Qi. When Qi is weak (Qi Deficiency) or stuck (Qi Stagnation), disease can develop.

A healthy Shen is nourished by the Heart, Blood, and Yin, while a disturbance in Shen is usually due to Heart, Blood or Yin Deficiency or Excessive Heat (Xie and Preast 2007e).

Prenatal Jing deficiency results in many congenital diseases. Postnatal Jing is generally depleted through chronic diseases, excessive behaviors, overworking, lack of sleep, and chronic dehydration (Xie and Preast 2007e).

In TCVM, blood is formed from Da Qi (air), Gu Qi, Ying Qi, and Jing (Xie and Preast 2007e). Diseases of the blood center around Blood Deficiency, defined by the organ involved and blockage (Stagnation) of blood flow.

Different organs are responsible for the formation and propagation of various body fluids. Jin Ye disease is dependent on the fluid involved but is generally a result of deficiencies.

Bian Zheng

Bian Zheng refers to the utilization of one or more of the diagnostic systems for pattern differentiation. This is where all the theories are put together to generate a TCVM diagnosis.

Bian Zheng for Veterinarians There are seven primary classification systems used when obtaining a TCVM diagnosis: Eight Principles, Triple Heater Patterns, Meridian Patterns, Four Levels, Zang-Fu Physiology, Qi–Blood–Body Fluid Patterns, and Six Phases.

- *Eight Principles*: Diseases divided into four pattern pairs: Exterior versus Interior, Hot versus Cold, Excess versus Deficiency, and Yang versus Yin (Xie and Preast 2007b). This categorization is applicable to all disease conditions.
- *Triple Heater Patterns*: Diseases are categorized by their location within the three parts (Jiao) of the body: Upper Jiao (Heart and Spleen), Middle Jiao (Spleen and Stomach), and Lower Jiao (Kidney and Liver). Applicable to many water-metabolism and Damp-Heat conditions (Xie and Preast 2007b).
- *Meridian Patterns*: Pattern differentiation is based on the affected meridian or channel.

Primarily used for musculoskeletal and infectious conditions (Xie and Preast 2007b,f).

- *Four Levels*: Divides the immune system into four levels: Wei Qi, Qi, Ying Qi, and Xue (Marsden 2015). Pattern differentiation is based on the level of the immune system affected. Wei Qi is the most superficial layer, basically the skin or outer barrier, and is generally attacked by Wind. Qi are the internal organs or systemic immune system (Marsden 2015). Attacks to the Qi level result in high fevers, thirst, sweating, and bounding pulses. Ying Qi is the plasma, while Xue is the blood. Attacks reaching both levels cause serious illness such as that seen with septicemia, hemorrhage, immune-mediated thrombocytopenia, and autoimmune hemolytic anemia (Marsden 2015).
- *Zang-Fu pathology*: Diseases associated with a specific Zang-Fu organ and classified as Deficient or Excess. This classification is applicable to most disease conditions (see Tables 3.7–3.11 for examples).
- *Qi–Blood–Body Fluid Patterns*: Vital substances are needed to nourish and support the Zang-Fu organs. Disease patterns are based on the fluid being affected. These diagnoses are most applicable to chronic internal and endocrine diseases (Xie and Preast 2007e).
- *Six Phases*: Patterns are divided into Yin and Yang and subsequently divided into inner, middle, and outer levels: Tai Yang (Greater Yang), Shao Yang (Lesser Yang), Yang Ming (Bright Yang), Tai Yin (Greater Yin), Shao Yin (Lesser Yin), and Jue Yin (Terminal Yin) (Xie and Preast 2007b,g). These diagnoses are applicable to most diseases affecting the immune system, central nervous system, and many musculoskeletal disorders (Marsden 2015). The Six Phases correlate to the Zang-Fu organs, often allowing for a Zang-Fu diagnosis as well.

Tongue and Pulse Diagnosis

The importance of an accurate tongue and pulse diagnosis in aiding the Bian Zheng cannot be stressed enough. These two attributes are critical for the TCVM diagnosis and proper herb selection. Table 3.14 provides a brief look into the complexity and intricacies of tongue and pulse diagnosis.

In general terms the tongue is evaluated by its size, shape, color, and presence of a coating. Tongue diagnosis is actually very nuanced and complicated. For example, specific areas of the tongue correspond with certain Zang-Fu organs, making the diagnoses even more specific.

Typically the femoral artery is used for pulse diagnosis in dogs and cats (Marsden 2015). The pulse is evaluated using the practitioner's fingertips. Special names are ascribed to the type of pulse based on the depth, intensity, tone, and rhythm, all of which are affected by things like vessel wall tone, vessel diameter, and heart rate. As with the tongue, pulse diagnosis is really complex. Unlike the tongue, unless the pet only has one pelvic limb, both femoral pulses should be palpated. Frequently the left and right pulses differ. In fact the left pulse is associated with Yin and Blood, while the right pulse is associated with Yang and Qi. Similar to the tongue, different areas of the femoral pulse also correspond to different Zang-Fu organs, again helping to home in on the diagnosis.

Classifications

TCVM Classifications

The organization of both individual Chinese herbs (CH) and Chinese herbal formulas (CF) is complex. CH and CF are mainly classified by their primary TCVM effect (Table 3.15). Individual herbs are further characterized by their taste (Table 3.16), thermal properties (Table 3.17), direction (Table 3.18), Zang-Fu channel and organ affinity (Table 3.19), source (Table 3.20), and adverse effects (Table 3.21) (Chen and Chen 2012a).

TCVM Classifications for Veterinarians

CH are divided into multiple categories based on their actions. Those categories are further subdivided. For example, heat-clearing herbs include the following subcategories: Heat-Clearing and

Table 3.14 Examples of tongue and pulse characteristics with associated TCVM conditions (Scott 1994; Xie and Preast 2007a; Chen et al. 2012).

Tongue		Pulse	
Description	TCVM conditions	Description	TCVM conditions
Pale	Blood deficiency, Qi deficiency	Taut	LIV Qi stagnation, blood stasis
Lavender	LIV Qi stagnation, blood stasis	Thin	LIV blood deficiency, Yin deficiency, blood deficiency
Flabby	SP Qi deficiency, dampness	Rapid, forceful	Heat, damp heat
Wet	SP Qi deficiency, dampness	Rapid	Heat (excess or deficiency)
Dark red	Stasis type of heat	Slow	Cold
Purple	Qi or blood stasis, LIV Qi stagnation, cold	Weak and thready	Deficiency
Yellow	Heat	Forceful	Excess
Swollen	Dampness, Qi deficiency, Yang deficiency, SP Qi deficiency	Wiry	Stagnation, pain, liver disease, phlegm
Small and thin	Qi or blood deficiency, KID Jing deficiency	Slippery	Phlegm, dampness, food stagnation
Yellow and dull	SP Qi deficiency, damp	Soft	Qi deficiency, cold
Swollen and pale	KID Yang deficiency	Choppy	Blood deficiency, Qi deficiency, blood stagnation
Swollen and red	Heat	Deep and wiry	Qi contained
Cracked and red	Yin deficiency	Deep	Interior condition, Qi deficiency
White	LU Qi deficiency	Middle to deep	Interior but not severe
Dark	KID Yin deficiency	Superficial	Excess

LIV, Liver; SP, Spleen; KID, Kidney; LU, Liver.
Source: Lisa P. McFaddin.

Table 3.15 Examples of individual Chinese herbs classified by TCVM categories (Freeman 2001a,b, 2002; Mitchell 2006; Chen and Chen 2012a). Both the Chinese and English names are provided.

Exterior releasing	Bai Zhi (Angelica Root); Bo He (Mint)
Heat clearing	Huang Qin (Scutellaria); Sheng Di Huang (Rehmannia Root)
Downward draining	Da Huang (Rhubarb Root); Huo Ma Ren (Hemp Seed)
Wind-damp dispelling	Du Huo (Pubescent Angelica Root); Mu Gua (Papaya)
Aromatic damp-dissolving	Cang Zhu (Atractylodes); Huo Po (Magnolia Bark)
Water-regulating and damp-resolving	Fu Ling (Poria); Yi Yi Ren (Coix Seeds)
Interior warming	Gan Jiang (Dried Ginger); Rou Gui (Cinnamon Bark)
Qi-regulating	Chen Pi (Citrus Peel); Xiang Fu (Cyperus)
Digestive	Shan Zha (Hawthorn Berry); Mai Ya (Barley Sprouts)
Antiparasitic	Guan Zhong (Dryopteris Root); Shi Jun Zi (Rangoon Creeper Fruit)
Stop bleeding	Da Ji (Japanese Thistle); Zi Zhu (Callicarp Leaf)
Blood-invigorating and stasis-removing	Dan Shen (Salvia Root); Jiang Huang (Turmeric)
Phlegm-resolving and coughing/wheezing-relieving	Jie Geng (Platycodon Root); Xing Ren (Apricot Seed)
Shen-calming	Suan Zao Ren (Spiny Date Seed); Zhu Sha (Cinnabar)
Liver-calming and wind-extinguishing	Di Long (Earthworm); Tian Ma (Tall Gastrodia Tuber)
Orifice opening	Bing Pan (Borneol); Shi Chang Pu (Acorus)
Tonics	Dang Gui (Angelica Root); Ren Shen (Ginseng Root)
Astringent	Fu Pen Zi (Rubus); Shan Zhu Yu (Cornus)
Emetic	Chang Shan (Dichroa Root); Gua Di (Melon Pedicle)
Topical	Da Suan (Garlic Bulb); Liu Huang (Sulfur)

Source: Lisa P. McFaddin.

Table 3.16 Examples of individual Chinese herbs classified by different taste properties (Freeman 2001a,b, 2002; Mitchell 2006; Chen and Chen 2012b). Both the Chinese and English names are provided.

Acrid	Ma Huang (Ephedra); Gui Zhi (Cinnamon Twigs)
Sweet	Gan Cao (Licorice Root); Huang Qi (Astragalus Root)
Sour	Wu Wei Zi (Schisandra Fruit); Bai Ji (Chinese Orchid)
Salty	Mang Xiao (Mirabilite); Lu Tong (Sweetgum Fruit)
Bland	Fu Ling (Poria Sclerotium); Zhu Ling (Polyporus)
Bitter	Da Huang (Rhubarb Root and Rhizome); Xing Ren (Apricot Kernel)
Astringent	Wu Wei Zi (Schisandra Fruit); Fu Xiao Mai (Triticum Seed)

Source: Lisa P. McFaddin.

Table 3.17 Examples of individual Chinese herbs classified by their thermal properties (Freeman 2001a,b, 2002; Mitchell 2006; Chen and Chen 2012a). Both the Chinese and English names are provided.

Cold or cool	Huang Qin (Baical Scullcap Root); Ban Lan Gen (Woad Root)
Hot or warm	Fu Zhi (Aconite Root); Gan Jiang (Ginger Root)
Neutral	Fu Ling (Poria Sclerotium)

Source: Lisa P. McFaddin.

Table 3.18 Examples of plant parts and types, as well as individual Chinese herbs classified by their direction (Freeman 2001a,b, 2002; Mitchell 2006; Chen and Chen 2012a). Both the Chinese and English names are provided.

Upward	Flowers; rapidly growing plants; Qiang Huo (Notopterygium Root)
Downward	Roots; minerals; Du Huo (Angelica Root)
Inward	Fu Zi (Acontie); Gan Jiang (Dried Ginger)
Outward	She Xiang (Musk); Shi Chang Pu (Acorus)

Source: Lisa P. McFaddin.

Table 3.19 Examples of individual Chinese herbs classified by their Zang-Fu organs and channel affiliations (Freeman 2001a,b, 2002; Mitchell 2006; Chen and Chen 2012a). Both the Chinese and English names are provided.

Direct effect		Indirect effect	
Herb example	**Zang-Fu channel**	**Herb example**	**Zang-Fu channel**
Xing Ren (Apricot Kernel)	Lung channel	Bu Gu Zhi (Psoralea seed)	Spleen channel Kidney channel
Ban Xia (Cooked Pinellia Rhizome)	Stomach channel	Fu Pen Zi (Chinese raspberry)	Kidney channel
Zhu Ling (Polyporus Sclerotium)	Urinary bladder	Xu Duan (Teasel root)	Liver channel Kidney channel

Source: Lisa P. McFaddin.

Table 3.20 Examples of individual Chinese herbs classified by their source (Freeman 2001a,b, 2002; Mitchell 2006; Chen and Chen 2012b). Both the Chinese and English names are provided.

Plants	Bai Dou Kou (Round Cardamon Fruit); Bu Gu Zhi (Psoralea seed)
Insects	Di Long (Earthworm); Sang Piao Xiao (Mantis egg case)
Minerals	Hua Shi (Talc)

Source: Lisa P. McFaddin.

Fire-Purging (Shi Gao, Gypsum); Heat-Clearing and Dampness-Drying (Huang Qin, Scutellaria); Heat-Clearing and Blood-Cooling (Sheng Di Huang, Rehmannia); Heat-Clearing and Toxin-Eliminating (Jin Yin Hua, Honeysuckle Flower); and Deficiency Heat Clearing (Qing Hao, Sweet Wormwood) (Freeman 2001a,b; Mitchell 2006; Chen and Chen 2012a). Additional examples of these categories and subcategories, as well as specific herb examples and their TCVM and biomedical effects, can be found in Table 3.15.

Table 3.21 Examples of individual Chinese herbs classified by their potential risk of adverse effects (AE) (Freeman 2001a,b, 2002; Mitchell 2006; Chen and Chen 2012b). Both the Chinese and English names are provided.

Risk of AE	Description	Examples
Superior	Few to no side effects with excellent therapeutic benefit	Gan Cao (Licorice Root); Ren Shen (Ginseng)
Medium	Potential for side effects while still having therapeutic value. Professional supervision and careful monitoring required during administration	Bai Shao (White Peony); Dang Gui (Angelica Root)
Inferior	Higher chance of side effects and/or toxicity. Most herbs still have therapeutic value, but careful herbal preparation and monitoring is critical	Da Huang (Rhubarb Root and Rhizome); Fu Zi (Aconite Root)

Source: Lisa P. McFaddin.

Taste Properties for Veterinarians

Each CH has its own taste which both contributes to and affects the therapeutic actions of the herb. The taste of a complete CF is dependent on the individual components. Taste is divided into acrid, sweet, sour, salty, bitter, neutral, and astringent (see Table 3.16 for example herbs).

Acrid herbs are characterized as dispersing, moving, drying, and pungent. They help induce sweating, dispel pathogens, and disperse and move Qi and Blood (Freeman 2001a,b; Chen and Chen 2012a). They should be used with caution in patients with Qi Deficiency, Yin Deficiency, Body Fluid Deficiency, and excessive sweating (Freeman 2001a,b; Chen and Chen 2012a). Examples include Gui Zhi (Cinnamon Twigs), Bo He (Mint), Chen Pi (Citrus Peel), and Hong Hua (Safflower Flower) (Freeman 2001a,b; Chen and Chen 2012a).

Sweet herbs are considered tonifying, harmonizing, moderating, and cloying (Freeman 2001a,b; Chen and Chen 2012a). The TCVM therapeutic actions include tonifying and harmonizing (balancing) herbal formulas, as well as reducing pain (Chen et al. 2012). Sweet herbs should be used with caution in patients with Spleen Deficiency and Damp signs (Freeman 2001a,b; Chen and Chen 2012a). Examples include Gan Cao (Licorice Root), Huang Qi (Astragalus Root), Da Zao (Jujube Fruit), and Ren Shen (Ginseng) (Freeman 2001a,b; Chen and Chen 2012a; Chen et al. 2012).

Sour herbs are known to stabilize and bind (Freeman 2001a,b; Chen and Chen 2012a). They help stop perspiration, stop bleeding, bind diarrhea, nourish Stomach Yin (improving appetite), and stop muscle spasms due to body fluid deficiency (Freeman 2001a,b; Chen and Chen 2012a). Examples include Wu Wei Zi (Schisandra Fruit), Xian He Cao (Agrimony), Shi Liu Pi (Pomagranate Rind), Wu Mei (Black Plum), and Bai Shao (White Peony) (Freeman 2001a,b; Mitchell 2006; Chen and Chen 2012a).

Bitter herbs are known to sedate, purge, dry damp, and eliminate heat (Freeman 2001a,b; Chen and Chen 2012a). TCVM therapeutic actions include draining heat downward to relieve constipation, pulling Lung Qi downward relieving wheezing and regulating breathing, clearing heat caused by infections, and draining damp and clearing heat (Chen et al. 2012). Bitter herbs should be used with caution in large quantities and patients with Yin or Body Fluid Deficiency (Freeman 2001a,b; Chen and Chen 2012a). Examples include Da Huang (Rhubarb Root and Rhizome), Xing Ren (Apricot Kernel), Zhi Zi (Gardenia Fruit), Huang Lian (Coptis Root), and Cang Zhu (Red Atractylodes Rhizome) (Freeman 2001a,b; Mitchell 2006; Chen and Chen 2012a).

Salty herbs are known to purge excess, soft hardness, and open kidney channels (Freeman 2001a,b; Chen and Chen 2012a). TCVM therapeutic actions include treating constipation, softening hardness to treat masses, and treating kidney disorders (Chen et al. 2012). Examples include Mang Xiao (Mirabilite), Mu Li (Oyster Shell), and Lu Tong (Sweetgum Fruit) (Freeman 2001a,b; Mitchell 2006; Chen and Chen 2012a).

Bland herbs have little to no taste and are often used as diuretics to drain edema and improve urinary function (Freeman 2001a,b; Chen and Chen 2012a). Examples include Fu Ling (Poria Sclerotium) and Zhu Ling (Polyporus) (Freeman 2001a,b; Mitchell 2006; Chen and Chen 2012a).

Astringent herbs are like sour herbs. They help stabilize, bind, and reduced/prevent Body Fluid loss (Chen and Chen 2012a). TCVM therapeutic actions include preventing Lung Qi leakage to treat cough, binding the intestines to resolve diarrhea, and stopping spontaneous sweating (Chen et al. 2012). Examples include Wu Wei Zi (Schisandra Fruit), Chi Shi Zhi (Halloysite), and Fu Xiao Mai (Triticum Seed) (Freeman 2001a,b; Mitchell 2006; Chen and Chen 2012a).

Western Classifications

CH can also be classified from a Western medicine perspective based on their pharmacologic effects. Extensive research has been conducted on the beneficial and detrimental effects of individual herbs.

As an example, let's take a closer look at Bai Shao (*Paeonia lactiflora* or White Peony). Bai Shao is classified in TCM as a blood tonic with the following Chinese therapeutic actions: nourishes Blood and preserves Yin; calms Liver Yang and Wind by nourishing the Liver; and relieves pain by supporting the Liver (Chen and Chen 2012a). Bai Shao has shown positive effects on:

1) Cardiovascular system by lowering blood pressure (Zhong Guo Yao Li Xue Tong Bao 1986).
2) Endocrine system by lowering blood glucose levels (Zhong Xi Yi Jie He Za Zhi 1986).
3) Gastrointestinal system by reducing intestinal spasms, reducing gastric acid secretion, and relieving constipation (Zhong Yi Za Zhi 1983, 1987; Zhong Yao Zhi 1983).
4) Immune system by reducing fevers and decreasing inflammation, and by having some antibacterial properties (Zhong Yao Zhi 1993; Xin Zhong Yi 1989).
5) Neurologic system through the reduction of pain and by acting as a central nervous system suppressant (Shang Hai Zhong Yi Yao Za Zhi 1983; Zhong Yao Tong Bao 1985).
6) Respiratory system through the reduction of cough and wheezing (Hu Nan Zhong Yi Za Zhi 1986; Zhong Yi Za Zhi 1987).

Based on its beneficial effects Bai Shao has potential herb–drug interactions with anticoagulants and with antiplatelet, diabetic, and sedative medications (Zhong Yao Tong Bao 1985; Chen 1998/1999; Chen and Chen 2012a).

At first glance, it may appear that TCVM and Western therapeutic effects have nothing in common, but the reality is this is all one medicine. Bai Shao is known to "soften" the liver, allowing Qi to move and drain more easily, as well as improving liver blood flow (Chen and Chen 2012a). Draining and moving Qi relieves cough, often due to liver Qi Stagnation (Marsden 2014a). Improved Qi flow improves spasms in both smooth muscle (intestinal tract) and skeletal muscle, which reduces pain (Marsden 2014a). Improved liver blood flow improves blood flow to the periphery, supporting all systems including neurologic, respiratory, endocrine, gastrointestinal, and immune, and encourages vasodilation and reduced blood pressure. Vasodilation also helps expel pathogens, i.e. improving immune system function (Marsden 2014a).

Herbal Monographs

Herbal monographs are used to completely describe a specific herb, both Eastern and Western. The American Botanical Council (www.abc.herbalgram.org) requires that herbal monographs contain the following information: nomenclature, parts used, constituents, range of applications and uses, contraindications, adverse effects, herb–drug interactions, dosage recommendations, and mechanisms of action.

Chinese herbal monographs differ slightly from traditional herbal monographs in that the Pinyin (Chinese name), thermal and taste properties, channels entered, and Chinese therapeutic actions are also included. The following demonstrates the information commonly found in Chinese herbal monographs (Figure 3.4).

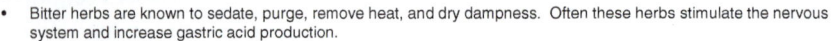

Herbal Monograph

PinYin: DanShen
Scientific Name: Salvia miltiorrhiza
English Name: Salvia Root
Source: Root of the plant
Properties: Bitter, Cold
- Bitter herbs are known to sedate, purge, remove heat, and dry dampness. Often these herbs stimulate the nervous system and increase gastric acid production.
- Cool herbs are often used to treat warm or hot diseases.

Channels Entered: Heart, Pericardium, Liver
Chemical Composition:
- >30 lipophilic (predominately diterpene chinone) compounds
- >50 hydrophillic (predominately phenolic acids) compounds

Chinese Therapeutic Actions:
- *Blood-Invigorating and Stasis-Removing Herbs*
- Regulates and Activates Blood circulation
- Disperses Blood stasis
- Cools the Blood
- Diminishes Swellings and Sores
- Nourishes the Blood
- Calms the Shen
- Stimulated Breast Milk Production

Pharmacological Effects:
Cardiovascular
- Most known for its effects on coronary heart disease, especially the treatment of angina pectoris.
- Reduces the negative effects of acute ischemic strokes (i.e speeds short-term recovery).
- Improvement of macro-and microcirculation.
- Coronary artery dilation.
- Prevention of myocardial ischemia.
- Prevention of reperfusion injury to the myocardium following an ischemic event.
- Protection of the brain following an ischemic event and reperfusion injury.
- Inhibition of cardiac hyperplasia secondary to angiotensin II.
- Inhibition of DNA synthesis of non-cardiomyocyte cells in the damaged heart.
Hematologic
- Antioxidant through scavenging oxygen free radicals.
- Platelet aggregation inhibition.
- Stimulation of NO production by endothelial cells.
- Reduction of hyperlipidemia is believed to be through oxidative changes to LDL resulting in reduced uptake by macrophages.
Veterinary Medicine
- Anticoagulant properties (interferes with extrinsic coagulation pathway, affects antithrombin III activity, inhibits platelet aggregation, and promotes fibrinolysis).
- Antioxidant properties (primarily as a free radical scavenger).
- Hypotensive properties (reduces peripheral vascular resistance and ACE inhibitor).
- GI protective properties (increases gastric mucosal blood flow and delays onset of aspirin-induced gastric lesions).
- Hepatic protective properties (especially in cases of chronic hepatitis and hepatic fibrosis).
- Antineoplastic properties.

Cautions and Contraindications:
- Do not use with Li Lu
- Use caution in patients with hematuria, hemoptysis, and hypermenorrhea.

Herb-Drug Interactions:
- Anticoagulants and Antiplatelet Drugs
- Digoxin

Toxicology: No reported fatalities

Figure 3.4 Herbal monograph of Dan Shen (Chen and Chen 2012a). Source: Lisa P. McFaddin.

Formula Components

Chinese herbal formulas have historically been created using a metaphorical hierarchy, which balances the formula, maximizes its effects, and minimizes side effects (Yi and Chang 2004; Chen and Chen 2012a). All CF contain four types of individual herbs: King Herb, Deputy Herb, Assistant Herb, and Envoy Herb (Yi and Chang 2004; Chen and Chen 2012a).

The **King or Chief Herb**, often found in the highest quantity within the formula, has the greatest effect or action on the imbalance being treated (Yi and Chang 2004; Chen and Chen 2012a). The **Deputy Herb** assists the King Herb with the primary goal but also assists in treating additional problems (Yi and Chang 2004; Chen and Chen 2012a). The **Assistant Herb** helps the King and Deputy herbs but also counteracts potential adverse effects associated with the first two herbs (Yi and Chang 2004; Chen and Chen 2012a). Assistant herbs may have an opposite effect of the King and/or Deputy herbs to balance the formula. Finally, the **Envoy Herb** focuses the formula on a specific segment of the body, organ, channel, or set of channels while harmonizing the formula (Yi and Chang 2004; Chen and Chen 2012a).

As an example, let's examine a commonly used CF, Si Miao San (Four Marvels Powder). Si Miao San is a simple, but extremely powerful, herbal formula which contains four individual herbs: Huang Bo, Yi Yi Ren, Cang Zhu, and Huai Niu Xi. The inclusion of each ingredient supports the herbal hierarchy described above. Huang Bo (Phellodendron Bark) is the King Herb which dries Damp, clears Heat, and clears inflammation from the gastrointestinal tract (Chen et al. 2012). Yi Yi Ren (Coix Seed) is the Deputy Herb which drains Damp, discharges pus, and supports the Spleen (Chen et al. 2012). Cang Zhu (Atractylodes rhizome) is the Assistant Herb which warms, supports, and protects the Spleen (Chen et al. 2012). Huai Niu Xi (Achryanthes root) is the Envoy Herb which moves Blood and acts as a mild Astringent (Chen et al. 2012).

The Chinese therapeutic effects of Si Miao San include Clearing Heat, Expelling Damp, Tonifying, and Moving (Chen et al. 2012). The Western therapeutic effects include aiding in the treatment of inflammatory disorders (cholangiohepatitis, colitis, pancreatitis, gastritis, cystitis, arthritis, vaginitis, anal sacculitis, sinusitis, dermatitis, pododermatitis, allergic dermatitis, otitis externa, pyoderma, seborrhea oleosa, perianal fistulas, inflammatory bowel disease, stomatitis, gingivitis, and conjunctivitis), degenerative myelopathy, immune-mediated thrombocytopenia, jaundice, hepatic lipidosis, diabetes mellitus, hyperadrenocorticism, hypoadrenocorticism, epilepsy, neoplasia, and lumbosacral pain (Chen et al. 2012; Marsden 2014b). The herb should be stopped if diarrhea develops and/or worsens.

Formula TCVM Classifications

As previously mentioned, CF are mainly classified by their Chinese therapeutic actions. The sum of the individual herbs within a formula creates the primary objectives for which the herb is used. The most common TCVM therapeutic categories for CF include Exterior-Releasing Formulas, Downward Draining Formulas, Harmonizing Formulas, Exterior- and Interior-Releasing Formulas, Heat-Clearing Formulas, Summer-Heat-Dispelling Formulas, Interior-Warming Formulas, Tonic Formulas, Shen-Calming Formulas, Orifice-Opening Formulas, Astringent Formulas, Qi-Regulating Formulas, Blood-Regulating Formulas, Wind-Expelling Formulas, Dryness-Relieving Formulas, Damp-Dispelling Formulas, Wind-Damp Dispelling Formulas, Phlegm-Dispelling Formulas, Reducing, Guiding, and Dissolving Formulas, Antiparasitic Formulas, Emetic Formulas, and Formulas that Treat Abscesses and Sores (Chen and Chen 2012a; Chen et al. 2012).

There are less involved TCVM classification systems for CF. The College of Integrative Therapies groups herbs by those treating Blood Disorders, Dampness and Phlegm, Qi Deficiency,

Qi Stagnation, Shao-Yang Disharmony, Wind Invasion, Yang Rising, and Yin and Yang Deficiency (Marsden 2014a). Natural Path Veterinary Herbal Formulas categorizes formulas by those which Transform Phlegm, Drain Damp, Tonify, Extinguish Wind, Clear Heat, and Move.

Tables 3.22 and 3.23 highlight the individual herbal components, TCVM indications, and Western indications for two commonly used Chinese herbal formulas in veterinary medicine: Ba Wei Di Huang Wan (BWDHW) and Xiao Yao San (XYS). BWDHW is often used to address common ailments associated with aging by supporting the kidney (Marsden 2014a). In Chinese medicine dwindling kidney resources are associated with cognitive decline and limiting lifespan. XYS is primarily used to aid in liver disorders and anxiety by supporting the liver and improving circulation (Marsden 2014c).

TCVM Therapeutic Classifications for Veterinarians

CF are further broken down into general categories and subclasses. For example, tonifying formulas, which supplement and support Qi, Blood, Yin, Yang, Jing and/or Body Fluids, include Qi Tonics, Blood Tonics, Qi and Blood Tonics, Yin Tonics, Yang Tonics, and Yin and Yang Tonics (Chen et al. 2012; Marsden 2014a). Qi Tonics, such as Zhong Yi Qi Tang (Tonify the Middle and Augment the Qi Decoction), typically treat Spleen and Lung Qi Deficiencies. Blood tonics, like Dang Gui Shao Yao San (Angelica and Peony Combination), treat Blood Deficiencies especially those affecting the Heart and Liver. Qi and Blood Tonics, such as Ba Zhen Tang (Eight-Treasure Decoction), treat a combination of Qi and Blood Deficiencies. Yin Tonics, like Zhi Bai Di Huang Wan (Anemarrhena, Phellodendron, and Rehmannia Pill), treat Yin Deficiencies, especially those affecting the Liver and Kidney. Yang Tonics, such as Ba Wei Di Huang Wan (Rehmannia 8), treat Kidney Yang Deficiencies. Yin and Yang Tonics, like Di Huang Yin Zi (Rehmannia Decoction), treat Yin and Yang Deficiencies.

Formula Western Classifications

CF can also be classified by their Western therapeutic effects (Table 3.24). The administration of CF based solely on the Western diagnosis is not advisable. The same TCVM diagnosis is often used for two very different Western diseases. For example, the TCVM diagnosis of Damp Heat may be applied to a patient with acute pancreatitis and a patient with a urinary tract infection (UTI), depending on the TCVM exam findings. In both cases the TCVM treatment principles would be to drain Damp and clear Heat. The same herb may not be appropriate for both patients. The pancreatitis patient may benefit from Si Miao San while the UTI patient may require San Ren Tang and respond poorly to the more potent Si Miao San formula.

Chinese Herbal Therapy Treatment Strategies

CH and CF are chosen based on the Chinese medical diagnosis (Hao and Lin 2003). The CH or CF is then matched to the specific symptoms exhibited by the patients (Hao and Lin 2003). Whatever the problem, the herb causing the opposite effect is chosen. For example, to treat Yin Deficiency a Yin-Tonic is chosen; to treat Damp Heat an herb or formula which clears Heat and drains Damp is chosen; or to treat Blood Deficiency a Blood-Tonic is chosen.

Regulation

The regulation of herbs and herbal formulas is mainly influenced by their categorization (drug, botanical drug, dietary supplement, or food additive) and target consumer (human or animal). Depending on the marketing and label claim, an herb or herbal formula may meet the definition of a drug, herbal drug, or dietary supplement.

Drugs

The modern definition of the word "drug" is based on the United States Federal Food, Drug and Cosmetic Act (FDCA), section 201(g). Drugs are defined as substances used to

Table 3.22 The formula ingredients, TCVM indications, and Western indications for Ba Wei Di Huang Wang (Rehmannia Eight) (Mitchell 2006; Chen et al. 2012; Chen and Chen 2012a; Marsden 2014a). Both the Chinese and English names are provided for the individual herbs. The TCVM properties of the individual herbs are also described. For the Western indications both the body system being treated and example conditions are provided.

Formula ingredients	
Sheng Di Huang (Rehmannia Root)	Heat-clearing and blood-cooling herb: warms and nourishes kidney Yin and blood Qi-tonifying herb: nourishes spleen, stomach, and lung Yin
Shan Yao (Chinese Yam)	Qi-tonifying herb: nourishes spleen, stomach, and lung Yin
Shan Zhu Yu (Cornus)	Astringent herb: tonifies liver and kidney; nourishes LIV blood and Yin
Fu Ling (Poria)	Water-regulating and damp-dissolving herb: supports the spleen and drains damp from the middle burner
Ze Xie (Water Plantain)	Water-regulating and damp-dissolving herb: promotes urination in the lower burner
Mu Dan Pi (Moutan)	Heat-clearing and blood-cooling herbs:clears heat and drains fire from the liver
Gui Zhi (Cinnamon Bark)	Exterior-releasing wind-cold herb: warms Yang eliminating water or phlegm stagnation; promotes blood circulation
Fu Zi (Prepared Aconite root)	Interior-warming herbs: warms kidney Yang which improves urine concentration ability and cools mild heart fire

TCVM indications
Tonify Qi
Tonifying kidney Qi Grasping Lung Qi
Tonify and nourish Yin
Kidney Yin deficiency
Kidney Yang deficiency
Kidney Qi deficiency
Dampness accumulation
Blood deficiency

Western indications	
Body system	**Example conditions**
Behavior	Nocturnal restlessness; cognitive dysfunction
Cardiopulmonary	Asthma; chronic cough (geriatric pets)
Endocrine	Diabetes mellitus (feline, late stage); hypothyroidism
Gastrointestinal	Constipation
Musculoskeletal	Lower back weakness or stiffness; muscle atrophy; stiffness; arthritis; degenerative joint disease
Neurologic	Paresis; back pain; hindlimb weakness; degenerative myelopathy
Ophthalmologic	Cataracts (especially with diabetes mellitus)
Urogenital	Urinary incontinence; mild to moderate azotemia; chronic renal failure

Source: Lisa P. McFaddin.

Table 3.23 The formula ingredients, TCVM indications, and Western indications for Xiao Yao San (Happy Wanderer) (Mitchell 2006; Chen et al. 2012; Chen and Chen 2012a; Marsden 2014c). Both the Chinese and English names are provided for the individual herbs. The TCVM properties of the individual herbs are also described. For the Western indications both the body system being treated, and example conditions are provided.

Formula ingredients	
Chai Hu (Bupleurum)	Exterior releasing wind-heat herb: moves stagnant liver Qi
Dang Gui (Angelica)	Blood-tonifying herb: moves and tonifies liver blood and Yin
Bai Shao Yao (White Peony)	Blood-tonifying herb: moves and tonifies liver blood and Yin
Bo He (Mint)	Exterior-releasing wind-heat: clears liver heat
Bai Zhu (White Atractylodes)	Qi-tonifying herb: drains and dries damp from the spleen and stomach; supports Qi formation in the spleen and lung
Fu Ling (Poria)	Water-regulating and damp-dissolving herb: drains and dries damp from the spleen and stomach; supports Qi formation in the spleen and lung
Gan Cao (Licorice)	Qi-tonifying herb: drains and dries damp from the spleen and stomach; supports Qi formation in the spleen and lung
Sheng Jiang (Zingiber)	Exterior releasing wind-cold herb: disperses wind-cold; warms the middle

TCVM indications
Harmonize regulate and harmonize the liver and spleen
Disperse liver Qi
Relieve stagnation
Tonify spleen Qi
Nourish blood
Liver blood deficiency
Blood deficiency
Disharmonies between liver and spleen
Spleen deficiency
Liver Qi stagnation
Damp symptoms are not prominent

Western indications	
Body system	**Example conditions**
Behavior	Depression; irritability (secondary to liver Qi stagnation); separation anxiety; timidity; irritable bowel disease (stress-induced); insomnia; restlessness; territorial aggression; dominance aggression; fear aggression
Dermatology	Allergic dermatitis; seborrhea sicca; recurrent superficial pyoderma; generalized demodectic mange
Gastrointestinal	Inflammatory bowel disease; irritable bowel syndrome; abdominal distension; abdominal pain; constipation; vomiting; gastrointestinal ulceration; megacolon; lymphangiectasia (especially with low albumin); diarrhea
Hepatic	Mild liver enzyme elevations; congenital microhepatica; chronic active hepatitis; cirrhosis; low albumin
Neoplasia	Adenocarcinoma
Ophthalmologic	Keratoconjunctivitis sicca
Urogenital	Irregular menstruation; uterine bleeding; premenstrual syndrome

Source: Lisa P. McFaddin.

Table 3.24 New and traditional Chinese herbal formulas used in veterinary medicine based on the affected Western organ system (Marsden 2014a; Ma 2016). The Chinese and English names are provided, when applicable.

Body system	Chinese formula name	English formula name
Abdominal conditions	Xiao Chai Hu Tang	Minor Bupleurum combination
	Xiao Yao San	Happy Wanderer
	Yi Guan Jian	Glehnia and Rehmannia combination
Behavioral conditions	Bu Zhong Yi Qi Tang	Ginseng and Astragalus combination
	n/a	Heart Qi Tonic™
	Si Miao San	Four Marvels
	n/a	Shen Calmer™
	Xiao Yao San	Happy Wanderer
	Yi Guan Jian	Glehnia and Rehmannia combination
Cardiovascular conditions	Bu Zhong Yi Qi Tang	Ginseng and Astragalus combination
	n/a	Heart Qi Tonic
	Liu Jun Zi Tang	Six Gentlemen combination
Dermatologic conditions	n/a	Dandruff Formula™
	n/a	External Wind™
	Qing Ying Tang	Clear the Nutritive Level combination
	San Ren Tang	Three Seeds combination
	Si Miao San	Four Marvels
	Si Wu Xiao Feng Yin	Four Materials Eliminate Wind combination
Ear conditions	n/a	Ear Damp Heat™
	Long Dan Er Miao San	Gentiana and Two Marvels combination
	Si Wu Xiao Feng Yin	Four Materials Eliminate Wind combination
Endocrine disorders	n/a	Ophiopogon Formula
	Si Miao San	Four Marvels
	Xiao Chai Hu Tang	Minor Bupleurum combination
	Xue Fu Zhu Yu Tang	Persica and Achyranthes combination
	Zhi Bai Di Huang Wan	Anemarrhena, Phellodendron, and Rehmannia combination
Eye conditions	Long Dan Xie Gan Tang	Gentiana combination
	San Ren Tang	Three Seeds combination

(Continued)

Table 3.24 (Continued)

Body system	Chinese formula name	English formula name
Hepatic disorders	Xiao Chai Hu Tang	Minor Bupleurum combination
	Xiao Yao San	Happy Wanderer
	Xue Fu Zhu Yu Tang	Persica and Achyranthes combination
	Yi Guan Jian	Glehnia and Rehmannia combination
Gastrointestinal disorders	Bu Zhong Yi Qi Tang	Ginseng and Astragalus combination
	San Ren Tang	Three Seeds combination
	n/a	Stomach Happy™
	Wei Ling Tang	Harmonize the stomach with Poria Five Herbs combination
	n/a	Stomach Happy
	Yi Guan Jian	Glehnia and Rehmannia combination
Musculoskeletal conditions	n/a	Bone Healing™
	n/a	Coix Formula
	Si Miao San	Four Marvels
	Xiao Huo Luo Dan	Minor Invigorate the Collaterals combination
	Yi Yi Ren Tang	Coix combination
	You Gui Wan	Eucommia and Rehmannia combination
Neoplasia	n/a	Breast Stasis Formula
	n/a	Max's Formula
	n/a	Stasis Breaker™
	Xue Fu Zhu Yu Tang	Persica and Achyranthes combination
	n/a	Hoxsey and Boneset Formula
Neurologic conditions	n/a	Cervical Formula
	n/a	Double P II™
	Xiao Chai Hu Tang	Minor Bupleurum combination
	Chai Ge Jie Ji Tang	Bupleurum and Kudzu combination
	Si Miao San	Four Marvels
	Zhi Bai Di Huang Wan	Anemarrhena, Phellodendron and Rehmannia combination
Reproductive disorders	Ban Xia Bai Zhu Tian Ma Tang	Pinellia, Atractylodes and Gastrodia Combination
	Bu Zhong Yi Qi Tang	Ginseng and Astragalus combination
	Jin Gui Shen Qi Wan	Rehmannia Eight combination

Body system	Chinese formula name	English formula name
Respiratory conditions	n/a	Lily Combination™
	San Ren Tang	Three Seeds combination
	Xue Fu Zhu Yu Tang	Persica and Achyranthes combination
Systemic immune-mediated and infectious conditions	n/a	Blood Heat Formula
	Qing Ying Tang	Clear the Nutritive Level combination
	Si Miao San	Four Marvels
	Xiao Chai Hu Tang	Minor Bupleurum combination
	Yi Guan Jian	Glehnia and Rehmannia combination
Urinary and renal conditions		Crystal Stone Formula
	Long Dan Xie Gan Tang	Gentiana combination
	San Ren Tang	Three Seeds combination
	Shao Fu Zhu Yu Tang	Fennel Seed and Corydalis combination
	Zhi Bai Di Huang Wan	Anemarrhena, Phellodendron and Rehmannia combination

n/a, indicates when a name is not applicable.
Source: Lisa P. McFaddin.

diagnose, cure, treat, or prevent disease in both humans and animals, as well as alter the body's functions or structure (FDA 2021c).

The process through which both human and animal drugs receive Food and Drug Administration (FDA) approval is expensive, arduous, and a little strange. First, the drug must be classified for use in animals. Second, the drug must be new. Third, the new drug must prove in clinical trials it is both effective and safe. While the FDA states "new drugs and certain biologics must be proven safe and effective to FDA's satisfaction before companies can market them in interstate commerce," the FDA does not "develop or test products before approving them" (FDA 2020, 2021b). Instead,

"[the] manufacturers must...prove they are able to make the drug product according to federal quality standards. . .[and] FDA experts review the results of laboratory,

animal, and human clinical testing done by manufacturers. If FDA grants an approval, it means the agency has determined that the benefits of the product outweigh the known risks for the intended use" (FDA 2020, 2021b).

Botanical Drugs

The FDA defines a botanical drug as a product

"intended for use in the diagnosis, cure, mitigation, treatment or prevention of disease in humans. A botanical drug product consists of vegetable materials, which may include plant materials, algae, macroscopic fungi, or combinations thereof. A botanical drug product may be available as (but not limited to) a solution (e.g. tea), powder, tablet, capsule, elixir, topical, or injection. Botanical drug products often have unique features, for example, complex mixtures, lack of a distinct active ingredient, and substantial prior human use. Fermentation products and highly purified or chemically modified botanical substances are not considered botanical drug products" (FDA 2022c).

The Center for Drug Evaluation and Research (CDER), a division within the FDA, released *Botanical Drug Development Guidance for Industry* in 2016. The Guidance provides recommendations for submitting new herbal drug applications and suggestions on how to standardize over-the-counter (OTC) drug monograph system (CDER 2016). As of October 2022, there were only two approved botanical drugs, both for people, on the market. Additionally,

"[t]here are some botanical drugs, including cascara, psyllium, and senna, that are included in the over the counter (OTC) drug review. For a botanical drug substance to be included in an OTC monograph, there must be published data establishing a general recognition of safety and effectiveness, including the results of adequate and well-controlled clinical studies" (FDA 2022c).

Human Dietary Supplements

All herbs and herbal formulas marketed for human consumption are classified as dietary supplements. They are often referred to as herbal supplements or botanicals. The Dietary Supplement Health and Education Act (DSHEA) of 1994, an amendment to the United States Federal Food, Drug and Cosmetic Act (FDCA, Title 21), was created to provide standards for dietary supplements (DSHEA 1994). Dietary supplements were defined as substances which complement the diet and contain at least one of the following ingredients: a vitamin, a mineral, an herb, an amino acid, or a product which affects caloric intake (DSHEA 1994). Within the provisions established by DSHEA, dietary supplements were classified as a separate regulatory category of food, meaning dietary supplements were not considered food or drug.

Almost all dietary supplements are considered OTC. FDA approval is not required to market or sell the products. DSHEA further stipulates the FDA is only responsible for ensuring the safety of supplements if there is gross risk of illness, inadequate evidence regarding product safety, or a supplement is adulterated (DSHEA 1994).

The FDA does not regulate the development, manufacturing, or marketing of dietary supplements. In 2006 the FDA issued a guidance document called "Questions and Answers Regarding the Labeling of Dietary Supplements as Required by the Dietary Supplement and Nonprescription Drug Consumer Protection Act" (FDA 2009). All this really did was require manufacturers to include a domestic address or phone number so people could more easily report adverse reactions to the companies.

The FDA does specify what information pertaining to health claims can be made. Health claims assert a relationship between a particular substance and its ability to diagnose, treat, cure, or prevent disease. The FDA may approve health claims if there is enough scientific evidence supporting the correlation (FDA 2018).

Many dietary supplements tout claims pertaining to a specific function within the body ("probiotics improve gut health") or a general well-being claim associated with a nutrient deficiency ("vitamin D prevents rickets"). The FDA does not require pre-approval of these claims but does require notification from the manufacturer within 30 days of marketing the supplement (FDA 2009). The FDA also requires placement of a "disclaimer" on the product informing consumers the claim has not been evaluated by the FDA, and the dietary supplement is "not intended to diagnose, treat, cure, or prevent any disease" (FDA 2018).

The FDA requires manufacturers notify the FDA when a new dietary ingredient is included in a supplement. Companies must demonstrate the new ingredient is expected to be safe without risk of illness to individuals taking the supplement per label instructions (FDA 2018). Regulatory action can be taken by the FDA if the product is deemed unsafe after marketing.

The FDA also requires all manufacturers and distributors of herbs and herbal formulas register with the FDA. The FDA does not approve companies:

"Owners and operators of domestic and foreign food, drug, and most device facilities must register their facilities with FDA, unless an exemption applies. FDA does have authority to inspect regulated facilities to verify that they comply with applicable good manufacturing practice regulations" (FDA 2017).

In the December 2006 Draft Guidance, the FDA released a "Guidance for industry on complementary and alternative medicine (CAM) products and their regulation by the FDA" in response to an increasing number of CAM products and public confusion regarding the regulation of said products.

"This guidance makes two fundamental points: First, depending on the CAM therapy or practice, a product used in a CAM therapy or practice may be subject to regulation as a biological product, cosmetic, drug, device, or food (including food additives and dietary supplements) under the [Federal Food, Drug, and Cosmetic Act, the "Act"] or the [Public Health Service (PHS)] Act. For example, the PHS Act defines "biological product," and the Act defines (among other things): Cosmetic; Device; Dietary supplement; Drug, as well as "new drug" and "new animal drug"; Food; and Food additive. These statutory definitions cover some CAM products. Second, neither the Act nor the PHS Act exempts CAM products from regulation. This means, for example, if

a person decides to produce and sell raw vegetable juice for use in juice therapy to promote optimal health, that product is a food subject to the requirements for foods in the Act and FDA regulations, including the hazard analysis and critical control point (HACCP) system requirements for juices in 21 CFR part 120. If the juice therapy is intended for use as part of a disease treatment regimen instead of for the general wellness, the vegetable juice would also be subject to regulation as a drug under the Act" (FDA 2007).

In summary, depending on how the herbal product is marketed and labeled, it may be considered a dietary supplement, food, or drug. Dietary supplements receive very little to no FDA oversight. Food substances must meet the requirements defined by the Federal Food, Drug, and Cosmetic Act (FDCA, Title 21). If the herbal product is marketed or used to treat disease, then it is considered a "drug" and must meet the requirements defined by the FDCA (Title 21).

Animal Dietary Supplements

When DSHEA was enacted, the language only discussed the use of dietary supplements in humans, not animals. Initially, animal dietary supplements included ingredients like those found in equivalent human dietary supplements and were sold under the guidelines of DSHEA (Grassie 2002). In 1996 the FDA published the "Inapplicability of the dietary supplement health and education act to animal products" (Docket No. 95N-0308) stating DSHEA did not apply to animal products (Schultz 1996). The FDA's rationale was that DSHEA did not specifically reference animal products but did specifically reference human products. Additionally, many of the human supplement ingredients had not been studied in animals and may be unsafe for companion animal use (Schultz 1996). Finally, the administration of many human supplement ingredients to food animals may be unsafe for human consumption (Schultz 1996).

This decision had two major repercussions for veterinary medicine. First, any animal dietary supplement produced and marketed under DSHEA was now considered a drug and must meet the requirements established by the FDA to obtain drug approval. Secondly, animal dietary supplements were now classified as animal food and regulated under the FDCA (Title 21). Under the FDCA (Title 21) any supplement claiming or intended to be used for the treatment or prevention of disease is considered a drug and must be approved by the FDA. Any unapproved "drug" is subject to regulatory action by the FDA.

Many supplement ingredients used in people are not approved for use in animal feed. This gets even more complicated because many human dietary supplements are marketed with specific label claims for affecting functions within the body. Many pet parents assume the same applications hold true for animals, again making these supplements more like drugs. According to the National Animal Supplement Council (NASC) there are over 400 unapproved substances marketed for use in animals (Grassie 2002).

The FDCA (Title 21) does not require premarket FDA approval before new animal food is sold. The FDCA does require "that food for animals, like food for people, be safe to eat, produced under sanitary conditions, free of harmful substances, and truthfully labeled" (FDA 2021c).

In 2011 Congress amended the FDCA (Title 21) by passing the Food Safety Modernization Act (FASMA) which allowed the FDA

"to better protect public health by strengthening the food safety system and shifting the focus from *responding* to contamination of the food supply to *preventing* contamination. The law applies to food for people as well as food for animals, including pet food. FSMA requires animal food facilities to create and implement a food safety plan. In the first part of the plan, the facilities assess food safety hazards that are potentially associated with the animal food (this is called "hazard analysis"). In the second part, the facilities take steps, when necessary, to reduce or eliminate identified food safety hazards (these steps are called "preventive controls"). The above FSMA requirements apply to companies that must register as an animal food facility because they manufacture, process, pack, or hold animal food for consumption in the United States. Besides having to follow the requirements under FSMA, registered animal food facilities must also comply with current good manufacturing practices (unless an exemption applies). These practices provide baseline standards for manufacturing, processing, packing, and holding animal food to ensure it's safe for animals to eat" (FDA 2022a).

Hazard analysis critical control point (HACCP) is a recognized worldwide as a "management system in which food safety is addressed through the analysis and control of biological, chemical, and physical hazards from raw material production, procurement and handling, to manufacturing, distribution and consumption of the finished product" (FDA 2022b). In 2021 the FDA's Center for Veterinary Medicine (CVM) released *Hazard Analysis and Risk-Based Preventative Controls for Food for Animals Guidance for Industry*. The document outlines the requirements for developing a food safety plan (FSP) for facilities producing animal food (CVM 2022). An FSP was defined as a written plan outlining a systematic approach to identifying food safety hazards that can be controlled to prevent or minimize the likelihood of foodborne illness or injury (CVM 2022). An FSP and HACCP are similar, but as of 2021 the FDA has not mandated an HACCP system for animal food (CVM 2022). Development and utilization of an HACCP is a voluntary process for companies in the animal food industry.

The FDCA does require pre-market approval for animal food additives. Food additives are defined as "any substance that directly or indirectly becomes a component of a food or that affects a food's characteristics" (FDA 2021a,c). Substances generally recognized as safe (GRAS) are exempt from the pre-market approval requirements (FDA 2021a,c).

For a substance to be categorized as GRAS the FDA states "qualified experts must agree that the substance is safe when added to food" (FDA 2021c). This is accomplished by either a history of common safe use in food or scientific studies. A company itself can determine if a substance is GRAS by submitting the following to the FDA: description of the substance, how the substance will be used and in what species, and how the company determined the product was GRAS (FDA 2021a,c). After reviewing the company's information, the FDA determines if the GRAS standard has been met.

A substance may be considered GRAS in one setting but not in another. Additionally, food additives cannot be labeled GRAS if used for a medicinal purpose. In that case the substance is considered a drug and must meet the requirements for a new animal drug (FDA 2021c). All of this is to say it is often more complicated to get approval for a food additive than a food, and even more complex if trying to meet the GRAS standards.

The CVM is responsible for regulating animal food products, including many botanicals. Failure of a food to meet the requirements outlined in the FDCA (Title 21) results in the food (or in this case the botanical) classified as adulterated or misbranded. The reality is a lot of botanicals used in veterinary medicine are considered unapproved food additives or unapproved animal drugs, and the FDA could take regulatory action (Burns 2017). Often the regulation of botanicals is low on the priority list for FDA regulators.

To summarize, an herb or herbal formula marketed as a food, containing ingredients with known and approved nutritional value, does not need CVM pre-market approval. An herb or herbal formula marketed as a food with unknown or unapproved ingredients requires CVM pre-market approval.

A veterinary herb or herbal formula marketed as a drug (generally ones with health or medical claims on the label) technically requires pre-market approval as a drug. If marketed as a drug without CVM approval it is required to meet FDA drug approval requirements. If those requirements cannot be met, the CVM may allow continued sales as "unapproved drugs of low regulatory priority" (Knueven 2018). This exemption is generally granted when the CVM believes the product is safe for its intended use and the company is acting responsibly with respect to manufacturing and marketing. The CVM may require the company register with the FDA as a drug manufacturer and follow specific labeling requirements for animal supplements (Knueven 2018).

Making all this more complicated, animal food is regulated at the federal and state levels. State agriculture departments are often responsible for regulating animal feed. State feed control officials generally do not regulate animal supplements unless they are labeled as animal feed or food additives (Burns 2017).

Most states follow standard outlined by the Association of American Feed Control Officers (AAFCO). The AAFCO has been in existence since 1906. AAFCO members are individuals from various governmental agencies throughout North America responsible for the regulation of animal feed. The FDA is a member of AAFCO. AAFCO exists as an animal-feed think tank in which members discuss potential rules and regulations pertaining to animal food. The ideas and models created by the AAFCO members are shared with the member's respective governmental agencies which then create laws. The individuals comprising AAFCO can regulate animal feed requirements within their jurisdictions, but AAFCO is not a regulatory body (AAFCO 2014).

Most states have adopted the AAFCO model for pet food regulations within their own laws, making the AAFCO model the default standard. The AAFCO model discusses recommendations for pet food labeling, i.e. what is written on the back of the bag of food. The model also covers the minimum recommended nutritional requirements and nutrient profiles for cats and dogs based on life stage. The following statement is found on most cat and dog foods: "[Pet Food Product Name] is formulated to meet the nutritional levels established by the AAFCO Dog (or Cat) Food Nutrient Profiles for [pet life stage]" (AAFCO 2014). For additional information about AAFCO and its pet food recommendations visit https://www.aafco.org.

Production

Keep in mind the FDA does not approve manufacturing companies.

"Owners and operators of domestic and foreign food, drug, and most device facilities must register their facilities with FDA, unless an exemption applies. FDA does have authority to inspect regulated facilities to verify that they comply with applicable good manufacturing practice regulations" (FDA 2017).

There appears to be room for error when it comes to manufacturing and bottling herbs. This highlights the importance of utilizing and recommending herbal products from trusted sources. There are several factors to consider when selecting a manufacturer, including the existence of a seed-to-seal guarantee, adherence to good manufacturing practices (GMP), and the existence of quality control measures.

Seed to Seal

An herbal manufacturing company should be able to trace the exact location from which each herb within the formula was grown and/or manufactured, processed, and bottled. The growing conditions are critical and overexposure to pesticides and fertilizers may adversely affect the therapeutic benefits and contribute to toxicity. Whenever possible the use of organic herbs is preferred. Accountability for each step within the manufacturing process ensures purity, potency, and patient protection.

Good Manufacturing Practices

The World Health Organization (WHO 2015) defines GMP as "a system for ensuring that products are consistently produced and controlled according to quality standards." Often evaluation of the final product is not enough to prevent human health hazards from potentially contaminated and/or adulterated medications. GMP monitors all areas of production, including the starting ingredients, buildings, equipment, training of personnel, and personnel hygiene. GMP identifies key areas of risk during the manufacturing process that could result in the production of potentially toxic and/or ineffective products. Areas of potential risk include contamination of the original products/ingredients, mislabeling of containers, and inaccurate measurement of the active ingredient(s) (WHO 2015).

The FDA requires all registered companies manufacturing CH and CF, follow current good manufacturing practice (CGMP) regulations as outlined in CFR Title 21.

"The CGMP regulations for drugs contain minimum requirements for the methods, facilities, and controls used in manufacturing, processing, and packing of a drug product. The regulations make sure that a product is safe for use, and that it has the ingredients and strength it claims to have" (FDA 2021c,d).

Finding a company which meets and/or exceeds the manufacturing controls established by CGMP ensures product purity and safety. A list of recommended herbal companies can be found in the Veterinarians section of this chapter.

GMP for Veterinarians

Written protocols are integral to the production of safe and effective products. The WHO has its own international GMP guidelines (WHO 2015). Many countries have created their own requirements modeled after the WHO guidelines.

In the United States, Title 21 of the Code of Federal Regulations covers the CGMP guidelines for finished pharmaceuticals (FDA 2021c,d). The CGMP ensures minimum requirements are met during the manufacturing, processing, and packaging of drugs. CGMP also requires the correct labeling of products including ingredients, strength, and certification of the product's safety. The FDA will not approve a new or generic drug without proof of compliance with the CGMP. The CGMP guidelines include the following requirements (FDA 2021c,d).

- The buildings and facilities are the appropriate size, clean, have good lighting and ventilation, and have sanitation equipment for the facility and employees.
- The equipment is appropriate, clean, well maintained, and operated by well-trained personnel.
- Personnel are well trained in equipment operations, safety, sanitation, and proper handling of medicinal ingredients and end products.
- The raw materials (active and inactive ingredients) are not contaminated or adulterated.
- The raw materials are labeled correctly.
- The correct volume/weight of raw materials is used.
- Only approved materials are being used.
- In-process and end-product samples are correctly identified and meet specifications for physical and chemical properties.
- The water supply to the facility meets minimum requirements for safe use and consumption.
- Written protocols regarding manufacturing and control have been established by the facility.

- Packages of finished products are clearly labeled.
- All samples of raw, in-process, and end-product materials are saved and stored appropriately for a specified amount of time.
- The facility keeps adequate records of raw material purchasing and quality control information; specifications for the type of raw materials used; specifications for mixing of ingredients; quality control measures; labeling requirements; and equipment maintenance.
- Personnel safety and hygiene.
- Complaints and accidents.

Quality Control

Quality control should be performed on all herbs throughout the growth, cultivation, processing, bottling and storage stages. Quality control also includes ensuring the right species and plant parts are chosen.

Ideally herbs should be grown in organic soil in their indigenous regions, as this yields the best medicinal results. Companies responsible for the raw herb material, i.e. growing and harvesting, should follow good agricultural practice (GAP) and good handling practices (GHP). Both GAP and GHP

"are voluntary audits [performed by the US Department of Agriculture] that verify that fruits and vegetables are produced, packed, handled, and stored as safely as possible to minimize risks of microbial food safety hazards. GAP and GHP audits verify adherence to the recommendations made in the U.S. Food and Drug Administration's Guide to Minimize Microbial Food Safety Hazards for Fresh Fruits and Vegetables and industry recognized food safety practices" (USDA 2020).

Once the raw herbs arrive at the processing facility the materials should undergo visual, chemical, heavy metal, pesticide, and microbial testing. Many of these tests should be performed repeatedly throughout the manufacturing, bottling, and storage phases. Companies should keep extensive records on the control measures, including facility cleanliness, product storage, product identification, and safety testing (USDA 2020).

Facility sanitation and cleanliness should include routine testing for microbial and yeast contaminants within the processing plant itself. Records of the product storage temperature and humidity standards for raw and processed herbs should be kept. Unique product identification for raw and processed herbs (seed to seal) is critical. Finally, safety testing should be performed on raw and processed herbs with safety limits that meet or exceed those outlined by the United States Pharmacopeia (https://www.usp.org). Herbs should be tested for the presence of pesticides, heavy metals, and microbial, yeast and mold counts.

The technique used for preparing (roasting, baking, stir-frying, and other) and extracting (using varying temperatures and pressures) the herbs is dependent on the individual herb and essential to the efficacy and potency of the final product. Only companies following the highest standards of care should be used for veterinary herbal medicine. Poor-quality herbs may contain toxic substances or contaminants, pose potential health hazards, and may lack therapeutic effect.

Endangered Species

Endangered species are *not* used in veterinary Chinese herbal formulas. The Convention on International Trade in Endangered Species of Wild Fauna and Flora (CITES) "is an international agreement between governments [whose] aim is to ensure that international trade in specimens of wild animals and plants does not threaten their survival" (CITES 2021). CITES protects more than 37 000 species of plants and animals, alive or dead. Any flora or fauna protected by CITES cannot legally be imported into the United States.

Not only is China a member of CITES, but all Chinese herbal manufacturers exporting raw and processed herbs must receive approval from the General Administration of Quality Supervision, Inspection and Quarantine of the People's Republic of China (AQSIQ 2020). The AQSIQ requires the screening of all herbal products for heavy metals, pesticide residues, moisture, and bacteria as stipulated by the receiving country (Xie 2011, 2012). The FDA also often screens raw herbs upon entering the United States.

Labeling

Product labeling rules and regulations are just as confusing as those surrounding manufacturing. For the most part there are no federal standards regarding herb and herbal formula labeling. The product labels should include a list of all ingredients and the intended use of the product. Avoid using supplements which make medical claims on the label, i.e. "for use in the prevention or treatment of [insert disease or condition name]."

Selecting companies whose products have been evaluated for purity, microbial analysis, and adulterants, preferably by third party organizations, is recommended. For animal supplements, but not often botanicals, there are three well-known organizations: ConsumerLab, NASC, or the United States Pharmacopeia. To learn more about these companies, see Chapter 4.

Safety

Safety concerns should focus on two concepts: adverse effects and herb–drug interactions (HDIs).

Adverse Effects

Adverse effects, also known as side effects, are defined as any unwanted and harmful outcomes caused by a drug or supplement. There is a scale of severity associated with adverse effects from mild to severe. Severe adverse effects are considered a form of toxicity.

The incidence of adverse reactions associated with herbal therapy is very low (Xie 2011).

The most common adverse signs affect the gastrointestinal tract, causing nausea, vomiting, diarrhea, and inappetance. Because Chinese herbal formulas contain two or more individual herbs the importance of understanding the common characteristics of each herb, as well as their combined effects, cannot be overstated. This is especially true if a patient has an adverse effect. Keep in mind the herbs comprising an herbal formula are chosen to help enhance the effectiveness of the formula but also to mitigate each other's potential for adverse effects.

The presence of side effects suggests either the dose is too high or the TCVM diagnosis is incorrect (Marsden 2014a). Occasionally patients experience adverse effects for only 24–48 hours, after which time the unwanted signs resolve. A practitioner may elect to "wait it out" to see if the clinical signs improve. Often the practitioner will reduce the dose and slowly increase it back over time, monitoring carefully for the recurrence of adverse signs. Symptoms persisting for more than 24 hours are caused by either an underlying issue (i.e. a secondary disease process not appreciated until the primary issue was controlled) or a new issue (i.e. infection). The risk of side effects is reduced by ensuring the correct TCVM diagnosis is made, the correct dose and duration of treatment, and the best possible source for the CH and CF is chosen (Figure 3.5).

True toxicity from Chinese herbs and herbal formulas is uncommon. When toxicity does occur the cardiovascular, gastrointestinal, nervous, and hepatic systems are the most commonly affected (Xie 2011). As we learned in the preceding section the risk of toxicity from contaminants is low when a GMP-certified company is chosen. The FDA maintains a list of toxic herbs which are prohibited from use within the United States. Additionally, if the CH and CF are prepared and manufactured in the United States, even if the raw material is grown outside of the country, federally mandated end-use agreements prohibit the inclusion of known toxic materials (Xie 2011).

Often adverse effects can be mitigated by preparing (often cooking, baking, or frying) the herb prior to incorporation into the CF. For example, Fu Zi or Aconite is toxic when large amounts of the raw plant are ingested (Chen and Chen 2012a). Signs of Aconite toxicosis include nausea, vomiting, abdominal pain, diarrhea, limb and facial numbness or weakness, abnormal heart rhythms, low blood pressure, chest pain, and even death (Chan 2009). Processing the herb, usually through cooking, reduces the risk of toxicity by at least 200% (Chen and Chen 2012a). Toxicity is also reduced by careful use of only small amounts of the processed herb in patients with Cold, specifically Yang Deficiency, signs (Chen and Chen 2012a).

Herbal Toxicity for Veterinarians

Knowledge in Chinese herbal therapy is critical to ensure patients are treated safely and effectively. The foundation for this knowledge is best obtained through training programs, while continuing education reinforces and expands the practitioner's abilities to effectively utilize CHM. A professional library stocked with paper and digital references on CHM is also key. The monographs for Chinese herbs and herbal formulas generally have sections on toxicity discussing the median lethal dose (LD_{50}) and potential HDIs.

The chance of toxicity when properly using CH and CF is extremely low. First, the amount

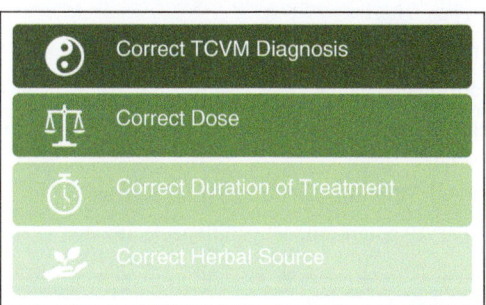

Figure 3.5 The steps used to reduce the risk of adverse effects in Chinese herbal therapy. Source: Lisa P. McFaddin.

of herb used, either by itself or within a formula, is so small there should never be enough herb to reach a toxic level. Secondly, the FDA bans the use of any plant with a significant risk of toxicity, such as Ma Huang (Ephedra) or Zhu Sha (Cinnabar). Finally, proper preparation of the raw materials further reduces the risk of toxicity, as with Fu Zi (Aconite). To increase practitioner awareness regarding potentially toxic CH, Table 3.25 describes several herbs with known toxic potential.

Herb–Drug Interactions

The likelihood of negative HDIs is generally low. Most of the cited negative HDIs arose from *in vivo* or *in vitro* testing without the support of clinical trials to back up their results. CH and CF are frequently used to combat the adverse effects associated with many traditional pharmaceuticals, which is a positive HDI (Xie 2011). Frequently HDIs are used to the clinician's advantage, allowing dose reduction, or even elimination, of a drug. The

Table 3.25 Chinese herbs with known toxic potential. Descriptions of the clinical signs of toxicity, as well as measures to reduce the risk of toxicity, are provided (Xie 2011; Chen and Chen 2012a; Marsden 2014a). The Chinese and English names are provided, when applicable.

Ban Xia (Pinellia)	CST	Cardiopulmonary: Palpitations, weak pulse, dyspnea, respiratory depression
		Gastrointestinal: Nausea, vomiting, abdominal pain, diarrhea
		Oral: Numbness, swelling, and pain of the mouth and throat, dry mouth, ptyalism
		Other: Hepatopathy, dizziness
	MRT	Avoid use in Yin-deficient patients
		Do not use with Wu Toi
		Use only prepared herb
		Monitor closely for signs of allergic reactions
Cang Er Zi (Xanthium Fruit)	CST	Gastrointestinal: Nausea, vomiting, abdominal pain, diarrhea, constipation, inappetance
		Neurologic: Seizures, loss of consciousness
		Other: Lethargy, dizziness, hepatopathy, shock
	MTR	Avoid use in Qi- and blood-deficient patients
		Use only prepared herb
		Use only lowest effective dose
		Avoid use during pregnancy
Da Ji (Euphoirbia)	CST	Dermatologic: Dermatitis, oral sores and swelling, conjunctivitis
		Gastrointestinal: Vomiting, abdominal pain, diarrhea
		Cardiovascular: Hypotension, dehydration, electrolyte imbalance
	MRT	Use only lowest effective dose
		Avoid long-term use
		Avoid in pregnancy or weak and debilitated patients

Fu Zi (Aconite)	CST	Cardiovascular: Arrhythmias, angina, hypotension
		Gastrointestinal: Nausea, vomiting, abdominal pain, diarrhea
		Neurologic: Numbness and weakness of the limbs, numbness of the face
	MRT	Use only prepared herb
		Do not use in hot patients, due to excess or deficiency
		Use lowest effective dose
		Do not use during pregnancy
Ma Huang (Ephedra)	CST	Cardiovascular:Hypertension, tachycardia
		Gastrointestinal: Nausea, vomiting, abdominal pain
		Neurologic: Restlessness, irritability, excitement, hypersensitivity
	MRT	Avoid use in pregnancy or weak or debilitated patients
		Use caution with patients with neurologic conditions
		Illegal to use in the United States
Qian Niu Zi (Morning glory seed)	CST	Cardiopulmonary: Tachycardia, cyanosis, respiratory distress, dizziness
		Gastrointestinal: Vomiting, abdominal pain, diarrhea, green watery stool with mucus
	MRT	Avoid use in pregnancy
		Avoid use in stomach Qi deficiency
Shi Jun Zi (Rangoon Creeper fruit)	CST	Gastrointestinal: Nausea, hiccups, vomiting, diarrhea, abdominal pain, cold extremities, hypotension
		Neurologic: Dizziness, vertigo
		Other: Allergic reactions
	MRT	Avoid use with hot teas
		Limit dosage and frequency of use per day
Zao Jiao (Chinese honey locust)	CST	Gastrointestinal: Nausea, vomiting, diarrhea, abdominal distension
		Neurologic: Irritability, weak extremities
	MRT	Avoid use in pregnancy or Qi- and Yin-deficient patients
		Use lowest effective dose
Zhu Sha (Cinnabar)	CST	Gastrointestinal: Abdominal pain, inappetance, diarrhea
		Neurologic: Agitation, tremors
		Other: Hepatotoxic, nephrotoxic
	MRT	Use only lowest effective dose
		Avoid long-term use
		Avoid in patients with preexisting hepatic or renal disease
		Avoid heat processing

CST, clinical signs of toxicity; MTR, methods for toxicity reduction.
Source: Lisa P. McFaddin.

practitioner must be aware of potential HDIs to avoid concurrent administration of Chinese herbs which may interfere with the efficacy of the pharmaceutical agent or herb itself.

One example of a potentially negative HDI involves the concurrent administration of Gan Cao with diuretics, like furosemide. Gan Cao, or Licorice, causes retention of sodium and water within the body, as well as increased renal potassium loss (Marsden 2014a). These effects can counteract the diuretic effects of furosemide. While the dose of Gan Cao in traditional Chinese veterinary herbal formulas is not high enough to truly affect blood sodium levels, practitioners should be aware of all potential HDIs.

HDIs for Veterinarians

Any effect, whether positive or negative, occurring because of the concurrent administration of Chinese herbal therapy and a pharmaceutical drug is considered an HDI. How the herbs and drugs move through the body (pharmacokinetics) and function within the body (pharmacodynamics) explain how and why HDIs may occur. Pharmacokinetics is the term used to describe how the HDI affects each substance's absorption, distribution, metabolism and elimination throughout the body (Chen 2013). Pharmacodynamics explains how the synergistic or antagonistic HDI affects each substance's mechanism of action (Chen 2013).

HDIs largely result in one of three outcomes: increased drug effectivity, decreased drug effectivity, or reduction of drug side effects (Marsden 2014a). An herb can increase or decrease drug effectiveness through pharmacokinetics and/or pharmacodynamics.

As an example, let's examine the pharmacokinetics of Hu Jiao and Dang Gui. Hu Jiao, or black pepper, improves mucosal blood flow enhancing drug absorption (Chen and Chen 2012b; Marsden 2014a). The polysaccharides found within Dang Gui, or Angelica rhizome, lubricates the intestines potentially inhibiting drug absorption (Chen and Chen 2012b; Marsden 2014a). Conversely, the same polysaccharides found within Dang Gui can protect the gut lining from irritation due to nonsteroidal anti-inflammatory administration (Chen and Chen 2012b; Marsden 2014a).

Alternatively, let's investigate the pharmacodynamics of Ma Huang, Gan Cao, and Sheng Jiang for clarification. Ma Huang, or Ephedra, increases sympathetic tone which when combined with other sympathomimetics, such as Sudafed, can result in toxicosis (Chen 2013). As mentioned earlier, Gan Cao, or licorice, increases sodium retention which could inhibit the effectiveness of furosemide (Chen and Chen 2012b; Marsden 2014a). Sheng Jiang, or fresh ginger, reduces nausea associated with many medications, especially chemotherapeutic agents (Chen and Chen 2012b; Marsden 2014a).

Herbs affecting the sympathetic nervous system, clotting, water retention, and insulin levels have the greatest risk of clinically significant HDIs (Chen 1998/1999, 2013). Table 3.26 highlights several common HDIs associated with CH and CF.

Formulations

When dispensing Chinese herbs ask yourself the following questions: Would an individual herb or herbal formula be most effective? What formulation would be most suitable for the patient? What is the correct dosing for the patient?

Individual Herb Versus Formula

There are times when single herbs are chosen or added to pre-made formulas, but for the most part herbal formulas are preferred. CF epitomize the saying "the sum is greater than the parts." While each herb has its own unique characteristics and beneficial properties, together herbal formulas exact a greater effect on the patient.

Formulation

Herbs are available in five forms: liquid extract, ground dried herb, granule, tablet, and teapill.

Table 3.26 Common herb–drug interactions divided by category (Xie 2011; Chen 2013; Marsden 2014a). Examples of individual herbs, their mechanisms of action, and incompatible drugs are provided.

Category	Herb examples	Mechanism of action	Incompatible drugs
Anticoagulant	Chuan Xiong (Szchuan Lovage Root) Dan Shen (Salvia Rhizome) Dang Gui (Angelica Root) Hong Hua (Safflower Flower) Tao Ren (Peach Seed)	Delay clotting through direct effects on platelets and/or the clotting cascade	Warfarin Enoxaparin Aspirin Dipyridamole Clopidogrel
Antidiabetic	Cang Zhu (Atractylodes Rhizome) Haung Qi (Astragalus Root) Shan Yao (Chinese Yam) Shi Gao (Gypsum) Zhi Mu (Anemarrhena Rhizome)	Decrease plasma glucose levels	Insulin Oral antidiabetic medications
Charred herbs	Da Huang (Rheum) Di Yu (Sanguisorba) Er Cha (Acacia) Hu Zhang (Polygonum) Wu Bei Zi (Rhus)	Herbs bind and reduce absorption of vitamin B	Vitamin B12 Vitamin B6 Vitamin B complex Niacinamide
Diuretic	Che Qian Zi Fu Ling (Poria) Ze Xie (Water Plantain Rhizome) Zhu Ling (Polyporus Sclerotium)	Increase loss of body fluid	Furosemide Spironolactone
Flavonoid containing	Chen Pi (Citrus Peel) Huang Qin (Scutellaria) Jin Yin Hua (Lonicera) Xuan Gu Hua (Inula)	Reduced herb effectiveness through chelation of metallic compounds	Aluminum hydroxide Calcium carbonite
Sympathomimetic	Ma Huang (Ephedra)	Increases sympathetic tone	Stimulants ADHD medication Antihypertensive drugs Antiepileptic drugs

Source: Lisa P. McFaddin.

For liquid extracts the bulk herbs are decocted in purified water or alcohol, creating a highly concentrated liquid extract (Brand 2018). Liquid extracts are the most bioavailable, or absorbed, but sometimes the least well tolerated by patients.

In ground dried herbs, the powdered granules are made either through fine milling or grinding of dried herb. This method is relatively inexpensive and easy to prepare compared to other preparations. Unfortunately, this preparation contains more inactive plant ingredients, like insoluble fiber. As a result, a higher dose is generally required to achieve the same affect. The larger quantity is less cost-effective for clients and often makes administration more difficult, depending on the amount needed.

Powdered granules are made by drying liquid extract. The liquid decoction is generally reduced through evaporation using a low temperature. The thickened liquid concentrate is sprayed into a tumbler which contains a fine powder (often a starch base or the ground herb itself). Through repeated churning of the concentrate and fine powder, a uniform powder is created. This final product, now called powdered granular extract or granules, has minimal clumping, an extended shelf-life, and contains less inactive plant ingredients making them approximately five times as potent as an equal quantity of the same dried herb or formula (Brand 2018). Granules may come as a loose powder or placed in pre-measured capsules.

Tablets are made by cooking, using steam and pressure, mixing, milling, and blending bulk herbs. The mixture is formed into tablets using cold compression. A binder, typically honey, is only used when necessary. Currently, only the Kan line of veterinary Chinese herbal formulas offers tableted versions of CF. Of note the tablets often require a higher dosing than that listed on the bottle.

Teapills are very small, darkly colored pills created by further condensing liquid extract and mixing it with a small amount of ground dried herb to create an herbal dough ball. The dough ball is cut into smaller pieces which are smoothed to create the pills.

Dosage

Dosing is ultimately up to the clinician. The clinician's dosage is based on the patient's TCVM diagnosis, weight, and herbal manufacturer. Each manufacturer has their own recommended dosing chart based on the herbal formula's strength and patient weight.

Like pharmaceutical agents there is often a dose range. To avoid adverse effects patients are often started on a lower dose then slowly increased to the most effective dose for the patient. Personally, I start with half to one-third of the projected final dose once daily, then slowly increase the herb to the full dose twice daily over three to nine days. Most herbal formulas are given twice daily, approximately every 12 hours.

Herbal Dosage for Veterinarians

The patient's TCVM diagnosis and response to therapy typically dictate the dose, frequency, and length of treatment. Some herbal formulas are meant for short-term use while others are used long term or lifelong. Each manufacturer has product books with suggested dosages, including frequency and length of treatment suggestions.

If an herbal formula is discontinued it should be done so gradually, often over 3–14 days. Sometimes CF are more beneficial at lower doses and do not need to be completely discontinued. A slow taper ensures the lowest effective dose is used.

Any potential side effects noted when starting the herbs often resolve on their own within 24 hours. Any symptoms which do not resolve are typically associated with an underlying disease process, either preexisting or concomitant. Because multiple TCVM diagnoses are often present at one time (think of TCVM disease conditions like layers of an onion or tree rings), treating the initial problem (for example an Excess condition) may reveal an underlying issue (such as a Deficiency) which needs to be addressed once the initial complaint resolves. Additionally, patients may develop a secondary problem unrelated to the initial complaint (for example an infection). If this occurs the new issue must be addressed to properly treat the patient. In both situations the CF may need to be reduced, temporarily stopped, or another herb may be added while continuing the initial herb.

In the extremely unlikely event that a patient experiences marked adverse effects or signs of toxicity, the veterinarian should be notified immediately. The herbal therapy may be stopped or adjusted depending on the patient's condition and CF in question.

The Why

Applications in Human Medicine

The National Institutes of Health (NIH) states one in five Americans use Chinese herbal products. The site references the study and use of Chinese herbal products to aid in the treatment of stroke, heart disease, mental disorders, and respiratory diseases (NCCIH 2021). The NIH expresses concern regarding the lack of scientific evidence, but no specifics are provided. The NIH National Center for Complementary and Integrative Health (NCCIH) has a dedicated section of their website providing summary fact sheets on a variety of herbs (https://nccih.nih.gov/health/herbsa-taglance.htm).

Applications in Veterinary Medicine

CHM is commonly used to aid in the treatment of dermatologic diseases, gastrointestinal disease, immune system disorders, immune system support, pain, and to do what drugs cannot (Liu et al. 2016; Bartholomew 2017; Guan et al. 2018; Chan 2019).

Personally, I view Chinese herbal medicine like apps for my phone: "there's an herb for that." In my opinion there is an herbal formula for almost every veterinary condition. A more detailed list of disorders, with supporting scientific studies, can be found in the Veterinarians section of this chapter.

Veterinary Research

Veterinary Chinese herbal therapy is a relatively well-studied treatment modality. A quick search on PubMed yields 310 articles for "veterinary Chinese herbal therapy," 154 articles for "Chinese herbal therapy canine," and 18 for "Chinese herbal therapy feline" as of February 2023. Presented below are the summaries of three veterinary CHM studies.

A Randomized and Controlled Study of the Efficacy of Yin Qiao San Combined with Antibiotics Compared to Antibiotics Alone for the Treatment of Feline Upper Respiratory Disease

Author(s): David Hirsch, DVM, MS; Deng Shan Shiau, PhD; Huisheng Xie, DVM, MS, PhD
Journal: *American Journal of Traditional Chinese Veterinary Medicine*
Date: 2017
Study design: Randomized clinical trial
Study hypothesis: The treatment of cats with upper respiratory tract infections (URI) with both antibiotics (Clavamox or doxycycline) and a Chinese herbal formula (Yin Qiao San) will result in faster resolution of clinical signs without adverse effects compared to cats treated with antibiotics alone.
Sample size: 50 cats from three different animal shelters in New Jersey and New York.

Materials and methods: Cats demonstrating one or more predefined signs of a URI were included in the study. Cats were randomly assigned to a treatment group (antibiotics only or Yin Qiao San plus an antibiotic) using a random number generator. Cats either received Clavamox or doxycycline as the antibiotic. There were 19 cats in the antibiotic-only group and 31 in the Yin Qiao San (YQS) + antibiotic group. Cats were observed for signs of conjunctivitis, sneezing and nasal discharge, lower respiratory signs, systemic signs, and oral cavity changes. A number value was assigned to each possible clinical sign within those categories. A total score

(Continued)

A Randomized and Controlled Study of the Efficacy of Yin Qiao San Combined with Antibiotics Compared to Antibiotics Alone for the Treatment of Feline Upper Respiratory Disease (Continued)

was obtained for each cat on days 0, 2, 4, 6, 8, and 10 following initiation of the treatment. A mean daily score for each group was obtained and analyzed using Wilcoxon tests.

Results

1) Significant reduction of clinical signs in the antibiotic-only group did not appear until days 6 and 8. By day 10 the mean clinical sign score increased, and there was no significant difference compared to the pretreatment values.
2) Significant reduction of clinical signs in the YQS + antibiotic group did not appear until day 4 and persisted through day 10.
3) There were no adverse effects noted in the YQS + antibiotic group.

Study conclusions: The use of YQS and antibiotics in cats with URIs resulted in faster and sustained resolution of their clinical signs compared to cats receiving antibiotics only.

Study limitations

1) There was a large discrepancy between the sample size of each treatment group.
2) There was no true control group: cats receiving no treatment.
3) Cats remained housed in the shelter throughout the study increasing their risk of exposure to other pathogens, and their stress levels likely remained elevated due to the shelter environment.
4) Technicians scoring the clinical signs were not blinded to the treatment groups.

L.P.M. conclusions: The use of Chinese herbal formulas, in conjunction with traditional Western therapies, may improve the clinical signs of cats with URIs without adverse effects. Further studies are needed to see if the effect is similar in owned cats not living in a shelter situation. Additional studies evaluating other possible Chinese herbal formulas should also be conducted.
(Hirsch et al. 2017)

A Randomized Controlled Study Comparing Da Xiang Lian Wan to Metronidazole in the Treatment of Stress Colitis in Shelter/Rescued Dogs

Author(s): Margaret Fowler, DVM, MS; Deng-Shan Shiau, PhD, and Huisheng Xie, DVM, PhD
Journal: *American Journal of Traditional Chinese Veterinary Medicine*
Date: 2017
Study design: Randomized clinical trial
Study hypothesis: The administration of a Chinese herbal formula, Da Xiang Lian Wan (DXLW), will be as effective as metronidazole in the resolution of diarrhea secondary to stress colitis.
Sample size: 56 dogs from shelters in Florida, South Carolina, and New Jersey.
Materials and methods: Dogs were included in the study if they were over five months of

age and had diarrhea typical of colitis (small volumes, frequent episodes, odiferous, and blood or mucus). A fecal sample was tested for parasitic ova and giardia (ELISA). A random number generator was used to assign dogs to either treatment group: metronidazole (27 dogs) or Da Xiang Lian Wan (DXLW, 29 dogs). The presence or absence of diarrhea was documented twice daily for each treatment group until two doses after resolution of the diarrhea or following 10 doses of the medication or herb. Successful treat was defined as diarrhea-free for 24 hours. Two-sample test was used for statistical analysis.

Results

1) Dogs in the metronidazole group had an 89% response rate within 10 doses of the medication, administered twice daily.
2) Dogs in the DXLW group had a 97% response rate within 10 doses of the herb, administered twice daily.
3) One dog in each group had an adverse reaction of vomiting.

Study conclusions: The administration of DXLW was as effective as metronidazole in the treatment of stress colitis in shelter dogs with minimal side effects.

Study limitations

1) There was no true control group.
2) The study was not blinded.

L.P.M. conclusions: Chinese herbal formulas offer an alternative treatment option for stress colitis in dogs. Further studies are needed to confirm efficacy, especially against placebo treatments, and with multiple formulas.

(Fowler et al. 2017)

Chinese Herbal Medicine for Dogs with Complete Cranial Cruciate Ligament Rupture: 181 Cases

Author(s): Jiu Wen, DVM, MS; Karen Johnston, DVM; and Dominic Gucciardo, DVM
Journal: *American Journal of Traditional Chinese Veterinary Medicine*
Date: 2016
Study design: Clinical trial
Study hypothesis: The use of a novel Chinese herbal supplement, HipGuard, would improve stifle joint healing in dogs with ruptured cranial cruciate ligaments.
Sample size: 181 companion dogs presenting to a local veterinarian from 2008 to 2012.
Materials and methods: Dogs were included in the study if they met the following criteria: lameness, pain on stifle palpation, cruciate ligament disease, cranial drawer sign, HipGuard consumption for more than one month with follow-up exams, and monitored for more than one year. Patients requiring surgery were removed from the study. Clinical evaluation included monthly physical exams for three months then every two to three months with a one-year follow-up exam. Baseline blood work, including complete blood count and chemistries, were performed intermittently for the first six months of supplementation. HipGuard was administered twice daily and tapered after resolution of clinical signs or continued long term. One-way analysis of variance was used for statistical analysis.

Results

1) 91.7% of the dogs had a good to excellent response to supplementation, defined as great improvement or resolution of presenting clinical signs.
2) 8.3% of the dogs did not respond to supplementation and required surgery.
3) The average healing time once supplementation was started was 4.7 months.
4) Overweight dogs were statistically more likely to require longer-term supplementation and were slower to respond.
5) Younger dogs appeared more likely to require surgery.
6) Labradors were over-represented in the nonresponder category.
7) No liver or kidney enzyme elevations noted while taking HipGuard.

(Continued)

Chinese Herbal Medicine for Dogs with Complete Cranial Cruciate Ligament Rupture: 181 Cases   (Continued)

8) Three dogs experienced self-limiting gastrointestinal side effects for the first few days therapy was started. The dose was lowered and slowly increased in these patients without further adverse effects.

Study conclusions: Dogs with cranial cruciate disease showed improvement in pain, lameness, and stifle instability within five months of starting HipGuard. The Chinese herbal supplement appears to be a safe and viable alternative to surgical correction for some dogs, especially if started soon after clinical signs appear.

Study limitations

1) No control group.
2) No comparative treatment groups: surgical, NSAIDs, etc.
3) Limited standardization in blood-work monitoring.
4) High chance for examiner bias.

L.P.M. conclusions: Cranial cruciate disease is a very common issue in canine patients with surgical correction not always a financially practical approach for owners. This study suggests the use of HipGuard as a safe and effect alternative to reduce pain and lameness, allowing self-healing of the stifle joint. (Wen et al. 2016)

Table 3.27 specifies many of the diseases and conditions for which CHM has shown a scientifically beneficial effect in veterinary medicine. The studies documenting these positive effects are also listed. This list is not all inclusive as new studies documenting the beneficial effects of CHM in veterinary medicine are being continually published. There are also abundant case studies demonstrating the successful use of CHM in veterinary patients. Individual case studies were not included in the table, focusing instead on clinical trials and some case series.

The How

Team Members

This section reviews the potential return on investment (ROI), how to effectively train the entire team, and how to promote and how to integrate CHM.

Return on Investment

ROI can be determined by evaluating client interest, veterinarian demand, hospital costs, applicability of the service, revenue stream, appointment scheduling, and pricing.

Table 3.27   Examples of studies demonstrating the efficacy of veterinary CHM in the treatment of multiple diseases and conditions as of February 2023.

System category	Disease conditions studied	Reference
Behavior	Anxiety	Arya et al. (2012)
Cardiovascular	Antihypertensive	Arya et al. (2012)
	Coagulation	Egger et al. (2016), Adelman et al. (2017), Liu and Ma (2020), Wong and Shiau (2020), Rodriguez et al. (2021)
	Vascular changes	Sun et al. (2015)
Dermatologic	Flea allergy dermatitis	Harris (2008)
	Otitis externa	McKee and Shiau (2019)
	Pyoderma	Bartholomew (2017)

System category	Disease conditions studied	Reference
Endocrine	Hyperadrenocorticism	Koh et al. (2017)
	Hyperthyroidism	Wilcox et al. (2009)
Gastrointestinal	Diarrhea	Fowler et al. (2017)
	Gastroprotective	Arya et al. (2012)
	Gut motility	Song et al. (2014)
	Inflammatory bowel disease	Chan (2019)
Immune system	Anti-inflammatory and antioxidant	Liao et al. (2008), Arya et al. (2012), Serrano et al. (2018)
	Antineoplastic	Wen and Johnson (2011), Wirth et al. (2014), Bartholomew and Xie (2018)
	Antiviral	He et al. (2013)
	Immune support	Xiujun et al. (2006), Song et al. (2008), Li and Hu (2010), Arya et al. (2012), Li et al. (2012a), Sivula (2012), He et al. (2013), Kong et al. (2014), Guan et al. (2018)
Musculoskeletal	Cruciate injury	Wen et al. (2016)
Neurologic	Epilepsy	Hayashi and Xie (2015), Dewey et al. (2020)
	Intervertebral disk disease	Cahyono (2015), Liu et al. (2016)
Reproductive	Anti-abortive	Zhong and Zhao (2013)
	Estrogen receptor	Li et al. (2012b)
	Fertility	Song et al. (2015)
Respiratory	Rhinitis	Makino et al. (2004)
	Upper respiratory infection	Hirsch et al. (2017)

Source: Lisa P. McFaddin.

Client Interest

Currently there are no studies documenting client interest or the popularity of TCVM. By evaluating trends in the general interest in TCM, client interest in veterinary alternative or integrative medicine, and pet health insurance client interest in CHM can be inferred.

General Interest The WHO included details about TCM for the first time in their 11th global compendium of the International Statistical Classification of Diseases and Related Health Problems (ICD) in August 2018 (WHO 2021). The purpose of the ICD is to influence the medical practices and standards for more than 100 countries (Cyranoski 2018). The WHO's recognition of the viability of TCM reflects the public's growing interest in alternative and integrative therapies for their own health.

Client Opinion Table 3.28 summarizes the pet owner demographics and statistics mentioned in the My Lessons section of the Introduction at the beginning of this book. Even if half of those owners are open to CHM, that is still 53.1 million potential patients.

A recent retrospective analysis performed by Shmalberg et al. (2019) assessed 161 referrals to an integrative medicine service in a veterinary teaching hospital in Florida. Of the sampled population, 76.4% received herbal supplements and 95.4% received acupuncture. The authors discovered dogs were much more likely to be treated compared to cats: 91.9% versus 8.1%, respectively (Shmalberg et al. 2019).

Table 3.28 Summary of the 2022 pet ownership and pet health insurance demographics in the United States discussed in the Introduction of the book (Burns 2018, 2022; MFAF 2018; APPA 2022; Nolen 2022; NAPHIA 2023).

- 83% of pets are owned by millennials (32%), generation X (24%), and baby boomers (27%)
- 69 million households owned dogs
- 45.3 million households owned cats
- Estimated over 81.1 million owned dogs
- Estimated over 60.7 million owned cats
- 68% of owners are interested in alternative treatment modalities for their pets
- 4.41 million pets have pet health insurance
- 82% of insurance pets are dogs

Source: Lisa P. McFaddin.

Pet Health Insurance Many pet insurance plans include coverage for integrative therapies, especially acupuncture (Woodley 2018). The presence of this type of coverage re-emphasizes the mainstream incorporation of these treatment modalities, as well as reflecting client demand.

Veterinarian Demand

In short there is a definite need for small animal veterinarians in general, as well as integrative veterinarians (see the Book Structure section of the Introduction and Chapter 1 for more specifics).

The expanding number of available Chinese herbal training courses over the past 10 years supports the increasing demand for veterinary training. While CHM certification is highly recommended, it is not required to practice veterinary CHM. Unfortunately, there are currently no concrete accounts of the number of certified and non-certified veterinarians practicing CHM in the country.

If we use the number of Chi University graduates only, ignoring the likelihood that some received acupuncture-only certification not CHM, there are approximately 7500 veterinarians currently practicing CHM in the United States. This represents a little under 4% of the total veterinarian population. Using the estimated 38.5 million potential integrative patients, there are over 5000 potential patients per veterinary Chinese herbalist. With these numbers I would say there is room for more practitioners.

Another way to examine the need in your specific area is to compare the number of general practitioners within a 5-, 10-, or 20-mile radius to the number of veterinarians advertising CHM. The search radius is dependent on your hospital's demographics. Most comparisons tend to follow the 5% trend, meaning no more than 5% of the surrounding hospitals are currently offering CHM. Ensuring your particular area is not saturated prevents the introduction of a redundant service.

Hospital Costs

Let's start by reviewing all the potential costs associated with introducing and offering CHM: veterinarian training, staff training, supplies and equipment, staffing, facilities, and advertising. Tables 3.29 and 3.30 demonstrate the different potential start-up costs, primarily dependent on the hospital's contribution toward the veterinarian's training and prior utilization of regular all-staff meetings. For more information on potential hospital costs refer to the Introduction at the beginning of this book.

Veterinarian Training

Course There are three main organizations offering training programs in the United States. All programs have the option to complete the entire course online. Only Chi University offers two on-site sessions lasting four days. Course completion time is 9–24 months depending on the program. However, keep in mind that most courses offer a problem-orientated approach, meaning veterinarians can usually start practicing herbal medicine, and generating revenue, while taking the course. Estimated cost reflects the average cost of all available courses. Additional information can be found in the Veterinarians section of this chapter (cost range, $2999–$495; average cost, $4871).

Table 3.29 Potential hospital start-up costs for CHM as of February 2023.

Category	Subcategories	Projected cost	
Veterinarian training	Course cost	$3020–8495	Average $5140
	Textbooks	$250–1550	Average $600
	Travel expenses	$0–3030	
	Time-off	$0–1737	
Staff training	Variable	$230–1396	
Supplies	Chinese herbal formulas	$34 per bottle	$34 per patient
	Measuring instruments	$45	
	Prescription vials	$65 for a box of 100	$0.65 per patient
Staffing	Variable	$\geq$$0	
Facilities	Overhead	$2–5 per minute for 30–60-minute appointments	$40–300 per patient
Advertising	Variable	$\leq$$420	

Source: Lisa P. McFaddin.

Table 3.30 Projected CHM start-up costs for eight hospital scenarios, with varying hospital contributions toward veterinary certification and staff training as of February 2023. The cost of veterinarian training is based on the averages presented Table 3.29. Staff training costs assume a 1.5-hour-long all-staff meeting, using national averages for employee numbers: eight non-DVMs and two DVMs (AVMA 2019; 2023). The cost of office supplies and lunch as estimated based on 10 employees attending the meeting. The overhead is based on an average of $3.5/minute. Missed revenue is calculated using the 2022 national mean revenue per hour for companion animal practices ($567/hour) (AVMA 2023). Advertising includes printed materials, digital advertisement, and community engaged.

Category	Projected expenses	Ex. 1	Ex. 2	Ex. 3	Ex. 4	Ex. 5	Ex. 6	Ex. 7	Ex. 8
Veterinarian training	Average course cost	$5140	$5140	$5140	n/a	$5140	$5140	$5140	n/a
	Average textbooks	$600	n/a	n/a	n/a	$600	n/a	n/a	n/a
	Travel expenses	$3030	n/a	n/a	n/a	$3030	n/a	n/a	n/a
	Additional time-off	$1737	$1737	n/a	n/a	$1737	$1737	n/a	n/a
Staff training	Office supplies	$30	$30	$30	$30	$30	$30	$30	$30
	Lunch	$200	$200	$200	$200	$200	$200	$200	$200
	Overhead	$315	$315	$315	$315	n/a	n/a	n/a	n/a
	Missed DVM revenue	$851	$851	$851	$851	n/a	n/a	n/a	n/a
Supplies	Herbal pharmacy	$680	$680	$680	$680	$680	$680	$680	$680
	Gram scale	$30	$30	$30	$30	$30	$30	$30	$30
	Reusable measuring spoons	$15	$15	$15	$15	$15	$15	$15	$15
	Prescription vials	$65	$65	$65	$65	$65	$65	$65	$65
Advertising		$420	$420	$420	$420	$420	$420	$420	$420
Total		$13113	$9483	$7746	$2606	$11947	$8317	$6580	$1440
Total without cost of supplies		$12323	$8693	$6956	$1816	$11157	$7527	$5790	$650

Source: Lisa P. McFaddin.

Textbooks Textbooks may not be required for the certification courses but are often highly recommended. The price range is based on a two- to five-book requirement (cost range, $250–1550; average cost, $600).

Travel Expenses The value provided reflects the total travel expenses based on two on-site sessions with four full days of training. Keep in mind selection of online only training would eliminate the costs associated with travel and room and board. Here is a breakdown of the costs:

- *Airfare*: Due to the global effects of the pandemic, the cost of a roundtrip domestic flight within the United States has been on a rollercoaster ride. As of January 2023, the average cost of a roundtrip domestic flight was $412 (BLS 2023; Trcek 2023). The $412 value was used when calculating the cost of airfare for two roundtrip flights (total cost, $824).
- *Lodging*: As of February 2023 the federal per diem rate for lodging on business trips is $98 per night (FederalPay.org 2023). The federal per diem rate was used for calculations, with four nights of lodging over two sessions (total cost, $784).
- *Car rental*: As of January 2023, the average weekly car rental price is $551 (French and Kemmis 2023). Rideshare and cabbing are extremely popular, but the variability in travel distances makes calculating an average cost impractical. It is suspected this cost would be comparable, if not lower, than that of a rental car. The total was calculated using five-day car rentals for two sessions (total cost, $1102).
- *Meals*: The federal per diem rate for business trip meals from October 2022 through September 2023 is $59 a day (FederalPay. org 2023). Most training programs provide at least one meal, as well as snacks. Meal expenditure is estimated to be $40/day for a total of eight days (total cost, $320).
- *Time Off*: Veterinarian paid time-off (PTO) for on-site courses only factors in as an added expense if additional PTO is provided outside of the contractual annual PTO. Clinics offer an average of 4.1 paid continuing education (CE) days per year (AAHA 2019). Allowing the veterinarian to use CE days for the onsite courses would not "cost" the hospital anything additional. There is also no additional cost if the hospital requires the veterinarian use their PTO for the onsite training. The clinic accrues an added expense if they agree to pay for the additional CE days. The price range provided represents a clinic offering 5–12 days of additional paid CE leave. The median pay for a full-time veterinarian, calculated by the US Bureau of Labor Statistics in 2022, was $100 370 or $48.26/hour (BLS 2022a). Each paid CE day was counted as eight hours. The total does not include potential lost revenue due to the veterinarian's absence, nor does it include relief veterinarian expenses. The average number of additional paid CE days was estimated to be 4.5 days (total cost, $1737).

Staff Training Team training expenses are highly variable and dependent on the preexistence of staff meetings and use of a staff meeting for training (compared to self-study). Refer to the Introduction of this book for a breakdown of these variables (cost range, $230–1396).

Supplies
- *Chinese herbal formulas:* The specific type and quantity of Chinese herbal formulas kept within the practice will be based on practitioner preference as well as the hospital's goal for inventory on-hand. Cost per patient for Chinese herbal formulas is based on the premise that each patient will receive at least one full bottle of herbs per appointment. The hospital cost for each Chinese herbal formula depends on the formulation (granules, tablets, or liquid extract) and bottle size (100 g, 4 oz, 300 tablets), ranging from $10 to $54, with an average of $34/bottle.

I would plan to start with 5–10 herbal formulas, one bottle of each. Keep in mind these are temporary hospital costs (total per patient, $34).

- *Measuring instruments:* A gram scale and reusable measuring spoons are necessary when mixing herbs and/or dispensing partial bottles of powder (total per patient, negligible).
- *Prescription vials:* Prescription vials, usually 10 dram or 40 dram, are necessary when splitting herbal bottles. On average a box of 100 vials costs $65. This expense may not be necessary if only full bottles are dispensed (total per patient, $0.65).

The supply cost is ultimately $0 per appointment. The CF are considered inventory not supplies, as their cost is expected to be recouped when sold to the client. Typically, herbal formulas are sold for 2–2.25 times the purchase price plus a dispensing fee. The cost of the gram scale and reusable measuring spoons is negligible when broken down by patient. Prescription vials will only be used for patients receiving a partial bottle of herbs. At most, the cost of the prescription vial would be $0.65 per patient. However, this cost will be recovered based on the formula markup and/or dispensing fee.

Staffing   Integrative appointments range from 30 to 60 minutes depending on the condition(s) being treated. Following the American Animal Hospital Association recommendations, a veterinary assistant (VA) or licensed technician (LT) should always restrain patients for physical examinations and procedures. A VA/LT is usually required for 15–20 minutes. Support staff assistance is not required while discussing plans with the client. During this time the VA/LT are free to assist other team members.

If the VA/LT is only needed for the examination, there is no difference in staffing cost for a CHM appointment compared to a traditional appointment. If the VA/LT is required to stay in the exam room for the entire appointment, the staff cost for the additional 15–45 minutes should be considered ($4.43–13.29 per patient). The provided expenses are based on a national average wage of $17.72/hour for veterinary technologists and technicians as of September 2022 (BLS 2022b).

Facilities   Facility expenses represent the costs needed to keep the doors open (aka overhead). Overhead includes rent or mortgage, utilities, administrative costs, and often employee costs divided by the minutes the practice is open (Stevenson 2016). The price per minute equals the amount of revenue needed just to break even. Overhead is extremely hospital specific, but the range tends to be $2–5/minute. The low end of the range in Table 3.30 represents the cost for a 30-minute appointment at a clinic with a $2/minute overhead, while the high end represents the cost for a 60-minute appointment at a clinic with a $5/minute overhead.

Designating a specific room, in a multi-exam room hospital, for integrative appointments minimizes the chances other associates will need the room for their appointments. However, there is then an added expense for designing the room and potential lost revenue if the room is not used regularly. The absence of a designated room theoretically reduces redecoration costs, but this can be disruptive for appointment flow if the treatment takes longer than the allotted time.

Advertising   There are numerous ways to advertise a new service. On average veterinary hospitals spend 0.7% of revenue on promotion and advertisement (AVMA 2019). Most of the advertising can be done with little to no additional expenditure. The Promotion section below discusses advertising ideas in further detail. The national median gross revenue for companion animal practices was $1.2 million in 2022 (AVMA 2023). Advertising costs are calculated assuming no more than 5% of the current advertising budget would be used for the promotion of the new service (estimated maximal cost, $420).

Start-Up Costs Table 3.29 summarizes projected start-up costs for CHM. Table 3.30 calculates potential start-up costs based on the degree of hospital contribution toward veterinarian and staff training. Different scenarios are presented in which the hospital covers all, some, or none of the expenses.

Applicability

As stated earlier CHM is versatile and beneficial for numerous conditions and ailments. As the clinician becomes more comfortable and confident in their CHM skills, the variety of cases for which CHM is recommended increases.

Revenue Stream

A well-trained and effective CHM practitioner can generate a relatively "recession proof" revenue stream. CF are very safe and many patients suffer from chronic conditions making CF ideal for long-term use. Online pharmacies do not legally carry the most used veterinary herb brands. Veterinary herbal manufacturers and distributors only sell through licensed practitioners and clinics. With each CF sold, either as a new prescription or refill, the income continues to build into the clinic over time.

Appointment Scheduling

There are four main factors to consider when planning CHM appointment protocols: appointment length; support staff availability; exam room availability; and follow-up appointment scheduling. There are other issues to consider when scheduling CHM appointments. For example, will CHM appointments be scheduled separately from traditional Western appointments, or will the appointment length be increased?

The initial integrative appointment is longer, 60 minutes, compared to follow-up appointments. Follow-up appointments should be scheduled for 30–50 minutes depending on the patient and if additional treatments are performed.

Keep the appointment positive. You want the pet to enjoy the experience. A relaxed pet is more easily treated. Avoid ancillary procedures which may cause stress: nail trims, anal gland expression, sanitary trims, anything with the ears, etc. Additional information on appointment scheduling can be found in the Introduction at the beginning of this book.

Pricing

An in-depth look into appointment pricing can be found in the Introduction. Here we discuss two pricing methods: current market fees and hospital cost-based pricing.

Current Market Fees There are no studies examining the average cost of veterinary integrative appointments. In general, clinicians practicing CHM also offer acupuncture, so one could apply the average cost of acupuncture appointments to all integrative appointment costs.

A study of five general practices within Central Florida found the price of acupuncture appointments ranged from $45 to $150, with a mean of $95.80 (Marks and Shmalberg 2015). The average length of these appointments was 47 minutes. According to the Nationwide® Purdue 2019 Veterinary Price Index, veterinary pricing increased by 21.1% between the end of 2014 and the end of 2018 (Purdue University 2019). Presuming services continued to increase by at least 5% annually, a 50-minute session would translate to $130 by January 2023.

Hospital Cost-Based Pricing Table 3.31 outlines the hospital cost per patient for 30- and 60-minute integrative appointments, respectively. The veterinarian training amortization per patient was calculated using the assumptions listed in Chapter 1. Supply assumptions were considered $0, as CF are considered inventory, and their cost (plus nominal expenses for applicable vials, scales, etc.) is recouped when the product is sold.

The formula for determining service fees is quite simple: Service Fee = Hospital Cost + Profit.

Table 3.31 Estimated hospital costs per patient for 30- and 60-minute integrative appointments as of February 2023. Start-up costs are taken from the totals in Table 3.30. Amortization is per patient and is based on the veterinarian seeing 952 integrative patients in two years. Overhead is calculated using $3.5/minute in a practice with two veterinarians. Multiple examples are provided with the variance determined by the total cost within each category. The total is rounded to the nearest whole number.

	Ex. 1	Ex. 2	Ex. 3	Ex. 4	Ex. 5	Ex. 6	Ex. 7	Ex. 8
30-Minute appointments								
Table 3.30 totals	$12 323	$8 693	$6 956	$1 816	$11 157	$7 527	$5 790	$650
Amortization	$12.94	$9.13	$7.31	$1.91	$11.72	$7.91	$6.08	$0.68
Overhead	$52.50	$52.50	$52.50	$52.50	$52.50	$52.50	$52.50	$52.50
Total	**$65**	**$62**	**$60**	**$54**	**$64**	**$60**	**$59**	**$53**
60-Minute appointments								
Table 3.30 totals	$12 323	$8 693	$6 956	$1 816	$11 157	$7 527	$5 790	$650
Amortization	$12.94	$9.13	$7.31	$1.91	$11.72	$7.91	$6.08	$0.68
Overhead	$105	$105	$105	$105	$105	$105	$105	$105
Total	**$118**	**$114**	**$112**	**$107**	**$117**	**$113**	**$111**	**$106**

Source: Lisa P. McFaddin.

The big question becomes how much profit? Table 3.32 illustrates the potential fee for integrative appointments based on hospital cost and variable markup percentages. It becomes readily apparent that the lower the hospital contribution, the higher the comparative profit.

Additional Considerations Many of my patients receive other treatments or diagnostics when they come in for their appointments. Frequently we adjust current medication regimens, run diagnostics (blood work, urinalysis, radiographs, etc.), discuss dietary and environmental modifications, and discuss nutrition and nutraceuticals, all of which increases revenue, average transaction charge (ATC), and DVM revenue per hour.

Offering integrative medicine also helps improve current client retention and drive new client acquisition. Marks and Shmalberg (2015) found 29% of new acupuncture and integrative patients returned for wellness and other services. Additionally, clients and surrounding veterinary practices are likely to refer patients once they see the benefit of CHM, especially in cases where Western medicine was not effective. Improving client retention and new client referrals help drive revenue.

Team Training

The concept of phase training is used when introducing acupuncture to the hospital team. A multi-media approach is used to assist with the training program and is outlined in Table 3.33.

Practice Manager's Role

To conquer this task the practice manager needs his or her own checklist which includes the following information:

- Schedule a date and time for the team training.
- Ensure all information pertaining to the new service is reviewed with the staff.
- Confirm all team members have completed the training.
- Certify all team members understand the information and can successfully educate clients.

Table 3.32 Potential 30- and 60-minute integrative appointment prices using hospital costs from Table 3.31 at varying percentage markups as of February 2023.

		Ex. 1	Ex. 2	Ex. 3	Ex. 4	Ex. 5	Ex. 6	Ex. 7	Ex. 8
30-Minute appointments									
Total hospital cost		**$66**	**$62**	**$61**	**$55**	**$65**	**$61**	**$59**	**$54**
Potential appointment price	40% Markup	$92	$87	$85	$77	$91	$85	$83	$76
	50% Markup	$99	$93	$92	$83	$98	$92	$89	$81
	60% Markup	$106	$99	$98	$88	$104	$98	$94	$86
	70% Markup	$112	$105	$104	$94	$111	$104	$100	$92
	80% Markup	$119	$112	$110	$99	$117	$110	$106	$97
60-Minute appointments									
Total hospital cost		**$118**	**$114**	**$112**	**$107**	**$117**	**$113**	**$111**	**$106**
Potential appointment price	40% Markup	$165	$160	$157	$150	$164	$158	$155	$148
	50% Markup	$177	$171	$168	$161	$176	$170	$167	$159
	60% Markup	$189	$182	$179	$171	$187	$181	$178	$170
	70% Markup	$201	$194	$190	$182	$199	$192	$189	$180
	80% Markup	$212	$205	$202	$193	$211	$203	$200	$191
	90% Markup	$224	$217	$213	$203	$222	$215	$211	$201
	100% Markup	$236	$228	$224	$214	$234	$226	$222	$212

Source: Lisa P. McFaddin.

Table 3.33 The breakdown of phase training steps and resources for the entire hospital team.

Phase 1: Background information	
Team training guide	The handout walks the practice manager and/or veterinarian through Phase 1 of the training
	A downloadable and editable copy of the handout is located on the companion website
Training presentation	The video covers background information on the modality
	PowerPoints can be downloaded, edited, and personalized from the companion website
	The document can be used as a PowerPoint or saved as an mp4 creating a personalized movie
Team training handout	The handout provides additional background information for the CSRs, VAs, and LTs to complement the knowledge gained from watching the training presentation
	A downloadable and editable copy of the handout is located on the companion website
Phase 2: Knowledge proficiency	
Quiz	A short quiz to ensure all team members have a good understanding of the service being offered
	A downloadable and editable copy of the handout is located on the companion website
	A key is provided

Phase 3: Expectations	
Training worksheets	A training checklist is provided for CSRs and VA/LTs with role-specific expectations and tasks for each staff member
	A recommended completion time is provided
	A downloadable and editable copy of the handout is located on the companion website
Phase 4: Client education	
Client scripts	Bullet point information and scripted examples used when discussing the therapy with clients
	A downloadable and editable copy of the handout is located on the companion website
Client education presentation	A short (5–7 minute) client educational video about the therapeutic modality
	PowerPoints can be downloaded, edited, and personalized from the companion website
	The document can be used as a PowerPoint or saved as an mp4 creating a personalized movie
Client education handout	An informational handout about the therapeutic modality written specifically for clients
	A downloadable and editable copy of the handout is located on the companion website

CSR, customer service representative; VA, veterinary assistant; LT, licensed technician.
Source: Lisa P. McFaddin.

Promotion

There are six common avenues of promotion for a veterinary integrative medicine (VIM) service: hospital website, social media, email blasts, mailers, in-hospital promotions, and client education.

Hospital Website

Advertise "Veterinary Chinese Herbal Medicine" in several locations on the website. On the made page insert "Now offering veterinary Chinese herbal medicine" with a link to success stories or client testimonials. Utilize the hospital website to advertise the VIM treatment under the "Services" section. Veterinarian biographs should include a description of the specialized training and professional initials. Create a veterinary CHM blog page discussing patient success stories.

Social Media

Utilize Facebook, Instagram, and/or Twitter to post facts, photographs, hashtags, and patient success stories. Include fun and intriguing facts about veterinary CHM. Clients love patient photos. Be sure to include ones with the herbal formulas they are taking. Create or utilize veterinary CHM-specific hashtags.

Email Blasts

Send fun mass emails to your clients introducing veterinary CHM. Consider monthly case presentations illustrating how the service has benefited patients. Almost everyone has at least one email address these days. Customer service representatives should be amassing client emails at the same rate as phone numbers.

Mailers

Mailers can be expensive and are largely unnecessary in this digital age. Mailers can be used to announce the introduction of CHM to existing clients. The mailer should include the name of the new service (Veterinary Chinese Herbal Medicine), a brief description of how veterinary CHM can help pet patients, the name of the doctor offering the service, a brief description of the training the doctor received, and one or more photographs of a pet taking veterinary CHM.

In-Hospital Promotions

Advertise veterinary CHM within the hospital using small promotions signs, informational signs, invoice teasers, and staff buttons. Small promotional signs can be placed in the waiting room and exam rooms. Include photos of pets and Chinese herbal formulas. Consider catch-phrases such as "Got Herbs?" or "We got an herb for that!"

Informational signs should include a brief description of how veterinary CHM can help pet patients, photographs of pets with their formulas, the name of the doctor offering the service, and a brief description of the training the doctor received.

Invoice teasers should consist of short phrases reminding and enticing owners regarding a new service offered at the practice. Examples include "Now Offering Veterinary Chinese Herbal Medicine"; "Curious if Chinese Herbal Medicine can help your pet?"; "Introducing Veterinary Chinese Herbal Medicine"; and "Would your pet benefit from Veterinary Chinese Herbal Medicine?"

Buttons can be made for the staff to wear with kitchy phrases reminding owners, in a fun way, of the new VIM service. Examples include "Got Herbs" and "Want to learn more about Veterinary Chinese Herbal Medicine?"

Client Education

Education is crucial to understanding the purpose and importance of any given treatment, as well as answering client questions and any concerns that may arise. The client handouts and videos solidify pet owner knowledge base reducing concerns and conveying value.

Integration

The key components for proper integration include availability of the service to the right patients; appropriate patient scheduling; appropriate support staff scheduling; and staff buy-in (understanding the benefits of the offered service).

Veterinarians

There are several factors to consider when veterinarians prepare to incorporate a VIM in their clinical repertoire: state requirements and restrictions, return on investment, course

availability, supplies and equipment, veterinary organizations, and continuing education.

State Requirements and Restrictions

Is CHM Considered the Practice of Veterinary Medicine?

Each state has its own veterinary provisions outlining what is and is not considered the practice of veterinary medicine. Currently no state specifically defines CHM as the practice of veterinary medicine. These rules can change, and careful review of your specific state requirements is recommended.

Does CHM Continuing Education Count Toward Licensure Continuing Education Requirements?

Currently no states require specific CE hours for veterinarians offering CHM nor do they specifically reference CHM CE. Some states limit the use of integrative medicine CE hours toward the annual CE requirement for license renewal. Most states permit the use of integrative CE if the lectures or webinars are performed by an approved provider. Review your specific state's requirements for further details. Table 1.14 in Chapter 1 lists each state's CE requirements and provides links for their Board of Veterinary Medicine on the companion website.

Are Your Assets Covered?

Check with your liability insurance to determine if you are covered when practicing CHM. Refer to the Introduction at the beginning of this book for additional information.

Return on Investment

Specifics are discussed in the Team Members section of this chapter.

Course Availability

Formal training in veterinary CHM is not required but highly encouraged. Training and certification provide the foundations of understanding as to how CHM can best help your veterinary patients. Completion of formal training and certification also help legitimize the modality. Pricing is accurate as of February 2023.

Veterinarians who are on the fence about committing to a full training course are encouraged to attend introductory lectures first. Familiarizing yourself with the information is a great way to determine if pursuing this modality is right for you and your practice. State and national veterinary conferences, as well as many online veterinary educational platforms (VIN, Vetfolio, DVM360 Flex, Vet Girl on the Run, and CIVT) frequently offer lectures on various integrative topics.

Chi University
- **Course name**: Veterinary Herbal Medicine Certification Set
- **Prerequisites**: License, in good standing, to practice veterinary medicine or third or fourth year veterinary student.
- **Description**
  - 165-hour American Association of Veterinary State Boards (AAVSB) Registry of Approved Continuing Education (RACE)-approved certification course in veterinary CHM.
  - The course introduces TCVM principles as applied to obtaining a successful diagnosis and the institution of appropriate herbal therapy. The use of CHM is taught by body systems.
  - Five modules consisting of 29–30 CE hours and five hours of wet lab demos. Modules are offered year-round and can be taken online or on-site in any order.
  - Students are eligible for the Certified Veterinary Chinese Herbalist certification endorsed by Chi University. Certification requirements include:
    o Successful completion of the program
    o Pass take-home exams for all modules
    o Submit three case reports.
- **Online training**: Online sessions are available for four months each.
- **On-site training**: On-site sessions are in Reddick, FL and last an average of four days each.

- **Completion time**: Approximately 20 months.
- **Cost**: $3850
  - Digital notes included
  - Free case consultation with Chi instructors
  - Separate cost for:
    o Chinese Herbal Fundamental Knowledge course
    o TCVM Fundamental Theories course
    o Printed notes
    o Herbal kits.
- **Contact information**
  - Address: 9650 W Hwy 318, Reddick, FL 32686, USA
  - Phone: (800) 860-1543
  - Website: www.chiu.edu.
  - Email: register@chiu.edu

College of Integrative Therapies (CIVT)
- **Course name**: Certification in Veterinary Chinese Herbal Medicine
- **Prerequisites**: License, in good standing, to practice veterinary medicine or third or fourth year veterinary student.
- **Description**
  - 180-hour non-RACE-approved certification course in veterinary CHM with the option to pursue a graduate diploma in veterinary CHM.
  - The course introduces TCVM principles as applied to obtaining a successful diagnosis and the institution of appropriate herbal therapy. The use of CHM is taught by body systems.
  - Certification requirements:
    o Complete all modules
    o Complete all module assessments
    o Forum participation
    o Case journal completion.
- **Online training**: Six online modules.
- **On-site training**: n/a
- **Completion time**: 12 months
- **Cost**: $3020
  - Digital copy of the notes
  - Case support from tutors
  - Access to online personalized tutors and mentoring.

- **Contact information**
  - Address: PO Box 352, Yeppoon, 4703 QLD, Australia
  - Phone: (304) 930-5684
  - Website: www.civtedu.org
  - Email: admin1@civtedu.org

College of Integrative Therapies (CIVT)

- **Course name**: Graduate Diploma Veterinary Chinese Herbal Medicine
- **Prerequisites**: License, in good standing, to practice veterinary medicine or third or fourth year veterinary student.
- **Description**
  - 1410-hour postdoctoral certification program in veterinary CHM nationally accredited under the Australian Qualifications Framework at the postgraduate level through nationally recognized training.
  - The program contains 112 hours of AAVSB RACE-approved CE.
  - The course builds upon the fundamentals taught in the certification course expanding the practitioner's knowledge base and skill regarding TCVM diagnoses and the appropriate application of Chinese herbal therapy.
  - Certification requirements:
    - ○ Complete all modules
    - ○ Complete all module assessments
    - ○ Forum participation
    - ○ Case log book completion
    - ○ Video recordings
    - ○ Telemedicine discussions with mentors
    - ○ Submission of two detailed case studies.

- **Online training**: Eight online modules.
- **On-site training**: n/a
- **Completion time**: 24 months
- **Cost**: $8495
  - Digital copy of the notes
  - Case support from tutors
  - Access to online personalized tutors and mentoring.
- **Contact information**
  - Address: PO Box 352, Yeppoon, 4703 QLD, Australia
  - Phone: (304) 930-5684

- Website: www.civtedu.org
- Email: admin1@civtedu.org

International Veterinary Acupuncture Society (IVAS)

- **Course name**: Certification in Veterinary Chinese Herbal Medicine
- **Prerequisites**: License, in good standing, to practice veterinary medicine or third or fourth year veterinary student.
- **Description**
  - 160-hour certification course in veterinary CHM.
  - The program contains 99 hours of AAVSB RACE-approved CE.
  - The course is conducted in conjunction with CIVT.
  - The course introduces TCVM principles as applied to obtaining a successful diagnosis and the institution of appropriate herbal therapy. The use of CHM is taught by body systems.
  - Certification requirements:
    - ○ Attendance and completion of all sessions
    - ○ Forum participation
    - ○ Submission of a case journal.

- **Online training**: Eight online modules.
- **On-site training**: n/a
- **Completion time**: 9 months
- **Cost**: $3448.85
  - Digital class notes provided
  - Online tutor support and mentoring.

- **Contact information**
  - Address: PO Box 271458, Fort Collins, CO 80527, USA
  - Phone: (970) 266-0666
  - Website: www.ivas.org
  - Email: office@ivas.org

International Veterinary Acupuncture Society (IVAS)

- **Course name**: Advanced Certification in Veterinary Chinese Herbal Medicine
- **Prerequisites**: License, in good standing, to practice veterinary medicine or third or fourth year veterinary student.
- **Description**

- 500+ hour certification course in veterinary CHM.
- The program contains 101 hours of AAVSB RACE-approved CE.
- The course is conducted in conjunction with CIVT.
- The course builds upon the fundamentals taught in the certification course expanding the practitioner's knowledge base and skill regarding TCVM diagnoses and the appropriate application of Chinese herbal therapy.
- Certification requirements:
  - Attendance and completion of all sessions
  - Forum participation
  - Submission of a case journal.

- **Online training**: Eight online modules.
- **On-site training**: n/a
- **Completion time**: 18 months

- **Cost**: $6887.35
  - Digital class notes provided
  - Online tutor support and mentoring
  - Herb samples.

- **Contact information**
  - Address: PO Box 271458, Fort Collins, CO 80527, USA
  - Phone: (970) 266-0666
  - Website: www.ivas.org
  - Email: office@ivas.org

Supplies

Table 3.34 lists the recommended starting supplies and suppliers when introducing veterinary CHM into the hospital. Figure 3.6 depicts the gram scale and reusable measuring spoons used in my hospital. Figure 3.7 shows the four most common herbal brands I use. Finally, Table 3.35

Table 3.34 Suggested starting supplies and approximate costs for CHM supplies as of February 2023. The hospital is assumed to start their herbal pharmacy with at least 10 different herbal formulas, carrying two different sizes or formulations of each herb. Five common formulas from A Time to Heal and Jing Tang are represented below to illustrate projected costs

A time to heal		Jing Tang		Cost
San Ren Tang	100 g	Hindquarter Weakness™	200 g	*Average $34/ bottle*
San Ren Tang	300 tablets	Hindquarter Weakness	200 caps	$680
Si Miao San	100 g	Liver Happy	200 g	
Si Miao San	300 tablets	Liver Happy	200 caps	
Xiao Chai Hu Tang	100 g	Max's Formula	200 g	
Xiao Chai Hu Tang	300 tablets	Max's Formula	200 caps	
Xiao Yao San	100 g	Tendon/Ligament™	200 g	
Xiao Yao San	300 tablets	Tendon/Ligament	200 caps	
Xue Fu Zhu Yu Tang	100 g	Wei Qi Booster™	200 g	
Xue Fu Zhu Yu Tang	300 tablets	Wei Qi Booster	200 caps	
Gram scale				$30
Reusable measuring spoons				$15
Prescription vials	The hospital will need to decide how the herbs will be sold: per bottle or parceled out. If bottles are opened and divided, prescription vials will be needed for distribution. One box of 100 count prescription vials (10 or 40 dram) is approximately $65			$65
Total cost				**$790**

Source: Lisa P. McFaddin.

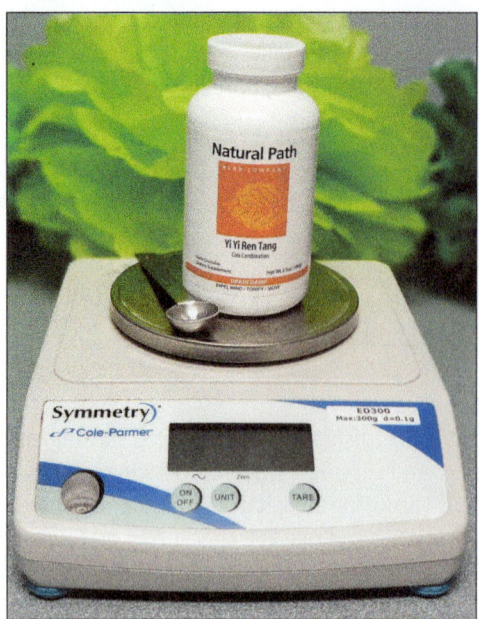

Figure 3.6 The gram scale and one of the reusable measuring spoons used at my hospital. Source: Lisa P. McFaddin.

provides the name of my two preferred herbal providers and the brands they offer.

Hospital remodeling and/or redecorating is generally not required. Additional storage space is required for the herbal bottles in the pharmacy or a separate area of the hospital.

Veterinary Organizations

A description of the most common veterinary organizations with a special interest in VIM and CHM are provided below. Table 3.36 summarizes the organizations' names, contact information, and membership dues.

American College of Veterinary Botanical Medicine (ACVBM)

- **Description**: Founded in 2014 to establish requirements for postdoctoral education and certification in veterinary botanical medicine. The goal was to create a diplomate status for the specialty of veterinary botanical medicine. Patrons can become supporting members through donations or apply to become members of the organizing committee. There is no annual CE requirement to maintain membership.
- **Membership benefits**: The ACVBM offers an annual CE conference.

American Holistic Veterinary Medical Association (AHVMA)

- **Description**: The AHVMA was founded in 1982 at the Western States Veterinary Conference with the goal of advancing integrative medicine through the education of integrative and non-integrative veterinarians, the introduction of integrative

Table 3.35 Commonly used veterinary Chinese herbal medicine suppliers and brands.

Supplier	Brands	Available formulation
A Time to Heal 140 Webster Road, Shelburne, VT 05482 (802) 497-2375 www.atimetohealherbs.com admin@atimetohealherbs.com	Natural Path	• Granular extracts • Liquid extracts
	Kan Essentials	• Tablet • Liquid extract
	Evergreen	• Granular extracts
Dr. Xie's Jing Tang Herbal 9700 West Hwy 318, Reddick, FL 32686 (866) 700-8772 www.tcvmherbal.com help@tcvmherbal.com	Jing Tang	• Granular powder, loose • Granular powder, capsules • Tea pills • Concentrated biscuits

Source: Lisa P. McFaddin.

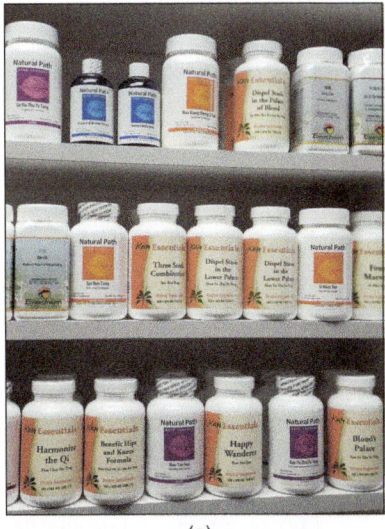

(a)

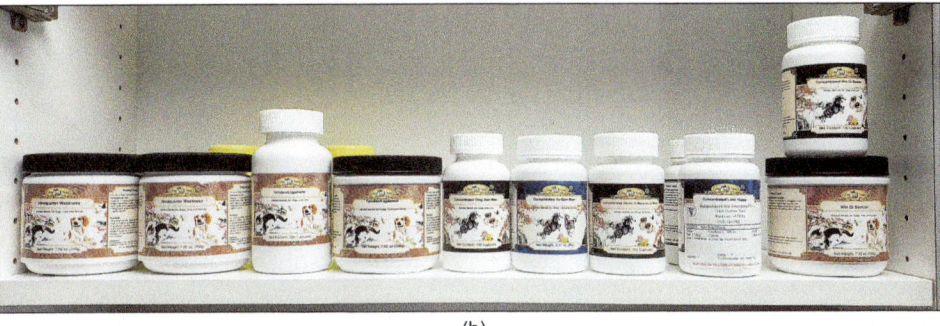

(b)

Figure 3.7 The four most used brands of veterinary Chinese herbal formulas used in my hospital: Natural Path, Kan Essentials, Evergreen, and Jing Tang. Source: Lisa P. McFaddin.

medicine to veterinary students, the promotion of research, and representation in the AVMA House of Delegates. There is no annual CE requirement to maintain membership.

- **Membership benefits**
  - Free subscription to the *AHVMA Journal*, a peer-reviewed journal.
  - Online resources for client education.
  - Searchable member directory.
  - Discounted vaccination titers through Kansas State University (KSU) Diagnostic Lab.
  - Free access to the Natural Medicines Database, an online resource for

supplements, natural medicines, and integrative therapies.
  - Reduced cost for the AHVMA annual conference.

College of Integrative Veterinary Therapies (CIVT)

- **Description**: An online organization open to all licensed animal health providers interested in integrative medicine. There are two membership options: full membership for veterinarians and associate membership for registered animal health professionals. CIVT strives to promote all aspects of evidence-based integrative medicine through online

Table 3.36 Veterinary associations and organizations with a special interest in veterinary integrative medicine and CHM as of February 2023.

Organization	Contact information	Membership dues
American College of Veterinary Botanical Medicine (ACVBM)	cyndvm@gmail.com	None
American Holistic Veterinary Medical Association (AHVMA)	PO Box 630, Abingdon, MD 21009 (410) 569-0795 office@ahvma.org	$300/year
College of Integrative Veterinary Therapies (CIVT)	PO Box 352, Yeppoon, 4703 QLD Australia (303) 800-5460 membership@civtedu.org	$185/year
Veterinary Botanical Medicine Association (VBMA)	6410 Highway 92, Acworth, GA 30102 office@vbma.org	$85/year
World Association of Traditional Chinese Veterinary Medicine (WATCVM)	WATCVM and AATCVM PO Box 141324, Gainesville, FL 32614 (844) 422-8286 support@aatcvm.org	$85/year

Source: Lisa P. McFaddin.

education and discussion forums. CIVT provides financial support to veterinary students interested in studying integrative medicine. CIVT also helps fund integrative medicine research. There is no annual CE requirement to maintain membership.

- **Membership Benefits**
  - Access to the online electronic library.
  - Access to the electronic *Journal of Integrative Veterinary Therapies.*
  - Three free CE webinars annually.
  - 20% discount on all webinars.
  - Discounts on specific CIVT courses.
  - Searchable member directory.
  - Access to the Natural Medicines Databases and the American Botanical Council Library.

Veterinary Botanical Medicine Association (VBMA)

- **Description**: Founded by Susan Wynn, DVM, CVA, CVCH, AHG in 2002. The VBMA comprises veterinarians and herbalists interested in promoting the responsible application of herbal therapies for animals.

There is no annual CE requirement to maintain membership.

- **Membership benefits**
  - VBMA members receive daily email discussion threads detailing real-life case questions and expert practical advice.
  - Weekly and monthly emails are also shared highlighting herbs commonly used in veterinary medicine.
  - Free subscription to the biannual online *Journal of Veterinary Botanical Medicine.*
  - Access to Herbal Wiki, an online herbal materia medica.
  - Access to additional educational articles, websites, and videos.
  - Discounted cost for telemedicine conferences and webinars.
  - Searchable member directory.
  - The VBMA offers an annual conference and multiple webinars.

World Association of Traditional Chinese Veterinary Medicine (WATCVM)

- **Description**: The WATCVM promotes the education, research, and practice of TCVM throughout the world. The WATCVM provides financial support to veterinary students interested in studying TCVM as well as establishing student organizations within veterinary schools. The WATCVM funds TCVM research programs. There is no annual CE requirement to maintain membership.

- **Membership benefits**
  - Access to online case discussion forums.
  - Free subscription to the *American Journal of Traditional Chinese Veterinary Medicine,* a peer-reviewed journal.
  - Access to the quarterly online TCVM newsletter.
  - Access to the online TCVM library.
  - Discounted TCVM conferences.
  - Access to the online classified ads.
  - Assistance with scientific writing as well as research design of grant proposals.
  - Dual membership in WATCVM and American Association of TCVM (AATCVM).
  - The WATCVM and AATCVM offer an annual International Conference on TCVM

Reference Books

The following is a list of recommended TCVM and veterinary CHM books as of February 2023. A summary of each book is provided.

Application of Traditional Chinese Veterinary Medicine in Exotic Animals
- Author: Zhiqiang Yang and Huisheng Xie, DVM, MS, PhD
- Summary: Proceedings from the 13th Annual International TCVM Conference discussing the introduction and implementation of TCVM therapies for exotic animals.

Chinese Herbal Formulas for Veterinarians
- Authors: John Chen, PhD, Pharm D, OMD, Lac, Tina Chen, MS, Lac, Signe Beebe, DVM, and Michael Salewski, DVM
- Summary: Monographs of Chinese herbal formulas used in veterinary medicine organized by their TCVM category. Each monograph discusses the nomenclature, formula composition, dosage, Chinese therapeutic

actions, clinical manifestations, veterinary clinical applications, veterinary modifications, cautions and contraindications, pharmacologic effects, human clinical studies and research, toxicology, suggested acupuncture therapies, and often additional author comments.

Chinese Medical Herbology and Pharmacology
- Authors: John Chen, PhD, Pharm D, OMD, Lac and Tina Chen, MS, Lac
- Summary: Monographs of Chinese herbs organized by their TCM category. Each monograph discusses the nomenclature, Chinese therapeutic actions, dosages, cautions and contraindications, chemical composition, pharmacologic effects, clinical studies and research, herb–drug interactions, toxicology, and often additional author comments.

Chinese Veterinary Herbal Handbook: 216 Most Commonly Used Veterinary Herbal Formulas
- Authors: Huisheng Xie, DVM, MS, PhD, Lauren Frank, DVM, CVA, Vanessa Preast, DVM, CVA, and Lisa Trevisanello, DVM, CVA
- Summary: The third edition is an earlier version of the *Clinical Manual of Veterinary Herbal Medicine* functioning as a faster reference guide. Focuses on formulas carried by Jing Tang Herbal.

Clinical Application of Different TCM Schools and Thoughts in Veterinary Practice
- Authors: Huisheng Xie, DVM, MS, PhD and Aituan Ma, DVM, PhD, MS
- Summary: Proceedings from the 18th Annual International TCVM Conference discussing the different TCVM schools and theories and TCVM therapy for infectious and inflammatory diseases, behavioral disorders, and other conditions.

Clinical Manual of Chinese Veterinary Herbal Medicine: 178 Commonly Used Veterinary Herbal Formulas
- Authors: Huisheng Xie, DVM, MS, PhD and Aituan Ma, DVM, PhD, MS

- Summary: A quick reference book covering the safe use of CHM in veterinary patients with an emphasis on practical information on commonly used Chinese herbal formulas as well as formula selection using TCVM and Western diagnoses. Scientific studies focusing on the referenced herbal formulas are provided. Focuses on formulas carried by Jing Tang Herbal.

Essential Guide to Chinese Herbal Formulas: Bridging Science and Tradition in Integrative Veterinary Medicine
- Author: Steve Marsden, DVM, ND, MSOM, Lac, Dipl.CH., RH(AHG)
- Summary: A quick reference book covering the safe use of CHM in veterinary patients with an emphasis on practical information on commonly used Chinese herbal formulas as well as formula selection using TCVM and Western diagnoses. Focuses on formulas carried by A Time to Heal Herbs.

Four Paws Five Directions: A Guide to Chinese Medicine for Cats and Dogs
- Author: Cheryl Schwartz, DVM
- Summary: An introduction to TCVM in veterinary medicine focusing on TCVM theory and acupuncture. Additional therapies are briefly covered: food therapy, herbal supplements, nutritional supplements, environmental modifications. The disease processes are organized by body system and the Five Element Theory.

Integrating Complementary Medicine into Veterinary Practice
- Authors: Robert S. Goldstein, VMD, Paula Jo Broadfoot, DVM, Richard E. Plamquist, DVM, Karen Johnstons, DVM, Jiu Jia Wen, DVM, Barbara Fougère, BSc, BVMS (Hons), BHSc (comp Med), MODT, MHSc (Herb Med), CVA (IVAs), CVBM, CVCP, and Margo Roman, DVM
- Summary: A comprehensive review of multiple integrative therapies, including CHM, acupuncture, homotoxicology, nanopharmacology, homotoxicology, and therapeutic nutrition. The book aims to educate

veterinary practitioners on the validity, effectiveness, and incorporation of each modality within daily practice.

Kan Essentials Chinese Herbal Formula Guide
- Author: Steve Marsden, DVM, ND, MSOM, Lac, Dipl.CH., RH(AHG)
- Summary: Product booklet discussing the clinical uses and dosing for the Kan Essentials herbal formulas.

Manual of Natural Veterinary Medicine: Science and Tradition
- Authors: Susan G. Wynn, DVM and Steve Marsden, DVM, ND, MSOM, Lac, Dipl. CH., RH(AHG)
- Summary: A quick reference book discussing the integrative therapy options for numerous diseases in veterinary medicine. The book is organized by Western conditions. For each category the potential TCVM diagnoses and treatment options are then discussed in succinct detail. A must-have for all integrative veterinarians.

Natural Path Herb Company Guide to Chinese Veterinary Herbal Medicine for Small Animals
- Author: Steve Marsden, DVM, ND, MSOM, Lac, Dipl.CH., RH(AHG)
- Summary: Product booklet discussing the clinical uses and dosing for the Natural Path herbal formulas.

Practical Guide to Traditional Chinese Veterinary Medicine: Emergencies and Five Element Syndromes
- Authors: Huisheng Xie, DVM, MS, PhD, Lindsey Wedemeyer, MA, VetMB, MRCVS, and Cheryl L Chrisman, DVM, MS, EdS, DACVIM (Neurology)
- Summary: The first of a four volume series discussing the practical use of TCVM in veterinary medicine. The book breaks down the TCVM pattern diagnosis and treatment options (acupuncture, Chinese herbal formulas, Tui-na, food therapy, and environmental changes) for common small animal emergencies. The book is organized using the Five Elements Theory of disease as it relates to emergent disorders.

Practical Guide to Traditional Chinese Veterinary Medicine: Exotic, Zoo, and Farm Animals

- Authors: Huisheng Xie, DVM, MS, PhD and Harvey E Ramirez
- Summary: The final book of a four volume series discussing the practical use of TCVM in veterinary medicine. The book breaks down the TCVM pattern diagnosis and treatment options (acupuncture, Chinese herbal formulas, Tui-na, food therapy, and environmental changes) for exotic, zoo, and farm animals.

Practical Guide to Traditional Chinese Veterinary Medicine: Small Animal Practice

- Authors: Huisheng Xie, DVM, MS, PhD, Lindsey Wedemeyer, MA, VetMB, MRCVS, Cheryl L Chrisman, DVM, MS, EdS, DACVIM (Neurology), and Lisa Trevisanellow, DrMEDVET
- Summary: The second of a four volume series discussing the practical use of TCVM in veterinary medicine. The book breaks down the TCVM pattern diagnosis and treatment options (acupuncture, Chinese herbal formulas, Tui-na, food therapy, and environmental changes) for common small animal diseases. The book is organized by the Western medical diagnoses and then further divided into the possible TCVM diagnoses for each disease process.

Traditional Chinese Veterinary Medicine Approach to Gastrointestinal and Hepatobiliary Diseases

- Authors: Liting Cao, DVM, PhD and Huisheng Xie, DVM, PhD
- Summary: Proceedings from the 22nd Annual International TCVM Conference discussing the use of TCVM for the treatment of gastrointestinal and hepatobiliary diseases.

Traditional Chinese Veterinary Medicine Approach to Veterinary Dermatological and Immune-Mediated Diseases

- Authors: Aituan Ma, DVM, PhD, MS, Cui Liu, DVM, PhD, Chang Yu, DVM, MS, and Huisheng Xie, DVM, MS, PhD

- Summary: Proceedings from the 21st Annual International TCVM Conference discussing the use of TCVM for the treatment of dermatologic and immune-mediated diseases.

Traditional Chinese Veterinary Medicine: Empirical Technique to Scientific Validation

- Authors: Zhiqiang Yang and Huisheng Xie, DVM, MS, PhD
- Summary: Proceedings from the 1st Annual International TCVM Conference discussing the scientific study of TCVM, including basic scientific research, small animal specific studies, exotic animal specific studies, large animal specific studies, and pediatric and geriatric medicine.

Traditional Chinese Veterinary Medicine for the Diagnosis and Treatment of Kidney and Water Element Disorders

- Authors: Aituan Ma, DVM, PhD, MS and Huisheng Xie, DVM, MS, PhD
- Summary: Proceedings from the 23rd Annual International TCVM Conference discussing the use of TCVM for the treatment of kidney and water element disorders.

Traditional Chinese Veterinary Medicine for Geriatric Medicine and Palliative Care

- Authors: Huisheng Xie, DVM, MS, PhD and Aituan Ma, DVM, PhD, MS
- Summary: Proceedings from the 19th Annual International TCVM Conference discussing the use of TCVM for geriatric medicine and palliative care.

Traditional Chinese Veterinary Medicine for Neurologic Diseases

- Authors: Huisheng Xie, DVM, MS, PhD, Cheryl L Chrisman, DVM, MS, EdS, DACVIM (Neurology), and Lisa Trevisanellow, DrMEDVET
- Summary: Proceedings from the 13th Annual International TCVM Conference discussing the use of TCVM for a variety of neurologic conditions.

Traditional Chinese Veterinary Medicine from Dragon Legend to Modern Practice
- Authors: Xiuhuii Zhong, Aituan Ma, DVM, PhD, MS, Lisa Trevisanellow, DrMEDVET, and Qingbo Wang
- Summary: Proceedings of the 14th Annual International TCVM Conference discussing the use of TCVM for the treatment of liver, gastrointestinal, equine specific, and exotic animal specific diseases. A variety of other topics are also covered, including the longitudinal muscle system, platelet-rich plasma in aquapuncture, and the adverse effects of CHM and acupuncture.

Traditional Chinese Veterinary Medicine: Fundamental Principles
- Authors: Huisheng Xie, DVM, MS, PhD and Vanessa Preast, DVM, CVA
- Summary: The quintessential introduction to TCVM theory with self-study quizzes, case examples, and practical application of TCVM therapies for small animal and equine patients.

Traditional Chinese Veterinary Medicine for Pain, Lameness, Neurological and Endocrine Disorders
- Authors: Huisheng Xie, DVM, MS, PhD and Aituan Ma, DVM, PhD, MS
- Summary: Proceedings from the 20th Annual International TCVM Conference discussing the use of TCVM for the treatment of pain, lameness, neurologic disorders, endocrine disorders, infertility, and other conditions.

Xie's Chinese Veterinary Herbology
- Authors: Huisheng Xie, DVM, MS, PhD and Vanessa Preast, DVM, CVA
- Summary: A practical guide covering the theory and application of veterinary CHM. The book is organized into three sections: herbal materia medica, herbal formulas, and clinical applications.

Promotion

Information regarding the hospital's promotion of CHM can be found in the Team Members section.

Integration

Key components for proper integration include availability, scheduling, and staff buy-in. Availability means offering the service to the right patient. Scheduling refers to appropriate patient and support staff scheduling. Staff buy-in ensures all team members understand the benefits of the offered service.

Conclusion

Veterinary CHM is a well-studied and increasingly popular therapeutic modality. The effects and benefits of CHM are numerous for veterinary patients. This chapter and companion website describe in detail how CHM can be successfully introduced into daily practice, as well as provide practical tools for implementation.

Acknowledgments

I would like to thank Dr. Steve Marsden for reviewing this chapter for content. Steve Marsden, DVM, ND, MSOM, Grad Dip Vet Acup, Grad Dip CVHM, Dipl/AC, Dipl/CH, CVA, AHG has received a doctorate in Naturopathic Medicine, an MSc in Oriental Medicine, and licensure in acupuncture and Diplomat status in Chinese herbology. He has treated both companion animals and people in Canada. Dr. Marsden is a world-renowned practitioner, instructor, lecturer, and author on multiple integrative medicine subjects, including CHM, acupuncture, and veterinary spinal manipulation. He has lectured for the CIVT, IVAS, Tufts Veterinary School, the Association of Veterinary Acupuncturists of Canada, and numerous national veterinary conferences. He is the co-author of the *Manual of Natural Veterinary Medicine*.

References

AAFCO (Association of American Feed Control Officers) (2014). *AAFCO Methods for Substantiating Nutritional Adequacy of Dog and Cat Foods*. https://www.aafco.org/wp-content/uploads/2023/01/Pet_Food_Report_2013_Annual-Appendix_C.pdf (accessed 5 May 2020).

AAHA (American Animal Hospital Association) (2019). *Compensation and Benefits*, 9e. Denver, CO: AAHA Press.

Adelman, L., Olin, S., Egger, C., and Stokes, J. (2017). The effect of oral Yunnan Baiyao on periprocedural hemorrhage and coagulation parameters in dogs undergoing nasal biopsy: a randomized controlled blinded study. *American Journal of Traditional Chinese Veterinary Medicine* 12 (2): 29–38.

APPA (Americn Pet Products Association) (2022). Pet industry market size and ownership statistics. https://www.americanpetproducts.org/news/News-Public-Relations/pet-industry-market-size-trends-ownership-statistics#:~:text=2021%2D2022%20APPA%20National%20Pet,U.S.%20households%20owned%20a%20pet (accessed 23 February 2023).

AQSIQ (General Administration of Quality Supervision, Inspection and Quarantine of the People's Republic of China) (2020). AQSIQ. www.aqsiq.net (accessed 17 December 2021).

Arya, V., Kashyap, C., and Thakur, N. (2012). Phytopharmacological properties and clinical applications of Crataegus Oxyacantha (Crataegus Laevigata). *American Journal of Traditional Chinese Veterinary Medicine* 7 (2): 23–31.

AVMA (American Veterinary Medical Association) (2019). Economic state of the veterinary profession. https://www.avma.org/news/press-release/AVMA-2019-Economic-State-of-the-Veterinary-Profession-Report-now-available. (accessed 26 July 2021).

AVMA (American Veterinary Medical Association) (2023). *2023 AVMA Report on the Economic State of the Veterinary Profession*. Schaumburg, IL: AVMA.

Bao, Z.Y.T. (1985). Bai Shao. *Journal of Chinese Herbology* 10 (6): 43.

Bao, Z.G.Y.L.X.T. (1986). Bai SHao. *Journal of Chinese Herbal Pharmacology* 2 (5): 26.

Bartholomew, M. (2017). A controlled in-vitro study comparing efficacy of two commercial antibiotic topical compounds and two Chinese herbal medicine topicals against bacteria cultured from 31 canine pyoderma cases. *American Journal of Traditional Chinese Veterinary Medicine* 12 (2): 17–28.

Bartholomew, M. and Xie, H. (2018). The use of traditional Chinese veterinary medicine in the treatment of 5 cases of neoplastic bone disease. *American Journal of Traditional Chinese Veterinary Medicine* 13 (1): 45–56.

BLS (Bureau of Labor Statistics) (2022a). Occupational outlook handbook: veterinarians 2022 median pay. https://www.bls.gov/ooh/healthcare/veterinarians.htm (accessed 18 February 2023).

BLS (Bureau of Labor Statistics) (2022b). Occupational outlook handbooks: veterinary technologists and technicians median pay 2020. https://www.bls.gov/ooh/healthcare/veterinary-technologists-and-technicians.htm (accessed 18 February 2023).

BLS (Bureau of Labor Statistics) (2023). News Release: Consumer Price Index January 2023. https://www.bls.gov/news.release/pdf/cpi.pdf (accessed 18 February 2023).

Brand, E. (2018). Maximizing the clinical efficacy of granule preparations: understanding dosage, regional trends and unforeseen challenges. *Chinese Medical Times* 3 (3): 1–6.

Burns, K. (2017). Assessing pet supplements. https://www.avma.org/javma-news/2017-01-15/assessing-pet-supplements (accessed 4 February 2021).

Burns, K. (2018). Pet ownership stable, veterinary care variable. https://www.avma.org/javma-news/2019-01-15/pet-ownership-stable-veterinary-care-variable (accessed 11 August 2021).

Burns, K. (2022). New report takes a deep dive into pet ownership. https://www.avma.org/news/new-report-takes-deep-dive-pet-ownership (accessed 6 November 2022).

Cahyono, T. (2015). The use of Chinese herbal medicine and acupuncture for neurological disease unresponsive to Western medications in 94 small animal cases. *American Journal of Traditional Chinese Veterinary Medicine* 10 (12): 43–61.

CDER (Center for Drug Evaluation and Research) (2016). Botanical Drug Development Guidance for Industry. https://www.fda.gov/media/93113/download (accessed 3 May 2021).

Chan, T. (2009). Aconite poisoning. *Journal of Clinical Toxicology* 47: 279–285.

Chan, M.J.Y. (2019). Efficacy of Chinese herbal medicine for the rescue treatment of refractory or intermittent idiopathic inflammatory bowel disease in canine patients: a retrospective study. *American Journal of Traditional Chinese Veterinary Medicine* 14 (1): 21–31.

Chen, J. (1998/1999). Recognition and prevention of herb–drug interactions. *Medical Acupuncture* 10 (2): 9–13.

Chen, J. (2013). *Concurrent Use of Herbal Medicines and Pharmaceuticals: Pharmacodynamic Interactions*. College of Integrative Veterinary Therapies.

Chen, J.K. and Chen, T.T. (2012a). *Chinese Medical Herbology and Pharmacology*. City of Industry, CA: Art of Medicine Press.

Chen, J.K. and Chen, T.T. (2012b). Part 1, Overview. In: *Chinese Medical Heerbology and Pharmacology*, 1–29. City of Industry, CA: Art of Medicine Press.

Chen, J.K., Chen, T.T., Beebe, S., and Salewski, M. (2012). *Chinese Herbal Formulas for Veterinarians*. City of Industry, CA: Art of Medicine Press.

CITES (Convention on International Trade in Endangered Species of Wild Fauna and Flora) (2021). CITES. https://cites.org/eng/disc/what.php (accessed 17 December 2021).

Clemmons, R. (2015). *Feeding According to TCM*. Reddick, FL: Jing Tang Publishing.

CVM (Center for Veterinary Medicine) (2022). Hazard Analysis and Risk-Based Preventative Controls for Food for Animals Guidance for Industry. https://www.fda.gov/media/110477/download (accessed 2 May 2023).

Cyranoski, D. (2018). Why Chinese medicine is heading for clinics around the world. *Nature* 561: 448–450.

Dewey, C., Gridley, A., and Fletcher, A. (2020). Evaluation of the Chinese herbal formula Di Tan Tang as an oral add-on therapy for dogs with presumptive refractory idiopathic epilepsy: an open-label investigation in 8 dogs. *American Journal of Traditional Chinese Veterinary Medicine* 15 (2): 1–6.

DSHEA (1994). Dietary Supplement Health and Education Act (DSHEA) of 1994 Public Law 103-417. https://ods.od.nih.gov/About/DSHEA_Wording.aspx#sec3 (accessed 2 February 2021).

Egger, C., Gibbs, D., Wheeler, J. et al. (2016). The effect of Yunnan Baiyao on platelet activation, buccal mucosal bleeding time, prothrombin time, activated partial thromboplastic time, and thromboelastography in health dogs: a randomized, controlled, blinded study. *American Journal of Traditional Chinese Veterinary Medicine* 11 (2): 27–36.

FDA (Food and Drug Administration) (2009). Guidance for Industry: Questions and Answers Regarding the Labeling of Dietary Supplements as Required by the Dietary Supplement and Nonprescription Drug Consumer Protection Act; Availability. https://www.federalregister.gov/documents/2009/09/01/E9-21094/guidance-for-industry-questions-and-answers-regarding-the-labeling-of-dietary-supplements-as (accessed 3 February 2021).

FDA (Food and Drug Administration) (2007). Complementary and Alternative Medicine

Products and their Regulation by the Food and Drug Administration: Draft Guidance for Industry. https://www.fda.gov/regulatory-information/search-fda-guidance-documents/complementary-and-alternative-medicine-products-and-their-regulation-food-and-drug-administration (accessed 6 May 2020).

FDA (Food and Drug Administration) (2017). Is it really FDA Approved? https://www.fda.gov/consumers/consumer-updates/it-really-fda-approved (accessed 4 February 2021).

FDA (Food and Drug Administration) (2018). Label Claims for Conventional Foods and Dietary Supplements. https://www.fda.gov/food/food-labeling-nutrition/label-claims-conventional-foods-and-dietary-supplements (accessed 3 February 2021).

FDA (Food and Drug Administration) (2020). The Ins and Outs of Extra-Label Drug Use in Animals: A Resource for Veterinarians. https://www.fda.gov/animal-veterinary/resources-you/ins-and-outs-extra-label-drug-use-animals-resource-veterinarians (accessed 2 February 2021).

FDA (Food and Drug Administration) (2021a). Animal Food & Feeds: Product Regulation. https://www.fda.gov/animal-veterinary/animal-food-feeds/product-regulation (accessed 20 February 2021).

FDA (Food and Drug Administration) (2021b). Animal Medicinal Drug Use Clarificaiton Act of 1994 (AMDUCA). https://www.fda.gov/animal-veterinary/guidance-regulations/animal-medicinal-drug-use-clarification-act-1994-amduca (accessed 24 January 2022).

FDA (Food and Drug Administration) (2021c). CFR - Code of Federal Regulations Title 21. https://www.accessdata.fda.gov/scripts/cdrh/cfdocs/cfcfr/CFRSearch.cfm?CFRPart=211&showFR=1. (accessed 16 December 2021).

FDA (Food and Drug Administration) (2021d). Facts About the Current Good Manufacturing Practices (CGMPs). http://www.fda.gov/Drugs/DevelopmentApprovalProcess/Manufacturing/ucm169105.htm (accessed 17 December 2021).

FDA (Food and Drug Administration) (2022a). FDA's Regulation of Pet Food. https://www.fda.gov/animal-veterinary/animal-health-literacy/fdas-regulation-pet-food#drug (accessed 2 May 2023).

FDA (Food and Drug Administration) (2022b). Hazard Analysis Critical Control Point (HACCP). https://www.fda.gov/food/hazard-analysis-critical-control-point-haccp/haccp-principles-application-guidelines#:~:text=HACCP%20is%20a%20management%20system,consumption%20of%20the%20finished%20product (accessed 2 May 2023).

FDA (Food and Drug Administration) (2022c). What is a botanical drug? https://www.fda.gov/about-fda/center-drug-evaluation-and-research-cder/what-botanical-drug (accessed 3 May 2023).

FederalPay.org (2023). FY 2023 Federal Per Diem Rates October 2022–September 2023. https://www.federalpay.org/perdiem/2023 (accessed 18 February 2023).

Fowler, M., Shiau, D.-S., and Xie, H. (2017). A randomized controlled study comparing Da Xiang Lian Wan to metronidazole in the treatment of stress colitis in shelter/rescued dogs. *American Journal of Traditional Chinese Veterinary Medicine* 12 (1): 45–54.

Freeman, J. (2001a). East/West herbal energetics part I. *Canadian Journal of Herbalism* 22 (2): 2–11.

Freeman, J. (2001b). East/West herbal energetics part II. *Canadian Journal of Herbalism* 24 (4): 12–22.

Freeman, J. (2002). East/West herbal energetics part III. *Canadian Journal of Herbalism* 23 (3): 6–18.

French, S. and Kemmis, S. (2023). Rental Car Pricing Statistics: 2023. https://www.nerdwallet.com/article/travel/car-rental-pricing-statistics#:~:text=The%20average%20weekly%20rental%20price,in%20advance%2C%20it%20was%20%24513 (accessed 18 February 2023).

Grassie, L. (2002). Update on Animal Dietary Supplements. https://www.nasc.cc/historical-summary (accessed 4 February 2021).

Guan, Y., Chen, J., Zhou, S. et al. (2018). A randomized and controlled study of the effect of Echinacea Purpurea on canine parvovirus and distemper virus antibody levels in dogs. *American Journal of Traditional Chinese Veterinary Medicine* 13 (2): 13–18.

Hao, W. and Lin, Z. (2003). Discussion of the methodologies employed in the Shanghuan Lun for pattern differentiation and formula making. *Journal of Traditional Chinese Medicine* 72: 21–26.

Harris, L. (2008). Treatment of a dog with flea allergy dermatitis with the Chinese herbal formula external wind. *American Journal of Traditional Chinese Veterinary Medicine* 3 (1): 57–59.

Hayashi, A. and Xie, H. (2015). Review of current research on Chinese herbal medicine for epilepsy. *American Journal of Traditional Chinese Veterinary Medicine* 10 (1): 31–42.

He, C.-L., Wan, Y.-F., He, X.-L. et al. (2013). Antiviral and immune enhancing effects of Xian Ren Zhang (Haworth) polysaccharides in vitro and in vivo. *American Journal of Traditional Chinese Veterinary Medicine* 8 (2): 23–30.

Hirsch, D., Shiau, D.S., and Xie, H. (2017). A randomized and controlled study of the efficacy of Yin Qiao San combined with antibiotics compared to antibiotics alone for the treatment of feline upper respiratory disease. *American Journal of Traditional Chinese Veterinary Medicine* 12 (2): 39–47.

Knueven, D. (2018). An introduction to supplements: evidence-based nutritional therapies. Illinois State Veterinary Medical Association. https://www.isvma.org/wp-content/uploads/2018/10/AnIntroductiontoSupplements EvidenceBasedNutritionalTherapies. pdf

Koh, R., Xie, H., and Cuypers, M. (2017). The therapeutic effect of acupuncture and Chinese herbal medicine in 12 dogs with hyperadrenocorticism. *American Journal of Traditional Chinese Veterinary Medicine* 12 (1): 55–68.

Kong, C., Zhong, X., Ma, A., and Zhao, Z. (2014). A randomized blinded double controlled experimental study of the effects of Gan Lian Yu Ping Feng on antibody titers and nonspecific immune indexes in chickens vaccinated against infectious laryngotracheitis virus. *American Journal of Traditional Chinese Veterinary Medicine* 9 (1): 39–49.

Li, R. and Hu, S. (2010). Evaluation of Zhe Ba Wei to enhance the humoral immune response. *American Journal of Traditional Chinese Veterinary Medicine* 5 (2): 7–13.

Li, R., Zhai, L., and Hu, S. (2012a). Enhancement of the immune responses of mice to ovalbumin by oral administration of Bai Zhu (Atractylodes). *American Journal of Traditional Chinese Veterinary Medicine* 7 (2): 15–22.

Li, Y., Wu, L., Yuan, L., and Hu, S. (2012b). Estrogen, ginsenosides Rb1 and Rg1 exhibit adjuvant activities via estrogen receptors. *American Journal of Traditional Chinese Veterinary Medicine* 7 (1): 17–25.

Liao, H., Banbury, L., and Leach, D. (2008). Antioxidant activity of 45 Chinese herbs and the relationship with their TCM characteristics. *Evidence-based Complementary and Alternative Medicine* 5 (4): 429–434.

Liu, J. and Ma, A. (2020). A randomized, blinded, controlled study on the effects of preoperative oral adnministration of Yunnan Baiyao for the mitigation of blood loss in dogs undergoing effective spay/neuter surgeries. *American Journal of Traditional Chinese Veterinary Medicine* 15 (2): 7–16.

Liu, C.M., Holyoak, G.R., and Lin, C.T. (2016). Acupuncture combined with Chinese herbs for the treatment in hemivertebral French bulldogs with emergent paraparesis. *Journal of Traditional and Complementary Medicine* 6 (4): 409–412.

Ma, A. (2016). *Clinical Manual of Chinese Veterinary Herbal Medicine*. Gainesville: Ancient Art Press.

Makino, T., Ito, Y., Sasaki, S.-Y. et al. (2004). Preventative and curative effects of

Gyokujeifu-san, a formula of traditional Chinese medicine, on allergic rhinitis induced with Japanese cedar pollens in guinea pigs. *Biological and Pharmaceutical Bulletin* 27 (4): 554–558.

Marks, D. and Shmalberg, J. (2015). Profitability and financial benefits of acupuncture in small animal private practice. *American Journal of Traditional Chinese Veterinary Medicine* 10 (1): 43–48.

Marsden, S. (2014a). *Essential Guide to Chinese Herbal Formulas: Bridging Science and Tradition in Integrative Veterinary Therapies.* College of Integrative Veterinary Therapies.

Marsden, S. (2014b). Si Miao San (Four marvels combination). In: *Essential Guide to Chinese Herbal Formulas: Bridging Science and Tradition in Integrative Veterinary Medicine,* 128–134. College of Integrative Veterinary Therapies.

Marsden, S. (2014c). Xiao Yao San (Rambling ease powder, easy wanderer). In: *Eassential Guide to Chinese Herbal Formulas: Bridging Science and Tradition in Integrative Veterinary Medicine,* 155–157. College of Integrative Veterinary Therapies.

Marsden, S. (2015). *Lecture Notes and Videos: Nutritional Strategies in Chinese Herbal Medicine - Building on the Success of Herbs with Diet Change.* Online, 135–137. College of Integrative Therapies.

McKee, M. and Shiau, D.-S. (2019). A randomized and controlled comparative study to determine the effectiveness of Long Dan Xie Gan in combination with Osurnia for the treatment of acute canine otitis externa. *American Journal of Traditional Chinese Veterinary Medicine* 14 (2): 13–22.

MFAF (Michelson Found Animals Foundation) (2018). Furred lines: Pet trends. https://www. prnewswire.com/news-releases/furred-lines-pet-trends-2019-300741947.html. (accessed 26 July 2021).

Mitchell, D. (2006). Fundamentals of Chinese Herbology. *Proceedings of the North American Veterinary Conference* (7–11 January 2006), Orlando, Florida. Small animal and exotics book 2, Volume 20.

NAPHIA (North American Pet Health Insurance Association) (2023). Industry Data. https:// naphia.org/industry-data/#my-menu (accessed 18 February 2023).

NCCIH (National Center for Complementary and Integrative Health) (2021). Herbs at a Glance. https://www.nccih.nih.gov/health/ herbsataglance (accessed 17 Decenber 2021).

Nolen, R.S. (2022). Pet owner ship rate stabilizes as spending increases. https://www.avma.org/ news/pet-ownership-rate-stabilizes-spending-increases (accessed 22 February 2023).

Ou, B., Huang, D., Hampsch-Woodill, M., and Flanagan, J. (2003). When east meets west: the relationship between yin–yang and antioxidation–oxidation. *Federation of American Societies for Experimental Biology* 17 (2): 127–129.

Purdue University (2019). Veterinary price index. https://assets.ctfassets.net/440y9b545yd9/5IsP 0OgjAls6CbaXWvTDuS/81213899998ebb624 d418b7521448a0a/FINAL_Nationwide-Purdue_2019-Veterinary-Price-Index.pdf (accessed 11 November 2023).

Rodriguez, A., Shiau, D.S., and Levinson, K. (2021). Preoperative oral administraiton of Yunnan Baiyao and its effects of coagulation parameters in tick-borne disease and/or heartworm seropositive dogs: a pilot study. *American Journal of Traditional Chinese Veterinary Medicine* 16 (2): 23–30.

Schultz, W. (1996). Inapplicability of the dietary supplement health and education act to animal products. *Food and Drug Administration Federal Register* 61 (78): 17706–17708.

Scott, J. (1994). An introduction to pulse diagnosis. *Journal of Chinese Medicine* 14: 1–20.

Serrano, A., Ros, G., and Nieto, G. (2018). Bioactive compounds and extracts from traditional herbs and their potential anti-inflammatory health effects. *Medicine (Basel)* 5 (3): 76.

Shmalberg, J., Xie, H., and Memon, M. (2019). Canine and feline patients referred exclusively for acupuncture and herbs: a two-year retrospective analysis. *Journal of Acupuncture and Meridian Studies* 12 (5): 145–150.

Sivula, N. (2012). Research and clinical applications of Ren Shen (Ginseng). *American Journal of Traditional Chinese Veterinary Medicine* 7 (2): 33–37.

Song, D., Song, J., and Song, X. (2008). Traditional Chinese veterinary medicine immunology and its application in the treatment of canine and feline diseases. *American Journal of Traditional Chinese Veterinary Medicine* 3 (1): 23–29.

Song, D. et al. (2014). Four randomized, controlled and blinded studies comparing the effects of Cu Yun Guan Zhu Ye and estradiol on the vagina, uterus and ovaries of mice. *American Journal of Traditional Chinese Veterinary Medicine* 9 (1): 51–63.

Song, D., Liu, J., Song, X. et al. (2015). Randomized, controlled in-vitro and in-vivo experimental studies of the effects of the Chinese herbal medicine Mu Bing Xiao Huang on intestinal peristalsis of rabbits. *American Journal of Traditional Chinese Veterinary Medicine* 10 (1): 15–24.

Stevenson, P. (2016). How to set practice service fees. https://cliniciansbrief.com/article/how-set-practice-service-fees (accessed 10 June 2020).

Sun, X., Yang, Z., Dong, H. et al. (2015). A randomized controlled study of the effects of Hong Hua (Carthamus) extracts on skin microvascular vasomotion at acupoint Pi-shu and NO and ET-1 production from microvascular endothelial cells in a murine model. *American Journal of Traditional Chinese Veterinary Medicine* 10 (1): 25–29.

Trcek, L. (2023). This is How Much Flight Prices Increase in 2023 (+FAQs). https://www.travelinglifestyle.net/this-is-how-much-flight-prices-increase-in-2023 (accessed 18 February 2023).

USDA (US Department of Agriculture) (2020). Good Agricultural Practices (GAP) Audits. https://www.ams.usda.gov/services/auditing/gap-ghp (accessed 17 Decenber 2020).

Wen, J. and Johnson, K. (2011). Long-term follow-up of canine mammary gland neoplasia in eight dogs treated with surgery and a new Chinese herbal formula. *American Journal of Traditional Chinese Veterinary Medicine* 6 (1): 27–31.

Wen, J., Johnson, K., and Gucciardo, D. (2016). Chinese herbal medicine for dogs with complete cranial cruciate ligament rupture: 181 cases. *American Journal of Traditional Chinese Veterinary Medicine* 11 (1): 41–48.

WHO (World Health Organization) (2015). Medicines: Good manufacturing practices. https://www.who.int/news-room/questions-and-answers/item/medicines-good-manufacturing-processes (accessed 17 December 2021).

WHO (World Health Organization) (2021). ICD-11 for Mortality and Morbidity Statistics. https://icd.who.int/browse11/l-m/en (accessed 18 December 2021).

Wilcox, D.L., Liu, H., Ma, Y. et al. (2009). Comparison of the Chinese herbal formula Hai Zao Yu Hu Tang and methimazole for the treatment of feline hyperthyroidism. *American Journal of Traditional Chinese Veterinary Medicine* 4 (1): 27–38.

Wirth, K., Kow, K., Salute, M.E. et al. (2014). In vitro effects of Yunnan Baiyao on canine hemangiosarcoma cell lines. *Veterinary and Comparative Oncology* 14 (3): 281–294.

Wong, C. and Shiau, D.-S. (2020). The effectiveness of integrativing Gui Pi Tang with conventional medicine in the treatment of thrombocytopenia in dogs: a retrospective study. *American Journal of Traditional Chinese Veterinary Medicine* 15 (2): 39–52.

Woodley, K. (2018). Pet insurance for holistic and integrative practice. https://ivcjournal.com/pet-insurance-integrative-practices (accessed 11 August 2021).

Xie, H. (2011). Toxicity of Chinese veterinary herbal medicines. *American Journal of Traditional Chinese Veterinary Medicine* 6 (2): 45–53.

Xie, H. (2012). Chinese veterinary herbal medicine: history, scientific validation and regulations. *American Journal of Traditional Chinese Veterinary Medicine* 7 (1): 1–5.

Xie, H. (2015). *Dr. Xie's Lecture Notes*, 1–176. Reddick, FL: Jing Tang Publishing.

Xie, H. and Preast, V. (2007a). Diagnostic methods. In: *Traditional Chinese Veterinary Medicine: Fundamental Principles*, 249–303. Reddick, FL: Chi Institute Press.

Xie, H. and Preast, V. (2007b). Diagnostic systems and pattern differentiation. In: *Traditional Chinese Veterinary Medicine: Fundamental Principles*, 305–468. Reddick, FL: Chi Institute Press.

Xie, H. and Preast, V. (2007c). Etiology and pathology. In: *Traditional Chinese Veterinary Medicine: Fundamental Principles* (ed. F.L. Reddick), 209–248. Chi Institute Press.

Xie, H. and Preast, V. (2007d). Five element theory. In: *Traditional Chinese Veterinary Medicine: Fundamental Principles*, 27–62. Reddick, FL: Chi Institute Press.

Xie, H. and Preast, V. (2007e). Qi, Shen, Jing, blood, and body fluid. In: *Traditional Chinese Veterinary Medicine: Fundamental Principles*, 69–100. Reddick, FL: Chi Institute Press.

Xie, H. and Preast, V. (2007f). The meridians. In: *Traditional Chinese Veterinary Medicine: Fundamental Principles*, 149–204. Reddick, FL: Chi Institute Press.

Xie, H. and Preast, V. (2007g). Yin and Yang. In: *Traditional Chinese Veterinary Medicine: Fundamental Principles*, 1–24. Reddick, FL: Chi Institute Press.

Xie, H. and Preast, V. (2007h). Zang-Fu Physiology. In: *Traditional Chinese Veterinary Medicine: Fundamental Principles*, 105–114. Reddick, FL: Chi Institute Press.

Xiujun, W., Hanru, L., and Shining, G. (2006). Clinical application and research of Si Qu Tang: a review. *American Journal of Traditional Chinese Veterinary Medicine* 1 (1): 22–29.

Yi, X.Z. (1989). Bai Shao. *New Chinese Medicine* 21 (3): 51.

Yi, Y.-D. and Chang, I.-M. (2004). An overview of traditional Chinese herbal formulae and a proposal of a new code system for expressing the formula titles. *Evidence Based Complementary and Alternative Medicine* 1 (2): 125–132.

Zhi, S.H.Z.Y.Y.Z. (1983). Bai Shao. *Shanghai Journal of Chinese Medicine and Herbology* 4: 14.

Zhi, Z.Y. (1983). Bai Shao. *Chinese Herbology Journal* 183.

Zhi, Z.Y.Z. (1983). Bai Shao. *Journal of Chinese Medicine* 8: 79.

Zhi, H.N.Z.Y.Z. (1986). Bai Shao. *Journal of Integrated Chinese and Western Medicine* 10: 593.

Zhi, Z.X.Y.J.H.Z. (1986). Bai Shao. *Journal of Integrative Chinese and Western Medicine* 10: 593.

Zhi, Z.Y.Z. (1987). Bai Shao. *Journal of Chinese Medicine* 9: 66.

Zhong, X. and Zhao, Y. (2013). Anti-abortive effects of Bao Tai Wu You, Tai Shan Pan Shi and Bai Zhu San in a murine model. *American Journal of Traditional Chinese Veterinary Medicine* 8 (2): 31–39.

4

Nutraceuticals

Introduction

Veterinary nutraceuticals, or animal health supplements, are a great resource for veterinarians and pet owners. Nutraceuticals aid in the prevention and treatment of multiple conditions. The regulation of nutraceuticals is complex. It is critical veterinarians have an adequate framework for the appropriate selection and administration of nutraceuticals to ensure they are used safely and effectively. The introduction of nutraceuticals into veterinary practice can be beneficial for both the patient and the health of the practice. The successful incorporation and utilization of nutraceuticals does not end with the veterinarian's training. Ongoing training of the support staff and client education are also crucial. This chapter discusses the what, why, and how for effective integration of nutraceuticals within your practice.

The What

Word Origin

Nutraceutical is a portmanteau (linguistic blend of two words to create a new one) of the words "nutrition" and "pharmaceutical" invented by Dr. Stephen DeFelice in 1989 (Kalra 2003).

Definition

Currently there is no cohesive definition for the word "nutraceutical." The definition depends on the country, organization, or person defining it. The Food and Drug Administration (FDA) does not recognize the word in any legal documents. Some veterinarians prefer the term "animal health supplements," especially because the word "supplement" is a term recognized by the FDA. For the purposes of this chapter, the term "veterinary nutraceutical" (VN) will be used interchangeably with the

Integrative Medicine in Veterinary Practice, First Edition. Lisa P. McFaddin.
© 2024 John Wiley & Sons, Inc. Published 2024 by John Wiley & Sons, Inc.
Companion website: www.wiley.com/go/mcfaddin/integrativemedicine

term "animal health supplement" (AHS). VN and AHS will be defined as product(s) isolated or derived from a food source(s) used to support healthy biological processes within animals. VN and AHS are not drugs so they cannot treat, diagnose, prevent, or cure disease.

Human History

The use of dietary ingredients to supplement health originated in Greece and China. Hippocrates himself can be viewed as a proponent of dietary supplements having said "let food be thy medicine and medicine be thy food" (Wikipedia 2019). The popularity of health foods combined with increasing interest in medicinal plants throughout the twentieth century accelerated the development of nutraceuticals in the United States (Heinrich 2009).

The Dietary Supplement Health and Education Act (DSHEA) of 1994, an amendment to the United States Federal Food, Drug and Cosmetic Act (FDCA), was created to provide standards for dietary supplements (DSHEA 1994). Dietary supplements were defined as substances which complement the diet and contain at least one of the following ingredients: a vitamin, a mineral, an herb, an amino acid, or a product which affects caloric intake (DSHEA 1994). Within the provisions established by DSHEA dietary supplements were classified as a separate regulatory category from food. As a result dietary supplements are considered neither food nor drug.

Almost all dietary supplements are available over the counter (OTC). FDA approval is not required to market or sell these products. DSHEA further stipulates the FDA is only responsible for ensuring the safety of supplements if there is gross risk of illness, inadequate evidence regarding product safety, or a supplement is adulterated (DSHEA 1994).

The FDA does not regulate the development, manufacturing, or marketing of dietary supplements. In 2006 the FDA issued a guidance document, "Questions and Answers Regarding the Labeling of Dietary Supplements as Required by the Dietary Supplement and Nonprescription Drug Consumer Protection Act," that requires manufacturers include an address or phone number for the reporting of adverse reactions (FDA 2009).

The FDA does specify what health claims can be made by a supplement manufacturer. Health claims assert a relationship between a particular substance and its ability to diagnose, treat, cure, or prevent disease. The FDA may approve health claims that are adequately substantiated with scientific and clinical evidence (FDA 2018).

Many dietary supplements tout claims pertaining to a specific function within the body (e.g. probiotics improve gut health) or a general well-being claim associated with a nutrient deficiency (e.g. vitamin D prevents rickets). The FDA does not require pre-approval of these claims but does require notification from the manufacturer within 30 days of marketing the supplement (FDA 2009). The FDA also requires placement of a "disclaimer" on the product informing consumers the claim has not been evaluated by the FDA, and the dietary supplement is "not intended to diagnose, treat, cure, or prevent any disease" (FDA 2018).

The FDA requires manufacturers notify the FDA when a new dietary ingredient is included in a supplement. Companies must demonstrate the new ingredient is expected to be safe without risk of illness to individuals taking the supplement per label instructions (FDA 2018). Regulatory action can be taken by the FDA if the product is deemed unsafe after marketing.

The current regulations of human dietary supplements fall short of providing full guidance, oversight, and consumer confidence. Safety, purity, and efficacy of human nutraceuticals are often in question. This highlights the importance of prescribing and taking supplements from trusted sources with independent testing.

Veterinary History

Unlike the other integrative therapies discussed in this book, the history of supplement use in veterinary medicine is not well documented. A relatively recent study by Elrod and Hofmeister (2019) surveyed 126 veterinarians about their knowledge and use of nutraceuticals at continuing education (CE) sessions at the University of Georgia College of Veterinary Medicine from 2012 to 2015. This showed that 66% of the participating veterinarians "strongly agree[d] they knew what nutraceuticals were," 55% agreed "they knew how nutraceuticals work and could apply them to their patients," 51% "agreed that they regularly recommend[ed] nutraceuticals to patients," 60% "recommend[ed] nutraceuticals in combination with conventional drugs for their patients," and 79% rarely or sometimes "recommend[ed] nutraceuticals alone for their patients"; 73% of veterinarians recommended nutraceuticals before the onset of disease, and 52% used nutraceuticals when other therapies failed. Over half of the veterinarians (53%) reported their clients asked for information about nutraceuticals (Elrod and Hofmeister 2019). The most recommended nutraceuticals were omega-3 fatty acids (94%) and glucosamine/chondroitin (93%) products, with osteoarthritis as the most common condition for which nutraceutical therapy was recommended (Elrod and Hofmeister 2019).

The history of veterinary nutraceutical use is best described through the most important scientific, regulatory, and product developments. Before delving into the evolution of nutraceuticals, we need to first understand the relevant terminology and how these products differ from drugs.

Terminology

The world of nutraceuticals comes with its own vocabulary. A basic understanding of these terms is crucial, allowing effective communication amongst professionals and with clients. A summary of common terms is provided below.

Adulterated food: "Food packaged or held under unsanitary conditions, food or ingredients that are filthy or decomposed, and food that contains any poisonous or deleterious substance, or other contaminant" (FDA 2021a).

Amino acids: Organic nitrogen-containing compounds. Of the hundreds of identified amino acids, 20 are used to make up almost every protein found in plants and animals.

Antioxidants: Synthetic or natural substances which prevent or delay cell damage. Antioxidants are considered a type of free radical scavenger.

Dietary ingredient: "A vitamin, mineral, herb or other botanical, amino acid, dietary substance for use by man to supplement the diet by increasing the total dietary intake or a concentrate, metabolite, constituent, extract, or combinations of the preceding substances" (FDA 2021c).

Dietary supplement (aka food supplement): Substances which complement the diet and contain at least one of the following ingredients: a vitamin, a mineral, an herb, an amino acid, or a product which affects caloric intake (FDA 2021d).

Drug: A substance used to diagnose, cure, treat, or prevent disease in both humans and animals, as well as alter the body's functions or structure (FDA 2021c).

Food additive: Substances added to food with the direct or indirect result of becoming part of the food or altering the properties of the food itself (FDA 2021c).

Free radicals: Unstable molecules naturally created during cell metabolism or formed due to toxins, radiation, or pollutant. Free radicals accumulate within tissues and cause cell damage.

Free radical scavengers: Substances which stabilize or neutralize free radicals to prevent harmful chain reactions and resultant cell damage.

Functional foods: Foods that have additional health benefits beyond basic nutritional requirements. This is a contentious term, as most foods have a function or purpose.

Microbiome: A group of microorganisms, their genes, and surrounding environmental conditions in a defined area (Marchesi and Ravel 2015).

Microbiota: A group of microorganisms in a defined environment (Marchesi and Ravel 2015). Most often used to describe the bacteria within the gastrointestinal tract.

Mineral: An inorganic substance required in various quantities by the body for normal growth, nutrition, and development.

Veterinary nutraceutical (aka animal health supplement): A product isolated or derived from a food source used to support normal biological processes within animals. They are not drugs so they cannot treat, diagnose, prevent, or cure disease.

Vitamin: Organic compounds which cannot be synthesized by the body and are required in small doses for normal growth, nutrition, and development (Hand et al. 2010).

Regulation

Veterinary Drugs Defined

The modern definition of the word "drug" is based on the United States FDCA, section 201(g). Drugs are defined as substances used to diagnose, cure, treat, or prevent disease in both humans and animals, as well as alter the body's functions or structure (FDA 2021c). The word "medicine" pertains specifically to substances, including drugs, which are used to treat disease.

Initially veterinarians could only use and prescribe drugs approved for use in animals. The Animal Medical Drug Use Clarification Act (AMDUCA) of 1994 allowed veterinarians to use both human and animal drugs in an "extra-label" or "off-label" manner provided the following provisions were met.

1) A valid veterinary–client–patient relationship exists, and no animal-specific alternative exists; or
2) An animal-specific alternative exists, but the drug does not contain the necessary ingredients, appropriate dosage, or suitable concentration; or
3) The available animal-specific drug is ineffective (FDA 2020, 2021b).

AMDUCA does not allow the use of human alternative medications in food animals if an animal-approved alternative exists.

The process through which animal drugs receive FDA approval is expensive and arduous. First, the drug must be classified for use in animals. Second, the drug must be new. Third, the new drug must prove in clinical trials it is both effective and safe. While the FDA states "new drugs and certain biologics must be proven safe and effective to FDA's satisfaction before companies can market them in interstate commerce," the FDA does not "develop or test products before approving them" (FDA 2020, 2021b). Instead,

> "[the] manufacturers must…prove they are able to make the drug product according to federal quality standards. . . (and] FDA experts review the results of laboratory, animal, and human clinical testing done by manufacturers. If FDA grants an approval, it means the agency has determined that the benefits of the product outweigh the known risks for the intended use" (FDA 2020, 2021b).

DSHEA and Veterinary Medicine

When DSHEA was enacted, the language only discussed the use of dietary supplements in humans, not animals. Initially animal dietary supplements included ingredients like those found in equivalent human dietary supplements and were sold under the guidelines of DSHEA (Grassie 2002). In 1996 the FDA published the "Inapplicability of the dietary supplement health and education act to animal products" (Docket No. 95N-0308) stating DSHEA did not apply to animal products (Schultz 1996). The FDA's rationale was that DSHEA did not specifically reference animal products but did specifically reference human products. Additionally, many of the human supplement ingredients had not been studied in animals and may be unsafe for companion animal use (Schultz 1996). Finally, the administration of many human supplement ingredients to food animals may render them unsafe for human consumption (Schultz 1996).

This decision had two major repercussions for veterinary medicine. First, any animal dietary supplement produced and marketed under DSHEA was now considered a drug and must meet the requirements established by the FDA to obtain drug approval. Secondly, animal dietary supplements were now classified as animal food and regulated under the FDCA.

Under the FDCA any supplement claiming or intended to be used for the treatment or prevention of disease is considered a drug and must be approved by the FDA. Any unapproved "drug" is subject to regulatory action by the FDA.

Many supplement ingredients used in people are not approved for use in animal feed. This gets even more complicated because many human dietary supplements are marketed with specific label claims for affecting functions within the body. Many pet parents assume the same applications hold true for animals, again making these supplements more like drugs. According to the National Animal Supplement Council (NASC) there are over 400 unapproved substances marketed for use in animals (Grassie 2002).

Animal Food

The FDCA does not require pre-market FDA approval before new animal food is sold. The FDCA does require "that food for animals, like food for people, be safe to eat, produced under sanitary conditions, free of harmful substances, and truthfully labeled" (FDA 2021c).

In 2011 Congress amended the FDCA by passing the Food Safety Modernization Act (FASMA) which allowed the FDA

"to better protect public health by strengthening the food safety system and shifting the focus from *responding* to contamination of the food supply to *preventing* contamination. The law applies to food for people as well as food for animals, including pet food. FSMA requires animal food facilities to create and implement a food safety plan. In the first part of the plan, the facilities assess food safety hazards that are potentially associated with the animal food (this is called "hazard analysis"). In the second part, the facilities take steps, when necessary, to reduce or eliminate identified food safety hazards (these steps are called "preventive controls"). The above FSMA requirements apply to companies that must register as an animal food facility because they manufacture, process, pack, or hold animal food for consumption in the United States. Besides having to follow the requirements under FSMA, registered animal food facilities must also comply with current good manufacturing practices (unless an exemption applies). These practices provide baseline standards for manufacturing, processing, packing, and holding animal food to ensure it's safe for animals to eat" (FDA 2022a).

The Hazard Analysis Critical Control Point (HACCP) is a worldwide-recognized

"management system in which food safety is addressed through the analysis and control of biological, chemical, and physical hazards from raw material production, procurement and handling, to manufacturing, distribution and consumption of the finished product" (FDA 2022b).

In 2021 the FDA's Center for Veterinary Medicine (CVM) released a "Hazard Analysis and Risk-Based Preventative Controls for Food for Animals Guidance for Industry." The document outlines the requirements for developing a food safety plan (FSP) for facilities producing animal food (CVM 2022). An FSP was defined as a written plan outlining a systematic approach to identifying food safety hazards that can be controlled to prevent or minimize the likelihood of foodborne illness or injury (CVM 2022). An FSP and HACCP are similar, but as of 2021 the FDA has not mandated an HACCP system for animal food (CVM 2022). Development and utilization of an HACCP is a voluntary process for companies in the animal food industry.

Animal Food Additives

The FDCA does require pre-market approval for animal food additives. Food additives are defined as "any substance that directly or indirectly becomes a component of a food or that affects a food's characteristics" (FDA 2021a,c). Substances generally recognized as safe (GRAS) are exempt from the pre-market approval requirements (FDA 2021a,c).

For a substance to be categorized as GRAS the FDA states "qualified experts must agree that the substance is safe when added to food" (FDA 2021c). This is accomplished by either a history of common safe use in food or scientific studies. A company itself can determine if a substance is GRAS by submitting the following to the FDA: description of the substance, how the substance will be used and in what species, and how the company determined the product was GRAS (FDA 2021a,c). After reviewing the company's information, the FDA determines if the GRAS standard has been met.

A substance may be considered GRAS in one setting but not in another. Additionally, food additives cannot be labeled GRAS if used for a medicinal purpose. In that case the substance is considered a drug and must meet the requirements for a new animal drug (FDA 2021c).

The CVM is responsible for regulating animal food products, including many nutraceuticals. Failure of a food to meet the requirements outlined in the FDCA may result in the food (or in this case VN) being classified as adulterated or misbranded. The reality is a lot of nutraceuticals used in veterinary medicine are considered unapproved food additives or unapproved animal drugs, and the FDA could take regulatory action (Burns 2017). To date, the regulation of animal supplements has been low on the FDA regulators' priority list.

To summarize, a VN marketed as a food, containing ingredients with known and approved nutritional value, does not need CVM pre-market approval. A VN marketed as a food with unknown or unapproved ingredients requires CVM pre-market approval.

A VN marketed as a drug (generally ones with health or medical claims on the label) technically requires pre-market approval as a drug. A VN marketed as a drug without CVM approval is required to meet FDA drug approval requirements. If those requirements cannot be met the CVM may allow continued sales as "unapproved drugs of low regulatory priority" (Knueven 2018). This exemption is generally granted when the CVM believes the product is safe for its intended use and the company is acting responsibly with respect to manufacturing and marketing. The CVM may require the company register with the FDA as a drug manufacturer and follow specific labeling requirements for the VN (Knueven 2018).

Keep in mind the FDA does not approve manufacturing companies.

"Owners and operators of domestic and foreign food, drug, and most device facilities must register their facilities with FDA, unless an exemption applies. FDA does have authority to inspect regulated facilities to verify that they comply with applicable good manufacturing practice regulations" (FDA 2017b).

Complementary and Alternative Medicine Products

The FDA may consider some human dietary supplements, specifically herbal products, complementary and alternative medicine (CAM) products. The 2006 FDA Draft Guidance for CAM products was created

"in response to an increasing number of CAM products and public confusion regarding the regulation of said products. This guidance makes two fundamental points: first, depending on the CAM therapy or practice, a product used in a CAM therapy or practice may be subject to regulation as a biological product, cosmetic, drug, device, or food (including food additives and dietary supplements) under the [Federal Food, Drug, and Cosmetic Act, the 'Act'] or the [Public Health Service (PHS)] Act. For example, the PHS Act defines "biological product," and the Act defines (among other things): Cosmetic; Device; Dietary supplement; Drug, as well as "new drug" and "new animal drug;" Food; and Food additive. These statutory definitions cover some CAM products. Second, neither the Act nor the PHS Act exempts CAM products from regulation. This means, for example, if a person decides to produce and sell raw vegetable juice for use in juice therapy to promote optimal health, that product is a food subject to the requirements for foods in the Act and FDA regulations, including the hazard analysis and critical control point (HACCP) system requirements for juices in 21 CFR part 120. If the juice therapy is intended for use as part of a disease treatment regimen instead of for the general wellness, the vegetable juice would also be subject to regulation as a drug under the Act" (FDA 2007).

State Regulation

State agriculture departments are often responsible for regulating animal feed. State feed control officials generally do not regulate VN unless they are labeled as animal feed or food additives (Burns 2017).

Most states follow standards outlined by the Association of American Feed Control Officers (AAFCO). The AAFCO has been in existence since 1906. AAFCO members are individuals from various governmental agencies throughout North America responsible for the regulation of animal feed. The FDA is a member of AAFCO. AAFCO exists as an animal-feed think tank in which members discuss potential rules and regulations pertaining to animal food. The ideas and models created by the AAFCO members are shared with the member's respective governmental agencies which then create laws. The individuals comprising AAFCO can regulate animal feed requirements within their jurisdictions, but AAFCO is not a regulatory body (AAFCO 2014).

Most states have adopted the AAFCO model for pet food regulations within their own laws, making the AAFCO model the default standard. The AAFCO model discusses recommendations for pet food labeling, i.e. what is written on the packaging. The model also covers the minimum recommended nutritional requirements and nutrient profiles for cats and dogs based on life stage. The following statement is found on most cat and dog foods: "[Pet Food Product Name] is formulated to meet the nutritional levels established by the AAFCO Dog (or Cat) Food Nutrient Profiles for [pet life stage]" (AAFCO 2014). For additional information about AAFCO and its pet food recommendations, visit https://www.aafco.org.

Production

The regulation of VN is confusing and does not inspire confidence among practitioners or consumers. A product is classified as an approved food, unapproved and unauthorized food, an unapproved but authorized drug, or an unapproved and unauthorized drug. Unfortunately, there are numerous misleading, and sometimes unsafe, human and animal products on the market. This makes safety and efficacy the primary concerns when considering VN.

It is ultimately up to the veterinarian to ensure the products they recommend are safe and effective. It is also the responsibility of the entire team to communicate to the client the rationale and precautions for each recommended VN.

There are several factors to consider, and questions to ask, when selecting a manufacturer: First, can the source materials be traced? Secondly, does the company follow good manufacturing practices (GMP)? Thirdly, what quality control measures are utilized? Fourthly, how accurate is the product labeling? Finally, does the company have a "seal of approval"?

Tracing Source Materials

The manufacturing company should be able to trace the exact source where each ingredient is grown/cultivated/isolated and/or manufactured, processed, and bottled. In the case of plant and animal-based products, growing and habitat conditions are critical. Processing contamination or inappropriate storage may limit therapeutic benefits or contribute to adverse effects. Accountability for each step within the manufacturing process ensures purity, potency, and patient protection.

Good Manufacturing Practice

The World Health Organization (WHO 2015) defines GMP as "a system for ensuring that products are consistently produced and controlled according to quality standards." Often evaluation of the final product is not enough to prevent human health hazards from potentially contaminated and/or adulterated medications. GMP monitors all areas of production, including the starting ingredients, buildings, equipment, training of personnel, and personnel hygiene. GMP identifies key areas of risk during the manufacturing process that could result in the production of potentially toxic and/or ineffective products. Areas of potential risk include contamination of the original products/ingredients; mislabeling of containers; and inaccurate measurement of the active ingredient(s) (WHO 2015).

The FDA requires all registered companies follow current good manufacturing practice (CGMP) regulations as outlined in CFR Title 21.

> "The CGMP regulations for drugs contain minimum requirements for the methods, facilities, and controls used in manufacturing, processing, and packing of a drug product. The regulations make sure that a product is safe for use, and that it has the ingredients and strength it claims to have" (FDA 2021c,d).

Finding a company which meets and/or exceeds the manufacturing controls established by CGMP ensures product purity and safety.

GMP for Veterinarians

Written protocols are integral to the production of safe and effective products. The WHO has its own international GMP guidelines (WHO 2015). Many countries have created their own requirements modeled after the WHO guidelines.

In the United States, Title 21 of the Code of Federal Regulations covers the CGMP guidelines for finished pharmaceuticals (FDA 2021c,d). The CGMP ensures minimum requirements are met during the manufacturing, processing, and packaging of drugs. CGMP also requires the correct labeling of products including ingredients, strength, and certification of the product's safety. The FDA will not approve a new or generic drug without proof of compliance with the CGMP. The CGMP guidelines include the following (FDA 2021c,d).

- The buildings and facilities are the appropriate size, clean, have good lighting and ventilation, and have sanitation equipment for the facility and employees.
- The equipment is appropriate, clean, well maintained, and operated by well-trained personnel.

- Personnel are well trained in equipment operations, safety, sanitation, and proper handling of medicinal ingredients and end products.
- The raw materials (active and inactive ingredients) are not contaminated or adulterated.
- The raw materials are labeled correctly.
- The correct volume/weight of raw materials is used.
- Only approved materials are being used.
- In-process and end-product samples are correctly identified and meet specifications for physical and chemical properties.
- The water supply to the facility meets minimum requirements for safe use and consumption.
- Written protocols regarding manufacturing and control have been established by the facility.
- Packages of finished products are clearly labeled.
- All samples of raw, in-process, and end-product materials are saved and stored appropriately for a specified amount of time.
- The facility keeps adequate records of raw material purchasing and quality control information; specifications for the type of raw materials used; specifications for mixing of ingredients; quality control measures; labeling requirements; equipment maintenance; personnel safety and hygiene; and complaints and accidents.

Quality Control

Quality control should be performed on all ingredients throughout the manufacturing, processing, bottling, and storage stages. At the processing facility the materials should undergo visual, chemical, heavy metal, pesticide, and microbial testing.

Quality Control for Veterinarians

Herbs or botanicals should ideally be grown in organic soil in their indigenous regions, as this yields the best medicinal results. Companies responsible for the raw materials (i.e. growing

and harvesting) should follow good agricultural practice (GAP) and good handling practices (GHP). Both GAP and GHP

> "are voluntary audits [performed by the U.S. Department of Agriculture] that verify that fruits and vegetables are produced, packed, handled, and stored as safely as possible to minimize risks of microbial food safety hazards. GAP & GHP audits verify adherence to the recommendations made in the U.S. Food and Drug Administration's Guide to Minimize Microbial Food Safety Hazards for Fresh Fruits and Vegetables and industry recognized food safety practices" (USDA 2020).

Many of these tests should be performed repeatedly throughout the manufacturing, bottling, and storage phases. Companies should keep extensive records on the control measures. This includes monitoring the facilities, storage, product identification methods, and safety testing. Facility sanitation and cleanliness should involve routine testing for microbial and yeast contaminants within the processing plant itself (USDA 2020), Product storage includes defining and maintaining temperature and humidity standards for raw and processed materials (USDA 2020). Unique product identification for raw materials (source tracing) is essential. Finally, safety testing should be performed on materials throughout the production, bottling and storage stages using safety limits that meet or exceed those outlined by the United States Pharmacopeia (USP, https://www.usp.org). Herbs should be tested for the presence of pesticides, heavy metals, or unsafe microbials, yeast and mold counts (USDA 2020).

Labeling

Product labeling rules and regulations are just as confusing as those surrounding VN manufacturing. For the most part there are no federal standards regarding VN labeling. The product labels should include a list of all ingredients and the intended use of the product. Avoid using supplements which make medical claims on the label, i.e. "for use in the prevention or treatment of [insert disease or condition name]."

Seal of Approval

Once should preferentially select companies whose products have been certified by trusted outside organizations such as ConsumerLab, National Animal Supplement Council (NASC) or the USP. This helps ensure products are safe and contain the materials as advertised. A brief description of each company, and their role in VN, are provided below. Table 4.1 summarizes the name, contact information, and purpose of each company.

ConsumerLab

ConsumerLab (CL) was established in 1999 as a trusted source for product review and ratings for vitamins and supplements. Individual products are purchased, tested, and reviewed by CL. During the review process CL determines the accuracy of the vitamin or supplement's label claim, product purity, dosage recommendations, safety, and side-effect data (CL 2022). The company then ranks the product alongside similar products. CL typically chooses what products to test, but manufacturers and distributors can pay to participate in their quality certification program (QCP). Products are evaluated in a similar fashion at the company's expense. The results are proprietary to the manufacturer. Products which "pass" are awarded the CL seal. The seal is a registered certification mark authorized by CL indicating the product's ingredients have been tested for quality, its use has been laboratory tested by experts, and more information about the product can be found on CL's website. To learn more about CL visit their website: www.consumerlab.com.

National Animal Supplement Council

The NASC, established in 2001, is a nonprofit organization dedicated to promoting and improving companion animal and horse health in the United States through the standardization and regulation of animal health supplements.

> "[The] NASC and its member companies work cooperatively with state, federal and international government officials to

Table 4.1 Organizations monitoring and providing seals of approval for veterinary nutraceuticals (VN) as of 2023.

Name	Contact information	Public information
ConsumerLab (CL)	www.consumerlab.com	Paid subscription allowing access to all products reviewed by CL. Available information includes CL's testing results, rankings, and links to relevant research about the products
National Animal Supplement Council (NASC)	PO Box 5168, Sun City West, AZ 83576 (760) 751-3360 https://www.nasc.cc	Provides a free list of member companies (suppliers, manufacturers, and distributors) of VN who have undergone quality audits by outside facilities
United States Pharmacopeia (USP)	www.usp.org	Provides a free list of verified supplements, brands, and retailers. Paid access to the online Dietary Supplement Compendium (provides >970 monographs, regulatory guidelines, and additional reference material)

Source: Lisa P. McFaddin.

create a legislative and regulatory environment that provides a framework that is **fair**, **reasonable**, **responsible**, and nationally **consistent.** Such an environment of safety, accuracy and quality serves the interests of NASC's members by ensuring that ethical manufacturing and labeling practices are complied with throughout the industry" (NASC 2022).

Veterinarians, retailers, distributors, manufacturers, and raw material suppliers can become members of the NASC. The NASC has voluntary paid programs in place to help ensure the highest quality standards are met for suppliers and manufacturers of animal health supplements: "The NASC Quality Seal identifies products from companies that are committed to quality, vigilance, and continuous improvement to promote the well-being of companion animals and horses" (NASC 2022). A supplement with the NASC Quality Seal indicates the company adheres to NASC guidelines, has passed an audit by an independent facility, adheres to NASC's stringent labeling requirements, has documented quality control and production procedures, has had the ingredients of the supplement reviewed by the NASC Scientific Advisory Committee, is subject to random product testing, and participates in NASC's Adverse Event Reporting System (NAERS) which monitors issues in real time (NASC 2022). To learn more about NASC visit their website: www.nasc.cc.

United States Pharmacopeia

Founded in 1820, the USP is an independent global nonprofit nongovernmental organization which aims to improve global health through establishing quality, purity, potency, and identity standards for medicine, food, ingredients, and dietary supplements. The USP is a volunteer organization whose Council of Experts and Expert Committee comprise people from academia, healthcare, governmental agencies, veterinary medicine, pharmaceutical industry, complementary and alternative medicine, dietary supplement industry, and retail pharmacies (USP 2022).

The USP publishes an annual pharmacopeia (compendium of drug information) with the National Formulary (USP-NF) for the United States.

"An article [drug, supplement, or herb] of commerce that is recognized in the USP–NF complies with USP–NF standards when it meets all of the requirements stated in the article's monograph, applicable General chapters, and the General Notices (with monograph requirements superseding those of the General chapters and General Notices, in any cases where requirements differ). Applicable standards apply at all times in the life of an article, from production to expiration. Thus, any official article is expected to meet the compendial standards if tested, and any official article actually tested as directed in the relevant monograph must meet such standards to demonstrate compliance. Frequency of testing and sampling are left to the preferences or direction of those performing compliance testing, and other users of USP–NF, including manufacturers, buyers, or regulatory authorities" (USP 2009).

The USP-NF has a role in US Federal Law. According to the FDCA any drug (human or animal) with a name recognized in the USP-NF must comply with current compendial standards (including identification, strength, quality, purity, and labeling) at all times (FDA 2021c). Drugs that do not comply are considered misbranded, adulterated, or both by the FDA, and regulatory action can be taken.

Human and animal dietary supplements are not required by Federal Law to meet USP-NF standards. To improve supplement safety and efficacy, the USP created a voluntary standardization and verification program. As part of this program, the USP publishes the *Dietary*

Supplements Compendium which contains monographs and quality standards for the production of dietary supplements. Manufacturers of both raw materials and final products can use these standards to ensure product safety, efficacy, and purity. Products which have met the USP standards and passed verification standards are awarded the USP Verified Mark (USP 2022). Products with the USP Verified Mark on the label are known to contain the actual ingredients listed on the label (including potency and quantity), are free of harmful contaminants, will be absorbed within the body as expected, and are made by companies following GMP according to the FDA and USP guidelines. To learn more about USP visit their website: www.usp.org.

Safety

Safety concerns surrounding VN should focus on two concepts: adverse effects (AEs) and VN–drug interactions.

Adverse Effects

AEs, also known as side effects, are defined as any unwanted and harmful outcomes caused by a drug or supplement. AEs are possible with any drug, supplement, herb, and even food used for veterinary patients. AEs associated with VN are often uncommon and mild. The severity of the AE is highly dependent on the supplement used. There is a scale of severity associated with AEs from mild to severe. Severe AEs are considered a form of toxicity. AEs can occur secondary to the active ingredient, inactive ingredient, or contaminant within the VN (Boothe 2020).

AEs are very uncommon when following the 4Rs rule: right VN, right patient, right patient purpose, and right dose. The *right VN* refers to using trusted manufacturers of VN (see the preceding section for further information). The *right patient* means the practitioner should ensure the use of VN is appropriate for the patient (consider age, existing medical conditions, and concurrent medications,

supplements, or herbs). The *right purpose* refers to the reason for using the VN, i.e. whether this supplement will help or hinder this patient. For example, a senior dog with arthritis and chronic diarrhea may not respond favorably to the addition of fish oil which may exacerbate the diarrhea. The *right dose* is just that: does the recommended amount of VN match the patient's needs? Sometimes a lower or even higher dosage is required. Additionally, the recommended treatment length should be considered.

An in-depth review of potential AEs associated with all VNs is beyond the scope of this book. Here were examine the AEs associated with two categories of VN: omega-3 fatty acids and cannabinoid oil. In general, AEs associated with VN are mild but ultimately dependent on the supplement in question. Omega-3 fatty acid side effects are uncommon, but if they do occur are typically mild, and dose dependent. Documented AEs associated with omega-3 fatty acids include gastrointestinal signs (decreased appetite, diarrhea, or vomiting), altered platelet function, altered immune function, and reduction of blood sugar (Lenox and Bauer 2013). Interestingly, the last two AEs may benefit the patient but are considered an AE as they are not the intended effect of the VN. Table 4.2 summarizes several documented AEs associated with omega-3 fatty acids in animals.

Cannabinoid (CBD) oil is generally very safe but has relatively common, though mild and often self-resolving, AEs. The most common AEs include sedation, slower heart rate, and increased hunger (Kogan et al. 2019). Table 4.3 summarizes several documented AEs associated with CBD oil in animals.

The sheer spectrum of VN makes it difficult to make generalization about VN, especially when many of the ingredients and products have not been adequately teste for safety and efficacy. The best recommendation is to research each supplement before recommending and administering it to patients. Good resources for investigating supplement safety can be found in Table 4.1.

Table 4.2 Studies documenting the category and details of adverse effects associated with omega-3 fatty acid administration in veterinary patients.

Category	Details	Study
Altered platelet function	Decreased platelet aggregation	Saker et al. (1998)
Gastrointestinal effects	Vomiting, diarrhea, pancreatitis	Fritsch et al. (2010a)
Altered immune function	Delayed hypersensitivity reaction	Hall et al. (2003), Wander et al. (1997)
	Affected lymphocyte function	Hall et al. (1999), LeBlanc et al. (2007)
Glycemic effects	Improved glucose control	Wilkins et al. (2004)

Source: Lisa P. McFaddin.

When following the 4Rs the chance of toxicity is extremely rare. Toxicity is typically a result of inadvertent overconsumption of veterinary or human supplements. For example, a five-year-old female spayed Bernese Mountain dog was euthanized when she suffered multiorgan damage (including coagulopathy, pancreatitis, peritonitis, pneumonia, liver damage, vasculitis, and acute kidney injury) following the ingestion of 200 veterinary joint supplements (Nobels and Khan 2015).

Just because there are no documented AEs or toxicities does not mean either is not possible. Many people, clients, and veterinarians do not take the time to report AEs. Additionally, the reporting process can be confusing, especially if the contact information is not provided on the packaging and the company does not have a system in place for receiving AE reports.

Chinese herbal medicine (CHM) and Western herbal medicine are often inappropriately lumped into the VN category (refer to Chapters 3 and 11, respectively, for specific information about safety, including AEs, toxicity, and herb–drug interactions).

Veterinary Nutraceutical–Drug Interaction

A *veterinary nutraceutical–drug interaction* (VNDI) occurs any time a VN interacts with a drug. There are positive and negative VNDIs. Probiotics and antibiotics are an example of a positive VNDI. Probiotics are commonly recommended for people and veterinary patients when taking antibiotics to prevent or minimize the risk of antibiotic-associated diarrhea. Numerous human studies, in adults and children, have proven the concurrent administration of probiotics with antibiotics

Table 4.3 Studies documenting the category and details of adverse effects associated with cannabinoid (CBD) oil administration in veterinary patients.

Behavioral	Sedation	Kogan et al. (2019), Vaughn et al. (2020)
	Licking and head shaking (after administration)	Deabold et al. (2019)
Cardiovascular	Hypotension	Kogan et al. (2019)
	Slow heart rate	Vaughn et al. (2020)
Gastrointestinal	Increased hunger	Kogan et al. (2019), Vaughn et al. (2020)
	Diarrhea	Kogan et al. (2019), Vaughn et al. (2020)
Hematologic changes	Elevated alkaline phosphatase	Gamble et al. (2018)

Source: Lisa P. McFaddin.

(generally not at the same time, though the timing of administration is an area of great debate in human and veterinary medicine) reduces the risk (and often prevents) antibiotic-associated diarrhea (Pattani et al. 2013; Guo et al. 2019b). This is a great example of how a VN can be used to combat an AE caused by a traditional pharmaceutical: antibiotics killing off good gut bacteria leading to diarrhea, and probiotics repopulating the gut with healthy bacteria preventing or reducing diarrhea.

There are also potentially negative VNDIs. The concurrent administration of St. John's Wort and tricyclic antidepressants (such as amitriptyline) can reduce the effectiveness of the antidepressants (Johne et al. 2002).

VNDI for Veterinarians

How the VN and drugs move through the body (pharmacokinetics) and function within the body (pharmacodynamics) explain how and why herb–drug interactions may occur. Pharmacokinetics is the term used to describe how the nutraceutical–drug interaction affects each substance's absorption,

distribution, metabolism, and elimination throughout the body (Chen 2013), while pharmacodynamics explains how the synergistic or antagonistic nutraceutical–drug interaction affects each substance's mechanism of action (Chen 2013).

An herb can increase or decrease drug effectiveness through pharmacokinetics and/or pharmacodynamics. VNDI pharmacokinetics involves affecting drug or VN mechanism of absorption, distribution, metabolism, and excretion (ADME). ADMEs are typically divided into four gene superfamilies (comprising >1000 proteins): cytochrome P450 (*CYP*), uridine diphosphate-glucuronosyltransferase (*UGT*), adenosine triphosphate-binding cassette (*ABC*), and organic anion-transporting polypeptide (*OATP*), as depicted in Figure 4.1 (Zanger and Schwab 2013; Asher et al. 2017). CYP drug metabolism enzymes and UGT-conjugating enzymes increase the drug's water solubility, increasing drug excretion (Asher et al. 2017). ABC drug uptake and efflux transporters and OATP drug transporters move drugs and their metabolites throughout the body (Asher et al. 2017). For example, St.

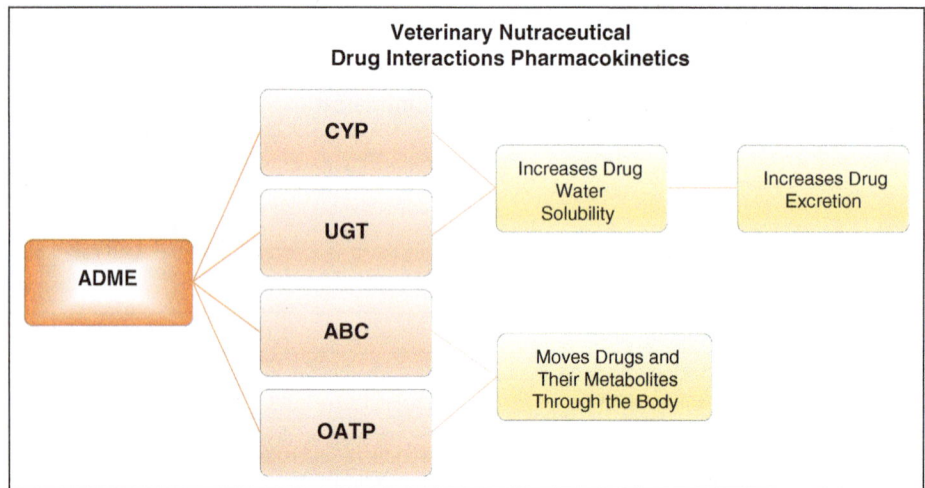

Figure 4.1 Schematic representation of the four main proteins affecting veterinary nutraceutical absorption, distribution, metabolism, and excretion (ADME) (Zanger and Schwab 2013; Asher et al. 2017). These protein superfamilies are responsible for most of the documented veterinary nutraceutical–drug interactions. CYP, cytochrome P450; UGT, uridine diphosphate-glucuronosyltransferase; ABC, adenosine triphosphate-binding cassette; OATP, organic anion transporting polypeptide. Source: Lisa P. McFaddin.

John's Wort can significantly reduce the bioavailability of digoxin by altering P-glycoprotein activity (an ABC transporter) resulting in increased drug elimination (Gurley et al. 2008).

Less commonly, VNDIs affect the pharmacodynamics. This is more likely to occur if the VN has a direct effect on the drug's mechanism of action (Asher et al. 2017). One example would be the potentially enhanced sedative effects when combining valerian root and alprazolam, both of which function as central nervous system (CNS) suppressants (Boothe 2020). It should be noted a literature search performed by Kelber et al. (2014) of available human and animal pharmacodynamic studies of valerian root could not verify potential interactions with any drug Another example is the multiple potential nutraceutical–drug interactions associated with St. John's Wort, outlined in Table 4.4.

The lack of AE event reporting and confusion regarding VN names limits the amount of available VNDI information. The shortage of VNDI studies mirrors the lack of AE and toxicity studies. More research, especially randomized (ideally double-blinded) clinical trials, is needed to ensure the efficacy and safety of VN. Problematically, many of the VNDI studies are performed *in vitro*, in laboratory species, extrapolated from human medicine, or the studies are not validated.

The absence of a standardized and federally mandated method for reporting VN AEs prohibits easy collection of AE and VNDI data. The numerous names used to market VNs confounds the practitioner's ability to research, track, and predict VNDIs (Boothe 2020). Additionally, most VNs contain more than one active ingredient, making it difficult to determine which ingredient is primarily responsible for a potential VNDI.

There are several online resources available to veterinarians to research VNDIs, as described in Table 4.5. Links to the websites are available on the companion website. Additionally, two comprehensive books, *Nutraceuticals in Veterinary Medicine* and *Safety of Dietary Supplements for Horses, Dogs, and Cats*, covering almost everything you would want to know about VNs, including VNDIs, was published in 2019.

Veterinary Nutraceutical Efficacy

Efficacy refers the ability of the VN to produce the desired effect. Efficacy is based on understanding the chemistry, how the substance is metabolized, distributed, and eliminated within the body (pharmacokinetics), and

Table 4.4 Examples of researched drug interactions associated with St. John's Wort (*Hypericum perforatum*).

Drug	Interaction	References
Benzodiazepine	Decreased half-life	George et al. (2003), Markowitz et al. (2003)
Cyclosporin, tacrolimus	Decreased efficacy Increased clearance	Roby et al. (2000); Henderson et al. (2002) Mai et al. (2004)
Oral contraceptives	Decreased efficacy	Henderson et al. (2002)
Digoxin	Increases excretion	Dürr et al. (2000), Mueller et al. (2004b), Gurley et al. (2008)
Procainamide	Increased bioavailability No effect on metabolism	Dasgupta et al. (2007)
Theophylline	Increased clearance	Nebel et al. (1999)
Tricyclic antidepressants	Decreased efficacy	Johne et al. (2002)
Warfarin	Prolonged effects	Roby et al. (2000), Henderson et al. (2002)

Source: Lisa P. McFaddin.

Table 4.5 Online resources with reliable information about veterinary nutraceuticals as of 2023.

ConsumerLab (CL)	Description	Paid subscription allowing access to all products reviewed by CL. Available information includes CL's testing results, rankings, and links to relevant research about the products
	Website	www.consumerlab.com
Food and Drug Administration (FDA)	Description	General information about human dietary supplements
	Website	https://www.fda.gov/food/dietary-supplements
	Description	Links to information about the FDA's regulation of pet food
	Website	https://www.fda.gov/animal-veterinary/animal-health-literacy/fdas-regulation-pet-food
Medscape: Drug-Interactions Checker	Description	Free resource to check for interactions between drugs, over-the-counter drugs, and herbal supplements
	Website	https://reference.medscape.com/drug-interactionchecker
National Animal Supplement Council (NASC)	Description	Provides a free list of member companies (suppliers, manufacturers, and distributors) of VN who have undergone quality audits by outside facilities
	Website	https://www.nasc.cc
National Center for Complementary and Integrative Health (NCCIH)	Description	General information about human dietary supplements
	Website	https://www.nccih.nih.gov/health/dietary-and-herbal-supplements
Nutraceuticals Word: Pet Nutraceuticals	Description	Free online magazine covering nutraceuticals used in companion animals
	Website	https://www.nutraceuticalsworld.com/knowledge-center/market-segments/pet-nutraceuticals
United States Pharmacopeia (USP)	Description	Free list of verified supplements, brands, and retailers. Access to the online Dietary Supplement Compendium (contains >970 monographs, regulatory guidelines, and additional reference material) is not free
	Website	www.usp.org

Source: adapted from (Boothe 2020).

mechanism of action (pharmacodynamics). All these factors determine the dose (how much) and frequency (how often) of administration.

This information may be very limited for any given VN, and the available information may be based on *in vitro* (in a test tube) testing or empirical (based primarily on clinical experience) data. Many supplements have multiple ingredients making evidence-based dosing difficult. It is the veterinarian's responsibility to ensure they research the VN to determine the best dosage and frequency for their patients.

It is important practitioners prescribing VN familiarize themselves with the products they are recommending, paying close attention to the pharmacokinetics and pharmacodynamics. VN can really help patients but, like any drug, the products must be used responsibly.

Classifications

A universal VN classification system does not exist, and it seems as if almost every practitioner has their own method. For the purposes of this chapter, I will divide VN into the following categories: vitamins, minerals, microbiome therapy, joint supplements, amino acids, antioxidants and free radical scavengers, and botanicals. These are each reviewed in detail in the following sections.

Vitamins

Vitamins are a group of organic compounds which cannot be synthesized by the body and are required in small doses for normal growth, nutrition, and development (Hand et al. 2010). Vitamins are classified as either water-soluble (vitamins B and C) or fat-soluble (vitamins A, D, E, and K). A quick reference summarizing the primary uses for each vitamin is provided in Table 4.6.

Vitamins can be administered individually (e.g. vitamin E capsules), in a combination formula (e.g. B complex), or as a multivitamin. Vitamins are either made from synthetic vitamins or wholefood products. The vitamins within both formulations are chemically (structurally) the same, but the ease with which the nutrients are absorbed and incorporated into the body often differs. Synthetic supplements require additives to stabilize and improve absorption of the vitamins (Yetley 2007). Personally, I prefer using wholefood vitamins whenever possible.

Vitamin A

Vitamin A (aka retinol) is a fat-soluble vitamin involved in the development and function of the retina, skin, bone, and immune system

(Pubchem 2004). Vitamin A has also been shown to inhibit carcinogenesis (cancer formation) (Pubchem 2004). Supplementation in veterinary medicine is primarily used to treat hypovitaminosis A and certain dermatologic conditions (VDH 2017d). AEs associated with oversupplementation include keratoconjunctivitis sicca (dry eye), elevated liver enzymes, and elevated blood lipids (VDH 2017d). There are no documented drug interactions (VDH 2017d). The molecular structure of vitamin A is depicted in Figure 4.2.

Vitamin B

The most common B vitamins used in veterinary medicine are vitamin B complex, vitamin B3 (niacin, and its metabolite niacinamide), vitamin B6 (pyridoxine), and vitamin B12 (cyanocobalamin). As the most used, vitamin B12 is described in more detail. Cyanocobalamin is a water-soluble vitamin with multiple important primary functions including hematopoiesis (production of blood cells and platelets), neural metabolism, cell growth and reproduction, food

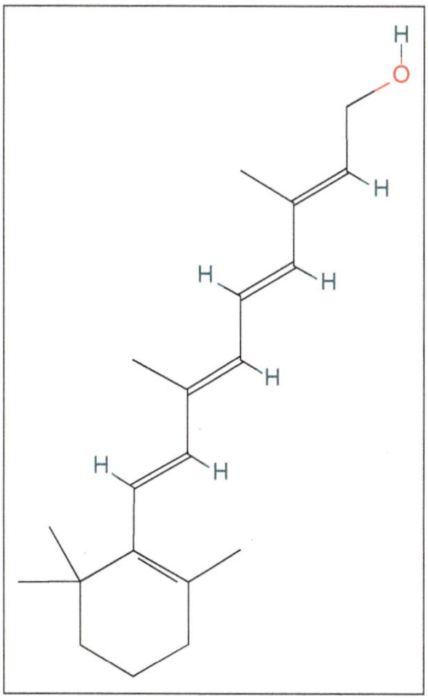

Table 4.6 The primary therapeutic uses of vitamins in veterinary medicine.

Vitamin A	Vitamin A deficiency; dermatologic conditions
Vitamin B	Dependent on the type. *Example*: vitamin B12 is used to treat cobalamin deficiency
Vitamin C	Vitamin C deficiency; inflammatory disorders
Vitamin D	Low calcium
Vitamin E	Dermatologic conditions; hepatobiliary (liver and gallbladder) disorders
Vitamin K	Vitamin K deficiency; coumarin toxicity; anticoagulant rodenticide toxicity

Source: Lisa P. McFaddin.

Figure 4.2 Molecular structure of vitamin A (retinol), $C_{20}H_{30}O$. Source: PubChem, https://pubchem.ncbi.nlm.nih.gov/compound/445354#section=3D-Conformer, September 16, 2004.

metabolism, and choline synthesis with folic acid (PubChem 2005c). The primary veterinary indication is cobalamin deficiency. There are no known AEs associated with oversupplementation. Vitamin B12 is known to interact with the concurrent administration of colchicine, chloramphenicol, and some chemotherapeutic agents (VDH 2017e). The molecular structure of vitamin B12 is depicted in Figure 4.3.

Vitamin C

Vitamin C (aka ascorbic acid) is a water-soluble vitamin which functions as a potent antioxidant (PubChem 2011). Vitamin C is also known to aid in fighting bacterial infections, functions as a cofactor for collagen synthesis and tissue repair, and is involved in carbohydrate and iron metabolism and synthesis of lipids and proteins (PubChem 2011). Supplementation is primarily used to treat vitamin C deficiencies and

certain inflammatory disorders (VDH 2017f). Oversupplementation can lead to the formation of calcium oxalate uroliths (bladder stones) (VDH 2017f). Potential drug interactions include reduced copper absorption in the gut and interaction with anticoagulants (VDH 2017f). The molecular structure of vitamin C is depicted in Figure 4.4.

Vitamin D

Vitamin D (aka cholecalciferol) is a fat-soluble steroid hormone which maintains blood calcium and phosphorus levels as well as regulating bone calcification (PubChem 2005b). Vitamin D is most used in the treatment of hypocalcemia (VDH 2019). Oversupplementation can lead to development of hypervitaminosis D (VDH 2019). Potential drug interactions include thiazide diuretics, cholestyramine, corticosteroids, and calcitriol (VDH 2019). The molecular structure of vitamin D is depicted in Figure 4.5.

Vitamin E

Vitamin E (α-tocopherol) is a fat-soluble vitamin with a multitude of primary functions. Vitamin E is a potent antioxidant and membrane

Figure 4.3 Molecular structure of vitamin B12 (cyanocobalamin), $C_{63}H_{88}CoN_{14}O_{14}P$. Source: PubChem, https://pubchem.ncbi.nlm.nih.gov/compound/5311498#section=2D-Structure, September 16, 2004.

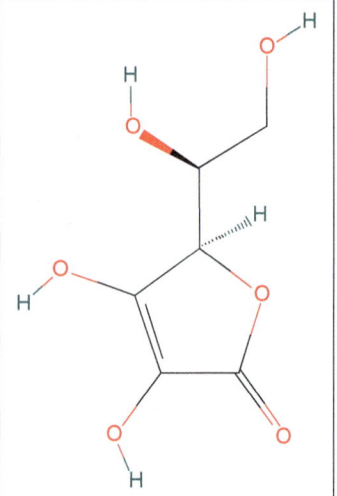

Figure 4.4 Molecular structure of vitamin C (ascorbic acid), $C_{63}H_{88}CoN_{14}O_{14}P$. Source: PubChem, https://pubchem.ncbi.nlm.nih.gov/compound/54670067#section=2D-Structure, December 16, 2005.

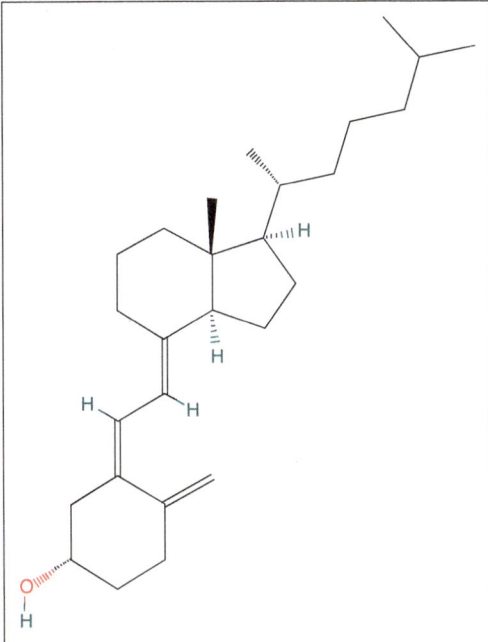

Figure 4.5 Molecular structure of vitamin D (cholecalciferol), $C_{27}H_{44}O$. Source: PubChem, https://pubchem.ncbi.nlm.nih.gov/ compound/5280795, September 16, 2004.

stabilizer, inhibits cyclooxygenase (COX) activity, decreases prostaglandin production, and inhibits tumor growth by interfering with angiogenesis and suppressing vascular endothelial growth factor (VEGF) gene transcription (PubChem 2005d). Vitamin E is commonly used to treat dermatologic and hepatobiliary (liver and gallbladder) disorders (Center 2004; Kapun et al. 2014). In rare instances vitamin E

administration has been associated with anaphylactoid reactions (VDH 2019). Vitamin E may interact with anticoagulants and vitamin A (VDH 2019). The molecular structure of vitamin E is depicted in Figure 4.6.

Vitamin K

Vitamin K is a fat-soluble vitamin which functions as a cofactor for clotting (PubChem 2005e). Supplementation is indicated to treat vitamin K deficiency and coumarin and anticoagulant rodenticide toxicity (VDH 2017g). Injectable vitamin K_1 can cause pain and swelling at the injection site (VDH 2017g). Vitamin K_1 should not be administered by intravenous injection. Vitamin K_3 can be nephrotoxic (cause kidney injury) and is not recommended in veterinary patients (VDH 2017g). Potential drug interactions have been documented with cephalosporins, salicylates, chloramphenicol, tetracycline, erythromycin, neomycin, sulfa drugs, and metronidazole (VDH 2017g). The molecular structure of vitamin K_1 is depicted in Figure 4.7.

Minerals

Minerals are a group of inorganic substances required in various quantities by the body for normal growth, nutrition, and development. The most common minerals supplemented in veterinary medicine include calcium, iron, zinc, aluminum, magnesium, and potassium. A quick reference summarizing the primary uses for each mineral is provided in Table 4.7.

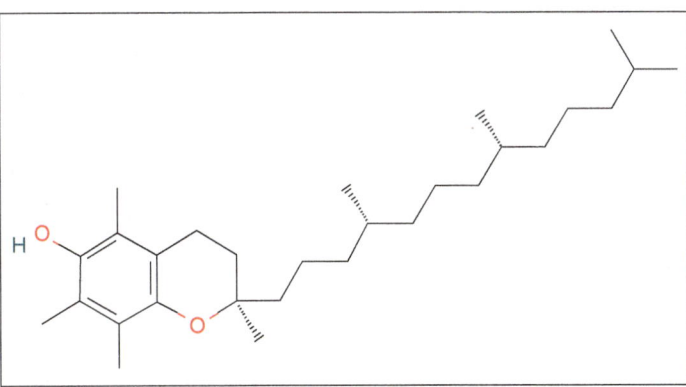

Figure 4.6 Molecular structure of vitamin E (alpha-tocopherol), $C_{29}H_{50}O_2$. Source: PubChem, https://pubchem.ncbi.nlm.nih. gov/compound/14985# section=2D-Structure, June 24, 2005.

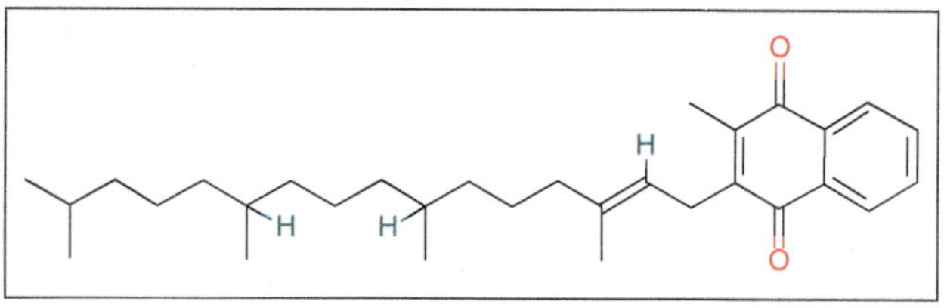

Figure 4.7 Molecular structure of vitamin K_1, $C_{20}H_{30}O$. Source: PubChem, https://pubchem.ncbi.nlm.nih.gov/compound/5280483#section=2D-Structure, March 25, 2005.

Table 4.7 The primary therapeutic uses of minerals in veterinary medicine.

Aluminum	High phosphorus; duodenal ulcers; gastroesophageal reflux; esophagitis; stress-induced gastric ulceration and hemorrhage; antidiarrheal
Calcium	Low calcium; high potassium; high magnesium; muscle spasms caused by insect bites and stings; cardiac asystole
Iron	Iron deficiency anemia
Magnesium	Excessive gastric acid; gastroesophageal reflux; esophagitis; stress-induced gastric irritation; laxative
Potassium	Low potassium
Zinc	Dermatologic conditions

Source: Lisa P. McFaddin.

There are several well-documented mineral–drug interactions. For example, patients taking potassium bromide need to be careful if changing the dog's diet because fluctuations in the salt (sodium chloride) levels can affect blood bromide levels. Also, patients taking doxycycline should avoid giving the medication with cheese as calcium can decrease absorption.

The use of multivitamins and minerals in healthy pets eating AAFCO-compliant commercial food is controversial, with most practitioners and nutritionists considering the practice unnecessary and potentially harmful, depending on the vitamin source and chance for overdose (Freeman 2017). Many integrative practitioners advocate for wholefood multivitamin supplementation in healthy pets. There is concern that the degree of processing required to create commercial food diminishes the bioavailability of many micronutrients (Knueven 2018).

Aluminum

Aluminum hydroxide is the most used formulation for binding dietary phosphorus and altering the pH of the gastrointestinal tract (VDH 2018). Aluminum hydroxide is used to treat hyperphosphatemia, duodenal ulcers, gastroesophageal reflux, esophagitis, stress-induced gastric ulceration/hemorrhage, and as an antidiarrheal (VDH 2018). Oversupplementation has been associated with constipation, hypophosphatemia, and gastric acid rebound (VDH 2018). Known drug interactions include fluoroquinolones, tetracyclines, iron, digoxin, diazepam, naproxen, aspirin, and potentially any enteric-coated medication (VDH 2018).

Calcium

The most used formulations of calcium include calcium acetate, calcium borogluconate, calcium carbonate, calcium chloride, calcium citrate, calcium gluconate, and calcium lactate. Calcium has many important primary functions within the body, including maintaining the integrity of the nervous, muscular and skeletal systems, and of cell membranes, maintaining vascular permeability, stimulating enzyme activation and maintaining normal physiologic function (VDH 2017a). Calcium is used to treat hypocalcemia, hyperkalemia, hypermagnesemia, muscle spasms induced by insect bites and stings, and cardiac asystole (VDH 2017a). Intravenous administration can cause negative cardiovascular effects (VDH 2017a). Irritation at the site of intramuscular injection and gastrointestinal irritation are other potential AEs (VDH 2017a). Calcium is known to interact with bisphosphonate, cardiac glycosides, ceftriazone, iron, levothyroxine, tetracyclines, and fluoroquinolones (VDH 2017a).

Iron

Iron is most administered as ferrous sulfate or iron dextran. Iron is present in all cells within the body, assisting enzymes and hemoglobin/myoglobin with everyday function (VDH 2017b). Iron is primarily used to correct iron deficiency anemia. Adverse effects associated with administration include gastrointestinal upset (pain, constipation, dark stool, and nausea), hypersensitivity reactions to injections, and hemosiderosis (VDH 2017b). Iron is known to interact with antacids, aluminum hydroxide, chloramphenicol, penicillamine, quinolone antibiotics, tetracycline antibiotics, vitamin C, and thyroxine (VDH 2017b).

Magnesium

Magnesium is typically administered as magnesium carbonate, magnesium hydroxide, magnesium oxide, and magnesium sulfate heptahydrate. Magnesium has many critical functions within the body, including adjusting gastric pH, acting as an enzyme cofactor, assisting with cellular energy production, regulating blood glucose levels, and regulating blood pressure (NIH 2020). Supplementation is used to treat excessive gastric acid (antacid), gastroesophageal reflux, esophagitis, stress-induced gastric irritation, and as a laxative (VDH 2017c). Oversupplementation may lead to diarrhea (VDH 2017c). Magnesium may interact with fluoroquinolones, tetracyclines, digoxin, diazepam, naproxen, aspirin, and potentially any enteric-coated medication (VDH 2017c).

Potassium

Potassium is typically administered as potassium chloride, potassium gluconate or potassium phosphate. As an intracellular cation potassium is crucial in maintaining normal cell tone, nerve conduction, contraction of smooth/skeletal/cardiac muscle, cell energy production, blood pressure, enzyme function and renal function (VDH 2020). Supplementation is used to treat hypokalemia. Potential AEs include gastrointestinal upset (nausea, vomiting, gas, pain, and diarrhea), hyperkalemia, and irritation to veins or tissues during injection (VDH 2020). Potassium may interact with potassium-sparing diuretics and nonsteroidal anti-inflammatory drugs (NSAIDs) (VDH 2020).

Zinc

Zinc is typically administered as zinc acetate, zinc gluconate, zinc sulfate, and zinc methionine. Zinc is responsible for maintaining normal cellular function, integrity, and growth (VDH 2017h). Additionally, zinc is a potent antioxidant and enzyme cofactor, as well as assisting with energy metabolism and immune system function (VDH 2017h). Zinc is primarily used to treat dermatologic conditions (VDH 2017h). Gastrointestinal upset (nausea, vomiting, and inappetance) can be seen with normal use and oversupplementation (VDH 2017h). Zinc may interact with copper, fluoroquinolones, tetracyclines, calcium, iron, D-penicillamine, and ursodiol (VDH 2017h).

Microbiome Therapy

The vast community of organisms living in the gastrointestinal tract of all animals, including humans, plays a crucial role in the health of the entire body, both locally at the level of the gut (nutrient digestion and absorption) and systemically (energy metabolism, immune modulation, brain health, and even joint health) (Mimee et al. 2016; Cintio et al. 2020). This system of symbiotic organisms has its own set nomenclature. The term "microbiome" refers to the bacteria, other organisms, their genes, and their environment throughout the gastrointestinal tract. Each segment of bowel contains a slightly different microenvironment with its own organisms, called the microbiota (Wernimont et al. 2020). Together all components of the microbiome aid digestion and absorption of dietary nutrients. Interestingly, the variety of microbiomes is very similar between cats and dogs (Wernimont et al. 2020).

Microbiome therapy (MT) focuses on improving a patient's microbiome to promote health and aid in the treatment of certain conditions. MT can be broken down into three main therapeutic categories, additive, subtractive, and modulatory (Figure 4.8) (Mimee et al. 2016). Additive therapies involve the supplementation of the gut with live microbial strains (e.g. probiotics) or entire microbiota (e.g. fecal transplants) (Mimee et al. 2016). Subtractive therapies focus on the elimination of pathogenic (harmful) bacteria (Mimee et al. 2016). In veterinary medicine this is primarily accomplished through the administration of gut-targeted antibiotics, such as metronidazole and tylosin, not the use of nutraceuticals. Finally, modulatory therapies focus on the administration of non-living substances which promote the growth and repopulation of desired gut microbes, e.g. prebiotics (Mimee et al. 2016).

The most common forms of MT used in veterinary medicine are prebiotics, probiotics, synbiotics, non-pathogenic yeast, and fecal transplants, as shown in Figure 4.8. Probiotics and prebiotics are considered the first generation of microbiome therapy, with the other therapies representing the next generation of MT (Mimee et al. 2016).

Prebiotics

Prebiotics are fermentable nutrients that feed the beneficial gut microbiota and promote overall health. These are specialized ingredients which selectively increase the quantity and quality of the "good" bacteria in the large intestinal tract. Technically, any fermentable food substance (carbohydrate, protein, amino acid, or fat) can function as a prebiotic (Wernimont et al. 2020). Most prebiotics are a subset of naturally occurring carbohydrates called oligosaccharides (Gibson et al. 2010).

Prebiotics are typically produced using wholefoods (and in uncommon cases arthropod exoskeletons) or synthetically from lactose, sucrose, or starch. The most produced oligosaccharides are derived from lactose (galacto-oligosaccharides, GOS) and fructose (fructo-oligosaccharides, FOS) (Gibson et al. 2010). GOS and FOS feed large intestinal bacteria, contribute to their repopulation (aka fat, happy, and fertile bacteria), and the fermentation of GOS and FOS generates different types of short-chain fatty acids (SCFAs) (Gibson et al. 2010). Other bacterial species

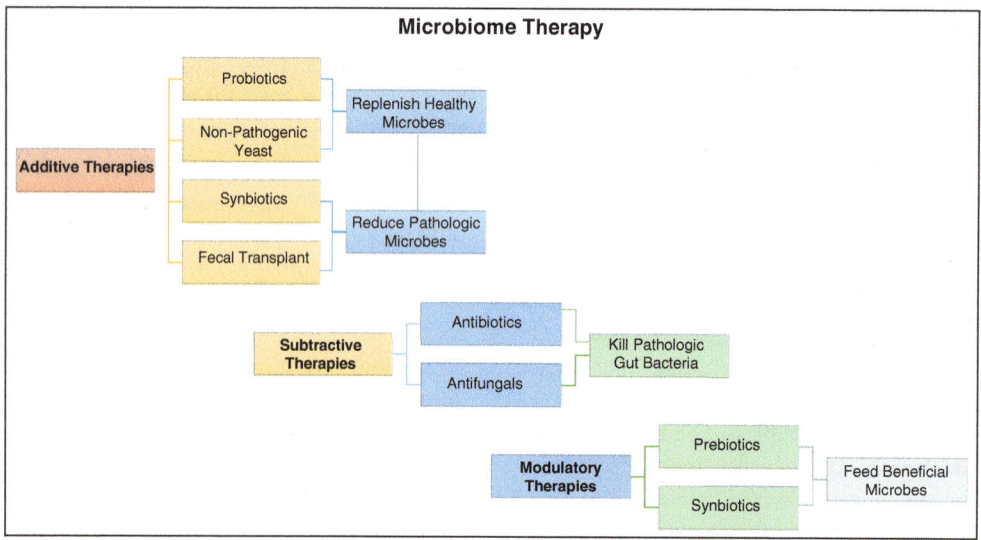

Figure 4.8 Algorithmic summary of the three categories of microbiome therapy, the most used modalities within each category, and the primary goal(s) of treatment. Source: Lisa P. McFaddin.

happily munch on these by-products creating different types of SCFA. The acid production lowers the pH of the gut, further encouraging the growth of healthy bacteria, while hindering the survival of unhealthy (pathologic) gut bacteria.

The SCFAs absorbed by the gut enter the bloodstream and cause positive effects throughout the body (Gibson et al. 2010). Figure 4.9 summarizes the mechanisms of action by which prebiotics exert their positive effects. Human studies have shown prebiotics, and their resulting SCFAs, improve gut health, mood and brain function, heart health, immune function, and assist with weight loss (Todesco et al. 1991; Moro et al. 2006; Gaman and Kuo 2008; Gao et al. 2009; Langen and Dieleman 2009; Candela et al. 2011; den Beston et al. 2013; Whelan 2013).

Prebiotics and SCFAs have demonstrated improvements in the gut microbiota populations in cats and dogs (Garcia-Mazcorro et al. 2017; Makielski et al. 2018; Wernimont et al. 2020). Unfortunately, the results were not statistically significant, likely due to small sample sizes. Additional studies evaluating prebiotics are limited and have yet to support the positive systemic effects documented in people (Abecia et al. 2010; Schmitz et al. 2012; Sergi et al. 2016).

Prebiotics for Veterinarians While there is no official definition for prebiotics, the International Scientific Association of Probiotics and Prebiotics (ISAPP) defines prebiotics as a "selectively fermented ingredient that results in specific changes in the composition and/or activity of the gastrointestinal microbiota, thus conferring benefit upon host health" (ISAPP 2021a). The ISAPP created criteria for classifying compounds as a prebiotic. The compound must be resistant to the acidic gastric pH, cannot be hydrolyzed by mammalian enzymes, cannot be absorbed within the gastrointestinal tract, can be fermented by the microbiota, and improves the growth and/or activity of the microbiota improving host health (ISAPP 2021a).

The most common prebiotics are a group of complex sugar molecules called oligosaccharides, comprising FOS , GOS, and mannose-containing oligosaccharides called mannan-oligosaccharides (MOS). FOS and inulin are classified as fructans, or fructose polymers (Gibson et al. 2010) Oligosaccharides are resistant to gastric acid and mammalian enzymes, allowing them to reach the large intestine unchanged (Gibson et al. 2010)..

Once in the large intestine, bacteria ferment the oligosaccharides creating SCFAs, such as lactic acid and acetic acid. Other bacteria cross-feed and use these substrates to create another type of acid (butyrate) (Gibson

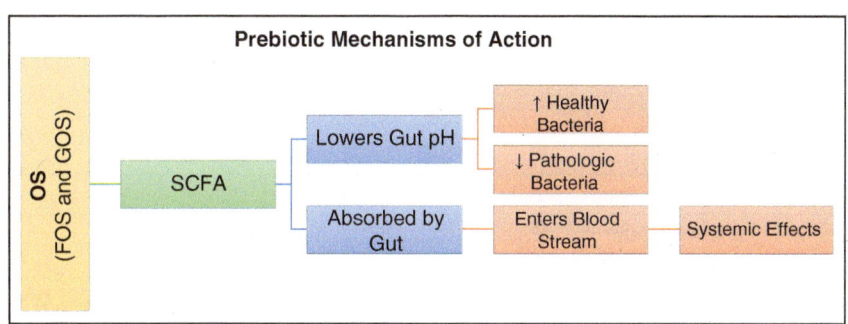

Figure 4.9 Algorithmic summary of prebiotic mechanisms of action. Fermentation of oligosaccharides (OS) (primarily fructo-oligosaccharide and galacto-oligosaccharide) produces various short-chain fatty acids (SCFA). SCFA lower the pH of the gastrointestinal tract increasing healthy gut bacteria and decreasing pathologic gut bacteria. SCFA are also absorbed by the gut, entering the bloodstream and causing multiple systemic beneficial effects (Gibson et al. 2010; ISAPP, 2021a). Source: Lisa P. McFaddin.

et al. 2010). The generation of more acids within the large intestine decreases the gut pH (butyrogenic effect), changing the composition and population of the gut microbiota (Gibson et al. 2010).

SCFAs are also the means through which prebiotics improve overall health. SCFAs are small enough to diffuse through the gut and enter the peripheral circulation (den Beston et al. 2013). As mentioned earlier, SCFAs have been shown to have many positive effects throughout the body in both laboratory animals and people, as outlined in Table 4.8.

Multiple veterinary studies have shown that prebiotics improve the type of bacteria comprising the gut microbiotia (Abecia et al. 2010; Schmitz et al. 2012; Garcia-Mazcorro et al. 2017). Unfortunately, these studies failed to demonstrate improvement in the clinical signs associated with chronic gastrointestinal diseases, such as irritable bowel syndrome and food-responsive chronic enteropathy. In all cases the sample sizes were small, affecting the statistical analysis. At this point the systemic improvements seen with increased SCFA production in people and laboratory animals can only be extrapolated to dogs and cats. Further studies are needed to prove the beneficial systemic effects of prebiotics in companion animals.

Probiotics

Probiotics change and improve the gut microbiota while also improving overall health (Schmitz and Suchodolski 2016). Human, laboratory animal, and bench-top tests (*in vivo* and *in vitro*) have demonstrated probiotics help repopulate the gut with healthy bacteria by displacing the pathologic bacteria, preventing pathologic bacteria from attaching to the gut lining, and by killing pathologic gut bacteria (Schmitz and Suchodolski 2016). Probiotics kill pathologic bacteria by producing their own antibacterial substances and encourage the host's immune system to attack them (Jones and Versalovic 2009). Figure 4.10 summarizes the mechanisms of action by which probiotics exert their positive effects.

Veterinary studies have shown probiotics exert a positive effect on the immune system and are effective in the resolution of certain causes of acute and chronic diarrhea in both dogs and cats (Bybee et al. 2011; Schmitz et al. 2012). Bacteria belonging to the genera *Lactobacillus*, *Bifidobacterium*, and *Enterococcus*

Table 4.8 Several studies supporting the beneficial effects of short-chain fatty acids (SCFA).

Body system	Beneficial effect	Supporting research
Cellular function	Improved lipid, glucose, and cholesterol metabolism	Todesco et al. (1991), Gao et al. (2009), den Beston et al. (2013)
	Improved immune system function	
	Increased intestinal calcium absorption	Teramoto et al. (2006)
	Increased rate of weight loss	Gao et al. (2009), den Beston et al. (2013)
Dermatologic	Reduced the clinical signs associated with atopic dermatitis	Moro et al. (2006)
Gastrointestinal	Improved symptoms associated with IBS and IBD	Langen and Dieleman (2009), Whelan (2013)
Neoplasia	Reduced the risk of colorectal cancer	Candela et al. (2011)
Neurologic	Improved cognition and mood	Gaman and Kuo (2008)

IBS, irritable bowel syndrome; IBD, inflammatory bowel disease.
Source: Lisa P. McFaddin.

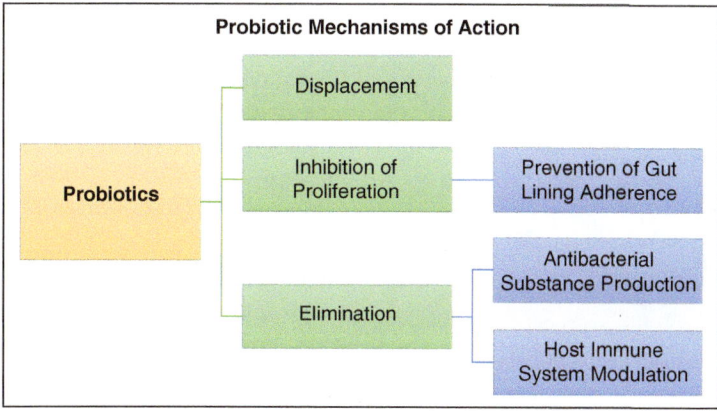

Figure 4.10 Algorithmic summary of probiotic mechanisms of action. Probiotics alter the gut microbiota through several mechanisms: displacement of pathologic gut bacteria, inhibition of proliferation of pathologic gut bacteria (by preventing their adherence to the intestinal lining), and elimination (through production of their own antimicrobial substances and stimulation/modulation of the host's immune system) (Schmitz and Suchodolski 2016; ISAPP 2021b). Source: Lisa P. McFaddin.

are the most commonly studied and utilized probiotics in veterinary medicine (Weese and Martin 2011; Schmitz and Suchodolski 2016; Jugan et al. 2017; Wernimont et al. 2020). Micrographs of these bacteria are depicted in Figures 4.11–4.13.

Some veterinarians believe the best probiotics originate from the host species, i.e. use feline-specific probiotics for cats and canine-specific for dogs. Most of the products on the market are not species specific, and there are no studies comparing the efficacy of generic with species-specific probiotics (Wernimont et al. 2020).

Probiotics for Veterinarians In 2013 an Expert Working Group under the ISAPP defined probiotics as "live microorganisms that, when administered in adequate amounts, confer a health benefit on the host" (ISAPP 2021b). As shown in Figure 4.10, probiotics alter the gut microbiota through several mechanisms: displacement, inhibition of proliferation, antimicrobial production, and host immune system

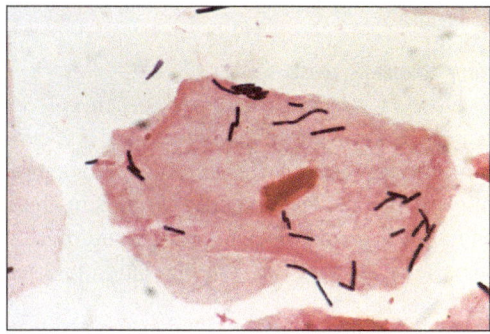

Figure 4.11 Micrograph image of *Lactobacillus* from a vaginal specimen, at a magnification of 63×. The bacteria appear as Gram-positive rods on epithelial cells. Source: Dr. Mike Miller, 1982/ Centers for Disease Control and Preventions (CDC).

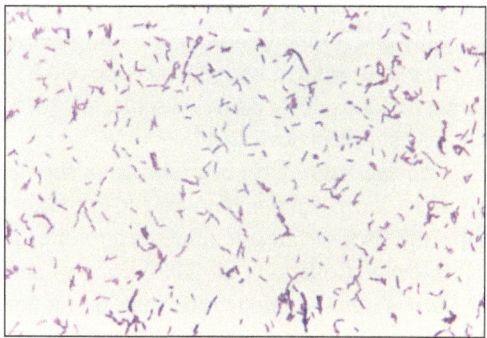

Figure 4.12 Micrograph image of *Bifidobacterium* on a blood agar plate, at a magnification of 1125×. The bacteria appear as Gram-positive rods. Source: Bobby Strong, 1972/Centers for Disease Control and Preventions (CDC).

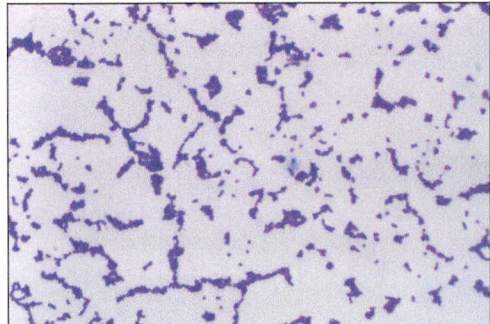

Figure 4.13 Micrograph image of *Enterococcus* which appear as small round Gram-positive cocci. Source: Dr. Richard Facklam, 1980/Centers for Disease Control and Preventions (CDC).

modulation. These mechanisms are often species dependent.

Lactobacillus probiotics have been shown to physically compete, exclude, and displace pathogenic bacteria within the gut, including *Escherichia coli* and *Salmonella* s (Lee et al. 2003). Probiotics can inhibit the proliferation of pathogenic bacteria by preventing attachment to the intestinal mucosa, interfering with mucus and mucin production, modulating the host's immune system, and creating their own antimicrobial agents (Jones and Versalovic 2009; Schmitz and Suchodolski 2016).

The formation of biofilms by some bacteria (especially *Lactobacillus* spp.) can physically interfere with pathogenic bacterial adherence (Lauková et al. 2004; Jones and Versalovic 2009). The biofilms and bacteria can also stimulate cytokine and antibody production and release by the gut-associated lymphatic tissue (GALT) (Jones and Versalovic 2009; Oelschlaeger 2010; Thomas and Versalovic 2010).

Bifidobacterium shave been shown *in vitro* to interfere with *Salmonella* spp., *Clostridium* spp., and *Escherichia coli* adherence to intestinal mucosa (Collado et al. 2007). *In vitro* and *in vitro* studies demonstrate that probiotics produce different antimicrobial substances (reuterin, fatty acids, lactic acid, and acetic acid) and downregulate gene expression for toxins or inactivate toxins commonly released by *Salmonella*, *E. coli*, and *C. perfringens*

(Castagliuolo et al. 1999; Saarela et al. 2000; Medellin-Peña et al. 2007; Jones and Versalovic 2009; Allaart et al. 2011; Bayoumi and Griffiths 2012).

Companion animal studies (*in vivo* and *in vitro*) have shown probiotics augment and stimulate the immune system by encouraging GALT cytokine release, simialr to the results seen in human studies (Benyacoub et al. 2003; Sauter et al. 2005, 2006; Schmitz et al. 2012; Rossi et al. 2014). Probiotics have also proven effective in controlling the clinical signs associated with certain canine and feline enteropathies, including acute infectious diseases, stress diarrhea, acute idiopathic diarrhea, and other chronic conditions (Kelley et al. 2009, 2012; Bybee et al. 2011; Arslan et al. 2012; Schmitz et al. 2015).

The best probiotic composition for canine and feline patients is still unknown (Schmitz and Suchodolski 2016). Given the species-specific attributes possessed by each bacterium, it is my opinion that a product with multiple bacterial strains is a better option compared to single-strain probiotics.

Synbiotics

Synbiotics are combination products containing both prebiotics and probiotics. The goal is synergy, i.e. the benefits will be greater when administrating both components at the same time (Schmitz and Suchodolski 2016). More research is needed to determine the true efficacy of these products.

Nonpathogenic Yeast

The use of yeasts, particularly *Saccharomyces boulardii*, as an alternative to probiotics is currently being investigated in human and veterinary medicine. Preliminary research in dogs suggests this may be a functional alternative for the treatment of chronic enteropathies (D'Angelo et al. 2018).

Fecal Transplants

Fecal transplants, stool transplants, fecal microbiota transplantation (FMT), and microbiome restorative therapy (MBRT) are often used interchangeably. All these terms refer to the insertion of feces from a healthy individual into the gastrointestinal tract of a diseased individual (Bojanova and Bordenstein 2016). Fecal and stool transplants are the transfer of unprocessed feces (stool), or portions of the feces, while FMT uses a more concentrated fecal solution (Bojanova and Bordenstein 2016).

The fecal material is collected from the healthy donor, mixed with saline or another solution, strained, and inserted directly into the gastrointestinal tract of the patient, typically through use of colonoscopy, endoscopy, sigmoidoscopy, or enema (FTF 2022). Unlike probiotics, FMT and fecal/stool transplants provide more than just beneficial gut bacteria. The microbiota consists of viruses, bacteria, fungi, archaea, protozoa, colonocytes (epithelial cells lining the large intestine), and commensal bacterial metabolites (compounds produced by healthy gut bacteria including SCFAs) (Bojanova and Bordenstein 2016).

FMT is believed to exert its effect through several mechanisms of action including repopulation, diversification, inhibition of proliferation, and elimination, as summarized in Figure 4.14 (Niederwerder 2018). FMT delivers an intact diversified population of healthy gut microorganisms directly into the colon improving the quantity and quality of the microbiota (Khoruts and Sadowsky 2018). The expanded microbiota improves nutrient utilization through more effective complex carbohydrate metabolism aiding digestion and nutrient absorption (Niederwerder 2018). Like probiotics, FMT prevent the proliferation and colonization of pathologic gut bacteria by interfering with their adherence and attachment to the colon (Khoruts and Sadowsky 2018). Also, like probiotics, FMT can eliminate pathologic bacteria through the production of antibacterial substances and improve the host's immune response (Khoruts and Sadowsky 2018).

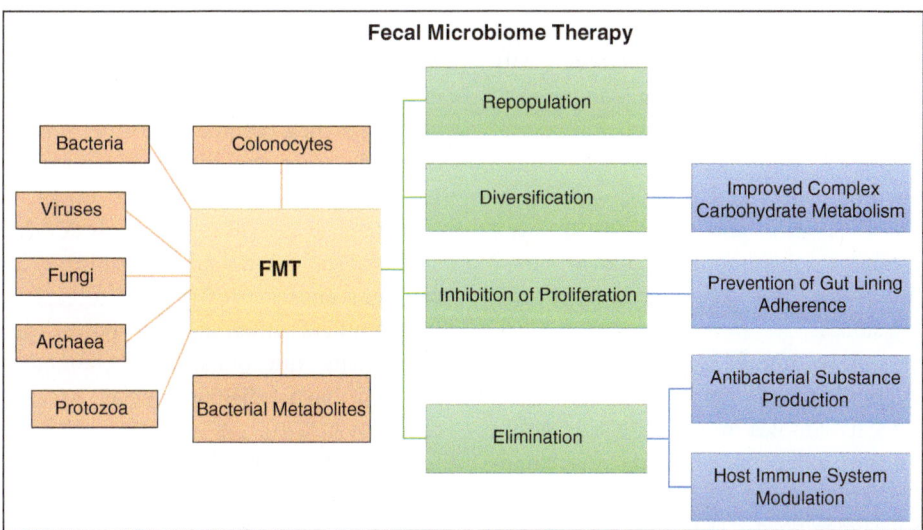

Figure 4.14 Algorithmic summary of fecal microbiome therapy (FMT) mechanisms of action. The microbiota within FMT stool samples consists of viruses, bacteria, fungi, archaea, protozoa, colonocytes (epithelial cells lining the large intestine), and commensal bacterial metabolites. FMT alters the gut health through several mechanisms: repopulation and diversification of the microbiota (leading to improved metabolism of complex carbohydrates), inhibition of proliferation of pathologic gut bacteria (by preventing their attachment and adherence to the intestinal lining), and elimination (through production of their own antimicrobial substances and stimulation/modulation of the host's immune system). Source: adapted from Khoruts and Sadowsky (2018).

Human FMT The earliest documented use of FMT in people dates to the fourth century in China (Zhang et al. 2012). Currently, FMT is most used to treat recurrent antibiotic-resistant *Clostridium difficile* infections in people (Borody and Khoruts 2011; Gupta et al. 2016; Kim and Gluck 2019). FMT has also been used with varying degrees of success as an adjunct treatment for inflammatory bowel disease, obesity, metabolic syndrome, and functional gastrointestinal disorders (Gupta et al. 2016; Kim and Gluck 2019).

As a newer mainstream therapy FMT is still experiencing growing pains, with the lack of standardization for donors as the primary issue. In a study review, Kim and Gluck (2019) outlined potential exclusion criteria for fecal donors. The ideal candidates were determined to be young to middle-age, healthy individuals free of communicable diseases (especially viral hepatitis, human immunodeficiency virus, and syphilis) and chronic illness (especially gastrointestinal, autoimmune, chronic pain, and neurologic conditions), who have not received antibiotics three to six months before stool collection (Kim and Gluck 2019). Universal donors are most used, compared to patient-directed donors. There are now several FDA-approved stool banks in the United States which collect and store samples to be used for FMT (Kim and Gluck 2019). Strict and frequent screening protocols are used to reduce the risk of infectious disease transmission.

Interestingly, sample preparation is relatively standardized amongst laboratories. Fresh fecal samples must be used within four hours of collection, while universal donor samples can be stored at −80 °C and delivered on dry ice when needed (Kim and Gluck 2019). Oral fecal microbiota capsules are also stored at −80 °C for up to six months (Kim and Gluck 2019). The most common adverse effects associated with FMT in people are bloating and loose stools for 24 hours after administration (Gupta et al. 2016; Kim and Gluck 2019).

Veterinary FMT The first recorded use of FMT in animals dates to seventeenth-century Italy involving rumen transfaunation (RT) (Niederwerder 2018). RT is the transfer of rumen contents (cud) from a donor to a recipient. RT is primarily used to treat indigestion and aid in postoperative recovery following left-displaced abomasum surgery (DePeters and George 2014). FMT use in small animals has become popularized over the last decade.

Niederwerder (2018) divides veterinary FMT use into three categories: prophylactic, therapeutic, and immunogenic. Prophylactic FMT is used as a preventative measure for patients with a high risk of exposure to gastrointestinal pathogens (think breeds at high risk of exposure to parvovirus or intestinal parasites). Therapeutic FMT is used to treat clinical illness. Immunogenic FMT increases the host's antibody production against specific gastrointestinal pathogens (infectious disease-causing agents) by exposing the gastric immune system to small doses of pathogens (think rectal vaccination) (Niederwerder 2018).

Therapeutic FMT is the most applied and studied treatment. Statistically significant benefits have been recognized in the treatment of acute diarrhea (compared to metronidazole), acute hemorrhagic diarrhea syndrome and parvovirus infection (Pereira et al. 2018; Chaitman et al. 2020; Gal et al. 2021). FMT case studies have documented improved clinical signs and/or resolution of disease in the treatment of inflammatory bowel disease, *C. difficile* infections, and chemotherapy-induced diarrhea (Bottero et al. 2017; Sugita et al. 2019, 2020).

Standardized protocols have not been established for donor selection or FMT administration (Niederwerder 2018). As with humans, the goal is to provide fecal material from healthy donors free of communicable diseases. Development of donor selection criteria and screening will improve FMT safety and efficacy in veterinary medicine.

Protocols must also be established for the standard volume of feces processed and administered, route of administration, frequency of administration, and duration of therapy (Niederwerder 2018). FMT can be administered orally (nasoduodenal intubation, enteroscopy, or oral capsule) or rectally (retention enema or colonoscopy) (Chaitman and Gaschen 2021). Depending on the technique, oral administration may be easier, but the sample must then travel to the colon and there is a higher chance of viable organism loss along the way (Chaitman et al. 2020). Regardless of the rectal technique used, the sample must be retained in the distal ileum, cecum, and colon for as long as possible to ensure maximal effect (i.e. give the microbes time to attach to the colonic wall) (Chaitman et al. 2020). Additionally, some practitioners recommend performing rectal ozone prior to FMT administration. While retention enemas are the most common technique, currently there are not enough data to support one route of administration over another.

There is limited information regarding potential or known adverse effects associated with FMT. Potential adverse effects include direct transmission of an infectious organism, increased gas, loose stool (likely transient), and weight gain (Chaitman et al. 2020).

Joint Supplements

Joint supplements are primarily used to aid in the resolution of clinical signs associated with osteoarthritis (OA) in both cats and dogs. OA is a form of chronic joint inflammation which leads to deterioration of the cartilage within the joint, causing stiffness, lameness, and pain. The prevalence of OA in dogs is approximately 20% in those over one year of age and 90% in those over five years of age (Johnston 1997; Johnson et al. 2020). Feline OA prevalence has been estimated to be between 16.5 and 91%, increasing with age (Clarke et al. 2005; Johnson et al. 2020).

Given the chronic nature of the disease a multimodal approach is generally taken to ensure the patient's comfort is improved and maintained. The most common treatments include weight management (nutritional), pain medications (nonsteroidal anti-inflammatory drugs, opioids, gabapentin, and amantadine), nutraceuticals, physical rehabilitation, and integrative therapies (spinal manipulation, acupuncture, cold laser, etc.) (Johnson et al. 2020).

The most frequently used and studied joint supplements include omega-3 fatty acids, glucosamine, chondroitin sulfate, and green-lipped mussels. Other commonly used supplements include methylsulfonylmethane, polysulfated glycosaminoglycan, avocado soybean unsaponifiables, undenatured type 2 collagen, curcumin, Boswellia, and eggshell membrane (ESM). Table 4.9 summarizes the source and primary effects of these supplements.

Less commonly used, but still useful, supplements include antler velvet, Devil's Claw, and astaxanthin. Most these supplements are available individually and as combination products. For the sake of brevity these supplements are not discussed in this chapter, but reliable information is readily available on the websites listed in Table 4.5.

Avocado Soybean Unsaponifiables

Avocado soybean unsaponifiables (ASU) is the remaining portion not used for soap (approximately 1%) after saponification of avocado and soybean oil (Christiansen et al. 2014). Saponification, or alkaline hydrolysis, is the formation of a soap through the reaction of a fat, oil, or lipid with an alkaline (basic) solution, such as sodium hydroxide or NaOH (Salehi et al. 2020). Multiple *in vitro* and *in vivo* human and animal studies have documented ASU's beneficial effects on OA, due to its anti-inflammatory, chondroprotective (protects joints), anticatabolic (prevents breakdown of proteins and muscle), and anabolic (helps build muscle) properties (Kut-Lasserre et al. 2001; Altinel et al. 2007, 2011; Lippiello et al. 2008; Boileau et al. 2009; Goudarzi et al. 2018). ASU appear safe (with no mentioned side effects) and effective as an adjunct therapy for the management of OA in dogs.

Table 4.9 The source and beneficial effects of the most used joint supplements in veterinary medicine as of January 2023.

Supplement name	Source	Beneficial effects
Avocado Soybean Unsaponafiables (ASU)	Avocado and soybean oil	Anti-inflammatory; protects cartilage; prevents muscle loss; helps build muscle
Boswellia	*Boswellia serrata* extract or resin	Anti-inflammatory; anti-arthritis; reduces pain
Chondroitin sulfate (CS)	Structural component of articular cartilage	Improves collagen elasticity; reduces joint pain
Curcumin	Turmeric spice	Anti-inflammatory; antioxidant; hepatoprotective; cholagogue; antiplatelet; anticancer
Eggshell membrane	Chicken eggs	Anti-inflammatory; chondroprotective; analgesic
Glucosamine	Articular cartilage	Reduce pain; improves cartilage formation and repair; reduces inflammation; reduces cartilage degradation
Green-Lipped Mussels (GLM)	*Perna canaliculus*	Anti-inflammatory; chondroprotective
Methylsulfonylmethane (MSM)	Dimethylsulfoxide (DMSO)	Anti-inflammatory; antioxidant; immunomodulatory; sulfur methylation
Omega-3 fatty acids	Fish, krill, and algal oil	Anti-oxidant; anti-inflammatory; anti-arrhythmogenic; improves heart function; reduces blood pressure; improves immune function; reduces weight loss; improves coat quality; improves dry eye
Polysulfated Glycosaminoglycans (PSGAGs)	Semisynthetic	Chondroprotectant
Undenatured Type II Collagen (UC-II)	Chicken sternum cartilage	Anti-inflammatory; analgesic; chondroprotective

Source: Lisa P. McFaddin.

A definitive dose range has not been established. Studies are needed to determine the safety and efficacy of ASU in the treatment of feline OA.

ASU for Veterinarians While several of the chemically active compounds within AUS are known (phystosterols, β-sitosterol, campesterol, stigmasterol, fat-soluble vitamins, and triterpene fatty acids), there are many unidentified active components (Christiansen et al. 2014; Grover and Samson 2016; Salehi et al. 2020). ASU are typically composed of one-third avocado and two-thirds soybean unsaponifiables (Christiansen et al. 2014). The sterol content is believed to be responsible for

ASU's beneficial effects on articular cartilage (Lippiello et al. 2008).

ASU minimize and prevent joint inflammation and damage by inhibiting inflammatory cytokine and matrix metalloproteinase (MMP) release, downregulating nitric oxide synthase and COX-2 expression, and inhibiting fibrinolysis (Kut-Lasserre et al. 2001; Lippiello et al. 2008; Boileau et al. 2009; Goudarzi et al. 2018). ASU also help repair damaged cartilage and joints through the stimulation of collagen and aggrecan synthesis and increasing transforming growth factor (TGF) production (Altinel et al. 2007, 2011; Lippiello et al. 2008; Salehi et al. 2020). The result is a reduction of pain and stiffness with improved mobility (Christiansen et al. 2014). Similar effects have been documented in canine joints, supporting the use of ASU for the management of canine OA (Altinel et al. 2007, 2011; Boileau et al. 2009).

Boswellia

Boswellia (aka Indian Frankincense) is an extracted resin from the *Boswellia serrata* tree (Figure 4.15). Boswellia has been used in Western, Chinese, and Ayurvedic medicine for the treatment of arthritis and other inflammatory conditions for years (Wynn and Fougère 2007). The active ingredient, boswellic acid, has been shown to reduce inflammation associated with rheumatoid arthritis, chronic bronchitis, asthma, and chronic inflammatory bowel disease in people (Yu et al. 2020). Additional studies suggest boswellic acid also reduces pain and improves clinical function in patients with arthritis (Kimmatkar et al. 2003; Shah et al. 2010; Gupta et al. 2011).

Limited studies also support the safety and efficacy of Boswellia as an adjunct treatment in the management in canine OA (Musco et al. 2019; Caterino et al. 2021; Martello et al. 2022). A definitive dose range has not been established. Studies are needed to determine the safety and efficacy of Boswellia in the treatment of feline OA.

Boswellia for Veterinarians The aromatic Boswellia resin contains multiple acids, most importantly acetyl-keto-β-boswellic acids (AKBA). AKBA has potent anti-inflammatory effects through the inhibition of the lipoxygenase (LOX) pathway (Sailer et al. 1996; Kimmatkar et al. 2003). Boswellia has also been shown to inhibit other proinflammatory mediators, such as prostaglandin, COX, nitric oxide (NO), and nuclear factor kappa B (NF-κB), prevent the degradation of collagen, and act as a dose-dependent modulate of cytochrome P450 (Dey et al. 2015; Comblain et al. 2016; Haroyan et al. 2018; Musco et al. 2019).

The veterinary literature documenting the efficacy and safety of Boswellia is limited but has promising results. Reichling et al. (2004) conducted a multicenter clinical trial investigating the use of Boswellia resin in the treatment of canine OA. There was a statistically significant improvement in lameness, pain, and gait after six weeks of therapy. Mild gastrointestinal signs (diarrhea and flatulence) were reported. Though all the results were not statistically significant, several randomized clinical trials support the use of Boswellia in the treatment of canine arthritis as part of a multi-ingredient nutraceutical regimen (Moreau et al. 2014; Caterino et al. 2021; Martello et al. 2022).

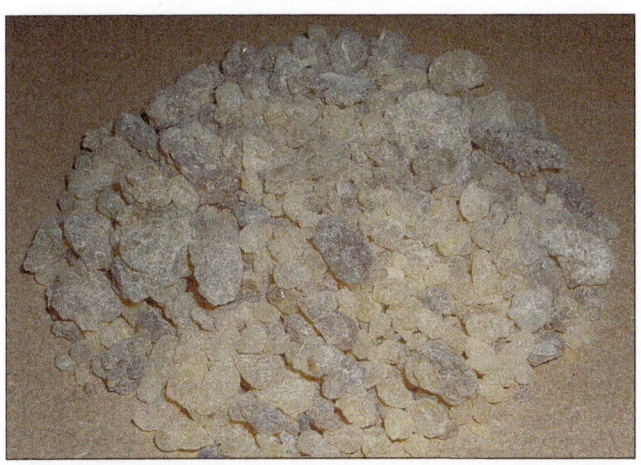

Figure 4.15 Photograph of resin from the *Boswellia serrata* tree, also known as Frankincense. Source: Gaius Cornelius/Wikimedia Commons/ Public domain.

Chondroitin Sulfate

Chondroitin sulfate is a produced within the body and is a structural component of articular cartilage (Jerosch 2011). Human studies have shown chondroitin sulfate improves collagen elasticity and reduces joint pain (Bucsi and Poór 1998; Anderson 1999; Michel et al. 2005; Iovu et al. 2008; Jerosch 2011). Several studies suggest the use of chondroitin sulfate, typically with glucosamine, reduce pain secondary to OA, though the results were not always statistically significant (Moreau et al. 2003; D'Altilio et al. 2007; McCarthy et al. 2007; Gupta et al. 2012). Further studies are necessary to confirm chondroitin sulfate's efficacy in the management of OA in veterinary patients.

Glucosamine and chondroitin sulfate are known to work together (synergistically), significantly improving weight-bearing and overall condition, while reducing pain scores, when co-administered (McCarthy et al. 2007). A "loading period," in which typically double the dose is given for two to six weeks, is needed for the supplement to take full effect (McCarthy et al. 2007).

Chondroitin Sulfate for Veterinarians Chondroitin sulfate (chemical structure depicted in Figure 4.16) is a naturally occurring glycosaminoglycan and a key component of the extracellular membrane (ECM). Chondroitin sulfate maintains a negative charge attracting water into the

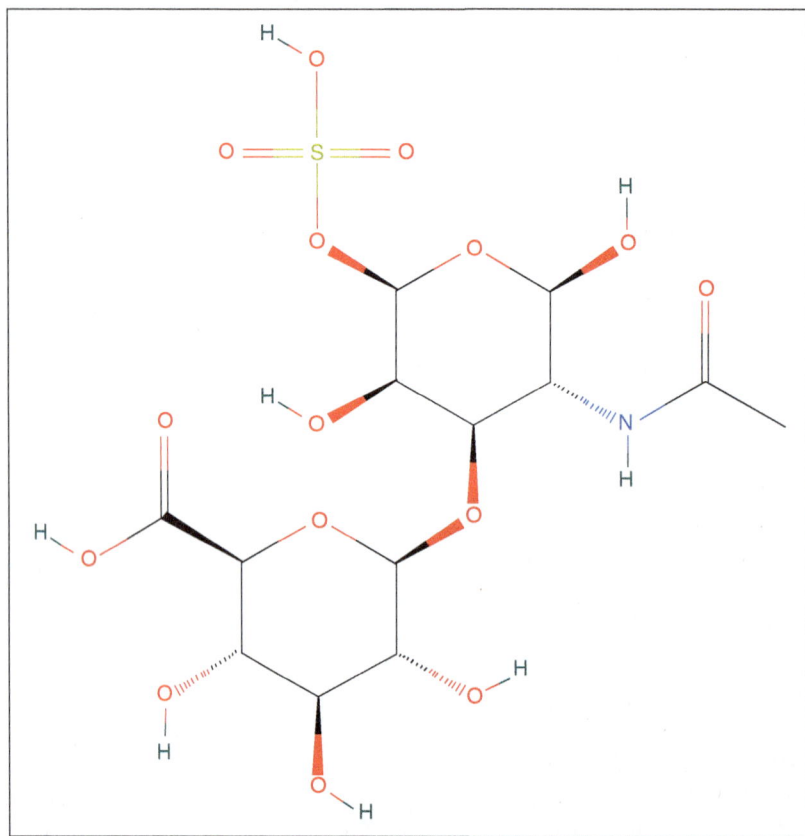

Figure 4.16 Chemical structure of chondroitin sulfate, (3R,4R)-2-[(2R,3S,4R,5R,6R)-3-acetamido-2,5-dihydroxy-6-(hydroxymethyl)oxan-4-yl]oxy-3,4-dihydroxy-3,4-dihydro-2H-pyran-6-carboxylic acid. Source: PubChem, https://pubchem.ncbi.nlm.nih.gov/compound/24766#section=2D-Structure, November 9, 2011.

joint, contributing to articular cartilage's ability to withstand high pressures and cyclic loading (Jerosch 2011).

Human and animal *in vivo* and *in vitro* studies indicate that the mechanism of action is multifactorial, but the full extent of its capabilities is likely unknown (Henrotin et al. 2010). Chondroitin sulfate exhibits potent chondroprotective (reducing chondrocyte apoptosis, promoting prostaglandin production, and reducing MMP) and anti-inflammatory properties (Uebelhart et al. 1998; Cho et al. 2004; Chou et al. 2005). Chondroitin sulfate has also been shown to stimulate the production of hyaluronic acid by synovial cells, boost chondrocyte metabolism, and encourage the synthesis of collagen and proteoglycan (David-Raoudi et al. 2009).

Numerous meta-analyses and randomized controlled trials have demonstrated chondroitin sulfate's efficacy in the reduction of pain and inflammation associated with OA in people, as well as slowing the progression of OA (Hochberg et al. 2008; Uebelhart 2008; Lee et al. 2009). Pharmacokinetic studies on humans and laboratory animals show good bioavailability following oral administration of chondroitin sulfate (Martel-Pelletier et al. 2010).

Unfortunately, results of clinical trials are not as clear-cut in veterinary medicine (Bhathal et al. 2017). There appear to be just as many trials and reviews suggesting chondroitin sulfate and glucosamine (often administered together) lack clinical evidence supporting their use or are ineffective, as there are touting their benefits (Bhathal et al. 2017; Scott et al. 2017) In a literature review by Bhathal et al. (2017), the authors describe in detail a potential design for a peer-review randomized clinical trial exploring the use of glucosamine and chondroitin sulfate in canines. As discussed by the authors, while glucosamine and chondroitin sulfate appear safe, further research is necessary to determine their efficacy in the management of canine (and feline) OA.

Glucosamine and chondroitin sulfate are often used together as joint supplements for both canine and feline patients. Co-administration may increase the bioavailability and efficacy (Beale 2004). Several studies suggest the combination of supplements reduces pain and lameness and improves weight-bearing (D'Altilio et al. 2007; Gupta et al. 2012; Vassalotti et al. 2017).

A loading period of two to six weeks is recommended for both glucosamine and chondroitin (Plumb 2015). Potential adverse effects for both products include hypersensitivity reactions and mild gastrointestinal effects, including flatulence and soft stools (Plumb 2015).

Curcumin

Turmeric, pictured in Figure 4.17, is a spice derived from the rhizome of the perennial *Curcuma longa* plant, a member of the ginger family (Priyadarsini 2014). Turmeric is used in both Western and Chinese herbal medicine for its anti-inflammatory, antioxidant, hepatoprotective, cholagogue (promotes bile flow), antiplatelet, and anticancer effects (Miquel et al. 2002; Wynn and Fougère 2007; Aggarwal and Harikumar 2009; Gupta et al. 2013; Hewlings and Kalman 2017; Withers et al. 2018).

Curcumin, a pigment in turmeric, is the primary compound responsible for turmeric's beneficial effects (Priyadarsini 2014). Multiple studies have demonstrated curcumin is effective, though the results were not always statistically significant, in controlling pain and reducing the inflammation associated with OA in people and dogs (Innes et al. 2003; Chandran and Goel 2012; Colitti et al. 2012; Panahi et al. 2014; Comblain et al. 2016; Daily et al. 2016).

Curcumin is very safe, well tolerated, and nontoxic even at high doses (Gupta et al. 2013). There is limited research available for the use of curcumin in feline patients. Curcumin can have a potent taste, making its use in cats difficult. Further research is needed to determine

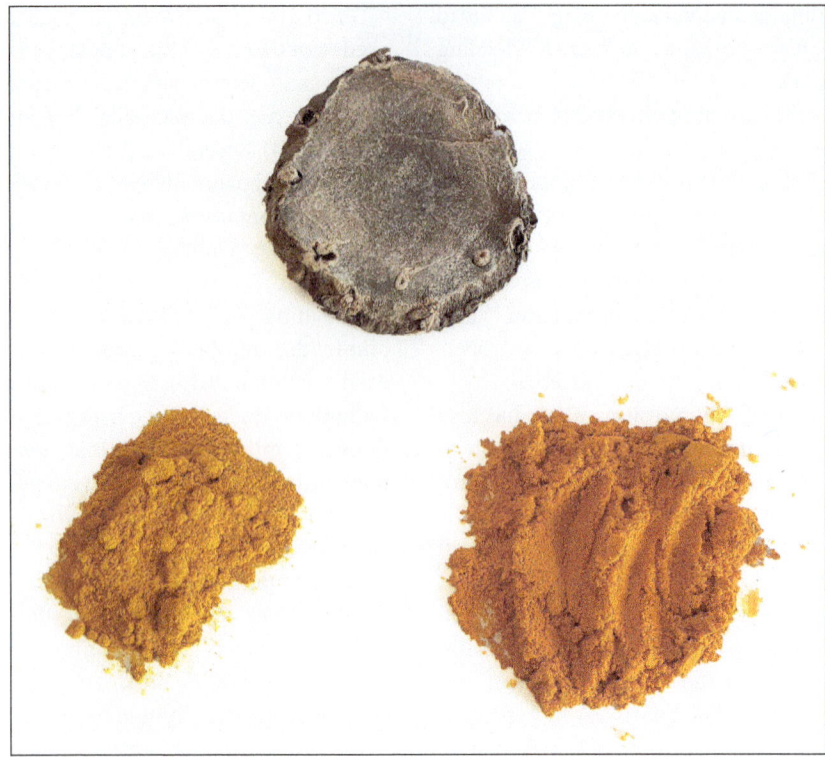

Figure 4.17 A slice of dried turmeric root (top), turmeric powder (bottom left), and a commercial curcumin supplement powder (bottom right). Source: Lisa P. McFaddin.

its safety, efficacy, and how best to administer to our feline patients.

Curcumin for Veterinarians Curcumin (difeuloylmethane) is the primary natural aromatic organic compound (phenol) found in the underground stem (rhizome) of *Curcuma longa* (turmeric). Turmeric contains 2–9% curcuminoids, including curcumin, demethoxycurcumin, disdemethoxycurcumin, and cyclic curcumin, with curcumin as the most abundant (Priyadarsini 2014). Curcumin, also known as diferuloylmethane or 1,7-bis(4-hydroxy-3-methoxyphenyl)-1,6-heptadiene-3,5-dione, is the primary polyphenol within turmeric (Hewlings and Kalman 2017).

Curcumin has been studied and used in people for the treatment of multiple cancers (colorectal, pancreatic, breast, prostate, multiple myeloma, lung cancer, and squamous cell carcinoma of the head and neck), inflammatory gastrointestinal disorders (inflammatory bowel disease, irritable bowel syndrome, peptic ulcers, and *Helicobacter pylori* infections), arthritis, uveitis, postoperative inflammation, inflammatory dermatologic conditions (vitiligo and psoriasis), Alzheimer's disease, cardiovascular diseases (acute coronary syndrome and atherosclerosis), diabetes, diabetic neuropathy, lupus nephritis, acquired immunodeficiency syndrome, biliary dyskinesia, hepatotoxicity, and recurrent respiratory tract infections (especially in children) (Aggarwal and Harikumar 2009; Gupta et al. 2013).

As mentioned previously, curcumin can be effective in reducing pain and inflammation in canine arthritis (Innes et al. 2003; Colitti et al. 2012; Comblain et al. 2016). *In vitro* studies show promise for the use of curcumin as an adjunct with chemotherapy or following chemotherapy for certain canine neoplasia (Levine et al. 2017; Withers et al. 2018). A recent *in vitro* study shows promise for the use of curcumin in the management of feline infectious peritonitis (FIP) (Ng et al. 2020). *In vivo*, ideally randomized clinical trials are needed to confirm efficacy for both neoplasia and FIP. Further studies are necessary to determine the efficacy of curcumin in in the treatment of other inflammatory conditions in both canines and felines.

Curcumin's antioxidant and anti-inflammatory properties are responsible for a majority of its multisystemic effects. *In vitro* and *in vivo* studies show this effect is achieved by enhancing markers of oxidative stress; increasing superoxide dismutase activity; reducing glutathione, malonedialdehyde, and lipid peroxide levels; scavenging free radicals including reactive oxygen species and reactive nitrogen species; and inhibiting LOX, COX, xanthine hydrogenase, and xanthine oxidase (Menon and Sudheer 2007; Sahebkar et al. 2015; Panahi et al. 2016). The antioxidant properties contribute to curcumin's anti-inflammatory abilities. The product is also able to block the activation of the inflammatory mediators tumor necrosis factor (TNF) and NF-κB (Hewlings and Kalman 2017). Oxidative stress reduction accounts for most of curcumin's ability to relieve OA symptoms (Panahi et al. 2016).

Unfortunately, curcumin has poor bioavailability due to poor absorption, rapid metabolism, and rapid elimination (Anand et al. 2007). To aid in absorption, curcumin is combined with black pepper, a source of piperine, which has been proven to increase bioavailability (Shoba et al. 1998). Curcumin is often mixed with a lipid source, usually medium-chain triglycerides, with the goal of improving absorption and delaying excretion (Feng et al. 2020). Due to the limited number of pharmacokinetic studies in companion animals, the human bioavailability and formulation recommendations are applied to companion animals. The dose range for curcumin in dogs is broad and often practitioner dependent.

Eggshell Membrane

Eggshell membrane (ESM) is the protective layer just inside the hard shell of a raw egg (the clear to slightly opaque film covering a hard-boiled egg – the one you hope to get under to easily peel off the shell in large satisfying chunks). ESM supplement is prepared by drying and grinding down the membrane without incorporation of the shell. ESM contains multiple ingredients which have the potential to reduce joint inflammation, protect joint cartilage from degradation (chondroprotective), and reduce the pain associated with arthritis, including type I collagen, CS, glucosamine, and hyaluronic acid (Wong et al. 1984; Ruff et al. 2009a).

Research in human and veterinary medicine is limited, but the results are promising. Several clinical trials have shown successful reduction of pain and improved flexibility in people with joint and connective tissue disorders, including OA (Ruff et al. 2009a,b; Danesch et al. 2014; Brunello and Masini 2016; Hewlings et al. 2019; Kiers and Bult 2021). As of March 2022, two clinical trials investigating the safety and efficacy of ESM in canines with OA showed mild improvement in mobility, lameness, and pain without evidence of adverse effects (Ruff et al. 2016; Muller et al. 2019). Currently there are no feline studies. Clearly further research is necessary confirming the effectiveness of ESM in the management of OA in veterinary patients.

ESM for Veterinarians   ESM is composed of protein, type I collagen, glycosaminoglycans (dermatan sulfate and chondroitin sulfate), sulfated glycoproteins (glucosamine), hyaluronic acid, sialic acid, semosine, isodemosine, ovotransferrin, lysyl oxidase, lysozyme, and β-*N*-acetylglucosaminidase (Baker and Balch 1962; Starcher and King 1980; Wong et al. 1984). A substantial amount of the dry matter weight of ESM comprises type I collagen (up to 25%), chondroitin sulfate (up to 2%), hyaluronic acid (up to 2%), and glucosamine (up to 1%) (Ruff et al. 2009a). These components work individually and synergistically contributing to the beneficial effects seen with ESM administration: anti-inflammatory, chondroprotecitve, and analgesic (Wedekind et al. 2017).

Glucosamine

Glucosamine is a structural component of articular cartilage. Articular cartilage, or hyaline cartilage, is the translucent, blue-hued cartilage covering the joint end of bones, comprising synovial joints (Pasquini et al. 2003). The tissue serves to reduce concussive forces and friction within the joint (Pasquini et al. 2003). Cartilage thickness is dependent on the joint location and function.

Glucosamine supplements can be obtained from natural (tissue-based) or synthetic sources. Human studies have shown glucosamine improves cartilage formation and repair, reduces inflammation, and reduces cartilage degradation (Anderson 1999; Michel et al. 2005; Iovu et al. 2008; Jerosch 2011). A study by Canapp et al. (1999) revealed dogs treated with glucosamine hydrochloride and chondroitin sulfate 21 days prior to chemically induced radiocarpal (wrist) joint OA had less evidence of joint inflammation and bony changes compared to untreated joints, supporting the chondroprotective nature of these supplements in canines.

Several studies suggest the use of glucosamine, typically with chondroitin sulfate, reduces pain and inflammation secondary to OA in canines, though the results were not always statistically significant (Moreau et al. 2003; D'Altilio et al. 2007; McCarthy et al. 2007; Gupta et al. 2012; Wenz et al. 2017; Martello et al. 2022). Further studies are necessary to confirm glucosamine's efficacy in the management of OA in veterinary patients.

Glucosamine supplementation is considered safe. Conflicting research suggests glucosamine may affect insulin sensitivity in people, leading to a theoretical issue for diabetics taking glucosamine, but this supplement–drug interaction has not been documented in people taking therapeutic doses (Monauni et al. 2000; Pouwels et al. 2001). Glucosamine has not been shown to affect blood glucose levels in healthy dogs and cats, but tests have not been conducted in diabetic patients (McNamara et al. 1996). Out of an abundance of caution most practitioners limit the use of glucosamine in diabetic patients, though this practice is likely unnecessary.

Glucosamine for Veterinarians Glucosamine salts are amino monosaccharides synthesized from glucose and present in the highest concentrations in connective tissue and cartilage (Jerosch 2011). Glucosamine, depicted in Figure 4.18, is a precursor to proteoglycans and glycosaminoglycans. Within articular cartilage glucosamine is involved in the production of multiple components of the ECM: hyaluronic acid, chondroitin sulfate, and collagen fibers (Jerosch 2011).

In vivo and *in vitro* studies have shown exogenous glucosamine stimulates chondrocyte production of proteoglycans and collagen (Varghese et al. 2007; Joshi et al. 2016). A study

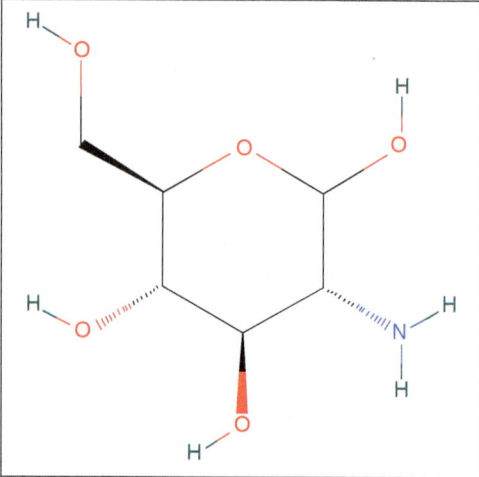

Figure 4.18 Chemical structure of glucosamine ($C_6H_{13}NO_5$; 2-amino-2-deoxy-D-glucopyranose). Source: PubChem, https://pubchem.ncbi.nlm.nih.gov/compound/439213#section=2D-Structure, June 24, 2005.

conducted by Gouze et al. (2006) found exogenous glucosamine did not increase chondrocyte production of ECM components, instead
exhibiting anti-inflammatory effects which
protected chondrocytes from cytokine damage
(i.e. chondroprotective). Additional *in vitro*
studies supported the chondroprotective theory through inhibition of lipoxidation and protein oxidation as well as inhibition of MMPs
and aggrecanases, cartilage cleavage enzymes
(Derfoul et al. 2007; Tiku et al. 2007; Eman
et al. 2019).

There are limited veterinary clinical trials
and systematic literature reviews evaluating
the efficacy of glucosamine. The available
studies yield conflicting results (Vandeweerd
et al. 2012; Bhathal et al. 2017). There are as
many trials and reviews suggesting chondroitin sulfate and glucosamine (often administered together) lack clinical evidence
supporting their use or are ineffective, as there
are touting their benefits (Bhathal et al. 2017;
Scott et al. 2017). In a literature review by
Bhathal et al. (2017), the authors describe in
detail a potential design for a peer-review randomized clinical trial exploring the use of glucosamine and chondroitin sulfate in canines.
As discussed by the authors, while glucosamine and chondroitin sulfate appear safe, further research is necessary to determine their
efficacy in the management of canine (and
feline) OA.

There are several glucosamine salts available
on the market: glucosamine sulfate and glucosamine hydrochloride. In people glucosamine sulfate appears to offer superior
bioavailability and clinical efficacy (Persiani
et al. 2005; Altman 2009). There are no veterinary studies comparing the bioavailability of
both formulations. Currently most veterinary
products contain glucosamine hydrochloride,
likely because this salt is less expensive to
manufacture (Altman 2009). Given the limited
pharmacokinetic data, the best dose for glucosamine in canine and feline pets is not well
documented (Bhathal et al. 2017). For now, following the manufacturer's recommended

dosing is advisable. Further research is needed
to determine which glucosamine salt has the
greatest efficacy, and the best dosing structure,
in veterinary patients.

Glucosamine and chondroitin sulfate are
often used together as joint supplements for
both canine and feline patients. Co-administration may increase the bioavailability and
efficacy (Beale 2004). Several studies suggest
the combination of supplements reduces pain
and lameness and improves weight-bearing
(D'Altilio et al. 2007; Gupta et al. 2012;
Vassalotti et al. 2017).

A loading period of two to six weeks is recommended for both glucosamine and chondroitin (Plumb 2015). Potential adverse effects
for both products include hypersensitivity reactions and mild gastrointestinal effects, including flatulence and soft stools (Plumb 2015).

Proteoglycans

Proteoglycans are one of the primary components of the ECM and found in all types of connective tissue. *Proteoglycans* comprise a core
protein with variable numbers of attached glycosaminoglycans (GAG) chains (Bliss 2013).
All GAGs, except hyaluronic acid, are covalently bonded to the core proteins (Frantz
et al. 2010).

Proteoglycans are classified by the core protein type, localization, and GAG composition.
The core protein length and amino acid composition vary. Localization and categorization
include intracellular, cell surface, pericellular
and basement membrane, and extracellular
proteoglycans (Frantz et al. 2010). GAG chains
consist of unbranched polysaccharide chains
made up of repeating disaccharide units
(Frantz et al. 2010; Iozzo and Schaefer 2015).
GAGs are either sulfated (chondroitin sulfate,
heparan sulfate, and keratan sulfate) or non-
sulfated (hyaluronic acid) (Frantz et al. 2010;
Iozzo and Schaefer 2015).

Proteoglycans are extremely hydrophilic,
often creating large aggregates which then
form a hydrogel matrix that can withstand
strong compressive forces (Frantz et al. 2010).

Proteoglycan aggregates may be firm, solidified, and reinforced by associated collagen fibrils (Bliss 2013).

Proteoglycan synthesis relies on the transcription and translation of the core protein followed by attachment of the GAG chains, and finally extracellular secretion of the mature *proteoglycan* (Iozzo and Schaefer 2015). *Proteoglycan* synthesis is a highly regulated process which can be altered by exposure to biochemical, biological, and pharmaceutical stimuli (Bliss 2013).

Green-Lipped Mussels

Green-lipped mussels (GLM), pictured in Figure 4.19, are shellfish native to New Zealand. Veterinary studies suggest GLM have anti-inflammatory and chondroprotective properties which, when administered alone or in combination with other nutraceuticals, help improve mobility and reduce pain associated with OA (Rainsford and Whitehouse 1980; Bierer and Bui 2002; Bui and Bierer 2003; Pollard et al. 2006; Servet et al. 2006; Gibson et al. 2010; Lascelles et al. 2010; Rialland et al. 2013). Not all clinical trials have documented a statistically significant improvement in pain and lameness following the administration of GLM, highlighting the need for further studies in companion animals, especially in the underrepresented feline population (Dobenecker et al. 2002).

GLM for Veterinarians GLM is typically processed using low-temperature techniques as heat can dramatically reduce its activity (Bierer and Bui 2002). GLM's mechanism of action is not fully understood but is believed to be due, at least in part, to its anti-inflammatory and chondromodulatory effects, reducing synovial inflammation and joint pain (Gibson et al. 1980; Miller and Ormrod 1980; Rainsford and Whitehouse 1980). GLM contains GAGs (specifically chondroitin sulfate), glutamine, omega-3 fatty acids, zinc, copper, manganese, vitamin E, and vitamin C (Murphy et al. 2003; Rialland et al. 2013). The presence of chondroitin sulfate likely contributes to GLM's chondroprotective effects (Bierer and Bui 2002).

The omega-3 fatty acid content, specifically eicosatetraenoic acid (ETA), is believed to be the primary compound responsible for GLM's anti-inflammatory properties (Treschow et al. 2007). Eicosapentaenoic acid (EPA) and docosahexaenoic acid (DHA) are present in low concentrations, suggesting these fatty acids contribute little to GLM's beneficial effects (Servet et al. 2006). ETA reduces inflammation by inhibiting arachidonic acid through the COX and LOX pathways, while also protecting the gastrointestinal tract (Rainsford and Whitehouse 1980; Bierer and Bui 2002).

GLM has been shown to improve weight-bearing, lameness, joint swelling, and pain scores (Bui and Bierer 2003; Servet et al. 2006; Rialland et al. 2013). Rialland et al. (2013) demonstrated dogs whose diets were supplemented with GLM for 30–90 days had increased plasma omega-3 levels and improved motor activity and peak vertical force. While GLM

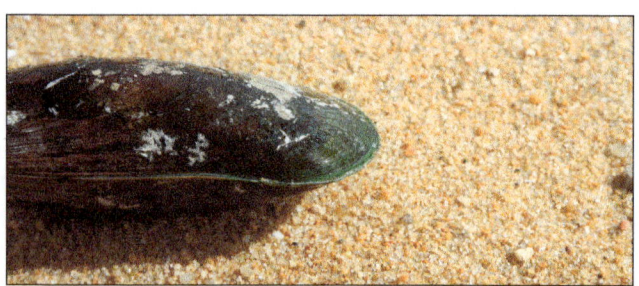

Figure 4.19 Photograph of a green-lipped mussel (*Perna canaliculus*) native to New Zealand. Source: Richard Giddins/Wikimedia Commons/CC BY 2.0.

affects COX and LOX, its use alone has not proven as effective at alleviating OA pain when compared to carprofen (Heilm-Bjŏrkman et al. 2009). Another study showed the degree of improvement was dependent on the size of the dog, i.e. the smaller the dog the greater the degree of improvement (Servet et al. 2006).

One study demonstrated that a diet supplemented with GLM, EPA, DHA, glucosamine, and chondroitin improved mobility in felines with OA, but the beneficial effects were not solely attributed to GLM (Lascelles et al. 2010). Further studies are necessary to confirm GLM's efficacy and dosage range in aiding the treatment of canine and feline OA.

Methylsulfonylmethane

Methylsulfonylmethane (MSM) is a naturally occurring organosulfur molecule but can also be synthesized easily in a laboratory setting. *In vitro* and *in vivo* human and laboratory animal studies have shown MSM has anti-inflammatory, antioxidant, immune modulatory, and sulfur methylation properties which reduce the clinical signs associated with OA, including pain reduction, cartilage preservation, improved range of motion and mobility, and reduce myalgia (Takashi et al. 2004; Usha and Naidu 2004; Kim et al. 2006, 2009; Butawan et al. 2017).

Currently there are no studies documenting the efficacy and safety of MSM in companion animals. MSM is commonly combined with glucosamine with or without chondroitin sulfate in commercially available canine and feline joint supplements. Justification for its use, dosage approximation, and safety are extrapolated from the relatively limited laboratory animal and human studies. While MSM may show promise in the management of OA, based on human and rodent studies, research is desperately needed in canine and feline patients to prove its efficacy and safety.

MSM for Veterinarians MSM is the first oxidized metabolite of dimethylsulfoxide (DMSO) (Kim et al. 2006). The chemical structure is depicted in Figure 4.20. DMSO, an organic form of sulfur, is a naturally occurring by-product of phytoplankton and algae decay (Brien et al. 2008). MSM is created synthetically by combining DMSO with hydrogen peroxide, yielding MSM and water (Kim et al. 2006).

Three randomized controlled trials in people confirmed MSM takes at least 12 weeks before a beneficial effect is seen (Usha and Naidu 2004; Kim et al. 2006; Debbie et al. 2011). Pharmacokinetic studies in people and rats show MSM is rapidly absorbed with more than 50% of the substance eliminated through the urine within 24 hours (Otsuki et al. 2002; Butawan et al. 2017). A randomized, double-blinded, placebo-controlled study in humans showed a synergistic effect on the management of the pain and joint immobility associated with OA when MSM was combined with glucosamine and chondroitin sulfate (Usha and Naidu 2004). While MSM administration appears safe, the sparse human research, and absent veterinary clinical trials, highlight the need for more information before routinely recommending this nutraceutical.

Omega-3 Fatty Acids

Omega-3 polyunsaturated fatty acids (PUFAs) are found in food, especially fish and flaxseed. As fish is the most common source, the term "fish oil" is often used synonymously with omega-3 fatty acids or omega-3s. The most utilized omega-3s in veterinary medicine are EPA and DHA. EPA and DHA are found in fish and seafood.

Omega-3s play many important roles within the body. They are vital to cell membrane structure and affect the function of cell

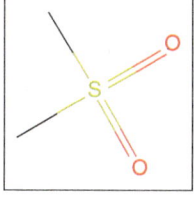

Figure 4.20 Chemical structure of methylsulfonylmethane (MSM), $C_2H_6O_2S$, aka dimethyl sulfone. Source: PubChem https://pubchem.ncbi.nlm.nih.gov/compound/6213#section=2D-Structure, September 16, 2004.

membrane receptors throughout the body (NIH 2021). They are critical to the function of multiple organs and tissues, especially the retina, brain, heart, blood vessels, lungs, immune system, and hormone (endocrine) system (NIH 2021).

The anti-inflammatory effects of omega-3s in canine and feline joints is well documented (Johnson et al. 2020). By reducing inflammation, omega-3s help restore range of motion and reduce pain. Additional veterinary studies have shown omega-3s are effective in aiding in the treatment of inflammatory skin disorders (atopy), cardiovascular disorders (arrhythmias, degenerative valve disease, anorexia caused by heart failure, and heart function), kidney disease, elevated lipid levels, inflammatory bowel disease, cognitive function, weight loss, and lymphoma survival time (with chemotherapy) (Hand et al. 2010; Bauer 2011; Magalhães et al. 2021). See Table 4.10 for examples of specific studies supporting the

Table 4.10 Studies investigating the beneficial effects of omega-3 fatty acids in veterinary medicine. The investigated body system, specific disease, species, and example studies are provided.

Body system	Diseases	Species	Studies
Cardiovascular	Arrhythmia	Canine	Smith et al. (2007), Laurent et al. (2008)
	Degenerative valve disease	Canine	Freeman et al. (1998, 2006), Nasciutti et al. (2021)
	Heart failure anorexia	Canine	Freeman et al. (1998)
	Heart function	Canine	Freeman (2010)
	Hyperlipidemia		Bauer (1995), de Albuquerque et al. (2021)
Cognition	Cognitive ability	Rat	Gamoh et al. (1999)
		Canine	Zicker et al. (2012)
Dermatologic	Allergic dermatitis	Feline	Lechowski et al. (1998)
	Atopy	Canine	Logas and Kunkle (1994), Mueller et al. (2004a, 2005), Saevik et al. (2004), Müller et al. (2016), Scott et al. (1997)
	Coat quality	Canine	Logas and Kunkle (1994), Combarros et al. (2020)
	Pruritis	Canine	Logas and Kunkle (1994), Nesbitt et al. (2003)
Gastrointestinal	Inflammatory bowel disease	Feline	Trepainer (2009), Lascelles et al. (2010)
Musculoskeletal	Osteoarthritis	Canine	Mehler et al. (2016), Fritsch et al. (2010a,b), James et al. (2010), Roush et al. (2010a,b), Moreau et al. (2013), Loef et al. (2019)
		Feline	Corbee et al. (2013)
Neoplasia	Lymphoma	Canine	Ogilvie et al. (2000)
Renal	Renal failure	Canine	Brown et al. (1998, 2000)
Respiratory	Asthma	Feline	Jérôme et al. (2010)
Ophthalmic	Development	Canine	Heinemann et al. (2005), Zicker et al. (2012)
	Keratoconjunctivitis sicca	Canine	Silva et al. (2018)

Source: Lisa P. McFaddin.

beneficial effects of omega-3 fatty acids as an adjunct treatment for a variety of conditions in veterinary medicine.

Currently there are more studies investigating the beneficial effects of omega-3s in canines compared to felines. The recommended dose is based on the species, size, and disease condition being treated, as well as the supplement type (including source and preparation) and manufacturer's recommendations. There are well-established dose ranges for canine patients, but further studies are needed to confirm the efficacy and dosage ranges for various feline conditions for which omega-3s are suspected to improve clinical outcome (Bauer 2006, 2011).

PUFAs for Veterinarians Companion animal diets, really diets for all mammals, must include essential fatty acids (EFAs), specifically PUFAs, which the body cannot synthesize itself (Bauer 2006). The presence of two or more double bonds between the carbons within the fatty acid chain separates PUFAs from saturated and monounsaturated fatty acids (NIH 2021). There are two families of essential PUFAs, omega-6 and omega-3. Omega-6 fatty acids have a carbon–carbon double bond six carbons from the methyl end of the fatty acid, as shown in Figure 4.21 (PubChem 2012a). Alternatively, omega-3 fatty acids have a carbon–carbon double bond three carbons from the methyl end, as shown in Figure 4.22 (PubChem 2012b).

Omega-6 and omega-3 fatty acids impact the structure of cell membranes through their integration into phospholipids. As a result, they directly affect cell membrane fluidity, flexibility, and permeability, as well as many cellular functions (specifically membrane-bound enzymes and cell signaling) (Higdon 2003). Dietary PUFA intake directly influences the omega-6 and omega-3 content within cell membranes (Higdon 2003).

Omega-6 Fatty Acids The parent fatty acid of omega-6 is linoleic acid which can be found in

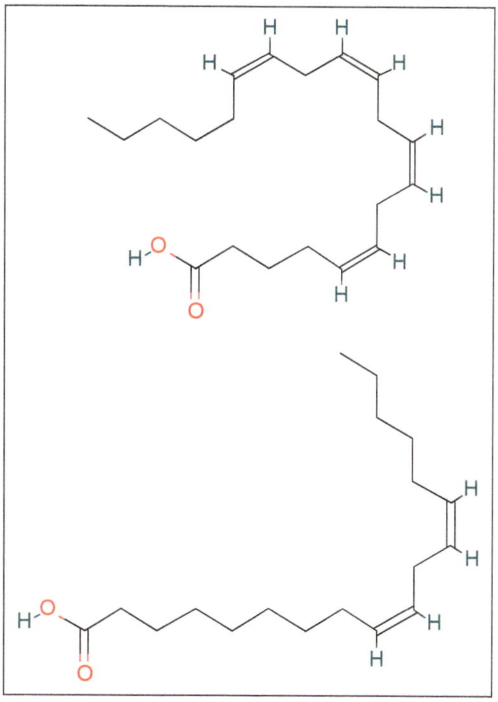

Figure 4.21 Chemical structure of omega-6 fatty acid (aka n-6 polyunsaturated fatty acid), $C_{38}H_{64}O_4$. Source: PubChem, https://pubchem.ncbi.nlm.nih.gov/compound/56842239, March 21, 2012.

vegetable oils (soybean, safflower, and corn oil), nuts (pine nuts, pecans, walnut, and Brazil nuts), seeds (hemp, sunflower, and sesame), vegetables (avocado), and meat (beef, chicken, pork, and eggs) (Higdon 2003; Whelan and Fritsche 2013). Linoleic acid can be elongated and desaturated into other bioactive omega-6 PUFAs, such as γ-linolenic acid and arachidonic acid (Higdon 2003; Whelan and Fritsche 2013). Arachidonic acid is then converted to bioactive eicosanoids like prostaglandins and leukotrienes, which are necessary for maintaining normal cell and tissue function and metabolism, but in excessive concentrations cause chronic inflammation and even cancer (Higdon 2003; Whelan 2013).

Diets low in linoleic acid lead to omega-6 fatty acid deficiencies in both dogs and cats. This condition is extremely uncommon, as almost all commercial diets contain adequate

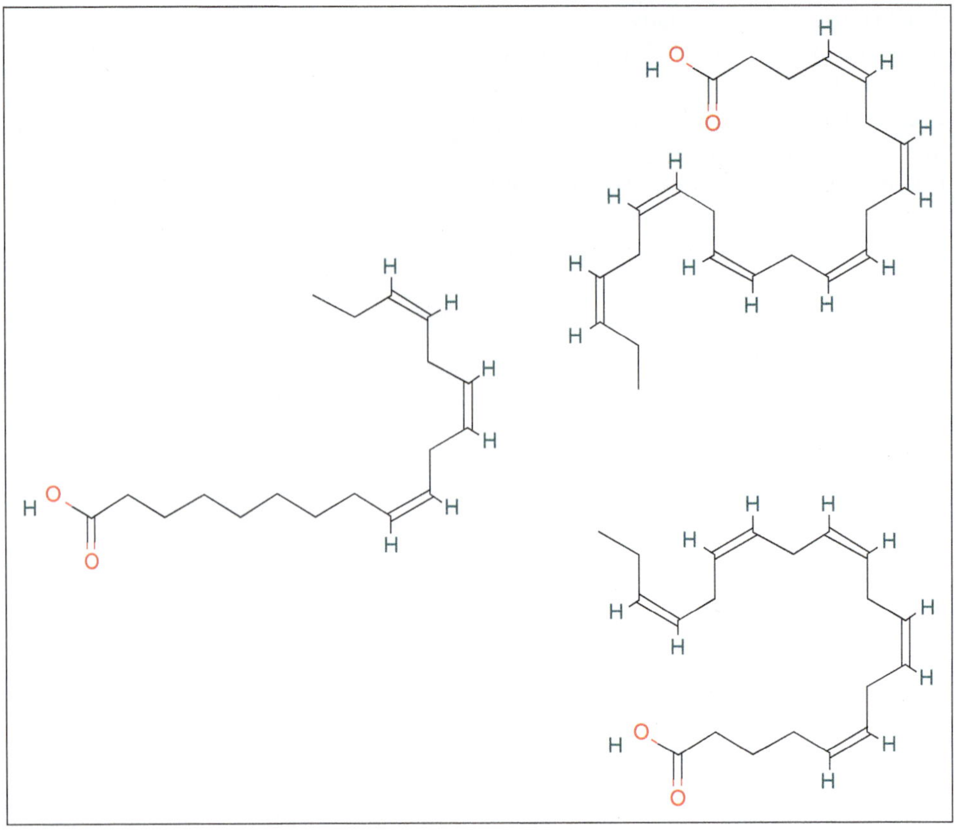

Figure 4.22 Chemical structure of omega-3 fatty acid (aka n-3 polyunsaturated fatty acid, Epanova), $C_{60}H_{62}O_6$. Source: PubChem, https://pubchem.ncbi.nlm.nih.gov/compound/56842239, March 21, 2012.

concentrations of omega-6 fatty acids (Biagi et al. 2004; Hand et al. 2010). The National Research Council (NRC) and the Association of American Feed Control Officials (AAFCO) have published the minimum requirements for all EFAs in commercially prepared cat and dog food. Refer to these references for current recommended minimum requirements.

Omega-6 deficiencies in canines typically present with dermatologic signs, such as dull coat, alopecia, and skin lesions (Biagi et al. 2004). Cats have limited D-6 desaturase activity, an enzyme that converts linoleic acid to arachidonic acid, making them more susceptible to omega-6 fatty acid deficiencies (Pawlosky et al. 1994). Cats fed diets low in linoleic acid have low growth rates, skin lesions, reduced platelet aggregation, reproductive

issues, and a propensity to develop hepatic lipidosis (Biagi et al. 2004; Bauer 2006).

Excessive PUFA intake can lead to potential gastrointestinal signs (vomiting, diarrhea, flatulence), pancreatitis (primarily in predisposed breeds), and steatitis (documented in cats with vitamin E deficiency) in animals (Momoi et al. 2001; Biagi et al. 2004). Overconsumption of omega-6 fatty acids has also been associated with increased expression of inflammatory markers and oxidative stress in chondrocytes and cartilage degradation, due to the overproduction of arachidonic acid (Loef et al. 2019).

Consumption of diets high in omega-6 (also known as a high omega-6/omega-3 ratio) in people has been associated with the development of chronic inflammatory conditions (cardiovascular disease, obesity, and nonalcoholic fatty liver disease) and an increased risk of certain cancers (D'Angelo et al. 2020). The typical standard American diet has an omega-6/omega-3 ratio of 10:1 to 25:1 (D'Angelo et al. 2020). Reducing the omega-6/omega-3 ratio (ideally 1:1 to 2:1) reduces systemic inflammation, the risk of obesity and other chronic inflammatory diseases, and the body's immediate inflammatory response following ingestion of a high-fat meal (DiNicolantonio and O'Keefe 2018).

The omega-6 to omega-3 ratio for cats and dogs recommended by the NRC has a huge range, 2.6:1 to 26:1 (NRC 2006). The *AAFCO recommends a maximum ratio of 30:1* (AAFCO 2016). Ratios higher than 10:1 have not shown beneficial effects, and in some cases lead to increased inflammatory markers in the blood (Scott et al. 1997; Kearns et al. 1999; Corbee et al. 2012). On the other hand, lowering the omega-6 to omega-3 ratio to 1.4:1, closer to the human ideal, has been shown to reduce cell-mediated immune response and PGE$_2$ production, while increasing blood lipid peroxidation levels and reducing vitamin E levels in dogs (Wander et al. 1997). Multiple studies have suggested an ideal EFA ratio is 5:1 to 6:1, with one study suggesting a ratio as

high as 10:1 for felines (Scott et al. 1997; Kearns et al. 1999; Biagi et al. 2004; Corbee et al. 2012).

Omega-3 Fatty Acids The parent fatty acid of omega-3 is the short-chain α-linolenic acid (ALA) which can be found in plant oils, such as flaxseed, walnut, canola, and soybean, and chia seeds (NIH 2021). Linoleic acid is converted to ALA in these plants through desaturation using the delta-15 desaturase enzyme (Calder 2013). Animals lack the delta-15 desaturase enzyme that make omega-3 EFAs, which must be supplied in the diet (Calder 2013). ALA serves as the precursor for long-chain omega-3 fatty acids, the most important of which are EPA and DHA, depicted in Figures 4.23 and 4.24 (Calder 2013).

The same enzymes which convert linoleic acid to arachidonic acid, delta-6 desaturase (D6D) and delta-5 desaturase (D5D), are used to convert ALA to EPA and DHA (Calder 2013). While D6D and D5D have an affinity for ALA and ETA, high linoleic acid blood levels (secondary to high dietary intake of omega-6 fatty acids) shift the enzymes' preference toward linoleic acid (Calder 2013). This limits the body's ability to self-produce EPA and DHA, requiring consumption in the diet.

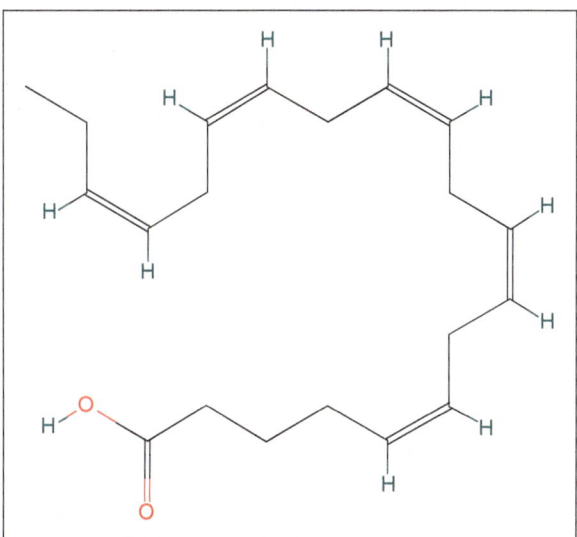

Figure 4.23 Molecular structure of eicosapentaenoic acid (aka EPA, timnodonic acid, icosapent, and icosapentaenoic acid), $C_{20}H_{30}O_2$. Source: PubChem, https://pubchem.ncbi.nlm.nih.gov/compound/446284, March 26, 2005.

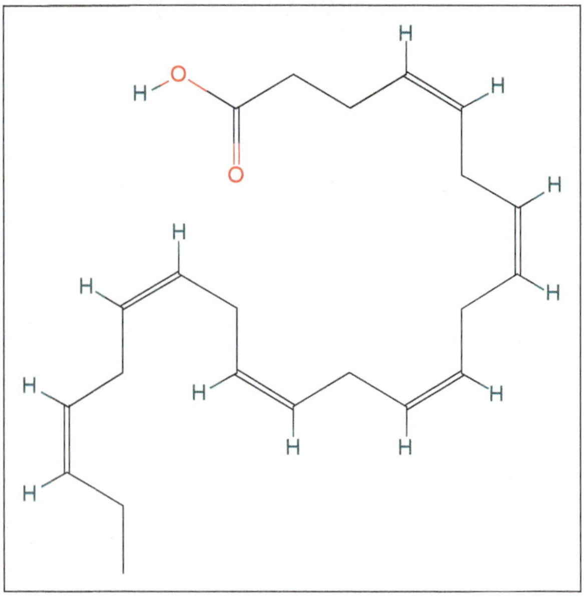

Figure 4.24 Molecular structure of docosahexaenoic acid (aka DHA, doconexent, and cervonic acid), $C_{22}H_{32}O_2$, Source: PubChem, https://pubchem.ncbi.nlm.nih.gov/compound/445580, September 16, 2004.

The 2016 AAFCO nutrient profiles require commercial cat and dog diets include the addition of ALA, EPA, and DHA (AAFCO 2016). AAFCO further established minimum percentage of dry matter for ALA and EPA plus DHA for dogs of all life stages. Despite these requirements, the dietary content of ALA, EPA, and DHA varies greatly between brands, with some diets containing very low concentrations (Dominguez et al. 2021).

The primary source of EPA and DHA, for both supplements and commercial diets, is from oily fish such as menhaden, anchovies, herring, mackerel, and krill (Higdon 2003; Dominguez et al. 2021). More recently, algal oil has been used as safe, bioavailable, and sustainable sources of long-chain omega-3 fatty acids (Dahms et al. 2019). Fish and krill primarily obtain long-chain omega-3 fatty acids from ingesting algae, which readily convert EPA to DHA using an alternate enzyme pathway (Pereira et al. 2004).

Omega-3 fatty acids are necessary to ensure normal animal growth and development, as well as the prevention of numerous chronic disease conditions (see Table 4.10). EPA and DHA exert their anti-inflammatory and cellular/tissue protective effects by interfering with the inflammatory cascade at multiple points:

decreasing the production of PGE_2 in cartilage; preventing arachidonic acid from binding with COX and LOX; decreasing the production of thromboxane A_2 and leukotrienes (thus suppressing cytokine release); and decreasing pro-matrix metalloproteinase expression in synovial fluid (Richardson et al. 1997; Lascelles et al. 2009; Roush et al. 2010a; Bauer 2011; Laflamme 2012). Many of these effects are not isolated to the joints, explaining the systemic benefit of omega-3 administration.

Omega-3 fatty acid supplementation in animals has been shown to reduce the expression of inflammatory markers and oxidative stress in chondrocytes, as well as reduce and delay cartilage degradation (Loef et al. 2019). Studies evaluating weight-bearing (force plate analysis), lameness scores, jumping abilities, and activity levels in dogs and cats confirm the beneficial effects of omega-3s in the treatment of OA (Roush et al. 2010a,b; Bauer 2011; Comblain et al. 2016). The concurrent administration of omega-3s with NSAIDs allows for the reduction or cessation of NSAIDs in dogs (Richardson et al. 1997; Comblain et al. 2016).

Omega-3 fatty acids are believed to reduce platelet activation and lower plasma coagulation factor levels (Vanschoonbeek et al. 2003).

No effect has been documented in people taking aspirin and omega-3 concurrently (Svaneborg et al. 2002). Prolonged clotting times have been noted in people taking omega-3s and warfarin (Buckley et al. 2004). Extrapolating from human research, care should be taken when recommending omega-3s to patients taking blood thinners. Omega-3s may also alter the bioavailability of lipophilic drugs (Goodman and Trepanier 2005).

Omega-3 fatty acids are susceptible to oxidation, which negatively affects their anti-inflammatory and antioxidant properties (Phung et al. 2020). The proper processing, refinement, and storage of fish oils is crucial to ensuring their purity and potency. Mildly oxidized omega-3s do not significantly alter their biochemical effects within the body (Ottestad et al. 2013). However, severely oxidized or rancid oils administered to laboratory animals, at higher than recommended doses, have shown deleterious effects including increasing newborn mortality and maternal insulin resistance in pregnant rats (Albert et al. 2016; Phung et al. 2020). To avoid these complications, ensure the product(s) you recommend are manufactured, refined, stored, and shipped appropriately. Additionally, veterinarians should review the manufacturer's quality assurance standards and product chemical analyses.

Polysulfated Glycosaminoglycans

Polysulfated glycosaminoglycans (PSGAG) are synthetic GAGs typically administered by either subcutaneous or intramuscular injection. PSGAGs can be administered by veterinary staff or by owners (once taught how to properly administer the injections). Veterinarians who practice acupuncture often use PSGAGs as a medium for aquapuncture, the injection of small volumes of sterile solutions into acupuncture points (see Chapter 1 for further information).

The dosage and frequency of administration for PSGAGs is well established. It is recommended the practitioner follow the manufacturer's recommendations with respect to dosage and administration. PSGAGs are administered in a tapering course starting multiple times a week and slowly lengthening to every three to four weeks as a long-term regimen. PSGAGs have shown improvement in signs associated with arthritis in dogs (Budsberg et al. 2007). There is currently one FDA-approved product for use in canines, Adequan.

Owner administration of subcutaneous PSGAGs has been shown to be well tolerated by dogs with mild, and typically self-resolving, side effects, including gastric upset, mild diarrhea, and pain at the injection site (Varcoe 2021). Further research is needed into the efficacy and safety of off-label use of Adequan in feline patients for the treatment of OA.

PSGAGs for Veterinarians

PSGAGs are a semi-synthetic compound composed of repeating disaccharide units and formulated by extracting GAGs from bovine tracheal cartilage (Elanco US Inc 2018). The GAG used in PGAGs is typically chondroitin sulfate with an additional three to four sulfate esters per disaccharide unit (Elanco US Inc 2018).

The exact mechanism of action is unknown but PSGAGs have been shown to increase the hydrophilic capacity of articular cartilage (improving cartilage elasticity), encourage chondrocyte synthesis of GAGs, and inhibit MMP production (anti-inflammatory effects) (Budsberg et al. 2007; Fujiki et al. 2007). Multiple *in vitro* studies and clinical trials have demonstrated PSGAGs safety and efficacy in the treatment of canine OA, though the results were not always statistically significant (de Haan et al. 1994; Sevalla et al. 2004; Budsberg et al. 2007; Fujiki et al. 2007; Elanco US Inc 2018). These studies suggest the administration of PGAGs led to a reduction in pain, improved mobility, and in some cases improved joint health.

Undenatured Type II Collagen

Undenatured type II collagen (UC-II) is a powdered, shelf-resistant supplement derived from chicken sternum cartilage (Gencoglu et al. 2020). Multiple studies have demonstrated improvement in the signs and symptoms associated with canine OA following daily administration of UC-II (Deparle et al. 2005; D'Altilio et al. 2007). UC-II functions as an anti-inflammatory and pain reducer, and protects joints and cartilage (chondroprotective) (Bagi et al. 2017).

UC-II is considered very safe and well tolerated with no adverse effects noted in the human and canine studies (Deparle et al. 2005; Marone et al. 2010). UC-II can safely be administered with other joint supplements, such as glucosamine and chondroitin sulfate (D'Altilio et al. 2007).

Current canine dose ranges are based on dosing used in previous studies. Furter studies are necessary to solidify UC-II's role as a "go-to" arthritis supplement for canines. In an unpublished abstract Blair and Bonavaud (2017) studied feline palatability and tolerance of UC-II. No clinical change was noted following administration, but the supplement was tolerated well without adverse effects. Further research is needed to investigate the efficacy and safety of UC-II in feline patients.

Additional studies are necessary to document UC-II's efficacy in the management of feline OA.

UC-II for Veterinarians The development of OA is multifactorial, including aging, chronic repetitive stress, injury, mechanical stress, genetics, and comorbidities (Gencoglu et al. 2020). All these changes lead to the development of inflammation and, eventually, structural changes within the joint. Joint inflammation is propagated by the synthesis of inflammatory mediators by joint and immune cells. These biochemical mediators include cytokines (TNF and interleukins-1, -6, -7, and -8), leukotriene inhibitory factor, proteases, PGE_2, inducible nitric oxide synthase (NOS), and leukotriene B4 (Amin et al. 2000; Abramson et al. 2001; Pelletier et al. 2001; Sandell and Aigner 2001). These compounds

stimulate the release of other proinflammatory molecules including MMPs, which play a critical role in collagen degradation and cartilage destruction (Nagase and Kashiwagi 2003; Mehana et al. 2019). Unsurprisingly, inhibition of these inflammatory mediators reduces OA progression and alleviates pain.

UC-II has been shown to induce oral tolerance, a process by which the immune system does not respond to orally administered antigens (Bagchi et al. 2002; Broere et al. 2008). UC-II activates immune cells, specifically T-cells, once it is taken up by the lymphoid tissue (called Peyer's patches) within the small intestine (Bagchi et al. 2002; Tong et al. 2009). The T-cells are transformed into T regulatory (Treg) cells which target type II collagen (Tong et al. 2009). Once Treg cells find damaged type II collagen within articular cartilage, they trigger the release of anti-inflammatory cytokines (including transforming growth factor-β, interleukin-4, and interleukin-10), reducing joint inflammation and initiating cartilage repair collagen (Tong et al. 2009).

Several studies have demonstrated UC-II's anti-inflammatory, analgesic, and chondroprotective properties in people with chronic OA and rheumatoid arthritis (Bagchi et al. 2002; Crowley et al. 2009; Lugo et al. 2013). Previous studies have shown UC-II is effective in reducing pain and lameness, as well as improving mobility in arthritic dogs (Deparle et al. 2005; D'Altilio et al. 2007; Bagchi et al. 2002; Gupta et al. 2012; Prabhoo and Billa 2018).

Collagen

As the main structural protein in connective tissue, collagens are one of the most plentiful and important proteins in the body, comprising approximately 30% of the total protein mass in mammals (Ricard-Blum 2011). All collagen is composed of amino acids linked together to form polypeptides, called α-chains. Three α-chains are bound together forming a triple helix or tropocollagen, as shown in Figure 4.25 (Bliss 2013). Within the α-chains every third amino acid is glycine. The most common collagen sequences are glycine-proline-X or glycine-X-hydroxyproline, where X can be any one of 17 different amino acids (Wu et al. 2021).

Collagen synthesis primarily occurs within fibroblasts, but extracellular synthesis can also occur. Transcription and translation of the α-chain genes within the cell create a pre-pro-polypeptide (Wu et al. 2021). The pre-pro-polypeptide becomes a procollagen following post-translational modifications within the endoplasmic reticulum (Wu et al. 2021). The procollagen is excreted from the cell in secretory vesicles following additional modifications within the Golgi apparatus. Once in the extracellular space collagen peptidase enzymes cleave the ends of the procollagen creating a tropocollagen (Wu et al. 2021).

The three α-chains may be identical, creating a homotrimer, or different, forming a heterotrimer. Mammals have 34 α-chain varieties, creating 28 distinct collagen types (Ricard-Blum 2011). The individual α-chains are numbered with Arabic numerals.

Collagens contain at least one triple helix and represent a diverse group of extracellular matrix glycoproteins with a tendency to form supramolecular systems (Exposito et al. 2010). Collagens are classified into several groups, but for the purposes of the musculoskeletal system the fibrillar collagens are the most important.

Type I, II, III, V, XI, XXIV, and XXVII collagens constitute the fibrillar collagen family. Type I and II are the most common collagen proteins found within the musculoskeletal system (Exposito et al. 2010). Type I collagen is found within skin, tendon, ligaments, blood vessels, organs, and bone. Type I collagen are heterotrimers arranged in long, thin cross-linked fribrils which create a structural and mechanical matrix (Exposito et al. 2010). This scaffolding increases the tensile strength of the tissue in which it is found.

Type II collagen is found in cartilage, particularly hyaline cartilage. The chemical structure of a type II collagen fragment is depicted in Figure 4.26. Type II collagen are homotrimers forming cross-linked fibrils arranged in a three-dimensional matrix which traps proteoglycan aggregates (Exposito et al. 2010). Type II collagen increases cartilage's resistance to deformation and increases tensile strength (Bliss 2013).

Amino Acids

Amino acids are organic nitrogen-containing compounds. Plants and animals synthesize proteins from amino acids. There are roughly 20 primary amino acids involved in protein synthesis in mammals (Hou and Wu 2018). Protein is a vital nutrient, serving many functions in the body including acting as a source of energy, carrying oxygen and other compounds in the blood, and ensuring muscle growth and tissue repair.

These 20 amino acids are divided into essential and nonessential. The body cannot manufacture essential amino acids (EAAs) or cannot synthesize enough EAAs to maintain health (Hou and Wu 2018). As such EAAs must be obtained from the diet. EAAs are not stored in the body for significant periods of time, necessitating repeated ingestion (Hou and Wu 2018).

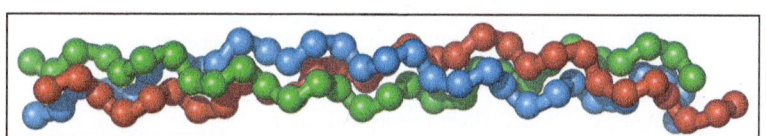

Figure 4.25 Cartoon model of the collagen triple helix (aka tropocollagen). Source: J.W. Schmidt/ Wikipedia/CC BY SA 3.0.

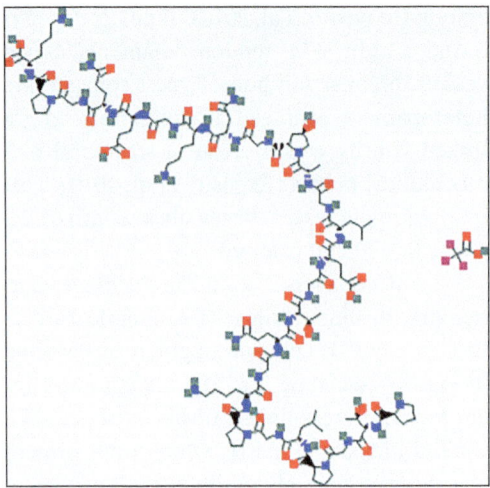

Figure 4.26 Chemical structure of a collagen type II fragment, $C_{108}H_{175}F_3N_{32}O_{39}$. Source: PubChem, https://pubchem.ncbi.nlm.nih.gov/compound/145707600, December 12, 2019.

Nonessential amino acids (NEAAs) are produced by the body in sufficient amounts and do not need to be supplemented through the diet.

Dogs have 10 EAAs: arginine, histidine, isoleucine, leucine, lysine, methionine, phenylalanine, threonine, tryptophan, and valine (Hand et al. 2010). Cats require the same EAAs plus taurine for a total of 11 EAAs (Hand et al. 2010). Commercial dog and cat foods, which meet or exceed AAFCO's nutritional requirements, contain enough EAAs to meet their basic metabolic requirements (AAFCO 2014). EAA supplements are most commonly used because a pet requires a higher concentration of an EAA than that provided in the diet (e.g. taurine supplementation in cats with certain types of heart disease) or higher concentrations of the EAA cause a beneficial effect (e.g. tryptophan given as a calming agent).

The most common EAAs used in veterinary medicine are arginine, lysine, taurine, and tryptophan. NEAAs are typically given to correct a deficiency or cause a beneficial effect. The most common NEAAs used in veterinary medicine include carnitine, glutamine, and theanine. Table 4.11 summarizes the primary supplementation uses for these amino acids. More detailed information is provided in the following sections.

Arginine

Arginine is an EAA involved in numerous processes critical for canine and feline health, including the formation of NO, synthesis of creatine, and maintenance of the body's nitrogen balance (Albaugh et al. 2017). NO is particularly important in the cardiovascular and immune systems, helping regulate blood pressure and immune defense mechanisms,

Table 4.11 The primary essential amino acids (EAA) and nonessential amino acids (NEAA) used in veterinary medicine, as well as their most important beneficial effects as of January 2023.

Amino acid	EAA vs. NEAA	Supplementation use
Arginine	EAA	Immune stimulation
Carnitine	NEAA	Weight loss; dilated cardiomyopathy[a]; hepatic lipidosis[a]
Glutamine	NEAA	Not commonly used
Lysine	EAA	Prevention and treatment of herpesvirus
Taurine	EAA (cats)	Dilated cardiomyopathy[a]; hepatic lipidosis[a]
Theanine	NEAA	Reduce anxiety and stress
Tryptophan	EAA	Reduce anxiety and stress

[a] Carnitine and taurine are typically used together to treat these conditions.
Source: Lisa P. McFaddin.

respectively (McRae 2016). Creatine is an amino acid which supplies energy to cells, particularly aiding in muscle contraction.

The term "nitrogen balance" reflects the difference between the amount of nitrogen (or protein) taken in and the amount lost (JAMA 1947). A positive nitrogen balance indicates more nitrogen (protein) is taken in than lost and muscle mass can be maintained or increased (aka anabolic state). Conversely, a negative nitrogen balance occurs when more nitrogen is lost than ingested leading to muscle wasting (aka catabolic state) (Dickerson 2016).

Human studies have demonstrated that arginine supplementation has beneficial effects on blood pressure regulation, athletic performance, and immunostimulant (Popovic et al. 2007; Zuchi et al. 2010; Dong et al. 2011; Gui et al. 2014; Kang et al. 2014; McRae 2016; Viribay et al. 2020). Canine studies are limited, with most of the available research involving terminal studies using canines as human models. Several studies have demonstrated the administration of L-arginine is cardioprotective and prevents post-ischemic (loss of oxygen supply) injury to the heart and lungs, through activation of NO (Sato et al. 1995; Ray et al. 1999; Chu et al. 2004; Soós et al. 2004).

A few feline studies have examined the effects of L-arginine on the immune system and suggest L-arginine has the potential for mild to moderate immunomodulatory properties in healthy cats (Rutherfurd-Markwick et al. 2013; Paßlack et al. 2020). L-arginine supplementation was found to be safe, without adverse effects, in both dogs and cats. Further research is needed into the practical veterinary applications of L-arginine supplementation.

Arginine for Veterinarians L-Arginine, an L-isomer of arginine depicted in Figure 4.27, is the most common form used in supplements. L-Arginine serves as a substrate for NOS which produces NO. The NO produced by the NOS in the vascular endothelium helps regulate smooth muscle relaxation (vasodilation) and is responsible for reducing blood pressure (Zuchi

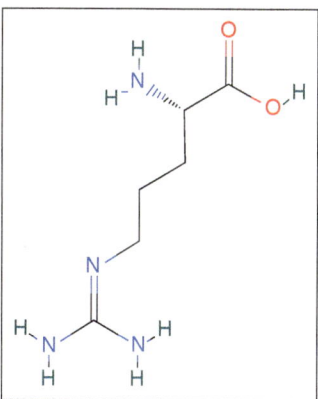

Figure 4.27 Molecular structure of arginine, $C_6H_{14}N_4O_2$. Source: PubChem, https://pubchem.ncbi.nlm.nih.gov/compound/6322, September 16, 2004.

et al. 2010). L-Arginine supplementation significantly reduces systolic and diastolic blood pressure in hypertensive adults (Dong et al. 2011; Gui et al. 2014).

NO also aids the immune system through its involvement in cell signaling and oxidative bactericidal responses (Popovic et al. 2007). L-Arginine supplementation has a positive immunostimulatory effect by increasing T-helper cell development (Popovic et al. 2007; Kang et al. 2014).

Arginine is not only vital for normal cell growth but has also been shown to be a rate-limiting step in the replication of malignant cells (Albaugh et al. 2017). The use of arginine in cancer management is a controversial topic in human oncology, with several studies touting the benefits of arginine deprivation while others supporting its supplementation (Albaugh et al. 2017). An *in vitro* study of canine lymphoma and osteosarcoma cell lines showed promise when using arginase to kill neoplastic cell lines, though further studies, including *in vivo* and clinical trials, are necessary to demonstrate efficacy and safety (Wells et al. 2013)

Carnitine

Carnitine is an NEAA found in mammalian protein, with beef containing the highest concentrations (Wynn 2001). Carnitine plays a pivotal role in energy production within the body.

Carnitine deficiencies occur most often due to problems with reabsorption or excessive loss of carnitine usually through the urine (Sanderson et al. 2001). Carnitine deficiency in dogs has been linked to the development of a specific type of heart disease (dilated cardiomyopathy, DCM) and muscle disorders (lipid storage myopathies) (Kittleson et al. 1997; Shelton et al. 1998).

Carnitine supplementation is most used in people as a weight loss supplement (with conflicting data regarding efficacy) and to improve cognition in people with dementia and Alzheimer's disease (Passeri et al. 1990; Sano et al. 1992; Villani et al. 2000; Pooyandjoo et al. 2016). Excess carnitine supplementation can lead to nausea and diarrhea in both people and animals.

Carnitine is most commonly used in companion animals to treat carnitine deficiency, as an aid in feline weight loss, as an adjunct treatment for DCM (used in conjunction with taurine, even in patients with normal carnitine levels), as an adjunct treatment for hepatic lipidosis in cats (along with taurine), and may help with some age-related changes (Kittleson et al. 1997; Center et al. 2000, 2012; Sanderson 2006; Hall and Jewell 2012; Floerchinger et al. 2015).

Carnitine for Veterinarians L-Carnitine, depicted in Figure 4.28, is the biologically active form of the amino acid synthesized from lysine and methionine (PubChem 2022d). Carnitine

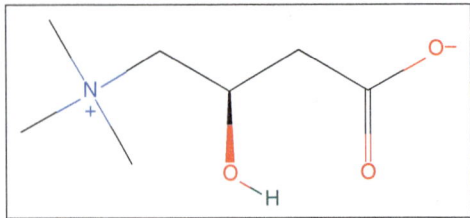

Figure 4.28 Molecular structure of L-carnitine, $C_7H_{15}NO_3$. Source: PubChem, https://pubchem.ncbi.nlm.nih.gov/compound/10917, June 1, 2005.

carries long-chain fatty acids (called acylcarnitine) into the mitochondria where they are oxidized, generating energy. Once inside the mitochondria, carnitine serves as a cofactor for the movement of acetyl-coenzyme A (CoA) out of the mitochondria, which enhances the rate of fatty acid oxidation (Wynn 2001).

As discussed, carnitine, along with taurine, is commonly used as adjunct treatment for DCM (Sanderson 2006). Supplementation is also used to counteract the effects of carnitine loss with age, often due to renal disease, which can lead to reduced serum fatty acid levels and increased systemic inflammation through oxidative damage (Kittleson et al. 1997; Hall and Jewell 2012). Unlike the results seen with people, carnitine did not improve cognitive abilities in dogs (Hall and Jewell 2012).

Carnitine has been shown to encourage weight loss in both cats and dogs by increasing energy utilization through heightened oxidation of fatty acids (Center et al. 2012; Floerchinger et al. 2015). Decreased fatty acid oxidation is one of the primary factors in the development of hepatic lipidosis in cats (Ibrahim et al. 2003). Carnitine and taurine are frequently given to cats with hepatic lipidosis to speed recovery by increasing fatty acid oxidation. Carnitine supplementation has not been shown to prevent hepatic lipidosis (Ibrahim et al. 2003).

Glutamine

Glutamine, while an NEAA, is the most abundant free amino acid in circulation. Glutamine is produced by the body and found in many foods, especially eggs, beef, milk, tofu, white rice, and corn (Lenders et al. 2009). Glutamine is required for proper cellular function and the production of protein and other amino acids (PubChem 2017).

Glutamine supplementation in people is primarily used to support the immune system (especially after surgery, major injuries or during chronic infections) and gastrointestinal system (serves as an energy source for intestinal cells and maintains the intestinal mucosal barrier which reduces bacterial translocation), and to potentially improve muscle gain and exercise performance (De-Souza and Greene 1998; Castell 2003; Fan et al. 2009; Legault et al. 2015; Cruzat et al. 2018; Shariatpanahi et al. 2019). There is now an FDA-approved form of oral L-glutamine powder used to reduce pain episodes in patients with sickle cell disease and treatment for sickle cell anemia (FDA 2017a).

Short-term supplementation in people appears safe but long-term use may negatively affect amino acid absorption and utilization (Holecek 2013). There are limited studies investigating the use of enteral glutamine in dogs and cats, and the results have been mixed.

Glutamine for Veterinarians Glutamine exists in two forms, L-glutamine and D-glutamine. L-Glutamine, depicted in Figure 4.29, is the most common form found in food and supplements (PubChem 2017).

Internal stores of glutamine become rapidly depleted during illness (Cruzat et al. 2018). Glutamine is necessary for intermediary metabolism, nitrogen exchange between

tissues and organs, pH homeostasis, supporting the immune system (particularly by serving as a source of energy for immune cells), and the synthesis of nucleotides, antioxidants and other substances needed to maintain cellular integrity and function (Cruzat et al. 2018).

Marks et al. (1999) found there was no reduction in intestinal permeability in cats treated with methotrexate and supplemented with enteral glutamine compared to those without supplementation. A trial conducted by Ohno et al. (2009) showed enteral glutamine supplementation in dogs following anesthesia and distal gastrectomy reduced the time needed to restore normal small intestinal contractions, significantly shortening the period of dysmotility compared to nonsupplemented patients.

In these studies, adverse effects associated with glutamine supplementation were considered minimal. Additional studies are needed to determine the efficacy and usefulness of glutamine supplementation.

Lysine

Lysine is an EAA found in mammalian meat, seafood, fish, and select vegetables (potatoes, peppers, and leeks), fruits (avocado, dried apricots, and pears), legumes (soy, kidney beans, and chickpeas), and nuts/seeds macadamia, pumpkin seeds, and cashews (O'Brien 2018). Lysine is crucial for normal protein and carnitine synthesis within the body (Tomé and Bos 2007).

Lysine has historically been used to prevent or treat herpesvirus outbreaks in people and cats (Wright 1994; Maggs et al. 2003). However, a systematic review of previous studies performed by Bol and Bunnik (2015) indicated lysine was not effective in the prevention or treatment of feline herpesvirus. At this point many veterinarians, me included, continue to use lysine for feline herpesvirus flare-up as anecdotally improvement is often seen.

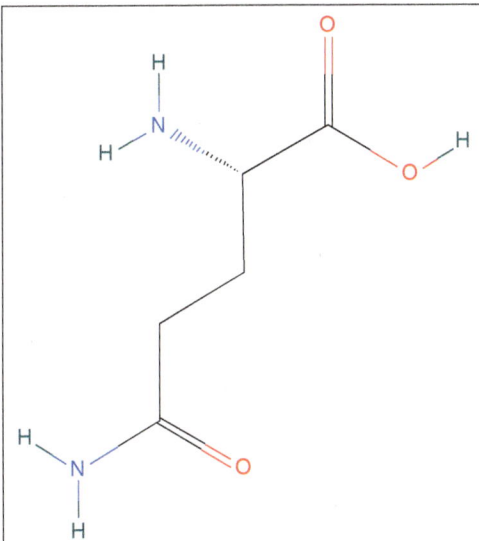

Figure 4.29 Molecular structure of glutamine, $C_5H_{10}N_2O_3$. Source: PubChem, https://pubchem.ncbi.nlm.nih.gov/compound/5961, September 16, 2004.

Lysine for Veterinarians The isomer L-lysine, depicted in Figure 4.30, is the most common form used in supplements (PubChem 2022f).

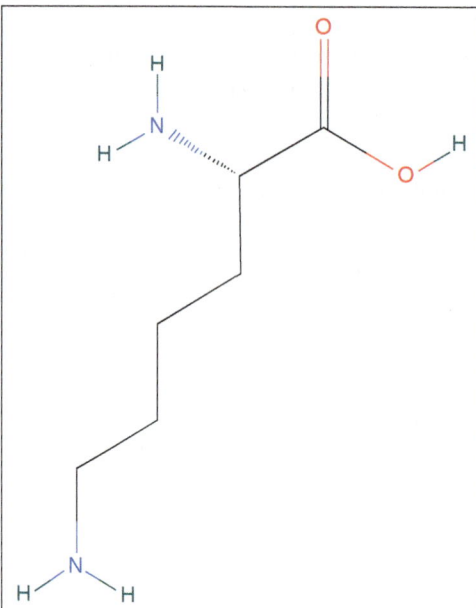

Figure 4.30 Molecular structure of lysine, $C_6H_{14}N_2O_2$. Source: PubChem, https://pubchem.ncbi.nlm.nih.gov/compound/5962, September 16, 2004.

L-Lysine supplementation has historically been used in people to prevent or treat cold sores, reduce anxiety, and improve calcium absorption and retention (Singh et al. 2011). Previous *in vitro* studies suggested L-lysine would inhibit the synthesis of arginine-rich proteins by the herpes simplex virus (HSV), preventing viral replication (Wright 1994).

A literature review by Mailoo and Rampes (2017) indicated L-lysine was ineffective in the prevention and treatment of HSV. The authors did note that higher doses (three times the recommended dose) improved patient comfort without resolution of the outbreak. L-Lysine is extremely safe, with no known toxicity in people or animals, suggesting that higher dosages may be a viable palliative treatment during a HSV flare-up (Braverman et al. 2009).

L-Lysine, especially when given in combination with L-arginine, has been shown to reduce anxiety and basal cortisol levels in healthy adults experiencing excessive levels of stress and anxiety (Smriga et al. 2007). Additionally,

early studies suggests L-lysine supplementation may help prevent and treat osteoporosis through increased dietary calcium absorption through the intestinal tract and reduced renal loss of calcium (Civitelli et al. 1992).

Veterinary use of L-lysine centers on preventing and treating feline herpesvirus type 1 (FHV-1). Initial *in vitro* studies confirmed arginine promoted FHV-1 replication, while high doses of lysine interfered with viral replication (Maggs et al. 2000). Despite Bol and Bunnik (2015), practitioners continue to prescribe the supplement. I suspect this is for two reasons. First, lysine is extremely safe, suggesting the risk of recommendation is minimal. Second, like people, cats on lysine supplementation anecdotally feel better even if viral replication is not halted.

Taurine

Taurine, depicted in Figure 4.31, is an NEAA for dogs and an EAA for cats. Taurine is naturally found in high concentrations in meat, fish, and dairy. Taurine is found in high concentrations in the brain, retina, muscle, and organs (Ripps and Shen 2012).

Taurine has multiple functions in the body including maintaining hydration status and electrolyte balance within the cells, aiding in digestion (helps form bile salts), regulating calcium levels within the cells, supporting the central nervous system and eyes, and regulating the immune system and antioxidant functions (Ripps and Shen 2012). Taurine supplementation is most used in people as an

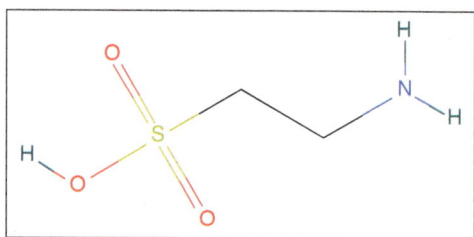

Figure 4.31 Molecular structure of taurine, $C_2H_7NO_3S$. Source: PubChem, https://pubchem.ncbi.nlm.nih.gov/compound/1123#section=2D-Structure, September 16, 2004.

adjunct treatment for diabetes, to improve cardiovascular function (lower blood pressure, lower cholesterol, reduce the risk of death from heart disease), increase athletic performance (protects muscle cells from damage and oxidative stress), and as an antioxidant (Militante and Lombardini 2002; Franconi et al. 2006; Abebe and Mozaffari 2011; Balshaw et al. 2012; Murakami 2014; PubChem 2022i).

Taurine supplementation in people has been used to aid in the treatment of cystic fibrosis and hypertension and as an antioxidant (PubChem 2022i). Taurine deficiency in companion animals leads to a specific type of heart disease called dilated cardiomyopathy. Taurine deficiency can also cause kidney dysfunction, developmental abnormalities, and severe retinal damage (Ripps and Shen 2012). Taurine supplementation is most used in companion animals for the treatment of taurine deficiency, as an adjunct to DCM treatment (with carnitine), and as an adjunct treatment for hepatic lipidosis (with carnitine) in cats (Kittleson et al. 1997; Ibrahim et al. 2003; Sanderson 2006).

Theanine

Theanine is a nonprotein NEAA commonly found in the plant species *Camellia*, specifically green tea or *Camellia sinensis* (Cartwright et al. 1954). L-Theanine, the active and most common form of theanine, comprises 1–2% of the dry weight of green tea (Cartwright et al. 1954). L-Theanine is responsible for the calming properties induced by green tea consumption (Juneja et al. 1999; Kakuda 2002). Commercially available L-theanine is either extracted from green tea or made synthetically.

L-Theanine is most used as a natural calming aid in people. Similarly, L-theanine is utilized in companion animals to reduce anxiety and stress, especially in separation anxiety, noise phobias, and inter-cat or inter-dog aggression (Pike et al. 2015; Araujo et al. 2018; Dramard et al. 2018).

Theanine for Veterinarians   L-Theanine, depicted Figure 4.32, is the most common bioavailable

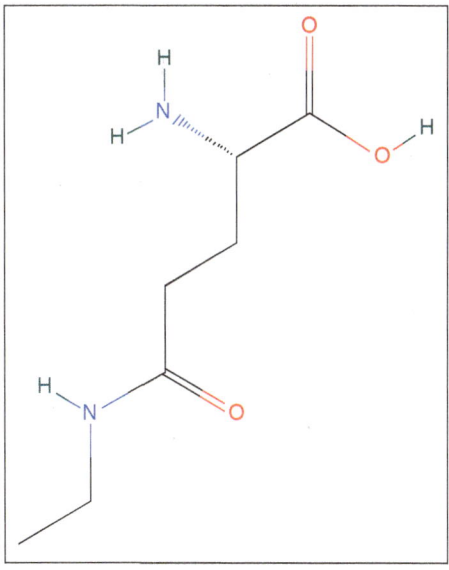

Figure 4.32   Molecular structure of L-theanine, $C_7H_{14}N_2O_3$. Source: PubChem, https://pubchem.ncbi.nlm.nih.gov/compound/439378, September 16, 2004.

form of theanine (PubChem 2022e). It can cross the blood–brain barrier within one hour after administration and remains in the plasma and brain for a few hours (Juneja et al. 1999). Human studies determined the relaxation effects of L-theanine are due to the generation of alpha waves in the brain (Juneja et al. 1999; Nobre et al. 2008). The greatest concentration of alpha waves (8–12 Hz) occurs during a relaxed, awake, and alert state. L-Theanine also helps reduce the body's physiological responses to stress, i.e. regulating blood pressure, heart rate, and cortisol secretion (Kimura et al. 2007).

In vivo studies have shown L-theanine exerts its effects primarily through its relationship with glutamate. Theanine is a natural analog and antagonist of glutamate, the primary excitatory neurotransmitter in the brain. L-Theanine can interfere with glutamate receptors and transporters, providing a neuroprotective effect (Kakuda 2002). Additionally, L-theanine increases gamma-aminobutryric acid (GABA) activity, a calming neurotransmitter, contributing to its calming effects (Kimura and Murata 1971).

Araujo et al. (2018) confirmed that the administration of L-theanine reduced fear levels in dogs typically scared of unfamiliar people. Pike et al. (2015) discovered L-theanine was effective in reducing dogs' overall responses to thunderstorms (drooling, clinging to owners, pacing, panting, and hiding) and increased the speed with which dogs returned to normal behavior following cessation of the storm.

Dramard et al. (2018) showed L-theanine was effective in reducing anxiety and stress in cats with several behavioral issues (inappropriate urination and defecation, fear aggression, hypervigilance, and self-barbering) as early as 15 days after supplementation. The application of L-theanine for feline lower urinary tract disease should be investigated as well. Side effects were not noted with L-theanine administration in either dogs or cats.

Tryptophan

Tryptophan is an EAA involved in protein synthesis and the production of several important bioactive substances in the body, including serotonin, melatonin, and vitamin B3 (niacin) (Höglund et al. 2019; PubChem 2022j). Serotonin is a neurotransmitter which affects mood and the body's stress response. Melatonin is a hormone produced by the brain which helps regulate our sleep–wake cycle. Vitamin B3 (niacin) is used to turn food into energy and keep the nervous system, digestive system, and skin healthy.

Tryptophan is typically obtained in the food, with chicken, eggs, cheese, fish, peanuts, pumpkin seeds, sesame seeds, milk, turkey, and soy having the highest concentrations (Friedman 2018). Synthetic tryptophan is also commercially available.

Tryptophan is most used in people to treat insomnia and other sleep disorders, anxiety and depression, and to improve overall emotional well-being (Paredes et al. 2009; Le Floc'h et al. 2011; Friedman 2018). Side effects with supplementation are uncommon but do occur, typically involving the gastrointestinal tract (heartburn, stomach pain, belching, vomiting, nausea, diarrhea, and inappetance) (Friedman 2018; Tinsley 2021). Headaches, dry mouth, and sexual dysfunction are also seen. In rare instances people can experience drowsiness, lightheadedness, blurred vision, muscle pain, skin rashes, cramping, difficulty breathing, fatigue, eosinophilia-myalgia syndrome, and even death (Friedman 2018; Tinsley 2021). Tryptophan–drug interactions may occur with any medication which increases serotonin levels.

Tryptophan is most used in veterinary medicine as a calming agent for both cats and dogs (DeNapoli et al. 2000; Kato et al. 2012; Landsberg et al. 2016; Naarden and Corbee 2019). Tryptophan supplementation in companion animals has been found to be very safe with minimal side effects.

Tryptophan for Veterinarians Tryptophan, depicted in Figure 4.33, serves as a substrate for the production of serotonin (5-hydroxytryptamine or 5-HT) in the brain and the gut, as well as melatonin in the pineal gland (Gao et al. 2018; Höglund et al. 2019). Tryptophan is catabolized and transformed into bioactive

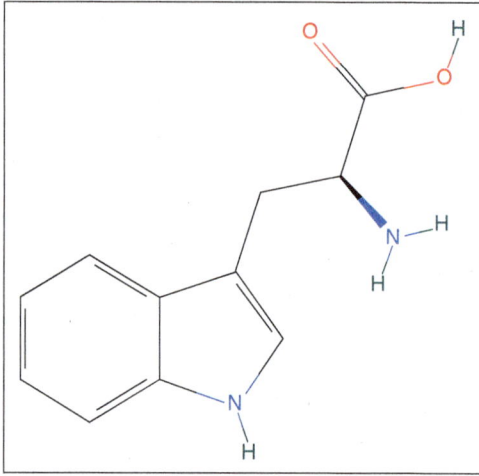

Figure 4.33 Molecular structure of L-tryptophan, $C_{11}H_{12}N_2O_2$. Source: PubChem, https://pubchem.ncbi.nlm.nih.gov/compound/6305, September 16, 2004.

substances through the kynurenic pathway (PubChem 2022j). These reactions are affected by the body's stress response to various insults. Tryptophan degradation also plays a role in the regulation of immune responses during infection, inflammation, and pregnancy (Le Floc'h et al. 2011; Gao et al. 2018).

Changes to the diet and gut microbiota have been shown to affect tryptophan's bioavailability in people (Reilly et al. 1997; Gao et al. 2018). Tryptophan depletion influences mood disorders in people affecting serotonin levels (Reilly et al. 1997; Le Floc'h et al. 2011). Interestingly, low tryptophan levels have been documented in many individuals diagnosed with anxiety and depression (Friedman 2018). This becomes a chicken and egg situation, begging the question which came first: low tryptophan levels or anxiety and depression?

Studies investigating the efficacy of tryptophan as an anxiolytic in companion animals have had mixed results. DeNapoli et al. (2000) noted modest improvement in dominance aggression when dogs were fed tryptophan-enriched high-protein diets or a low-protein diets without tryptophan supplementation. Dogs with territorial aggression fed a low-protein diet enriched with tryptophan also experienced reduced aggression. Kato et al. (2012) found a diet supplemented with α-casozepine and L-tryptophan seemed to improve the dogs' ability to deal with stress and reduce anxiety-related behaviors.

While Templeman et al. (2018) cited no behavioral differences between dogs fed a tryptophan-enriched diet compared to those fed a control diet, when exposed to familiar and unfamiliar people. Another study by Templeman et al. (2019) found breed differences in the required amount of dietary tryptophan. Additionally, the dietary tryptophan requirements for all dogs in the study was higher than the current AAFCO and NRC recommendations (NRC 2006; AAFCO 2014).

For cats tryptophan has been added to prescription urinary diets formulated to minimize and ideally prevent the recurrence of feline idiopathic cystitis (FIC). A study conducted by Naarden and Corbee (2019) revealed no statistical difference in the rate of recurrence of FIC symptoms (defined as having at least two of the following signs: stanguria, periuria, hematuria, dysuria, and pollakiuria) between the tryptophan-enhanced and regular diet. Similarly, Miyaji et al. (2015) found feeding cats a prescription diet enriched with tryptophan raised plasma tryptophan levels but had no effect on plasma cortisol levels. Alternatively, Landsberg et al. (2016) discovered cats fed a diet supplemented with L-tryptophan and α-casozepine had reduced stress responses when placed in an unfamiliar location, but the supplementation did not improve their reactions when exposed to unfamiliar people. While tryptophan may hold promise in reducing stress and anxiety, as well as helping pets cope with stressful situations more readily, further research is necessary for efficacy confirmation.

Antioxidants and Free Radical Scavengers

Antioxidants are synthetic or natural substances which prevent or delay cell damage. Free radical scavengers protect cells from damage caused by free radicals. Free radicals are unstable molecules naturally created during cell metabolism. Free radicals can build up over time within the cell and cause damage. Antioxidants are a type of free radical scavenger. Going forward, I will refer to antioxidants specifically but highlight when/if the substance also functions as a free radical scavenger.

Free radicals are created by damaged tissues and by the immune cells responding to the area of inflammation (Manzanares et al. 2012). There are two types of free radicals: reactive oxygen species (ROS) and reactive nitrogen species (RNS). Cellular damage causes free radical formation which causes more damage, leading to more free radical formation and creating a self-perpetuating cycle. Cancer is an extreme example and consequence of this cycle.

All animals have an inherent (endogenous) antioxidant defense system consisting of substances (enzymes, proteins, and vitamins) within and outside of the cell that attack and attempt to inactivate ROS and RNS (Chan 2019). If the amount of oxidative stress (i.e. quantity of ROS and RNS) overwhelms the endogenous antioxidant system, irreparable damage can occur to molecules and tissues within the body. This is where the theory of antioxidant supplementation comes into play. By providing the body with additional outside (exogenous) sources of antioxidants, damage from free radicals should be reduced and ideally stopped.

Fruits and vegetables have high antioxidant content. The United States Government recommends all people eat a diet high in fruits and vegetables in part because research suggests these individuals have a lower risk of certain diseases (NCCIH 2013). The National Center for Complementary and Integrative Health (NCCIH) and the National Institutes of Health (NIH) do not recommend antioxidant supplementation, citing a lack of scientific evidence supporting their efficacy and potential risk for adverse effects and drug interactions (NCCIH 2013).

Large, randomized, placebo-controlled trials investigating the use of antioxidant supplements in human medicine have yielded overwhelmingly inconclusive or negative results (Harvard School of Public Health 2022). For an in-depth look into the NCCIH's and Harvard's recommendations, refer to their websites.

Proponents of antioxidant supplements are very vocal, as evidenced by the countless advertisements for antioxidant-rich berries, drinks, food, and supplements plastering our televisions and the internet. Personally, I feel antioxidants can be very useful, but like anything else there is no magic pill to cure everything.

Antioxidant nutraceuticals are utilized regularly in veterinary medicine, but the supporting evidence, like that in human medicine, is conflicting. Part of the problem is the general lack of available research. Hagen et al. (2019) measured blood levels for oxidative stress (oxidative biomarkers) in sick dogs receiving antioxidant supplements (combination of *N*-acetylcysteine, *S*-adenosylmethionine, silybin, and vitamin E) compared to those without supplementation. The authors found no statistical difference in oxidative biomarker levels between the two groups. In contrast, Sechi et al. (2017) found long-term dietary supplementation with antioxidants improved cellular metabolism and reduced free radicals in dogs.

Despite these conflicting results the most commonly used antioxidants in veterinary medicine include astaxanthin, coenzyme Q10, curcumin, milk thistle, *N*-acetylcysteine, omega-3 fatty acid, quercetin, resveratrol, *S*-adenosylmethionine, and vitamins C and E. Table 4.12 summarizes the beneficial effects of commonly used antioxidant supplements in veterinary medicine. Curcumin, omega-3 fatty acids and vitamins C and E are discussed in earlier sections. The remaining antioxidants are discussed in more detail in the following sections.

Astaxanthin

Astaxanthin is a red pigment commonly found in certain algae (*Haematococcus pluvialis*, *Chlorella zofingiensis*, and *Chlorococcum*) and yeast (*Phaffia rhodozyma*) and is responsible for giving salmon, shrimp, and other seafood their reddish color (Higuera-Ciapara et al. 2006). The FDA has approved astaxanthin as a color and food additive for specific uses in certain animal feed, primarily salmonid (FDA 2022c). *Haematococcus pluvialis* is the preferred source for astaxanthin due to its high percentage of the pigment per dry matter and superior absorption compared to synthetic astaxanthin (Higuera-Ciapara et al. 2006).

Astaxanthin, as a very potent antioxidant, has multiple biological activities and health benefits in people and animals, and is a common human nutritional supplement (Rao et al. 2014). Astaxanthin supplementation is most used in people for its beneficial effects in cardiovascular

Table 4.12 The most used antioxidant supplements in veterinary medicine with the primary beneficial effects as of January 2023.

Antioxidant	Source	Beneficial effects
Astaxanthin	Algae and yeast	Immune modulating; immune stimulant; improves exercise performance; reduces exercise fatigue; anti-inflammatory
Coenzyme Q10	Oily fish, organ meat, whole grains	Cardiac and skeletal muscle protectant
Curcumin	Turmeric spice	Anti-inflammatory; antioxidant; hepatoprotective; cholagogue; antiplatelet; anticancer
Glutathione	Mammalian tissue	Semen extender; increases antitumor effects of chemotherapeutic agents
Milk thistle	*Silybum marianum*	Hepatoprotectant; supports the immune system
N-Acetylcysteine	Synthetic	Acetaminophen toxicity; reduces respiratory inflammation in chronic bronchitis; supports the immune system in feline immunodeficiency virus
Omega-3 fatty acid	Fish, flaxseed	Cardioprotectant; anti-arrhythmogenic; improves cognitive abilities; lowers blood lipid levels; improves epidermis and coat quality; reduces gut inflammation; improves renal function; decreases lung inflammation; protects ocular development; improves dry eye
Quercetin	Dietary (fruits/vegetables)	Antitumor activity; anti-inflammatory; analgesic
Resveratrol	Plants (grapes, berries, peanuts)	Immune supporting and stimulating; anti-aging; helps kill cancer cells
S-Adenosyl methionine (SAMe)	Within the body synthetic	Hepatoprotective; improves cognitive function; delays cognitive decline
Vitamin C	Dietary (fruits/Vegetables)	Immune stimulating; improves collagen synthesis and tissue repair; improves lipid and protein synthesis
Vitamin E	Dietary (plant-based oil, nuts and seeds, fruits/vegetables)	Improves cell health; anti-inflammatory; inhibits tumor growth; improves hepatic and gallbladder function; supports the skin

Source: Lisa P. McFaddin.

disease prevention, immune modulation and stimulation, gastric ulcer resolution (especially caused by *Helicobacter pylori* infections), anti-diabetic, reduction of ocular inflammation, anticancer activity, and skin protection activity (Tanaka et al. 1995; Jyonouchi et al. 2000; Uchiyama et al. 2002; Chew and Jean 2004; Higuera-Ciapara et al. 2006; Suzuki et al. 2006; Kamath et al. 2008; Park et al. 2010; Fassett and Coombes 2011; Augusti et al. 2012; Davinelli et al. 2018; Pereira et al. 2021).

While companion animal research is limited, there have been several well-designed trials supporting the use of astaxanthin as an immune modulatory and stimulating agent (Chew et al. 2011; Park et al. 2013). Astaxanthin may also be useful in improving exercise performance and mitigating exercise-induced fatigue in canine athletes (Zanghi et al. 2015). Astaxanthin consumption in food and supplement form is considered very safe for animals and people with no significant adverse effects reported in the literature (Stewart et al. 2008; Rao et al. 2014; Turck et al. 2020).

Astaxanthin for Veterinarians Astaxanthin, depicted in Figure 4.34, is classified as a fat-soluble xanthophyll and nonprovitamin A carotenoid (PubChem 2005a). The unique molecular structure of astaxanthin allows the pigment to function outside and inside cells (Rao et al. 2014). Astaxanthin has a myriad of biological activities, including inhibition of oxidation (antioxidant) and lipid peroxidation, and is anti-inflammatory and antidiabetic (by reducing the oxidative stress caused by hyperglycemia) (Naguib 2000; Uchiyama et al. 2002; Suzuki et al. 2006; Kamath et al. 2008; Park et al. 2010; Rao et al. 2014; Sztretye et al. 2019; Wu et al. 2019).

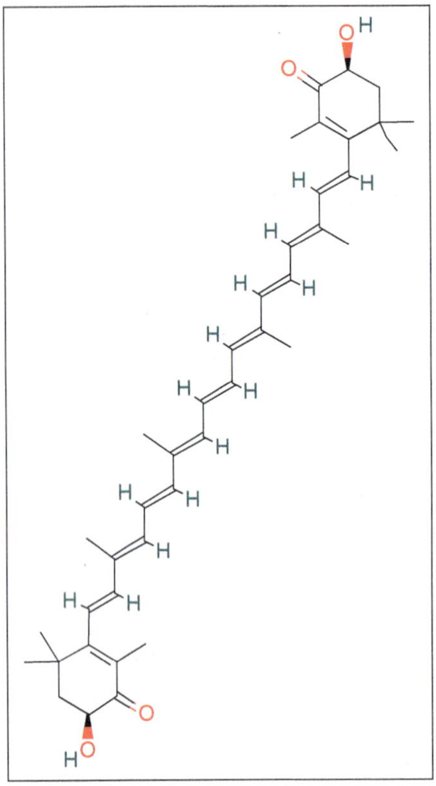

Figure 4.34 The molecular structure of astaxanthin, $C_{40}H_{52}O_4$. Source: PubChem, https://pubchem.ncbi.nlm.nih.gov/compound/5281224, June 24, 2005.

Veterinary research, while limited, has proven its potent antioxidant effects in companion animals. Chew et al. (2011) demonstrated astaxanthin improved cell-mediated and humoral immune responses and reduced DNA damage in beagles. Plasma astaxanthin levels were dose dependent, with peak absorption occurring six weeks after supplementation was initiated. Park et al. (2013) determined that astaxanthin supplementation reduced age-related oxidative and inflammatory damage and enhanced mitochondrial function in female beagles of all ages, though the effect was greater in geriatric compared to young dogs. Zanghi et al. (2015) found feeding astaxanthin to canine athletes increased plasma triglyceride levels before exercise and prevented exercise-induced plasma glucose depletion, indicating supplementation may improve exercise performance and reduce fatigue.

Animal studies suggest that bioavailability is increased when astaxanthin is ingested in the form of *Haematococcus* (Rao et al. 2014). Consumption with dietary oils has also been shown to increase absorption (Rao et al. 2014).

Coenzyme Q10

Coenzyme Q10 (CoQ10) is a ubiquitous molecule found within every cell membrane and is commonly ingested in the diet (Snood and Keenaghan 2022). The primary dietary sources of CoQ10 are oily fish (salmon, tuna), organ meat (liver), and whole grains (Saini 2011). This vitamin-like molecule provides energy to cells, ensures proper organ function, assists chemical reactions, and acts as an antioxidant (Snood and Keenaghan 2022).

CoQ10 supplementation has been used successfully in people to reduce the symptoms associated with moderate-to-severe heart failure and other adverse cardiovascular events (Jafari et al. 2018). CoQ10 has also shown promise in the reduction of frequency of migraine headaches (Sándor et al. 2005).

CoQ10 is used most as an adjunct in the treatment of certain types of heart disease and muscle disorders, primarily in the dog

(Sattawaphaet 2018). CoQ10 likely has a lot more to offer our companion animals, but further research is necessary to best assess its role in veterinary medicine.

CoQ10 supplementation, even at very high doses, has been shown to be very safe in dogs and people, with few to no side effects (Yerramilli-Rao et al. 2012). CoQ10 is fat-soluble and best absorbed when ingested with an oil or fat (Saini 2011).

Coenzyme Q10 for Veterinarians CoQ10, depicted in Figure 4.35, is also known as ubiquinone. It is a fat-soluble vitamin-like molecule found within every cell membrane (PubChem 2022b). CoQ10 supplements are available in the oxidized form (ubiquinone) or the reduced form (ubiquinol). The bioavailability in people and animals is dependent on the carrier lipids and preservatives used (López-Lluch et al. 2019).

CoQ10 has a pivotal role in the transfer of electrons within the mitochondrial oxidative respiratory chain and adenosine triphosphate (ATP) production (Schniertshauer et al. 2016). CoQ10 functions as an antioxidant, increases the production of superoxide dismutase (another antioxidant), reduces lipid peroxidation levels, and preserves NO which improves blood flow and protects blood vessels (Kędziora-Kornatowska et al. 2010; Cordero et al. 2012; Schniertshauer et al. 2016; Snood and Keenaghan 2022).

Human studies demonstrate CoQ10 can improve heart cell function and left ventricular contractility in heart failure patients (Jafari et al. 2018). CoQ10 has also been shown to improve endothelial function in patients with other forms of heart disease and type 2 diabetes (Zozina et al. 2018).

The available veterinary research is limited. CoQ10 has shown promise as an adjunct treatment in dogs with myxomatous degenerative mitral valve disease (Sattawaphaet 2018). CoQ10 may be useful in the prevention and treatment of cardiac arrest patients (Ren et al. 1994). The use of CoQ10 in the treatment of myopathies is primarily based on case studies, extrapolation of data from other species, and *in vitro* testing. Randomized prospective clinical trials are necessary to confirm the applications and efficacy of CoQ10 supplementation.

Glutathione

Glutathione (GSH) is composed of three amino acids (cysteine, glutamic acid, and glycine) and is found in most mammalian tissue. GSH functions as an antioxidant, improves metabolic detoxification, and helps regulate the immune system within the body (Pizzorno 2014; Minich and Brown 2019). The effects of GSH and its deficiencies are well studied. Many age-related changes in people (neurologic degeneration, mitochondrial dysfunction, and cancer) have been linked to suboptimal or low levels of GSH (Franco et al. 2007; Ballatori et al. 2009).

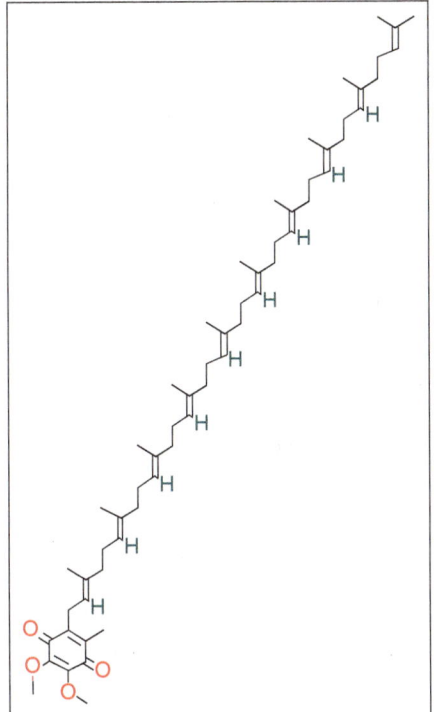

Figure 4.35 The molecular structure of coenzyme Q10, $C_{59}H_{90}O_4$. Source: Pubchem, https://pubchem.ncbi.nlm.nih.gov/compound/5281915, March 26, 2005.

GSH supplementation studies are relatively limited in people, often yielding conflicting results. Some studies have raised concerns regarding the usefulness of GSH supplementation. Allen and Bradley (2011) found no improvement in oxidative stress biomarkers in subjects given GSH for four weeks, while other studies indicate GSH supplement (in oral, nebulized, transdermal, and topical formulations) may aid in the treatment of certain chronic neurologic, cardiovascular, and respiratory conditions, cystic fibrosis, autism, chronic otitis media, nail biting, and in reducing lipoprotein (LDL) cholesterol (Testa et al. 2001; Arosio et al. 2002; Bishop et al. 2005; Kern et al. 2011; Pizzorno 2014; Campolo et al. 2017).

GSH research in companion animals is limited. Currently there are no studies investigating the systemic effects of GSH supplementation in companion animals. Research is focused on how the administration of other antioxidants affect endogenous GSH levels (Hill et al. 2005; Viviano and VanderWielen 2013). Clinical trials examining the efficacy of GSH supplementation are necessary to gauge its usefulness as a nutraceutical.

Glutathione for Veterinarians GSH, depicted in Figure 4.36, is a tripeptide composed of cysteine, glycine, and glutamic acid (Pizzorno 2014; PubChem 2022c). Its primary roles are to reduce oxidative stress, maintain redox balance, promote the activity of other antioxidants, activate enzymes, support the synthesis and repair of DNA, proteins, and prostaglandins, and support and regulate the immune system (Minich and Brown 2019).

As stated previously, companion animal GSH research is limited. Several veterinary studies have shown GSH added to freezing extenders improved canine semen quality post-thaw and sperm longevity (Monteiro et al. 2009; Lucio et al. 2016; Del Prete et al. 2018). Małek et al. (2021) confirmed the use of doxorubicin conjugated with GSH-stabilized gold nanoparticles improved the chemotherapeutic agent's antitumor and cytotoxic effects. Obviously further research is necessary to determine the safety and efficacy of GSH supplementation.

Milk Thistle

Milk thistle (aka silymarin), pictured in Figure 4.37, is an herbal supplement derived from the *Silybum marianum* plant. This phytochemical has been used as a functional food for more than 2000 years to treat a variety of liver conditions (Delmas et al. 2020). More recently, silymarin has been used to aid in the treatment of alcoholic liver disease, drug- and toxin-induced liver disease, gallbladder disease, conditions affecting bile production and flow, liver cancer, and viral hepatitis (Frederico et al. 2017; Tighe et al. 2020). Silymarin has also been used to minimize the effects of Alzheimer's disease and other neurologic conditions causing cognitive decline, as a

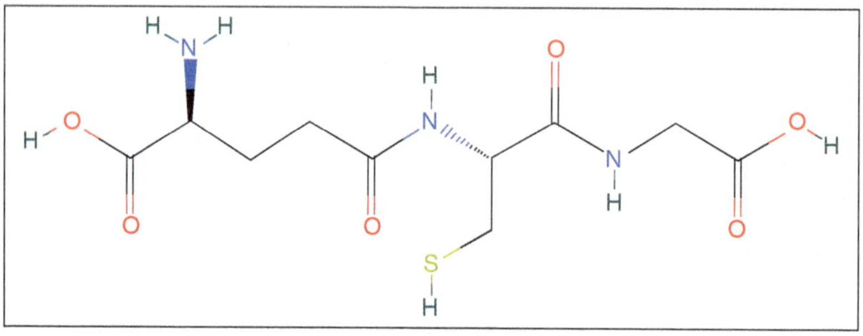

Figure 4.36 Molecular structure of glutathione, $C_{10}H_{17}N_3O_6S$. Source: PubChem, https://pubchem.ncbi.nlm.nih.gov/compound/124886#section=2D-Structure, June 8, 2005.

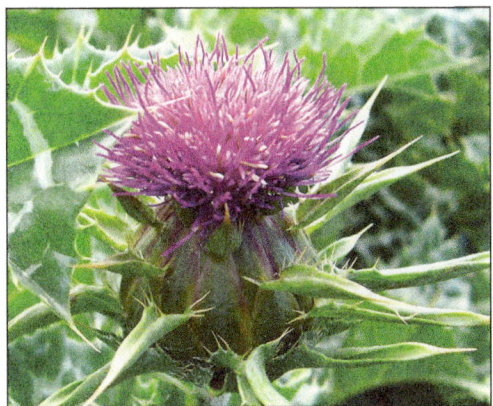

Figure 4.37 Photograph of the milk thistle (*Silybum marianum*) plant. Source: Fir0002/ Wikimedia Commons/CC BY-SA 3.0.

chemopreventative and chemosensitizer, and as an antiviral agent (Guo et al. 2019a; Liu et al. 2019; Delmas et al. 2020). Silymarin is most used in companion animals as a liver protectant and to aid in the treatment of a wide range of liver conditions (Webster and Copper 2009; Marchegiani et al. 2020).

According to the NCCIH, a division of the NIH, silymarin is well tolerated and safe at recommended doses (NCCIH 2020). If adverse effects do occur, they are generally mild and involve the gastrointestinal tract. Allergic reactions have been documented in people allergic to related plants such as ragweed, daisy, chrysanthemum, and marigold (NCCIH 2020). The NCCIH also recommends people with type 2 diabetes use caution as silymarin may lower blood glucose levels (NCCIH 2020). The safety and efficacy of silymarin in companion animals has, thus far, been similar.

Milk Thistle for Veterinarians   The milk thistle supplement is created using a lipophilic extract from the seed of the *Silybum marianum* plant. The active ingredients, collectively known as silymarin, are three isomer flavonolignans, silybin, silydianin, and silychristin (Abenavoli et al. 2010). The most biologically active component, silybin, comprises 50–70% of silymarin (Abenavoli et al. 2010).

Silymarin functions as an antioxidant (reduces free radical production and lipid peroxidation), antifibrotic, hepatoregenerative, choleretic, anti-hepatotoxin, immunomodulatory agent, and as an anti-inflammatory (Abenavoli et al. 2010; Tighe et al. 2020).

The phytochemical has poor bioavailability primarily because of its lipophilic nature, reducing solubility (Tighe et al. 2020). Different formulations have been created for human and animal supplements, all with an attempt to improve bioavailability (Yan-ui et al. 2006). Silymarin exhibits negligible inhibition of cytochrome P450 enzymes, even at supratherapeutic doses, suggesting drug–herb interactions are unlikely at therapeutic doses (Tighe et al. 2020).

The hepatoprotective effects of silymarin are well studied in companion animals, especially when combined with *S*-adenosylmethionine and other potent antioxidants, vitamin E and *N*-acetylcysteine (Webster and Copper 2009; Avizeh et al. 2010; Skorupski et al. 2011; Au et al. 2012). The antioxidant and anti-inflammatory properties of silymarin have also proven effective in the management of canine sepsis, acute systemic inflammation, and gentamicin-induce nephrotoxicity (Varzi et al. 2007; Soltanian et al. 2020).

N-Acetylcysteine

N-Acetylcysteine (NAC) is a synthetic and modified form of the amino acid cysteine (PubChem 2022a). NAC supplementation has multiple functions, including GSH biosynthesis, detoxification, free radical scavenger, and as a powerful antioxidant (Mokhtari et al. 2017). NAC has been well studied and proven to be very safe (Mokhtari et al. 2017).

NAC plays a major role in liver and kidney detoxification, including treating people with acetaminophen overdose, liver and kidney infection, chronic liver or kidney diseases, and liver cancer (Green et al. 2013; Mokhtari et al. 2017). NAC has been used for over 30 years to treat acetaminophen toxicity in cats (St. Omer and McKnight 1980; Gaunt et al. 1981).

NAC has a well-established safety profile in humans and animals. If adverse effects are noted, signs typically involve the gastrointestinal tract (nausea, vomiting) (Tenório et al. 2021).

N-Acetylcysteine for Veterinarians NAC, depicted in Figure 4.38, is metabolized into cysteine within the body (PubChem 2022a). Cysteine, a nonessential amino acid created from methionine and serine, is a precursor of GSH (PubChem 2022a). Much of NAC's antioxidant abilities are derived from its ability to stimulate GSH synthesis, along with glutamic acid and glycine (Minich and Brown 2019).

While NAC is best known for its role in treating nephrotoxicity and hepatotoxicity, NAC has been used for multiple conditions in people. NAC is a mucolytic agent and can be used to reduce the frequency and severity of symptoms associated with chronic bronchitis (Stey et al. 2000). NAC has been used as an adjunct treatment for gynecological issues, such as polycystic ovary syndrome, premature birth, recurrent pregnancy loss, and infertility (Mokhtari et al. 2017). NAC has been shown to aid in the treatment of a variety of other inflammatory conditions, including ulcerative colitis, chronic obstructive pulmonary disease, and asthma (Mokhtari et al. 2017). NAC has been used to improve muscle performance primarily through its role as a free radical scavenger (Kirksick and Willoughby 2005). NAC has also been useful in the management of several psychiatric and neurodegenerative conditions (Moreira et al. 2007; Martínez-Banaclocha 2016; Ooi et al. 2018).

Limited *in vitro* and *in vivo* research has yielded conflicting results regarding the use of NAC for the management of chronic bronchitis and feline immunodeficiency virus (FIV) (Mortola et al. 1998; Reinero et al. 2011). Further studies are needed to determine applicability and efficacy. Interestingly, a pharmacokinetic study conducted by Buur et al. (2013) found the current dosing recommendations for the cat may be too low for acute conditions but should be adequate for chronic disease. Further investigation is needed to confirm the correct dose as historical recommendations were extrapolated form human dosing. NAC has proven useful as an adjunct treatment for a variety of inflammatory canine diseases, including minimizing myocardial ischemia and reperfusion injury following cardiac arrest, lung injury secondary to cardiopulmonary bypass, parvovirus infections, and otitis externa (Fischer et al. 2003; Qu et al. 2013; Gaykwad et al. 2017; May et al. 2019).

Adverse effects are uncommon, and their occurrence is dependent on the formulation used (oral, intravenous, or inhalant) and the dosage (Tenório et al. 2021). The formulation chosen depends on the condition being treated. Intravenous administration is typically used for acetaminophen toxicity and patients unable to take oral medication. Inhaled therapy is most often used to treat respiratory conditions.

Quercetin

Quercetin, refer to Figure 4.39, and quercetin-type molecules are the most abundant flavonoids in most fruits and vegetables (Li et al. 2016; PubChem 2022g). Quercetin has many biological functions, including anti-inflammatory, antioxidant, psychostimulant, inhibition of lipid peroxidation, inhibition of platelet aggregation, inhibition of capillary

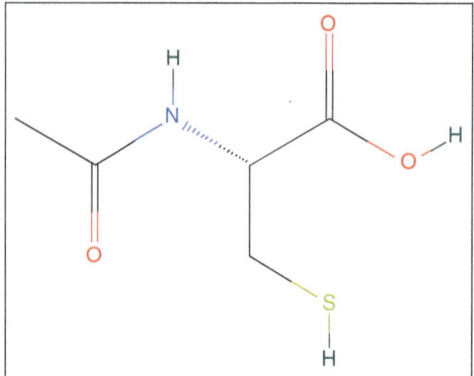

Figure 4.38 Molecular structure of *N*-acetylcysteine, $C_5H_9NO_3S$. Source: PubChem, https://pubchem.ncbi.nlm.nih.gov/compound/12035#section=2D-Structure, September 16, 2004.

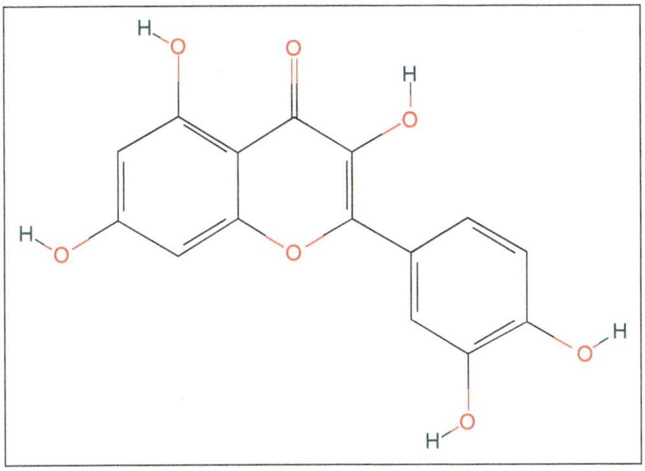

Figure 4.39 Molecular structure of quercetin, $C_{15}H_{10}O_7$. Source: PubChem, https://pubchem.ncbi.nlm.nih.gov/compound/5280343, September 16, 2004.

permeability, and stimulation of mitochondrial biogenesis (Davis et al. 2009; Li et al. 2016).

Multiple randomized clinical trials in people have shown quercetin is effective in reducing the rate of upper respiratory tract infections, allergic respiratory disease, and food allergies (Nieman et al. 2009; Heinz et al. 2010; Mlcek et al. 2016). Quercetin is very safe with few to no side effects (Li et al. 2016).

Veterinary studies are extremely limited and typically involve *in vitro* investigations. These studies do suggest quercetin may be used as an adjunct treatment for certain canine neoplasms and to reduce pain and inflammation associated with osteoarthritis (Britti et al. 2017; Ryu et al. 2019). Randomized clinical trials are needed to confirm quercetin's efficacy and safety in companion animals.

Resveratrol

Resveratrol is a phytoalexin, a chemical defense mechanism produced by certain plant tissues to protect themselves from parasites, bacteria, and environmental stressors (PubChem 2022h). Resveratrol is found in over 70 edible plants, including grapes (especially abundant in the seeds and skin), berries, and peanuts (Burns et al. 2002). Resveratrol is also found in red wine, prompting the French paradox, the theory that regular red wine consumption by the French population contributes to the comparatively low incidence of cardiovascular disease despite a high daily intake of saturated fat (Renaud and Lorgeril 1992).

The medical profession initially questioned the efficacy of resveratrol, but more recent evidence suggests the supplement has great potential primarily due to its antioxidant properties (Vang et al. 2011). Resveratrol also possesses anti-inflammatory, anti-apoptotic (prevents cell death), cardioprotective, neuroprotective, hepatoprotective, antineoplastic properties, and anti-obesity properties (Faghihzadeh et al. 2015; Galiniak et al. 2019; Ferreira et al. 2020; Hecker et al. 2021). *In vitro* and *in vivo* studies suggest resveratrol has a positive effect on the cardiovascular, hepatic, endothelial, immune, and metabolic systems (Faghihzadeh et al. 2015; Breuss et al. 2019; Malaguarnera 2019; Springer and Moco 2019). Resveratrol also helps regulate lipid and glucose metabolism, providing potentially beneficial effects for diabetic and obese patients (Zhou et al. 2022).

While veterinary studies are limited, preliminary evidence suggests resveratrol may support the immune system, delaying signs of aging, and improve cancer cell death (Cheng et al. 2013, 2014; Carlson et al. 2018; Mathew et al. 2018). Resveratrol supplementation is well tolerated by humans and animals with only mild gastrointestinal signs noted at higher doses (Breuss et al. 2019). Resveratrol is readily absorbed following ingestion but has been shown to degrade quickly, negatively affecting its bioavailability (Park and Pezzuto 2015).

Resveratrol for Veterinarians Resveratrol, depicted in Figure 4.40, is a polyphenol phytoestrogen (PubChem 2022h). Resveratrol first became popular because of its antiglycation properties. Glycation is the covalent attachment of a sugar to a protein or lipid, forming advanced glycation end products (AGEs). AGEs were first identified when cooking proteins and sugars together. This process, called the Maillard reaction, is often used to enhance the color, flavor, aroma and texture of food. Consumption of external (or exogenous) AGEs lead to an increase in serum AGE levels (Kim et al. 2017).

Endogenous AGEs occur spontaneously over time from a small proportion of intestinally absorbed sugars. The excessive accumulation of AGEs can lead to cellular and tissue damage through their interactions with the ECM. AGEs can cross-link with collagen and elastic fibers within the ECM reducing tissue elasticity, interfere with intracellular proteins and increase oxidative stress affecting cellular function, or less commonly affect cell receptors (RAGE) triggering the inflammatory cascade (Kim et al. 2017). The accumulation of AGEs is one of the hallmarks of aging in humans and animals (Kim et al. 2017). The antiglycation (or anti-AGE) properties of resveratrol have been well studied in humans and nonprimate animals (Galiniak et al. 2019).

In vitro canine studies demonstrated resveratrol has pro-apoptotic effects against certain canine cancer cells (Carlson et al. 2018). *In vitro* and *in vivo* studies suggest resveratrol beneficially affects the canine immune system through stimulation of phagocytosis, oxidative burst, and the production of leukocytes and cytokines (Mathew et al. 2018). Feline studies focus on the protective effects of resveratrol against arsenic toxicity, specifically its ability to ameliorate oxidative damage in the lungs, kidneys, and brain (Cheng et al. 2013, 2014).

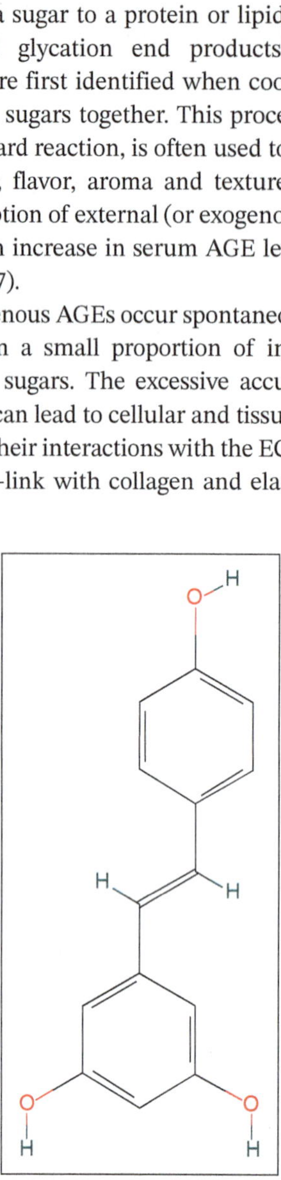

S-Adenosyl-L-methionine

S-Adenosyl-L-methionine (SAMe) is made within the body, from the amino acid methionine, and synthetically. SAMe plays a key role in normal cellular function and survival (Lu 2000).

In people, SAMe is primarily used as an adjunct treatment for chronic liver disease, psychiatric disorders (especially depression and anxiety) and Alzheimer's disease (Guo et al. 2015; Galizia et al. 2016; Sharma et al. 2017). Numerous studies have confirmed the safety of administration but the efficacy is still questioned, highlighting the need for further research (Guo et al. 2015; Galizia et al. 2016).

SAMe is primarily used in veterinary medicine as an adjunct treatment for acute and chronic liver disease and liver toxicity (Webster and Copper 2009). SAMe also shows promise as a dietary aid for the management of age-related mental impairment, specifically canine cognitive dysfunction (Rème et al. 2008).

Figure 4.40 Molecular structure of resveratrol, $C_{14}H_{12}O_3$. Source: PubChem, https://pubchem.ncbi.nlm.nih.gov/compound/445154, March 25, 2005.

SAMe for Veterinarians Methionine is converted into its active form, SAMe, by the enzyme methionine adenosyltransferase (Lu 2000). The molecular structure of SAMe is depicted in Figure 4.41. SAMe is involved in transmethylation, transsulfuration, and polyamine synthesis (Lu 2000).

SAMe restores liver glutathione reserves and decreases liver damage (Guo et al. 2015). SAMe is believed to relieve depressive symptoms by increasing the synthesis of monoamine neurotransmitters (Galizia et al. 2016).

Several studies have confirmed SAMe's status as an effective and safe liver protectant for acute and chronic hepatopathies in both the dog and the cat (Webb et al. 2003; Center et al. 2008; Webster and Copper 2009; Skorupski et al. 2011; Marchegiani et al. 2020). In an *in vitro* study using canine hepatocytes, Au et al. (2012) concluded SAMe and silymarin reduced cytokine production (specifically PGE_2, interleukin-8, and macrophage chemotactic protein-1) and prevented NF-κB translocation, thus inhibiting inflammation and oxidative stress. Interestingly, Center et al. (2005) found the concurrent administration of prednisolone and SAMe appeared to inhibit the pro-oxidant effects of prednisolone but did not negate the development of vacuolar hepatopathy.

Over a decade ago Linnebank et al. (2010) discovered patients with Alzheimer's disease had lower levels of SAMe within the cerebrospinal fluid (CSF). Multiple studies have confirmed supplementation with SAMe (combined with other antioxidants) maintained and often improved cognitive function and mood in patients with Alzheimer's (Chan et al. 2008; Remington et al. 2008, 2015). In a randomized, double-blind, placebo-controlled trial by Rème et al. (2008), the SAMe-supplemented dogs had a 50% reduction in their mental impairment scores compared to the placebo group after eight weeks of therapy.

Botanicals

Botanicals encompass any substance obtained from a plant or plant part. Included within this category is Ayurvedic medicine, flower essences (dilute liquid extracts of plants, typically stored in an alcohol base), nutraceuticals,

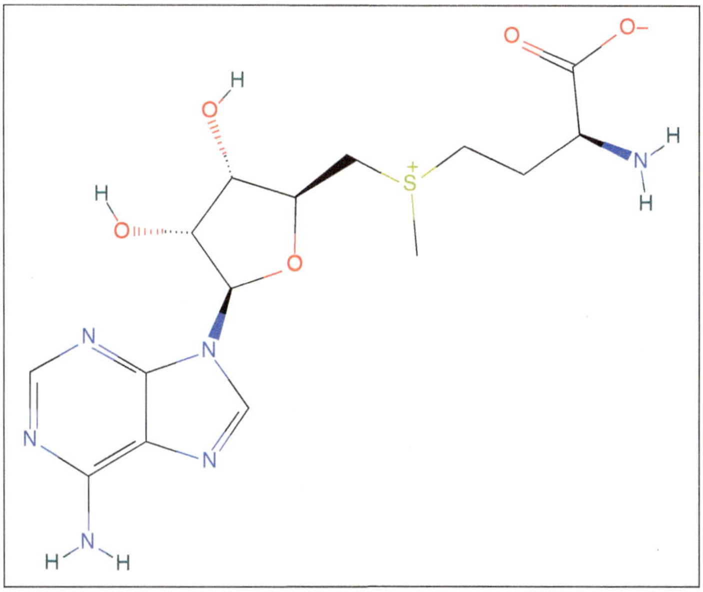

Figure 4.41 Molecular structure of *S*-adenosyl-L-methionine, $C_{15}H_{22}N_6O_5S$. Source: PubChem, https://pubchem.ncbi.nlm.nih.gov/compound/34755#section=2D-Structure, September 16, 2004.

Chinese herbal medicine, and Western herbal medicine (see Chapters 3 and 11, respectively, for further information on these latter two modalities).

The most common botanicals used in VN include Boswellia, cannabinoids, curcumin, milk thistle, mushrooms, and valerian. Less commonly used botanicals include Ashwagandha, Devil's Claw, *Ginkgo biloba*, Magnolia, Phellodendron, and St. John's Wort. Table 4.13 summarizes the beneficial effects of each botanical. Additional detail is provided about the most used botanicals in the following sections; Boswellia, curcumin and milk thistle are discussed in earlier sections.

Cannabidiol

Cannabidiols (CBD) are a non-intoxicating substance derived from *Cannabis sativa*. Figure 4.42 shows a photograph of the cannabis plant, also

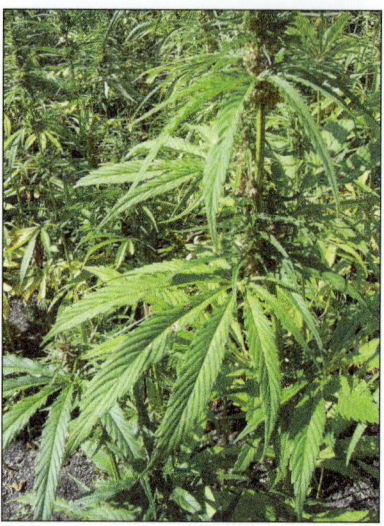

Figure 4.42 Photograph of the *Cannabis sativa* plant, also known as the hemp or marijuana plant. Source: Nabokov/Wikimedia Commons/ Public domain.

Table 4.13 The common/scientific names and beneficial effects of regularly used botanicals in veterinary nutraceuticals as of January 2023.

Common name	Scientific name	Beneficial effects
Ashwagandha	*Withania somnifera*	Anti-inflammatory; antioxidant; immune modulating; antitumor; adaptogen
Boswellia	*Boswellia serrata*	Anti-inflammatory; analgesic; antibacterial; antidiarrheal
Cannabinoids	*Cannabis sativa*	Analgesic; anxiolytic; antiepileptic; improves cognition; antitumor
Curcumin	*Curcuma longa*	Anti-inflammatory; antioxidant; hepatoprotective; cholagogue; antiplatelet; anticancer
Devil's claw	*Harpagophytum procumbens*	Anti-inflammatory; analgesic
Ginkgo	*Ginkgo biloba*	Anti-inflammatory; improves cognition
Magnolia	*Magnolia officinalis*	Anxiolytic
Milk thistle	*Silybum marianum*	Hepatoprotectant; supports the immune system
Mushrooms	Reishi, Turkey Tail, Shiitake, and Maitake	Immune stimulating; antitumor
Phellodendron	*Phellodendron amurense*	Anxiolytic
St. John's Wort	*Hypericum perforatum*	Antidepressant; anxiolytic; anti-inflammatory
Valerian root	*Valeriana officinalis*	Sedative; anxiolytic

Source: Wynn and Fougère (2007) with permission of Elsevier.

known as hemp or marijuana. CBD oil is most prescribed to treat epilepsy in people. The legality of using CBD products in veterinary medicine is confusing and often state dependent. CBD products are typically used in companion animals to help manage OA-related pain, behavioral issues, cognitive decline, epilepsy, and delay the growth of certain cancers (McGrath et al. 2019; Brioschi et al. 2020; Henry et al. 2020; Verrico et al. 2020; Corsetti et al. 2021).

Hemp versus Marijuana

The genus *Cannabis*, in the flowering plant family of Cannabaceae, has three primary species: *Cannabis sativa, Cannabis indica*, and *Cannabis ruderalis* (Pollio 2016). *Cannabis sativa* is the most cultivated species. Hemp and marijuana are *not* different species or strains of *Cannabis*. They are broad colloquial classifications of *C. sativa* adopted by our culture but not considered legitimate scientific nomenclature (Pollio 2016). Technically there are numerous cultivars (a variety of plant cultivated by selective breeding) of both hemp and marijuana (van Bakel et al. 2011).

Hemp and marijuana are legally distinguished by their concentrations of tetrahydrocannabinol (THC), the psychoactive ingredient of marijuana. The Agricultural Improvement Act of 2018 defined hemp as "the plant *Cannabis sativa* L. and any part of that plant, including the seeds thereof and all derivatives, extracts, cannabinoids, isomers, acids, salts, and salts of isomers, whether growing or not, with a delta-9 tetrahydrocannabinol concentration of not more than 0.3% on a dry weight basis" (H.R.2. 2018).

Hemp is *C. sativa* containing <0.3% THC, and marijuana is *C. sativa* containing >0.3% THC.

CBD for Veterinarians *Cannabis sativa* contains more than 540 phytochemicals including cannabinoids (or phytocannabinoids), terpene, and phenolic compounds (Andre et al. 2016). Cannabinoids, which include both CBD and THC, are the most well studied of the compounds. CBD is the primary cannabinoid of interest given its high concentration within the plant and therapeutic potential, and because of THC's psychoactive properties and risk of toxicity in many veterinary patients. Extensive effort, time, and money has been poured into the metabolic engineering of hemp to increase the CBD content while minimizing the THC levels (Deguchi et al. 2020).

To understand the beneficial effects of CBD we must first review the endocannabinoid system (ECS). The ECS consists of endogenous cannabinoids (endocannabinoids), cannabinoid receptors, and their enzymes (responsible for synthesis and degradation of endocannabinoids) (Lu and Mackie 2016). The ECS is a neuromodulatory system involved in metabolic homeostasis and behavior (Woods 2007; Lu and Mackie 2016). Disturbances within the ECS have been associated with certain chronic inflammatory conditions, infertility, obesity, diabetes, cardiovascular disease, gastrointestinal disorders, anxiety, neurologic conditions, psychiatric disorders, and migraines (Lu and Mackie 2016; Borowska et al. 2018; VanDolah et al. 2019).

Endocannabinoids are lipids, whose precursors are found within lipid membranes. They are liberated when needed, released into the extracelluar space, and then interact with cannabinoid receptors (Lu and Mackie 2016). The primary endocannabinoids are anandamide and 2-arachidonylglycerol (VanDolah et al. 2019).

Cannabinoid receptors have been found in the brain, liver, and peripheral adipose tissue (Woods 2007). The primary receptors are G protein-coupled receptors, CB_1 and CB_2 (Howlett et al. 2002). CB_1 receptors are principally found in the central nervous system, as well as the peripheral nervous system (Mackie 2005). CB_2 receptors are primarily expressed on immune cells, microglial cells, in the vascular system, and under certain pathologic conditions (such as nerve injury) in the peripheral nervous system (Howlett et al. 2002; Lu and Mackie 2016). Activation of these receptors causes a myriad of effects, including inhibition of neurotransmitter release or synaptic function, modulation of cytokine release, alteration of cellular physiology and motility, and triggering of gene transcription (Howlett et al. 2002).

There are a variety of endocannabinoid enzymes used to synthesize and degrade endocannabinoids. The enzyme is dependent on the specific endocannabinoid and its location of action (Lu and Mackie 2016).

Phytocannabinoid research has exploded because of their ability to modulate the ECS. THC exerts its intoxicating effects by acting as a CB_1 receptor agonist (Borgelt et al. 2013). Alternatively, CBD has a variety of pharmacological actions including inhibiting endocannabinoid reuptake, activating certain endocannabinoid receptors, and stimulating serotonin receptors (Lu and Mackie 2016; VanDolah et al. 2019). CBD has no psychoactive properties because of its lack of effect on the cannabinoid receptors (Fasinu et al. 2016).

A distinction should be made between hemp seed oil, hemp oil, and CBD oil. Hemp seed oil consists of oils extracted from the seeds of hemp plants (Callaway 2004). The oil is rich in omega-6 and omega-3 fatty acids, γ-linolenic acids, and other antioxidants, while containing little to no CBD and no THC (Callaway 2004). Hemp seed oil is frequently used as a nutritional supplement.

Hemp oil and CBD oil are often lumped together. Both are derived from the flowers and leaves of the hemp plant. The oil is rich in CBD, β-caryophyllene, other phytocannabinoids, and terpenoids with <0.3% THC (by dry weight) (VanDolah et al. 2019). Hemp and CBD oils are both primarily used for medicinal purposes.

There is a disproportionate amount of research devoted to studying THC and CB_1 receptors compared to CBD. Despite the limited number of randomized clinical trials, CBD and hemp oil have been investigated and used for the treatment of seizures, chronic pain, migraines, chronic inflammation, depression, and anxiety in people (Fasinu et al. 2016; Donvito et al. 2018; VanDolah et al. 2019).

Comparatively, the efficacy and safety of CBD oil for the treatment of epilepsy has been studied the most (Arzimanoglou et al. 2020). In a review by Donvito et al. (2018), the authors concluded there is overwhelming preclinical evidence supporting the antinociceptive effects of CBD in treating inflammatory and neuropathic pain in rodents, and clinical trials should be conducted to determine the efficacy in people. Additionally, Epidiolex, a purified CBD oral solution, was approved by the FDA in June 2018 for the treatment of seizures in people. Several patients in the Epidiolex safety studies had elevated liver enzymes (VanDolah et al. 2019). As a result, the FDA recommend doctors run liver function tests before starting Epidiolex as well as one and three months into treatment.

VanDolah et al. (2019) acknowledge safety studies have not been conducted on "full-spectrum" phytocannabinoid products. In a review of safety studies by Iffland and Grotenhermen (2017), the authors concluded CBD had a favorable profile in human and animal studies. Adverse effects were often mild, including tiredness, diarrhea, and changes in appetite and weight. The authors did highlight the need for additional studies establishing toxicological parameters for CBD.

Product purity is one of the biggest concerns when considering CBD and hemp oil. Bonn-Miller et al. (2017) analyzed 84 human CBD and hemp oil products purchased online. The CBD and THC content was accurately labeled in only 26 of the products. Moreover, 26% of the products contained less CBD than advertised (Bonn-Miller et al. 2017). These findings highlight the importance of using trusted sources to ensure only high-quality and accurately labeled products are recommended for our veterinary patients.

Because CBD is highly lipophilic it is most supplied as an oil or alcoholic formulation (Millar et al. 2020). The bioavailability of CBD in people is estimated to be 6% (Millar et al. 2018). The substance is generally eliminated faster than it is absorbed in the gastrointestinal tract due to precipitation (Millar et al. 2018). Route of administration and administration with food have been shown to improve bioavailability. Suspensions designed to be administered via oral or oromucosal routes have faster times to peak plasma concentration and maximum concentrations (C_{max}) (Millar et al. 2018). CBD oil administered to healthy adults with a high-fat/high-calorie meal have a fourfold increase in bioavailability compared to fasted subjects (Itin et al. 2019). CBD-infused oils also have better pharmacokinetic profiles in dogs (Bartner et al. 2018). Additionally, CBD should

be protected from light, stored at room temperature, and dissolved in medium-chain triglyceride oil to prevent degradation within the bottle (Millar et al. 2018).

A pharmacokinetic study in dogs conducted by Gamble et al. (2018) revealed a half-life of 4.2 hours without side effects. Deabold et al. (2019) demonstrated that CBD supplementation every 12 hours in dogs achieved an adequate C_{max} with few to no side effects. In the same study cats were shown to absorb and eliminate CBD differently with lower serum concentration and mild adverse effects, including increased self-grooming and head-shaking.

CBD use in veterinary medicine is not currently well studied. Preliminary studies have shown CBD is effective in the management of OA-related pain, behavioral issues, cognitive decline, neoplastic cell proliferation, and epilepsy (McGrath et al. 2019; Brioschi et al. 2020; Henry et al. 2020; Verrico et al. 2020; Zadik-Weiss et al. 2020; Corsetti et al. 2021).

The Legality of Hemp

The Controlled Substances Act (CSA) of 1970 classified the *Cannabis sativa* plant as a Schedule I controlled substance which included "drugs, substances, or chemicals defined as drugs with no currently accepted medical use and a high potential for abuse" (DEA 2021). In short, cannabis was declared federally illegal.

The Agricultural Improvement Act of 2018 (the 2018 Farm Bill) removed cannabis plants and their derivatives which contain less than 0.3% THC (aka hemp) from the CSA, making those products federally legal (H.R.2. 2018). The 2018 Farm Bill also declared the FDA maintained the authority to regulate cannabis or cannabis-derived compounds under the Food, Drug and Cosmetic Act (FDCA) and section 351 of the Public Health Service Act (H.R.2. 2018; FDA 2021c).

Several states have passed their own hemp bills, legalizing the production of cannabis plants with less than 0.3% THC. States also regulate the cultivation, preparation, and manufacturing of hemp products. A few states permit the conditional use of cannabis with more than 0.3% THC (aka marijuana), decriminalized its use, or allowed the use of medical marijuana for *people only*. These state laws do not apply to veterinary medicine, and in the eyes of the Federal Government marijuana is still considered illegal.

Despite the reclassification of hemp and its derivatives, CBD products are typically excluded. On the off chance a CBD product meets the requirements of hemp, it is subject to FDA regulations established by the FDCA, as well as state regulations.

(Continued)

The Legality of Hemp   **(Continued)**

CBD products cannot be sold as dietary supplements and are exempt from the protections afforded by the Dietary Supplement Health and Education Act (DSHEA) of 1994. This is because any substance used as an active ingredient in an approved drug product under the FDCA is excluded from the definition of dietary supplement. While the FDA has not approved marketing applications for pharmaceutical cannabis, the FDA has approved one cannabis-derived and three cannabis-related drug products for people. These products are treated as pharmaceuticals and require a prescription from a licensed healthcare provider. This means there are numerous unapproved CBD products marketed for the treatment of certain medical conditions.

> The existence of FDA-approved CBD products precludes the legal use of CBD products as dietary supplements.

Many states have their own regulations and exemptions regarding the use of CBD products. Unfortunately states legislatures frequently do not consider veterinary medicine when creating these laws. As a result, veterinarians and their patients are often excluded from these exemptions, making the legal use of CBD products even more confusing. Every practitioner should review their states laws and consult their state veterinary board before recommending, carrying, and/or dispensing CBD products.

> Review your state laws and consult your state veterinary board before recommending, carrying, or dispensing CBD products.

Mushrooms

Medicinal mushrooms (MMs) have been used for hundreds of years in traditional Chinese medicine and other Asian countries. There are more than 100 species of MM, but the four most used species, depicted in Figures 4.43–4.46, are reishi (*Ganoderma lucidum*), turkey tail (*Trametes versicolor* or *Coriolus versicolor*), shiitake (*Lentinus edodes*), and maitake (*Grifola frondosa*) (PDQ 2022).

MMs possess approximately 130 different medicinal functions. MMs are primarily known for their effects on the immune system and cancer development (oncogenesis). MMs are approved for use as an adjunct treatment for many cancers in both China and Japan (PDQ

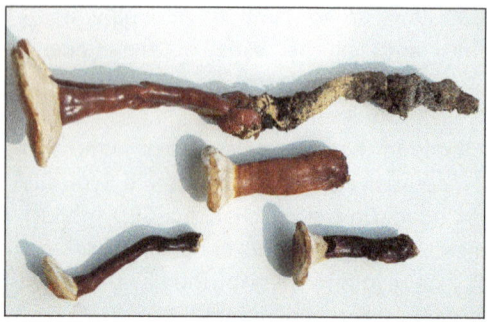

Figure 4.43   Photograph of reishi (*Ganoderma lucidum*) mushrooms. Source: Аимаина хикари/Wikimedia Commons/Public domain.

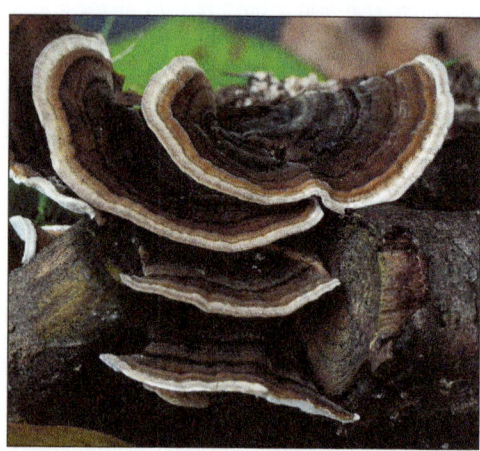

Figure 4.44   Photograph of turkey tail (*Coriolus versicolor*) mushrooms. Source: Michael Linnenbach/Wikimedia Commons/CC BY-SA 4.0.

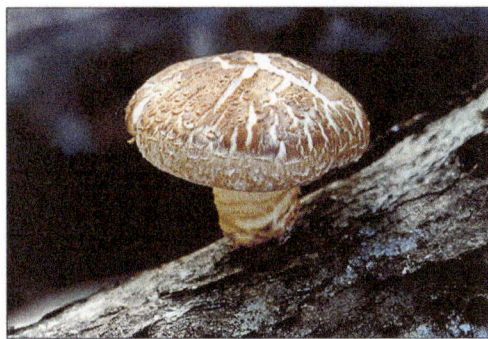

Figure 4.45 Photograph of a shiitake (*Lentinus edodes*) mushroom. Source: Keith Weller, 2005. https://www.ars.usda.gov/oc/images/photos/nov05/k3024-9/ (last accessed under June 08, 2023).

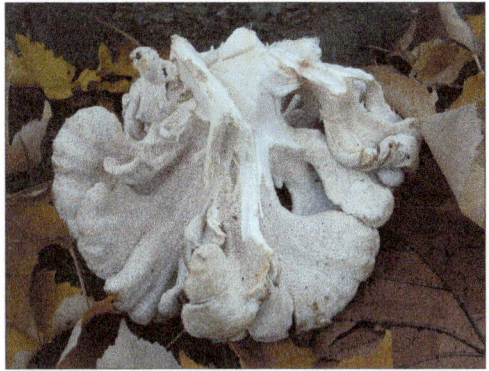

Figure 4.46 Photograph of a maitake (*Grifola frondosa*) mushroom. Source: Sinisa Radic/ Wikimedia Commons/vCC BY-SA 4.0.

2022). MMs also function as antioxidants, free radical scavengers, and cardiovascular protectants, and are antihypercholesterolemic, antiviral, antibacterial, antiparasitic, antifungal, detoxifying, hepatoprotective, and antidiabetic (Wasser 2014; PDQ 2022).

Adverse effects are uncommon when MMs are used appropriately (i.e. correct species and dosing). If adverse effects do occur, they typically involve mild gastrointestinal upset (Jeitler et al. 2020). The primary concern with veterinary patients is palatability. Depending on the formulation, some canine and feline patients refuse to ingest MMs even when mixed with food.

MMs are primarily used in veterinary medicine to stimulate the immune system and for their antitumor effects. Their use is primarily based on data extrapolated from *in vitro* and *in vivo* studies on laboratory animals and available human clinical trials. Further research is necessary to confirm the efficacy and safety of MMs in veterinary patients.

MMs for Veterinarians The immunostimulant properties of MMs are primarily derived from their high concentrations of high-molecular-weight polysaccharides (β-glucan) (Akramiene et al. 2007). Mushroom proteins, protein-conjugate complexes, terpenes, terpenoids, and likely many unclassified substances also contribute to their efficacy (Zhao et al. 2020). MMs exert a direct effect on the patient's innate immune system, activating the complement system, enhancing macrophage and natural killer cell function, and activating a multitude of immune receptors (Akramiene et al. 2007; PDQ 2022).

The mechanisms through which MMs prevent oncogenesis are unclear, but angiogenesis inhibition appears to play a key role. Unfortunately, there are limited human clinical trials, and many of the existing trials yield conflicting results (Jeitler et al. 2020).

Not all of the bioactive compounds, and their mechanisms of action, have been classified. Further research is needed to understand the pharmacokinetics, pharmacodynamics, nutrigenomics, and potential drug interactions for each bioactive compound within MM (Money 2016; Zhao et al. 2020).

MMs are most often used as an immunostimulant and antineoplastic supplement in canine and feline patients. Veterinary studies investigating MMs are extremely limited. A study by Griessmayr et al. (2008) found there was no beneficial response in dogs with lymphoma given a maitake PETfraction as a single-agent treatment. A pilot study conducted by Brown and Reetz (2012) demonstrated the administration of turkey tail mushrooms (*Coriolus versicolor*) significantly delayed the metastasis of splenic hemangiosarcoma following splenectomy. A follow-up study by Gedney et al. (2022) compared the survival time of dogs with splenic hemangiosarcoma who received doxorubicin versus doxorubicin with a supplement containing *C. versicolor* (I'm-Yunity) following splenectomy. The authors found the administration of the MM did not improve survival time (Gedney et al. 2022). Clearly more research is needed to determine the applicability and efficacy of MMs in companion animals.

Valerian Root

Valerian root (VR) is the root of the flowering plant *Valeriana officinalis*, depicted in Figure 4.47. The plant was originally native to Asia and Europe but is now commonly grown in the United States. VR has been used for hundreds of years as an herbal remedy to promote sleep and reduce anxiety. The exact mechanisms of action are unknown.

While the available *in vitro* and *in vivo* studies suggest VR is efficacious, additional clinical trials are clearly needed for confirmation. VR appears to be safe and well tolerated with few,

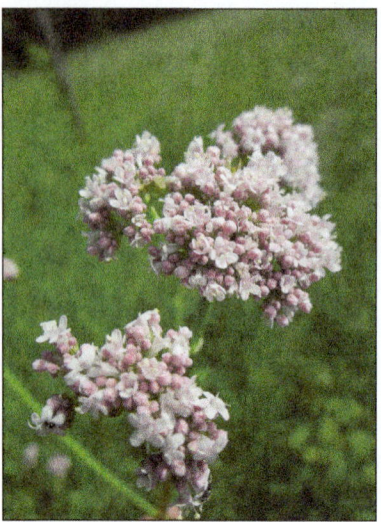

Figure 4.47 Photograph of the *Valeriana officinalis* flower. Source: AnRo0002/Wikimedia Commons/ CC0 1.0.

if any, side effects and no clinically relevant herb–drug interactions (Kelber et al. 2014).

VR is primarily used to reduce anxiety in veterinary patients. Mild sedation is a potential, and generally desired, side effect of its use. VR veterinary research is extremely limited, and most of the information is extrapolated from *in vitro* and laboratory animal or human *in vivo* studies.

VR for Veterinarians The roots and rhizomes contain numerous bioactive compounds, including sesquiterpenes of the volatile oil, valepotriates, flavonoids, triterpenes, lignans, and alkaloids (Houghton 1999; Goppel and Franz 2004). The sesquiterpenes (valerenic acid and its derivatives, valeranone, valeranal, and kessyl esters) and valepotritates (valtrate, didrovaltrate, acebaltrate, and isovaleroxyhydroxyvaltrate) are the primary constituents (Houghton 1999; Goppel and Franz 2004).

Presumably the numerous bioactive substances exert a combination of effects. VR has been shown to affect GABA, adenosine, barbiturate, serotonin, and benzodiazepine receptors, as well as inhibiting excessive activity in the amygdala (Houghton 1999; Dietz et al. 2005). For example, valerenic acid increases GABA levels within the brain by inhibiting enzyme-induced breakdown and preferentially binding to specific $GABA_A$ receptors causing sedation and reducing anxiety (Houghton 1999; Benke et al. 2009; Murphy et al. 2010). Valepotriates are prodrugs whose mechanisms of action are poorly understood, but they appear to contribute to VR's anxiolytic properties (Houghton 1999). Additionally, many of the flavonoids elicit anxiolytic, sedating, and sleep-enhancing effects as well (Fernández et al. 2004).

VR has been effective in the management of insomnia, anxiety, obsessive-compulsive disorders, Parkinson's disease, Alzheimer's disease, and brain ischemia (Fernández-San-Martín et al. 2010; Murphy et al. 2010; Pakseresht et al. 2011; Wang et al. 2014; Jung et al. 2015). There are still questions regarding the efficacy of

VR, especially with respect to its anxiolytic and sleep-enhancing properties. A meta-analysis carried out by Nunes and Sousa (2011) suggested there was insufficient evidence to recommend the use of VR for anxiety and only limited evidence supporting its use for insomnia.

A study by Bol et al. (2017) investigating the olfactory responsiveness of cats to VR found 50% of cats expressed interest in the VR compared to three other herbs. VR is most used for anxiety (separation, noise-phobia, travel, and aggression) in dogs and cats. Anecdotal evidence suggests VR is very safe in companion animals, with sedation being a desired and occasionally side effect reported by owners. Randomized clinical trials are needed to definitively assess the efficacy of VR in cats and dogs.

The Why

Applications in Human Medicine

According to the Council for Responsible Nutrition (CRN) 2019 Consumer Survey on Dietary Supplements, of the 2006 people age 18 years and older living in the United States polled, 77% reported consuming dietary supplements. The vast majority, 81%, were 35–54 years of age (CRN 2019). The 10 most popular supplements in this study included multivitamins, vitamin D, vitamin C, protein, calcium, vitamin B or B complex, omega-3 fatty acids, green tea, magnesium, probiotics, iron, vitamin E, and turmeric (Kamiński et al. 2020).

In a 2020 ConsumerLab.com survey of 9800 people taking dietary supplements, the most popular supplements were vitamin D, magnesium, and fish oil (Murphy 2020). Throughout 2020 the sale of collagen, magnesium, and cannabidiol increased the most compared to other supplements; while sales of curcumin, cinnamon, CoQ10, and coconut oil were reduced (Murphy 2020).

People appear to take dietary supplements for one of four reasons: perceived nutrient deficit (not filled by diet alone), maintenance of health, prevention of disease, and treatment of disease (Kamiński et al. 2020). Interestingly, using the National Health and Nutrition Examination Survey (NHANES) data from 1999 to 2010 and the National Death Index mortality data, Chen et al. (2019) concluded the overall risk of mortality was not lowered by the consumption of dietary supplements among 30 899 US adults.

The NIH's Dietary Supplement Label Database (DSLD) collects information on dietary supplement labels. As of April 2022 the DSLD contained information on 143 369 labels, up from 60 000 in 2011 (NIH 2022). Given the sheer magnitude of supplements and their potential applications, it is difficult to conduct efficacy and safety studies for every supplement on the market. Fortunately, dietary supplements as a whole are relatively safe, though the potential risk for supplement–drug interactions is relatively high (Ronis et al. 2018).

Applications in Veterinary Medicine

At least 33% of US households with dogs, and 30% of households with cats, use VN (Burns 2017). According to Grand View Research (GVR) the global pet supplement market size in 2019 was $637.6 million, with 43.34% of the market share in North America (GVR 2020). There will be a predicted 6.4% compound annual rate of growth between 2020 and 2027. GVR further suggests socioeconomic aspects, increased pet adoption, and increased humanization were the key factors driving market growth (GVR 2020).

According to the American Kennel Club (AKC) the four most popular canine nutraceuticals are glucosamine, fish oil, antioxidants (e.g. vitamin C, vitamin E, and coenzyme Q10), and probiotics (Reisen 2020). The most popular client reasons for using canine nutraceuticals included joint pain, mobility issues, arthritis, improving coat quality and skin, skin allergies, heart health, supporting the pet as he/she ages, and gastrointestinal issues (Reisen 2020).

The VN market is growing, with 90% of veterinarians selling at least one VN (Boothe 2020). There are still many veterinarians with general concerns regarding the safety and efficacy of VN, especially given the overall lack of regulation. There are numerous well-designed studies available proving the effectiveness of many VN for specific conditions. There are also measures we can take to ensure the products we recommend are backed by scientific data and meet third-party quality standards (think NASC Quality Seal). When used appropriately VN can help our patients.

Ultimately, the decision to recommend VN is up to the practitioner. Prior to dispensing a VN, practitioners must ask themselves a number of questions: Would this patient benefit from a VN? Is there scientific evidence supporting the use of a specific VN (or a combination supplement) for this condition? Are adverse effects or VNDIs expected? What is the best source (i.e. manufacturer and formulation) for this VN? These considerations are summarized in Figure 4.48.

Once the veterinarian decides to prescribe a VN the hospital team should understand the "what" and "why" of the supplement the veterinarian is recommending. This knowledge will help team members re-explain to clients why the veterinarian recommended a particular VN (because you know there are always more questions at checkout). Remember client education and communication is crucial to ensuring our patients receive the best possible care at home.

Veterinary Nutraceutical Research

VN are a relatively well-studied treatment modality. As of July 2022, a search on PubMed. gov using the key terms "veterinary nutraceuticals," "veterinary supplements," "canine nutraceuticals," "canine supplements," "feline neutraceuticals," and "feline supplements" yielded over 12 000 free full articles. While there appear to be a lot of studies, there are a lot of different supplements on the market. There are also a lot of conditions for which these supplements are being used. This makes the number of studies for each supplement–condition combination comparatively low. Presented below are the summaries of three VN studies.

Figure 4.48 Factors and questions the veterinarian should consider when utilizing and prescribing veterinary nutraceuticals (VN): Will this supplement benefit the patient? Is there evidence-based medicine supporting the use of the supplement for this condition? Are there potential adverse effects or VN–drug interactions (VNDI)? What is the best manufacturer and formulation for the patient? Source: Lisa P. McFaddin.

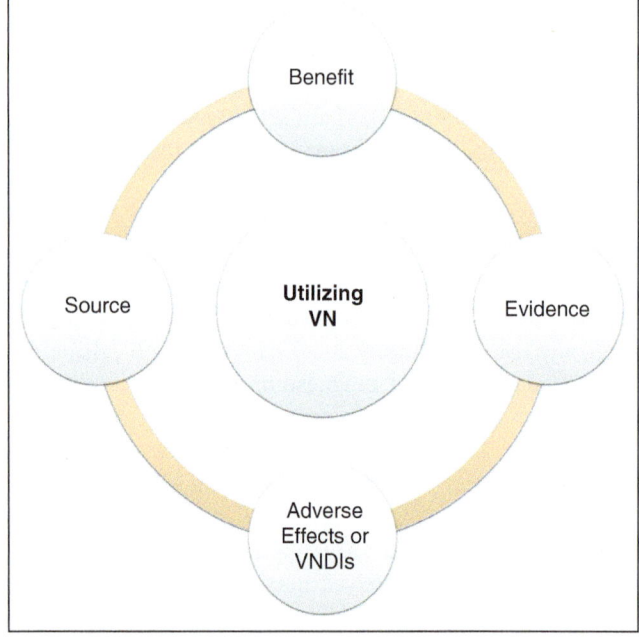

Effects of a Nutritional Supplement in Dogs Affected by Osteoarthritis

Authors: Nadia Musco, Giuseppe Vassalotti, Vincenzo Mastellone, Laura Cortese, Giorgia Rocca, Maria Molinari, Serena Calabró, Raffaella Tudisco, Monica Cutringelli, and Pietro Lombardi

Journal: *Veterinary Medicine and Science*

Date: 2019

Study design: Double-blind randomized controlled trial

Study hypothesis: The administration of a joint supplement (Dinamic™) to dogs with osteoarthritis (OA) would reduce the clinical signs associated with OA. Dinamic contained 10% glucosamine, 1.25% chondroitin sulfate, *Ribes nigrum*, 3% Krill flour, Shiitake (*Lentinus edodes*) mushroom, *Equisetum arvense*, *Boswellia serrata*, *Curcuma longa*, and Devil's Claw (*Harpagophytum procumbens*)

Sample size: 20 client-owned mix breed dogs

Materials and methods: Dogs were enrolled in the study based on radiographic evidence of mild OA (cartilage damage), a history of intermittent mild lameness, and pain in the affected joint. Study participants did not have other medical conditions. Dogs were randomly assigned to two groups: control and treatment. Dogs received no medications or supplements for two months prior to the start of the experiment. Dogs were dosed once daily with the supplement for 90 days. Patients were evaluated and scored on lameness, pain on manipulation and palpation, range of motion, and joint swelling before starting treatment and monthly thereafter. A complete blood count (CBC), chemistry panel, reactive oxygen metabolites, interleukin (IL)-6, and tumor necrosis factor alpha (TNF-α) were measured on fasted blood samples before starting treatment and then monthly. Statistical analysis was performed using one-way analysis of variance.

Results

1) Lameness, pain, range of motion, and joint swelling significantly improved in the treatment groups.
2) No adverse effects noted on the blood results between the treatment and control group.
3) Alkaline phosphatase (ALP) and cholesterol were significantly lower in the treatment group.
4) Hematologic indicators of oxidative stress were significantly decreased in the treatment group.
5) Hematologic indicators of antioxidant potential were significantly increased in the treatment group.

Study conclusions: Administration of Dinamic improved the clinical signs and hematologic evidence of inflammation associated with OA during the 90-day treatment without evidence of adverse effects.

Study limitations

1) Lameness, mobility, and pain measurements were subjective, and examiners were not blinded to the treatment group.
2) The supplement contained multiple ingredients making it impossible to determine which product or products had the most effect.
3) No placebo control group.
4) Small sample sizes.
5) Patients had arthritis affecting different joints, and often had multiple joints involved, all of which affects weight-bearing abilities.

L.P.M. conclusion: The supplement, Dinamic, appeared to improve the clinical condition of dogs with arthritis. The length of effect was

(Continued)

Effects of a Nutritional Supplement in Dogs Affected by Osteoarthritis (Continued)

confusingly described. The time necessary to see a beneficial effect was unclear. The results suggest this supplement may be useful in a multimodal approach to OA management, but additional studies are needed.

(Musco et al. 2019)

Cannabis sativa L. May Reduce Aggressive Behavior Toward Humans in Shelter Dogs

Authors: Sara Corsetti, Simona Borruso, Livia Malandrucco, Valentina Spallucci, Laura Maragliano, Rafaella Perino, Pietro D'Agostino, and Eugenia Natoli
Journal: *Scientific Reports*
Date: 2021
Study design: Clinical trial
Study hypothesis: Cannabidiol (CBD) oil will reduce aggressive behavior toward people in shelter dogs.
Sample size: 24 shelter dogs with a variety of severe preexisting behavioral issues diagnosed by the shelter veterinarian.
Materials and methods: Dogs were divided in a nonrandom fashion into two groups: those receiving CBD oil daily and those receiving a placebo daily. CBD oil was an extract from *Cannabis sativa* that did not contain THC. Behavioral data was collected for three hours before starting and on day 15 and day 45, and 15 days after stopping treatment. The same two observers monitored the dog's behavior without interacting with them. Statistical analysis was performed using Friedman test and Mann–Whitney U test.

Results

1) Dogs receiving CBD oil showed reduced aggression, but the difference was not statistically significant.

2) There was no difference between the two groups with respect to other behavioral issues and signs of stress.

Study conclusions: CBD shows promise for reducing aggression in shelter dogs, despite the nonsignificant findings.

Study limitations

1) Choosing dogs with a specific type of behavioral issue, i.e. separation anxiety or aggression, instead of multiple issues may have been easier to see if CBD exerted an effect.
2) Small sample size.
3) No quality or purity testing performed on the CBD oil used.
4) Only one dose of CBD oil was used.

L.P.M. conclusion: This study should be viewed as a starting point for investigating the positive behavioral effects of CBD oil in canines. Large sample sizes are needed, as well as standardization of the types of behavioral issues. Given CBD oil's notoriously poor bioavailability, testing responses to varying doses would be useful as well.

(Corsetti et al. 2021)

Prospective Randomized Clinical Trial Assessing the Efficacy of Denamarin for Prevention of CCNU-Induced Hepatopathy in Tumor-Bearing Dogs

Authors: K.A. Skorupski, G.M. Hammond, A.M. Irish, M.S. Kent, T.A. Guerrero, C.O. Rodriguez, and D.W. Griffin

Journal: *Journal of Veterinary Internal Medicine*

Date: 2011

Study design: Randomized clinical trial

Study hypothesis: Administration of Denamarin to dogs undergoing chemotherapy with CCNU (lomustine) would lower aminotransferase (ALT) activity compared to dogs not receiving Denamarin.

Sample size: 50 client-owned dogs with histologic or cytologic diagnosis of lymphoma (LSA), mast cell tumors (MCT), or histiocytic sarcoma (HS). Dogs with a previous history of elevated ALT and/or hepatopathy were excluded.

Materials and methods: Dogs were randomly assigned to one of two treatment groups. Group A dogs received Denamarin at the time of the first dose of CCNU. Denamarin was administered daily on an empty stomach using the manufacturer's recommended dosing throughout the study. Group B received CCNU without Denamarin. CCNU treatments were repeated no more than every four weeks. Liver function hematologic testing, i.e. ALT, aspartate aminotransferase (AST), alkaline phosphatase (ALKP), gamma-glutamyl transferase (GGT), total bilirubin, albumin, cholesterol, and blood urea nitrogen (BUN), was performed before starting CCNU and at each dose of CCNU. Study was concluded once they completed the recommended CCNU doses. Dogs with normal ALT values at the time of the last CCNU dose did not have follow-up blood work. Dogs with elevated ALT levels at the time of the last CCNU dose continued ALT monitoring until the value normalized or for up to six months. Data was evaluated using multiple statistical analyses.

Results

1) Age, sex, breed distribution, and weight were not significant between the two groups.
2) Tumor types were not significantly different between the two groups.
3) 84% of dogs receiving CCNU alone had elevated ALT values.
4) 68% of dogs receiving CCNU and Denamarin had elevated ALT values.
5) Dogs receiving CCNU alone had significantly higher ALT, AST, ALP, and bilirubin values compared to the CCNU and Denamarin group.
6) Dogs receiving CCNU alone were significantly more likely to have treatment delays or cessation due to ALT elevations.

Study conclusions: The administration of Denamarin with CCNU reduces the level of liver enzyme elevations and increases the chances the patient will complete the CCNU course.

Study limitations

1) Type and severity of neoplasia was not standardized.
2) Use of steroids prior to the study was allowed.
3) Denamarin is a combination product, so unable to determine if SAMe, milk thistle, or the combination was responsible for the beneficial effects.

L.P.M. conclusion: CCNU commonly causes increased liver enzymes in dogs. The concurrent use of Denamarin appears safe and effective in reducing the ALT elevations and ensuring dogs receive the requisite number of CCNU treatments.

(Skorupski et al. 2011)

The How

Team Members

This section reviews the potential return on investment (ROI), how to effectively train the entire team, how to promote, and how to integrate VN into daily practice.

Return on Investment

The ROI concepts discussed in the other chapters do not traditionally apply to VN. VN are commodities or goods purchased by the hospital from a vendor or manufacturer with the intent to turn around and sell the product to the client. The concepts of client interest, veterinarian demand, and staff are still important and deserve consideration.

Client Interest

As stated previously, the global pet supplement market is huge and relatively recession proof. According to the eighth edition of *Pet Supplements in the U.S.* (Market Research 2021), despite COVID-19 pet supplement sales rose 21%, bringing in close to $800 million in 2020. The exponential increase in sales was attributed to clients' increasing interest in their pet's health and wellness, increased contact proximity and time with their pets during lockdown, and increased need for "calming supplements" to combat anxiety and stress for both humans and their pets (Research and Markets 2021).

Veterinarian Demand

A survey of 126 veterinarians (sampled between 2012 and 2015) showed they were open to discussing the use of VN with clients when the veterinarians were familiar with the VN, felt there was a benefit with use, and believed the products were safe (Elrod and Hofmeister 2019). VN were most commonly discussed for the treatment of OA, with glucosamine/ chondroitin and omega-3 fatty acids being recommended the most (Elrod and Hofmeister 2019). The bottom line is clients are interested in VN, and it is up to the veterinarian (and the entire hospital team) to educate our clients. Personally, I would rather my clients hear the information from me than Dr. Google.

Veterinarian Training

There are currently no true training courses specifically on VN. Most major veterinary conferences offer lectures on various VN, usually by disease condition (like VN for joints or liver health, etc.). Some organizations and companies offer online training at no cost or for a small fee.

Staff Training

Team training expenses are highly variable and dependent on the preexistence of staff meetings and use of a staff meeting for training (compared to self-study). Refer to the Introduction at the beginning of this book for a breakdown of these variables (cost range, $230–1295).

Additional Considerations

The veterinarian will likely recommend a VN during a traditional or integrative appointment. Special VN scheduling protocols are not necessary, and there are no additional staffing or facility costs. VN can be used as a gateway to discuss, offer and incorporate other VIM services. Hospital remodeling, unless more pharmacy space is required, is generally not needed. Pricing is typically based on either the manufacturer's suggested retail price or the hospital's normal pricing strategy.

Team Training

The concept of phase training is used when introducing veterinary integrative medicine (VIM) to the hospital team. A multi-media approach is used to assist with the training program as outlined in Table 4.14.

Table 4.14 The breakdown of phase training steps and resources for the entire hospital team.

Phase 1: Background information	
Team training guide	The handout walks the practice manager and/or veterinarian through Phase 1 of the training
	A downloadable and editable copy of the handout is located on the companion website
Training presentation	The video covers background information on the modality
	PowerPoints can be downloaded, edited, and personalized from the companion website
	The document can be used as a PowerPoint or saved as an mp4 creating a personalized movie
Team training handout	The handout provides additional background information for the CSRs, VAs, and LTs to complement the knowledge gained from watching the training presentation
	A downloadable and editable copy of the handout is located on the companion website
Phase 2: Knowledge proficiency	
Quiz	A short quiz to ensure all team members have a good understanding of the service being offered
	A downloadable and editable copy of the handout is located on the companion website
	A key is provided
Phase 3: Expectations	
Training worksheets	A training checklist is provided for CSRs and VA/LTs with role-specific expectations and tasks for each staff member
	A recommended completion time is provided
	A downloadable and editable copy of the handout is located on the companion website
Phase 4: Client education	
Client scripts	Bullet point information and scripted examples used when discussing the therapy with clients
	A downloadable and editable copy of the handout is located on the companion website
Client education presentation	A short (5–7 minute) client educational video about the therapeutic modality
	PowerPoints can be downloaded, edited, and personalized from the companion website
	The document can be used as a PowerPoint or saved as an mp4 creating a personalized movie
Client education handout	An informational handout about the therapeutic modality written specifically for clients
	A downloadable and editable copy of the handout is located on the companion website

CSR, customer service representative; VA, veterinary assistant; LT, licensed technician.

Practice Manager's Role

To conquer this task the pratice manager needs his or her own checklist which includes the following information:

- Schedule a date and time for the team training.
- Ensure all information pertaining to the new service is reviewed with the staff.
- Confirm all team members have completed the training.
- Certify all team members understand the information and can successfully educate clients.

Promotion

There are six common avenues of promotion for a VIM service: hospital website, social media, email blasts, mailers, in-hospital promotions, and client education.

Hospital Website

Advertise "Veterinary Nutraceuticals" in several locations on the website. On the made page insert "Now offering [supplement brand or specific supplement name]" with a link to success stories or client testimonials. Create a VN blog page discussing patient success stories using various supplements.

Social Media

Utilize Facebook, Instagram, and/or Twitter to post facts, photographs, hashtags, and patient success stories. Include fun and intriguing facts about VN. Clients love patient photos. Be sure to include ones with the VN they are taking. Create or utilize VN specific hashtags.

Email Blasts

Send fun mass emails to your clients introducing VN. Consider monthly case presentations illustrating how VN have benefited patients. Almost everyone has at least one email address these days. . Customer service representatives should be amassing client emails at the same rate as phone numbers.

Mailers

Mailers can be expensive and are largely unnecessary in this digital age, especially when discussing products for sale.

In-Hospital Promotions

Advertise VN within the hospital using promotional signs. Promotional signs are often provided by the manufacturer and can be placed in the waiting room and exam rooms.

Client Education

Education is crucial for clients to understand the purpose and importance of any product being given to their pet. The client handouts and videos solidify pet owner knowledge base surrounding VN as a whole, reducing concerns and conveying value.

Integration

The key components for proper integration include deciding what products to carry or recommend (veterinarian dependent), availability of the products, and staff buy-in.

Veterinarians

There are several factors to consider when veterinarians prepare to incorporate a VIM in their clinical repertoire: state requirements and restrictions, return on investment, supplies, veterinary organizations, and CE.

State Requirements and Restrictions
Is Prescribing VN Considered the Practice of Veterinary Medicine?

Technically if VN are used to treat or prevent disease, then they are being used as a drug, and would constitute the practice of veterinary medicine. Given the legal landmine surrounding the regulation, or lack thereof, of VN refer to your state's veterinary board and laws for specific information. Links for state boards and regulations are provided on the companion website.

Does Nutraceutical Continuing Education Count Toward Licensure Continuing Education Requirements?

If the CE is Registry of *Approved* Continuing Education (RACE) approved, then yes.

Are Your Assets Covered?

Check with your liability insurance company if you have question regarding the recommendation of VN. Refer to the Introduction at the beginning of this book for additional information.

Course Availability

As discussed in the Team Members section, there are currently no online or on-site courses specifically for VN. Many major conferences often offer RACE-approved lectures on VN, and some veterinary organizations or manufacturers offer paid or free online CE discussing various VN. Learning about VN is often a self-driven endeavor with your drug representatives, the Veterinary Information Network (VIN) and PubMed being your best resources.

Supplies

The only supplies needed are the inventory of the VN the hospital is going to carry. The practice manager and veterinarians should discuss their desired stock.

Veterinary Organizations

A description of the most common veterinary organizations with a special interest in VIM and VN is provided. Table 4.15 lists the contact names, contact information, and membership dues for these organizations.

American Holistic Veterinary Medical Association (AHVMA)

- **Description**: The AHVMA was founded in 1982 at the Western States Veterinary Conference with the goal of advancing integrative medicine through the education of integrative and non-integrative veterinarians, the introduction of integrative medicine to veterinary students, the promotion of research, and representation in the AVMA House of Delegates. There is no annual CE requirement to maintain membership.
- **Membership benefits**
  - Free subscription to the *AHVMA Journal*, a peer-reviewed journal.
  - Online resources for client education.
  - Searchable member directory.
  - Discounted vaccination titers through Kansas State University (KSU) Diagnostic Lab.
  - Free access to the Natural Medicines Database, an online resource for supplements, natural medicines, and integrative therapies.

Table 4.15 Veterinary associations and organizations with a special interest in integrative medicine and veterinary nutraceuticals.

Organization	Contact information	Membership dues
American Holistic Veterinary Medical Association (AHVMA)	PO Box 630, Abingdon, MD 21009 (410) 569-0795 office@ahvma.org	$300/year
College of Integrative Veterinary Therapies (CIVT)	PO Box 352, Yeppoon, 4703 QLD, Australia (303) 800-5460 membership@civtedu.org	$185/year
Veterinary Botanical Medicine Association (VBMA)	6410 Highway 92, Acworth, GA 30102 office@vbma.org	$85/year

– Reduced cost for the AHVMA annual conference.

College of Integrative Veterinary Therapies (CIVT)

- **Description**: An online organization open to all licensed animal health providers interested in integrative medicine. There are two membership options: full membership for veterinarians and associate membership for registered animal health professionals. CIVT strives to promote all aspects of evidence-based integrative medicine through online education and discussion forums. CIVT provides financial support to veterinary students interested in studying integrative medicine. CIVT also helps fund integrative medicine research. There is no annual CE requirement to maintain membership.
- **Membership benefits**
  - Access to the online electronic library.
  - Access to the electronic *Journal of Integrative Veterinary Therapies*.
  - Three free CE webinars annually.
  - 20% discount on all webinars.
  - Discounts on specific CIVT courses.
  - Searchable member directory.
  - Access to the Natural Medicines Databases and the American Botanical Council Library.

Veterinary Botanical Medicine Association (VBMA)

- **Description**: Founded by Susan Wynn, DVM, CVA, CVCH, AHG in 2002. The VBMA comprises veterinarians and herbalists interested in promoting the responsible application of herbal therapies for animals. No required annual CE to maintain membership.
- **Membership benefits**
  - VBMA members receive daily email discussion threads detailing real-life case questions and expert practical advice.
  - Weekly and monthly emails are also shared highlighting herbs commonly used in veterinary medicine.
  - Free subscription to the biannual online *Journal of Veterinary Botanical Medicine*.
  - Access to Herbal Wiki, an online herbal materia medica.
  - Access to additional educational articles, websites, and videos.
  - Discounted cost for telemedicine conferences and webinars.
  - Searchable member directory.
  - The VBMA offers an annual conference and multiple webinars.

Reference Materials

The following is a list of recommended veterinary integrative medicine books, many of which discuss nutraceutical use as of January 2023. A summary of each book is also provided.

Canine Nutrigenomics: The New Science of Feeding Your Dog for Optimum Health
- Authors: Jean Dodds, DVM and Diana Laverdure
- Summary: An in-depth discussion into the study of how nutrition affects gene expression in canines.

Clinical Nutrition: Veterinary Clinics of North America Small Animal Practice
- Authors: Dottie Laflamme, DVM, PhD, DACVN and Debra Zoran, DVM, PhD, DACVIM
- Summary: A condensed summary covering the foundation of small animal nutrition, its practical applications to everyday life, and the nutritional management of common canine and feline diseases.

Dr. Pitcairn's Complete Guide to Natural Health for Dogs and Cats
- Authors: Richard Pitcairn, DVM, PhD and Susan Pitcairn
- Summary: An introduction into the applications of integrative pet care for owners.

Healing with Whole Foods: Asian Traditions and Modern Nutrition
- Author: Paul Pitchford
- Summary: An in-depth look into the applications of Chinese food therapy with traditional Chinese medicine descriptions of common food items and a multitude of recipes for various human diseases.

Integrating Complementary Medicine into Veterinary Practice

- Authors: Robert S. Goldstein, VMD, Paula Jo Broadfoot, DVM, Richard E. Plamquist, DVM, Karen Johnstons, DVM, Jiu Jia Wen, DVM, Barbara Fougère, BSc, BVMs (Hons), BHSc (comp Med), MODT, MHSc (Herb Med), CVA (IVAs), CVBM, CVCP, and Margo Roman, DVM
- Summary: A comprehensive review of multiple integrative therapies including: Chinese herbal medicine, acupuncture, homotoxicology, nanopharmacology, homotoxicology, and therapeutic nutrition. The book aims to educate veterinary practitioners on the validity, effectiveness, and incorporation of each modality within daily practice.

Manual of Natural Veterinary Medicine: Science and Tradition

- Authors: Susan G. Wynn, DVM and Steve Marsden, DVM, ND, MSOM, Lac, Dipl. CH., RH(AHG)
- Summary: A quick reference book discussing the integrative therapy options for numerous diseases in veterinary medicine. The book is organized by Western conditions. For each category the potential TCVM diagnoses and treatment options are then discussed in succinct detail. A must-have for all integrative veterinarians.

Nutraceuticals in Veterinary Medicine

- Authors: Ramesh Gupta, Ajay Srivastava, and Rajiv Lall
- Summary: An in-depth look into veterinary nutraceuticals evaluating common ingredients, classifications, applications, utilization, safety and toxicity data, recent trends in research and product development, and regulation.

Nutrient Requirements of Dogs and Cats

- Author: National Research Council
- Summary: A detailed description of the nutrient requirements for dogs and cats based on age and lifestyle, as well as nutrient metabolism and diseases related to nutritional deficiencies.

Principles and Practice of Phytotherapy: Modern Herbal Medicine

- Authors: Kerry Bone and Simon Mills
- Summary: An introduction to the theories and applications of Western herbal medicine for the human practitioner. The book contains 50 evidence-based monographs.

Safety of Dietary Supplements for Horses, Dogs, and Cats

- Author: National Research Council
- Summary: An in-depth discussion centered on the safety and efficacy of dietary supplements as well as current laws and regulations.

Veterinary Herbal Medicine

- Authors: Susan Wynn, DVM, DACVN and Barbara Fougère, BSc, BVMS (Hons), MODT, BHSc (Comp Med), CVA (IVAS), CVCP, CV Herb Med, MHSc (Herb Med)
- Summary: Comprehensive reference book on veterinary Western herbal medicine. The book is divided into five sections covering the history of Western herbal medicine, controversies surrounding Western herbal medicine, materia medica, clinical uses within veterinary medicine, and appendices. This book is a must-have for all veterinarians practicing western herbal medicine.

Promotion

Information regarding the hospital's promotion of VN can be found in the Team Members section.

Integration

Key components for proper integration for the veterinarian primarily revolve around their knowledge of the available products or supplements, efficacy, applicability, safety, and potential drug interactions. Staff buy-in, and a general understanding of the category of VN, ensures all team members understand the benefits of the products.

Conclusion

Veterinary nutraceuticals (VN) are an ever-expanding and evolving therapeutic option for our companion animals. It is important the entire hospital team is aware of the regulatory issues surrounding VN production. Safety and efficacy concerns should always be considered before recommending or prescribing a VN. The potential effects and benefits of VN are numerous for veterinary patients. This chapter and companion website describe in detail how VN can be successfully introduced into daily practice, as well as provide practical tools for implementation.

Acknowledgments

I would like to thank Dr. Brendan Boostrom, DVM, MS, DACVIM (Oncology) for reviewing the chapter for content. Dr. Boostrom is a Board-Certified Veterinary Oncologist at MedVet Northern Virginia. He has authored and co-authored multiple publications in the *Journal of Veterinary Internal Medicine*, the *Journal of Veterinary Ophthalmology*, and *Veterinary Comparative Oncology*.

References

AAFCO (Association of American Feed Control Officers) (2014). AAFCO Methods for Substantiating Nutritional Adequacy of Dog and Cat Foods. https://www.aafco.org/wp-content/uploads/2023/01/Model_Bills_and_Regulations_Agenda_Midyear_2015_Final_Attachment_A.__Proposed_revisions_to_AAFCO_Nutrient_Profiles_PFC_Final_070214.pdf (accessed 5 May 2020).

AAFCO (Association of American Feed Control Officials) (2016). 2016 AAFCO Midyear Meeting Committee Reports. https://www.aafco.org/Portals/0/SiteContent/Meetings/Midyear/2016/2016_Midyear_Committee_Reports_w_cover.pdf (accessed 9 March 2022).

Abebe, W. and Mozaffari, M. (2011). Role of taurine in the vasculature: an overview of experimental and human studies. *American Journal of Cardiovascular Disease* 1 (3): 293–311.

Abecia, L., Hoyles, L., Khoo, C. et al. (2010). Effects of a novel galactooligosaccharide on the faecal microbiota of inflammatory bowel disease cats during a randomized, double-blind, cross-over feeding study. *International Journal of Probiotics and Prebiotics* 52 (2): 61–68.

Abenavoli, L., Raffaele Capasso, N.M., and Capasso, F. (2010). Milk thistle in liver dieases: past, present, future. *Phytotherapy* 24 (10): 1423–1432.

Abramson, S.B., Attur, M., Amin, A.R., and Clancy, R. (2001). Nitric oxide and inflammatory mediators in the perpetuation of osteoarthritis. *Current Rheumatology Reports* 3 (6): 535–541.

Aggarwal, B. and Harikumar, K. (2009). Potential therapeutic effects of curcumin, the anti-inflammatory agent, against neurodegenerative, cardiovascular, pulmonary, metabolic, autoimmune and neoplastic diseases. *International Journal of Biochemistry and Cell Biology* 41 (1): 40–59.

Akramiene, D., Kondrota, A., Didziapetriene, J., and Kevelaitis, E. (2007). Effects of beta-glucans on the immune system. *Medicina* 43 (8): 597–606.

Albaugh, V., Pinzon-Guzman, C., and Barbul, A. (2017). Arginine metabolism and cancer. *Journal of Surgical Oncology* 115 (3): 273–280.

Albert, B., Vickers, M.H., Gray, C. et al. (2016). Oxidized fish oil in rat pregnancy causes high newborn mortality and increases maternal insulin resistance. *American Journal of*

Physiology, Regulatory, Integrative and Comparative Physiology 311 (3): R497–R504.

de Albuquerque, P., De Marco, V., Vendramini, T.H.A. et al. (2021). Supplementation of omega-3 and dietary factors can influence the cholesterolemia and triglyceridemia in hyperlipidemic Schnauzer dogs: a preliminary report. *PLoS One* 16 (10): e0258058.

Allaart, J.G., van Asten, A.J.A.M., Vernooij, J.C.M., and Gröne, A. (2011). Effect of *Lactobacillus fermentum* on beta2 toxin production by *Clostridium perfringens*. *Applied and Environmental Microbiology* 77 (13): 4406–4411.

Allen, J. and Bradley, R. (2011). Effects of oral glutathione supplementation on systemic oxidative stress biomarkers in human volunteers. *Journal of Alternative and Complementary Medicine* 17 (9): 827–833.

Altinel, L., Saritas, Z.K., Kose, K.C. et al. (2007). Treatment with unsaponifiable extracts of avocado and soybean increases TGF-β1 and TGF-β2 levels in canine joint fluid. *Tohoku Journal of Experimental Medicine* 211 (2): 181–186.

Altinel, L., Sahin, O., Kose, K.C. et al. (2011). Healing of osteochondral defects in canine knee with avocado/soybean unsaponifiables: a morphometric comparative analysis. *Journal of the Turkish Joint Disease Foundation* 22 (1): 48–53.

Altman, R. (2009). Glucosamine therapy for knee osteoarthritis: pharmacokinetic considerations. *Expert Review of Clinical Pharmacology* 2 (4): 359–371.

Amin, A., Dave, M., Attur, M., and Abramson, S. (2000). COX-2, NO, and cartilage damage and repair. *Current Rheumatology Reports* 2: 447–453.

Anand, P., Kunnumakkara, A., Newman, R., and Aggarwal, B. (2007). Bioavailability of curcumin: problems and promises. *Molecular Pharmaceutics* 4 (6): 807–818.

Anderson, M. (1999). Oral chondroprotective agents. Part I. Common compounds. *Compendium on Continuing Education* 21: 601–609.

Andre, C., Hausman, J.-F., and Guerriero, G. (2016). *Cannabis sativa*: the plant of the thousand and one molecules. *Frontiers in Plant Science* 7: 19.

Araujo, J., de Rivera, C., Ethier, J.L. et al. (2018). Anxitane tablets reduce fear of human beings in a laboratory model of anxiety-related behavior. *Journal of Veterinary Behavior* 5 (5): 268–275.

Arosio, E., De Marchi, S., Zannoni, M. et al. (2002). Effect of glutathione infusion on leg arterial circulation, cutaneous microcirculation, and pain-free walking distance in patients with peripheral obstructive arterial disease: a randomized, double-blind, placebo-controlled trial. *Mayo Clinic Proceedings* 77 (8): 754–759.

Arslan, H., Aksu, D., Terzi, G., and Nisbet, C. (2012). Therapeutic effects of probiotic bacteria in parvoviral enteritis in dogs. *Revue De Medecine Veterinaire* 163 (2): 55–59.

Arzimanoglou, A., Brandl, U., Cross, J.H. et al. (2020). Epilepsy and cannabidiol: a guide to treatment. *Epileptic Disorders* 22 (1): 1–14.

Asher, G., Corbett, A., and Hawke, R. (2017). Common herbal dietary supplement–drug interactions. *American Family Physician* 96 (2): 101–107.

Au, A., Hasenwinkel, J., and Frondoza, C. (2012). Hepatoproctective effects of S-adenosylmethionine and silybin on canine hepatocytes in vitro. *Journal of Animal Physiology and Animal Nutrition* 97 (2): 331–341.

Augusti, P., Quatrin, A., Somacal, S. et al. (2012). Astaxanthin prevents changes in the activities of thioredoxin reductase and paraoxonase in hypercholesterolemic rabbits. *Journal of Clinical Biochemistry and Nutrition* 51 (1): 42–49.

Avizeh, R., Najafrzadeh, H., Razijalali, M., and Shirali, S. (2010). Evaluation of prophylactic and therapeutic effects of silymarin and N-acetylcysteine in acetaminophen-induced hepatotoxicity in cats. *Journal of Veterinary Pharmacology and Therapeutics* 33 (1): 95–99.

Bagchi, D., Misner, B., Bagchi, M. et al. (2002). Effects of orally administered undenatured type II collagen against arthritic inflammatory diseases: a mechanistic exploration. *International Journal of Clinical Pharmacology Research* 22 (3–4): 101–110.

Bagi, C., Berryman, E., Teo, S., and Lane, N. (2017). Oral administration of undenatured native chicken type II collagen (UC-II) diminished deterioration of articular cartilage in a rat model of osteoarthritis (OA). *Osteoarthritis and Cartilage* 25 (12): 2080–2090.

van Bakel, H., Stout, J.M., Cote, A.G. et al. (2011). The draft genome and transcriptome of *Cannabis sativa*. *Genome Biology* 12 (10): R102.

Baker, J. and Balch, D. (1962). A study of the organic material of hen's-egg shell. *Biochemical Journal* 82 (2): 352–361.

Ballatori, N., Krance, S.M., Notenboom, S. et al. (2009). Glutathione dysregulation and the etiology and progression of human diseases. *Biological Chemistry* 390 (3): 191–214.

Balshaw, T., Bampouras, T., Barry, T., and Sparks, S.A. (2012). The effect of acute taurine ingestion on 3-km running performance in trained middle-distance runners. *Amino Acids* 44 (2): 555–561.

Bartner, L., McGrath, S., Rao, S. et al. (2018). Pharmacokinetics of cannabidiol administered by 3 delivery methods at 2 different dosages to health dogs. *Canadian Journal of Veterinary Research* 82 (3): 178–183.

Bauer, J. (1995). Evaluation and dietary considerations in idiopathic hyperlipidemia in dogs. *Journal of the American Veterinary Medical Association* 206 (11): 1684–1688.

Bauer, J. (2006). Metabolic basis for the essential nature of fatty acids and the unique dietary fatty acid requirements of cats. *Journal of the American Veterinary Medical Association* 229 (11): 1729–1732.

Bauer, J. (2011). Therapeutic use of fish oils in companion animals. *Journal of the American Veterinary Medical Association* 239 (1): 1441–1451.

Bayoumi, M. and Griffiths, M. (2012). In vitro inhibition of expression of virulence genes responsible for colonization and systemic spread of enteric pathogens using *Bifidobacterium bifidum* secreted molecules. *International Journal of Food Microbiology* 156 (3): 255–263.

Beale, B. (2004). Use of nutraceuticals and chondroprotectants in osteoarthritic dogs and cats. *Veterinary Clinics of North America Small Animal Practice* 34 (1): 271–289.

Benke, D., Barberis, A., Kopp, S. et al. (2009). GABA A receptors as in vivo substrate for the anxiolytic action of valerenic acid, a major constituent of valerian root extracts. *Neuropharmacology* 56 (1): 174–181.

Benyacoub, J., Czarnecki-Maulden, G.L., Cavadini, C. et al. (2003). Supplementation of food with *Enterococcus faecium* (SF68) stimulates immune functions in young dogs. *Journal of Nutrition* 133 (4): 1158–1162.

den Besten, G., van Eunen, K., Groen, A.K. et al. (2013). The role of short-chain fatty acids in the interplay between diet, gut microbiota, and host energy metabolism. *Journal of Lipid Research* 54 (9): 2325–2340.

Bhathal, A., Spryszak, M., Louizos, C., and Frankel, G. (2017). Glucosamine and chondroitin use in canines for osteoarthritis: a review. *Open Veterinary Journal* 7 (1): 36–49.

Biagi, G., Mordenti, A.L., and Cocchi, M. (2004). The role of dietary omega-3 and omega-6 essential fatty acids in the nutrition of dogs and cats: a review. *Progress in Nutrition* 6 (2): 1–12.

Bierer, T.L. and Bui, L. (2002). Improvement of arthritic signs in dogs fed green-lipped mussel (*Perna canaliculus*). *Journal of Nutrition* 132 (6): 1634S–1636S.

Bishop, C., Hudson, V.M., Hilton, S.C., and Wilde, C. (2005). A pilot study of the effect of inhaled buffered reduced glutathione on the clinical status of patients with cystic fibrosis. *Chest* 127 (1): 308–317.

Blair, J. and Bonavaud, S. (2017). Palataility and tolerability of a novel joint supplement in the cat. *Journal of Feline Medicine and Surgery* 19: 961–969.

Bliss, S. (2013). Musculoskeletal structure and physiology. In: *Canine Sports Medicine and Rehabilitation* (ed. M.C. Zink and J.B. Van Dyke), 32–59. Oxford: Wiley-Blackwell.

Boileau, C., Martel-Pelletier, J., Caron, J. et al. (2009). Protective effects of total fraction of avocado/soybean unsaponifiables on the structural changes in experimental dog osteoarthritis: inhibition of nitric oxide synthase and matrix metalloproteinase-13. *BMC Arthritis Research and Therapy* 11 (2): R41.

Bojanova, D. and Bordenstein, S. (2016). Fecal transplants: what is being transferred? *PLoS Biology* 14 (7): e1002503.

Bol, S. and Bunnik, E. (2015). Lysine supplementation is not effective for the prevention or treatment of feline herpesvirus 1 infection in cats: a systematic review. *BMC Veterinary Research* 11: 284.

Bol, S., Caspers, J., Buckingham, L. et al. (2017). Responsiveness of cats (Felidae) to silver vine (*Actinidia polygama*), Tatarian honeysuckle (*Lonicera tatarica*), valerian (*Valeriana officinalis*) and catnip (*Nepeta cataria*). *BMC Veterinary Research* 13 (1): 70.

Bonn-Miller, M., Loflin, M.J.E., Thomas, B.F. et al. (2017). Labeling accuracy of cannabidiol extracts sold online. *Journal of the American Medical Association* 318 (17): 1708–1709.

Boothe, D. (2020). Nutraceuticals: Where we are today? *Western Veterinary Conference* (February 16–19), Las Vegas, Nevada.

Borgelt, L., Franson, K., Nussbaum, A., and Wang, G. (2013). The pharmacologic and clinical effects of medical cannabis. *Pharmacotherapy* 33 (2): 195–209.

Borody, T. and Khoruts, A. (2011). Fecal microbiota transplantation and emerging applications. *Nature Reviews Gastroenterology and Hepatology* 9 (2): 88–96.

Borowska, M., Czarnywojtek, A., Sawicka-Gutaj, N. et al. (2018). The effects of cannadinois on

the endocrine system. *Endokyrnologia Polska* 69 (6): 705–719.

Bottero, E., Benvenuti, E., and Ruggiero, P. (2017). Fecal microbiota transplantation (FMT) in 16 dogs with idiopathic IBD. *Veterinaria (Cremona)* 31 (1): 31–45.

Braverman, E., Pfeiffer, C., Blum, K., and Smayda, R. (2009). *The Healing Nutrients Within: Facts, Findings, and New Research on Amino Acids*, 3e. Laguna Beach, CA: Basic Health Productions.

Breuss, J., Atanasov, A., and Uhrin, P. (2019). Resveratrol and its effects on the vascular system. *International Journal of Molecular Sciences* 20 (7): 1523.

Brien, S., Prescott, P., Bashir, N. et al. (2008). Systematic review of the nutritional supplements dimethyl sulfoxide (DMSO) and methylsulfonylmethane (MSM) in the treatment of osteoarthritis. *Osteoarthritis and Cartilage* 16 (11): 1277–1288.

Brioschi, F., Di Cesare, F., Gioeni, D. et al. (2020). Oral transmucosal cannadidiol oil formulation as part of a multimodal analgesic regimen: effects on pain relief a and quality of life improvement in dogs affected by spontaneous osteoarthritis. *Animals* 10 (9): 1505.

Britti, D., Crupi, R., Impellizzeri, D. et al. (2017). A novel composite formulation of palmitoylethanolamide and quercetin decreases inflammation and relieves pain in inflammatory and osteoarthritic pain models. *BMC Veterinary Research* 13 (1): 229.

Broere, F., Wieten, L., Klein Koerkamp, E.I. et al. (2008). Oral or nasal antigen induces regulatory T cells that suppress arthritis and proliferation of arthritogenic T cells in joint draining lymph nodes. *Journal of Immunology* 181 (2): 899–906.

Brown, D. and Reetz, J. (2012). Single agent polysaccharopeptide delays metastases and improves survival in naturally occurring hemangiosarcoma. *Evidence-Based Complementary and Alternative Medicine* 2012: 384301.

Brown, S.A., Brown, C.A., Crowell, W.A. et al. (1998). Beneficial effects of chronic administration of dietary ω-3 polyunsaturated fatty acids in dogs with renal insufficiency. *Journal of Laboratory and Clinical Medicine* 131 (5): 447–455.

Brown, S.A., Brown, C.A., Crowell, W. et al. (2000). Effects of dietary polyunsaturated fatty acid supplementation in early renal insufficiency in dogs. *Journal of Laboratory and Clinical Medicine* 135 (3): 275–286.

Brunello, E. and Masini, A. (2016). NEM® brand eggshell membrane effective in the treatment of pain and stiffness associated with osteoarthritis of the knee in an Italian study population. *International Journal of Clinical Medicine* 7 (2): 169–175.

Buckley, M., Good, A., and Knapp, W. (2004). Fish oil interaction with warfarin. *Annals of Pharmacotherapy* 38 (1): 50–52.

Bucsi, L. and Poór, G. (1998). Efficacy and tolerability of oral chondroitin sulfate as a symptomatic slow-acting drug for osteoarthritis (SYSADOA) in the treatment of knee osteoarthritis. *Osteoarthritis and Cartilage* 6 (Suppl. A): 31–36.

Budsberg, S., Bergh, M., Reynolds, L., and Streppa, H. (2007). Evaluation of pentosan polysulfate sodium in the postoperative recovery from cranial cruciate injury in dogs: a randomized, placebo-controlled clinical trial. *Veterinary Surgery* 36 (3): 234–244.

Bui, L. and Bierer, T. (2003). Influence of green lipped mussels (*Perna canaliculus*) in alleviating signs of arthritis in dogs. *Veterinary Therapeutics* 4 (4): 397–407.

Burns, K. (2017). Assessing pet supplements. https://www.avma.org/javma-news/2017-01-15/assessing-pet-supplements (accessed 4 February 2021).

Burns, J., Yokota, T., Ashihara, H. et al. (2002). Plant foods and herbal sources of resveratrol. *Journal of Agriculture and Food Chemistry* 50 (11): 3337–3340.

Butawan, M., Benjamin, R., and Bloomer, R. (2017). Methylsulfonylmethane: applications and safety of a novel dietary supplement. *Nutrients* 9 (3): 290.

Buur, J., Pedro Diniz, K.R., KuKanich, B., and Tegzes, J. (2013). Pharmacokinetics of N-acetylcysteine after oral and intravenous administration to healthy cats. *American Journal of Veterinary Research* 74 (2): 290–293.

Bybee, S., Scorza, A., and Lappin, M. (2011). Effect of the probiotic *Enterococcus faecium* SF68 on presence of diarrhea in cats and dogs housed in an animal shelter. *Journal of Veterinary Internal Medicine* 25 (4): 856–860.

Calder, P. (2013). Omega-3 polyunsaturated fatty acids and inflammatory processes: nutrition or pharmacology? *British Journal of Clinical Pharmacology* 75 (3): 645–662.

Callaway, J.C. (2004). Hempseed as a nutritional resource: an overview. *Euphytica* 140: 35–72.

Campolo, J., Bernardi, S., Cozzi, L. et al. (2017). Medium-term effect of sublingual l-glutathione supplementation on flow-mediated dilation in subjects with cardiovascular risk factors. *Nutrients* 38: 41–47.

Canapp, S. Jr., McLaughlin, R.M. Jr., Hoskinson, J.J. et al. (1999). Scintigraphic evaluation of dogs with acute synovitis after treatment with glucosamine hydrochloride and chondroitin sulfate. *American Journal of Veterinary Research* 60 (12): 1552–1557.

Candela, M., Guidotti, M., Fabbri, A. et al. (2011). Human intestinal microbiota: cross-talk with the host and its potential role in colorectal cancer. *Critical Reviews in Microbiology* 37 (1): 1–14.

Carlson, A., Alderete, K.S., Grant, M.K.O. et al. (2018). Anticancer effects of resveratrol in canine hemangiosarcoma cell lines. *Veterinary Comparative Oncology* 16 (2): 253–261.

Cartwright, P., Roberts, E., and Wood, D. (1954). Theanine an amino acid of N-ethyl amide present in tea. *Journal of the Science of Food and Agriculture* 5: 597–599.

Castagliuolo, I., Riegler, M.F., Valenick, L. et al. (1999). *Saccharomyces boulardii* protease inhibits the effects of *Clostridium difficile* toxins A and B in human colonic mucosa. *Infection and Immunity* 67 (1): 302–307.

Castell, L. (2003). Glutamine supplementation in vitro and in vivo, in exercise and in immunodepression. *Sports Medicine* 33 (5): 323–345.

Caterino, C., Aragosa, F., Della Valle, G. et al. (2021). Clinical efficacy of Curcuvet and Boswellic acid combined with conventional nutraceutical product: an aid to canine osteoarthritis. *PLoS One* 16 (5): e0252279.

Center, S.A. (2004). Metabolic, antioxidant, nutraceutical, probiotic, and herbal therapies relating to the management of hepatobiliary disorders. *Veterinary Clinics of North America Small Animal Practice* 34 (1): 67–172.

Center, S.A., Harte, J., Watrous, D. et al. (2000). The clinical and metabolic effects of rapid weight loss in obese pet cats and the influence of supplemental oral L-carnitine. *Journal of Veterinary Internal Medicine* 14 (6): 598–608.

Center, S.A., Warner, K.L., McCabe, J. et al. (2005). Evaluation of the influence of S-adenosylmethionine on systemic and hepatic effects of prednisolone in dogs. *American Journal of Veterinary Research* 66 (2): 330–341.

Center, S.A., Randolph, J.F., Warner, K.L. et al. (2008). The effects of S-adenosylmethionine on clinical pathology and redox potential in the red blood cell, liver, and bile of clinical normal cats. *Journal of Veterinary Internal Medicine* 19 (3): 303–314.

Center, S.A., Warner, K.L., Randolph, J.F. et al. (2012). Influence of dietary supplementation with (L)-carnitine on metabolic rate, fatty acid oxidation, body condition, and weight loss in overweight cats. *American Journal of Veterinary Research* 73 (7): 1002–1015.

Chaitman, J. and Gaschen, F. (2021). Fecal microbiota transplantation in dogs. *Veterinary Clinics of North America Small Animal Practice* 51 (1): 219–233.

Chaitman, J., Ziese, A.-L., Pilla, R. et al. (2020). Fecal microbial and metabolic profiles in dogs with acute diarrhea receiving either fecal microbiota transplantation or oral metronidazole. *Frontiers in Veterinary Science* 7: 192.

Chan, D. (2019). Where did immunonutrition go? *European Veterinary Emergency and Critical Care Congress*, 6–8 June 2019, Tallinn, Estonia.

Chan, A., Paskavitz, J., Remington, R. et al. (2008). Efficacy of a vitamin/nutriceutical formulation for early-stage Alzheimer's disease: a 1-year, open-label pilot study with an 16-month caregiver extension. *American Journal of Alzheimer's Disease and Other Dementias* 56 (9): 571–585.

Chandran, B. and Goel, A. (2012). A randomized, pilot study to assess the efficacy and safety of curcumin in patients with active rheumatoid arthritis. *Phytotherapy Research* 26 (11): 1719–1725.

Chen, J. (2013). *Concurrent Use of Herbal Medicines and Pharmaceuticals: Pharmacodynamics Interactions*. College of Integrative Veterinary Therapies.

Chen, F., Du, M., Blumberg, J.B. et al. (2019). Association among dietary supplement use, nutrient intake, and mortality among US adults: a cohort study. *Annals of Internal Medicine* 170 (9): 604–613.

Cheng, Y., Xue, A., Yao, C. et al. (2013). Resveratrol ameliorates the oxidative damage induced by arsenic trioxide in the feline lung. *Journal of Veterinary Medical Science* 75 (9): 1139–1146.

Cheng, Y., Xue, J., Jiang, H. et al. (2014). Neuroprotective effect of resveratrol on arsenic trioxide-induced oxidative stress in feline brain. *Human and Experimental Toxicology* 33 (7): 737–747.

Chew, B. and Jean, P. (2004). Carotenoid action on the immune response. *Journal of Nutrition* 134 (1): 257S–261S.

Chew, B., Mathison, B.D., Hayek, M.G. et al. (2011). Dietary astaxanthin enhances immune response in dogs. *Veterinary Immunology and Immunopathology* 140 (3–4): 199–206.

Cho, S.Y., Sim, J.-S., Jeong, C.S. et al. (2004). Effects of low molecular weight chondroitin sulfate on type II collagen-induced arthritis in DBA/1J mice. *Biological and Pharmaceutical Bulletin* 27 (1): 47–51.

Chou, M.M., Vergnolle, N., McDougall, J.J. et al. (2005). Effects of chondroitin and glucosamine sulfate in a dietary bar formulation on inflammation, interleukin-1β, matrix metalloprotease-9, and cartilage damage in arthritis. *Experimental Biology and Medicine* 230 (4): 255–262.

Christiansen, B., Bhatti, S., Goudarzi, R., and Emami, S. (2014). Management of osteoarthritis with avocado/soybean unsaponifiables. *Cartilage* 6 (1): 30–44.

Chu, Y., Wu, Y.C., Chou, Y.C. et al. (2004). Endothelium-dependent relaxation of canine pulmonary artery after prolonged lung graft preservation in University of Wisconsin solution: role of L-arginine supplementation. *Journal of Heart and Lung Transplant* 23 (5): 592–598.

Cintio, M., Scarsella, E., Sgorlon, S. et al. (2020). Gut microbiome of healthy and arthritic dogs. *Veterinary Sciences* 7 (3): 92.

Civitelli, R., Villareal, D.T., Agnusdei, D. et al. (1992). Dietary L-lysine and calcium metabolism in humans. *Nutrition* 8 (2): 400–405.

CL (ConsumerLab) (2022). Quality Certification Program. https://www.consumerlab.com/quality-certification-program (accessed 30 January 2022).

Clarke, S.P., Mellor, D., Clements, D.N. et al. (2005). Prevalence of radiographic signs of degenerative joint disease in a hospital population of cats. *Veterinary Record* 157 (25): 793–799.

Colitti, M., Gaspardo, B., Della Pria, A. et al. (2012). Transcriptome modification of white blood cells after dietary administration of curcumin and non-steroidal anti-inflammatory drug in osteoarthritic affected dogs. *Veterinary Immunology and Immunopathology* 147 (3–4): 136–146.

Collado, M., Grześkowiak, L., and Salminen, S. (2007). Probiotic strains and their combination inhibit in vitro adhesion of pathogens to pig intestinal mucosa. *Current Microbiology* 55 (3): 260–265.

Combarros, D., Castilla-Castaño, E., Lecru, L.A. et al. (2020). A prospective, randomized, double blind, placebo-controlled evaluation of the effects of an n-3 essential fatty acids supplement (Agepi® ω3) on clinical signs, and fatty acid concentrations in the erythrocyte membrane, hair shafts and skin surface of dogs. *Prostaglandins, Leukotrienes, and Essential Fatty Acids* 159: 102140.

Comblain, F., Serisier, S., Barthelemy, N. et al. (2016). Review of dietary supplements for the management of osteoarthritis in dogs in studies from 2004 to 2014. *Journal of Veterinary Pharmacology and Therapeutics* 39 (1): 1–15.

Corbee, R.J., Booij-Vrieling, H.E., van de Lest, C.H.A. et al. (2012). Inflammation and wound healing in cats with chronic gingivitis/stomatitis after extraction of all premolars and molars were not affected by feeding of two diets with different omega-6/omega-3 polyunsaturated fatty acid ratios. *Journal of Animal Physiology and Animal Nutrition* 96 (4): 671–680.

Corbee, R., Barnier, M.M.C., van de Lest, C.H.A., and Hazewinkel, H.A.W. (2013). The effect of dietary long-chain omega-3 fatty acid supplementation on owner's perception of behaviour and locomotion in cats with naturally occurring osteoarthritis. *Journal of Animal Physiology and Animal Nutrition* 97 (5): 846–853.

Cordero, M., Cano-García, F.J., Alcocer-Gómez, E. et al. (2012). Oxidative stress correlates with headache symptoms in fibromyalgia: coenzyme Q_{10} effect on clinical improvement. *PLoS One* 7 (4): e35677.

Corsetti, S., Borruso, S., Malandrucco, L. et al. (2021). *Cannabis sativa* L. may reduce aggressive behavior towards humans in shelter dogs. *Scientific Reports* 11 (1): 2773.

CRN (Council for Responsible Nutrition) (2019). Dietary supplement use reaches all time high. https://www.crnusa.org/newsroom/dietary-supplement-use-reaches-all-time-high (accessed 1 June 2021).

Crowley, D.C., Francis, C.L., Prachi, S., et al. (2009). Safety and efficacy of undenatured type II collagen in the treatment of osteoarthritis of the knee: a clinical trial. *International Journal of Medical Sciences* 6 (6): 312–321.

Cruzat, V., Rogero, M.M., Keane, K.N. et al. (2018). Glutamine: metabolism and immune function, supplementation and clinical translation. *Nutrients* 10 (11): 1564.

CVM (Center for Veterinary Medicine) (2022). Hazard Analysis and Risk-Based Preventative Controls for Food for Animals Guidance for Industry. https://www.fda.gov/media/110477/ download (accessed 2 May 2023).

Dahms, I., Bailey-Hall, E., Sylvester, E. et al. (2019). Safety of a novel feed ingredient, algal oil containing EPA and DHA, in a gestation–lactation–growth feeding study in Beagle dogs. *PLoS One* 14 (6): e0217794.

Daily, J., Yang, M., and Park, S. (2016). Efficacy of turmeric extracts and curcumin for alleviating the symptoms of joint arthritis: a systematic review and meta-analysis of randomized clinical trials. *Journal of Medicinal Food* 19 (8): 717–729.

D'Altilio, M., Peal, A., Alvey, M. et al. (2007). Therapeutic efficacy and safety of undenatured type II collagen singly or in combination with glucosamine and chondroitin in arthritic dogs. *Toxicology Mechanisms and Methods* 17 (4): 189–196.

Danesch, U., Seybold, M., Rittinghausen, R. et al. (2014). NEM brand eggshell membrane effective in the treatment of pain associated with knee and hip osteoarthritis: results from a six center, open label German clinical study. *Journal of Arthritis*, 3(3), 136.

D'Angelo, S., Fracassi, F., Bresciani, F. et al. (2018). Effect of *Saccharomyces boulardii* in dogs with chronic enteropathies: double-blinded, placebo-controlled study. *Veterinary Research* 182 (9): 258.

D'Angelo, S., Motti, M.L., and Meccariello, R. (2020). ω-3 and ω-6 polyunsaturated fatty acids, obesity and cancer. *Nutrients* 12 (9): 2751.

Dasgupta, A., Hovanetz, M., Olsen, M. et al. (2007). Drug–herb interaction: effect of St John's wort on bioavailability and metabolism of procainamide in mice. *Archives of Pathology and Laboratory Medicine* 131 (7): 1094–1098.

David-Raoudi, M., Deschrevel, B., Leclercq, S. et al. (2009). Chondroitin sulfate increases hyaluronan production by human synoviocytes through differential regulation of hyaluronan synthases: role of p38 and Akt. *Arthritis and Rheumatism* 60 (3): 760–770.

Davinelli, S., Nielsen, M.E., and Scapagnini, G. (2018). Astaxanthin in skin health, repair, and disease: a comprehensive review. *Nutrients* 10 (4): 522.

Davis, J., Murphy, E., and Carmichael, M. (2009). Effects of the dietary flavonoid quercetin upon performance and health. *Current Sports Medicine Reports* 8 (4): 206–213.

DEA (Drug Enforcement Administration) (2021). Drug Scheduling. https://www.dea .gov/drug-information/drug-scheduling (accessed 18 July 2021).

Deabold, K., Schwark, W., Wolf, L., and Wakshlag, J. (2019). Single-dose pharmacokinetics and preliminary safety assessment with use of CBD-rich hemp nutraceutical in healthy dogs and cats. *Animals* 9 (10): 832.

Debbie, E., Agar, G., Fichman, G. et al. (2011). Efficacy of methylsulfonylmethane supplementation on osteoarthritis of the knee: a randomized controlled study. *BMC Complementary and Alternative Medicine* 11: 50.

Deguchi, M., Kane, S., Potlakayala, S. et al. (2020). Metabolic engineering strategies of industrial hemp (*Cannabis sativa* L.): a brief review of the advances and challenges. *Frontiers in Plant Science* 11: 580621.

Del Prete, C., Ciani, F., Tafuri, S. et al. (2018). Effect of superoxide dismutase, catalase, and glutathione peroxidase supplementation in the extender on chilled semen of fertile and hypofertile dogs. *Journal of Veterinary Science* 19 (5): 667–675.

Delmas, D., Xiao, J., Vejux, A., and Aires, V. (2020). Silymarin and cancer: a dual strategy in both chemoprevention and chemosensitivity. *Molecules* 25 (9): 2009.

DeNapoli, J., Dodman, N.H., Shuster, L. et al. (2000). Effect of dietary protein content and tryptophan supplementation on dominance aggression, territorial aggression, and hyperactivity in dogs. *Journal of the American Veterinary Medical Association* 217 (4): 504–508.

Deparle, L., Gupta, R.C., Canerdy, T.D. et al. (2005). Efficacy and safety of glycosylated undenatured type-II collagen (UC-II) in therapy of arthritic dogs. *Journal of Veterinary Pharmacology and Therapeutics* 28 (4): 385–390.

DePeters, E. and George, L. (2014). Rumen transfaunation. *Immunology Letters* 162 (2A): 69–76.

Derfoul, A., Miyoshi, A., Freeman, D., and Tuan, R. (2007). Glucosamine promotes chondrogenic phenotype in both chondrocytes and mesenchymal stem cells and inhibits MMP-13 expression and matrix degradation. *Osteoarthritis and Cartilage* 15 (6): 646–655.

De-Souza, D. and Greene, L. (1998). Pharmacological nutrition after burn injury. *Journal of Nutrition* 128 (5): 797–803.

Dey, D., Chaskar, S., Athavale, N., and Chitre, D. (2015). Acute and chronic toxicity, cytochrome p450 enzyme inhibition, and HERG channel blockade studies with a polyherbal, ayurvedic formulation for inflammation. *Biomedical Research International* 2015: 971982.

Dickerson, R. (2016). Nitrogen balance and protein requirements for critically ill older patients. *Nutrients* 8 (4): 226.

Dietz, B., Mahady, G., Pauli, G., and Farnsworth, N. (2005). Valerian extract and valerenic acid are partial agonists of the 5-HT5a receptor in vitro. *Molecular Brain Research* 138 (2): 191–197.

DiNicolantonio, J.J. and O'Keefe, J.H. (2018). Importance of maintaining a low omega-6/omega-3 ratio for reducing inflammation. *Open Heart* 5 (2): e000946.

Dobenecker, B., Beetz, Y., and Kienzle, E. (2002). A placebo-controlled double-blind study on the effect of nutraceuticals (chondroitin sulfate and mussel extract) in dogs with joint diseases as perceived by their owners. *Journal of Nutrition* 132 (6 Suppl. 2): 1690S–1691S.

Dominguez, T., Kaur, K., and Burri, L. (2021). Enhanced omega-3 index after long- versus short-chain omega-3 fatty acid supplementation in dogs. *Veterinary Medicine and Science* 7 (2): 370–377.

Dong, J.-Y., Qin, L.-Q., Zhang, Z. et al. (2011). Effect of oral l-arginine supplementation on blood pressure: a meta-analysis of randomized, double-blind, placebo-controlled trials. *American Heart Journal* 162 (6): 959–965.

Donvito, G., Nass, S.R., Wilkerson, J.L. et al. (2018). The endogenous cannabinoid system: a budding source of targets for treating inflammatory and neuropathic pain. *Neuropsychopharmacology* 43 (1): 52–79.

Dramard, V., Kern, L., Hofmans, J. et al. (2018). Effect of l-theanine tablets in reducing stress-related emotional signs in cats: an open-label field study. *Irish Veterinary Journal* 71: 21.

DSHEA (1994). Dietary Supplement Health and Education Act (DSHEA) of 1994 Public Law 103–417. https://ods.od.nih.gov/About/DSHEA_Wording.aspx#sec3 (accessed 2 February 2021).

Dürr, D., Stieger, B., Kullak-Ublick, G.A. et al. (2000). St John's Wort induces intestinal P-glycoprotein/MDR1 and intestinal and hepatic CYP3A4. *Clinical Pharmacology and Therapeutics* 68 (6): 598–604.

Elanco US Inc. (2018). Adequan Canine. https://dailymed.nlm.nih.gov/dailymed/drugInfo.cfm?setid=b0fbf2e7-5a2a-4fa2-957c-3d4693a891fe (accessed 14 March 2022).

Elrod, S. and Hofmeister, E. (2019). Veterinarians' attitudes towards use of nutraceuticals. *Canadian Journal of Veterinary Research* 83 (4): 291–297.

Eman, A., Winter, T., Aukema, H.M., and Miller, D.W. (2019). Effects of various dietary supplements on inflammatory processes in primary canine chondrocytes as a model of osteoarthritis. *Canadian Journal of Veterinary Research* 83 (3): 206–217.

Exposito, J.-Y., Valcourt, U., Cluzel, C., and Lethias, C. (2010). The fibrillar collagen family. *International Journal of Molecular Science* 11 (2): 407–426.

Faghihzadeh, F., Hekmatdoost, A., and Adibi, P. (2015). Resveratrol and liver: a systematic review. *Journal of Research in Medical Sciences* 20 (8): 797–810.

Fan, Y.-p., Yu, J.-c., Kang, W.-m., and Zhang, Q. (2009). Effects of glutamine supplementation on patients undergoing abdominal surgery. *Chinese Medical Sciences Journal* 24 (1): 55–59.

Fasinu, P., Phillips, S., Sohly, M.E., and Walker, L. (2016). Current status and prospects for cannabidiol preparations as new therapeutic agents. *Pharmacotherapy* 36 (7): 781–796.

Fassett, R. and Coombes, J. (2011). Astaxanthin: a potential therapeutic agent in cardiovascular disease. *Marine Drugs* 9 (3): 447–465.

FDA (Food and Drug Administration) (2007). Complementary and Alternative Medicine Products and their Regulation by the Food and Drug Administration: Draft Guidance for Industry. https://www.fda.gov/regulatory-information/search-fda-guidance-documents/complementary-and-alternative-medicine-products-and-their-regulation-food-and-drug-administration (accessed 6 May 2020).

FDA (Food and Drug Administration) (2009). Guidance for Industry: Questions and Answers Regarding the Labeling of Dietary Supplements as Required by the Dietary Supplement and Nonprescription Drug Consumer Protection Act; Availability. https://www.federalregister.gov/documents/2009/09/01/E9-21094/guidance-for-industry-questions-and-answers-regarding-the-labeling-of-dietary-supplements-as (accessed 3 February 2021).

FDA (Food and Drug Administration) (2017a). FDA approved L-glutamine powder for the treatment of sickle cell disease. https://www.fda.gov/drugs/resources-information-approved-drugs/fda-approved-l-glutamine-powder-treatment-sickle-cell-disease (accessed 25 June 2022).

FDA (Food and Drug Administration) (2017b). Is it really FDA Approved? https://www.fda.gov/consumers/consumer-updates/it-really-fda-approved (accessed 4 February 2021).

FDA (Food and Drug Administration) (2018). Label Claims for Conventional Foods and Dietary Supplements. https://www.fda.gov/food/food-labeling-nutrition/label-claims-conventional-foods-and-dietary-supplements (accessed 3 February 2021).

FDA (Food and Drug Administration) (2020). The Ins and Outs of Extra-Label Drug Use in Animals: A Resource for Veterinarians. https://www.fda.gov/animal-veterinary/resources-you/ins-and-outs-extra-label-drug-use-animals-resource-veterinarians (accessed 2 February 2021).

FDA (Food and Drug Administration) (2021a). Animal Food and Feeds: Product Regulation. https://www.fda.gov/animal-veterinary/animal-food-feeds/product-regulation (accessed 20 February 2021).

FDA (Food and Drug Administration) (2021b). Animal Medicinal Drug Use Clarificaiton Act of 1994 (AMDUCA). https://www.fda.gov/animal-veterinary/guidance-regulations/animal-medicinal-drug-use-clarification-act-1994-amduca (accessed 24 January 2022).

FDA (Food and Drug Administration) (2021c). CFR - Code of Federal Regulations Title 21. https://www.accessdata.fda.gov/scripts/cdrh/cfdocs/cfcfr/CFRSearch.cfm?CFRPart=211&showFR=1. (accessed 16 December 2021).

FDA (Food and Drug Administration) (2021d). Facts About the Current Good Manufacturing Practices (CGMPs). http://www.fda.gov/Drugs/DevelopmentApprovalProcess/Manufacturing/ucm169105.htm (accessed 17 December 2021).

FDA (Food and Drug Administration) (2022a). FDA's Regulation of Pet Food. https://www.fda.gov/animal-veterinary/

animal-health-literacy/fdas-regulation-pet-food#drug (accessed 2 May 2023).

FDA (Food and Drug Administration) (2022b). Hazard Analysis Critical Control Point (HACCP). https://www.fda.gov/food/guidance-regulation-food-and-dietary-supplements/hazard-analysis-critical-control-point-haccp#:~:text=HACCP%20is%20a%20management%20system,consumption%20of%20the%20finished%20product (accessed 2 May 2023).

FDA (Food and Drug Administration) (2022c). Summary of Color Additives for Use in the United States in Foods, Drugs, Cosmetics, and Medical Devices. https://www.fda.gov/industry/color-additive-inventories/summary-color-additives-use-united-states-foods-drugs-cosmetics-and-medical-devices#part82 (accessed 4 July 2022).

Feng, J., Huang, M., Chai, Z. et al. (2020). The influence of oil composition on the transformation, bioaccessibility, and intestinal absorption of curcumin in nanostructured lipid carriers†. *Food and Function* 11 (6): 5223–5239.

Fernández, S., Wasowski, C., Paladini, A.C., and Marder, M. (2004). Sedative and sleep-enhancing properties of linarin, a flavonoid-isolated form *Valeriana officinalis*. *Pharmacology Biochemistry and Behavior* 77 (2): 399–404.

Fernández-San-Martín, M.I., Masa-Font, R., Palacios-Soler, L. et al. (2010). Effectiveness of valerian on insomnia: a meta-analysis of randomized placebo-controlled trials. *Sleep Medicine* 11 (6): 505–511.

Ferreira, A.C., Serejo, J.S., Durans, R. et al. (2020). Dose-related effects of resveratrol in different models of pulmonary arterial hypertension: a systematic review. *Current Cardiology Reviews* 16 (3): 231–240.

Fischer, U.M., Cox, C.S. Jr., Allen, S.J. et al. (2003). The antioxidant N-acetylcysteine preserves myocardial function and diminishes oxidative stress after cardioplegic arrest. *Journal of Thoracic and Cardiovascular Surgery* 126 (5): 1483–1488.

Floerchinger, A.M., Jackson, M.I., Jewell, D.E. et al. (2015). Effect of feeding a weight loss food beyond a caloric restriction period on body composition and resistance to weight gain in dogs. *Journal of the American Veterinary Medical Association* 247 (4): 375–384.

Franco, R., Schoneveld, O., Pappa, A., and Panayiotidis, M. (2007). The central role of glutathione in the pathophysiology of human diseases. *Archives of Physiology and Biochemistry* 113 (4–5): 234–258.

Franconi, F., Loizzo, A., Ghirlanda, G., and Seghieri, G. (2006). Taurine supplementation and diabetes mellitus. *Current Opinion in Clinical Nutrition and Metabolic Care* 9 (1): 32–36.

Frantz, C., Stewart, K., and Weaver, V. (2010). The extracellular matrix at a glance. *Journal of Cell Science* 123: 4195–4200.

Frederico, A., Dallio, M., and Loguercio, C. (2017). Silymarin/Silybin and chronic liver disease: a marriage of many years. *Molecules* 22 (2): 191.

Freeman, L. (2010). Beneficial effects of omega-3 fatty acids in cardiovascular disease. *Journal of Small Animal Practice* 51 (9): 462–470.

Freeman, L.M. (2017). Dietary Supplements for Pets: Harmful or Helpful? https://vetnutrition.tufts.edu/2017/03/dietary-supplements-for-pets-harmful-or-helpful (accessed 20 February 2021).

Freeman, L.M., Rush, J.E., Kehayias, J.J. et al. (1998). Nutritional alterations and the effect of fish oil supplementation in dogs with heart failure. *Journal of Veterinary Internal Medicine* 12 (6): 440–448.

Freeman, L., Rush, J., and Markwell, P. (2006). Effects of dietary modification in dogs with early chronic valvular disease. *Journal of Veterinary Internal Medicine* 20 (5): 1116–1126.

Friedman, M. (2018). Analysis, nutrition, and health benefits of tryptophan. *International Journal of Tryptophan Research* 11: 1178646918802282.

Fritsch, D.A., Allen, T.A., Dodd, C.E. et al. (2010a). A multicenter study of the effect of dietary supplementation with fish oil omega-3 fatty acids on carprofen dosage in dogs with osteoarthritis. *Journal of the American Veterinary Medical Association* 236 (5): 535–539.

Fritsch, D.A., Allen, T.A., Dodd, C.E. et al. (2010b). Dose-titration effects of fish oil in osteoarthritic dogs. *Journal of Veterinary Internal Medicine* 24 (5): 1020–1026.

FTF (Fecal Transplant Foundation) 2022. What is FMT? https://thefecaltransplantfoundation. org/what-is-fecal-transplant (accessed 9 February 2022).

Fujiki, M., Shineha, J., Yamanokuchi, K. et al. (2007). Effects of treatment with polysulfated glycosaminoglycan on serum cartilage oligomeric matrix protein and C-reactive protein concentrations, serum matrix metalloproteinase-2 and -9 activities, and lameness in dogs with osteoarthritis. *American Journal of Veterinary Research* 68 (8): 827–833.

Gal, A., Barko, P.C., Biggs, P.J. et al. (2021). One dog's waste is another dog's wealth: a pilot study of fecal microbiota transplantation in dogs with acute hemorrhagic diarrhea syndrome. *PLoS One* 16 (4): e0250344.

Galiniak, S., Aebisher, D., and Bartusik-Aebisher, D. (2019). Health benefits of resveratrol administration. *Journal of the Polish Biochemical Society and of the Polish Academy of Sciences* 66 (1): 13–21.

Galizia, I., Oldani, L., Macritchie, K. et al. (2016). S-adenosyl methionine (SAMe) for depression in adults. *Cochrane Database of Systematic Reviews* (10): CD011286.

Gaman, A. and Kuo, B. (2008). Neuromodulatory processes of the brain–gut axis. *Neuromodulation* 11 (4): 249–259.

Gamble, L.-J., Boesch, J.M., Frye, C.W. et al. (2018). Pharmacokinetics, safety, and clinical efficacy of cannabidiol treatment in osteoarthritic dogs. *Frontiers in Veterinary Science* 5: 165.

Gamoh, S., Hashimoto, M., Sugioka, K. et al. (1999). Chronic administration of docosahexaenoic acid improves reference memory-related learning ability in young rats. *Neuroscience* 93 (1): 237–241.

Gao, Z., Yin, J., Zhang, J. et al. (2009). Butyrate improves insulin sensitivity and increases energy expenditure in mice. *Diabetes* 58 (7): 1509–1517.

Gao, J., Xu, K., Liu, H. et al. (2018). Impact of the gut microbiota on intestinal immunity mediated by tryptophan metabolism. *Frontiers in Cellular and Infection Microbiology* 8: 13.

Garcia-Mazcorro, J., Barcenas-Walls, J., Suchodolski, J., and Steiner, J. (2017). Molecular assessment of the fecal microbiota in healthy cats and dogs before and during supplementation with fructo-oligosaccharides (FOS) and inulin using high-throughput 454-pyrosequencing. *PeerJ* 5: e3184.

Gaunt, S., Baker, D., and Green, R. (1981). Clinicopathologic evaluation N-acetylcysteine therapy in acetaminophen toxicosis in the cat. *American Journal of Veterinary Research* 42 (11): 1982–1984.

Gaykwad, C., Garkhal, J., Chethan, G.E. et al. (2017). Amelioration of oxidative stress using N-acetylcysteine in canine parvoviral enteritis. *Journal of Veterinary Pharmacology and Therapeutics* 41 (1): 68–75.

Gedney, A., Salah, P., Mahoney, J.A. et al. (2022). Evaluation of the anti-tumour activity of *Coriolus versicolor* polysaccharopeptide (I'm-Yunity) alone or in combination with doxorubicin for canine splenic hemangiosarcoma. *Veterinary Comparative Oncology* 20 (3): 688–696.

Gencoglu, H., Orhan, C., Sahin, E., and Sahin, K. (2020). Undenatured type II collagen (UC-II) in joint health and disease: a review on the current knowledge of companion animals. *Animals* 10 (4): 697.

George, D., Schwarz, U., Wilkinson, G., and Kim, R. (2003). Coordinate induction of both cytochrome P4503A and MDR1 by St John's wort in healthy subjects. *Clinical Pharmacology and Therapeutics* 73 (1): 41–50.

Gibson, R., Gibson, S., Conway, V., and Chappell, D. (1980). *Perna canaliculus* in the treatment of arthritis. *Practitioner* 224 (1347): 955–960.

Gibson, G., Scott, K.P., Rastall, R.A., and Tuohy, K.M. (2010). Dietary prebiotics: current status and new definition. *Food Science and Technology Bulletin Functional Foods* 7 (1): 1–19.

Goodman, L. and Trepanier, L. (2005). Potential drug interactions with dietary supplements. *Compendium* 27 (10): 780–790. http://vetfolio-vetstreet.s3.amazonaws.com/mmah/80/99d0ebe0d44abcbe44070451d2df3a/filePV_27_10_780.pdf.

Goppel, M. and Franz, G. (2004). Stability control of valerian ground material and extracts: a new HPLC-method for the routine quantification of valerenic acids and lignans. *Pharmazie* 59 (6): 446–452.

Goudarzi, R., Reid, A., and McDougall, J. (2018). Evaluation of the novel avocado/soybean unsaponifiable Arthrocen to alter joint pain and inflammation in a rat model of osteoarthritis. *PLoS One* 13 (2): e0191906.

Gouze, J.-N., Gouze, E., Popp, M.P. et al. (2006). Exogenous glucosamine globally protects chondrocytes from the arthritogenic effects of IL-1β. *Arthritis Research and Therapy* 8 (6): R173.

Grassie, L. (2002). Update on Animal Dietary Supplements. https://www.nasc.cc/historical-summary (accessed 4 February 2021).

Green, J., Heard, K., Reynolds, K., and Albert, D. (2013). Oral and intravenous acetylcysteine for treatment of acetaminophen toxicity: a systematic review and meta-analysis. *Western Journal of Emergency Medicine* 14 (3): 218–226.

Griessmayr, P., Gauthier, M., Barber, L., and Cotter, S. (2008). Mushroom-derived maitake PETfraction as a single agent for the treatment of lymphoma in dogs. *Journal of Veterinary Internal Medicine* 21 (6): 1409–1412.

Grover, A. and Samson, S. (2016). Benefits of antioxidant supplements for knee osteoarthritis: rationale and reality. *Nutrition Journal* 15: 1.

Gui, S., Jia, J., Niu, X. et al. (2014). Arginine supplementation for improving maternal and neonatal outcomes in hypertensive disorder of pregnancy: a systematic review. *Journal of the Renin–Angiotensin–Aldosterone System* 15 (1): 88–96.

Guo, T., Chang, L., Xiao, Y., and Liu, Q. (2015). S-adenosyl-L-methionine for the treatment of chronic liver disease: a systematic review and meta-analysis. *PLoS One* 10 (3): e0122124.

Guo, H., Co, H., Cui, X. et al. (2019a). Silymarin's inhibition and treatment effects for Alzheimer's disease. *Molecules* 24 (9): 1748.

Guo, Q., Goldenberg, J.Z., Humphrey, C. et al. (2019b). Probiotics for the prevention of pediatric antibiotic-associated diarrhea. *Cochrane Database of Systematic Reviews* (4): CD004827.

Gupta, P., Samarakoon, S., Chandola, H., and Ravishankar, B. (2011). Clinical evaluation of *Boswellia serrata* (Shallaki) resin in the management of Sandhivata (osteoarthritis). *Ayu* 32 (4): 478–482.

Gupta, R., Canerdy, T.D., Lindley, J. et al. (2012). Comparative therapeutic efficacy and safety of type-II collagen (uc-II), glucosamine and chondroitin in arthritic dogs: pain evaluation by ground force plate. *Journal of Animal Physiology and Animal Nutrition* 96 (5): 770–777.

Gupta, S., Patchva, S., and Aggarwal, B. (2013). Therapeutic roles of curcumin: lessons learned from clinical trials. *AAPS Journal* 15 (1): 195–218.

Gupta, S., Allen-Vercoe, E., and Petrof, E. (2016). Fecal microbiota transplant: in perspective. *Therapeutic Advances in Gastroenterology* 9 (2): 229–238.

Gurley, B.J., Swain, A., Williams, D.K. et al. (2008). Gauging the clinical significane of P-glycoprotein-mediated herb–drug interactions: comparative effects of St. John's wort, Echinacea, clarithromycin, and rifampin on digoxin pharmacokinetics. *Molecular Nutrition and Food Research* 52 (7): 772–779.

GVR (Grand View Research) (2020). *Pet Supplements Market Size, Share & Trends Analysis Report by Pet Type (Cats, Dogs), by Distribution Channel (Offline, Online), by Region (North America, Europe, APAC, CSA,*

MEA), and Segment Forecasts, 2020–2027. Consumer F&B.

H.R.2 (2018). Agricultural Improvement Act of 2018, Public Law Number 115–334. https://www.congress.gov/bill/115th-congress/house-bill/2 (accessed 17 July 2022).

de Haan, J., Goring, R., and Beale, B. (1994). Evaluation of polysulfated glycosaminoglycan for the treatment of hip dysplasia in dogs. *Veterinary Surgery* 23 (3): 177–178.

Hagen, D., Ekena, J., Geesaman, B., and Viviano, K. (2019). Antioxidant supplementation during illness in dogs: effect on oxidative stress and outcome, an exploratory study. *Journal of Small Animal Practice* 60 (9): 543–550.

Hall, J. and Jewell, D. (2012). Feeding healthy beagles medium-chain triglycerides, fish oil, and carnitine offsets age-related changes in serum fatty acids and carnitine metabolites. *PLoS One* 7 (11): e49510.

Hall, J., Wander, R., Du, J.G.S., and Jewell, D. (1999). Effect of dietary n-6-to-n-3 fatty acid ratio on complete blood and total white blood cell counts, and T-cell subpopulations in aged dogs. *American Journal of Veterinary Research* 6 (3): 319–327.

Hall, J.A., Tooley, K.A., Gradin, J.L. et al. (2003). Effects of dietary n-6 and n-3 fatty acids and vitamin E on the immune response of healthy geriatric dogs. *American Journal of Veterinary Research* 64 (6): 762–772.

Hand, M., Thatcher, C.D., Remillard, R.L. et al. (2010). *Small Animal Clinical Nutrition*, 5e. Topeka, KS: Mark Morris Institute.

Haroyan, A., Mukuchyan, V., Mkrtchyan, N. et al. (2018). Efficacy and safety of curcumin and its combination with boswellic acid in osteoarthritis: a comparative, randomized, double-blind, placebo-controlled study. *BMC Complementary and Alternative Medicine* 18 (1): 7.

Harvard School of Public Health (2022). The Nutrition Source: Antioxidants. https://www.hsph.harvard.edu/nutritionsource/antioxidants (accessed 2 July 2022).

Hecker, A., Schellnegger, M., Hofmann, E. et al. (2021). The impact of resveratrol on skin wound healing, scarring, and aging. *International Wound Journal* 19 (1): 9–28.

Heilm-Björkman, A., Tulamo, R.-M., Salonen, H., and Raekallio, M. (2009). Evaluating complementary therapies for canine osteoarthritis part I: green-lipped mussel (*Perna canaliculus*). *Evidence-based Complementary and Alternative Medicine* 6 (3): 365–373.

Heinemann, K.M., Waldron, M.K., Bigley, K.E. et al. (2005). Long-chain (n-3) polyunsaturated fatty acids are more efficient than alpha-linolenic acid in improving electroretinogram responses of puppies exposed during gestation, lactation, and weaning. *Journal of Nutrition* 135 (8): 1960–1966.

Heinrich, M. (2009). Nutraceutical. https://www.britannica.com/science/nutraceutical (accessed 2 February 2021).

Heinz, S., Henson, D.A., Austin, M.D. et al. (2010). Quercetin supplementation and upper respiratory tract infection: a randomized community clinical trial. *Pharmacological Research* 62 (3): 237–242.

Henderson, L., Yue, Q.Y., Bergquist, C. et al. (2002). St John's wort (*Hypericum perforatum*): drug interactions and clinical outcomes. *British Journal of Clinical Pharmacology* 54 (4): 349–356.

Henrotin, Y., Mathy, M., Sanchez, C., and Lambert, C. (2010). Chondroitin sulfate in the treatment of osteoarthritis: from in vitro studies to clinical recommendations. *Therapeutic Advances in Musculoskeletal Disease* 2 (6): 335–348.

Henry, J.G., Shoemaker, G., Prieto, J.M. et al. (2020). The effect of cannabidiol on canine neoplastic cell proliferation and mitogen-activated protein kinase activation during autophagy and apoptosis. *Veterinary and Comparative Oncology* 19 (2): 253–265.

Hewlings, S. and Kalman, D. (2017). Curcumin: a review of its effects on human health. *Food* 6 (10): 92.

Hewlings, S., Kalman, D., and Schneider, L. (2019). A randomized, double-blind, placebo-controlled, prospective clinical trial evaluating water-soluble chicken eggshell membrane for improvement in joint health in adults with knee osteoarthritis. *Journal of Medicinal Food* 22 (9): 875–884.

Higdon, J. (2003). Essential Fatty Acids. https://lpi.oregonstate.edu/mic/other-nutrients/essential-fatty-acids#sources (accessed 6 March 2022).

Higuera-Ciapara, I., Félix-Valenzuela, L., and Goycoolea, F.M. (2006). Astaxanthin: a review of its chemistry and applications. *Critical Reviews in Food Science and Nutrition* 46 (2): 185–196.

Hill, A., Rogers, Q., O'Neill, S., and Christopher, M. (2005). Effects of dietary antioxidant supplementation before and after oral acetaminophen challenge in cats. *American Journal of Veterinary Research* 66 (2): 196–204.

Hochberg, M., Zhan, M., and Lagenberg, P. (2008). The rate of decline of joint space width in patients with osteoarthritis of the knee: a systematic review and meta-analysis of randomized placebo-controlled trials of chondroitin sulfate. *Current Medical Research and Opinion* 24 (11): 3029–3035.

Höglund, E., Øverli, Ø., and Winberg, S. (2019). Tryptophan metabolic pathways and brain serotonergic activity: a comparative review. *Frontiers in Endocrinology* 10: 158.

Holecek, M. (2013). Side effects of long-term glutamine supplementation. *Journal of Parenteral and Enteral Nutrition* 37 (5): 607–616.

Hou, Y. and Wu, G. (2018). Nutritionally essential amino acids. *Advances in Nutrition* 9 (6): 849–851.

Houghton, P. (1999). The scientific basis for the reputed activity of valerian. *Journal of Pharmacy and Pharmacology* 51 (5): 505–512.

Howlett, A., Barth, F., Bonner, T.I. et al. (2002). International Union of Pharmacology XXVII: classification of cannabinoid receptors. *Pharmacology Reviews* 54 (2): 161–202.

Ibrahim, W., Bailey, N., Sunvold, G.D., and Bruckner, G.G. (2003). Effects of carnitine and taurine on fatty acid metabolism and lipid accumulation in the liver of cats during weight gain and weight loss. *American Journal of Veterinary Research* 64 (10): 1265–1277.

Iffland, K. and Grotenhermen, F. (2017). An update on safety and side effects of cannabidiol: a review of clinical data and relevant animal studies. *Cannabis and Cannabinoid Research* 2 (1): 139–154.

Innes, J., Fuller, C.J., Grover, E.R. et al. (2003). Randomised, double-blind, placebo-controlled parallel group study of P54FP for the treatment of dogs with osteoarthritis. *Veterinary Record* 152 (15): 457–460.

Iovu, M., Dumais, G, and du Souich (2008). Anti-inflammatory activity of chondroitin sulfate. *Osteoarthritis and Cartilage* 16 (Suppl. 3): S14–S18.

Iozzo, R. and Schaefer, L. (2015). Proteoglycan form and function: a comprehensive nomenclature of proteoglycans. *Matrix Biology* 42: 11–55.

ISAPP (International Scientific Association of Probiotics and Prebiotics) (2021a). Prebiotics. https://isappscience.org/for-scientists/resources/prebiotics (accessed 20 February 2021).

ISAPP (International Scientific Association of Probiotics and Prebiotics) (2021b). Probiotics. https://isappscience.org/for-scientists/resources/probiotics (accessed 8 February 2021).

Itin, C., Domb, A., and Hoffman, A. (2019). A meta-opinion: cannabinoids delivered to oral mucosa by a spray for systemic absorption are rather ingested into gastro-intestinal tract: the influences of fed/fasting states. *Expert Opinion on Drug Delivery* 16 (10): 1031–1035.

Jafari, M., Mousavi, S., Asgharzadeh, A., and Yazdani, N. (2018). Coenzyme Q10 in the treatment of heart failure: a systematic review of systematic reviews. *Indian Heart Journal* 70 (Suppl. 1): S111–S117.

JAMA (1947). Nitrogen balance. *Journal of the American Medical Association* 133 (4): 247.

Jeitler, M., Michalsen, A., Frings, D. et al. (2020). Significance of medicinal mushrooms in integrative oncology: a narrative review. *Frontiers in Pharmacology* 11: 580656.

Jérôme, L., Cambier, C., Chandler, T. et al. (2010). Prophylactic effects of omega-3 polyunsaturated fatty acids and luteolin on airway hyperresponsiveness and inflammation in cats with experimentally-induced asthma. *Veterinary Journal* 184 (1): 111–114.

Jerosch, J. (2011). Effects of glucosamine and chondroitin sulfate on cartilage metabolism in OA: outlook on other nutrient partners especially omega-3 fatty acids. *International Journal of Rheumatology* 2011: 969012.

Johne, A., Schmider, J., Brockmöller, J. et al. (2002). Decreased plasma levels of amitriptyline and its metabolites on comedication with an extract from St. John's Wort (*Hypericum perforatum*). *Journal of Clinical Psychopharmacology* 22 (1): 46–54.

Johnson, K., Lee, A., and Swanson, K. (2020). Nutrition and nutraceuticals in the changing management of osteoarthritis in dogs and cats. *Journal of the American Veterinary Medical Association* 256 (12): 1353–1341.

Johnston, S. (1997). Osteoarthritis: joint anatomy, physiology, and pathobiology. *Veterinary Clinics of North America: Small Animal Practice* 27 (4): 699–723.

Jones, S. and Versalovic, J. (2009). Probiotic *Lactobacillus reuteri* biofilms produce antimicrobial and anti-inflammatory factors. *BMC Microbiology* 9: 35.

Joshi, V., Alam, S., Dimri, U., and Kumar, V. (2016). Veterinary nutraceuticals: an alternative medicine. *Indian Dairyman* 68: 90–93.

Jugan, M., Rudinsky, A., Parker, V., and Gilor, C. (2017). Use of probiotics in small animal veterinary medicine. *Journal of the American Veterinary Medical Association* 250 (5): 519–528.

Juneja, L., Chu, D.-C., Okubo, T. et al. (1999). l-Theanine: a unique amino acid of green tea and its relaxation effect in humans. *Trends in Food Science and Technology* 10 (6–7): 199–204.

Jung, H.Y., Yoo, D.Y., Nam, S.M. et al. (2015). Valerenic acid protects against physical and psychological stress by reducing the turnover of serotonin and norepinephrine in mouse hippocampus-amygdala region. *Journal of Medicinal Food* 18 (12): 1333–1339.

Jyonouchi, H., Sun, S., Iijima, K., and Gross, M.D. (2000). Antitumor activity of astaxanthin and its mode of action. *Nutrition and Cancer* 36 (1): 59–65.

Kakuda, T. (2002). Neuroprotective effects of the green tea components theanine and catechins. *Biological and Pharmaceutical Bulletin* 25 (12): 1513–1518.

Kalra, E. (2003). Nutraceutical: definition and introduction. *AAPS PharmSci* 5 (3): E25.

Kamath, B.S., Srikanta, B.M., Dharmesh, S.M. et al. (2008). Ulcer preventive and antioxidative properties of astaxanthin from *Haematococcus pluvialis*. *European Journal of Pharmacology* 590 (1–3): 387–395.

Kamiński, M., Kręgielska-Narożna, M., and Bogdański, P. (2020). Determination of the popularity of dietary supplements using Google search rankings. *Nutrients* 12 (4): 908.

Kang, K., Shu, X.-L., Zhong, J.-X., and Yu, T.-T. (2014). Effect of L-arginine on immune function: a meta-analysis. *Asia Pacific Journal of Clinical Nutrition* 23 (3): 351–359.

Kapun, A.P., Salobir, J., Levart, A. et al. (2014). Vitamin E supplementation in canine atopic dermatitis: improvement of clinical signs and effects on oxidative stress markers. *Veterinary Record* 175 (22): 560.

Kato, M., Miyaji, K., Ohtani, N., and Ohta, M. (2012). Effects of prescription diet on dealing with stressful situations and performance of anxiety-related behaviors in privately owned anxious dogs. *Journal of Veterinary Behavior* 7 (1): 21–26.

Kearns, R.J., Hayek, M.G., Turek, J.J. et al. (1999). Effect of age, breed and dietary omega-6 (n-6): omega-3 (n-3) fatty acid ratio on immune function, eicosanoid production, and lipid peroxidation in young and aged dogs. *Veterinary Immunology and Immunopathology* 69 (2–4): 165–183.

Kędziora-Kornatowska, K., Czuczejko, J., Motyl, J. et al. (2010). Effects of coenzyme Q10 supplementation on activities of selected antioxidative enzymes and lipid peroxidation in hypertensive patients treated with indapamide. A pilot study. *Archives of Medical Science* 6 (4): 513–518.

Kelber, O., Niever, K., and Kraft, K. (2014). Valerian: no evidence for clinically relevant interactions. *Evidence-based Complementary and Alternative Medicine* 2014: 879396.

Kelley, R., Minikhiem, D., Kiely, B. et al. (2009). Clinical benefits of probiotic canine-derived *Bifidobacterium animalis* strain AHC7 in dogs with acute idiopathic diarrhea. *Veterinary Therapeutics* 10 (3): 121–130.

Kelley, R., Levy, K., Mundell, P., and Hayek, M. (2012). Effects of varying doses of a probiotic supplement fed to healthy dogs undergoing kenneling stress. *Journal of Applied Research in Veterinary Medicine* 10 (3): 205–216.

Kern, J.K., Geier, D.A., Adams, J.B. et al. (2011). A clinical trial of glutathione supplementation in autism spectrum disorders. *Medical Science Monitor* 17 (12): CR677–CR682.

Khoruts, A. and Sadowsky, M. (2018). Understanding the mechanisms of faecal microbiota transplantation. *Nature Reviews Gastroenterology and Hepatology* 13 (9): 508–516.

Kiers, J. and Bult, J. (2021). Mildly processed natural eggshell membrane alleviates joint pain associated with osteoarthritis of the knee: a randomized double-blind placebo-controlled study. *Journal of Medicinal Food* 24 (3): 292–298.

Kim, K. and Gluck, M. (2019). Fecal microbiota transplantation: an update on clinical practice. *Clinical Endoscopy* 52 (2): 137–143.

Kim, L.S., Axelrod, L.J., Howard, P. et al. (2006). Efficacy of methylsulfonylmethane (MSM) in osteoarthritis pain of the knee: a pilot clinical trial. *Osteoarthritis and Cartilage* 14 (3): 286–294.

Kim, Y.H., Kim, D.H., Lim, H. et al. (2009). The anti-inflammatory effects of methylsulfonylmethane on lipopolysaccharide-induced inflammatory responses in murine macrophages. *Biological and Pharmaceutical Bulletin* 32 (4): 651–656.

Kim, C.-S., Park, S., and Kim, J. (2017). The role of glycation in the pathogenesis of aging and its prevention through herbal products and physical exercise. *Journal of Exercise Nutrition and Biochemistry* 21 (3): 55–61.

Kimmatkar, N., Thawani, V., Hingorani, L., and Khiyani, R. (2003). Efficacy and tolerability of *Boswellia serrata* extract in treatment of osteoarthritis of knee: a randomized double blind placebo controlled trial. *Phytomedicine* 10 (1): 3–7.

Kimura, R. and Murata, T. (1971). Influence of alkylamides of glutamic acid and related compounds on the central nervous system. I. Central depressant effect of theanine. *Chemical and Pharmaceutical Bulletin* 19 (6): 1257–1261.

Kimura, K., Ozeki, M., Juneja, L., and Ohira, H. (2007). l-Theanine reduces psychological and physiological stress responses. *Biological Psychology* 74 (1): 39–45.

Kirksick, C. and Willoughby, D. (2005). The antioxidant role of glutathione and N-acetyl-cysteine supplements and exercise-induced oxidative stress. *Journal of the International Society of Sports Nutrition* 2 (2): 38–44.

Kittleson, M.D., Keene, B., Pion, P.D., and Loyer, C. (1997). Results of the multicenter spaniel trial (MUST): taurine- and carnitine-responsive dilated cardiomyopathy in American cocker spaniels with decreased plasma taurine concentration. *Journal of Veterinary Internal Medicine* 11 (4): 204–211.

Knueven, D. (2018). An introduction to supplements: evidence-based nutritional therapies. Illinois State Veterinary Medical Association. https://www.isvma.org/wp-content/uploads/2018/10/AnIntroduction toSupplementsEvidenceBasedNutritional Therapies.pdf

Kogan, L., Schoenfeld-Tacher, R., Hellyer, P., and Rishniw, M. (2019). US Veterinarians' knowledge, experience, and perception regarding the use of cannabidiol for canine medical conditions. *Frontiers in Veterinary Science* 5: 338.

Kut-Lasserre, C., Miller, C.C., Ejeil, A.L. et al. (2001). Effect of avocado and soybean unsaponifiables on gelatinase A (MMP-2), stromelysin 1 (MMP-3), and tissue inhibitors of matrix metalloproteinase (TIMP-1 and TIMP-2) secretion by human fibroblasts in culture. *Journal of Periodontology* 72 (12): 1685–1694.

Laflamme, D. (2012). Nutritional care for aging cats and dogs. *Veterinary Clinics of North America: Small Animal Practice* 42 (4): 769–791.

Landsberg, G., Milgram, B., Mougeot, I. et al. (2016). Therapeutic effects of an alpha-casozepine and L-tryptophan supplemented diet on fear and anxiety in the cat. *Journal of Feline Medicine and Surgery* 19 (6): 594–602.

Lascelles, B.D.X., King, S., Roe, S. et al. (2009). Expression and activity of COX-1 and 2 and 5-LOX in joint tissues from dogs with naturally occurring coxofemoral joint osteoarthritis. *Journal of Orthopaedic Research* 27 (9): 1204–1208.

Lascelles, B.D.X., DePuy, V., Thomson, A. et al. (2010). Evaluation of a therapeutic diet for feline degenerative joint disease. *Journal of Veterinary Internal Medicine* 24 (3): 487–495.

Lauková, A., Stompfová, V., and Ouwehand, A. (2004). Adhesion properties of enterococci to intestinal mucus of different hosts. *Veterinary Research Communications* 28 (8): 647–655.

Laurent, G., Moe, G., Hu, X. et al. (2008). Long chain n-3 polyunsaturated fatty acids reduce atrial vulnerability in a novel canine pacing model. *Cardiovascular Research* 77 (1): 89–97.

Le Floc'h, N., Otten, W., and Merlot, E. (2011). Tryptophan metabolism, from nutrition to potential therapeutic applications. *Amino Acids* 41 (5): 1195–1205.

LeBlanc, C., Dietrich, M.A., Horohov, D.W. et al. (2007). Effects of dietary fish oil and vitamin E supplementation on canine lymphocyte proliferation evaluated using a flow cytometric technique. *Veterinary Immunology and Immunopathology* 119 (3–4): 180–188.

Lechowski, R., Sawosz, E., and Kluciński, W. (1998). The effect of the addition of oil preparation with increased content of n-3 fatty acids on serum lipid profile and clinical condition of cats with miliary dermatitis. *Zentralblatt für Veterinärmedizin, Reihe A* 45 (6–7): 417–424.

Lee, Y.-K., Puong, K.-Y., Ouwehand, A., and Salminen, S. (2003). Displacement of bacterial pathogens from mucus and Caco-2 cell surface by lactobacilli. *Journal of Medical Microbiology* 52 (10): 925–930.

Lee, Y., Woo, J.-H., Choi, S.J. et al. (2009). Effect of glucosamine or chondroitin sulfate on the osteoarthritis progression: a meta-analysis. *Rheumatology International* 30 (2): 357–363.

Legault, Z., Bagnall, N., and Kimmerly, D.S. (2015). The influence of oral L-glutamine supplementation on muscle strength recovery and soreness following unilateral knee extension eccentric exercise. *International Journal of Sports Nutrition and Exercise Metabolism* 25 (5): 417–426.

Lenders, C.M., Liu, S., Wilmore, D.W. et al. (2009). Evaluation of a novel food composition database that includes glutamine and other amino acids derived from gene sequencing data. *European Journal of Clinical Nutrition* 63 (12): 1433–1439.

Lenox, C. and Bauer, J. (2013). Potential adverse effects of omega-3 fatty acids in dogs and cats. *Journal of Veterinary Internal Medicine* 27 (2): 217–226.

Levine, C., Bayle, J., Biourge, V., and Wakshlag, J. (2017). Cellular effects of a turmeric root and rosemary leaf extract on canine neoplastic cell lines. *BMC Veterinary Research* 13 (1): 388.

Li, Y., Yao, J., Han, C. et al. (2016). Quercetin, inflammation and immunity. *Nutrients* 8 (3): 167.

Linnebank, M., Popp, J., Smulders, Y. et al. (2010). S-adenosylmethionine is decreased in the cerebrospinal fluid of patients with

Alzheimer's disease. *Neurodegenerative Diseases* 7 (6): 373–378.

Lippiello, L., Nardo, J., Harlan, R., and Chiou, T. (2008). Metabolic effects of avocado/soy unsaponifiables on articular chondrocytes. *Evidence-Based Complementary and Alternative Medicine* 5 (2): 191–197.

Liu, C.-H., Jassey, A., Hsu, H.-Y., and Lin, L.-T. (2019). Antiviral activities of silymarin and derivatives. *Molecules* 24 (8): 1552.

Loef, M., Schoones, J.W., Kloppenburg, M., and Ioan-Facsinay, A. (2019). Fatty acids and osteoarthritis: different types, different effects. *Joint, Bone, Spine* 86 (4): 451–458.

Logas, D. and Kunkle, G. (1994). Double-blinded crossover study with marine oil supplementation containing high-dose icosapentaenoic acid for the treatment of canine pruritic skin disease. *Veterinary Dermatology* 5 (3): 99–104.

Looijer-van Langen, M.A.C. and Dieleman, L.A. (2009). Prebiotics in chronic intestinal inflammation. *Inflammatory Bowel Diseases* 15 (3): 454–462.

López-Lluch, G., Del Pozo-Cruz, J., Sánchez-Cuesta, A. et al. (2019). Bioavailability of coenzyme Q10 supplements depends on carrier lipids and solubilization. *Nutrition* 57: 133–140.

Lu, S. (2000). S-adenosylmethionine. *International Journal of Biochemistry and Cell Biology* 32 (4): 391–395.

Lu, H.-C. and Mackie, K. (2016). An introduction to the endogenous cannabinoid system. *Biological Psychiatry* 79 (7): 516–525.

Lucio, C.F., Silva, L.C.G., Regazzi, M. et al. (2016). Effect of reduced glutathione (GSH) in canine sperm cryopreservation: in vitro and in vivo evaluation. *Cryobiology* 72 (2): 135–140.

Lugo, J.P., Saiyed, Z.M., Lau, F.C., et al. (2013). Undenatured type II collagen (UC-II®) for joint support: a randomized, double-blind, placebo-controlled study in healthy volunteers. *Journal of the International Society of Sports Nutrition* 10 (48): 1–12.

Mackie, K. (2005). Distribution of cannabinoid receptors in the central and peripheral nervous system. In: *Cannabinoids. Handbook of Experimental Pharmacology*, vol. 168 (ed. R.G. Pertwee), 299–325. Berlin, Heidelberg: Springer.

Magalhães, T.R., Lourenço, A.L., Gregório, H., and Queiroga, F.L. (2021). Therapeutic effect of EPA/DHA supplementation in neoplastic and non-neoplastic companion animal diseases: a systematic review. *In Vivo* 35 (3): 1419–1436.

Maggs, D., Collins, B., Thorne, J., and Nasisse, M. (2000). Effects of L-lysine and L-arginine on in vitro replication of feline herpesvirus type-1. *American Journal of Veterinary Research* 61 (12): 1474–1478.

Maggs, D., Nasisse, M., and Kass, P. (2003). Efficacy of oral supplementation with L-lysine in cats latently infected with feline herpesvirus. *American Journal of Veterinary Research* 64 (1): 37–42.

Mai, I., Bauer, S., Perloff, E.S. et al. (2004). Hyperforin content determines the magnitude of the St John's Wort–cyclosporine drug interaction. *Clinical Pharmacology and Therapeutics* 76 (4): 330–340.

Mailoo, V. and Rampes, S. (2017). Lysine for herpes simplex prophylaxis: a review of the evidence. *Integrative Medicine: A Clinician's Journal* 16 (3): 42–46.

Makielski, K., Cullen, J., O'Connor, A., and Jergens, A. (2018). Narrative review of therapies for chronic enteropathies in dogs and cats. *Journal of Veterinary Internal Medicine* 33 (1): 11–22.

Malaguarnera, L. (2019). Influence of resveratrol on the immune response. *Nutrients* 11 (5): 946.

Małek, A., Taciak, B., Sobczak, K. et al. (2021). Enhanced cytotoxic effect of doxorubicin conjugated to glutathione-stabilized gold nanoparticles in canine osteosarcoma: in vitro studies. *Molecules* 26 (12): 3487.

Manzanares, W., Dhaliwal, R., Jiang, X. et al. (2012). Antioxidant micronutrients in the critically ill: a systematic review and meta-analysis. *Critical Care* 16 (2): R66.

Marchegiani, A., Fruganti, A., Gavazza, A. et al. (2020). Evidences on molecules most frequently included in canine and feline complementary feed to support liver function. *Veterinary Medicine International* 2020: 9185759.

Marchesi, J. and Ravel, J. (2015). The vocabulary of microbiome research: a proposal. *Microbiome* 3: 31.

Market Research (2021). *Pe* Packaged Facts.

Markowitz, J.S., Donovan, J.L., DeVane, C.L. et al. (2003). Effect of St John's Wort on drug metabolism by induction of cytochrome P450 3A4 enzyme. *Journal of the American Medical Association* 290 (11): 1500–1504.

Marks, S.L., Cook, A.K., Reader, R. et al. (1999). Effects of glutamine supplementation of an amino acid-based purified diet on intestinal mucosal integrity in cats with methotrexate-induced enteritis. *American Journal of Veterinary Research* 60 (6): 755–763.

Marone, P.A., Lau, F.C., Gupta, R.C. et al. (2010). Safety and toxicological evaluation of undenatured type II collagen. *Toxicology Mechanisms and Methods* 20 (4): 175–189.

Martello, E., Bigliati, M., Adami, R. et al. (2022). Efficacy of a dietary supplement in dogs with osteoarthritis: a randomized placebo-controlled, double-blind clinical trial. *PLoS One* 17 (2): e0263971.

Martel-Pelletier, J., Tat, S.K., and Pelletier, J.-P. (2010). Effects of chondroitin sulfate in the pathophysiology of the osteoarthritic joint: a narrative review. *Osteoarthritis and Cartilage* 18 (Suppl. 1): S7–S11.

Martínez-Banaclocha, M. (2016). Cysteine network (CYSTEINET) dysregulation in Parkinson's disease: role of N-acetylcysteine. *Current Drug Metabolism* 17 (4): 368–385.

Mathew, L.M., Woode, R.A., Axiak-Bechtel, S.M. et al. (2018). Resveratrol administration increases phagocytosis, decreases oxidative burst, and promoted pro-inflammatory cytokine production in healthy dogs. *Veterinary Immunology and Immunopathology* 203: 21–29.

May, E., Ratliff, B., and Bemis, D. (2019). Antibacterial effect of N-acetylcysteine in combination with antimicrobials on common canine otitis externa bacterial isolates. *Veterinary Dermatology* 30 (6): 531–e161.

McCarthy, G., O'Donovan, J., Jones, B. et al. (2007). Randomised double-blind, positive-controlled trial to assess the efficacy of glucosamine/chondroitin sulfate for the treatment of dogs with osteoarthritis. *Veterinary Journal* 174 (1): 54–61.

McGrath, S., Bartner, L.R., Rao, S. et al. (2019). Randomized blinded controlled clinical trial to assess the effect of oral cannabidiol administration in addition to conventional antiepileptic treatment on seizure frequency in dogs with intractable idiopathic epilepsy. *Journal of the American Veterinary Medical Association* 254 (11): 1301–1308.

McNamara, P., Barr, S., and Erb, H. (1996). Hematologic, hemostatic, and biochemical effects in dogs receiving an oral chondroprotective agent for thirty days. *American Journal of Veterinary Research* 57 (9): 1390–1394.

McRae, M. (2016). Therapeutic benefits of l-arginine: an umbrella review of meta-analyses. *Journal of Chiropractic Medicine* 15 (3): 184–189.

Medellin-Peña, M.J., Wang, H., Johnson, R. et al. (2007). Probiotics affect virulence-related gene expression in *Escherichia coli* O157:H7. *Applied and Environmental Microbiology* 73 (13): 4259–4267.

Mehana, E.-S., Khafaga, A., and El-Blehi, S. (2019). The role of matrix metalloproteinases in osteoarthritis pathogenesis: an updated review. *Life Sciences* 234: 116786.

Mehler, S.J., May, L.R., King, C. et al. (2016). A prospective, randomized, double blind, placebo-controlled evaluation of the effects of eicosapentaenoic acid and docosahexaenoic acid on the clinical signs and erythrocyte membrane polyunsaturated fatty acid concentrations in dogs with osteoarthritis. *Prostaglandins, Leukotrienes and Essential Fatty Acids* 109: 1–7.

Menon, V. and Sudheer, A. (2007). Antioxidant and anti-inflammatory properties of curcumin. *Advances in Experimental Medicine and Biology* 595: 105–125.

Michel, B.A., Stucki, G., Frey, D. et al. (2005). Chondroitins 4 and 6 sulphate in osteoarthritis of the knee: a randomized controlled trial. *Arthritis and Rheumatism* 52 (3): 779–786.

Militante, J. and Lombardini, J. (2002). Treatment of hypertension with oral taurine: experimental and clinical studies. *Amino Acids* 23 (4): 381–393.

Millar, S., Stone, N., Yates, A., and O'Sullivan, S. (2018). A systematic review on the pharmacokinetics of cannabidiol in humans. *Frontiers in Pharmacology* 9: 1365.

Millar, S., Maguire, R., Yates, A., and O'Sullivan, S. (2020). Towards better delivery of cannabidiol (CBD). *Pharmaceuticals* 13 (9): 219.

Miller, T. and Ormrod, D. (1980). The anti-inflammatory activity of *Perna canaliculus* (NZ green lipped mussel). *New Zealand Medical Journal* 92 (667): 187–193.

Mimee, M., Citorik, R.J., and Lu, T.K. (2016). Microbiome therapeutics: advances and challenges. *Advanced Drug Delivery Reviews* 105 (Pt A): 44–54.

Minich, D. and Brown, B. (2019). A review of dietary (phyto)nutrients for glutathione support. *Nutrients* 11 (9): 2073.

Miquel, J., Bernd, A., Sempere, J.M. et al. (2002). The curcuma antioxidants: pharmacological effects and prospects for future clinical use. A review. *Archives of Gerontology and Geriatrics* 34 (1): 37–46.

Miyaji, K., Kato, M., Obtani, N., and Ohta, M. (2015). Experimental verification of the effects on normal domestic cats by feeding prescription diet for decreasing stress. *Journal of Applied Animal Welfare Science* 18 (4): 355–362.

Mlcek, J., Jurikova, T., Skrovankova, S., and Sochor, J. (2016). Quercetin and its anti-allergic immune response. *Molecules* 21 (5): 623.

Mokhtari, V., Afsharian, P., Shahhoseini, M. et al. (2017). A review of various uses of N-acetylcysteine. *Cell Journal* 19 (1): 11–17.

Momoi, Y., Goto, Y., Tanide, K. et al. (2001). Increase in plasma lipid peroxide in cats fed a fish diet. *Journal of Veterinary Medical Science* 63 (12): 1293–1296.

Monauni, T., Zenti, M.G., Cretti, A. et al. (2000). Effects of glucosamine infusion on insulin secretion and insulin action in humans. *Diabetes* 49 (6): 926–935.

Money, N.P. (2016). Are mushrooms medicinal? *Fungal Biology* 120 (4): 449–453.

Monteiro, J.C., Gonçalves, J.S.A., Rodrigues, J.A. et al. (2009). Influence of ascorbic acid and glutathione antioxidants on frozen-thawed canine semen. *Reproduction in Domestic Animals* 44 (Suppl. 2): 359–362.

Moreau, M., Dupis, J., Bonneau, N., and Desnoyers, M. (2003). Clinical evaluation of a nutraceutical, carprofen and meloxicam for the treatment of dogs with osteoarthritis. *Veterinary Research* 152 (11): 323–329.

Moreau, M., Troncy, E., Del Castillo, J.R.E. et al. (2013). Effects of feeding a high omega-3 fatty acids diet in dogs with naturally occurring osteoarthritis. *Journal of Animal Physiology and Animal Nutrition (Berl)* 97 (5): 830–837.

Moreau, M., Lussier, B., Pelletier, J.-P. et al. (2014). A medicinal herb-based natural health product improves the condition of a canine natural osteoarthritis model: a randomized placebo-controlled trial. *Research in Veterinary Science* 97 (3): 574–581.

Moreira, P.I., Harris, P.L.R., Zhu, X. et al. (2007). Lipoic acid and N-acetyl cysteine decrease mitochondrial-related oxidative stress in Alzheimer disease patient fibroblasts. *Journal of Alzheimers Disease* 12 (2): 195–206.

Moro, G., Arslanoglu, S., Stahl, B. et al. (2006). A mixture of prebiotic oligosaccharides reduces the incidence of atopic dermatitis during the first six months of age. *Archives of Disease in Childhood* 91 (10): 814–819.

Mortola, E., Okuda, M., Ohno, K. et al. (1998). Inhibition of apoptosis and virus replication in feline immunodeficiency virus-infected cells by N-acetylcysteine and ascorbic acid.

Journal of Veterinary Medical Science 60 (11): 1187–1193.

Mueller, R.S., Fieseler, K.V., Fettman, M.J. et al. (2004a). Effect of omega-3 fatty acids on canine atopic dermatitis. *Journal of Small Animal Practice* 45 (6): 293–297.

Mueller, S.C., Uehleke, B., Woehling, H. et al. (2004b). Effect of St John's Wort dose and preparations on the pharmacokinetics of digoxin. *Clinical Pharmacology and Therapeutics* 75 (6): 546–557.

Mueller, R.S., Fettman, M.J., Richardson, K. et al. (2005). Plasma and skin concentrations of polyunsaturated fatty acids before and after supplementation with n-3 fatty acids in dogs with atopic dermatitis. *American Journal of Veterinary Research* 66 (5): 868–873.

Müller, M.R., Linek, M., Lowenstein, C. et al. (2016). Evaluation of cyclosporine-sparing effects of polyunsaturated fatty acids in the treatment of canine atopic dermatitis. *Veterinary Journal* 210: 77–81.

Muller, C., Enomoto, M., Buono, A. et al. (2019). Placebo-controlled pilot study of the effects of an eggshell membrane-based supplement on mobility and serum biomarkers in dogs with osteoarthritis. *Veterinary Journal* 253: 105379.

Murakami, S. (2014). Taurine and atherosclerosis. *Amino Acids* 46 (1): 73–80.

Murphy, J. (2020). Top vitamins and supplements in 2020. https://www.mdlinx.com/article/top-vitamins-and-supplements-in-2020/1x034atzR5XSk5FHhFg0Mt (accessed 1 June 2021).

Murphy, K., Mann, N.J., and Sinclair, A.J. (2003). Fatty acid and sterol composition of frozen and freeze-dried New Zealand green lipped mussel (*Perna canaliculus*) from three sites in New Zealand. *Asia Pacific Journal of Clinical Nutrition* 12 (1): 50–60.

Murphy, K., Kubin, Z., Shepherd, J., and Ettinger, R. (2010). *Valeriana officinalis* root extracts have potent anxiolytic effects in laboratory rats. *Phytomedicine* 17 (8–9): 674–678.

Musco, N., Vassalotti, G., Mastellone, V. et al. (2019). Effects of a nutritional supplement in dogs affected by osteoarthritis. *Veterinary Medicine and Science* 5 (3): 325–335.

Naarden, B. and Corbee, R. (2019). The effect of a therapeutic urinary stress diet on the short-term recurrence of feline idiopathic cystitis. *Veterinary Medicine and Science* 6 (1): 32–38.

Nagase, H. and Kashiwagi, M. (2003). Aggrecanases and cartilage matrix degradation. *Arthritis Research and Therapy* 5 (2): 94–103.

Naguib, Y.M. (2000). Antioxidant activities of astaxanthin and related carotenoids. *Journal of Agricultural and Food Chemistry* 48 (4): 1150–1154.

NASC (National Animal Supplement Council) (2022). Our Mission. https://www.nasc.cc/about-our-mission (accessed 30 January 2022).

Nasciutti, P.R., Moraes, A.T., Santos, T.K. et al. (2021). Protective effects of omega-3 fatty acids in dogs with myxomatous mitral valve disease stages B2 and C. *PLoS One* 16 (7): e0254887.

NCCIH (National Center for Complementary and Integrative Health) (2013). Antioxidants: In Depth. https://www.nccih.nih.gov/health/antioxidants-in-depth (accessed 2 July 2022).

NCCIH (National Center for Complementary and Integrative Health) (2020). Milk Thistle. https://www.nccih.nih.gov/health/milk-thistle (accessed 3 March 2021).

Nebel, A., Schneider, B., Baker, R., and Kroll, D. (1999). Potenital metabolic interaction between St John's Wort and theophylline. *Annals of Pharmacology* 33 (4): 502.

Nesbitt, G., Freeman, L.M., and Hannah, S.S. (2003). Effect of n-3 fatty acid ratio and dose on clinical manifestations, plasma fatty acids and inflammatory mediators in dogs with pruritus. *Veterinary Dermatology* 14 (2): 67–74.

Ng, S.W., Selvarajah, G.T., Hussein, M.Z. et al. (2020). In vitro evaluation of curcumin-encapsulated chitosan nanoparticles against feline infectious peritonitis virus and pharmacokinetics study in cats. *BioMed Research International* 2020: 3012198.

Niederwerder, M. (2018). Fecal microbiota transplantation as a tool to treat and reduce susceptibility to disease in animals. *Veterinary Immunology and Immunopathology* 206: 65–72.

Nieman, D.C., Henson, D.A., Maxwell, K.R. et al. (2009). Effects of quercetin and EGCG on mitochondrial biogenesis and immunity. *Medicine and Science in Sports and Exercise* 41 (7): 1467–1475.

NIH (National Institutes of Health) (2020). Magnesium Fact Sheet for Health Professionals. https://ods.od.nih.gov/factsheets/Magnesium-HealthProfessional/#:~:text=Magnesium%20is%20a%20cofactor%20in,%2C%20oxidative%20phosphorylation%2C%20and%20glycolysis (accessed 20 February 2021).

NIH (National Institutes of Health) (2021). Omega-3 Fatty Acids Fact Sheet for Health Professionals. https://ods.od.nih.gov/factsheets/Omega3FattyAcids-HealthProfessional (accessed 28 February 2022).

NIH (National Institutes of Health) (2022). Dietary Supplement Label Database (DSLD). https://dsld.od.nih.gov (accessed 23 July 2022).

Nobels, I. and Khan, S. (2015). Multiorgan dysfunction syndrome secondary to joint supplement overdosage in a dog. *Canadian Veterinary Journal* 56 (4): 361–364.

Nobre, A., Rao, A., and Owen, G. (2008). l-Theanine, a natural constituent in tea, and its effect on mental state. *Asia Pacific Journal of Clinical Nutrition* 17 (Suppl. 1): 167–168.

NRC (National Research Council) (2006). *Nutrient Requirements of Dogs and Cats*. Washington, DC: National Academies Press.

Nunes, A. and Sousa, M. (2011). Use of valerian in anxiety and sleep disorders: what is the best evidence. *Acta Médica Portuguesa* 24 (4): 961–966.

O'Brien, S. (2018). 4 Impressive Health Benefits of Lysine. https://www.healthline.com/nutrition/lysine-benefits (accessed 26 June 2022).

Oelschlaeger, T. (2010). Mechanisms of probiotic actions: a review. *International Journal of Medical Microbiology* 300 (1): 57–62.

Ogilvie, G.K., Fettman, M.J., Mallinckrodt, C.H. et al. (2000). Effect of fish oil, arginine, and doxorubicin chemotherapy on remission and survival time for dogs with lymphoma: a double-blind, randomized placebo-controlled study. *Cancer* 88 (8): 1916–1928.

Ohno, T., Mochiki, E., Ando, H. et al. (2009). Glutamine decreases the duration of postoperative ileus after abdominal surgery: an experimental study of conscious dogs. *Digestive Diseases and Sciences* 54 (6): 1208–1213.

Ooi, S.L., Green, R., and Pak, S. (2018). N-acetylcysteine for the treatment of psychiatric disorders: a review of current evidence. *BioMed Research International* 2018: 2469486.

Otsuki, S., Qian, W., Ishihara, A., and Kabe, T. (2002). Elucidation of dimethylsulfone metabolism in rat using a ^{35}S radioisotope tracer method. *Nutrition Research* 22: 313–322.

Ottestad, I., Retterstøl, K., Myhrstad, M.C.W. et al. (2013). Intake of oxidised fish oil does not affect circulating levels of oxidised LDL or inflammatory markers in healthy subjects. *Nutrition, Metabolism and Cardiovascular Diseases* 23 (1): e3–e4.

Pakseresht, S., Boostani, H., and Sayyah, M. (2011). Extract of valerian root (*Valeriana officinalis* L.) vs. placebo in treatment of obsessive-compulsive disorder: a randomized double-blind study. *Journal of Complementary and Integrative Medicine* https://doi.org/10.2202/1553-3840.1465.

Panahi, Y., Rahimnia, A.-R., Sharafi, M. et al. (2014). Curcuminoid treatment for knee osteoarthritis: a randomized double-blind placebo-controlled trial. *Phytotherapy Research* 28 (11): 1625–1631.

Panahi, Y., Alishiri, G., Parvin, S., and Sahebkar, A. (2016). Mitigation of systemic oxidative stress by curcuminoids in osteoarthritis: results of a randomized controlled trial. *Journal of Dietary Supplements* 13 (2): 209–220.

Paredes, S., Barriga, C., Reiter, R.J., and Rodríguez, A.B. (2009). Assessment of the potential role of tryptophan as the precursor of serotonin and melatonin for the aged sleep–wake cycle and immune function: *Streptopelia risoria* as a model. *International Journal of Tryptophan Research* 2: 23–26.

Park, E.-J. and Pezzuto, J.M. (2015). The pharmacology of resveratrol in animals and humans. *Biochimica et Biophysica Acta* 1852 (6): 1071–1113.

Park, J.S., Chyun, J.H., Kim, Y.K. et al. (2010). Astaxanthin decreased oxidative stress and inflammation and enhanced immune response in humans. *Nutrition and Metabolism* 7: 18.

Park, J.S., Mathison, B.D., Hayek, M.G. et al. (2013). Astaxanthin modulates age-associated mitochondrial dysfunction in healthy dogs. *Journal of Animal Science* 91 (1): 268–275.

Pasquini, C., Spurgeon, T., and Pasquini, S. (2003). *Anatomy of Domestic Animals: Systemic and Regional Approach*, 10e. Pilot Point, TX: Sudz Publishing.

Passeri, M., Cucinotta, D., Bonati, P.A. et al. (1990). Acetyl-L-carnitine in the treatment of mildly demented elderly patients. *International Journal of Clinical Pharmacology Research* 10 (1–2): 75–79.

Paßlack, N., Kohn, B., and Zentek, J. (2020). Effects of arginine and ornithine supplementation to a high-protein diet on selected cellular immune variables in adult cats. *Journal of Veterinary Internal Medicine* 34 (2): 852–856.

Pattani, R., Palda, V., Hwang, S., and Shah, P. (2013). Probiotics for the prevention of antibiotic-associated diarrhea and *Clostridium difficile* infection among hospitalized patients: systematic review and meta-analysis. *Open Medicine* 7 (2): e56–e67.

Pawlosky, R., Barnes, A., and Salem, N. Jr. (1994). Essential fatty acid metabolism in the feline: relationship between liver and brain production of long-chain polyunsaturated fatty acids. *Journal of Lipid Research* 35 (11): 2032–2040.

PDQ (PDQ Integrative, Alternative, and Complementary Therapies Editorial Board) (2022). Medicinal Mushrooms (PDQ®): Health Professional Version. https://www.ncbi.nlm.nih.gov/books/NBK401261 (accessed 19 July 2022).

Pelletier, J.-P., Martel-Pelletier, H., and Abramson, S.B. (2001). Osteoarthritis, an inflammatory disease. *Arthritis and Rheumatism* 44 (6): 1237–1247.

Pereira, S.L., Leonard, A.E., Huang, Y.-S. et al. (2004). Identification of two novel microalgal enzymes involved in the conversion of the ω3-fatty acid, eicosapentaenoic acid, into docosahexaenoic acid. *Biochemical Journal* 384 (Pt 2): 357–366.

Pereira, G.Q., Gomes, L.A., Santos, I.S. et al. (2018). Fecal microbiota transplantation in puppies with canine parvovirus infection. *Journal of Veterinary Internal Medicine* 32 (2): 707–711.

Pereira, C.P.M., Souza, A.C.R., Vasconcelos, A.R. et al. (2021). Antioxidant and anti-inflammatory mechanisms of action of astaxanthin in cardiovascular diseases (review). *International Journal of Molecular Medicine* 47 (1): 37–48.

Persiani, S., Roda, E., Rovati, L.C. et al. (2005). Glucosamine oral bioavailability and plasma pharmacokinetics after increasing doses of crystalline glucosamine sulfate in man. *Osteoarthritis and Cartilage* 13 (12): 1041–1049.

Phung, A.S., Bannenberg, G., Vigor, C. et al. (2020). Chemical compositional changes in over-oxidized fish oils. *Foods* 9 (10): 1501.

Pike, A., Horwitz, D., and Lobprise, H. (2015). An open-label prospective study of the use of l-theanine (Anxitane) in storm-sensitive client-owned dogs. *Journal of Veterinary Behavior* 10 (4): 324–331.

Pizzorno, J. (2014). Glutathione! *Integrative Medicine: A Clinician's Journal* 13 (1): 8–12.

Plumb, D. (2015). *Plumb's Veterinary Drug Handbook*, 8e. Ames, IA: Wiley Blackwell.

Pollard, B., Guilford, W., Ankenbauer-Perkins, K., and Hedderley, D. (2006). Clinical efficacy and tolerance of an extract of green-lipped mussel (*Perna canaliculus*) in dogs presumptively diagnosed with degenerative joint disease. *New Zealand Veterinary Journal* 54 (3): 114–118.

Pollio, A. (2016). The name *Cannabis*: a short guide for nonbotanists. *Cannabis and Cannabinoid Research* 1 (1): 234–238.

Pooyandjoo, M., Nouhi, M., Shab-Bidar, S. et al. (2016). The effect of (L-)carnitine on weight loss in adults: a systematic review and meta-analysis of randomized controlled trials. *Obesity Reviews* 17 (10): 970–976.

Popovic, P.J., Zeh, H. III, and Ochoa, J.B. (2007). Arginine and immunity. *Journal of Nutrition* 137 (6 Suppl. 2): 1681S–1686S.

Pouwels, M., Jacobs, J.R., Span, P.N. et al. (2001). Short-term glucosamine infusion does not affect insulin sensitivity in humans. *Journal of Clinical Endocrinology and Metabolism* 86 (5): 2099–2103.

Prabhoo, R., and Billa, G. (2018). Undenatured collagen type II for the treatment of osteoarthritis: a review. *International Journal of Research in Orthopaedics* 4 (5): 684–689.

Priyadarsini, K.I. (2014). The chemistry of curcumin: from extraction to therapeutic agent. *Molecules* 19 (12): 20091–20112.

PubChem (2004). Retinol. https://pubchem.ncbi.nlm.nih.gov/compound/445354 (accessed 20 February 2021).

PubChem (2005a). Astaxanthin. https://pubchem.ncbi.nlm.nih.gov/compound/5281224 (accessed 2 July 2022).

PubChem (2005b). Cholecalciferol. https://pubchem.ncbi.nlm.nih.gov/compound/5280795 (accessed 20 February 2021).

PubChem (2005c). Cyanocobalamin. https://pubchem.ncbi.nlm.nih.gov/compound/5311498 (accessed 20 February 2021)

PubChem (2005d). DL-alpha-Tocopherol. https://pubchem.ncbi.nlm.nih.gov/compound/2116 (accessed 20 February 2021).

PubChem (2005e). Vitamin K. https://pubchem.ncbi.nlm.nih.gov/compound/5280483 (accessed 20 February 2021).

PubChem (2011). Ascorbic Acid. https://pubchem.ncbi.nlm.nih.gov/compound/54670067 (accessed 20 February 2021).

PubChem (2012a). Compound Summary for CID 56842208, Omega-6 Fatty Acids. https://pubchem.ncbi.nlm.nih.gov/compound/56842208 (accessed 5 March 2022).

PubChem (2012b). Compound Summary for CID 56842239, Omega-3 Fatty Acids. https://pubchem.ncbi.nlm.nih.gov/compound/56842239 (accessed 5 March 2022).

PubChem (2017). Glutamine. https://pubchem.ncbi.nlm.nih.gov/compound/5961 (accessed 25 June 2022).

PubChem (2022a). Acetylcysteine. https://pubchem.ncbi.nlm.nih.gov/compound/12035 (accessed 10 July 2022).

PubChem (2022b). Coenzyme Q10. https://pubchem.ncbi.nlm.nih.gov/compound/5281915 (accessed 5 July 2022).

PubChem (2022c). Glutathione. https://pubchem.ncbi.nlm.nih.gov/compound/124886#section=2D-Structure (accessed 5 July 2022).

PubChem (2022d). Levocarnitine. https://pubchem.ncbi.nlm.nih.gov/compound/10917 (accessed 25 June 2022).

PubChem (2022e). L-Theanine. https://pubchem.ncbi.nlm.nih.gov/compound/439378 (accessed 28 June 2022).

PubChem (2022f) Lysine. https://pubchem.ncbi.nlm.nih.gov/compound/5962 (accessed 26 June 2022).

PubChem (2022g). Quercetin. https://pubchem.ncbi.nlm.nih.gov/compound/5280343 (accessed 10 July 2022).

PubChem (2022h). Resveratrol. https://pubchem.ncbi.nlm.nih.gov/compound/445154 (accessed 10 July 2022).

PubChem (2022i). Taurine. https://pubchem. ncbi.nlm.nih.gov/compound/1123 (accessed 28 June 2022).

PubChem (2022j). Tryptophan. https://pubchem .ncbi.nlm.nih.gov/compound/6305 (accessed 28 June 2022).

Qu, X., Li, Q., Waang, X. et al. (2013). N-acetylcysteine attenuates cardiopulmonary bypass-induced lung injury in dogs. *Journal of Cardiothoracic Surgery* 8: 107.

Rainsford, K. and Whitehouse, M. (1980). Gastroprotective and anti-inflammatory properties of green lipped mussel (*Perna canaliculus*) preparation. *Arzneimittel-Forschung* 30 (12): 2128–2132.

Rao, A.R., Moi, P.S., Ravi, S., and Aswathanarayana, R.G. (2014). Astaxanthin: sources, extraction, stability, biological activities and its commercial applications. A review. *Marine Drugs* 12 (1): 128–152.

Ray, E., Landis, M., and Miller, W. (1999). Effects of dietary l-arginine on the reactivity of canine coronary arteries. *Vascular Medicine* 4 (4): 211–217.

Reichling, J., Schmökel, H., Fitzi, J. et al. (2004). Dietary support with Boswellia resin in canine inflammatory joint and spinal disease. *Schweizer Archiv für Tierheilkunde* 146 (2): 71–79.

Reilly, J., McTavish, S., and Young, A. (1997). Rapid depletion of plasma tryptophan: a review of studies and experimental methodology. *Journal of Psychopharmacology* 11 (4): 381–382.

Reinero, C., Lee-Fowler, T.M., Dodam, J.R. et al. (2011). Endotracheal nebulization of N-acetylcysteine increases airway resistant in cats with experimental asthma. *Journal of Feline Medicine and Surgery* 13 (2): 69–73.

Reisen, J. (2020). Four Popular Dog Supplements. https://www.akc.org/expert-advice/nutrition/popular-dog-supplements (accessed 1 June 2021).

Rème, C.A., Dramard, V., Kern, L. et al. (2008). Effect of S-adenosylmethionine tablets on the reduction of age-related mental decline in dogs: a double-blinded, placebo-controlled trial. *Veterinary Therapeutics* 9 (2): 69–82.

Remington, R., Chan, A., Paskavitz, J., and Shea, T.B. (2008). Efficacy of a vitamin/nutriceutical formulation for moderate-stage to later-stage Alzheimer's disease: a placebo-controlled pilot study. *American Journal of Alzheimers Disease and Other Dementias* 24 (1): 27–33.

Remington, R., Bechtel, C., Larsen, D. et al. (2015). A phase II randomized clinical trial of a nutritional formulation for cognition and mood in Alzheimer's disease. *Journal of Alzheimers Disease* 45 (2): 395–405.

Ren, Z., Ding, W., Su, Z. et al. (1994). Mechanisms of brain injury with deep hypothermic circulatory arrest and protective effects of coenzyme Q10. *Journal of Thoracic and Cardiovascular Surgery* 108 (1): 126–133.

Renaud, S. and de Lorgeril, M. (1992). Wine, alcohol, platelets, and the French paradox for coronary heart disease. *Lancet* 339 (8808): 1523–1526.

Rialland, P., Bichot, S., Lussier, B. et al. (2013). Effect of a diet enriched with green-lipped mussel on pain behavior and functioning in dogs with clinical osteoarthritis. *Canadian Journal of Veterinary Research* 77 (1): 66–74.

Ricard-Blum, S. (2011). The collagen family. *Cold Spring Harbor Perspectives in Biology* 3 (1): a004978.

Richardson, D., Schoenherr, W., and Zicker, S. (1997). Nutritional management of osteoarthritis. *Veterinary Clinics of North America: Small Animal Practice* 27 (4): 883–911.

Ripps, H. and Shen, W. (2012). Review: taurine: a "very essential" amino acid. *Molecular Vision* 18: 2673–2686.

Roby, C., Anderson, G.D., Kantor, E. et al. (2000). St John's Wort: effect on CYP3A4 activity. *Clinical Pharmacology and Therapeutics* 67 (5): 451–457.

Ronis, M., Pedersen, K., and Watt, J. (2018). Adverse effecs of nutraceuticals and dietary supplements. *Annual Review of Pharmacology and Toxicology* 58: 583–601.

Rossi, G., Pengo, G., Caldin, M. et al. (2014). Comparison of microbiological, histological, and immunomodulatory parameters in response to treatment with either combination therapy with prednisone and metronidazole or probiotic VSL#3 strains in dogs with idiopathic inflammatory bowel disease. *PLoS One* 9 (4): e94699.

Roush, J.K., Cross, A.R., Renberg, W.C. et al. (2010a). Evaluation of the effects of dietary supplementation with fish oil omega-3 fatty acids on weight bearing in dogs with osteoarthritis. *Journal of the American Veterinary Medical Association* 236 (1): 67–73.

Roush, J.K., Dodd, C.E., Fritsch, D.A. et al. (2010b). Multicenter veterinary practice assessment of the effects of omega-3 fatty acids on osteoarthritis in dogs. *Journal of the American Veterinary Medical Association* 236 (1): 59–66.

Ruff, K., DeVore, D., Leu, M., and Robinson, M. (2009a). Eggshell membrane: a possible new natural therapeutic for joint and connective tissue disorders. Results from two open-label human clinical studies. *Clinical Interventions in Aging* 4: 234–240.

Ruff, K., Winkler, A., Jackson, R.W. et al. (2009b). Eggshell membrane in the treatment of pain and stiffness from osteoarthritis of the knee: a randomized, multicenter, double-blind, placebo-controlled clinical study. *Clinical Rheumatology* 28 (8): 907–914.

Ruff, K., Kopp, K.J., Von Behrens, P. et al. (2016). Effectiveness of NEM® brand eggshell membrane in the treatment of suboptimal joint function in dogs: a multicenter, randomized, double-blind, placebo-controlled study. *Veterinary Medicine* 7: 113–121.

Rutherfurd-Markwick, K., Hendriks, W., Morel, P., and Thomas, D. (2013). The potential for enhancement of immunity in cats by dietary supplementation. *Veterinary Immunology and Immunopathology* 3–4 (15): 333–340.

Ryu, S., Park, S., Lim, W., and Song, G. (2019). Quercetin augments apoptosis of canine osteosarcoma cells by disrupting mitochondrial membrane potential and regulating PKB and MAPK signal transduction. *Journal of Cellular Biochemistry* 120 (10): 17449–17458.

Saarela, M., Mogensen, G., Fondén, R. et al. (2000). Probiotic bacteria: safety, functional and technological properties. *Journal of Biotechnology* 84 (3): 197–215.

Saevik, B.K., Bergvall, K., Holm, B.R. et al. (2004). A randomized, controlled study to evaluate the steroid sparing effect of essential fatty acid supplementation in the treatment of canine atopic dermatitis. *Veterinary Dermatology* 15 (3): 137–145.

Sahebkar, A., Serbanc, M., Ursoniuc, S., and Banach, M. (2015). Effect of curcuminoids on oxidative stress: a systematic review and meta-analysis of randomized controlled trials. *Journal of Functional Foods* 18: 898–909.

Sailer, E.R., Subramanian, L.R., Rall, B. et al. (1996). Acetyl-11-keto-beta-boswellic acid (AKBA): structure requirements for binding and 5-lipoxygenase inhibitory activity. *British Journal of Pharmacology* 117 (4): 615–618.

Saini, R. (2011). Conenzyme Q10: the essential nutrient. *Journal of Pharmacy and BioAllied Sciences* 3 (3): 466–467.

Saker, K., Eddy, A., Thatcher, C., and Kalnitsky, J. (1998). Manipulation of dietary (n-6) and (n-3) fatty acids alters platelet function in cats. *Journal of Nutrition* 128 (12 Suppl): 2645S–2647S.

Salehi, B., Rescigno, A., Dettori, T. et al. (2020). Avocado–soybean unsaponifiables: a panoply of potentialities to be exploited. *Biomolecules* 10 (1): 130.

Sandell, L. and Aigner, T. (2001). Articular cartilage and changes in arthritis: cell biology of osteoarthritis. *Arthritis Research and Therapy* 3 (2): 107–113.

Sanderson, S.L. (2006). Taurine and carnitine in canine cardiomyopathy. *Veterinary Clinics of North America Small Animal Practice* 36 (6): 1325–1343.

Sanderson, S.L., Osborne, C.A., Lulich, J.P. et al. (2001). Evaluation of urinary carnitine and taurine excretion in 5 cystinuric dogs with carnitine and taurine deficiency. *Journal of Veterinary Internal Medicine* 15 (2): 94–100.

Sándor, P.S., DiClemente, L., Coppola, G. et al. (2005). Efficacy of coenzyme Q10 in migraine prophylaxis: a randomized controlled trial. *Neurology* 64 (4): 713–715.

Sano, M., Bell, K., Cote, L. et al. (1992). Double-blind parallel design pilot study of acetyl levocarnitine in patients with Alzheimer's disease. *Archives of Neurology* 49 (11): 1137–1141.

Sato, H., Zhao, Z.Q., McGee, D.S. et al. (1995). Supplemental L-arginine during cardioplegic arrest and reperfusion avoids regional postischemic injury. *Journal of Thoracic and Cardiovascular Surgery* 110 (2): 302–314.

Sattawaphaet, W. (2018). Effects of coenzyme Q10 supplementation on cardiac troponin I level, heart rate variability, and echocardiographic profiles in canine with myomatous degenerative mitral valve disease. *Thai Journal of Veterinary Medicine* 48 (3): 443–452.

Sauter, S., Allenspach, K., Gaschen, F. et al. (2005). Cytokine expression in an ex vivo culture system of duodenal samples from dogs with chronic enteropathies: modulation by probiotic bacteria. *Domestic Animal Endocrinology* 29 (4): 605–622.

Sauter, S., Benyacoub, J., Allenspach, K. et al. (2006). Effects of probiotic bacteria in dogs with food responsive diarrhoea treated with an elimination diet. *Journal of Animal Physiology and Animal Nutrition* 90 (7–8): 269–277.

Schmitz, S. and Suchodolski, J. (2016). Understanding the canine intestinal microbiota and its modification by pro-, pre- and synbiotics: what is the evidence? *Veterinary Medicine and Science* 2 (2): 71–94.

Schmitz, S., Garden, O., Weling, D., and Allenspach, K. (2012). Gene expression of selected signature cytokines of T cell subsets in duodenal tissues of dogs with and without inflammatory bowel disease. *Veterinary Immunology and Immunopathology* 146 (1): 87–91.

Schmitz, S., Glanemann, B., Garden, O.A. et al. (2015). A prospective, randomized, blinded, placebo-controlled pilot study on the effect of *Enterococcus faecium* on clinical activity and intestinal gene expression in canine food-responsive chronic enteropathy. *Journal of Veterinary Internal Medicine* 29 (2): 533–543.

Schniertshauer, D., Müller, S., Mayr, T. et al. (2016). Accelerated regeneration of ATP level after irradiation in human skin fibroblasts by coenzyme Q10. *Photochemistry and Photobiology* 92 (3): 488–494.

Schultz, W. (1996). Inapplicability of the dietary supplement health and educaiton act to animal products. *Food and Drug Administration Federal Register* 61 (78): 17706–17708.

Scott, D.W., Miller, W.H. Jr., Reinhart, G.A. et al. (1997). Effect of an omega-3/omega-6 fatty acid-containing commercial lamb and rice diet on pruritis in atopic dogs: results of a single-blinded study. *Canadian Journal of Veterinary Research* 61: 145–153.

Scott, R., Evans, R., and Conzemius, M. (2017). Efficacy of an oral nutraceutical for the treatment of canine osteoarthritis. A double-blind, randomized, placebo-controlled prospective clinical trial. *Veterinary and Comparative Orthopaedics and Traumatology* 30 (5): 318–323.

Sechi, S., Fiore, F., Chiavolelli, F. et al. (2017). Oxidative stress and food supplementation with antioxidants in therapy dogs. *Canadian Journal of Veterinary Research* 81 (3): 206–216.

Sergi, S., Martínez-Subiela, S., Cerdà-Cuéllar, M. et al. (2016). Oral chondroitin sulfate and prebiotics for the treatment of canine inflammatory bowel disease: a randomized, controlled clinical trial. *BMC Veterinary Research* 12: 49.

Servet, E., Biourge, V., and Marniquet, P. (2006). Dietary intervention can improve clinical signs in osteoarthritic dogs. *Journal of Nutrition* 136 (7 Suppl): 1995S–1997S.

Sevalla, K., Todhunter, R., Vernier-Singer, M., and Budsberg, S. (2004). Effect of polysulfated glycosaminoglycan on DNA content and proteoglycan metabolism in normal and osteoarthritic canine articular cartilage explants. *Veterinary Surgery* 29 (5): 407–414.

Shah, M.R., Mehta, C.S., Shukla, V.D. et al. (2010). A clinical study of Matra Vasti and an ayurvedic indigenous compound drug in the management of Sandhigatavata (Osteoarthritis). *Ayu* 31 (2): 210–217.

Shariatpanahi, Z., Eslamian, G., Ardehali, S.H., and Baghestani, A.-R. (2019). Effects of early enteral glutamine supplementation on intestinal permeability in critically ill patients. *Indian Journal of Critical Care Medicine* 23 (8): 356–362.

Sharma, A.P.G., Gerberg, P., Bottiglieri, T. et al. (2017). S-Adenosylmethionine (SAMe) for neuropsychiatric disorders: a clinician-oriented review of research. *Journal of Clinical Psychiatry* 78 (6): e656–e667.

Shelton, G.D., Nyhan, W.L., Kass, P.H. et al. (1998). Analysis of organic acids, amino acids, and carnitine in dogs with lipid storage myopathy. *Muscle and Nerve* 21 (9): 1202–1205.

Shoba, G., Joy, D., Joseph, T. et al. (1998). Influence of piperine on the pharmacokinetics of curcumin in animals and human volunteers. *Planta Medica* 64 (4): 353–356.

Silva, D.A., Nai, G.A., Giuffrida, R. et al. (2018). Oral omega 3 in different proportions of EPA, DHA, and antioxidants as adjuvant in treatment of keratoconjunctivitis sicca in dogs. *Arquivos Brasileiros de Oftalmologia* 81 (5): 421–428.

Singh, M., Rao, D.M., Pande, S., and Battu, S. (2011). Medicinal uses of L-lysine: past and future. *International Journal of Research in Pharmaceutical Sciences* 2 (4): 637–642.

Skorupski, K., Hammond, G.M., Irish, A.M. et al. (2011). Prospective randomized clinical trial assessing the efficacy of Denamarin for prevention of CCNU-induced hepatopathy in tumor-bearing dogs. *Journal of Veterinary Internal Medicine* 25 (4): 838–845.

Smith, C.E., Freeman, L.M., Rush, J.E. et al. (2007). Omega-3 fatty acids in Boxer dogs with arrhythmogenic right ventricular cardiomyopathy. *Journal of Veterinary Internal Medicine* 21 (2): 265–273.

Smriga, M., Ando, T., Akutsu, M. et al. (2007). Oral treatment with L-lysine and L-arginine reduces anxiety and basal cortisol levels in healthy humans. *Biomedical Research* 28 (2): 85–90.

Snood, B. and Keenaghan, M. (2022). Conenzyme Q10. https://www.ncbi.nlm.nih.gov/books/NBK531491 (accessed 23 March 2021).

Soltanian, A., Mosallanejad, B., Jalali, M.R. et al. (2020). Comparative evaluation of therapeutic effects of silymarin and hydrocortisone on clinical and hematological alterations, and organ injury (liver and heart) in a low-dose canine lipopolysaccharide-induced sepsis model. *Veterinary Research Forum* 11 (3): 235–241.

Soós, P., Andrasi, T., Buhmann, V. et al. (2004). Myocardial protection after systemic application of L-arginine during reperfusion. *Journal of Cardiovascular Pharmacology* 43 (6): 782–788.

Springer, M. and Moco, S. (2019). Resveratrol and its human metabolites: effects on metabolic health and obesity. *Nutrients* 11 (1): 143.

St. Omer, V. and McKnight, E. (1980). Acetylcysteine for treatment of acetaminophen toxicosis in the cat. *Journal of the American Veterinary Medical Association* 176 (9): 911–913.

Starcher, B. and King, G. (1980). The presence of desmosine and isodesmosine in eggshell membrane protein. *Connective Tissue Research* 8 (1): 53–55.

Stewart, J.S., Lignell, A., Pettersson, A. et al. (2008). Safety assessment of astaxanthin-rich microalgae biomass: acute and subchronic toxicity studies in rats. *Food and Chemical Toxicology* 46 (9): 3030–3036.

Stey, C., Steurer, J., Bachmann, S. et al. (2000). The effect of oral N-acetylcysteine in chronic bronchitis: a quantitative systematic review. *European Respiratory Journal* 16: 253–262.

Sugita, K., Yanuma, N., Ohno, H. et al. (2019). Oral faecal microbiota transplantation for the treatment of *Clostridium difficile*-associated diarrhoea in a dog: a case report. *BMC Veterinary Research* 15 (1): 11.

Sugita, K., Shima, A., Takahashi, K. et al. (2020). Successful outcome after a single endoscopic fecal microbiota transplantation in a Shiba dog with non-responsive enteropathy during the treatment with chlorambucil. *Journal of Veterinary Medical Science* 83 (6): 984–989.

Suzuki, Y., Ohgami, K., Shiratori, K. et al. (2006). Suppressive effects of astaxanthin against rat endotoxin-induced uveitis by inhibiting the NF-kappaB signaling pathway. *Experimental Eye Research* 82 (2): 275–281.

Svaneborg, N., Kristensen, S.D., Hansen, L.M. et al. (2002). The acute and short-time effect of supplementation with the combination of n-3 fatty acids and acetylsalicylic acid on platelet function and plasma lipids. *Thrombosis Research* 105 (4): 311–316.

Sztretye, M., Dienes, B., Gonczi, M. et al. (2019). Astaxanthin: a potential mitochondrial-targeted antioxidant treatment in diseases and with aging. *Oxidative Medicine and Cellular Longevity* 2019: 3849692.

Takashi, H., Ueno, S., Kumamoto, S., and Yoshikai, Y. (2004). Suppressive effect of methylsulfonylmethane (MSM) on type II collagen-induced arthritis in DBA/1J mice. *Japanese Pharmacology and Therapeutics* 32 (7): 421–427.

Tanaka, T., Makita, H., Ohnishi, M. et al. (1995). Chemoprevention of rat oral carcinogenesis by naturally occurring xanthophyll's, astaxanthin and canthaxanthin. *Cancer Research* 55: 4059–4064.

Templeman, J.R., Davenport, G.M., Cant, J.P. et al. (2018). The effect of graded concentrations of dietary tryptophan on canine behavior in response to the approach of a familiary or unfamiliar individual. *Canadian Journal of Veterinary Research*, 82(4), 294–305.

Templeman, J.R., Mansilla, W., Fortener, L., and Shoveller, A. (2019). Tryptophan requirements in small, medium, and large breed adult dogs using the indicator amino acid oxidation technique. *Journal of Animal Science* 97 (8): 3274–3285.

Tenório, M.C.D.S., Graciliano, N.G., Moura, F.A. et al. (2021). N-Acetylcysteine (NAC): impacts on human health. *Antioxidants* 10 (6): 967.

Teramoto, F., Rokutan, K., Sugano, Y. et al. (2006). Long-term administration of 4G-beta-D-galactosylsucrose (lactosucrose) enhances intestinal calcium absorption in young women: a randomized, placebo-controlled 96-wk study. *Journal of Nutritional Science and Vitaminology (Tokyo)* 52 (5): 337–346.

Testa, B., Testa, D., Mesolella, M. et al. (2001). Management of chronic otitis media with effusion: the role of glutathione. *Laryngoscope* 111 (8): 1486–1489.

Thomas, C.M. and Versalovic, J. (2010). Probiotics–host communication: modulation of signaling pathways in the intestine. *Gut Microbes* 1 (3): 148–163.

Tighe, S., Akhtar, D., Igbal, U., and Ahmed, A. (2020). Chronic liver disease and silymarin: a biochemical and clinical review. *Journal of Clinical and Translational Hepatology* 8 (4): 454–458.

Tiku, M., Narla, H., Jain, M., and Yalamanchili, P. (2007). Glucosamine prevents in vitro collagen degradation in chondrocytes by inhibiting advanced lipoxidation reactions and protein oxidation. *Arthritis Research and Therapy* 9 (4): R76.

Tinsley, G. (2021). What is Tryptophan? https://www.healthline.com/health/tryptophan (accessed 30 June 2022).

Todesco, T., Rao, A.V., Bosello, O., and Jenkins, D.J. (1991). Propionate lowers blood glucose and alters lipid metabolism in healthy subjects. *American Journal of Clinical Nutrition* 54 (5): 860–865.

Tomé, D. and Bos, C. (2007). Lysine requirement through the human life cycle. *Journal of Nutrition* 137 (6 Suppl. 2): 1642S–1645S.

Tong, T., Zhao, W., Wu, Y.-Q. et al. (2009). Chicken type II collagen induced immune balance of main subtype of helper T cells in mesenteric lymph node lymphocytes in rats with collagen-induced arthritis. *Inflammation Research* 59 (3): 367–377.

Trepainer, L. (2009). Diopathic inflammatory bowel disease in cats: rational treatment selection. *Journal of Feline Medicine and Surgery* 11 (1): 32–38.

Treschow, A., Hodges, L.D., Wright, P.F.A. et al. (2007). Novel anti-inflammatory omega-3 PUFAs from the New Zealand green-lipped mussel, *Perna canaliculus. Comparative Biochemistry and Physiology Part B: Biochemistry and Molecular Biology* 147 (4): 645–656.

Turck, D., Castenmiller, J., de Henauw, S. et al. (2020). Safety of astaxanthin for its use as a novel food in food supplements. *EFSA Journal* 18 (2): e05993.

Uchiyama, K., Naito, Y., Hasegawa, G. et al. (2002). Astaxanthin protects beta-cells against glucose toxicity in diabetic db/db mice. *Redox Report* 7 (5): 290–293.

Uebelhart, D. (2008). Clinical review of chondroitin sulfate in osteoarthritis. *Osteoarthritis and Cartilage* 16 (Suppl. 3): S19–S21.

Uebelhart, D., Thonar, E., Zhang, J., and Williams, J. (1998). Protective effect of exogenous chondroitin 4,6-sulfate in the acute degradation of articular cartilage in the rabbit. *Osteoarthritis and Cartilage* 6 (Suppl. A): 6–13.

USDA (United States Department of Agriculture) (2020). Good Agricultural Practices (GAP) Audits. https://www.ams. usda.gov/services/auditing/gap-ghp (accessed 17 Decenber 2020).

Usha, P. and Naidu, M. (2004). Randomised, double-blind, parallel, placebo-controlled study of oral glucosamine, methylsulfonylmethane and their combination in osteoarthritis. *Clinical Drug Investigations* 24 (6): 353–363.

USP (United States Pharmacopeia) (2009). General Notices and Requirements. https:// www.uspnf.com/sites/default/files/usp_pdf/ EN/USPNF/generalNoticesandRequirements Final.pdf. (accessed 5 February 2021).

USP (United States Pharmacopeia) (2022). USP. usp.org (accessed 30 January 2022)

Vandeweerd, J.-M., Coisnon, C., Clegg, P. et al. (2012). Systematic review of efficacy of nutraceuticals to alleviate clinical signs of osteoarthritis. *Journal of Veterinary Internal Medicine* 26 (3): 448–456.

VanDolah, H., Bauer, B., and Mauck, K. (2019). Clinician's guide to cannabidiol and hemp oils. *Mayo Clinic Proceedings* 94 (9): 1840–1851.

Vang, O., Ahmad, N., Baile, C.A. et al. (2011). What is new for an old molecule? Systematic review and recommendations on the use of resveratrol. *PLoS One* 6 (6): e19881.

Vanschoonbeek, K., de Maat, M.P.M., and Heemskerk, J.W.M. (2003). Fish oil consumption and reduction of arterial disease. *Journal of Nutrition* 133 (3): 657–660.

Varcoe, G., Tomlinson, J., and Manfredi, J. (2021). Owner perceptions of long-term systemic use of subcutaneous administration of polysulfated glycosaminoglycan. *Journal of the American Animal Hospital Association* 57 (5): 205–211.

Varghese, S., Theprungsirikul, P., Sahani, S. et al. (2007). Glucosamine modulates chondrocyte proliferation, matrix synthesis, and gene expression. *Osteoarthritis and Cartilage* 15 (1): 59–68.

Varzi, H.N., Esmailzadeh, S., Morovvati, H. et al. (2007). Effect of silymarin and vitamin E on gentamicin-induced nephrotoxicity. *Journal of Veterinary Pharmacology and Therapeutics* 30 (5): 477–481.

Vassalotti, G., Musco, N., Lombardi, P. et al. (2017). Nutritional management of search and rescue dogs. *Journal of Nutritional Science* 6: e44.

Vaughn, D., Kulpa, J., and Paulionis, L. (2020). Preliminary investigation of the safety of escalating cannabinoid doses in healthy dogs. *Frontiers in Veterinary Science* 7: 51.

VDH (Veterinary Drug Handbook) (2017a). Calcium Salts. https://www.vin.com/ members/cms/project/defaultadv1.

aspx?pId=13468&id=7978572 (accessed 20 February 2021).

VDH (Veterinary Drug Handbook) (2017b). Iron Salts. https://www.vin.com/members/cms/project/defaultadv1. aspx?pId=13468&id=8091856 (accessed 20 February 2021).

VDH (Veterinary Drug Handbook) (2017c). Magnesium Salts. https://www.vin.com/members/cms/project/defaultadv1. aspx?pId=13468&id=7893210 (accessed 20 February 2021).

VDH (Veterinary Drug Handbook) (2017d). Vitamin A. https://www.vin.com/members/cms/project/defaultadv1.aspx?pId=13468&id=8606339 (accessed 20 February 2021).

VDH (Veterinary Drug Handbook) (2017e). Vitamin B12. https://www.vin.com/members/cms/project/defaultadv1.aspx?pId=13468&id=7314892 (accessed 20 February 2021).

VDH (Veterinary Drug Handbook) (2017f) Vitamin C. https://www.vin.com/members/cms/project/defaultadv1.aspx?pId=13468&id=7168959 (accessed 20 February 2021).

VDH (Veterinary Drug Handbook) (2017g). Vitamin K. https://www.vin.com/members/cms/project/defaultadv1.aspx?pId=13468&id=7660643 (accessed 20 February 2021).

VDH (Veterinary Drug Handbook) (2017h). Zinc Salts. https://www.vin.com/members/cms/project/defaultadv1.aspx?pId=13468&id=8690373 (accessed 20 February 2021).

VDH (Veterinary Drug Handbook) (2018). Aluminum Hydroxide. https://www.vin.com/members/cms/project/defaultadv1. aspx?pId=13468&id=8622949. (accessed 20 February 2021).

VDH (Veterinary Drug Handbook) (2019). Vitamin D. https://www.vin.com/members/cms/project/defaultadv1.aspx?pId=3468&id=7169310 (accessed 20 February 2021).

VDH (Veterinary Drug Handbook) (2020). Potassium Salts. https://www.vin.com/members/cms/project/defaultadv1. aspx?pId=13468&id=8708936 (accessed 20 February 2021).

Verrico, C.D., Wesson, S., Konduri, V. et al. (2020). A randomized, double-blind, placebo-controlled study of daily cannabidiol for the treatment of canine osteoarthritis pain. *Pain* 161 (9): 2191–2202.

Villani, R., Gannon, J., Self, M., and Rich, P. (2000). L-carnitine supplementation combined with aerobic training does not promote weight loss in moderately obese women. *International Journal of Sport Nutrition and Exercise Metabolism* 10 (2): 199–207.

Viribay, A., Burgos, J., Fernández-Landa, J. et al. (2020). Effects of arginine supplementation on athletic performance based on energy metabolism: a systematic review and meta-analysis. *Nutrients* 12 (5): 1300.

Viviano, K.R. and VanderWielen, B. (2013). Effect of N-acetylcysteine supplementation on intracellular glutathione, urine isoprostanes, clinical score, and survival in hospitalized ill dogs. *Journal of Veterinary Internal Medicine* 27 (2): 250–258.

Wander, R., Hall, J.A., Gradin, J.L. et al. (1997). The ratio of dietary (n-6) to (n-3) fatty acids influences immune system function, eicosanoid metabolism, lipid peroxidation and vitamin E status in aged dogs. *Journal of Nutrition* 127 (6): 1198–1205.

Wang, C., Xiao, Y., Yang, B. et al. (2014). Isolation and screened neuroprotective active constituents from the roots and rhizomes of *Valeriana amurensis. Fitoterapia* 96: 48–55.

Wasser, S. (2014). Medicinal mushroom science: current perspectives, advances, evidences, and challenges. *Biomedical Journal* 37 (6): 345–356.

Webb, C., Twedt, D., Fettman, M., and Mason, G. (2003). S-adenosylmethionine (SAMe) in a feline acetaminophen model of oxidative injury. *Journal of Feline Medicine and Surgery* 5 (2): 69–75.

Webster, C. and Copper, J. (2009). Therapeutic use of cytoprotective agents in canine and feline hepatobiliary disease. *Veterinary Clinics of North America: Small Animal Practice* 39 (3): 631–652.

Wedekind, K.J., Ruff, K.J., Atwell, C.A. et al. (2017). Beneficial effects of natural eggshell membrane (NEM) on multiple indices of arthritis in collagen-induced arthritic rats. *Modern Rheumatology* 27 (5): 838–848.

Weese, J. and Martin, H. (2011). Assessment of commercial probiotic bacterial contents and label accuracy. *Canadian Veterinary Journal* 52 (1): 43–46.

Wells, J.W., Evans, C.H., Scott, M.C. et al. (2013). Arginase treatment prevents the recovery of canine lymphoma and osteosarcoma cells resistant to the toxic effects of prolonged arginine deprivation. *PLoS One* 8 (1): e54464.

Wenz, W., Hornung, C., Cramer, C. et al. (2017). Effect of glucosamine sulfate on osteoarthritis in the cruciate-deficient canine model of osteoarthritis. *Cartilage* 8 (2): 173–179.

Wernimont, S.M., Radosevich, J., Jackson, M.I. et al. (2020). The effects of nutrition on the gastrointestinal microbiome of cats and dogs: impact on health and disease. *Frontiers in Microbiology* 11: 1266.

Whelan, K. (2013). Mechanisms and effectiveness of prebiotics in modifying the gastrointestinal microbiota for the management of digestive disorders. *Proceedings of the Nutrition Society* 72 (3): 288–298.

Whelan, J. and Fritsche, K. (2013). Linoleic acid. *Advances in Nutrition* 4 (3): 311–312.

WHO (World Health Organization) (2015). Medicines: Good manufacturing practices. https://www.who.int/news-room/questions-and-answers/item/medicines-good-manufacturing-processes (accessed 17 December 2021).

Wikipedia (2019). Chinese food therapy. https://en.wikipedia.org/wiki/Chinese_food_therapy (accessed December 2019).

Wilkins, C., Long, R.C. Jr., Waldron, M. et al. (2004). Assessment of the influence of fatty acids on indices of insulin sensitivity and myocellular lipid content by use of magnetic resonance spectroscopy in cats. *American*

Journal of Veterinary Research 65 (8): 1090–1099.

Withers, S.S., York, D., Johnson, E. et al. (2018). In vitro and in vivo activity of liposome-encapsulated curcumin for naturally occurring canine cancers. *Veterinary and Comparative Oncology* 16 (4): 571–579.

Wong, W., Hendrix, M.J., von der Mark, K. et al. (1984). Collagen in the egg shell membranes of the hen. *Developmental Biology* 104 (1): 28–36.

Woods, S. (2007). The endocannabinoid system: mechanisms behind metabolic homeostasis and imbalance. *American Journal of Medicine* 120 (2 Suppl. 1): S9–S17.

Wright, E. (1994). Clinical effectiveness of lysine in treating recurrent aphthous ulcers and herpes labialis. *General Dentistry* 42 (1): 40–42.

Wu, D., Xu, H., Chen, J., and Zhang, L. (2019). Effects of astaxanthin supplementation on oxidative stress. *International Journal for Vitamin and Nutrition Research* 90 (1–2): 179–194.

Wu, M., Cronin, K., and Crane, J. (2021). *Biochemistry, Collagen Synthesis*. Treasure Island, FL: StatPearls.

Wynn, S. (2001). Carnitine: Nutrition Reference. https://www.vin.com/members/cms/project/defaultadv1.aspx?pid=373&id=4743749&f5=1 (accessed 7 March 2021).

Wynn, S. and Fougère, B. (2007). *Veterinary Herbal Medicine*. St. Louis, MO: Elsevier.

Yan-ui, X., Yun-mei, S., Zhi-pend, C., and Qi-neng, P. (2006). Preparation of silymarin proliposome: a new way to increase oral bioavailability of silymarin in beagle dogs. *International Journal of Pharmaceutics* 319 (1–2): 162–168.

Yerramilli-Rao, P., Beal, M.F., Watanabe, D. et al. (2012). Oral repeated-dose toxicity studies in coenzyme Q10 in beagle dogs. *International Journal of Toxicology* 31 (1): 58–69.

Yetley, E. (2007). Multivitamin and multimineral dietary supplements: definitions, characterization, bioavailability, and drug interactions. *American Journal of Clinical Nutrition* 85 (1): 269S–276S.

Yu, G., Xiang, W., Zhang, T. et al. (2020). Effectiveness of Boswellia and Boswellia extract for osteoarthritis patients: a systematic review and meta-analysis. *BMC Complementary Medicine and Therapies* 20 (225): 1–16.

Zadik-Weiss, L., Ritter, S., Hermush, V. et al. (2020). Feline cognitive dysfunction as a model for Alzeimer's disease in the research of CBD as a potential treatment. A narrative review. *Journal of Cannabis Research* 2 (1): 43.

Zanger, U. and Schwab, M. (2013). Cytochrome P450 enzymes in drug metabolism: regulation of gene expression, enzyme activities, and impact of genetic variation. *Pharmacology and Therapeutics* 138 (1): 103–141.

Zanghi, B., Middleton, R., and Reynolds, A. (2015). Effects of postexercise feeding of a supplemental carbohydrate and protein bar with or without astaxanthin from *Haematococcus pluvialis* to exercise-conditioned dogs. *American Journal of Veterinary Research* 76 (4): 338–350.

Zhang, F., Luo, W., Shi, Y. et al. (2012). Should we standardize the 1,700-year-old fecal microbiota transplantation? *American Journal of Gastroenterology* 107 (11): 1755–1756.

Zhao, S., Gao, Q., Rong, C. et al. (2020). Immunomodulatory effects of edible and medicinal mushrooms and their bioactive immunoregulatory products. *Journal of Fungi* 6 (4): 269.

Zhou, Q., Wang, Y., Han, X. et al. (2022). Efficacy of resveratrol supplementation on glucose and lipid metabolism: a meta-analysis and systematic review. *Frontiers in Physiology* 13: 795980.

Zicker, S., Jewell, D., Yamka, R., and Milgram, N. (2012). Evaluation of cognitive learning, memory, psychomotor, immunologic, and retinal functions in healthy puppies fed foods fortified with docosahexaenoic acid-rich fish oil from 8 to 52 weeks of age. *Journal of the American Veterinary Medical Association* 241 (5): 583–594.

Zozina, V., Covantev, S., Goroshko, O.A. et al. (2018). Coenzyme Q10 in cardiovascular and metabolic diseases: current state of the problem. *Current Cardiology Reviews* 14 (3): 164–174.

Zuchi, C., Ambrosio, G., Lüscher, T., and Landmesser, U. (2010). Nutraceuticals in cardiovascular prevention: lessons from studies on endothelial function. *Cardiovascular Therapeutics* 28 (4): 187–201.

5

Ozone Therapy

Introduction

Ozone therapy, a relatively new therapeutic modality in veterinary medicine, is defined as the introduction of medical-grade ozone gas into or onto the body with the intent to treat or cure a specific disease condition. The administration of ozone (alone or in solution) intravenously, subcutaneously, rectally, or topically can aid in the treatment of most chronic inflammatory and infectious conditions. Ozone should not be administered through inhalation unless percolated (bubbled) through oil first.

The introduction of ozone therapy into a veterinary practice can be beneficial for both the patient and the health of the practice. The successful incorporation and utilization of veterinary ozone therapy (VOT) does not end with the veterinarian's training. Support staff training and client education are crucial. This chapter will discuss the what, why, and how for the effective integration of VOT within your practice.

The What

Word Origin

Ozone is derived from the Greek work *ozein*, meaning odorous.

Definition

The introduction of medical-grade ozone gas into or onto the body with the intent to treat or cure a specific disease condition. Ozone is administered (alone or in solution) intravenously, subcutaneously, rectally, or topically, but never through inhalation (unless percolated through oil).

Human History

Ozone therapy is a relatively new therapeutic modality, having become popular within the last 40 years. Ozone was discovered, but not

Integrative Medicine in Veterinary Practice, First Edition. Lisa P. McFaddin.
© 2024 John Wiley & Sons, Inc. Published 2024 by John Wiley & Sons, Inc.
Companion website: www.wiley.com/go/mcfaddin/integrativemedicine

recognized as a form of oxygen, by the Dutch chemist Martinus van Marum in 1785 when an odd odor was noted following the sparking of electricity above water (Toth and Hillger 2022). In 1839, the German-Swiss chemist Christian Friedrich Schönbein isolated the gas, naming it ozone (Toth and Hillger 2022). Schönbein is often considered the father of ozone therapy.

Ozone was used in the mid to late 1800s to disinfect operating rooms and sterilize surgical instruments, purify drinking water, in the treatment of diphtheria, and purify blood in test tubes in Europe (Elvis and Ekta 2011; Naik et al. 2016). Nicola Tesla patented the first ozone generator in the United States in 1896 (Elvis and Ekta 2011). Two years later the Institute for Oxygen Therapy opened in Berlin, specializing in the injection of ozone into the body (Naik et al. 2016).

During the early twentieth century ozone was primarily used topically to treat infected wounds, chronic middle-ear infections, and during dental procedures (Stoker 1902; Elvis and Ekta 2011; Naik et al. 2016). The popularity of ozone therapy in the treatment of systemic inflammatory and infectious diseases blossomed in Europe throughout the mid-twentieth century (AEPROMO 2015). Ozone therapy was similarly used in the United States in the mid to late 1980s, focusing on the treatment of chronic infectious and inflammatory disorders (Elvis and Ekta 2011). The International Ozone Institute (IOI), now known as the International Ozone Association (IOA), was founded in 1971. The American Academy of Ozone Therapy was founded in 2010.

The use of medical ozone therapy is still considered controversial, with many Western medicine practitioners and organizations vehemently opposing its use. In 2019 the Food and Drug Administration (FDA) amended the label requirements for devices producing ozone in Title 21, Part 801.415 (FDA 2022). The FDA stated

"[o]zone is a toxic gas with no known useful medical application in specific, adjunctive, or preventive therapy. For ozone to be effective as a germicide, it must be present in a concentration far greater than that which can be safely tolerated by man and animals.

It goes on to say any device producing ozone above a certain concentration, designed to be used in a hospital setting or around ill people, or used to treat a medical condition 'for which there is no proof of safety and effectiveness' would be considered 'adulterated or misbranded'" (FDA 2022).

Veterinary History

The first published research involving ozone therapy in veterinary medicine involved laboratory animals, starting in the late 1980s (Shulz 1986). Ozone research in veterinary medicine has been limited over the past 50 years, with a rise in interest (based on the frequency and number of species studied) during the last 20 years.

VOT is considered a niche modality with very few veterinarians offering the therapy throughout the continental United States. Veterinarians trained to use ozone properly find the therapy crucial to everyday practice especially when treating infection, cancers, and anything causing inflammation.

Like human medicine, the use of VOT remains controversial among veterinarians. As of September 2022, there are no veterinary associations or organizations dedicated to VOT, and training courses (both hands-on and virtual) for veterinarians is limited.

Terminology

The world of ozone therapy comes with its own vocabulary. A basic understanding of these terms is crucial, allowing effective communication amongst professionals and with clients. A summary of common terms is provided below.

Alcohol: An organic compound containing one or more hydroxyl (oxygen–hydrogen) groups bound to a carbon atom (Vitz et al. 2022)

Aldehyde: An organic compound containing a carbon double bonded to an oxygen atom (carbonyl group), single bonded with a hydrogen atom, and single bonded with another atom or groups of atoms (March and Brown 2020).

Allodynia: A form of neuropathic pain in which nonpainful stimuli cause pain.

Analgesia: The inability to feel pain. An analgesic is a substance or drug which reduces or relieves pain.

Antigens: A foreign substance or toxin causing an immune response (and often antibody production) in the body.

Apoptosis: Cell death.

Atmosphere: Layers of gas surrounding the Earth maintained in place by gravity.

Atom: Smallest unit of ordinary matter of a chemical element (Trefil et al. 2022). Atoms contain a nucleus (composed of one or more positive protons and a number of neutral neutrons) and one or more negatively charged electrons.

Autohemotherapy: Removal, infusion with ozone, and re-injection of patient's own blood in an aseptic technique.

Carbonyl group: An organic compound composed of a carbon atom double bonded to an oxygen atom (LibreTexts 2022b).

Carboxyl group: An organic compound composed of a carbon atom double bonded to an oxygen atom and single bonded to a hydroxyl group (OH) (Helmenstine 2020).

Carboxylic acid: An organic compound with acidic properties (aka organic acid) containing a carboxyl group attached to another atom or chain of molecules (Helmenstine 2020).

Cell-mediated immunity: Part of the adaptive immune response not reliant on the production of antibodies. Cell-mediated immunity takes longer to respond, occurs within tissues, and is primarily driven by T cells, divided into helper T cells (which function to activate other immune cells) and killer or cytotoxic T cells (which directly kill cells containing the pathogen).

Corona discharge: An electrical discharge caused by the exposure of a fluid or gas (air) surrounding a conductor carrying a high voltage (ME 2022).

Covalent bond: A chemical bond involving the sharing of an electrons, forming electron pairs, between atoms (Ouellette and Rawn 2014).

Dipolar: An electrically neutral compound or molecule which carries both a positive and negative charge.

Dismutation (aka disproportionation): A reaction in which a chemical undergoes oxidation and reduction (redox reaction). Ozone dismutation refers to the breakdown of two ozone molecules (O_3) into three oxygen molecules (O_2).

Double bond: A covalent bond in which two electron pairs are shared between two atoms (Ouellette and Rawn 2014).

Glycolysis: The enzymatic breakdown of glucose releasing energy and pyruvic acid.

Hydrocarbon: An organic compound exclusively composed of hydrogen and carbon atoms.

Hyperalgesia: A form of neuropathic pain in which there is an abnormally increased sensitivity to pain.

Humoral immunity: Part of the adaptive immune response driven by B cells, involving the production of antigen-specific antibodies by effector B cells (plasma cells). Humoral immunity provides the immune system with a memory of the antigen through the production of memory B cells, allowing quick neutralization of the antigen if seen in the future.

Hypoxia: Low levels of oxygen within tissues.

Insufflation: Blowing a substance (gas, liquid, or powder) into a body cavity.

In vitro (Latin for "within the glass"): Studies performed outside of a living organism. Most commonly microorganisms, tissue cultures, and cells are studied in petri dishes and/or test tubes.

In vivo (Latin for "in glass"): Studies performed within living organisms, not tissue extracts or cells.

Ketone: An organic compound containing a carbon atom covalently bonded to an oxygen atom (carbonyl group), while also bonded to two other carbon-containing molecules (Brown 2022).

Lymphocytes: A type of white blood cell involved in the immune system, formed in the bone marrow, and found in blood and lymph tissue. T cells, B cells, and natural killer cells are types of lymphocytes.

Lysis: Rupture of a cell.

Macrophage: A type of white blood cell involved in the immune system, found within almost all tissues, which directly engulfs (ingests) and destroys (digests) pathogens.

Molecule: Smallest part of a substance that maintains the physical and chemical properties of the substance, consisting of two or more atoms (LibreTexts 2022a).

Neuropathic pain: Pathologic pain caused by damage or injury to nerves responsible for transferring information from the body (peripheral nervous system) to the spinal cord or brain (central nervous system).

Nociception: Detection and communication of noxious stimuli by the nervous system.

Nociceptive pain: Physiologic pain caused by damage to the body and is typically well localized and temporary.

Noxious stimulus: A signal which is damaging or threatening to normal tissue.

Oxidation: The loss of electrons and increase in charge (becomes more positive) (Wiley 2002).

Oxidizing agent (aka oxidant or oxidizer): A substance that removes or accepts electrons from a reducing agent during a redox reaction (Wiley 2002).

Oxygen: An element with the atomic symbol O. Oxygen gas is colorless, odorless, tasteless, and noncombustible (but does promote the burning of combustible materials) (PubChem 2022a).

Ozone: An inorganic molecule composed of three oxygen atoms, O_3, which create a colorless to pale blue volatile gas with a distinct odor (PubChem 2022b).

Ozonide: A chemical compound formed by the reaction of ozone with another compound (Hassan et al. 2020).

Ozone generator (aka ozonator): A device designed to create ozone from either room air or pure oxygen gas using primarily an electrical discharge (corona) or ultraviolet (UV) light.

Ozonolysis (aka Criegee mechanism): The process by which ozone interacts with and breaks apart (cleaves) the double bonds in hydrocarbons (OCP 2022).

Pain: The sensation and emotional experience associated with tissue damage (perceived or actual).

Pathogen: A broad term referring to an organism (bacteria, fungus, virus, or other microorganism) or agent (cancer, chemical, organic or inorganic material) which causes disease.

Percolating: Filtering of a liquid or gas slowly through a porous substance, such as a filter or surface.

Phagocytosis: Ingestion (engulfing) of a large particle by a cell using its plasma membrane, creating an internal compartment within the cell.

Prolotherapy (aka nonsurgical ligament and tendon reconstruction and regenerative joint injection): The injection of a small volume of a sterile irritant into a painful joint, tendon, or ligament with the goal of stimulating the body's natural healing ability, stabilizing the weakened tissues, and reducing pain (Hauser et al. 2016; AOAPRM 2020).

Reactive oxygen species (ros): Highly reactive and unstable molecules containing oxygen which react with other molecules in a cell; examples include singlet oxygen, peroxides, super-oxides, and hydroxyl radicals (Shields et al. 2021).

Redox reaction (aka oxidation–reduction reaction): A chemical reaction during which the oxidation state of the involved compounds changes, i.e. the gain and loss of electrons (Wiley 2002).

Reducing agent (aka reductant): A substance that donates electrons to an oxidizing agent during a redox reaction (Wiley 2002).

Reduction: The gaining of electrons and subsequent decrease in charge (becomes more negative) (Wiley 2002).

Rheological properties: The ability of a material to change shape, distort, or change its flow.

Single bond: A covalent bond in which one electron pair is shared between two atoms (Ouellette and Rawn 2014).

Stratosphere: Second layer of the atmosphere existing 6–30 miles above the Earth's surface.

Stratospheric ozone: Layer of ozone located within the stratosphere, responsible for absorbing much of the harmful UV radiation from the sun (EPA 2022a). Considered the "good ozone."

Troposphere: First layer of the atmosphere starting at the Earth's surface and extending upward 6–7 miles.

Tropospheric ozone: Ozone found within the troposphere which contributes to air pollution, aka the "bad ozone" (EPA 2022a).

Ultraviolet (UV) light or radiation: A form of invisible light energy (aka electro-magnetic radiation) with a wavelength shorter than that of visible light (10–400 nm) but longer than that of X-rays (FDA 2020). Sunlight is the primary source of UV radiation. There are three main forms of UV radiation, in order of decreasing wavelengths: UVA, UVB, and UVC. The stratospheric ozone layer filters the amount and type of UV radiation reaching the Earth's surface, absorbing all UVC and some UVB radiation (FDA 2020). UV radiation reaching the Earth's surface can penetrate different layers of the skin depending on their wavelength, with UVA (longest wavelength) penetrating to the middle skin layer (dermis) and UVB (shorter wavelength) penetrating the outer skin layer (dermis) (EPA 2022a).

Ozone Basics

Ozone Production

Ozone, depicted in Figure 5.1, is an inorganic molecule composed of three oxygen atoms, O_3 (PubChem 2022b). Ozone is a colorless to pale blue explosive gas with a characteristic odor (PubChem 2022b). Ozone occurs naturally (atmospheric) and can be made synthetically.

Atmospheric Ozone

Naturally generated ozone is typically found in the upper atmosphere (stratosphere) and lower atmosphere (troposphere), as shown in

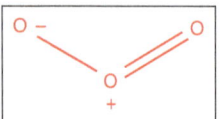

Figure 5.1 Molecular structure of ozone or triatomic oxygen, O_3. Source: Pubchem, https://pubchem.ncbi.nlm.nih.gov/compound/24823, August 1, 2005.

Figure 5.2. Stratospheric ozone, located 6–30 miles above the Earth's surface, is formed when dioxygen, O_2, interacts with UV light (EPA 2022a). This "ozone layer" creates a protective barrier around the planet, reducing the amount of harmful UV radiation reaching the surface (EPA 2022a). A small percentage of stratospheric ozone is transported down to the tropospheric layer.

Most of the tropospheric ozone is generated from O_2 reacting with sunlight and natural gases or air pollutants, such as volatile organic compounds (VOC) and nitrogen oxides (NO_x) (NOAA CSL 2010; EPA 2022a). Tropospheric ozone contributes to smog. Smog is a form of air pollution causing the sky to appear brown or gray, reducing air quality, and is not considered beneficial (EPA 2022b). Tropospheric ozone does not significantly influence the concentration of stratospheric ozone.

Ozone is an unstable and highly reactive molecule; its formation is quickly balanced by its destruction due to chemical reactions with

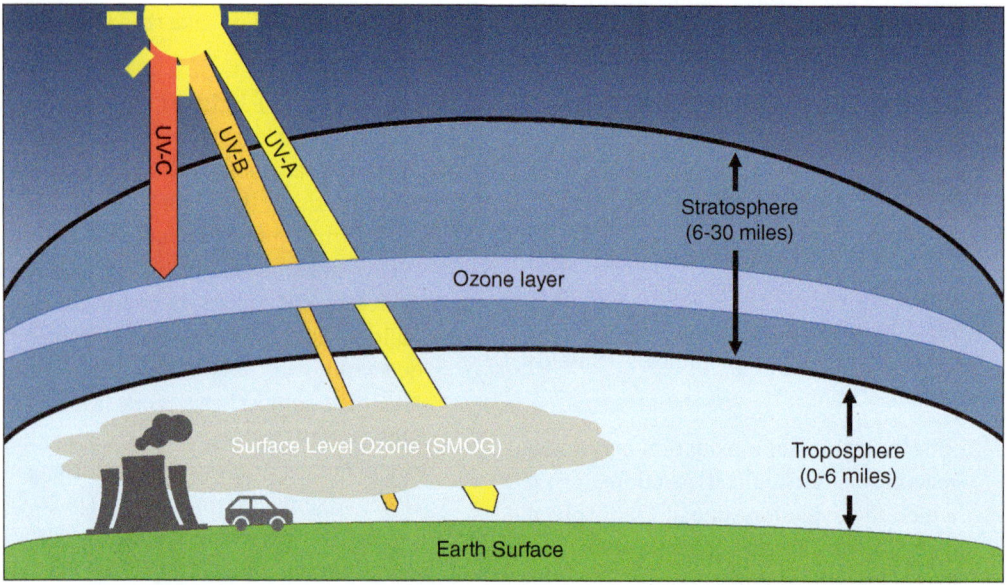

Figure 5.2 A schematic representation of ozone within the atmosphere. The ozone layer is located within the stratosphere, 6–30 miles above the Earth's surface. Ozone is formed when an oxygen molecule (O_2) interacts with ultraviolet (UV) light. The ozone layer protects the earth from harmful UV-C and most UV-B radiation. Ozone within the troposphere is generated from O_2 reacting with sunlight, natural gas, and air pollutants which contributes to smog, a form of air pollution. Source: Lisa P. McFaddin.

other substances (NOAA CSL 2010). Ozone concentrations are heavily dependent on the saturation of reactive gases, sunlight intensity, location within the atmosphere, temperature, and other factors (NOAA CSL 2010). The existence of atmospheric ozone highlights the dichotomy of this molecule's beneficial (protective ozone layer) and negative (smog) attributes. The United States Environmental Protective Agency (EPA) developed the phrase "good up high – bad nearby" to help people remember that the ozone layer in the stratosphere is good for the planet, while high levels of ozone near the surface are bad for health (EPA 2003).

Atmospheric Ozone for Veterinarians

Stratospheric ozone is generated through a two-step chemical process. Step 1 requires UV radiation to break apart one O_2 molecule, producing two oxygen atoms, O_2 + UV radiation = 2 O (NOAA CSL 2010). Step 2 involves the binding of one oxygen atom and one O_2 molecule into a single O_3 molecule, $O + O_2 = O_3$ (NOAA CSL 2010). The overall reaction is $3O_2$ molecules + UV radiation = $2O_3$ molecules.

Ozone Generator

An ozone generator (aka ozonator) is a device designed to create ozone from room air or pure oxygen gas using either an electrical discharge (corona), UV light, plasma, or electrolysis (Rodriguez 2016). Room air can safely be used when the end product is applied as a disinfectant. Only pure oxygen gas should be used for medical applications of ozone therapy in people and animals. Room air contains 80% nitrogen which can form the potentially toxic gases nitrous oxide and nitric oxide when passed through the generators (Shallenberger 2011).

Corona discharge (aka electrosynthesis) is the most common power source used to create medical ozone (Shallenberger 2011). Oxygen gas is exposed to an electric spark which separates the oxygen atoms allowing a percentage of the atoms to recombine as ozone, as illustrated in Figure 5.3. Electrosynthesis produces the

highest concentration of ozone gas, up to 15% by volume (Shallenberger 2011; Rodriguez 2016).

The instability of ozone causes the O_3 molecules to interact and break down into more stable O_2 molecules relatively quickly, in a process called dismutation, as shown in Figure 5.3 (Shallenberger 2011). In a glass container 50% of the ozone will dismutate every 45 minutes; plastic containers result in 50% dismutation every 30 minutes (Shallenberger 2011). This means ozone must be generated and used as needed. Ozone solutions (aside from ozonated oils) cannot be mixed up and sent home with clients to use later.

The concentration of ozone is typically measured in microgram per milliliter (µg/ml). The maximum concentration used in veterinary medicine is generally 5% or 70 µg/ml (Shoemaker 2005). The desired ozone concentration is dependent on the method of administration and condition being treated. The practitioner should utilize an ozone analyzer to ensure the accuracy of the ozone concentration produced by the generator (Shallenberger 2011; Rodriguez 2016).

Ozone Generators for Veterinarians

Ozone generators using corona discharge contain two electrodes separated by a gas-filled gap, as shown in Figure 5.3. One of the electrodes contains an electric insulator (dielectric). As oxygen gas is passed through the generation cell (creating the gas-filled gap) an alternating current (AC) voltage is applied (ME 2022). The electrical discharge causes some of the O_2 molecules to dissociate into oxygen atoms. The oxygen atoms recombine with the non-dissociated O_2 molecules forming O_3 (Rodriguez 2016). This process also produces heat and light, requiring a cooling system to prevent overheating. The ozone concentration increases the longer the gas is exposed to the electrical charge.

While the concept of ozone generation is similar among the various types of ozonators (O_2 + energy source = O_3), non-eletrosynthesis ozone generators produce lower ozone

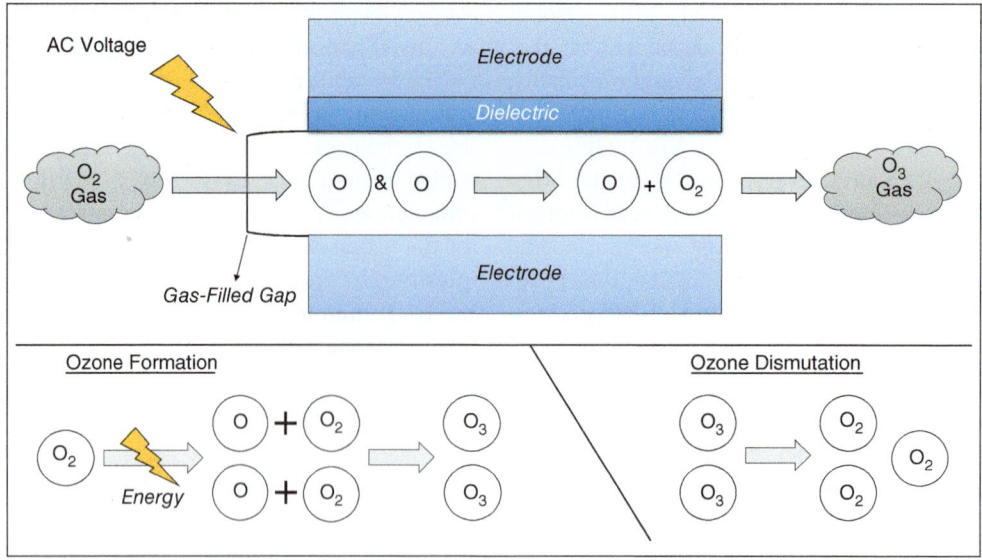

Figure 5.3 A schematic representation of a corona discharge ozone generator and the formation and dismutation of ozone. The generator contains two electrodes separated by a gas-filled gap. One of the electrodes contains an electric insulator (dielectric). As oxygen gas passes through the generation cell, an alternating current (AC) voltage is applied, and the electrical discharge causes some of the oxygen (O_2) molecules to dissociate into oxygen (O) atoms. The oxygen atoms recombine with non-dissociated oxygen molecules forming ozone (O_3). Ozone molecules are unstable and break down into more stable oxygen (O_2) molecules quickly. Source: Lisa P. McFaddin.

concentrations. UV ozone generators use UVC radiation (wavelength <240 nm) with peak effects seen at 160–185 nm (Summerfelt 2003; Claus 2021). UVC-generated ozone typically has a maximum concentration of 2%, with the wavelength and quantity of energy transmitted having the greatest effect on concentration (Summerfelt 2003).

Like corona discharge generators, plasma (aka cold plasma) ozone generators rely on electricity to create ozone. Cold plasma generators contain two neon tubes, one with a dielectric, separated by a gas-filled gap (Huang et al. 2022). Application of a low-level current between the two noble gas tubes creates an electrostatic plasma field which ionizes oxygen forming ozone. Cold plasma generators produce ozone concentrations similar to those of corona discharge generators without the production of heat (Huang et al. 2022). The tradeoff is that cold plasma generators are typically larger and more expensive than other ozone

generators. Ozone production is primarily dependent on the discharge power of the two neon tubes (Huang et al. 2022).

Electrolytic ozone generators use water as the starting substrate and lead dioxide or boron-doped diamonds as a catalyst, splitting water molecules into hydrogen (H), oxygen (O_2), and ozone (Stanley 2004). The hydrogen is then extracted leaving ozone concentrations of between 20 and 30% (Stanley 2004).

Ozonators used in veterinary medicine should be compact and, at the bare minimum, contain an oxygen input, oxygen flow meter, ozone generator cell, cooling system, high voltage transmitter, power supply, ozone destructor, ozone output, method for controlling ozone production, a method for measuring ozone production, and means to calibrate the ozone production (Rodriguez 2016). Each variable is critical for producing and delivering the correct concentration and quantity of ozone every time. An in-depth discussion of these attributes is beyond the scope of this book, but information is readily available in the References section of this chapter.

Administration Techniques

When performing VOT the practitioner must consider the following variables: the ozone concentration, formulation, volume to be administered, route of administration, and frequency of administration. All these factors are primarily dependent on the condition being treated, summarized in Figure 5.4.

Formulation

VOT can be administered as a gas (aka oxygen/ozone mixture, OOM) or percolated with saline, water, or oil. OOM is obtained directly from the ozone generator in a syringe or specialized bag. OOM can be used systemically or topically. OOM must be administered as soon as possible after it is generated. As mentioned earlier, ozone will degrade and become inactive quickly. A delay in administration reduces the efficacy of the therapy.

Ozone dissolves easily, and can be percolated into 0.9% sterile sodium chloride (NaCl) and used systemically (intravenous or subcutaneous) and topically (Shoemaker 2005; Roman 2013; Rodriguez 2016; Newkirk 2020). Ozone dissolves easily in water creating a "stable magnetic matrix" due to the dipolar (electrically neutral) nature of both water and ozone (Shallenberger 2011). When properly diffused, ozonated water can maintain efficacy for up to 10 hours at room temperature and up to 24 hours in the refrigerator (Shallenberger 2011). Ozonated water can be used systemically (through consumption) or topically (Shoemaker 2005).

Most often olive oil or sunflower oil are used for ozonated oil. The percolation process is very time-consuming, taking at least 24–36 hours of continuous ozone infusion to properly saturate the oil (Shallenberger 2011). Practitioners may elect to make their own ozonated oil or utilize pre-manufactured products. Ozonated oils can remain efficacious for up to six months when stored at either room temperatures or refrigerated (Ugazio

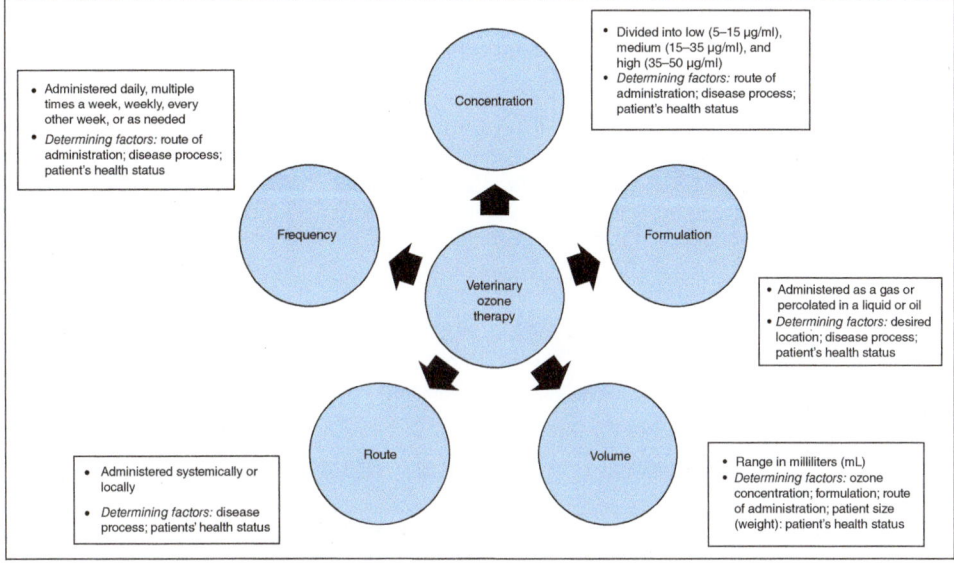

Figure 5.4 The primary variables to consider when administering veterinary ozone therapy (VOT). The key information and primary determining factors for each variable are summarized (Shoemaker 2005; Roman 2013; Rodriguez 2016; Newkirk 2020). Source: Lisa P. McFaddin.

et al. 2020). Ozonated oil has the consistency of petroleum jelly. It can be used topically (skin or gums) or systemically (inhaled) (Shoemaker 2005; Roman 2013; Rodriguez 2016; Newkirk 2020).

Route of Administration

Figures 5.5 and 5.6 summarize the most common methods of systemic and local administration. Systemic administration can be divided into injections and insufflations. A brief description of the methods of administration and most common uses for each administration type is provided below.

VOT Injection Techniques

The route of injection can be further subdivided into intravenous (MATH, MinorAH), intra-articular, intradermal, intramuscular, and subcutaneous. Intravenous injection of OOM is not recommended due to the increased risk of embolism, myocardial infarction (heart attack), or even death (Rodriguez 2016).

Intra-Articular Injection Intra-articular ozone administration is a form of prolotherapy used

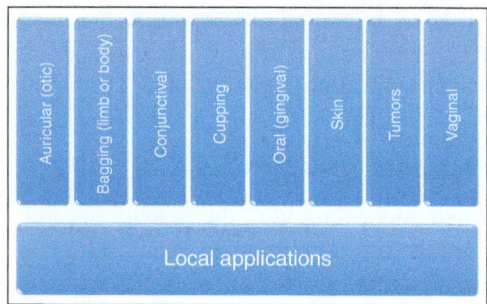

Figure 5.6 The common methods and locations for local veterinary ozone therapy (VOT) administration (Shoemaker 2005; Roman 2013; Rodriguez 2016; Newkirk 2020). Source: Lisa P. McFaddin.

to reduce the pain and inflammation associated with degenerative joint diseases and intra-articular ligament damage (Kozat and Okman 2019). Prolotherapy (aka nonsurgical ligament and tendon reconstruction and regenerative joint injection) is the injection of a small volume of a sterile irritant into a painful joint, tendon, or ligament with the goal of stimulating the body's natural healing ability, stabilizing weakened tissues, and reducing pain (Hauser et al. 2016; AOAPRM 2020). The concentration and volume of OOM injected

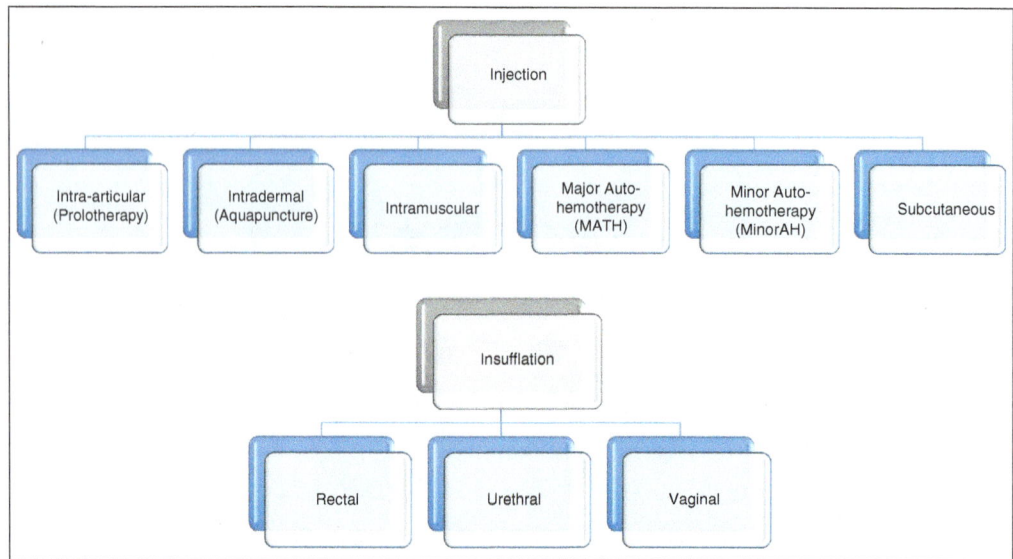

Figure 5.5 A summary of the common methods of systemic veterinary ozone therapy (VOT) administration (Shoemaker 2005; Roman 2013; Rodriguez 2016; Newkirk 2020). Source: Lisa P. McFaddin.

into and around the joint is dependent on the patient's condition and weight (Rodriguez 2016). This technique can also be used for intervertebral disk protrusions, with injection of ozone around the dorsal spinous processes and joints between the vertebrae (Shoemaker 2005).

Intramuscular Injection A small volume (1–1.5 ml) of OOM is injected directly into a specific muscle. This technique aids in the treatment of musculoskeletal disorders, such as myalgia (muscle pain) and osteoarthritis (Rodriguez 2016).

Intradermal Injection Aquapuncture, using ozone, is a form of intradermal ozone administration. Aquapuncture is the injection of a sterile liquid into specific acupuncture points. See Chapter 1 for further information.

Major Autohemotherapy (MATH) Depending on patient size, between 5 and 150 ml of blood is removed and aseptically stored in a syringe or transfusion bag with an anticoagulant, typically 0.8% sodium citrate (Shoemaker 2005; Rodriguez 2016). An equal volume of OOM is slowly added and mixed with the blood, and the mixture is re-administered intravenously to the patient (Rodriguez 2016). MATH is most used to aid in the treatment of severe infectious diseases (such as canine parvovirus, leptospirosis, canine viral hepatitis, canine distemper virus, and tick-borne diseases), circulatory disorders, and systemic immune deficiencies (Rodriguez 2016; Kozat and Okman 2019).

Minor Autohemotherapy (MinorAH) Like MATH, a small volume of blood is removed in an anticoagulant (often heparin)-coated syringe, ozonated, and re-injected intramuscularly into the patient (Rodriguez 2016). MinorAH is used to aid in the treatment of chronic dermatologic conditions (such as atopy, seasonal allergies, chronic pyoderma, flea allergy dermatitis, contact dermatitis, ringworm, and demodectic mange), general immune support, and as an adjunct for cancer therapy (Rodriguez 2016; Kozat and Okman 2019).

Subcutaneous Injection A small volume of OOM or a large volume of ozonated 0.9% NaCl can be injected into the subcutaneous tissue (Rodriguez 2016). Subcutaneous OOM is used to aid in the treatment of arthritis, severe dermatitis, and for general immune modulation (Rodriguez 2016). Subcutaneous saline can be used for any acute or chronic condition causing dehydration, especially chronic renal disease.

VOT Insufflation Techniques

Insufflation is the act of blowing a substance (gas, powder, or liquid) into a body cavity, with rectal and vaginal insufflation being the most common.

Rectal Insufflation This is one of the most common administration techniques in VOT. A specific volume of OOM, based on patient size and condition, is administered rectally using an ozone syringe and an appropriately sized red rubber catheter with generous amounts of water-soluble lubricant (Rodriguez 2016). Many practitioners recommend bubbling the OOM through water to humidify it prior to administration (Shoemaker 2005; Roman 2013).

Pressure should be applied to the external anal sphincter during insufflation to prevent leakage of the OOM. Enema retention times vary from as fast as 30 seconds up to 10 minutes. Some sources recommend tucking the tail, to aid in retention.

Rectal insufflation takes advantage of the highly vascular mucous membrane that is the rectum, allowing for fast absorption of ozone (Rodriguez 2016). Additionally, there is direct uptake into the caudal mesenteric vessels, delivering ozone promptly to the liver and pancreas (Roman 2013). Rectal insufflation can be used for a wide variety of conditions including whole body administration, chronic kidney disease, chronic liver disease, immune-mediated diseases (generalized and especially of the gastrointestinal tract), osteoarthritis, gastrointestinal tract infections, antibiotic-associated diarrhea, colitis, pancreatitis, and if there are conditions where percolated saline administration may be detrimental (low blood pressure, low body temperature, heart failure) (Roman 2013; Rodriguez 2016).

Urethral Insufflation Either OOM or ozonated saline can be placed directly into the urethra and urinary bladder using a urinary catheter. The volume and concentration are dependent on the patient's size and condition. Urethral insufflation is most used for the treatment of chronic bladder inflammation (cystitis) and infection (Shoemaker 2005; Rodriguez 2016).

Vaginal Insufflation Like rectal insufflation, a syringe with a specific volume of OOM can be insufflated into the vagina using a sterile intra-vaginal or smaller red rubber catheter and sterile lubricant (Rodriguez 2016; Kozat and Okman 2019). After administration digital pressure can be used to prevent escape of the OOM for the desired amount of time, typically 5–10 minutes (Rodriguez 2016). Alternatively, the catheter can be attached directly to the ozone generator allowing a continuous infusion of OOM for approximately five minutes (Rodriguez 2016; Kozat and Okman 2019). As with rectal insufflation, many practitioners recommend humidifying the OOM prior to administration (Shoemaker 2005; Roman 2013).

VOT Local Techniques

Local applications are primarily used to treat nonsystemic issues. Most commonly, ozonated oil or saline is used. The formulation is dependent on the area and condition being treated. OOM is applied topically using limb or body bagging (placing portions of the body in an air-tight bag attached to an ozone generator) and cupping (using glass cups attached to the ozone generator). Figure 5.6 lists the most common methods and areas local VOT is applied. Topical VOT can be used to aid in the treatment of infections, chronic

inflammation, ulcers (skin and corneal), and certain cancers (Shoemaker 2005; Roman 2013; Rodriguez 2016; Newkirk 2020).

Mechanisms of Action

Ozone does not function like a drug, but instead stimulates biological systems. Ozone (O_3) is a potent oxidizing agent (oxidant) capable of reacting with both inorganic and organic compounds. An oxidant is a substance that removes or accepts electrons from a reducing agent during a redox reaction (Wiley 2002). When exposed to tissue, ozone breaks down into an oxygen molecule (O_2) and a reactive oxygen atom (O). The single oxygen atom oxidizes organic compounds in tissues or microbial agents (viruses, bacteria, yeast, fungi, and protozoa). These chemical reactions and resultant molecules are responsible for ozone's beneficial effects (Naik et al. 2016). Ozone's effects can be divided into four broad categories: antimicrobial, immune-stimulating, anti-inflammatory and analgesic, and the stimulation of oxygen metabolism (anti-hypoxic) (Naik et al. 2016).

Antimicrobial Effects

Numerous studies have proven the antimicrobial effects of ozone, including antibacterial, antifungal, and antiviral. Many review articles mention ozone's antiprotozoal activity, but the data are limited and conflicting.

Ozone exerts its antimicrobial and antifungal effects primarily by disrupting the integrity of the cell walls and disrupting crucial intracellular functions (Elvis and Ekta 2011). *In vitro* and *in vivo* studies have shown ozone can kill and prevent the growth of multiple Gram-negative, Gram-positive, aerobic, and anaerobic bacteria, including *Escherichia coli, Salmonella* sp., *Staphylococcus aureus, Bacillus subtilis, Porphyromonas* species, and *Actinobacillus actinomycetemcomitans*, as well as disrupt and prevent the formation of biofilms (Thanomsub et al. 2002; Estrela et al. 2006; Kshitish and Laxman 2010; Suh et al. 2019; Cagini et al. 2020; Anzolin et al. 2020).

In vitro studies have shown ozone can kill, disrupt colonization, and prevent the growth of some dermatophytes (ringworm species, *Microsporum gypseum* and *Trichophyton rubrum*) and *Candida* species (Kshitish and Laxman 2010; Ouf et al. 2016; Zargaran et al. 2017; Monzillo et al. 2020).

In vitro and *in vivo* studies suggest ozone can be used to kill a variety of viral infections including adenovirus, influenza A, respiratory syncytial virus (RSV), and coronavirus (including SARS-CoV-2 or COVID-19) (Blanchard et al. 2020; Cagini et al. 2020; Cattel et al. 2021; Chirumbolo et al. 2021; Budi et al. 2022). Unfortunately, much

of the viral research centers on *in vitro* studies involving nonmedical (i.e. disinfectant) applications. There are a few promising *in vivo* studies focusing on medical ozone therapy for certain viral infections (especially COVID-19), but further research is necessary (Budi et al. 2022).

Immune Stimulation

Ozone has a positive and broad effect on the immune system, including increased sensitivity and production of immune cells and antibodies (Naik et al. 2016) (see Figure 5.7 for the complex and intermingled effects ozone has on the immune system).

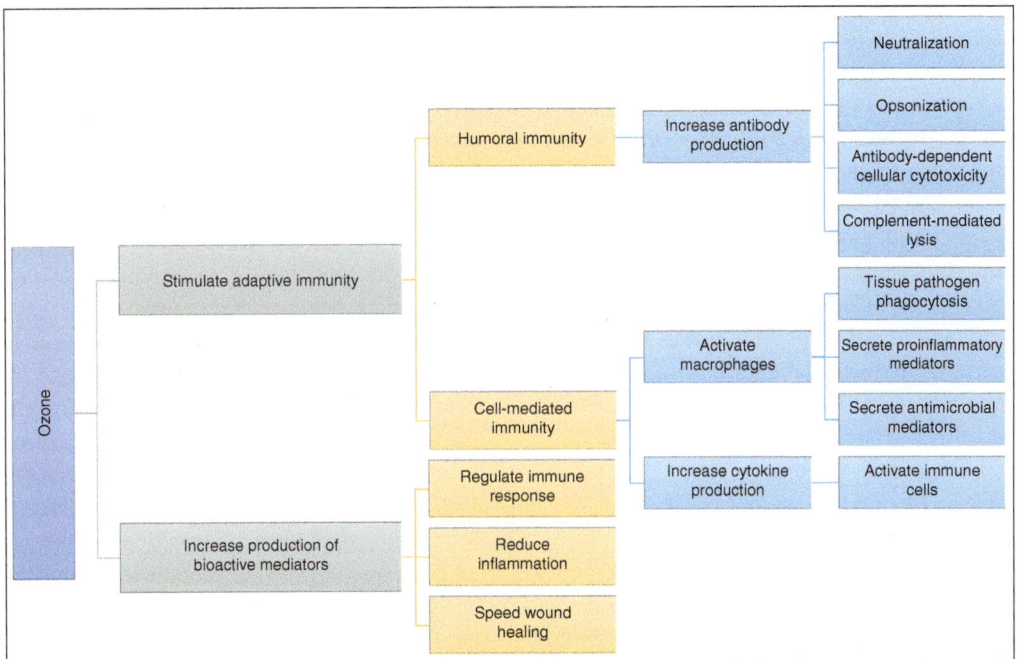

Figure 5.7 An algorithmic summary of the effects of ozone on the immune system through stimulation of the adaptive immune response and increased production of bioactive mediators. Activation of the humoral immune response occurs through increased antibody production. Antibodies serve four primary functions: neutralization (binding pathogens and preventing them from entering or damaging cells), opsonization (coating pathogens to stimulate phagocytosis by macrophages and other immune cells), antibody-dependent cellular cytotoxicity (ADCC, bridging target cells or pathogens with effector cells causing lysis or apoptosis), and complement-mediated lysis (activation of the complement cascade resulting in lysis of the organism or infected cell) (Forthal 2014). Activation of the cell-mediated immune response occurs through activation of macrophages and cytokine production. Macrophages kill pathogens through phagocytosis, as well as stimulate the secretion of proinflammatory and antimicrobial mediators (Hirayama et al. 2018). Cytokines activate B cells, macrophages, and killer T cells (Alberts et al. 2002). Ozone increases the production of bioactive mediators, including interferon, tumor necrosis factor (TNF), leukotrienes, and interleukin-2, which regulates the immune response, reduces inflammation, and speeds wound healing (Elvis and Ekta 2011; Gupta and Mansi 2012; Naik et al. 2016). Source: Lisa P. McFaddin.

Anti-Inflammatory and Analgesic

Ozone therapy has been shown to decrease the production of, and help the body regulate, chemicals causing pain and inflammation (Naik et al. 2016). The chemicals produced when ozone interacts with tissues and body fluid improve hormone production, neurotransmitter release, and overall metabolism, all of which help reduce pain and inflammation and improve blood flow (Seyam et al. 2018).

Anti-Hypoxic Effects

Tissues with low oxygen levels are considered hypoxic, especially when levels are low enough to negatively affect function. Ozone is a super-oxygenator, and has been shown to increase blood circulation and oxygen tissue delivery, and improve cellular energy production (Elvis and Ekta 2011; Naik et al. 2016). Increasing tissue oxygen levels improves overall cell and tissue health, supports the immune system, and can help reduce inflammation (and thus pain).

Oxygen utilization is typically decreased systemically in patients with cancer and cardiovascular diseases. Patients with chronic pain generally have local tissue oxygen deprivation. All of these conditions require an influx of oxygen and, almost more importantly, an improvement in oxygen utilization to heal.

Mechanisms of Action for Veterinarians

Without getting too much into the weeds, we need to briefly examine the chemistry behind therapeutic ozone, starting with ozonolysis. Ozonolysis is also known as the Criegee mechanism, named after the chemist who first described the chemical reactions. Ozone readily cleaves the double bonds found in hydrocarbons, initially generating unstable intermediate compounds called Criegee intermediates (CIs) or primary ozonides (Hassan et al. 2020). The CIs undergo additional chemical reactions creating a mixture of three possible secondary ozonides, classified as peroxides, which are more stable than the primary ozonides (OCP 2022). The secondary ozonides undergo additional reactions forming aldehydes, ketones, alcohols, or carboxylic acids (Hassan et al. 2020).

Within the body ozone rapidly reacts with fluids (plasma, lymph, urine, saliva, and water) and tissue. Many of these substances are composed of polyunsaturated fatty acids (PUFAs). Ozone plus PUFAs create hydrogen peroxide (H_2O_2) and a variety of lipid ozonation products (LOP), depending on the type of PUFA to which it is exposed (Bocci et al. 2011). The most relevant LOPs are 4-hydroxynonenal (4-HNE) and *trans*-4-hydroxyhexenal (4-HHE) (Bocci et al. 2011).

Hydrogen peroxide, the quintessential reactive oxygen species (ROS), has also been described as an ozone messenger (de Sire et al. 2021). ROS were historically considered toxic to tissues, causing critical cell damage. More studies have shown ROS can be beneficial or detrimental, function as indicators of oxidative stress, and serve as immune system mediators (Bocci et al. 2011; Shields et al. 2021; de Sire et al. 2021).

Ozonlysis of phospholipids and lipoproteins is nonspecific and nonselective, leading to the question: what is preventing ozone from killing healthy cells? Typically, the oxidative stress caused by ozone-generated ROS is neutralized by endogenous free radical scavengers, such as superoxide dismutase, glutathione peroxidase, catalase, and NADPH quinone-oxidoreductase (de Sire et al. 2021). As a result, ozone creates small and short-lived oxidative stressors which can induce the transcription of genes responsible for the production of endogenous antioxidants, improving local perfusion, enhancing tissue oxygen delivery, and supporting the immune system (Smith et al. 2017).

Antimicrobial

Bacterial cell walls are primarily composed of peptidoglycans, a mesh-like network of polysaccharide strands cross-linked with short peptide bridges and intermingled with other peptides (Dörr et al. 2019). The entire bacterial cell envelope is ripe with hydrocarbons and double bonds. Exposing bacteria to ozone causes oxidation and cleavage of these double bonds (ozonolysis), damaging the cytoplasmic membrane (Elvis and Ekta 2011). The secondary ozonides cause further intracellular damage through oxidation of organelles (Gupta and Mansi 2012). The result of these poorly functioning and perforated bacteria is cell death.

Fungal cell walls contain glucans, glycoproteins, and chitin (Kang et al. 2018). Ozonolysis of fungi causes oxidation of the phospholipids and lipoproteins, as well as inhibition of germ tube formation, disruption of existing biofilms, and direct damage to the DNA and RNA (Elvis and Ekta 2011; Zargaran et al. 2017).

Basic viral architecture includes a capsid, virus attachment protein, and its genetic material (DNA or RNA), and occasionally a viral envelope (Louten 2016). Viral envelopes, when present, are the outermost layer of the virus and comprise a lipid membrane (Louten 2016). Viral capsids are made of one or more repeating viral protein subunits surrounding a nucleic acid genome (Louten 2016). Virus attachment proteins are embedded in the outermost layer of the virus and enable the virus to attach to the plasma membrane of a host cell (Louten 2016).

Viruses exposed to ozone undergo oxidation, with the development of secondary peroxides, causing capsid damage, interference of viral replication, and prevention of viral adherence to the host cell (Elvis and Ekta 2011; Gupta and Mansi 2012). The immune-stimulating properties of ozone amplify its antiviral effects through increased clearance of viral particles by the immune system.

Immune Stimulating

Ozone has been shown to stimulate both arms of the adaptive immune response – the humoral and cell-mediated immune systems – as summarized in Figure 5.7 (Elvis and Ekta 2011). Ozone has been shown to stimulate the production of antibodies (immunoglobulins), activate macrophages, and increase the production of cytokines (further stimulating the activation of other immune cells) (Elvis and Ekta 2011; Gupta and Mansi 2012; Naik et al. 2016). Additionally, there is an increase in the production of bioactive mediators, such as interferon,

---

A Quick Review of the Adaptive Immune System

Humoral immunity, driven by B-cell lymphocytes, relies on the production of antibodies in response to the presence of antigens within the extracellular fluid (Dornell 2021). Naive B cells produce memory B cells and effector B cells in the presence of antigens. Memory B cells are long-lived and drive the secondary immune response, circulating within the body ready to quickly produce antigen-specific antibodies if the same antigen is encountered in the future (Dornell 2021). Effector B cells (aka plasma cells) are short-lived and secrete antigen-specific antibodies (Dornell 2021).

Cell-mediated immunity, primarily driven by T-cell lymphocytes, does not rely on the production of antibodies (Dornell 2021).

T-cell activation, maturation, and differentiation is dependent on the presentation of antigens bound to major histocompatibility complex (MHC) class I and II proteins on the surface of antigen-presenting cells within tissues (Wieczorek et al. 2017). Naive T cells differentiate into helper T cells and killer T cells when activated by MHC class II and I, respectively (Wieczorek et al. 2017). Helper T cells function to stimulate other immune cells (B cells, macrophages, and killer T cells) through the release of cytokines (Alberts et al. 2002). Killer or cytotoxic T cells lyse target cells eliminating the antigen-presenting pathogens (Dornell 2021).

Source: adapted from Dornell (2021).

Can the Immune System Produce Its Own Ozone?

Interestingly, there is a controversial immunologic hypothesis that natural immune cells, especially neutrophils, can generate oxidants, including ozone, from singlet oxygen and water (Babior et al. 2003; Kettle and Winterbourn 2005; Onyango 2016). It is further theorized that this "biological ozone" acts a chemical switch in the modulation of oxidative stress and inflammation, affecting both the immune and circulatory systems (Chirumbolo et al. 2021).

Source: adapted from Chirumbolo et al. (2021).

A Review of Pain Terminology

As of 2020, the International Association for the Study of Pain (IASP) defined pain as "[a]n unpleasant sensory and emotional experience associated with, or resembling that associated with, actual or potential tissue damage" (Raja et al. 2020; IASP 2021). The committee also added [s]ix key notes and etymology:

1) Pain is always a personal experience that is influenced to varying degrees by biological, psychological, and social factors.
2) Pain and nociception are different phenomena. Pain cannot be inferred solely from activity in sensory neurons.
3) Through their life experiences, individuals learn the concept of pain.
4) A person's report of an experience as pain should be respected.
5) Although pain usually serves an adaptive role, it may have adverse effects on function and social and psychological well-being. Verbal description is only one of several behaviors to express pain; inability to communicate does not negate the possibility that a human or a nonhuman animal experiences pain (Raja et al. 2020; IASP 2021).

While pain is always subjective and must involve cognitive awareness, nociception is the process through which the nervous system initially recognizes and then communicates noxious stimuli to the peripheral and central nervous system (Cramer et al. 2014; Raja et al. 2020). Historically, the mechanism of pain has been divided into four or five major processes: transduction, transmission, modulation, projection, and perception (IMCPDCIB 1987). Transduction is the process through which nociceptors area activated, typically through exposure to noxious stimuli (mechanical, chemical, or thermal). Transmission is the process by which sensory information is relayed from the peripheral nervous system to the central nervous system. Modulation occurs primarily within the spinal cord where the nociception is amplified or suppressed. Projection occurs when the signal travels from the spinal cord to the brain. Finally, perception refers to the cognitive integration of the sensory signals.

Transduction, transmission, modulation, and projection comprise nociception. Once the patient (human or animal) is consciously aware of the painful stimulus it is considered pain. This distinction allows for a better understanding of the pathophysiology of pain and the types of pain. For example, nociceptive pain is defined as "pain that arises from actual or threatened damage to non-neural tissue and is due to the activation of nociceptors" (IASP 2021). Nociceptive pain, also known as physiologic pain, is well localized, transient, and crucial for the protective physiologic reflex of avoidance. Nociceptive pain is what prevents us from continually touching the hot stove.

In contrast, neuropathic pain is defined as "pain caused by a lesion or disease of the somatosensory nervous system...Neuropathic pain is a clinical description (and not a diagnosis) which requires a demonstrable lesion or a disease that satisfies established neurological diagnostic criteria" (IASP 2021). Neuropathic pain is always considered pathologic. Neuropathic pain can lead to neuroplasticity (potentiation), making the connections and responses of nociceptive fibers stronger and more able to withstand change, leading to hyperalgesia (abnormally heightened sensitivity to pain) and allodynia (central pain sensitization in which nonpainful stimuli elicit pain).

tumor necrosis factor (TNF), leukotrienes, and interleukin-2, which helps regulate the immune response, reduce inflammation, and speed wound healing (Elvis and Ekta 2011; Gupta and Mansi 2012; Naik et al. 2016).

Anti-Inflammatory and Analgesic

Ozone exerts its anti-inflammatory effects primarily through the production of free radical scavengers and the suppression and regulation of inflammatory mediators. The oxidative stress caused by ozone increases activation of the transcriptional factor mediating nuclear factor-erythroid 2-related factor 2 (Nrf2) (Smith et al. 2017). Nrf2 is responsible for activating the transcription of antioxidant response elements (AREs). AREs increase the production of a number of antioxidant enzymes that function as free radical scavengers, including superoxide dismutase, glutathione peroxidase, glutathione S-transferase, catalase, heme oxygenase-1, NADPH-quinone-oxidoreductase, and heat shock proteins (Inal et al. 2011; Smith et al. 2017; Seyam et al. 2018). Ozone has been shown to decrease the production and regulate the function of inflammatory mediators such as interleukin (IL)-6, IL-8, TNF-α, prostaglandins, and bradykinin (de Sire et al. 2021). Ozone therapy also protects against mitochondria die-off due to excessive exposure to free radicals (Shallenberger 2011). Mitochondrial dysfunction has been linked to sensory processing and chronic pain (Flatters 2015).

The anti-inflammatory effects contribute to ozone's analgesic properties. Several studies have also shown ozone directly affects the modulation and perception of pain, at least in part by increasing the levels of circulating serotonin and endogenous opioids (Paoloni et al. 2009; Raeissadat et al. 2018; Ulusoy et al. 2019). This means ozone therapy has been shown to inhibit both nociception (sensory signals alerting the nervous system of exposure to a noxious stimulus) and pain (conscious awareness and interpretation of a noxious stimulus).

Anti-Hypoxic Effects

Ozone directly affects tissue perfusion through changes in the rheologic properties of erythrocytes, vasodilation, erythrocyte glycolysis, and increasing cell energy production (Clavo et al. 2004; Shallenberger 2011; Naik et al. 2016; de Sire et al. 2021). This leads to increased tissue oxygen saturation (PO_2), improved blood oxygen transportation, and improved aerobic cellular metabolism (Naik et al. 2016).

Rheologic Properties Whole blood is a non-Newtonian, two-phase liquid composed of cells and cellular components (erythrocytes, leukocytes, and platelets) suspended in plasma (Nader et al. 2019). The ability of whole blood's viscoelastic properties to change under shearing conditions is primarily dependent on the ability of erythrocytes to change shape and distort (rheologic properties) (Nader et al. 2019).

The effect of ozone on erythrocyte rheologic properties appears to be dose-dependent, with lower concentrations causing rigidization and higher concentrations improving membrane fluidity (Górnicki and Gutsze 2000). Improved erythrocyte elasticity eases blood flow in capillary vessels, increasing oxygen delivery to inflamed or damaged tissues (Gupta and Mansi 2012).

Interestingly, a recent *in vitro* study evaluating the effects of ozonation on hypoxia, hemolysis, and red blood cell morphology in patients with aortic dissection demonstrated therapeutic levels of ozone improved the oxygen content of erythrocytes but did not change their morphology (Deng et al. 2018). Further research is necessary to determine if ozone administered at therapeutic levels does affect erythrocyte rheology.

Vasodilation Ozone causes vasodilation through the increased production of nitric oxide, adenosine, and prostacyclin (de Sire et al. 2021). Ozone has also been shown to activate angiogenesis, further improving blood flow to tissues (Gupta and Mansi 2012).

Glycolysis Ozone can increase the speed of erythrocyte glycolysis, increasing cellular metabolism and energy production as well as increasing the levels of 2,3-diphosphoglycerate (Bocci 2004). 2,3-Diphosphoglycerate shifts the oxyhemoglobin dissociation curve to the right, positively affecting tissue PO_2 levels (Bocci 2004).

Cellular Metabolism Ozone therapy can increase adenosine triphosphate (ATP) production by 40% and increases the ratio of nicotinamide adenine dinucleotide (NAD) to NADH (Shallenberger 2011). Additionally, ozone therapy has a mitochondrial protective effect, reducing die-off through exposure to excessive free radicals (Shallenberger 2011).

Safety

When used correctly, ozone therapy is safe and effective. Like all therapeutic modalities, there are several precautions to consider concerning operator safety, equipment safety, administration safety, adverse effects, specific diseases, and certain medications and nutraceuticals. These precautions are summarized in Figure 5.8.

Operator Safety
Ozone should not be inhaled or breathed directly, as this can cause lung damage. Ozone should be administered in a well-ventilated area, especially if a bagging technique is used. Individuals may have increased sensitivity to ozone causing breathing issues or headaches (FDA 2022). The practice manager and veterinarian should be aware of potential employee and client hypersensitivities. Do not use open flames around oxygen or ozone generators (PubChem 2022a,b). Oxygen, while not flammable, can cause materials to ignite more easily and burn more rapidly (PubChem 2022a).

As mentioned earlier, the FDA does not support the use of medical ozone considering it a "toxic gas with no known useful medical application[s]" (FDA 2022). Inhalation of ozone can be very toxic to the lungs and extrapulmonary organs (Sagai and Bocci 2011). Depending on the dose and route of administration, known side effects include excessive tearing (epiphora), upper airway irritation, nasal irritation and inflammation (rhinitis), cough, headache, nausea, vomiting, shortness of breath, blood vessel swelling, poor circulation, various heart problems, and stroke (Elvis and Ekta 2011; Gupta and Mansi 2012; Naik et al. 2016; Rodriguez 2016). Complications associated with ozone therapy in people are uncommon when administered at 0.0007% (7 ppm or 7 µg/ml) per application (Sagai and Bocci 2011; Naik et al. 2016). When VOT is administered at the correct dosage and route it is considered safe, with very few side effects, and effective (Rodriguez 2016).

Pulmonary Ozone Toxicology for Veterinarians
Airway hypersensitivity and reactivity is one of the first signs noted following ozone inhalation (Sagai and Bocci 2011). Airway inflammation and even cell death can occur depending on the dosage and length of exposure (Sagai and Bocci 2011).

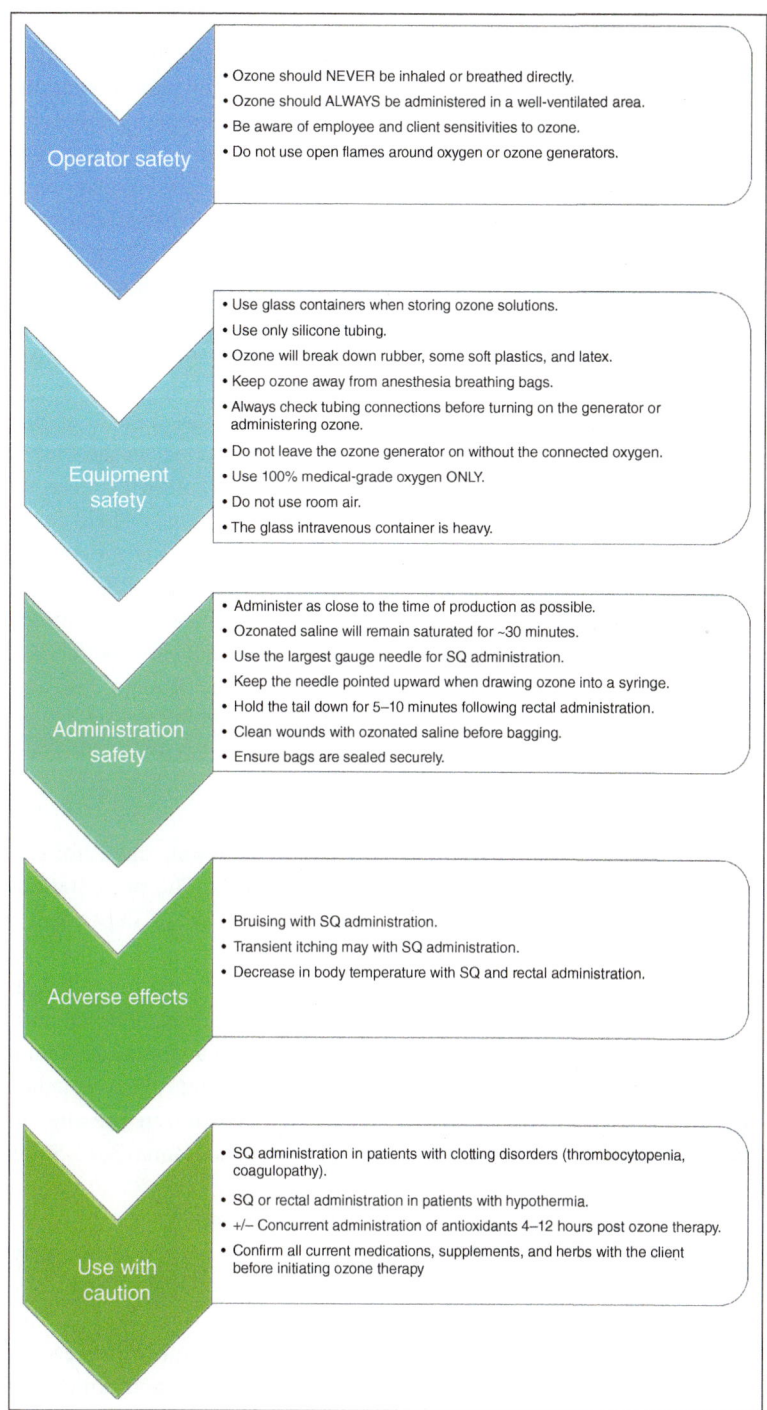

Operator safety

- Ozone should NEVER be inhaled or breathed directly.
- Ozone should ALWAYS be administered in a well-ventilated area.
- Be aware of employee and client sensitivities to ozone.
- Do not use open flames around oxygen or ozone generators.

Equipment safety

- Use glass containers when storing ozone solutions.
- Use only silicone tubing.
- Ozone will break down rubber, some soft plastics, and latex.
- Keep ozone away from anesthesia breathing bags.
- Always check tubing connections before turning on the generator or administering ozone.
- Do not leave the ozone generator on without the connected oxygen.
- Use 100% medical-grade oxygen ONLY.
- Do not use room air.
- The glass intravenous container is heavy.

Administration safety

- Administer as close to the time of production as possible.
- Ozonated saline will remain saturated for ~30 minutes.
- Use the largest gauge needle for SQ administration.
- Keep the needle pointed upward when drawing ozone into a syringe.
- Hold the tail down for 5–10 minutes following rectal administration.
- Clean wounds with ozonated saline before bagging.
- Ensure bags are sealed securely.

Adverse effects

- Bruising with SQ administration.
- Transient itching may with SQ administration.
- Decrease in body temperature with SQ and rectal administration.

Use with caution

- SQ administration in patients with clotting disorders (thrombocytopenia, coagulopathy).
- SQ or rectal administration in patients with hypothermia.
- +/− Concurrent administration of antioxidants 4–12 hours post ozone therapy.
- Confirm all current medications, supplements, and herbs with the client before initiating ozone therapy

Figure 5.8 An overview of the precautions necessary to ensure veterinary ozone therapy is performed safely and effectively. SQ, subcutaneous. Source: Lisa P. McFaddin.

Unlike other inhaled gases, ozone does not rely on a pressure gradient or diffusion to transport past the biofilm covering the alveoli (aka the alveolar lining layer or ALL) (Pryor et al. 1995). Instead, ozone instantaneously oxidizes the biomolecules present in the ALL, especially the PUFAs found in lung surfactants, creating ROS, predominantly peroxides and heterogenous LOPs (Pryor et al. 1995). As the antioxidant capability of the ALL is limited, mild to marked inflammation (dose and length of exposure dependent) occurs secondary to ozone inhalation (Sagai and Bocci 2011). Unfortunately, the body's response to inflammation within the airway perpetuates this inflammation by bringing more inflammatory mediators to the initial site of injury. Hypersensitivity reactions in human and animal models suggest an even stronger inflammatory response is seen in patients with known pulmonary conditions such as asthma, bronchitis, and chronic obstructive pulmonary disease (Sagai and Bocci 2011).

Equipment Safety

There are multiple factors to consider regarding the materials used when generating and administering ozone. Glass containers should be used to store ozone mixed with sterile solutions (i.e. saline) (Shallenberger 2011). Only silicon tubing should be used, as ozone will break down rubber, some soft plastics (e.g. thermoplastic elastomers, nitrile, and nylon), and latex (McFaddin III 2022). Ozone equipment should be kept away from anesthesia breathing bags (composed of black rubber). The silicone tubing connections should be checked before turning on the generator or administering ozone to prevent leakage (Shallenberger 2011). Ozone generators should never be left on when not connected to an oxygen supply. Only 100% medical-grade oxygen, never room air, should be used. Finally, the glass intravenous container used for ozonated saline is heavy. Ensure the stand is appropriately balanced to limit the risk of tipping over.

Administration Safety

As with the operator and equipment safety, there are several administration protocols to considers. Ozone should be administered as close to the time of production as possible (Shallenberger 2011). Ozonated saline will remain saturated for approximately 30 minutes (Shallenberger 2011). The largest gauge needle should be used for subcutaneous administration to limit the time ozonated saline remains in contact with the plastic intravenous line tubing (Roman 2013). When ozone gas is drawn into a syringe the needle should be pointed upward, as ozone is heavier than oxygen (Roman 2013). Following rectal ozone administration, the tail must be held down between the pelvic limbs (covering the anus) for 5–10 minutes to prevent rectal leakage of the ozone (Roman 2013). Consider cleaning wounds with ozonated saline before performing ozone bagging techniques (Roman 2013). Finally, ensure the bag is sealed securely to prevent ozone leakage (Roman 2013).

Adverse Effects

While uncommon, there are several possible adverse effects. The presentation and severity of the side effect is dependent on the route of administration, dose, and patient condition. Bruising or itching following subcutaneous administration, itching or inflammation following topical application, and reduction in body temperature following subcutaneous and rectal administration are the most common adverse effects (Roman 2013; Shoemaker 2005).

Use with Caution

Subcutaneous administration may cause bleeding in patients with clotting disorders (thrombocytopenia, coagulopathy). Care should be taken when administering rectal or subcutaneous ozone to hypothermic (cold) patients (Roman 2013).

Practitioners may recommend the concurrent administration of vitamin C or other antioxidants to reduce the risk of systemic free radical damage (Shoemaker 2005; Roman 2013). Antioxidants should not be administered within 4–12 hours of ozone therapy (Shoemaker 2005). Practitioners should also confirm all current medications, supplements, and herbs with the client before initiating ozone therapy.

The Why

Applications in Human Medicine

Despite the FDA's stance on ozone therapy, many human practitioners tout the safety and efficacy of this modality in the treatment of numerous conditions. Ozone therapy is primarily used to eliminate pathogens, restore oxygen metabolism, improve circulation, support the immune system, and stimulate an antioxidant response (Gupta and Mansi 2012). Much of the historical support for ozone therapy is based on *in vitro* testing, but more recently clinical trials have supported the efficacy and safety of ozone therapy for the treatment of specific disease processes. Table 5.1 summarizes the most common conditions for which ozone therapy is used in human medicine.

Applications in Veterinary Medicine

Ozone therapy is most used in veterinary medicine to aid in the treatment of chronic inflammatory and infectious conditions (Shoemaker 2005). The condition being treated determines the dose, route of application, and frequency of administration.

Veterinary Research

As a relatively new therapeutic modality, there is limited VOT research. As of November 2022, a quick search on PubMed yielded 352 articles for "veterinary ozone," 193 articles for "ozone canine," and 39 for "ozone feline." Unfortunately, many of these articles are published in countries with limited international exposure, not translated into English, or are poorly presented case studies (Orlandin et al. 2021).

Ozonated oil has been shown to be effective in the treatment of dermatomycosis in rabbits and plaque prevention in canines (Madan et al. 2010; Abreu-Villela et al. 2021). There are several studies which did not demonstrate a statistically significant antimicrobial

Table 5.1 Summary of the most common applications of medical ozone therapy in human medicine with the supporting research as of January 2023.

Body system	Specific disease processes	Supporting research
Dermal	Chronic wound healing	Fitzpatrick et al. (2018), Anzolin et al. (2020)
Musculoskeletal	Osteoarthritis; tendinopathies; myalgia; fibromyalgia	Raeissadat et al. (2018), Ulusoy et al. (2019), de Sire et al. (2021)
Neurologic	Intervertebral disk disease; lower back pain; cervical pain	Paoloni et al. (2009), de Sire et al. (2021)
Oral (dentistry)	Periodontal disease; infections; surgical healing; prosthodontics; restorative dentistry; orthodontics; orthopedics	Elvis and Ekta (2011), Gupta and Mansi (2012), Naik et al. (2016), Suh et al. (2019)
Infectious diseases	COVID-19	Cattel et al. (2021), Chirumbolo et al. (2021), Budi et al. (2022)
Wound healing	Chronic	Fitzpatrick et al. (2018), Anzolin et al. (2020)

Source: Lisa P. McFaddin.

improvement following ozone administration (Daud et al. 2011; Orlandin et al. 2021). Case studies have demonstrated the effective use of VOT in the treatment of chronic wounds in canine and feline patients, but clinical trials are necessary to confirm efficacy and safety (Kosachenco et al. 2018; Repciuc et al. 2020).

VOT, in the form of subcutaneous ozone and ozone retention enemas, may be recommended before fecal transplantation (microbiome restorative therapy) to remove existing colonic bacteria, disrupt the biofilm created by pathogenic bacteria, and increase colonic oxygen levels (Roman 2015). These recommendations are primarily based on clinical experience and case studies, requiring clinical trials to definitively support the effectiveness of this protocol.

Over the last 10 years, studies investigating ozone's role in food animal (bovine, caprine, and ovine) reproductive medicine has gained interest and shown promising results (Orlandin et al. 2021). As the focus of this book is on companion animal medicine, specific studies are not referenced in this chapter.

While there are various case reports in companion animals, the availability of randomized clinical trials, retrospective studies, or even case series is severely lacking (Shimizu et al. 2013; Kozat and Okman 2019; Orlandin et al. 2021). Most applications of VOT are based on data extrapolated from *in vitro*, laboratory animal, or human studies. Figure 5.9 summarizes the most common applications of VOT classified by the administration method.

As summarized by Orlandin et al. (2021), multiple factors can impact the clinical outcome of ozone therapy, including signalment (age, species, sex), species anatomic differences, blood composition, fecal pH and composition, intestinal microbiota, method of ozone preparation, method of ozone administration, and markers of oxidative stress. This underscores the importance (and necessity) of careful study design. Give the public's general interest in "natural" medicine, we will likely see a rise in veterinary ozone research in the near future.

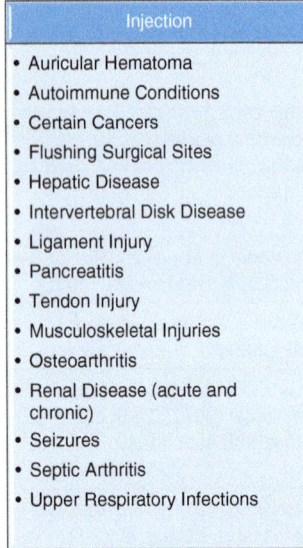
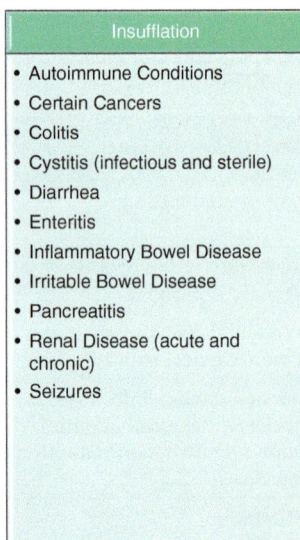
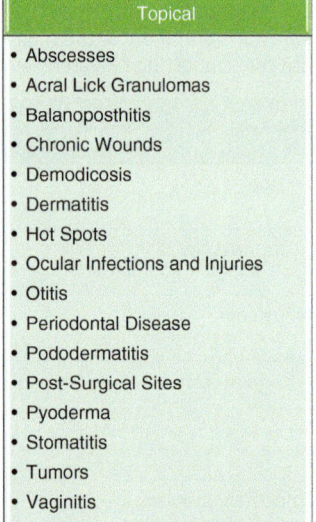

Injection	Insufflation	Topical
• Auricular Hematoma	• Autoimmune Conditions	• Abscesses
• Autoimmune Conditions	• Certain Cancers	• Acral Lick Granulomas
• Certain Cancers	• Colitis	• Balanoposthitis
• Flushing Surgical Sites	• Cystitis (infectious and sterile)	• Chronic Wounds
• Hepatic Disease	• Diarrhea	• Demodicosis
• Intervertebral Disk Disease	• Enteritis	• Dermatitis
• Ligament Injury	• Inflammatory Bowel Disease	• Hot Spots
• Pancreatitis	• Irritable Bowel Disease	• Ocular Infections and Injuries
• Tendon Injury	• Pancreatitis	• Otitis
• Musculoskeletal Injuries	• Renal Disease (acute and chronic)	• Periodontal Disease
• Osteoarthritis	• Seizures	• Pododermatitis
• Renal Disease (acute and chronic)		• Post-Surgical Sites
• Seizures		• Pyoderma
• Septic Arthritis		• Stomatitis
• Upper Respiratory Infections		• Tumors
		• Vaginitis

Figure 5.9 The most common conditions for which ozone therapy is used in veterinary medicine grouped by the route of administration (Shoemaker 2005; Roman 2013; Rodriguez 2016). Source: Lisa P. McFaddin.

The How

Team Members

This section reviews the potential return on investment (ROI), how to effectively train the entire team, how to promote, and how to integrate the integrative therapy.

Return on Investment

ROI can be determined by evaluating client interest, veterinarian demand, hospital costs, applicability of the service, appointment scheduling, and pricing.

Client Interest

Currently there are no studies documenting client interest or the popularity of VOT. By evaluating trends in client opinion and pet health insurance, interest in VOT can be inferred.

Client Opinion

Table 5.2 summarizes the pet owner demographics and statistics mentioned in the My Lessons section of the Introduction. Even if half of those owners are open to VOT, that is still 53.1 million potential patients.

Table 5.2 Summary of the 2022 pet ownership and pet health insurance demographics in the United States discussed in the Introduction of the book (Burns 2018, 2022; MFAF 2018; APPA 2022; Nolen 2022; NAPHIA 2023).

- 83% of pets are owned by millennials (32%), generation X (24%), and baby boomers (27%)
- 69 million households owned dogs
- 45.3 million households owned cats
- Estimated over 81.1 million owned dogs
- Estimated over 60.7 million owned cats
- 68% of owners are interested in alternative treatment modalities for their pets
- 4.41 million pets have pet health insurance
- 82% of insurance pets are dogs

Source: Lisa P. McFaddin.

Pet Health Insurance

Many pet insurance plans include coverage for integrative therapies, especially acupuncture (Woodley 2018). The presence of this type of coverage re-emphasizes the mainstream incorporation of these treatment modalities, as well as reflecting client demand.

Veterinarian Demand

A census of the number of veterinary hospitals offering VOT has not been performed but is expected to be low. A rough estimate, based on a brief internet search of hospitals advertising VOT in major cities throughout the continental United States, would be one to two clinics for each major city and surrounding suburbs. This suggests there is ample opportunity to introduce VOT into a practice without fear of an already saturated market. Another way to examine the need in your area is to compare the number of general practitioners within a 5-, 10-, or 20-mile radius to the number of clinics offering VOT. The search radius is dependent on your hospital's demographics.

Hospital Costs

Let us start by reviewing the potential costs associated with introducing and offering VOT: veterinarian training, staff training, supplies and equipment, staffing, facilities, and advertising. Table 5.4 demonstrates varying start-up costs, depending on the hospital's contribution toward the veterinarian's training and prior utilization of regular all-staff meetings. For more information on potential hospital costs, refer to the Introduction at the beginning of this book.

Veterinarian Training

Course Costs There are three main training programs in the United States. Two of the three offer online training options. Typical completion time is less than one month for online courses and two to four days for on-site sessions. Additional information can be found in the Veterinarians section of this chapter (cost range, $199–1300).

Textbooks Textbooks may not be required for the courses but are often recommended. The price range for one to two books is $50–250 (average cost, $192).

Travel Expenses Travel costs include airfare, lodging, car rental, and meals. The estimated pricing is based on one on-site sessions with two full days of training.

- *Airfare*: As of February 2023, the average round-trip domestic flight within the United States was $412 (BLS 2023; Trcek 2023). The $412 value was used when calculating the cost of airfare for three round-trip flights (total cost, $412).
- *Lodging*: As of February 2023 the federal per diem rate for lodging on business trips is $98 per night (FederalPay.org 2023). The federal per diem rate was used for calculations, with three nights of lodging for one session (total cost, $294).
- *Car rental*: As of January 2023, the average weekly car rental price is $551 (French and Kemmis 2023). Rideshare and cabbing are extremely popular, but the variability in travel distances makes calculating an average cost impractical. It is suspected this cost would be comparable, if not lower, than that of a rental car. The total was calculated using five-day car rentals for one session (total cost, $551).
- *Meals*: The federal per diem rate for business trip meals from October 2022 through September 2023 is $59 a day (FederalPay. org 2023). Meal expenditure was calculated for 2.5 days (total cost, $148).
- *Time Off*: Veterinarian paid time-off (PTO) for on-site courses only factors in as an added expense if additional PTO is provided outside of the veterinarian's contractual annual PTO. Clinics offer an average of 4.1 paid continuing education (CE) days per year (AAHA 2019). All the available ozone CE would fall within the average paid CE days and would not cost the clinic or veterinarian anything additional (total cost, $0).

Staff Training Team training expenses are highly variable and dependent on the preexistence of staff meetings and use of a staff meeting for training (compared to self-study). Refer to the Introduction at the beginning of the book for a breakdown of these variables (cost range, $230–1295).

Supplies Initial supplies for VOT include an ozone generator, oxygen source, oxygen regulator, and accessories (Shallenberger 2011). The approximate costs for each are provided below. Figures 5.10 and 5.11 depict some of the supplies commonly utilized when performing VOT.

Ozone Generator The price range for ozone generators is broad and dependent on the output capacity, anticipated concentration of ozone, presence of a built-in regulator, presence of a built-in ozone destruct, and the type of displace (cost range as of February 2023, $1000–10000).

Oxygen Source Having a small portable oxygen tank (with regulator, tubing, and valves) dedicated for ozone therapy is advisable (cost range as of February 2023, $300–600, does not include cost of refilling the oxygen within the tank).

Ozone Accessories Required accessories are determined by the practitioner goals and desired application methods but typically include fluid bubbler and mounting kit with stand (for ozonated saline), ear insufflator, cups (for dermal application), oil bubbler (for creating ozonated oils), limb bagging supplies, rectal catheters, ozone insufflation bags, ozone syringes, ozone fluid jars, luer locks, silicone tubing (size dependent on use), needles, syringes, and an ozone destruct (cost range as of February 2023, $300–1500).

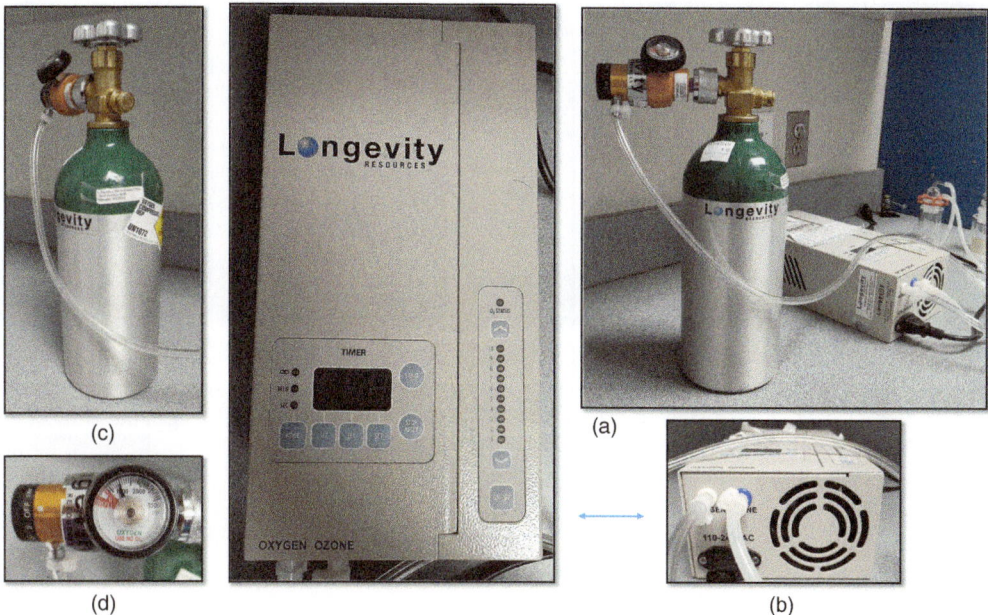

Figure 5.10   Images of basic essential ozone equipment. (a) An ozone generator connected to an oxygen source. (b) An ozone generator imaged from the top with control panel and from the side with the connections for the power supply, oxygen in, and ozone out. (c) Small oxygen tank serving as the oxygen source. (d) Oxygen regulator attached to the oxygen source. Source: Lisa P. McFaddin.

Staffing   VOT appointments range from 30 to 60 minutes depending on the condition(s) being treated. Following the American Animal Hospital Association (AAHA) recommendations a veterinary assistant or licensed technician (VA/LT) should restrain patients for physical examinations and procedures. On average a VA/LT is used in the exam room for approximately half of the appointment time. For VOT the VA/LT will likely be utilized for the length of the entire appointment, and the cost should be considered. The expenses presented in Tables 5.5–5.7 are based on needing a VA/LT to assist the doctor for an additional 15–45 minutes ($4.43–13.29 per patient). The provided expenses are based on a national average wage of $17.72 per hour for veterinary technologists and technicians as of September 2022 (BLS 2022).

Facilities   Facility expenses represent the costs needed to keep the doors open (aka

overhead). Overhead includes rent or mortgage, utilities, administrative costs, and often employee costs divided by the minutes the practice is open (Stevenson 2016). The price per minute equals the amount of revenue needed just to break even. Overhead is extremely hospital specific, but the range tends to be $2–5/minutes.

VOT should be performed in a room with good ventilation to prevent pulmonary (and non-pulmonary organ) irritation. There are pros and cons to having the owner present during VOT. The pros include owner education and awareness of the procedure and increased patient relaxation, while the cons include increased risk of client exposure to ozone gas and potentially heightened patient anxiety. Ultimately the decision to perform VOT with the client present is based on practitioner preference.

Designating a specific room for ozone also minimizes the chances other associates

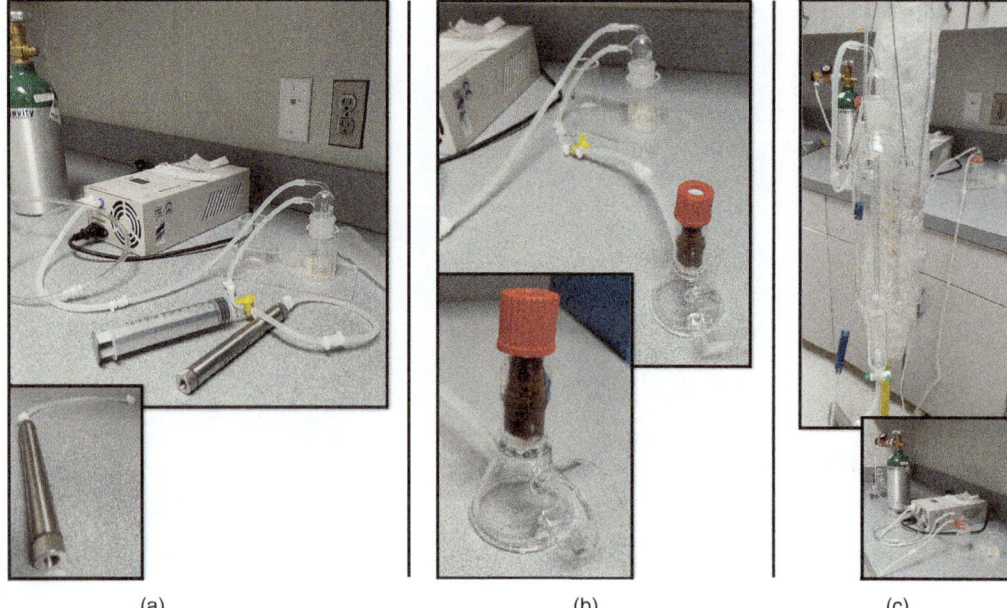

| (a) | (b) | (c) |

Figure 5.11 Images of common accessories utilized when performing veterinary ozone therapy. (a) Setup used for rectal ozone administration. Ozone is humidified using distilled water in a glass bubbler before filling the syringe. A three-way stopcock is used to direct the ozone to stay in the water chamber and tubing, fill the syringe, or flow through the destruct. The destruct (silver rod) is used to convert excess ozone back to oxygen preventing operator inhalation of ozone. (b) Setup used for ozone cupping. As with rectal ozone the gas is humidified prior to administration. A three-way stopcock is again used to direct the flow of the ozone. (c) Setup used for ozonated saline. Sterile saline is placed in the glass container (1000 ml glass super column). Tubing directs ozone from the generator to the super column (a glass trap is used to prevent backflow of ozone). Sterile intravenous fluid tubing is attached to the super column allowing administration of the ozonated saline to the patient. Source: Lisa P. McFaddin.

will need the room for their appointments. However, there is then an added expense for designing the room and potential lost revenue if the room is not used regularly. The absence of a designated room theoretically reduces redecoration costs, but this can be disruptive for appointment flow if the treatment takes longer than the allotted time.

Advertising There are numerous ways to advertise a new service. On average veterinary hospitals spend 0.7% of revenue on promotion and advertisement (AVMA 2019). Most of the advertisement can be done with little to no additional expenditure. The national median gross revenue for companion animal practices was $1.2 million in 2022 (AVMA 2023).

Advertising costs are calculated assuming no more than 5% of the current advertising budget would be used for promotion of the new service (estimated maximal cost, $420).

Start-Up Costs Table 5.3 summarizes projected start-up costs for VOT. Table 5.4 calculates potential start-up costs based on the degree of hospital contribution toward veterinarian and staff training. Different scenarios are presented in which the hospital covers all, some, or none of the expenses.

Applicability

As stated earlier, VOT is a versatile and beneficial modality with general applicability to chronic inflammatory and infectious conditions.

Table 5.3 Total potential hospital start-up costs and per patient expenses for veterinary ozone therapy (VOT) as of February 2023.

Category	Subcategories	Projected cost	
Veterinarian training	Course costs	$199–1300	Average $712
	Textbooks	$75–250	Average $192
	Travel expenses	$1405	
	Time-off	$0	
Staff training	Variable	$230–1396	
Supplies	Ozone generator	$1000–10 000	Average $3000
	Oxygen source	$300–600	Average $450
	Ozone accessories	$300–1500	Average $750
Staffing	Variable	$4.43–13.29	Average $8.86
Facilities	Overhead	$2–5 per minute for a 30–60-minute appointment	$60–300 per patient
Advertising	Variable	≤$420	

Source: Lisa P. McFaddin.

Appointment Scheduling

There are four main factors to consider when planning VOT appointment protocols: appointment length, support staff availability, exam room availability, and follow-up appointment scheduling.

There are other issues to consider when scheduling VOT appointments. For example, will VOT appointments be scheduled separately from traditional Western appointments, or will the appointment length need to be increased? Will vaccinations be given during the VOT appointment? Some practitioners prefer to separate vaccine administration from VOT sessions.

The initial and follow-up appointments range from 30 to 60 minutes. Appointment length is dependent on the patient, their condition, and route of administration. Appointment length may be shorter than 30 minutes if the follow-up appointment consists of treatment only, without an examination.

Keep the appointment positive. You want the pet to enjoy the experience. A relaxed pet is more easily treated. Avoid ancillary procedures which may cause stress: nail trims, anal gland expression, sanitary trims, anything with the ears, etc. Additional information on appointment scheduling can be found in the Introduction at hte beginning of this book.

Pricing

An in-depth look into appointment pricing can be found in the Introduction. Typically, we consider pricing using two methods: current market fees and hospital cost-based pricing. Currently there are no studies examining the current market fees for VOT.

Hospital Cost-Based Pricing Table 5.5 outlines the hospital cost per patient for 15-, 30-, and 60-minute VOT appointments, respectively. The veterinarian training amortization per patient was calculated using the assumptions listed in Chapter 1. Supply assumptions were based on the costs provided in Table 5.3 using the same guidelines for amortization applied to the training.

Now that we have the hospital costs, we can move toward determining the appropriate

Table 5.4 Projected veterinary ozone therapy (VOT) start-up costs for eight hospital scenarios, with varying hospital contributions toward veterinary certification and staff training as February 2023. The cost of veterinarian training is based on the averages presented Table 5.3. Staff training costs assume a 1.5-hour-long all-staff meeting, using national averages for employee numbers: eight non-DVMs and two DVMs (AVMA 2019, 2023). The cost of office supplies and lunch as estimated based on 10 employees attending the meeting. The overhead is based on an average of $3.5/minute. Missed revenue is calculated using the 2022 national mean revenue per hour for companion animal practices ($567/hour) (AVMA 2023). Advertising includes printed materials, digital advertisement, and community engaged.

Category	Projected expenses	Ex. 1	Ex. 2	Ex. 3	Ex. 4	Ex. 5	Ex. 6	Ex. 7	Ex. 8
Veterinarian training	Average course cost	$712	$712	$712	n/a	$712	$712	$712	n/a
	Average textbooks	$192	n/a	n/a	n/a	$192	n/a	n/a	n/a
	Travel expenses	$1405	$1405	n/a	n/a	$1405	$1405	n/a	n/a
	Average time-off	$0	$0	$0	$0	$0	$0	$0	$0
Staff training	Office supplies	$30	$30	$30	$30	$30	$30	$30	$30
	Lunch	$200	$200	$200	$200	$200	$200	$200	$200
	Overhead	$315	$315	$315	$315	n/a	n/a	n/a	n/a
	Missed revenue	$851	$851	$851	$851	n/a	n/a	n/a	n/a
Supplies	Ozone generator	$3000	$3000	$3000	$3000	$3000	$3000	$3000	$3000
	Oxygen source	$450	$450	$450	$450	$450	$450	$450	$450
	Ozone accessories	$750	$750	$750	$750	$750	$750	$750	$750
Advertising		$538	$538	$538	$538	$538	$538	$538	$538
Total		**$8880**	**$8789**	**$7384**	**$6672**	**$7277**	**$7085**	**$5680**	**$4968**

Source: Lisa P. McFaddin.

Table 5.5 Estimated hospital costs per patient for 15-, 30-, and 60-minute veterinary ozone therapy (VOT) appointments as of February 2023. Start-up costs are taken from the totals in Table 5.4. Amortization is per patient and is based on the veterinarian seeing 952 integrative patients in two years. Overhead is calculated using $3.5/minute in a practice with two veterinarians. Multiple examples are provided with the variance determined by the total cost within each category. The total is rounded to the nearest whole number.

	Ex. 1	Ex. 2	Ex. 3	Ex. 4	Ex. 5	Ex. 6	Ex. 7	Ex. 8
15-minute appointments								
Table 5.4 totals	$8880	$8789	$7384	$6672	$7277	$7085	$5680	$4968
Amortization	$9.33	$9.23	$7.76	$7.01	$7.64	$7.44	$5.97	$5.22
Overhead	$26	$26	$26	$26	$26	$26	$26	$26
Total	**$35**	**$35**	**$34**	**$33**	**$34**	**$33**	**$32**	**$31**
30-minute appointments								
Table 5.4 totals	$8880	$8789	$7384	$6672	$7277	$7085	$5680	$4968
Amortization	$9.33	$9.23	$7.76	$7.01	$9.10	$8.90	$7.43	$6.68
Overhead	$52.50	$52.50	$52.50	$52.50	$52.50	$52.50	$52.50	$52.50
Total	**$62**	**$62**	**$60**	**$60**	**$60**	**$60**	**$58**	**$58**
60-minute appointments								
Table 5.4 totals	$8880	$8789	$7384	$6672	$7277	$7085	$5680	$4968
Amortization	$9.33	$9.23	$7.76	$7.01	$9.10	$8.90	$7.43	$6.68
Overhead	$105	$105	$105	$105	$105	$105	$105	$105
Total	**$114**	**$114**	**$113**	**$112**	**$113**	**$112**	**$111**	**$110**

Source: Lisa P. McFaddin.

service cost. The formula to determine service fees is quite simple: Service Fee = Hospital Cost + Profit. The big question becomes how much profit? Table 5.6 illustrates the potential fee for 15-, 30-, and 60-minute VOT appointments, respectively, based on hospital cost and variable markup percentages. It becomes readily apparent that the lower the hospital contribution the higher the comparative profit.

Additional Considerations Patients receive other treatments or diagnostics when they come in for their treatments. The practitioner can adjust current medication regimens, run diagnostics (blood work, urinalysis, radiographs, etc.), discuss dietary and environmental modifications, and discuss nutrition and nutraceuticals, all of which increase revenue, average transaction per client (ATC), and veterinarian revenue per hour.

Team Training

The concept of phase training is used when introducing VOT to the hospital team. A multimedia approach is used to assist with the training program and is outlined Table 5.7.

Practice Manager's Role in Training

To conquer this task the pratice manager needs his or her own checklist which includes the following information:

- Schedule a date and time for the team training.
- Ensure all information pertaining to the new service is reviewed with the staff.
- Confirm all team members have completed the training.
- Certify all team members understand the information and can successfully educate clients.

Table 5.6 Potential 15-, 30-, and 60-minute veterinary ozone therapy (VOT) appointment prices using hospital costs from Table 5.5 at varying percentage markups as of February 2023.

		Ex. 1	Ex. 2	Ex. 3	Ex. 4	Ex. 5	Ex. 6	Ex. 7	Ex. 8
15-minute appointments									
Total hospital cost		$35	$35	$34	$33	$34	$33	$32	$31
Potential appointment price	40% Markup	$49	$49	$48	$46	$48	$46	$45	$43
	50% Markup	$53	$53	$51	$50	$51	$50	$48	$47
	60% Markup	$56	$56	$54	$53	$54	$53	$51	$50
	70% Markup	$60	$60	$58	$56	$58	$56	$54	$53
	80% Markup	$63	$63	$61	$59	$61	$59	$58	$56
	90% Markup	$67	$67	$65	$63	$65	$63	$61	$59
	100% Markup	$70	$70	$68	$66	$68	$66	$64	$62
30-minute appointments									
Total hospital cost		$62	$62	$60	$60	$60	$60	$58	$58
Potential appointment price	40% Markup	$87	$87	$84	$84	$84	$84	$81	$81
	50% Markup	$93	$93	$90	$90	$90	$90	$87	$87
	60% Markup	$99	$99	$96	$96	$96	$96	$93	$93
	70% Markup	$105	$105	$102	$102	$102	$102	$99	$99
	80% Markup	$112	$112	$108	$108	$108	$108	$104	$104
	90% Markup	$118	$118	$114	$114	$114	$114	$110	$110
	100% Markup	$124	$124	$120	$120	$120	$120	$116	$116
60-minute appointments									
Total hospital cost		$114	$114	$113	$112	$113	$112	$111	$110
Potential appointment price	40% Markup	$160	$160	$158	$157	$158	$157	$155	$154
	50% Markup	$171	$171	$170	$168	$170	$168	$167	$165
	60% Markup	$182	$182	$181	$179	$181	$179	$178	$176
	70% Markup	$194	$194	$192	$190	$192	$190	$189	$187
	80% Markup	$205	$205	$203	$202	$203	$202	$200	$198
	90% Markup	$217	$217	$215	$213	$215	$213	$211	$209
	100% Markup	$228	$228	$226	$224	$226	$224	$222	$220

Source: Lisa P. McFaddin.

Promotion

There are six common avenues of promotion for a veterinary integrative medicine (VIM) service: hospital website, social media, email blasts, mailers, in-hospital promotions, and client education.

Hospital Website

Advertise "Veterinary Ozone Therapy" or "Ozone Therapy" or "Medical Ozone" in several locations on the website main page, services, veterinarian's biography, and blog page. On the made page create a button or banner

Table 5.7 The breakdown of phase training steps and resources for the entire hospital team.

Phase 1: Background information	
Team training guide	The handout walks the practice manager and/or veterinarian through Phase 1 of the training
	A downloadable and editable copy of the handout is located on the companion website
Training presentation	The video covers background information on the modality
	PowerPoints can be downloaded, edited, and personalized from the companion website
	The document can be used as a PowerPoint or saved as an mp4 creating a personalized movie
Team training handout	The handout provides additional background information for the CSRs, VAs, and LTs to complement the knowledge gained from watching the training presentation
	A downloadable and editable copy of the handout is located on the companion website
Phase 2: Knowledge proficiency	
Quiz	A short quiz to ensure all team members have a good understanding of the service being offered
	A downloadable and editable copy of the handout is located on the companion website
	A key is provided
Phase 3: Expectations	
Training worksheets	A training checklist is provided for CSRs and VA/LTs with role-specific expectations and tasks for each staff member
	A recommended completion time is provided
	A downloadable and editable copy of the handout is located on the companion website
Phase 4: Client education	
Client scripts	Bullet point information and scripted examples used when discussing the therapy with clients
	A downloadable and editable copy of the handout is located on the companion website
Client education presentation	A short (5–7 minute) client educational video about the therapeutic modality
	PowerPoints can be downloaded, edited, and personalized from the companion website
	The document can be used as a PowerPoint or saved as an mp4 creating a personalized movie
Client education handout	An informational handout about the therapeutic modality written specifically for clients
	A downloadable and editable copy of the handout is located on the companion website

CSR, customer service representative; VA, veterinary assistant; LT, licensed technician. Source: Lisa P. McFaddin.

stating "Now offering veterinary ozone therapy" or "Now offering ozone therapy" or "Now offering medical ozone" with a link to success stories or client testimonials. Utilize the hospital website to advertise the VIM treatment under the "Services" section. On the veterinarian's biograph section include a description of the specialized training. Create a VOT blog page discussing patient success stories.

Social Media

Utilize Facebook, Instagram, and/or Twitter to post facts, photographs, hashtags, and patient success stories. Include fun and intriguing facts about VOT. Clients love patient photographs, especially when receiving VOT. Create or utilize VOT specific hashtags.

Email Blasts

Send fun mass emails to your clients introducing VOT. Consider monthly case presentations illustrating how the service has benefited patients. Almost everyone has at least one email address these days. Customer service representatives should be amassing client emails at the same rate as phone numbers.

Mailers

Mailers can be expensive and are largely unnecessary in this digital age. Mailers can be used to announce the introduction of VOT to existing clients. The mailer should include the name of the new service, a brief description of how VOT can help pet patients, the name of the doctor performing VOT, possibly a brief description of the training the doctor received, and possibly a photograph of a pet receiving VOT.

In-Hospital Promotions

Advertise VOT within the hospital using small promotional signs, informational signs, invoice teasers, and staff buttons. Small promotional signs can be placed in the waiting room and exam rooms. Include photographs of pets receiving VOT. Consider catchphrases such as "Got Ozone?"

Informational signs should include a brief description of how VOT can help pet patients, photographs of pets receiving VOT, name of the doctor performing VOT, and a brief description of the training the doctor received.

Invoice teasers should consist of short phrases reminding and enticing owners regarding a new service offered at the practice. Examples include "Now offering Veterinary Ozone Therapy"; "Curious If Medical Ozone Could Help Your Pet?"; "Introducing Veterinary Ozone Therapy"; and "Would Your Pet Benefit from Veterinary Ozone Therapy?"

Buttons can be made for the staff to wear with kitchy phrases reminding owners, in a fun way, of the new VIM service. Examples include "Got Ozone?" and "Want to learn more about Ozone Therapy?"

Client Education

Education is crucial to understanding the purpose and importance of any given treatment. The client handouts and videos solidify pet owner knowledge base, reducing concerns and conveying value.

Integration

The key components for proper integration include availability of the service to the right patients; appropriate patient scheduling; appropriate support staff scheduling; and staff buy-in (understanding the benefits of the offered service).

Veterinarians

There are several factors to contemplate when veterinarians are considering, and preparing to incorporate, a VIM in their clinical repertoire: state requirements and restrictions, return on investment, course availability, supplies and equipment, veterinary organizations, and continuing education.

State Requirements and Restrictions

Is VOT Considered the Practice of Veterinary Medicine?

While VOT is used to treat, correct, change, or resolve disease, VOT may or may not be considered the practice of veterinary medicine, especially given the FDA's current position on ozone therapy. Check your local state board for further information. Links to each state's veterinary board can be found on online.

Does VOT Continuing Education Count Toward Licensure Continuing Education Requirements?

Currently no states require specific CE hours for VOT. Some states limit the type and number of hours of integrative medicine CE. hours toward the annual CE requirement for license renewal. Review your specific state's requirements for further details.

Are Your Assets Covered?

Check with your liability insurance to determine if you are covered when practicing VOT. Refer to the Introduction of this book for additional information.

Return on Investment

Specifics are discussed in the Team Members section of this chapter.

Course Availability

While certification is not required, formal training is highly recommended. Training and certification provide the foundation for understanding how VOT can best help your veterinary patients. Completion of formal training also helps legitimize the modality. While the current training options are limited, major conferences may offer Registry of Approved Continuing Education (RACE)-approved lectures on VOT, and some veterinary organizations (such as the College of Integrative Veterinary Therapies or CIVT) offer paid webinars. These introductory lectures can provide a basic understanding regarding the mechanisms of action and practical applications of VOT, hopefully priming interested veterinarians to undergo more extensive training. Pricing is accurate as of February 2023.

Animal Wellness Academy

- **Course name**: Introduction to Ozone Therapy
- **Prerequisites**: Veterinarian membership required
- **Description**
  - Online course with a certificate of completion.
  - Geared toward veterinarians, veterinary technicians, and paraprofessionals.
  - Course discusses what ozone is, the pathophysiological effects on the body, practical applications, methods of administration, and clinical cases.
  - Quiz required for course completion.
- **Online training**: One lesson, course length not provided.
- **On-site training**: Two-day course.
- **Completion time**: None
- **Cost**: Veterinarian membership $50/month
- **Contact information**
  - Phone: 866-764-1212
  - Website: https://animalwellnessacademy. org/courses/introduction-to-ozone-therapy
  - Email: info@animalwellnessacademy.org

O$_3$ Vets

- **Course name**: Basic Veterinary Ozone Course
- **Prerequisites**: Veterinary or veterinary technician with a license in good standing
- **Description**
  - Online video course with a certificate of completion.
  - Geared toward veterinarians or veterinary technicians with little to no ozone therapy training.
  - Course covers the history, biochemistry, techniques, methods of administration, indications, contraindications, biological and clinical effects, ozone studies, prolotherapy and ozone, equipment needed, client education, ozone oils, ozone–UV combination therapy, clinical applications and observations, and hands-on therapy.
  - A mailed certificate is provided upon completion of the course and quizzes.
  - Participants have access to the course for one year with phone support.
- **Online training**: 14 video lessons and eight downloadable video protocols. The number of hours is not provided.
- **On-site training**: None
- **Completion time**: Up to one year
- **Cost**: $449
- **Contact information**

- Address: 105 Bridge St, Dimondale, MI 48821
- Phone: 517-925-8148
- Website:https://o3vets.com/products/online-basic-vet-ozone-course
- Email: info@O3vets.com

O₃ Vets

- **Course name**: Ozone Therapy Training
- **Prerequisites**: Veterinary or veterinary technicians with license in good standing
- **Description**
  - On-site course with a certificate of completion.
  - Geared toward veterinarians or veterinary technicians with little to no ozone therapy training.
  - Course covers the history, biochemistry, techniques, methods of administration, indications, contraindications, biological and clinical effects, ozone studies, prolotherapy and ozone, equipment needed, client education, ozone oils, ozone–UV combination therapy, clinical applications and observations, and hands-on therapy.
  - Hands-on experience with ozone generators, various routes of administration, and cadaver injections.
  - One-hour follow-up with clinic following training.

- **Online training**: None
- **On-site training**: Two-day course
- **Completion time**: Up to one year
- **Cost**: $899
- **Contact information**
  - Address: 105 Bridge St, Dimondale, MI 48821
  - Phone: 517-925-8148
  - Website:https://o3vets.com/products/online-basic-vet-ozone-course
  - Email: info@O3vets.com

Oxygen Healing Therapies

- **Course name**: Frank Shallenberger's Ozone Therapy Training and Certification Course: "The Essentials of Natural Medicine" Veterinarian Ozone Course

- **Prerequisites**: Veterinary with license in good standing. Dr. Frank Shallenberger's Ozone Therapy Training and Certification Course.
- **Description**
  - On-site course with a certificate of completion last offered 2018.
  - Course covered history of ozone therapy in people and animals, ozone chemistry and biochemistry, general applications, misconceptions of therapy, medical uses of ozone, methods of delivery, proper dosages, combining ozone therapy with other integrative and allopathic therapies, clinical applications, pitfalls of therapy, case presentations, and open discussions.
  - Hands-on wet lab.
  - Veterinarians can still take the Ozone Therapy Training Course and Certification, but the veterinary-specific course does not appear to be currently available.

- **Online training**: None
- **On-site training**: Two-day course plus two-day prerequisite course
- **Completion time**: Minimum four days
- **Cost**: $1300 for Ozone Therapy Training Course and Certification. Additional cost of the veterinary specific course was $1050.
- **Contact information**
  - Address: 1231 Country Club Drive, Carson City, NV 89703
  - Phone: 775-450-3766
  - Website: http://www.oxygenhealingtherapies.com/Shallenberger_Ozone_Therapy_Course_Details.htm
  - Email: ozonetherapies@gmail.com

Ûdemy

- **Course name**: Ozone Therapy: Most Needed Adjunct to Veterinary Medicine
- **Prerequisites**: Veterinarians and veterinary technicians. Licensing requirement not listed. Knowledge of veterinary medicine required. Knowledge of holistic medicine optional.
- **Description**
  - Online course introducing the benefits of ozone therapy in veterinary medicine.

– Course covers the mechanisms of action, methods of administration, and practical applications.

- **Online training**: Three sections and seven lectures, total of 7 hours 50 minutes.
- **On-site training**: None
- **Completion time**: Lifetime access
- **Cost**: $199
- **Contact information**
  – Website: https://www.udemy.com/course/ozone-therapy-most-needed-adjunct-to-veterinary-medicine

Supplies and Equipment

As mentioned in the Team Members section, the initial supplies for VOT include an ozone generator, oxygen source, oxygen regulator, and accessories (Shallenberger 2011). Initial equipment costs range from $1600 to $12100. Refer to the previous section for further details. There are several veterinary ozone suppliers, as well as human equipment which can be adapted for veterinary use. Most courses discuss their preferred suppliers which may include O_3vets (https://o3vets.com), Apoza (http://www.apoza.com/), Promolife (www.promolife.com), Longevity (https://www.ozonegenerator.com), and Herrmann Apparatebau (HAB, https://www.h-a-b.de/start), among others.

Hospital remodeling and/or redecorating is generally not required when offering VOT. Ozone generation and VOT must be performed in areas with excellent ventilation.

Veterinary Organizations

A description of the most common organizations with a special interest in ozone are provided below. Table 5.8 summarizes each organization's name, contact information, and membership dues.

American Academy of Ozonotherapy (AAO)

- **Description**: The AAO was founded in 2010 and is the only professional academy focused on ozonotherapy in the United States.

  The American Academy of Ozonotherapy (AAO) is an academy of health professionals dedicated to establishing standards for the art and science of Ozonotherapy, educating the public and other health professionals about the many uses of Ozonotherapy in medicine, and promoting research in Ozonotherapy. Our goal is to enhance the health and well being of people through this safe, inexpensive, and effective therapy. AAO is a proud member of the International Medical Ozone Federation (www.imeof.org), and adheres to the standards endorsed

Table 5.8 Veterinary associations and organizations with a special interest in veterinary ozone therapy (VOT) as of February 2023.

Organization	Contact information	Membership dues
American Academy of Ozonotherapy (AAO)	(888) 991-2268 Online contact us form	$300/year
American Holistic Veterinary Medical Association (AHVMA)	PO Box 630, Abingdon, MD 21009 (410) 569-0795 office@ahvma.org	$300/year
College of Integrative Veterinary Therapies (CIVT)	PO Box 352, Yeppoon, 4703 QLD, Australia (303) 800-5460 membership@civtedu.org	$185/year

Source: Lisa P. McFaddin.

by the IMEOF as described in the Madrid Declaration (see link below) (AAO 2015). General membership is open to all medical professionals who have taken or will take an approved ozone certification course. There is no annual CE requirement to maintain membership.

- **Membership benefits**
  - Discounted rates for the annual meetings and training seminars.
  - Access to members-only forum.
  - Listing on the international profile directory.
  - Access to the electronic newsletter.

American Holistic Veterinary Medical Association (AHVMA)

- **Description**: The AHVMA was founded in 1982 at the Western States Veterinary Conference with the goal of advancing integrative medicine through the education of integrative and non-integrative veterinarians, the introduction of integrative medicine to veterinary students, the promotion of research, and representation in the AVMA House of Delegates. There is no annual CE requirement to maintain membership.
- **Membership benefits**
  - Free subscription to the *AHVMA Journal*, a peer-reviewed journal.
  - Online resources for client education.
  - Searchable member directory.
  - Discounted vaccination titers through Kansas State University (KSU) Diagnostic Lab.
  - Free access to the Natural Medicines Database, an online resource for supplements, natural medicines, and integrative therapies.
  - Reduced cost for the AHVMA annual conference.

College of Integrative Veterinary Therapies (CIVT)

- **Description**: An online organization open to all licensed animal health providers interested in integrative medicine. There are two membership options: full membership for veterinarians and associate membership for registered animal health professionals. CIVT strives to promote all aspects of evidence-based integrative medicine through online education and discussion forums. CIVT provides financial support to veterinary students interested in studying integrative medicine. CIVT also helps fund integrative medicine research. There is no annual CE requirement to maintain membership.
- **Membership benefits**
  - Access to the online electronic library.
  - Access to the electronic *Journal of Integrative Veterinary Therapies*.
  - Three free CE webinars annually.
  - 20% discount on all webinars.
  - Discounts on specific CIVT courses.
  - Searchable member directory.
  - Access to the Natural Medicines Databases and the American Botanical Council Library.

Reference Books

The following is a list of my recommended integrative medicine and ozone books. A summary of each book is provided.

Integrating Complementary Medicine into Veterinary Practice

- Authors: Robert S. Goldstein, VMD, Paula Jo Broadfoot, DVM, Richard E. Plamquist, DVM, Karen Johnstons, DVM, Jiu Jia Wen, DVM, Barbara Fougère, BSc, BVMs (Hons), BHSc (comp Med), MODT, MHSc (Herb Med), CVA (IVAs), CVBM, CVCP, and Margo Roman, DVM
- Summary: A comprehensive review of multiple integrative therapies including Chinese herbal medicine, acupuncture, homotoxicology, nanopharmacology, homotoxicology, and therapeutic nutrition. The book aims to educate veterinary practitioners on the validity, effectiveness, and incorporation of each modality within daily practice.

Manual of Natural Veterinary Medicine:
Science and Tradition

- Authors: Susan G. Wynn, DVM and Steve Marsden, DVM, ND, MSOM, Lac, Dipl. CH., RH(AHG)
- Summary: A quick reference book discussing the integrative therapy options for numerous diseases in veterinary medicine. The book is organized by Western conditions. For each category the potential TCVM diagnoses and treatment options are reviewed in succinct detail. A must-have for all integrative veterinarians.

Ozone Therapy in Veterinary Medicine

- Author: Zully B. Zamora Rodriguez PhD, DMV
- Summary: A reference book discussing the human and veterinary history, mechanisms of action, toxicology, and practical applications of VOT. Divided into nine chapters, the author presents the information in a clear and concise manner. A must-have for practitioners interested in or practicing ozone therapy.

Principles and Applications of Ozone Therapy:
A Practical Guideline for Physicians

- Author: Frank Shallenberger, MD, HMD, ABAAM
- Summary: A quick reference guide for all medical professionals interested in and practicing ozone therapy. The book includes concise information regarding the mechanisms of action, clinical applications, and methods of administration. The book promotes the American Associations of Ozonotherapy.

Veterinary Ozone Treatment Guide

- Author: O_3 Vets
- Description: A digital quick reference organized by methods of administration discussing indications, dosages, necessary equipment and supplies, and protocols.

Promotion

Information regarding the hospital's promotion of VOT can be found in the Team Members section.

Integration

Key components for proper integration include availability, scheduling, and staff buy-in. Availability means offering the service to the right patient. Scheduling refers to appropriate patient and support staff scheduling. Staff buy-in ensures all team members understand the benefits of the offered service.

Conclusion

Ozone therapy is a newer therapeutic modality in veterinary medicine. Early research suggests ozone therapy is useful as an adjunct or primary method of treatment for chronic inflammatory and infectious conditions. This chapter and online resources describe in detail how VOT can be successfully introduced into daily practice, as well as provide practical tools for implementation.

Acknowledgments

I would like to thank Dr. Toni Connell for reviewing this chapter for content. Dr. Toni Connell, DVM, MBA, CVA is an integrative veterinarian, and former owner, at Independent Hill Veterinary Clinic. She is certified in veterinary acupuncture (CVA) through IVAS. Dr. Connell has undergone formal training in Chinese veterinary herbal medicine, veterinary homeopathy, and veterinary ozone therapy.

References

AAHA (American Animal Hospital Association) (2019). *Compensation and Benefits*, 9e. Denver, CO: AAHA Press.

AAO (American Academy of Ozonotherapy) (2015). AAOT. www.aaot.us (accessed 20 November 2022).

Abreu-Villela, P., Ferraro, M., Rodrigues, R.R. et al. (2021). Ozone therapy in the prevention of dental plaque formation in dogs. *Journal of Veterinary Dentistry* 38 (1): 18–23.

AEPROMO (Spanish Association of Medical Professionals in Ozone Therapy) (2015). Ozonetherapy history. https://aepromo.org/en/ozonotherapy-history/ (accessed 6 September 2022).

Alberts, B., Johnson, A., Lewis, J. et al. (2002). Helper T cells and lymphocyte activation. In: *Molecular Biology of the Cell*, 4e (ed. B. Alberts, A. Johnson, J. Lewis, et al.). New York: Garland Science.

Anzolin, A.P., da Silveira-Kaross, N.L., and Bertol, C.D. (2020). Ozonated oil in wound healing: what has already been proven? *Medical Gas Research* 10 (1): 54–59.

AOAPRM (American Osteopathic Association of Prolotherapy Regenerative Medicine) (2020). What is Prolotherapy. https://prolotherapycollege.org/ (accessed 29 October 2020).

APPA (American Pet Products Association) (2022). Pet industry market size and ownership statistics. https://www.americanpetproducts.org/research-insights/industry-trends-and-stats (accessed 23 February 2023).

AVMA (American Veterinary Medical Association) (2019). Economic state of the veterinary profession. https://www.avma.org/news/press-release/AVMA-2019-Economic-State-of-the-Veterinary-Profession-Report-now-available. (accessed 26 July 2021).

AVMA (American Veterinary Medical Association) (2023). *2023 AVMA Report on the Economic State of the Veterinary Profession.* Schaumburg, IL: AVMA.

Babior, B., Takeuchi, C., Ruedi, J. et al. (2003). Investigating antibody-catalyzed ozone generation by human neutrophils. *Proceedings of the National Academy of Sciences of the United States of America* 100 (6): 3031–3034.

Blanchard, E.L., Lawrence, J.D., Noble, J.A. et al. (2020). Enveloped virus inactivation on personal protective equipment by exposure to ozone. *medRxiv* https://doi.org/10.1101/2020.05.23.20111435.

BLS (Bureau of Labor Statistics) (2022). Occupational outlook handbooks: veterinary technologists and technicians median pay 2020. https://www.bls.gov/ooh/healthcare/veterinary-technologists-and-technicians.htm (accessed 18 February 2023).

BLS (Bureau of Labor Statistics) (2023). News Release: Consumer Price Index. https://www.bls.gov/news.release/pdf/cpi.pdf (accessed 18 February 2023).

Bocci, V. (2004). Ozone as Janus: this controversial gas can be either toxic or medially useful. *Mediators of Inflammation* 13 (1): 3–11.

Bocci, V., Zanardi, I., and Travagli, V. (2011). Oxygen/ozone as a medical gas mixture. A critical evaluation of the various methods clarifies positive and negative aspects. *Medical Gas Research* 1 (6): 1–9.

Brown, W. (2022). Ketone. https://www.britannica.com/science/ketone (accessed 29 September 2022).

Budi, D.S., Rofananda, I.F., Pratama, N.R. et al. (2022). Ozone as an adjuvant therapy for COVID-19: a systematic review and meta-analysis. *International Immunopharmacology* 110: 109014.

Burns, K. (2018). Pet ownership stable, veterinary care variable. https://www.avma.org/javma-news/2019-01-15/pet-ownership-stable-veterinary-care-variable (accessed 11 August 2021).

Burns, K. (2022). New report takes a deep dive into pet ownership. https://www.avma.org/news/new-report-takes-deep-dive-pet-ownership (accessed 6 November 2022).

Cagini, C., Mariniello, M., Messina, M. et al. (2020). The role of ozonized oil and a combination of tobramycin/dexamethasone eye drops in the treatment of viral conjunctivitis: a randomized clinical trial. *International Ophthlamology* 40 (12): 3209–3215.

Cattel, F., Giordano, S., Bertiond, C. et al. (2021). Ozone therapy in COVID-19: a narrative review. *Virus Research* 291: 198207.

Chirumbolo, S., Valdenassi, L., Simonetti, V. et al. (2021). Insights on the mechanisms of action of ozone in the medical therapy against COVID-19. *International Immunopharmacology* 96: 107777.

Claus, H. (2021). Ozone generation by ultraviolet lamps. *Photochemistry and Photobiology* 97, 3: 471–476.

Clavo, B., Pérez, J.L., López, L. et al. (2004). Effect of ozone therapy on muscle oxygenation. *Journal of Alternative and Complementary Medicine* 9 (2): 251–256.

Cramer, G., Darby, S.A., and Frysztak, R. (2014). Pain of spinal origin. In: *Clinical Anatomy of the Spine, Spinal Cord, and ANS*, 3e (ed. G.D. Cramer and S.A. Darby), 508–539. St. Louis, MO: Elsevier.

Daud, F.V., Ueda, S.M.Y., Navarini, A., and Mímica, L.M.J. (2011). The use of ozonized oil in the treatment of dermatophitosis caused by *Microsporum canis* in rabbits. *Brazilian Journal of Microbiology* 42 (1): 274–281.

Deng, L., Meng, W., Li, D. et al. (2018). The effect of ozone on hypoxia, hemolysis and morphological change of blood from patients with aortic dissection (AD): a preliminary in vitro experiment of ozonated autohemotherapy for treating AD. *American Journal of Translational Research* 10 (6): 1829–1840.

Dornell, J. (2021). Humoral vs Cell-Mediated Immunity. https://www.technologynetworks. com/immunology/articles/humoral-vs-cell-mediated-immunity-344829 (accessed 3 October 2022).

Dörr, T., Moynihan, P.J., and Mayer, C. (2019). Editorial: bacterial cell wall structure and dynamics. *Frontiers in Microbiology* 10: 2051.

Elvis, A. and Ekta, J. (2011). Ozone therapy: a clinical review. *Journal of Natural Sicence, Biology and Medicine* 21 (1): 66–70.

EPA (Environmental Protection Agency) (2003). Ozone: Good Up High - Bad Nearby. https:// www.epa.gov/sites/default/files/documents/gooduphigh.pdf (accessed 17 September 2022).

EPA (Environmental Protection Agency) (2022a). Ozone Pollution and Your Patients' Health. https://www.epa.gov/ ozone-pollution-and-your-patients-health/ what-ozone (accessed 13 September 2022).

EPA (Environmental Protection Agency) (2022b). Smog, Soot, and Other Air Pollution from Transportation. https://www.epa.gov/ transportation-air-pollution-and-climate-change/smog-soot-and-other-air-pollution-transportation#:~:text=What%20is%20 smog%3F,mostly%20of%20ground%20level%20 ozone (accessed 17 September 2022).

Estrela, C., Estrela, C.R., Decurcio, D.D.A. et al. (2006). Antimicrobial potential of ozone in an ultrasonic cleaning system against *Staphylococcus aureus. Brazilian Dental Journal* 17 (2): 134–138.

FDA (Food and Drug Administration) (2020). Ultraviolet (UV) Radiation. https://www.fda .gov/radiation-emitting-products/tanning/ ultraviolet-uv-radiation (accessed 17 September 2022).

FDA (Food and Drug Administration) (2022). CFR - Code of Federal Regulations Title 21; Part 801 - Labelling, Subpart H - Special Requirements for Specific Devices. https:// www.accessdata.fda.gov/scripts/cdrh/cfdocs/ cfcfr/CFRSearch.cfm?fr=801.415 (accessed 5 September 2022).

FederalPay.org (2023). FY 2023 Federal Per Diem Rates October 2022–September 2023. https:// www.federalpay.org/perdiem/2023 (accessed 18 February 2023).

Fitzpatrick, E., Holland, O.J., and Vanderlelie, J.J. (2018). Ozone therapy for the treatment of chronic wounds: a systematic review. *International Wound Journal* 15 (4): 633–644.

Flatters, S. (2015). The contribution of mitochondria to sensory processing and pain. *Progress in Molecular Biology and Translation Science* 131: 119–146.

Forthal, D.N. (2014). Function of antibodies. *Microbiology Spectrum Journal* 2 (4): 1–17.

French, S. and Kemmis, S. (2023). Rental Car Pricing Statistics:2023. https://www. nerdwallet.com/article/travel/car-rental-pricing-statistics#:~:text=The%20average%20 weekly%20rental%20price,in%20 advance%2C%20it%20was%20%24513 (accessed 18 February 2023).

Górnicki, A. and Gutsze, A. (2000). In vitro effects of ozone on human erythrocyte membranes: an EPR study. *Acta Biochimica Polonica* 47 (4): 963–971.

Gupta, G. and Mansi, B. (2012). Ozone therapy in periodontics. *Journal of Medicine and Life* 5 (1): 59–67.

Hassan, Z., Stahlberger, M., Rosenbaum, N., and Bräse, S. (2020). Criegee intermediates beyond ozonolysis: synthetic and mechanistic insights. *Angewandte Chemie International Edition* 60 (28): 15138–15152.

Hauser, R., Lackner, J., Steilen-Matias, D., and Harris, D. (2016). A systematic review of dextrose prolotherapy for chronic musculoskeletal pain. *Clinical Medicine Insights. Arthritis and Musculoskeletal Disorders* 9: 139–159.

Helmenstine, A.M. (2020). Definition of Carboxyl Group in Chemistry. https://www.thoughtco.com/definition-of-carboxyl-group-and-examples-604879 (accessed 29 September 2022).

Hirayama, D., Iida, T., and Nakase, H. (2018). The phagocytic function of macrophage-enforcing innate immunity and tissue homeostasis. *International Journal of Molecular Sciences* 19 (1): 92.

Huang, M., Hasan, M.K., Rathore, K. et al. (2022). Plasma generated ozone and reactive oxygen species for point of use PPE decontamination system. *PLoS One* 17 (2): e0262818.

IASP (Interntional Association for the Stuy of Pain) (2021). Terminology: Pain. https://www.iasp-pain.org/resources/terminology/#pain (accessed 10 October 2022).

IMCPDCIB (Institute of Medicine; Committee on Pain, Disability, and Chronic Illness Behavior) (1987). The anatomy and physiology of pain. In: *Pain and Disability: Clinical, Behavioral, and Public Policy Perspectives* (ed. M. Osterweis, A. Kleinman, and D. Mechanic). Washington, DC: National Academies Press.

Inal, M., Dokumacioglu, A., Özcelik, E., and Ucar, O. (2011). The effects of ozone therapy and coenzyme Q_{10} combination on oxidative stress markers in healthy subjects. *Irish Journal of Medical Science* 180 (3): 703–707.

Kang, X., Kirui, A., Muszyński, A. et al. (2018). Molecular architecture of fungal cell walls revealed by solid-state NMR. *Nature Communications* 9: 2747.

Kettle, A.J. and Winterbourn, C.C. (2005). Do neutrophils produce ozone? An appraisal of current evidence. *BioFactors* 24 (1–4): 41–45.

Kosachenco, D., Autônomo, M.V., Bárbara, D. et al. (2018). Therapeutic effect of ozone therapy in wound healing in dogs: cases report. *Revista Española Ozonoterapia* 8: 197–210.

Kozat, S. and Okman, E.N. (2019). Has ozone therapy a future in veterinary medicine? *Journal of Animal Husbandry and Dairy Science* 3 (3): 25–34.

Kshitish, D. and Laxman, V. (2010). The use of ozonated water and 0.2% chlorhexidine in the treatment of periodontitis patients: a clinical and microbiologic study. *Indian Journal of Dental Research* 21 (3): 341–348.

LibreTexts (2022a). 3.3: Molecules and Chemical Nomenclature. https://chem.libretexts.org/Bookshelves/Introductory_Chemistry/Beginning_Chemistry_(Ball)/03%3A_Atoms_Molecules_and_Ions/3.03%3A_Molecules_and_Chemical_Nomenclature (accessed 29 September 2022).

LibreTexts (2022b). The Carbonyl Group. https://chem.libretexts.org/Bookshelves/Organic_Chemistry/Supplemental_Modules_(Organic_Chemistry)/Aldehydes_and_Ketones/Properties_of_Aldehydes_and_Ketones/The_Carbonyl_Group#:~:text=A%20carbonyl%20group%20is%20a,contributing%20to%20smell%20and%20taste (accessed 29 September 2022).

Louten, J. (2016). Virus structure and classification. In: *Essential Human Virology*, 19–29. London: Academic Press.

Madan, K., Díaz Gómez, M.F., Castellanos, F., and Pérez, M. (2010). Ozonized citronellal formulations effects in the treatment of rabbits with dermatomycosis. *Revista CENIC* 41: 1–8.

March, J. and Brown, W. (2020). Aldehyde. https://www.britannica.com/science/aldehyde (accessed 29 September 2022).

McFaddin III, J.G. (2022). Ozone's effect on various materials. A discussion with a Senior Technical Representative for Avantor. [Interview] (29 October 2022).

ME (Michigan Engineering) (2022). Ozonators. https://encyclopedia.che.engin.umich.edu/ozonators (accessed 17 September 2022).

MFAF (Michelson Found Animals Foundation) (2018). Furred lines: Pet trends. https://www.prnewswire.com/news-releases/furred-lines-pet-trends-2019-300741947.html. (accessed 26 July 2021).

Monzillo, V., Lallitto, F., Russo, A. et al. (2020). Ozonized gel against four candida species: a pilot study and clinical perspectives. *Materials* 13 (7): 1731.

Nader, E., Skinner, S., Romana, M. et al. (2019). Blood rheology: key parameters, impact on blood flow, role in sickle cell disease and effects of exercise. *Frontiers in Physiology* 10: 1329.

Naik, S.V., Rajeshwari, K., Kohli, S. et al. (2016). Ozone: a biological therapy in dentistry. Reality or myth? *Open Dentistry Journal* 10: 196–206.

NAPHIA (North American Pet Health Insurance Association) (2023). Industry Data. https://naphia.org/industry-data/#my-menu (accessed 18 February 2023).

Newkirk, M. (2020). How ozone therapy helps dogs and cats. *Animal Wellness Magazine* (14 August).

NOAA CSL (National Oceanic and Atmospheric Administration, Chemical Sciences Laboratory) (2010). How is ozone formed in the atmosphere. https://csl.noaa.gov/assessments/ozone/2010/twentyquestions/Q2.pdf (accessed 13 September 2022).

Nolen, R.S. (2022). Pet ownership rate stabilizes as spending increases. https://www.avma.org/news/pet-ownership-rate-stabilizes-spending-increases (accessed 22 February 2023).

OCP (Organic Chemistry Portal) (2022). Ozonolysis. https://www.organic-chemistry.org/namedreactions/ozonolysis-criegee-mechanism.shtm (accessed 29 September 2022).

Onyango, A.N. (2016). Endogenous generation of singlet oxygen and ozone in human and animal tissues: mechanisms, biological significance, and influence of dietary components. *Oxidative Medicine and Cellular Longevity* 2016: 2398573.

Orlandin, J.R., Machado, L.C., Ambrósio, C.E., and Travaglib, V. (2021). Ozone and its derivatives in veterinary medicine: a careful appraisal. *Veterinary and Animal Science* 13: 100191.

Ouellette, R. and Rawn, J.D. (2014). Structure and bonding in organic compounds. In: *Organic Chemistry: Structure, Mechanism, and Synthesis* (ed. R. Ouellette and J.D. Rawn), 1–39. San Diego, CA: Elsevier.

Ouf, S.A., Moussa, T.A., Abd-Elmegeed, A.M., and Eltahlawy, S.R. (2016). Anti-fungal potential of ozone against some dermatophytes. *Brazilian Journal of Microbiology* 47 (3): 697–702.

Paoloni, M., Di Sante, L., Cacchio, A. et al. (2009). Intramuscular oxygen-ozone therapy in the treatment of acute back pain with lumbar disc herniation. *Spine* 34 (13): 1337–1344.

Pryor, W.A., Squadrito, G.L., and Friedman, M. (1995). The cascade mechanism to explain ozone toxicity: the role of lipid ozonation products. *Free Radical Biology and Medicine* 19 (6): 935–941.

PubChem (2022a). Oxygen. https://pubchem.ncbi.nlm.nih.gov/compound/977 (accessed 17 September 2022).

PubChem (2022b). Ozone. https://pubchem.ncbi.nlm.nih.gov/compound/24823 (accessed 5 September 2022).

Raeissadat, S.A., Rayegani, S.M., Sadeghi, F., and Rahimi-Dehgolan, S. (2018). Comparison of ozone and lidocaine injection efficacy vs dry needling in myofascial pain syndrome patients. *Journal of Pain Research* 11: 1273–1279.

Raja, S.N., Carr, D.B., Cohen, M. et al. (2020). The revised IASP definition of pain: concepts, challenges, and compromises. *Pain* 161 (9): 1976–1982.

Repciuc, C.C., Toma, C.G., Ober, C.A., and Oana, L.I. (2020). Management of surgical wound dehiscence by oxygen-ozone therapy in a FIV-positive cat: a case report. *Journal of the University of Veterinary Science Brno, Czech Republic* 89 (2): 189–194.

Rodriguez, Z.B.Z. (2016). *Ozone Therapy in Veterinary Medicine*. La Habana, Cuba: @ Collective of Authors.

Roman, M. (2013). Ozone Therapy: Beyond Oxygen 2013; The Most Needed Adjunct to Veterinary Medicine. Seminars to the Simposio Internacional de Ozonioterapia na Medicina Veterinaria, Brazil (25–27 August 2017). https://www.ibo3a.com.br/wp-content/uploads/2020/06/ANAIS-I-Simp%C3%B3sio-Internacional-de-Ozonioterapia-na-Medicina-Veterin%C3%A1ria-1.pdf

Roman, M. (2015). Ozone therapy used instead of antibiotics for microbiome restorative therapy yields successful outcomes for dogs and cats with fecal transplants. *Townsend Letter* 384–392. https://www.thefreelibrary.com/Ozone+therapy+used+instead+of+antibiotics+for+microbiome+restorative...-a0421522724.

Sagai, M. and Bocci, V. (2011). Mechanisms of action involved in ozone therapy: is healing induced via a mild oxidative stress? *Medical Gas Research* 1: 29.

Seyam, O., Smith, N.L., Reid, I. et al. (2018). Clinical utility of ozone therapy for musculoskeletal disorders. *Medical Gas Research* 8 (3): 103–110.

Shallenberger, F. (2011). *Principles and Applications of Ozone Therapy: A Practical Guideline for Physicians*. CreateSpace Independent Publishing Platform.

Shields, H., Traa, A., and Raamsdonk, K.V. (2021). Beneficial and detrimental effects of reactive oxygen species on lifespan: a comprehensive review of comparative and experimental studies. *Frontiers in Cell and Developmental Biology* 9: 628157.

Shimizu, N., Shimizu, N., and Washizu, M. (2013). Ozonetherapy for Dogs and Cats. https://lomr.org/wp-content/uploads/2013/11/Dogs-Cats.pdf (accessed 10 September 2020).

Shoemaker, J.M. (2005). Ozone Therapy: History, Physiology, Indications, Results. http://www.fullcircleequine.com/oz_therapy.pdf (accessed 12 September 2022).

Shulz, S. (1986). The role of ozone/oxygen in clindamycin-associated enterocolitis in the Djungarian hamster (*Phodopus sungorus sungorus*). *Laboratory Animals* 20 (1): 41–48.

de Sire, A., Agostini, F., Lippi, L. et al. (2021). Oxygen–ozone therapy in the rehabilitation field: state of the art on mechanisms of action, safety and effectiveness in patients with musculoskeletal disorders. *Biomolecules* 11 (3): 356.

Smith, N.L., Wilson, A.L., Gandhi, J. et al. (2017). Ozone therapy: an overview of pharmacodynamics, current research, and clinical utility. *Medical Gas Research* 7 (3): 212–219.

Stanley, B. (2004). Electrolytic ozone generation and its application in pure water systems. *Water Conditioning and Purification International Magazine* https://wcponline.com/2004/08/14/electrolytic-ozone-generation-application-pure-water-systems/.

Stevenson, P. (2016). How to set practice service fees. https://cliniciansbrief.com/article/how-set-practice-service-fees. (accessed 10 June 2020).

Stoker, G. (1902). Ozone in chronic middle-ear deafness. *Lancet* 160 (4131): 1187–1188.

Suh, Y., Patel, S., Kaitlyn, R. et al. (2019). Clinical utility of ozone therapy in dental and oral medicine. *Medical Gas Research* 9 (3): 163–167.

Summerfelt, S. (2003). Ozonation and UV irradiation: an introduction and examples of current applications. *Aquacultural Engineering* 28 (1–2): 21–36.

Thanomsub, B., Anupunpisit, V., Chanphetch, S. et al. (2002). Effects of ozone treatment on cell growth and ultrastructural changes in bacteria. *Journal of General and Applied Microbiology* 48 (4): 193–199.

Toth, G. and Hillger, D. (2022). Percursor era contributors to meteorology: Renaissance through World War I. https://rammb.cira.colostate.edu/dev/hillger/precursor.htm#schonbein (accessed 6 September 2022).

Trcek, L. (2023). This is How Much Flight Prices Increase in 2023 (+FAQs). https://www.travelinglifestyle.net/this-is-how-much-flight-prices-increase-in-2023 (accessed 18 February 2023).

Trefil, J., Bertsch, G. and McGrayne, S.B. (2022). Atom. https://www.britannica.com/science/atom (accessed 29 September 2022).

Ugazio, E., Tullio, V., Binello, A. et al. (2020). Ozonated oils as antimicrobial systems in topical applications. Their characterization, current applications, and advances in improved delivery techniques. *Molecules* 25 (2): 334.

Ulusoy, G.R., Bilge, A., and Öztürk, Ö. (2019). Comparison of corticosteroid injection and ozone injection for relief of pain in chronic lateral epicondylitis. *Acta Orthopaedica Belgica* 85 (3): 317–324.

Vitz, E., Moore, J.W., Shorb, J. et al. (2022). 8.14: Alcohols. https://chem.libretexts.org/Bookshelves/General_Chemistry/Book%3A_ChemPRIME_(Moore_et_al.)/08%3A_Properties_of_Organic_Compounds/8.14%3A_Alcohols (accessed 29 September 2022).

Wieczorek, M., Abualrous, E.T., Sticht, J. et al. (2017). Major histocompatibility complex (MHC) class I and MHC class II proteins: conformational plasticity in antigen presentation. *Frontiers in Immunology* 8: 292.

Wiley (2002). Redox Reactions. https://www.wiley.com/college/boyer/0470003790/reviews/redox/redox.htm (accessed 26 September 2022).

Woodley, K. (2018). Pet insurance for holistic and integrative practice. https://ivcjournal.com/pet-insurance-integrative-practices (accessed 11 August 2021).

Zargaran, M., Fatahinia, M., and Mahmoudabadi, A.Z. (2017). The efficacy of gaseous ozone against different forms of *Candida albicans. Current Medical Mycology* 3 (2): 26–32.

6

Photobiomodulation

Introduction

Photobiomodulation (PBM) is an emerging and effective treatment modality used primarily to aid in the treatment of skin wounds and pain. PBM uses light (most commonly red or near-infrared) to stimulate, heal, regenerate, and protect damaged tissue. The introduction of PBM into a veterinary practice can be beneficial for both the patient and the health of the practice. The successful incorporation and utilization of PBM is reliant upon effective education and training of the entire hospital team, as well as client education. This chapter discusses the what, why, and how for the effective integration of PBM within your practice.

The What

Word Origin

PBM is a portmanteau of the words "photo" (meaning light) and "biomodulation" (meaning modifying or changing a biological or biochemical process).

Definition

In 2015 Drs. Anders, Lanzafame, and Arany, with the support of the American Society for Laser Medicine and Surgery (ASLMS), defined PBM as

"a form of light therapy that utilizes non-ionizing forms of light sources, including lasers, LEDs, and broadband light, in the visible and infrared spectrum. It is a non-thermal process involving endogenous chromophores eliciting photophysical (i.e. linear and nonlinear) and photochemical events at various biological scales. This process results in beneficial therapeutic outcomes including but not limited to the alleviation of pain or inflammation, immunomodulation, and promotion of wound healing and tissue regeneration" (Anders et al. 2015).

The terms low-level laser/light therapy, cold laser, and PBM are often used interchangeably.

Integrative Medicine in Veterinary Practice, First Edition. Lisa P. McFaddin.
© 2024 John Wiley & Sons, Inc. Published 2024 by John Wiley & Sons, Inc.
Companion website: www.wiley.com/go/mcfaddin/integrativemedicine

Human History

The first well-documented use of light in the treatment of human disease dates to the eighteenth century. Niels Ryberg Finsen, a Danish physician, used red and blue light to treat multiple conditions, including lupus vulgaris (Nobel 1967). Finsen proved concentrated rays from sunlight could kill bacteria and stimulate tissue, winning him the Nobel Prize in Medicine and Physiology in 1903 (Nobel 1967).

In 1960, Theodore Maiman, an American engineer, created the first operational laser (*light amplification by stimulated emission of radiation*) by shining a high-powered flash lamp on silver-ended synthetic rods producing a narrow beam of monochromatic light with a wavelength of 694 nm (MAGLAB 2021). Despite unwarranted public concerns of lasers as death rays, most of the scientific community embraced the potential applications for lasers in all branches of science.

Mester et al. (1976) presented the first practical application of laser therapy in human medicine by demonstrating the positive effect of low-dose laser light on hair growth and wound healing. In 1979, Drs. Ellet Drake and Leon Goldman established the American Society for Laser Medicine and Surgery (ASLMS 2021). The ASLMS comprises biophysicists, biochemists, biomedical engineers, physicians and clinicians, and other scientists. The organization's primary goals are to educate those within the scientific and medical community, as well as laypersons, provide guidelines for the safe and effective use of lasers, and offer credentialing procedures (ASLMS 2021).

Throughout its history PBM has undergone several name changes reflecting our understanding of its mechanisms of action (MOA) and the evolution of its applications. Many of these names are still used by individuals (physicians and scientists alike) and can be found in the literature. Many use these terms interchangeably, though PBM is currently considered the most accurate descriptor. Alternate names include photobiostimulation, low-level laser or light therapy, low-power laser therapy, cold laser, and soft laser (Anders et al. 2015).

Veterinary History

The use of PBM in veterinary medicine took hold in the early 2000s, likely prompted by Food and Drug Administration (FDA) approval of the Class IIIb therapeutic laser in 2002 (FDA 2020). The Class IIIb laser was called a "cold laser" or "low-level laser therapy" because the units operated under 500 mW and did not generate heat when used. One of the first published recommendations for the use of PBM in veterinary rehabilitation was in 2005 (Millis et al. 2005).

FDA approval of the Class IV laser, in 2006, sparked further interest and broader practical applications of PBM in veterinary medicine (FDA 2020). The Class IV laser was initially referred to as "high-power laser therapy," as it operated at greater than 500 mW.

Historical and current veterinary PBM research has focused on the treatment of pain and wound repair. The incorporation of PBM is considered common practice in the treatment of many musculoskeletal conditions.

There are several professional organizations, which veterinarians can join, promoting the research and practical applications of PBM, as well as hosting annual or biannual conferences: the ASLMS, the North American Association of Photobiomodulation Therapy (NAALT), and the World Association of Laser Therapy (WALT).

Terminology

Photobiomodulation therapy (PBMT) comes with its own vocabulary. A basic understanding of these terms is crucial, allowing effective communication amongst professionals and with clients. A summary of common terms is provided below.

Absorption coefficient: Measure of the degree of electromagnetic radiation absorbed as the light passes through a substance (Patil and Dhami 2008).

Biophysics: A field of study using physics to better understand biological systems from cells to entire organisms, including the human body (Biophysical Society 2023).

Chromophore: An atom or group of atoms contributing to the color of a compound (Patil and Dhami 2008). Also described as the portion of a molecule responsible for its color.

Coherence: Waves of radiation have a fixed phase and frequency (Heiskanen and Hamblin 2018).

Conductivity: How well a specific material conducts electricity (Heiskanen and Hamblin 2018).

Diode: A semiconductor device with two terminals which allows electrons and energy to only flow in one direction (Heiskanen and Hamblin 2018).

Electromagnetic spectrum: All types of electromagnetic energy (NASA 2013).

Endogenous: Originating within an organism or body or something caused by internal factors.

Exogenous: Originating outside an organism or body or something caused by outside (external) factors.

Fluence: Energy delivered per unit area, measured in joules per square centimeter (J/cm^2) (JEDEC 2023).

Frequency: The rate at which something (in this case waves) passes during a specific period of time (JEDEC 2023). Frequency and wavelength are inversely proportional. Waves with shorter wavelengths have a higher frequency, while waves with lower frequencies have longer wavelengths.

Hertz (abbreviated Hz): A unit of frequency equal to one cycle per second (JEDEC 2023).

Irradiance: The flux of radiant energy per unit area, or the power divided by the area (W/cm^2) (de Freitas and Hamblin 2016). Often referred to as power density, but this is technically incorrect (Chung et al. 2012).

Joules (abbreviated J): A measurement of energy. More specifically the Système International (SI) unit of work (energy) created by the force of 1 newton acting through a distance of 1 meter (Britannica 2020). With respect to light, each photon contains a certain amount of energy measured in joules. Joules and photons have a proportional relationship: the more photons, the higher the joules (or energy) (JEDEC 2023).

Laser: An acronym for *l*ight *a*mplification by *s*timulated *e*mission of *r*adiation. A narrow beam of single frequency light emitted by a device which utilizes light, electrical energy, or electromagnetic energy as its source (NASA 2021).

LED (aka light-emitting diode): A semiconductor diode which produces light when a current flows through it (Edwards 2005).

Monochromatic: Containing one color.

Photoacceptor: A pigment that uses light (photons) as the first step in a photochemical reaction (Sineshchekov 1995).

Photobiomodulation (aka low-level laser or light therapy or cold laser therapy): The use of light (most commonly red or near-infrared) to stimulate, heal, regenerate, and protect damaged tissue (Hamblin 2017).

Photobiophysics: A branch of biophysics studying how light interacts with biological systems (Reusch 2013).

Photochemical reaction: A chemical reaction induced by the absorption of light energy (Reusch 2013).

Photochemistry: A branch of chemistry studying the chemical effects of light (Reusch 2013).

Photon: A particle of electromagnetic radiation with zero mass at rest, which carries energy proportional to the radiation frequency (Reusch 2013). For example, short wavelengths have high frequencies and high-energy photons.

Power: Rate of energy delivery measured in watts (W), where $1\,W = 1\,J/s$ (Patil and Dhami 2008).

Radiation: Energy which travels and spreads out through space (NASA 2013).

Semiconductor: A solid substance composed of an insulator and a metal which has conductivity (Heiskanen and Hamblin 2018).

Tissue penetration: How deep (or how many tissue layers) a beam of light can penetrate.

Visible light: A specific range of electromagnetic radiation, typically between 380 and 700 nm, visible to the human eye (Nagaraja 2021).

Wavelength: Distance between the peaks of a wave, usually measured in nanometers or nm (Patil and Dhami 2008).

Light Basics

Electromagnetic Spectrum

The electromagnetic (EM) spectrum includes all types of EM radiation. Radiation is defined as the energy, in the form of waves or particles, which travels and spreads out through space (NASA 2013). The EM spectrum includes radio waves, microwaves, infrared light, visible light, ultraviolet light, X-rays, and gamma rays. Each wave has their own unique wavelength, as illustrated in Figure 6.1.

Visible Light

Merriam-Webster dictionary defines light as "electromagnetic radiation (EMR) of any wavelength that travels in a vacuum with a speed of 186,000 miles per second" (Merriam-Webster 2021). Visible light, often used synonymously with the word "light," is the range of EMR visible to the human eye, typically between 380 and 700 nm (Nagaraja 2021).

Light travels in waves, and the distance between the peaks is called a wavelength, measured in nanometers or nm, as shown in Figure 6.2. The type or color of light is defined by its wavelength with every color having its own unique wavelength. Red light has a much longer wavelength compared to purple light, as depicted in Figure 6.3. Sunlight and white light comprise the full spectrum of visible light. Passing the light through a prism causes the different wavelengths to separate into all the colors of the rainbow, as shown in Figure 6.4 (Nagaraja 2021).

Laser and LED Basics

Lasers

A laser is a device which can convert light or electrical energy into a focused and high-energy beam (NASA 2021). Laser light is monochromatic (one color), contains a single light frequency (coherent), and does not spread out very far over long distances (NASA 2021). Figure 6.5 depicts six different line lasers which each project a single focused horizontal illuminated line.

Manufacturers of laser products sold in the United States must comply with all requirements in the Title 21 Code of Federal Regulations

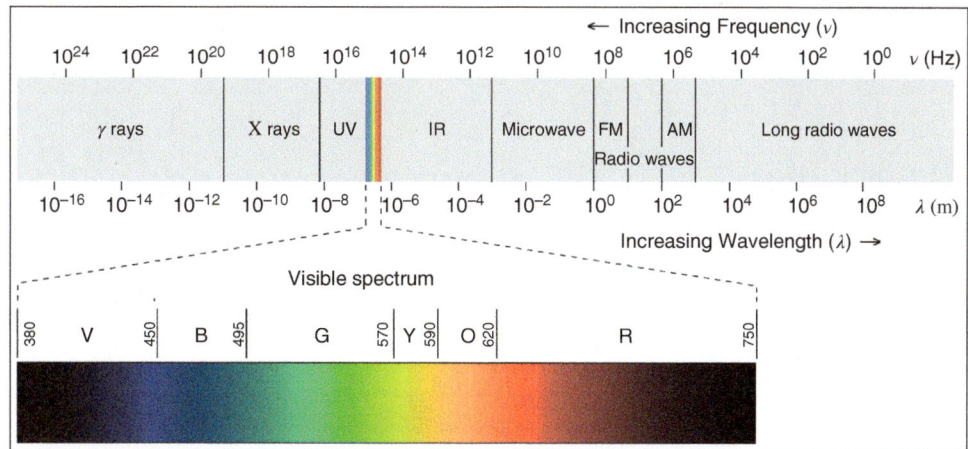

Figure 6.1 A schematic depiction of the distribution of electromagnetic waves with respect to frequency and wavelength, highlighting the visible part of the electromagnetic spectrum. Source: Gringer Phillip Ronan, February 19, 2013, https://upload.wikimedia.org/wikipedia/commons/3/30/EM_spectrumrevised.png.

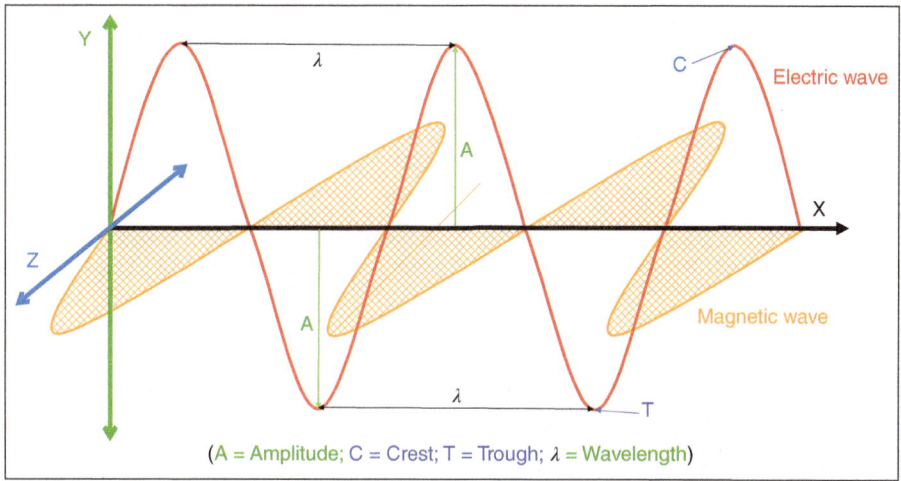

Figure 6.2 A graphical illustration of a light (electromagnetic) wave which contains oscillations of both an electric wave and a magnetic wave vibrating perpendicular to one another. The x-axis represents distance traveled and the propagation direction, the y-axis is the strength of the electric field, and the z-axis is the strength of the magnetic field. Most graphs of light waves contain only the x-axis and y-axis, focusing on the electrical component. The amplitude (A) is the distance from the central axis (equilibrium) to the tip of the crest (C) or trough (T) and is a measure of the energy (strength) carried by the wave. A wavelength (λ) is the distance from one crest or trough to the next crest or trough. The frequency is the number of wavelengths occurring during a set period. Source: Lisa P. McFaddin.

of the Federal Food, Drug, and Cosmetic Act (FFDCA), Subchapter J, Radiological Health (FDA 2023). Laser products used for medical purposes must also comply with medical device regulations established by the FDA Center for Devices and Radiological Health (CDRH) (FDA 2021, 2023).

The CDRH "regulates radiation-emitting electronic products (medical and non-medical) such as lasers, x-ray systems, ultrasound

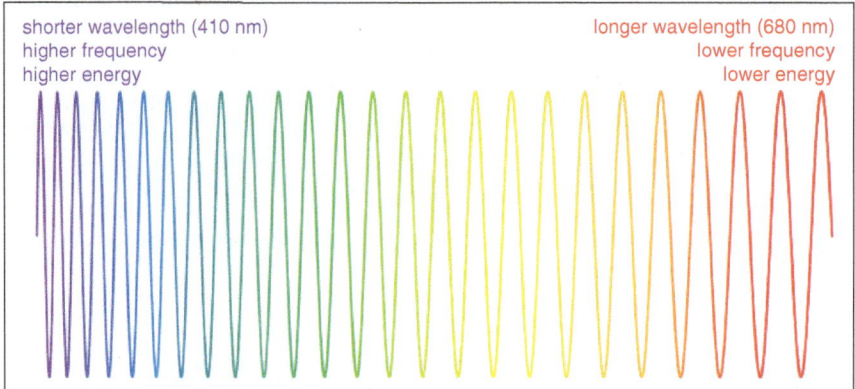

shorter wavelength (410 nm)
higher frequency
higher energy

longer wavelength (680 nm)
lower frequency
lower energy

Figure 6.3   A diagram depicting the differences in wavelength and frequency between the various colors comprising visible light. Violet has the shortest wavelength with the highest frequency, while red has the longest wavelength and shortest frequency. Source: DrSciComm, January 23, 2019, https://commons .wikimedia.org/wiki/File:VisibleWavelengths.png.

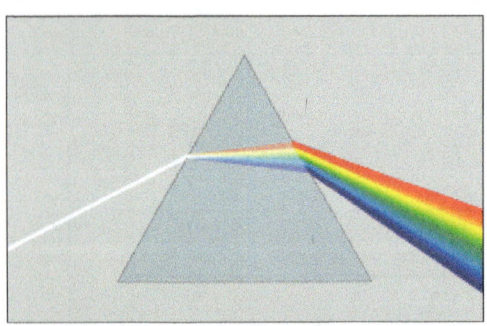

Figure 6.4   Illustration of the dispersion of light through a prism into the colors of the rainbow: red, orange, yellow, green, blue, indigo, and violet. Source: Joanjoc, February 11, 2005, CC BY-SA 3.0, https:// commons.wikimedia.org/w/index.php?curid=57730.

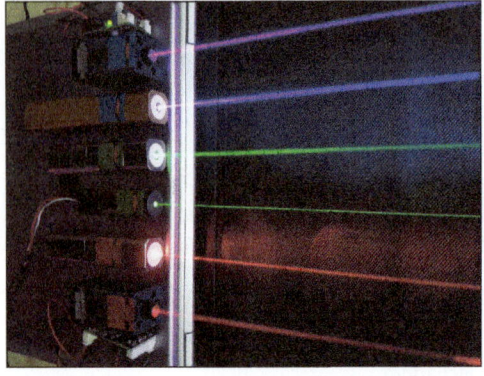

Figure 6.5   Photograph of multiple line lasers. From bottom to top there are two red lasers (635 and 660 nm), two green lasers (520 and 532 nm), and two blue lasers (405 and 445 nm). Source: 彭嘉傑/ Wikimedia Commons/CC BY 2.5.

equipment, microwave ovens and color televisions" (FDA 2022). Manufacturers of lasers used for medical use must comply with the following requirements: establishment registration, medical device listing, premarket notification or approval, investigational device exemption for clinical studies, quality system regulation, labeling requirements, and medical device reporting (FDA 2022).

Table 6.1 The FDA classification system for lasers. A description of each laser's hazard potential and product examples are provided (Harvard 2018; FDA 2021).

Class	Hazard potential	Product example
I	Non-hazardous under normal working conditions. Potential hazard if viewed with optical aids (magnifier, binocular, or telescope)	Laser printers CD players DVD players
II	Relatively low hazard, but hazard potential increases if viewed for prolonged periods of time or with optical aids. Output is $\leq 1\,mV$	Bar code scanners
IIIa	Transient hazard potential if viewed directly without protective eyewear. Risk increases with optical aids. Severity dependent on the power and size of the beam. Output dependent on the color but generally $\leq 5\,mV$	Laser pointers
IIIb	High and immediate hazardous potential to the skin and eyes if exposed to the direct beam. Output between 5 and $500\,mV$	Light show projectors Industrial lasers Research lasers Medical devices
IV	High and immediate hazardous potential to the skin and eyes if exposed to the direct or reflected beam. Possible fire risk. Output $>500\,mV$	Light show projectors Industrial lasers Research lasers Medical Devices

Source: Lisa P. McFaddin.

Lasers are classified based on their potential risk to the user (aka hazard potential), summarized in Table 6.1 (FDA 2021, 2023). Level I, II, and IIa are low risk. They emit very bright lights which trigger a person's natural blink reflex preventing injury because the person cannot stare directly at the beam of light for long periods of time (FDA 2021, 2023). Class IIIa and IIIb are medium-powered lasers, while class IV lasers are considered high-powered lasers. Classes IIIa, IIIb, and IV concentrate energy into a small area, pose a greater risk of thermal burns, and do not elicit a person's natural blink response (FDA 2021, 2023).

The most common lasers used for PBM in human and veterinary medicine are Class III and Class IV, falling within the red and near-infrared spectrum (Heiskanen and Hamblin 2018; Dompe et al. 2020). Refer to the Techniques and Protocols section for further information regarding the use of Class III versus Class IV lasers in veterinary medicine.

Lasers for Veterinarians

Lasers produce an artificial monochromatic, coherent, collimated, and polarized beam of light that is very thin, bright, and focused and which can travel long distances (NASA 2021). A laser is created by exciting electrons in a laser gain medium using light, electricity, or a chemical reaction as the energy source (Heiskanen and Hamblin 2018). A laser gain medium is material (glass, crystal, or gas) which can absorb energy (excite electrons) and amplify light (emit photons). Mirrors are used at either end of the laser cavity to bounce light back and forth, continuously stimulating the laser gain medium, creating more photons (Heiskanen and Hamblin 2018). One of the mirrors is partially reflective, allowing light (the laser beam) to escape the laser cavity, as illustrated in Figure 6.6.

Light-Emitting Diodes

Light-emitting diodes (LEDs) are very small light bulbs without filaments, which use less energy and last longer than traditional

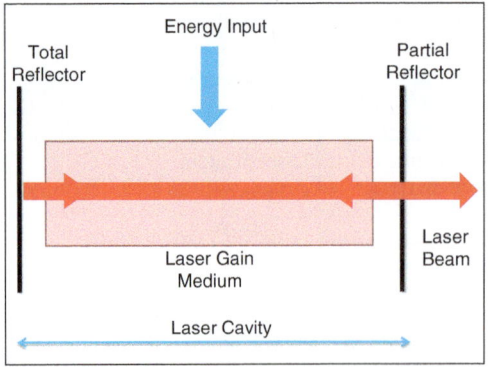

Figure 6.6 A simple schematic of a laser. The laser cavity contains two mirrors and a laser gain medium. One of the mirrors is completely reflective (total reflector) and one is partially reflective (partial reflector). An outside energy source (light, electricity, or chemical reaction) excites the electrons within the laser gain medium. When the electrons return to ground (normal) state, the electrons emit particles of light (photons). The presence of the two mirrors amplifies the light. The partial reflector allows a thin beam of monochromatic light (laser beam) to escape the laser cavity. Source: Lisa P. McFaddin, image adapted from Heiskanen and Hamblin (2018).

incandescent bulbs, and do not produce heat (Heiskanen and Hamblin 2018). LEDs come in a variety of sizes, shapes, and colors, as shown in Figure 6.7.

LEDs produce light through the movement of negative electrons and positive holes inside a semiconductor. Unlike lasers, the light produced by LEDs is not monochromatic and contains more than one frequency (non-coherent) (Heiskanen and Hamblin 2018). The most common LEDs used for PBM in human and veterinary medicine are in the red and near-infrared spectrum (Heiskanen and Hamblin 2018).

LEDs for Veterinarians

LEDs generate an artificial, narrow-spectrum and non-coherent beam of light. Most LEDs used in PBM contain a PIN semiconductor diode (see Figure 6.8). The PIN diode contains three regions: a positive or P-region, a negative or N-region, and an intrinsic layer of high resistivity (I-region) in between (Chung et al. 2012; Heiskanen and Hamblin 2018). Application of an electric potential to the semiconductor causes separation of the electrons in the N-region and holes in the P-region (Chung et al. 2012; Heiskanen and Hamblin 2018). The electrons and holes recombine in the I-region producing non-coherent light (electroluminescence). The wavelength (color) of the light depends on the energy gap and materials in the semiconductor (Chung et al. 2012; Heiskanen and Hamblin 2018). The direction of the electric field is from N to P (Chung et al. 2012; Heiskanen and Hamblin 2018).

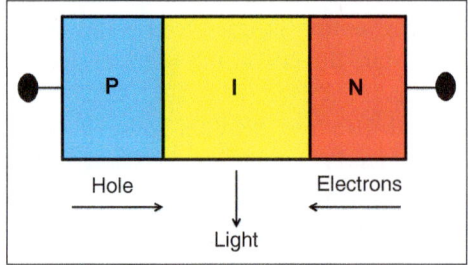

Figure 6.8 A schematic of a simple PN light-emitting diode (LED). The PIN diode contains three regions: a positive or P-region, a negative or N-region, and an intrinsic layer of high resistivity (I-region) in between. Application of an electric potential to the semiconductor causes separation of the electrons in the N-region and holes in the P-region. The electrons and holes recombine in the I-region producing non-coherent light (electroluminescence). Source: Lisa P. McFaddin, image adapted from Heiskanen and Hamblin (2018).

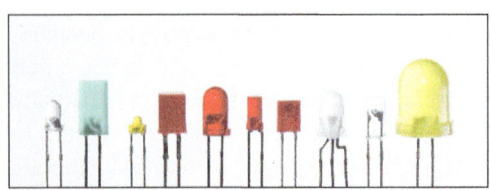

Figure 6.7 Light-emitting diodes (LEDs) come in a variety of colors, shapes, and sizes. The plastic covering is frequently the same color as the light produced. Source: Afrank99/Wikimedia Commons/ CC BY-SA 2.0.

Lasers versus LEDs

PBM is a noninvasive application of light from a low-power light source (typically laser or LED) with the intention of promoting tissue repair, reducing inflammation, and ultimately reducing pain (Chung et al. 2012). LED light has a narrow spectrum of color (not monochromic), is non-coherent (waves do not fully align), and its emissions do not generate heat (Heiskanen and Hamblin 2018). Laser PBM is still the more popular and researched modality in human and veterinary medicine, though practical applications and research into LED PBM has recently been gaining traction (Desmet et al. 2006; Kim and Calderhead 2011).

Photobiophysics and Photochemistry Basics

Background knowledge of photobiophysics and photochemistry are necessary to understand the theory and practical applications of PBM. Photobiophysics is a branch of biophysics (uses physics to understand biological systems) studying how light interacts with biological systems, while photochemistry is a branch of chemistry exploring the chemical effects of light (Reusch 2013).

The First Law of Photochemistry (aka the Grotthuss–Draper Law) states "light must be absorbed by a compound in order for a photochemical reaction to take place" (Reusch 2013). A photochemical reaction is a process involving the rearranging of molecules initiated by the absorption of energy in the form of light (Reusch 2013).

Within the body the compounds absorbing light are photoacceptors and chromophores (Sineshchekov 1995). Photoacceptors are technically a type of chromophore. They are pigments that use light (photons) as the first step in a photochemical reaction (Sineshchekov 1995). Chromophores are endogenous (originating within the body) or exogenous (originating outside of the body) materials which contribute to the color of a substance through the absorption of specific wavelengths of light (Sineshchekov 1995). Examples of endogenous chromophores include melanin, hemoglobin, protein, and bilirubin (Patil and Dhami 2008). Tattoo ink is an example of an exogenous chromophore.

Particles of light (photons) hitting the surface of the skin, and other tissue layers, can be reflected, transmitted, scattered, or absorbed, as illustrated in Figure 6.9 (Dederich 1991). During reflection the light bounces off the contact surface. Transmission is the passage of the laser beam through a substance without interacting (reflecting, scattering, or absorbing) with any of the molecules. Scattering occurs when photons deviate from their unidirectional path after striking an obstacle, such as molecules, organelles, cells, and collagen fibers (Patil and Dhami 2008). Scattering negatively affects absorption and how deep the laser beam can penetrate the tissue.

Only absorbed photons can produce an effect, according to the First Law of Photochemistry (Sutherland 2002). Absorbed photons can cause thermal, mechanical, and/or chemical changes to the chromophores (Patil and Dhami 2008).

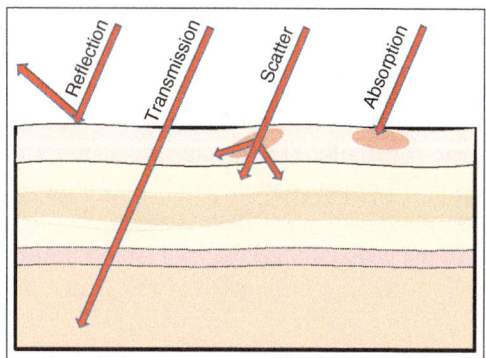

Figure 6.9 A schematic representation of the four possible outcomes during laser–tissue interaction: reflection, transmission, scatter, and absorption. Reflection and transmission do not contribute to the beneficial effects of PBM. Scatter reduces the depth of penetration but may increase absorption. Absorption is responsible for PBM's beneficial effects. Source: Lisa P. McFaddin.

Tissue Interaction for Veterinarians

Reflection and transmission are undesired effects. Reflection occurs when the beam passes between different media, such as glass, air, water, and even the surface of the skin (Patil and Dhami 2008). The photons bounce off the surface without penetrating or causing a biological effect (Fekrazad et al. 2011). The angle of reflection is opposite to that of the incident (emitted) wave. Light reflection, from the hair and skin, can be reduced by holding the probe as close to the skin as possible (Zein et al. 2018).

Transmission occurs in the absence of chromophores allowing all photons to pass through tissues without causing a photochemical reaction. Total transmission is the passage of the laser beam through the tissue without producing an effect (Patil and Dhami 2008). The wavelength of light and the type of target chromophores and photoacceptors affect the degree of transmission.

Scattering can have beneficial and negative effects. Scatter occurs when the laser beam passes through a non-homogeneous substance containing multiple size molecules, such as skin and its underlying tissues, causing the light wave to change direction (Fekrazad et al. 2011). The degree of scatter is dependent on the size of the molecules and wavelength of the laser (Patil and Dhami 2008). Longer wavelengths are less affected by scatter, while shorter wavelengths experience greater scatter (Wang et al. 1995). Scatter negatively affects tissue penetration (the greater the scatter, the less depth of penetration) but it may increase absorption (Patil and Dhami 2008).

Tissue penetration is dictated by absorption and scatter due to molecules and structures within the tissues (i.e. tissue type) (Wang et al. 1995). Peak penetration has been documented at the near-infrared (NIR) wavelength of 810 nm (Wang et al. 1995). Longer wavelengths are absorbed by water molecules which reduces tissue penetration (Wang et al. 1995). Tissue penetration contributes to the light source's potency and frequently the efficacy (Wang et al. 1995).

Multiple studies have shown lengthening the wavelength improves tissue penetration and clinical response up to a point, but beyond the maximal value the beneficial effects cease, and negative or inhibitory effects may be seen (Huang et al. 2011; Hamblin 2017). This "biphasic dose response" suggests there is an optimal dose or energy density (described as joules per centimeter squared or J/cm^2) for PBM (Huang et al. 2011).

Lasers versus LEDs

The superiority of lasers compared to LEDs and other forms of low-level light therapy (LLLT) is hotly contested. The basis of the argument boils down to coherence and tissue penetration. Laser light is coherent, meaning the waves have a fixed phase and frequency (Heiskanen and Hamblin 2018). Coherent laser light interacts with tissue differently than non-coherent light. Small imperfections in tissues cause interference patterns in laser light (aka "laser speckles") which more effectively interact with cellular components, specifically the mitochondria (Heiskanen and Hamblin 2018).

Lasers have greater tissue penetration (i.e. how deep into the body the laser light travels) compared to LEDs. Laser light is also well collimated, so the light beams do not diverge when traveling long distances. This means laser light can be focused on a specific area of the body.

Both lasers and LLLT have shown beneficial effects in human and veterinary medicine. At present there are more data available on the positive uses of lasers compared to other forms of light therapy. This is not to say LLLT does not have its place, but a majority of the PBM information available in veterinary medicine centers around lasers.

Parameters

There are several parameters to consider before purchasing a laser, planning a treatment protocol, or operating a laser. These factors include wavelength, power, dose, treatment time, and

Table 6.2 Important factors to keep in mind when working with therapeutic lasers in veterinary medicine.

Parameter	Description
Wavelength	• Distance between the peaks of a wave, usually measured in nanometers (nm) • Typically, wavelengths fall between 600 and 1000 nm (red and near-infrared spectrum) • **Determines the depth of tissue penetration** • Shorter wavelengths (600–700 nm) are used to treat superficial tissues and longer wavelengths (780–950 nm) are used for deeper tissues
Power	• Rate at which energy is delivered, expressed in watts (W) or milliwatts (mW) • **Determines treatment length** • 1 W equals 1 joule per second: 1 W = 1 J/s • Lower watt lasers (Class III, <500 mW) are best suited for superficial tissues, and higher watt lasers (Class IV, >500 mW) are typically used for conditions affecting deeper tissues • Refer to Figures 6.11 and 6.12 for examples of a Class IIIb and Class IV laser, respectively
Dose	• Laser's energy measured in joules (J) • Expressed as the amount of energy delivered over a surface area (J/cm²) • Range is dependent on the condition being treated, typically between 2 and 10 J/cm²
Treatment time	• Length of the treatment, measured in seconds
Treatment interval	• Length of time between treatments • Varies by condition: days to weeks • Effects are cumulative

treatment intervals. A brief explanation of each is provided in Table 6.2.

PBM Parameters for Veterinarians

The source of the light and dose are crucial to the efficacy and safety of PBM. The PBM parameters can be divided into the irradiation parameters and the dosage parameters, as shown in Figure 6.10. Irradiation parameters include wavelength, power, irradiance, frequency, pulse structure, cohesion, and polarization. Dosage parameters include energy, energy density, irradiation time, and treatment interval. Many researchers refer to the irradiation parameters as "the medicine" and the irradiation time as "the dose" (Chung et al. 2012; de Freitas and Hamblin 2016). Most veterinary PBM references refer to the energy density as "the dose."

Irradiation Parameters

Wavelength Most veterinary therapeutic lasers emit red (600–700 nm) or NIR (770–1000 nm) (Godbold 2014; Hamblin 2017; Fessehav 2020). Blue and green light have poor tissue penetration and are not typically used (Hamblin 2016); 600–1200 nm are the most common wavelengths used in veterinary medicine (Godbold 2014; Fessehav 2020). Photons in this portion of the NIR spectrum have better tissue penetration due to reduced absorption by water and non-targeted chromophores (Chung et al. 2012). Ultraviolet light (100–400 nm) is generally absorbed by melanin

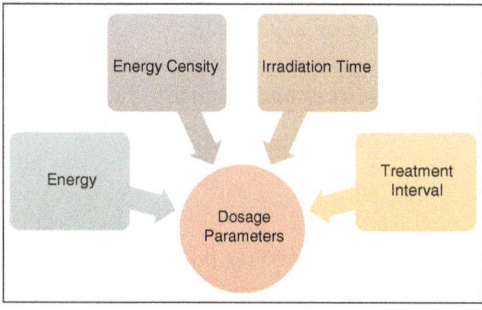

Figure 6.10 An algorithmic breakdown of the irradiation and dosage parameters in photobiomodulation. Source: Lisa P. McFaddin.

and proteins, while water absorbs light at the higher end of the spectrum (1400–10 000 nm) (Fessehav 2020).

Shorter wavelengths (600–700 nm) are used most often to treat superficial tissue injury (Zein et al. 2018). Helium–neon (HeNe) laser diodes produce wavelengths between 632 and 650 nm which can penetrate tissues 0.8–15 mm deep (Hagler 2019). Longer wavelengths (780–950 nm) are used to treat deeper tissues (Zein et al. 2018). Gallium arsenide (GaAs) and gallium aluminum arsenide (GaAlAs) diodes produce wavelengths between 820 and 904 nm which can penetrate tissues 10 mm to 5 cm deep (Hagler 2019).

Interestingly, PBM using wavelengths between 700 and 770 nm have not been found to produce beneficial effects (Karu 2010). The combination of multiple wavelengths during a particular PBMT is believed to increase its therapeutic effect, though definitive evidence supporting this claim is lacking (Zein et al. 2018).

Power   Power is the rate at which energy is generated or consumed. With respect to PBM, power is expressed in watts (W) or milliwatts (mW) (Chung et al. 2012). One watt equals one joule per second.

The lower the wattage, the longer the treatment time needed to penetrate deeper tissues (Downing 2017). Class III lasers are most used for superficial wounds due to their lower power (<500 mW) (Godbold 2014). Long treatment times are necessary when Class III lasers are used to treat musculoskeletal or deeper tissue conditions. Figure 6.11 depicts one model of a Class IIIb laser used in veterinary medicine.

Class IV lasers are most used to treat conditions affecting musculoskeletal and deep tissue conditions (Godbold 2014). Figure 6.12 depicts one model of a Class IV laser used in veterinary medicine.

Irradiance   Irradiance, also known as power density, is defined as the power divided by the spot size (Chung et al. 2012). Laser beams

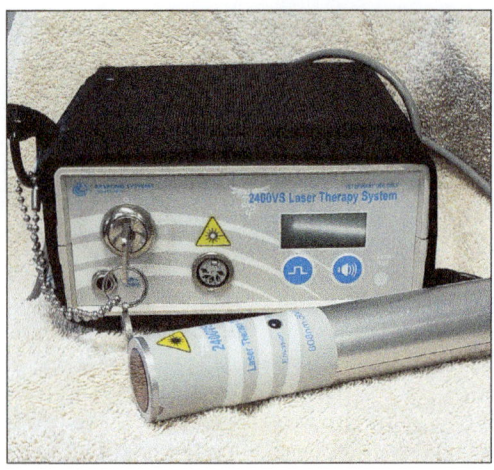

Figure 6.11   Example of a Class IIIb laser used in veterinary medicine. Source: Lisa P. McFaddin.

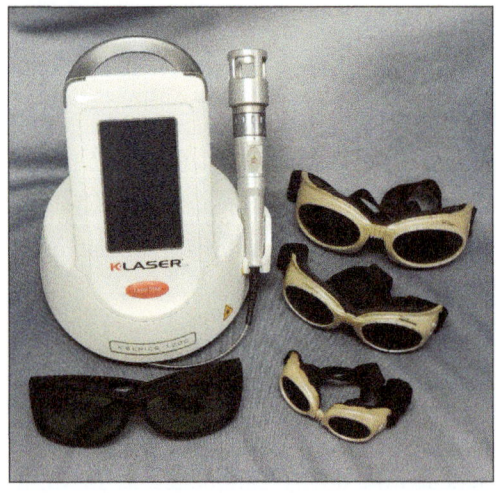

Figure 6.12   Example of a Class IV laser used in veterinary medicine. Source: Lisa P. McFaddin.

typically take on a Gaussian shape (think Bell curve) with peak irradiance in the center and decreases in irradiance farther from the center (Chung et al. 2012). Irradiance in the tail end increases as power increases (de Freitas and Hamblin 2016).

Frequency   Frequency is the number of times a laser pulses in one second, measured in Hertz (Hz) (Chung et al. 2012). Lower frequencies are typically used to treat acute conditions and wounds, while higher frequencies are used for chronic conditions and pain.

Some researchers recommend using pulsed frequency, in which the emission of laser photons is turned on and off depending on the body's biological responses, over traditional continuous wave emissions (Gaynor 2015). The applicability and efficacy of this approach is still up for debate.

Pulse Structure The pulse structure, also known as the emission mode or delivery system, can be categorized as a continuous wave (CW) or pulsed wave (PW). The pulse structure comprises the power (W), pulse frequency (Hz), pulse width (seconds), and duty cycle (a percentage) (Chung et al. 2012; de Freitas and Hamblin 2016). The peak power is measured in non-pulsed beams (CW), while the average power is calculated in pulsed beams (PW) (Chung et al. 2012; de Freitas and Hamblin 2016).

PW appears superior when used for the treatment of wound healing, and stroke management in people, while studies suggest CW is more effective for nerve regeneration in people (Hashmi et al. 2010). There is limited research comparing the efficacy of CW versus PW in veterinary medicine. One study by Kampa et al. (2020) found an 830 nm low-intensity laser had a higher mean output power, and deeper tissue penetration, in CW compared to PW when used on live canine tissue.

The selected pulse structure may be dependent on the ability of the laser being used and the condition being treated. Pre-programmed laser treatments, i.e. those created by the manufacturer, often use both CW and PW. A mixture of both pulse structures may be beneficial in stimulating different cell types during any given treatment, though further research is needed (Hashmi et al. 2010; Zein et al. 2018).

Coherence Laser beams have high coherence (i.e. a narrow spectral bandwidth), while LEDs are non-coherent but still have a narrow bandwidth (de Freitas and Hamblin 2016). Coherent light can produce laser speckle which appears to be a factor in PBM's effect on cells and subcellular organelles (Chung et al. 2012). The laser speckle pattern determines with what substances the laser will interact (Chung et al. 2012).

Polarization Both linear and circular polarization can affect scattering in tissue, but this property is often ignored when discussing the effects of PBM (de Freitas and Hamblin 2016).

Dose Parameters

Energy Measured in joules (J) and determined by power (W) multiplied by time (s) (de Freitas and Hamblin 2016). This is often used to describe the dose, but it ignores the relationship between irradiance and time (Chung et al. 2012).

Energy Density Defined as J/cm^2. This is most often referred to as "the dose" in veterinary PBM. Before determining the dose, the practitioner must know the goal of the treatment (analgesia, anti-inflammatory, wound healing, etc.), duration of the condition (acute vs. chronic), tissue depth (superficial or deep), and tissue type (skin, muscle, tendon, ligament, or bone) (Brunke 2018). There is no official consensus amongst veterinarians regarding the optimal dosage for specific disease conditions. There are numerous treatment tables available with guideline dose ranges for specific conditions. Table 6.3 combines a number of these references into one summary table.

Some sources recommend $2–6 J/cm^2$ for issues affecting superficial tissues and $6–12 J/cm^2$ for conditions affecting deeper tissues (Gaynor 2015). As a rule, most veterinary conditions can be treated with a dose of $1–15 J/cm^2$ (Hagler 2019). Chronic deep-seated conditions, such as lick granulomas, may require $15–20 J/cm^2$ (Johnson 2016). Other sources suggest using a non-contact method, with $2–8 J/cm^2$ for most wounds and $1–3 J/cm^2$ for postsurgical wounds recommended once daily for 7–10 days (Hagler 2019). The highest dose ($30–40 J/cm^2$) is recommended for the management of degenerative myelopathy (Miller et al. 2020).

Table 6.3 Veterinarian PBM energy density (or dose) recommendations based on the condition being treated (Mills and Gross 2014; Looney et al. 2018; Lopez and Brundage 2019; Wardlaw et al. 2019; Miller et al. 2020; Alves et al. 2022b).

Condition	Recommended energy density	
	Acute (J/cm^2)	Chronic (J/cm^2)
Arthralgia	4–6	4–8
Anti-inflammatory	1–6	4–8
Degenerative myelopathy	n/a	30–40
Intervertebral disk disease	4–6	4–6
Myalgia	2–4	4–8
Open wound	2–6	2–8
Osteoarthritis	n/a	8–10
Postoperative wound	1–3	n/a
Trigger points	10	10

Source: Lisa P. McFaddin.

Irradiation (Treatment) Time The irradiation or treatment time is expressed in seconds. Confusingly, this is often referred to as "the dose" for the PBM treatment. The required treatment time is dependent on the output power of the laser and the desired dose. To provide 1 J of energy from a laser emitting 500 mW the probe would need to be held in place for two seconds (Millis et al. 2005). To manually calculate the treatment time, multiply the relative area to be treated (in cm^2) by the desired dose (J/cm^2) and divide by the wattage (W) (Chung et al. 2012). Depending on the type of laser used the treatment time can be used as a guideline for how long the probe is moved in a pattern over the affected area or for point-to-point lasers how long the probe is held over each point. While most laser units have software with pre-programmed treatment time, the practitioner should still be able to calculate the treatment time, especially for specific non-programmed conditions.

Treatment Time Calculation

- Treatment size: size of a notecard (100 cm^2)

- Condition being treated: chronic inflammation

- Dose: 4 J/cm^2

- Power: Class IV laser with 4 W = 4 J/s

$$4\,J\,/\,cm^2 \times 100\,cm^2 = 400\,J$$

$$400\,J \div 4\,J\,/\,s = \mathbf{100\,s}$$

- Point-to-point laser: 100 cm^2 can be divided into 12 points = **~8 s/point**

Treatment Interval The length of time between treatments is highly condition and practitioner dependent. Further research is needed to determine the most beneficial treatment intervals for various conditions. Treatments may be performed daily, multiple times a week, weekly, every other week, every few weeks, or as needed. There is a cumulative effect with PBM, so in theory the closer together the treatments the sooner results should be seen.

Techniques and Protocols

Laser Probes
Different probes are available depending on the company and class of laser chosen. Probes are usually classified by their treatment diameter and the number of diodes. The treatment diameter refers to the size of the laser beam which correlates to the area of tissue being treated. The treatment area for most cold lasers is between that of a quarter (1.9 cm or 0.75 inch) and a silver dollar (2.65 cm or roughly 1 inch) (ColdLasers.org 2021). Lasers used for acupuncture or trigger point therapy have a much smaller beam and treatment diameter, allowing the delivery of laser photons to a very specific area. The probe may contain a single diode applicator or clusters of diodes.

The use of contact versus non-contact techniques and probes is based on the power of the laser. High-powered lasers typically use non-contact techniques as there is a greater potential of overheating the target tissues.

Delivery Mode

The two most common methods of laser light emission are CW and PW. CW emits light constantly until stopped – think turning on a light switch and walking away. PW emits light in a series of pulses – think repeatedly turning a light switch on and off. The pulse rate refers to the number of pulses per second, expressed as Hertz (Hz) (Godbold 2014).

Both CW and PW PBM can be effective. CW is best for delivering high amounts of laser photons to tissues quickly and is most often used to treat painful conditions (ColdLasers.org 2021). PW increases the treatment time because of the break between each pulse and is typically used for tissue healing and reducing inflammation (ColdLasers.org 2021). There are multiple types of pulsed lasers defined by their pulse repetition rates, energy density, durations, and mechanisms used to generate light in a pulsed manner (Hashmi et al. 2010). Superpulsed is the most common form. Superpulsed lasers generate very short pulses of laser energy, theoretically allowing deeper tissue penetration while limiting thermal tissue damage (Hashmi et al. 2010). Many pre-programmed laser protocols consist of a combination of CW and PW.

Techniques

For point-to-point laser units the desired treatment area is divided into a specific number of points. Usually, a treatment area is described in relation to a business card ($50\,cm^2$), credit card ($75\,cm^2$), or a notecard ($100\,cm^2$). The number of points per area is dependent on the size of the probe, but six points per $50\,cm^2$ is common. The probe is held in place, either above or touching the hair/skin, for a set period of time (seconds) depending on the treatment length.

Non-point-to-point units require continuous movement throughout the treatment period.

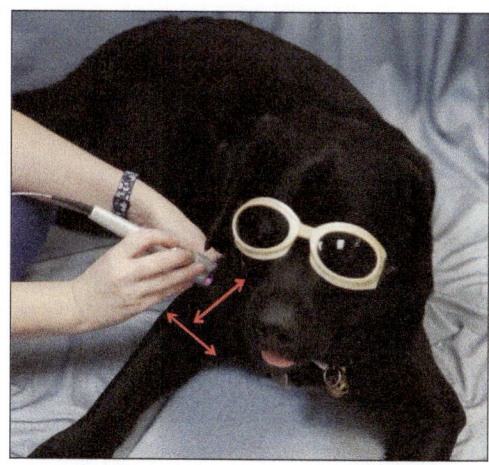

Figure 6.13 Demonstration of a gridding technique over the right elbow. The probe is slowly moved up and down, as well as side to side. The probe should be held perpendicular (90° angle) to the area being treated. Note the proper use of personal protective goggles for the patient. Source: Lisa P. McFaddin.

The two most described techniques include gridding and surrounding. In gridding, the area being treated is visually divided into smaller sections (approximately the size of the probe), and the probe is moved in a slow grid pattern (back and forth; up and down) over the entire area throughout the treatment interval (Figure 6.13). The technique ensures each section receives adequate laser photon exposure.

With the surrounding technique, the probe is slowly moved around the area of interest, as seen in Figure 6.14. This is most often used for wound healing and involves treating only the periphery of the wound (Niebaum 2013). With both gridding and surrounding the probe should be moved slowly enough to ensure each area receives an adequate number of photons but not long enough to cause thermal injury.

Regardless of the technique used, proper positioning is critical to a successful outcome. The probe must be held perpendicular (90° angle) to the target tissue (Brunke 2018). The 90° angle reduces reflection and scatter, maximizing tissue penetration (Dycus 2014).

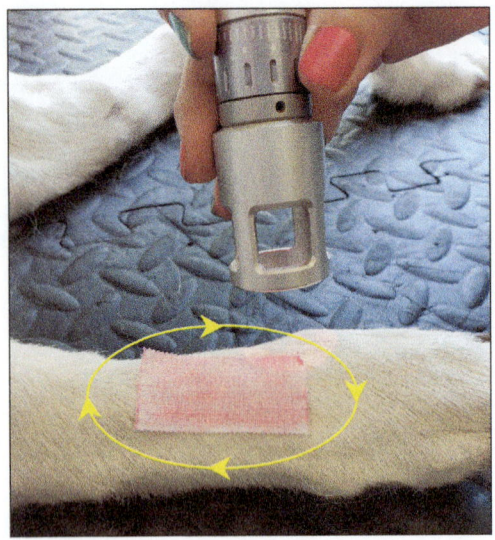

Figure 6.14 Demonstration of a surrounding technique on a wound. The wound is represented by the colored tape. The probe is slowly moved around the lesion. Note the probe is held perpendicular (90° angle) to the treatment area. Source: Lisa P. McFaddin.

Class III lasers often require the handpiece make direct contact with the skin throughout the duration of the treatment (Hagler 2019). Class IV lasers do not require direct contact delivery, but specific adaptors or handpieces may be available from the manufacturer allowing direct contact with the skin.

Between 50 and 99% of laser photons can be absorbed by animal hair (Niebaum 2013). Shaving, trimming, or parting the fur may be necessary depending on the patient's coat and desired treatment area (Hagler 2019; Hochman-Elam et al. 2020). Darker hair and skin absorb more photons. Increased movement of the probe may be required over areas with darker pigmentation to avoid excessive heating (Hagler 2019; Hochman-Elam et al. 2020). The presence of topical medications and solutions can increase systemic absorption and cause overheating of the skin (Niebaum 2013; Hagler 2019). These solutions and ointments should be removed before the application of PBM.

Some practitioners recommend icing the target area for 5–10 minutes before performing PBM (Rivera 2022). The primary physiologic effects of cryotherapy (icing) are vasoconstriction (narrowing of blood vessels) and reduction of inflammation (Ciolek 1985). This transient vasoconstriction decreases the amount of vascular protein and red blood cells delivered to a specific area (Johnson and Kellogg 2010). Red blood cells contain hemoglobin which, along with water and protein, are some of the most common chromophores (Prohaska and Hohman 2022). Thus, a reduction in blood supply can improve absorption of laser photons by the target tissue (Haslerud et al. 2017).

A new and novel PBM technique involving the application of a fluorescence light energy system has caught the attention of veterinarians. A topical photoconverter hydrogel is applied directly to the skin, and a blue light is used to activate the gel generating fluorescence (Marchegiani et al. 2019). The applied substance delivers fluorescent light energy to the target tissue without generating heat, and without being absorbed by the target tissue (Marchegiani et al. 2019). Most studies have been conducted *in vitro*, but a few *in vivo* veterinary studies have evaluated its use in the treatment of veterinary dermatologic conditions (Marchegiani et al. 2019, 2020, 2022). Further research is necessary to confirm the validity, efficacy, and practicality of this exciting emerging science.

Protocol

The treatment protocol is typically based on the condition being treated, the patient size, the skin and coat color, and the owner availability and compliance. Ultimately the veterinarian is responsible for determining the treatment protocol. Factors to consider when developing a treatment protocol should include the size of the treatment area, desired dose, treatment intervals, tissue safety, and post-treatment considerations.

Treatment Area

Unless PBM is being used for laser acupuncture, the treatment area should include the target tissue and the tissue immediately surrounding it. When treating wounds, the affected skin and healthy skin should be treated (Johnson 2016). Spinal cord injuries (surgical and non-surgical cases) should include the site of injury, two spinal cord segments above and below, and the surrounding paraspinal muscles (Gross 2014).

Dose

Almost all veterinary therapeutic lasers have software with pre-programmed protocols for the treatment of specific conditions. Depending on the age of the software, the user can often input at least some patient-specific information such as species, patient size, size and location of the target area or tissue, skin and coat color, and coat length (Godbold 2014). The veterinarian can also manually adjust the power and/or energy density (and as a result treatment time). The end goal is to maximize tissue penetration and treatment efficacy. Refer to Table 6.3 for veterinary-specific PBM energy density (dose) recommendations.

Treatment Intervals

Session frequency is highly practitioner, patient condition, and owner dependent. Daily to every other day treatments for one to three sessions are typically recommended for acute musculoskeletal conditions (Johnson 2016). For chronic musculoskeletal conditions daily to every other day sessions are suggested for the first week followed by treatments two to three times a week until symptoms resolve (Johnson 2016).

Quite often, postsurgical PBMT is performed as a single treatment immediately following surgery. Daily treatments are recommended for acute spinal cord conditions, including postoperative, throughout hospitalization (Hagler 2019). Treatments two to three times a week for four to six weeks are recommended for chronic spinal cord conditions (Hagler 2019).

Always remember the treatment intervals are based on owner compliance. If an owner cannot commit to daily treatments an alternative, yet still beneficial, PBM protocol should

be utilized. Open communication with the client regarding the pros and cons of augmented treatment schedules should be discussed.

Patient Restraint

Most patients enjoy, or at the very least tolerate, PBM treatments. PBM treatments can be described to clients as a "gentle warming sensation." This should be a positive experience. PBMT should be performed in a quiet setting with limited distraction and traffic. Minimal restraint is generally utilized. Pets who are wiggling too much may not receive the proper treatment and are at a higher risk of inadvertent ocular exposure to the laser by either scatter or direct transmission. Food can be a great distraction, especially for our canine patients, to help keep them still. Unless the hospital has a policy prohibiting it, having the client present may help keep the pet calm and still.

Occasionally patients dislike the beeping associated with a running laser, but this sound effect can usually be turned down or off. Though very uncommon, patients who will not tolerate eye coverings may need light sedation, especially when using the laser around the head. Use of sedation is at the veterinarian's discretion.

Patients, especially cats, may need to reposition themselves mid-treatment. Patience is necessary to ensure patients are calm and comfortable, and that proper probe positioning and scanning methods are utilized throughout the session. PBM on cats may need to be performed in the cat carrier, without the lid. Cats and small dogs may need to remain in their owner's laps throughout the treatment.

Safety

Refer to the Safety section of this chapter for information.

Post-Treatment Considerations

Patients with chronic sources of pain feel relief within 24–48 hours of treatment. Owners may need to be reminded to limit their pet's exercise for the first 24 hours to avoid overexertion and injury (Niebaum 2013). In rare instances patients may have a transient increase in their level of pain. The exact mechanism of action is unknown, but fortunately the pain appears to self-resolve within 48 hours (Niebaum 2013; Hagler 2019). Uncommonly patients may feel more tired or lethargic for up to 48 hours after treatment (Niebaum 2013).

Clients often want to know how they can tell PBMT is helping. Monitoring clinical improvement is dependent on the condition being treated. Progression of wound healing is relatively easy to benchmark, while the response for chronic musculoskeletal injuries may be more subtle. Clients should be instructed on what variables to look out for, including pain reduction, mood improvement, energy increase, lameness reduction or resolution, increased play, and behavior changes (e.g. sleeping on the couch or bed again).

Mechanisms of Action

The MOA are complex, multifaceted, and the full extent is not yet understood. For ease of explanation this chapter identifies two methods for understanding PBM's MOA: physiologic effects and therapeutic effects.

- *Physiologic MOA*: The interaction of light with damaged or diseased tissue causes changes at the molecular, cellular, and tissue level (Cheng et al. 2021). There is an initial interaction between light and cellular photoacceptors causing the activation of secondary mediators leading to changes in cell signaling, cellular metabolism, protein secretion, and shifts in gene expression (Heiskanen and Hamblin 2018). The result is the increased production of energy in the form of adenosine triphosphate (ATP), restoration of normal cell function, an increase in local circulation, a reduction of acute inflammation, a reduction of acute and chronic pain, an acceleration of wound healing, and an improvement in tissue regeneration (de Freitas and Hamblin 2016). Figure 6.15 summarizes the complex chain of physiologic reactions induced by PBM.
- *Therapeutic effects*: PBM has four major biological or therapeutic effects: pain reduction (analgesia), anti-inflammatory, immune-modulation, and aids tissue healing and regeneration, summarized in Figure 6.16 (Arany 2016).

Physiologic MOA for Veterinarians

There are an overwhelming number of interconnected factors and pathways which play into PBM's MOA. The complete mechanism is still not fully understood. For organizational purposes the mechanisms are categorized by their molecular, cellular, and tissue effects, outlined in Figure 6.17 (de Freitas and Hamblin 2016).

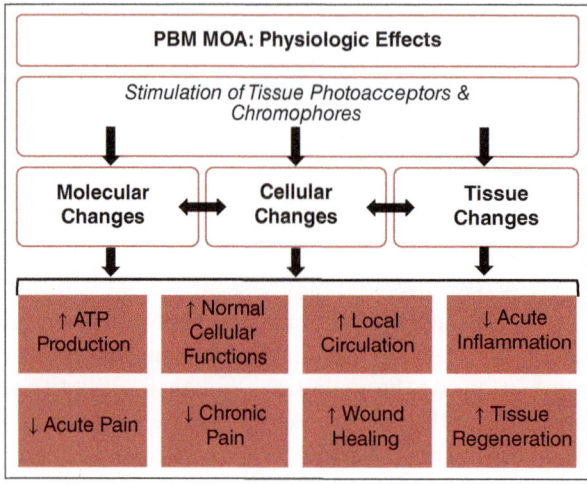

Figure 6.15 A summary of the multiple mechanisms of action involved in PBM when examining its physiologic effects. Therapeutic use of a monochromatic, coherent, collimated, and polarized laser stimulates photoaccceptors and chromophores within the tissues and cells causing effects at the molecular, cellular, and tissue level leading to a host of beneficial responses. Source: Lisa P. McFaddin.

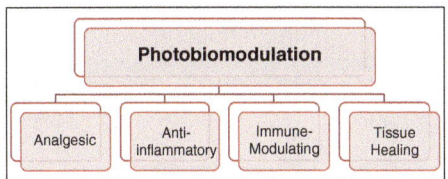

Figure 6.16 The four main biological effects (therapeutic mechanisms) seen following PBM therapy. Source: Lisa P. McFaddin.

Molecular Mechanisms
The primary categories of molecules involved in PBM include chromophores, signaling molecules, transcription factors, and effector molecules.

Chromophores Endogenous chromophores contribute color to a cell or tissue (Patil and Dhami 2008). The primary chromophores involved in the photochemistry and photobiology of PBM include cytochrome C oxidase, retrograde mitochondrial signaling, light-sensitive ion channels, and direct cell-free light-mediated effects on molecules, summarized in Table 6.4 (de Freitas and Hamblin 2016).

Cytochrome C Oxidase Mitochondria, known as the "powerhouse" of the cell, are highly dynamic organelles responsible for maintaining cellular homeostasis through the

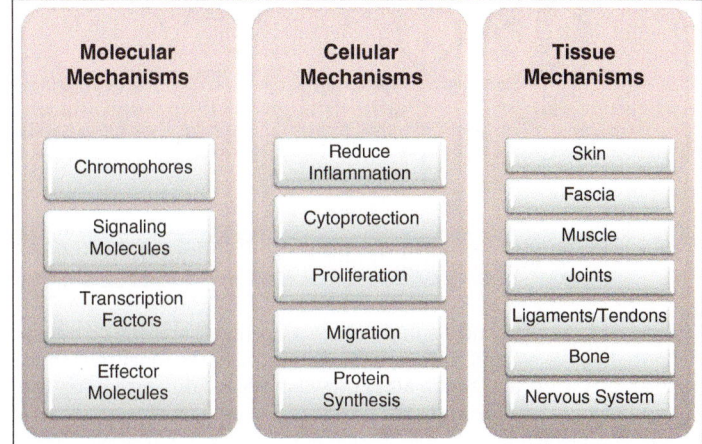

Figure 6.17 An algorithmic breakdown of the physiologic mechanisms of action involved in PBM. Source: Lisa P. McFaddin.

Table 6.4 Summary of the most common chromophores affected by PBM.

Name	Biological effects	Beneficial effects with PBM
CCO	Increases production of MMP, ATP, cAMP, and NO Regulates ROS production Increased CI, CII, and CIII activity	Increases mitochondrial energy production Increases mitochondrial metabolism
RMS	Adaptive response triggered by changes in cellular metabolism and intracellular calcium	Increases mitochondrial energy production Increases mitochondrial metabolism Stimulates protein synthesis Triggers gene upregulation
LSIC	Nonselective permeabilization of the cell membrane to calcium, sodium, and magnesium	± Contribute to laser-induced mast cell activation
Cell-free	TGF-β and Cu-Zn-SOD	Unknown

ATP, adenosine triphosphate; cAMP, cyclic adenosine monophosphate; CI, complex I of the METC; CII, complex II of the METC; CIII, complex III of the METC; CCO, cytochrome C oxidase; Cu-Zn-SOD, copper/zinc superoxide dismutase; LSIC, light sensitive ion channels; METC, mitochondrial electron transport chain; MMP, mitochondrial membrane potential; ROS, reactive oxygen species; RMS, retrograde mitochondrial signaling; TGF-β, transforming growth factor beta. Source: Lisa P. McFaddin.

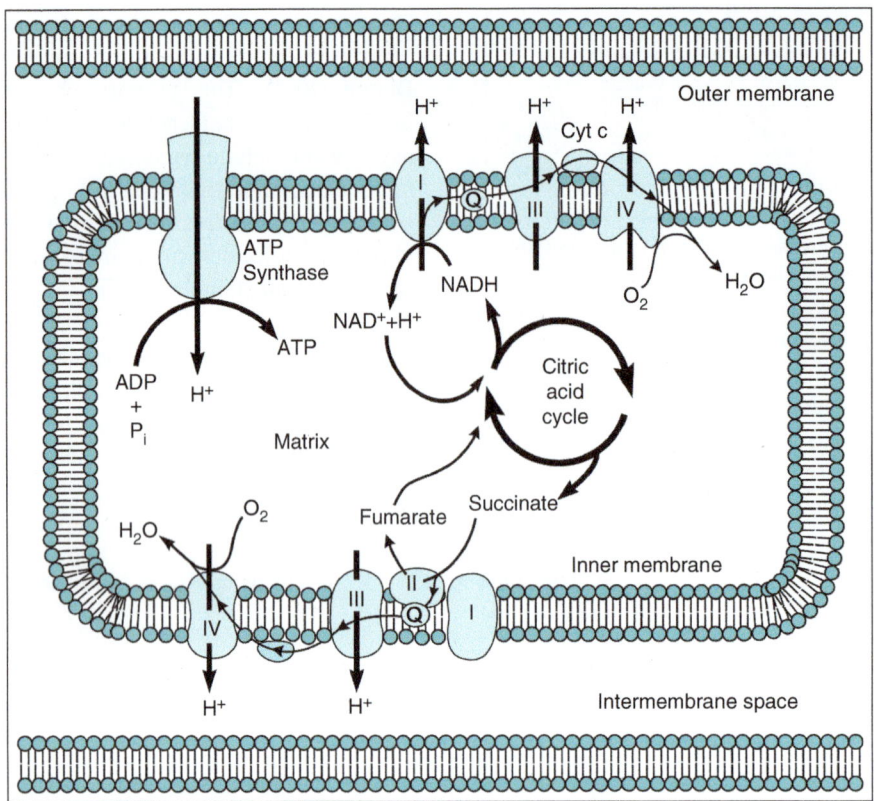

Figure 6.18 A schematic diagraph of the mitochondrial electron transport chain (METC). The METC is composed of five protein complexes (I–V) located in the inner mitochondrial membrane. The catabolism of glucose, fatty acids, and amino acids provides molecules which enter the tricarboxylic acid (TCA) cycle. The TCA cycle generates substrates for the METC, including nicotinamide adenine dinucleotide plus a hydrogen (NADH) and flavin adenine dinucleotide plus two hydrogens (FADH$_2$). NADH and FADH$_2$ each donate a pair of electrons to the METC though Complexes I and II, respectively. A pair of electrons from either Complex I or II is used to reduce ubiquinone (Q) to ubiquinol (QH$_2$). Complex III oxidizes QH$_2$ sending one electron to cytochrome C (Complex IV). For every electron cytochrome C receives, two protons (H$^+$) are pumped into the intermembrane space (IMS). Oxygen serves as a terminal electron acceptor, and is reduced to water, at Complex IV. Four electrons are required to reduce oxygen into water. This should cause four protons to be pumped into the IMS, but two protons are consumed. Only two H$^+$ are pumped into the IMS. The movement of protons creates the mitochondrial membrane potential which dissipates when H$^+$ reenters the mitochondrial matrix through Complex V (not labeled). This movement is coupled by the production of adenosine triphosphate (ATP) from adenosine diphosphate (ADP) (Nolfi-Donegan et al. 2020). Source: Fvasconcellos 22:35 September 9, 2007, https://commons.wikimedia.org/wiki/File:Mitochondrial_electron_transport_chain%E2%80%94Etc4.svg.

production of ATP and low levels of reactive oxygen species (ROS) (Siekevitz 1957; Nolfi-Donegan et al. 2020). The mitochondrial electron transport chain (METC) generates cellular ATP and ROS through oxdative phosphorylation using a series of electron transport reactions (Nolfi-Donegan et al. 2020). An in-depth review of the METC is beyond the scope of this chapter. Figure 6.18 provides a visual summary of ATP production using the METC, while Figure 6.19 depicts the generation of ROS.

Cytochrome C oxidase (CCO), known as Complex IV, is the terminal enzyme in the MECT, mediating the reduction of oxygen to water and promoting the formation of ATP (Nolfi-Donegan et al. 2020). CCO functions as

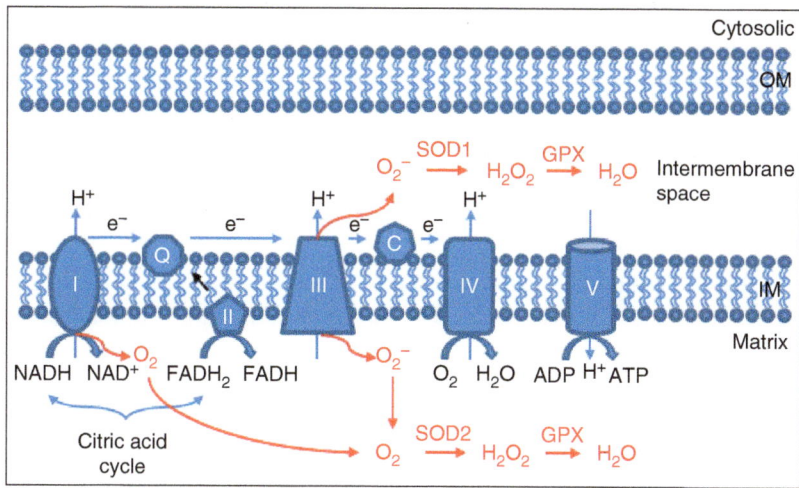

Figure 6.19 Schematic diagraph of the production of reactive oxygen species (ROS) within the mitochondrial electron transport chain (METC). Electrons (e−) donated from nicotinamide adenine dinucleotide plus one hydrogen (NADH) and flavin adenine dinucleotide plus two hydrogens (FADH$_2$) are passed through the MECT with the end goal of reducing oxygen to water. This creates a mitochondrial membrane potential stimulating the production of adenosine triphosphate (ATP) from adenosine diphosphate (ADP). Electrons can leak from Complexes I, II, and III leading to the reduction of oxygen to superoxide (O$_2$•−) which can then be dismutated to hydrogen peroxide (H$_2$O$_2$) by superoxide dismutase in the intermembrane space (IMS) and in the matrix (SOD1 and SOD2, respectively). Hydrogen peroxide can be further reduced to water by glutathione peroxidase (GPX). Superoxide and hydrogen peroxide are classified as ROS (Zhao et al. 2019; Nolfi-Donegan et al. 2020). OM, outer membrane; IM, inner membrane; Q, ubiquinone; C, cytochrome C (Li et al. 2013; Zhao et al. 2019; Nolfi-Donegan et al. 2020) Source: Xinyuan Li, March 19, 2013, http://www.jhoonline.org/content/6/1/19. https://commons.wikimedia.org/wiki/File:Production_of_mitochondrial_ROS,_mitochondrial_ROS.png.

a photoacceptor and transducer of photosignals when exposed to red and NIR spectra (Karu et al. 2005). PBM has been shown to increase electron availability to CCO which increases the mitochondrial membrane potential (MMP) and the production of ATP, cyclic adenosine monophosphate (cAMP), and ROS (Wu et al. 2014). cAMP is produced within the mitochondria by carbon dioxide/bicarbonate-regulated soluble adenylyl cyclase (sAC) in response to the presence of carbon dioxide. cAMP then activates protein kinase A (PKA) which helps regulate ATP production through the phosphorylation of mitochondrial proteins (Acin-Perez et al. 2009).

PBM also increases the activity of Complexes I, II, and III and the levels of nitric oxide (NO). CCO can have a direct effect on NO production through the reduction of nitrite to NO (Poyton and Ball 2011). NO, classified as an ROS,

functions to regulate mitochondrial respiration through its interactions with Complex V and CCO (Nolfi-Donegan et al. 2020).

ROS are short-lived chemical intermediaries that play critical roles in cell signaling, regulation of cell cycle progression, enzyme activation, and the synthesis of nucleic acid and protein (Zorov et al. 2014). PBM of normal cells can cause either an increase or decrease in the MMP compared to baseline. Both scenarios lead to a transient low-level increase in the generation of ROS, the beneficial effects of which remain to be seen (Hamblin 2017). While the exact mechanism is not known, PBM performed on damaged cells appears to reduce ROS and markers of oxidative stress (Hamblin 2017).

CCO has peak photochemical effects around 635 and 730 nm (Karu 2008, 2010). The primary beneficial effect seen with stimulation of CCO is an increase in mitochondrial energy production and metabolism, as well repairing mitochondrial dysfunction (Desmet et al. 2006).

Retrograde Mitochondrial Signaling Mitochondrial signaling, also known as retrograde regulation, is the cell's response to changes in the functional state of the mitochondria (Butow and Avadhani 2004). Traditional anterograde signals bring information from the nucleus and cytoplasm to the mitochondria. Retrograde signals, considered an adaptive response, are often triggered by metabolic changes or changes in intracellular calcium (Ca^{2+}) (Butow and Avadhani 2004).

As discussed above mitochondrial exposure to red and NIR light causes the absorption of light energy by CCO increasing the MMP. This in turn increases the synthesis of ATP and changes the concentration of ROS, Ca^{2+} and NO which leads to changes in the mitochondrial ultrastructure and ultimately communication with the cell nucleus (Karu 2008). The nucleus initiates retrograde cellular signaling propagating changes in ATP synthesis, the intracellular redox potential, pH, cAMP levels, protein synthesis, and gene upregulation (Karu 2008).

Light-Sensitive Ion Channels Transient receptor potential channels (TRPC) are light-sensitive calcium channels modulated by phosphoinositides (a type of cellular membrane phospholipid) (de Freitas and Hamblin 2016). TRPC are members of the family of light-gated G-protein coupled receptors known as opsins which are particularly responsive to blue and green light (Hamblin 2017). TRPC are pleiotropic cellular sensors responsive to a variety of external stimuli including light, heat, cold, pressure, taste, and smell. Activation of TRPC causes non-selective permeabilization of the cell membrane to calcium, sodium, and magnesium (Caterina and Pang 2016).

TRP vanilloid (TRPV1) is involved in the degranulation of mast cells and laser-induced mast cell activation (Caterina and Pang 2016).

Mast cells often congregate at the site of skin wounds, and there is evidence suggesting light stimulation of mast cells promotes wound healing (de Freitas and Hamblin 2016). The clinical application of light-sensitive ion channels remains open, especially in veterinary medicine where red and NIR wavelengths are primarily utilized.

Direct Cell-Free Light-Mediated Effects on Molecules There are some molecules which function as chromophores even without a cellular association. Their role in PBM's MOA is not fully understood. Examples include transforming growth factor (TGF)-β and copper/zinc superoxide dismutase (Cu-Zn-SOD) (de Freitas and Hamblin 2016).

Signaling Molecules Signaling molecules, also called ligands, are molecules which carry a message from cell to cell. Ligands bind to other molecules, often receptors on cell walls, triggering a chain of chemical reactions within the cell (Cooper 2000). The most common signaling molecules affected by PBM are ATP, cAMP, ROS, Ca^{2+}, and NO, summarized in Figure 6.20 (de Freitas and Hamblin 2016).

Adenosine Triphosphate An increased production of ATP is the most common and significant biological effect caused by PBM (Farivar et al. 2014). PBM-induced increases in ATP have been associated with enhanced muscle function and performance, improved cerebral blood flow and oxygen utilization, and enhanced wound healing (Ferraresi et al. 2016; Hamblin 2016; Tsai and Hamblin 2017).

Cyclic Adenosine Monophosphate PBM directly increases cAMP levels, which downregulates inflammation in part by inhibiting the synthesis of tumor necrosis factor (TNF) (de Freitas and Hamblin 2016; Dompe et al. 2020).

Reactive Oxygen Species ROS are beneficial in low concentrations but can be detrimental with

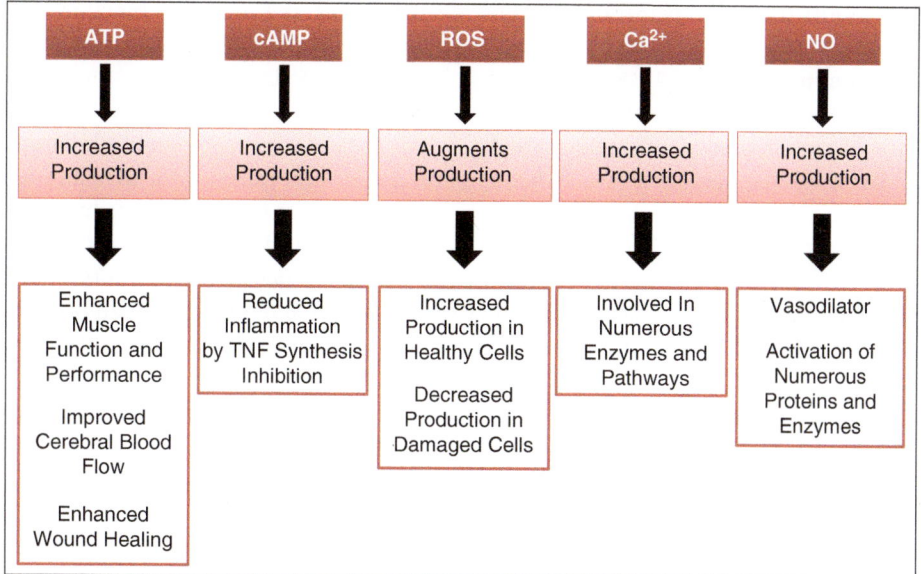

Figure 6.20 Common signaling molecules stimulated by PBM, the effects caused by PBM, and the therapeutic effects of the signaling moleculares. ATP, adenosine triphosphate; cAMP, cyclic adenosine monophosphate; ROS, reactive oxygen species; Ca^{2+}, calcium; NO, nitric oxide. Source: Lisa P. McFaddin.

chronic exposure to higher concentrations (Shields et al. 2021). Normal cells exposed to PBM experience an increase in the MMP and mitochondrial ROS production. PBM helps stabilize the MMP, reducing the production of ROS, in damaged cells and tissues which typically have preexisting oxidative stress, excitotoxicity, and/or inhibition of electron transport (de Freitas and Hamblin 2016).

Calcium   PBM leads to an increase in intracellular Ca^{2+} levels (de Freitas and Hamblin 2016). Ca^{2+} serves as a signaling molecule for a multitude of important enzymes and pathways necessary for normal cellular and tissue function (de Freitas and Hamblin 2016).

Nitric Oxide   PBM has been shown to increase NO production through multiple mechanisms. Exposure to NIR light causes the release of NO from human monocytes (Lindgård et al. 2006). Moriyama et al. (2005) discovered different NIR wavelengths have differential effects on the expression of nitric oxide synthase which

catalyzes the production of NO from L-arginine (Moriyama et al. 2005).

NO is an important vasodilator, forming cyclic guanosine monophosphate (cGMP) through the stimulation of guanylate cyclase. cGMP then directly affects Ca^{2+} concentrations through activation of protein kinase G. NO is also involved in the activation of iron-regulatory factors in macrophages and the modulation of certain proteins and enzymes (de Freitas and Hamblin 2016).

Transcription Factors   Transcription factors (TF) are proteins which control the rate of transcription of genetic information by binding to DNA-regulatory sequences. They function to increase or decrease gene transcription and protein synthesis, and change cellular function (Adcock and Caramori 2009). The TF most affected by PBM include nuclear factor (NF)κB, receptor activator of NFκB ligand (RNKL), hypoxia inducible factor (HIF-1α), Akt/GSK3/β-catenin pathway, Akt/mTOR/CyclinD1 pathway, extracellular signal-regulated kinase/forkhead box protein M1 (ERK/FOXM1), peroxisome prolif-erator-activated receptors (PPAR), and runt-related transcription factor 2 (RUNX2) (de Freitas and Hamblin 2016). They regulate the expression of genes related to inflammatory and stress-induced cellular responses which helps improve the ability of cells and tissue to heal and regenerate (de Freitas and Hamblin 2016).

Effector Molecules Effector molecules are small molecules which bind to a protein and regulate its biological activity (van den Bosch et al. 2020). The effector molecules most impacted by PBM include certain growth fac-tors, mediators of oxidative stress, cytokines, and heat shock proteins (de Freitas and Hamblin 2016). Figure 6.21 provides a sche-matic summary of the regulatory effect PBM exerts on effector molecules.

Growth Factors The growth factors known to increase following PBM include TGF-β, brain-derived neurotrophic factor (BDNF), vascular endothelial growth factor (VEGF), hepatocyte growth factor (HGF), basic fibroblast growth factor (bFGF), and keratinocyte growth factor (KGF) (de Freitas and Hamblin 2016). Table 6.5 summarizes the primary function of each growth factor as well as their primary thera-peutic effect following PBM.

Mediators of Oxidative Stress Inflammation results in local increases in ROS and reactive nitrogen species (RNS) which reduce the natu-ral antioxidant defense mechanisms and acti-vate certain transcription factors, increasing the production of proinflammatory cytokines, growth factors, chemokines, and adhesion molecules (de Freitas and Hamblin 2016). PBM has been shown to reduce oxidative stress through the reduction of ROS and RNS (Farivar et al. 2014; Hamblin 2017).

Cytokines PBM increases the release of both proinflammatory and anti-inflammatory cytokines and other inflammatory mediators including TNF, interleukins, histamine, TGF-β, prostaglandins, and eicosanoids (de Freitas and Hamblin 2016). In the presence of preexisting inflammation, PBM appears to downregulate anti-inflammatory cytokines and inflammatory mediators, contributing to the modality's anti-inflammatory effects (de Freitas and Hamblin 2016; Hamblin 2017).

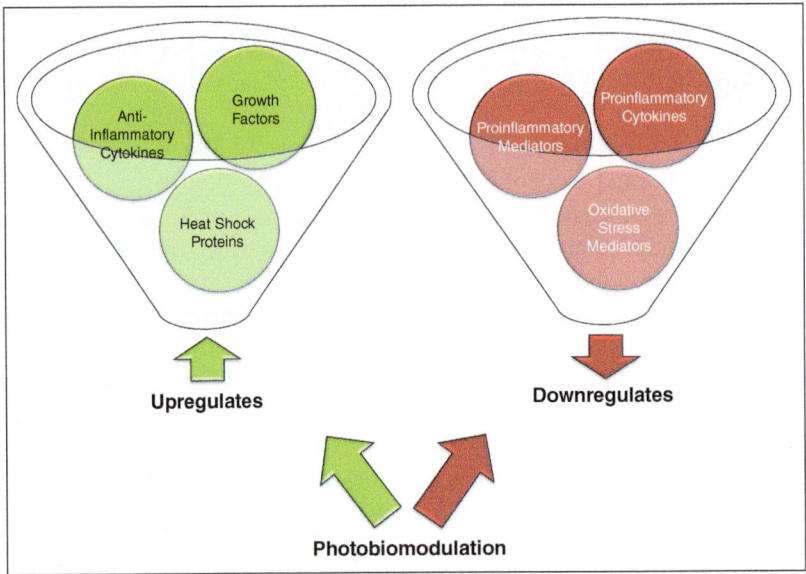

Figure 6.21 The regulatory effect of PBM on effector molecules. Source: Lisa P. McFaddin.

Table 6.5 The primary function, therapeutic effects, and supporting research for the main growth factors stimulated by PBM.

	Primary function	Therapeutic effect	Study
TGF-β	Stimulates collagen production Induces the expression of ECM components Inhibits MMP Stimulates cell migration, proliferation, and tissue repair following injury	Enhances healing of skin wounds and tendinous injuries by increasing synthesis of collagen and proteoglycans	Aliodoust et al. (2014)
BDNF	Modulates dendritic structure Potentiates synaptic transmission within the central nervous system	Neuroprotectant and promotes the development of dendrites	Meng and Xing (2013)
VEGF	Stimulates angiogenesis	Induces angiogenesis	Cury et al. (2013)
HGF	Regulates cell proliferation, motility, and development Anti-apoptotic and anti-inflammatory effects on hepatocytes during regeneration	May enhance liver regeneration following trauma	Araújo et al. (2013)
bFGF	Mitogen and chemoattractant for endothelial cells and fibroblasts Accelerates granulation tissue formation	Enhances would healing	Damante et al. (2009)
KGF	Induces re-epithelialization Proliferation and migration of epithelial cells Maintains normal epithelial structure		

bFGF, basic fibroblast growth factor; BDNF, brain-derived neurotrophic factor; ECM, extracellular matrix; HGF, hepatocyte growth factor; KGF, keratinocyte growth factor; MMP, matrix metalloproteinases; TGF-β, transforming growth factor β; VEGF, vascular endothelial growth factor. Source: Lisa P. McFaddin.

In the absence of inflammation, PBM upregulates proinflammatory cytokines and mediators to encourage tissue healing and remodeling (Wu et al. 2010; de Freitas and Hamblin 2016; Hamblin 2017).

Heat Shock Proteins   Heat shock proteins (HSP) are stress proteins involved in the maturation, stabilization and degradation of proteins, as well as apoptosis (Whitley et al. 1999). PBM has been shown to upregulate the production of HSP (Farivar et al. 2014; Tsai and Hamblin 2017).

Cellular Mechanisms
Cellular mechanisms describe how the laser photons interact with and directly affect the whole cell. The most common laser–cell interactions include reduction of inflammation, cytoprotection, proliferation, migration,

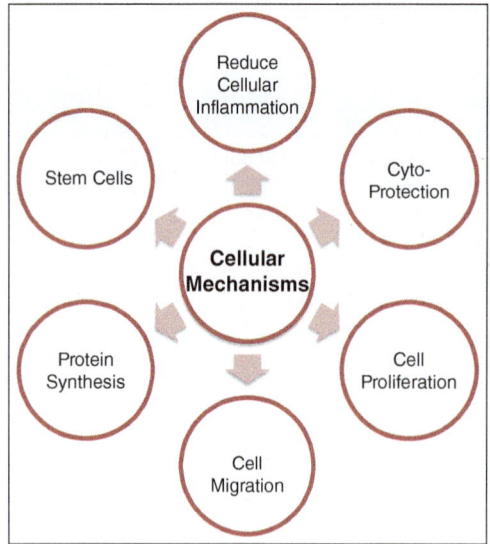

Figure 6.22 Schematic summary of the most common cellular mechanisms associated with PBM. Source: Lisa P. McFaddin.

protein synthesis, and stimulation of stem cells, illustrated in Figure 6.22 (de Freitas and Hamblin 2016).

Inflammation   PBM has been shown to reduce cellular inflammation by decreasing intracellular ROS accumulation, inhibiting the production of prostaglandin (PG)E2, and reducing the expression of cyclooxygenase 1 and 2 (COX-1 and COX-2), calcium-dependent phospholipase A2 (cPLA2), and secretory phospholipase A2 (sPLA2) (Lim et al. 2013). PBM can also stimulate monocyte response and augment the expression of cytokines and chemokines (Chen et al. 2014).

Cytoprotection   *In vitro* studies suggest PBM protects cells from damage due to toxin exposure and amyloid deposition (Eells et al. 2003; Wong-Riley et al. 2005; Liang et al. 2006; Zhang et al. 2012)

Proliferation   *In vitro* and *in vivo* studies have demonstrated PBM positively influenced the proliferation levels of keratinocytes, fibroblasts, vascular endothelial cells, osteoblasts, melanocytes, and human epidermal stem cells, all of which aid in wound healing (Szymanska et al. 2013; Amid et al. 2014; Esmaeelinejad et al. 2014; Sperandio et al. 2015).

Migration   *In vitro* studies determined PBM improves the migration of tenocytes, melanocytes, human epidermal stem cells, and embryonic nerve cells (Rochkind et al. 2009; Tsai et al. 2012; Liao et al. 2014; AlGhamdi et al. 2015).

Protein Synthesis   The direct effects of PBM on protein synthesis have been discussed previously.

Stem Cells   *In vitro* and *in vivo* studies confirm PBM induces stem cell migration, differentiation, proliferation, viability, and protein expression (Abrahamse 2012; Ginani et al. 2015).

Tissue Mechanisms

There are numerous *in vitro* and *in vivo* studies on humans and animals investigating the beneficial effects of PBM on different tissue types under various conditions (de Freitas and Hamblin 2016). For practical use the primary tissues of interest include skin, fascia, muscles, joints, ligaments and tendons, bones, and the nervous systems (central and peripheral) (Esmaeelinejad et al. 2014; Hamblin 2016; Dos Santos et al. 2019; Ramezani et al. 2020; Silva et al. 2020; Xiang et al. 2020; Alayat et al. 2022; Ferlito et al. 2022).

Molecular and cellular mechanisms are the primary method through which PBM elicits these beneficial effects. The end results are one or more of the four biological effects (Therapeutic MOA) described in the next section. The therapeutic and tissue mechanisms are so intertwined it is nearly impossible to talk about one without discussing the other.

Therapeutic MOA for Veterinarians

As mentioned previously, PBM has four primary therapeutic MOA, also called biological effects.

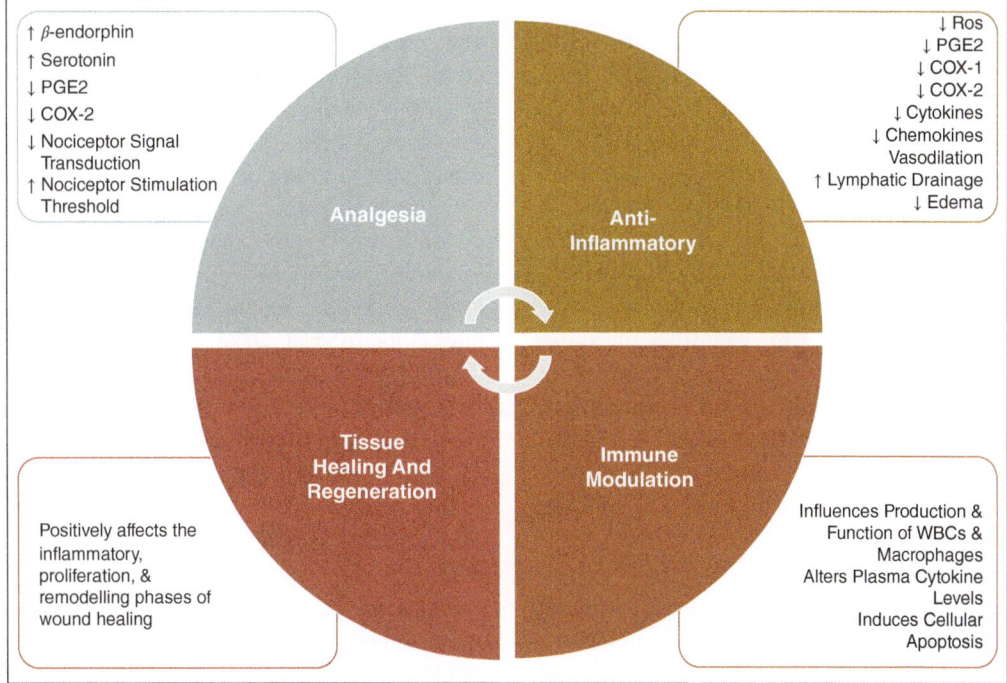

Figure 6.23 The four key biological effects or therapeutic mechanisms of action caused by PBM and the main methods through which each effect is achieved. PGE2, prostaglandin E2; COX-2, cyclooxygenase-2; ROS, reactive oxygen species; COX-1, cyclooxygenase-1; WBC, white blood cells. Source: Lisa P. McFaddin.

These effects are summarized in Figure 6.23 and discussed in further detail below.

Analgesia

PBM reduces pain through several processes: increasing β-endorphin and serotonin circulation, decreasing PGE2 and COX-2 levels, reducing nociceptor signal transduction and increasing nociceptor stimulation threshold (Mizutani et al. 2004; Bjordal et al. 2006; Aras et al. 2010). PBM likely exhibits other analgesic properties which have yet to be discovered and currently serve as a fascinating area of study.

Studies by Rogatko et al. (2017) and Renwick et al. (2018) show improved weight-bearing in dogs receiving LLLT, with varying wavelengths, following tibial plateau level osteotomy (TPLO). The application of PBM led to a reduction in postoperative pain which was directly responsible for improved weight-bearing (Rogatko et al. 2017; Renwick et al. 2018).

Not all studies successfully documented the analgesic effects of PBM. Kennedy et al. (2018) found LLLT did not yield beneficial effects on pain and pelvic limb function following TPLO. Additionally, Bennaim et al. (2017) found no difference in the recovery rates of non-ambulatory dogs, following hemilaminectomy, treated with PBM, physical rehabilitation plus sham PBM, or sham PBM.

Anti-inflammatory

As discussed previously PBM reduces inflammation by decreasing the levels of intracellular ROS, PGE2, COX-1, COX-2, cPLA2, sPLA, cytokines, and chemokines. Additionally, dilation of local blood and lymph vessels promotes the anti-inflammatory effects. A transient vasodilation increases local circulation and oxygenation of target tissues, activates the lymphatic drainage system, and reduces edema (Maegawa et al. 2000; Hamblin 2017).

The anti-inflammatory effects of PBM have been well studied in the treatment of various conditions in humans and animals (Hamblin 2017). Cold laser can typically be used for any condition ending in "-itis." As with analgesics, there are studies that do not support this theory. A study conducted by Stitch et al. (2014) did not support the use of LLLT in the management of pedal pruritus secondary to canine atopic dermatitis.

Refer to Table 6.7 for examples of studies conducted in companion animals documenting the efficacy of PBM in reducing inflammation for a variety of conditions. Keep in mind that pain often accompanies inflammation, so reducing one often improves the other.

Immune Modulation

PBM can have positive effects on the immune system of humans and animals through multiple pathways (Kneebone 2011). PBM has been shown to influence the proliferation and function of immune cells (lymphocytes, neutrophils, and macrophages), alter plasma cytokine levels (interleukins, growth factors, and TNF), and induce cellular apoptosis (Ganju et al. 1999; Alves et al. 2013; Dos Anjos et al. 2017; Mehani 2017).

Currently there are no studies evaluating the direct effects of PBM on the immune system of companion animals. There are several studies documenting this therapeutic effect in laboratory animals including conditions affecting the lungs, abdomen, wound healing, and snake bites (Ribeiro et al. 2009; de Lima et al. 2012; de Souza Costa et al. 2018; Reis et al. 2021).

Tissue Healing and Regeneration

PBM positively affects three of the four phases of wound healing: inflammation, proliferation, and remodeling. A refresher on the phases of wound healing is provided in the box.

Inflammation is controlled by stimulating the function of mast cells, local release of cytokines, chemokines, other biochemical mediators, and macrophage phagocytosis (Hawkins et al. 2005; Lopez and Brundage 2019; Mosca et al. 2019). PBM encourages the

---

A Brief Review of Wound Healing

Wound healing is divided into four overlapping phases: hemostasis, inflammation, proliferation, and remodeling (Figure 6.24). Refer to Chapter 7 for further information.

Hemostasis: Bleeding is generally halted within seconds to hours following injury (Landén et al. 2016). Initially vessels constrict reducing blood flow, followed quickly by platelets which attach to the subendothelium of the disrupted blood vessel wall plugging the hole.

Inflammation: The inflammatory phase generally lasts one to five days and occurs concurrently with hemostasis (Landén et al. 2016). The result is an increase in vascular permeability, vasodilation, chemotaxis, and the recruitment of more white blood cells, causing the classic signs of inflammation: redness, heat, swelling, and pain (Chen et al. 2018).

Proliferation: Approximately three days after injury monocytes recruited to the site differentiate into macrophages (Landén et al. 2016). The primary goals of the proliferative phase are to establish a new connective tissue matrix, lay down new vasculature, and form granulation tissue (Schultz et al. 2015).

Remodeling: The established granulation tissue is transitional and over 21 days to one year remodels and matures into functional scar tissue (Landén et al. 2016).

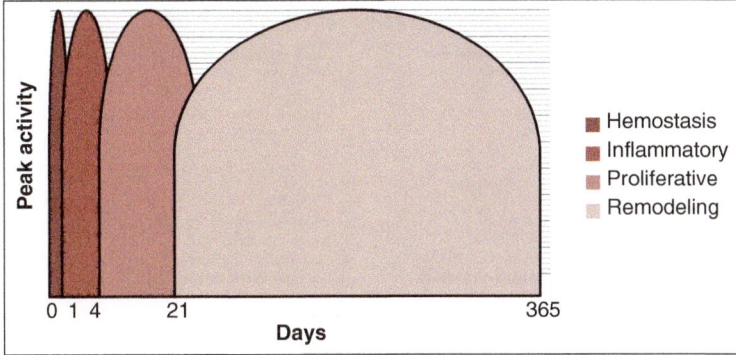

Figure 6.24 A graphic representation of the four phases of wound healing showing the approximate length of time, and peak activity, for each phase. Source: Lisa P. McFaddin.

proliferation and remodeling phases through the promotion of epithelial and endothelial migration, epithelial proliferation, angiogenesis, fibroblast matrix synthesis, and wound contraction (Arany 2016). Researchers speculate PBM also increases the production and activity of fibroblasts and macrophages, improves leukocyte movement, promotes collagen formation, and induces neovascularization (Chung et al. 2012), hastening wound healing and improving the tensile strength of the healing tissue (Hawkins et al. 2005). PBM has also been used to reduce scar tissue formation (Hagler 2019).

In a literature review by Lopez and Brundage (2019), the authors found daily laser exposure at the 600–800 nm range had the most consistent beneficial effects on wound healing in rodents. The authors also suggest further studies were necessary to determine the best wavelengths and treatment frequency for wound healing in other species (Lopez and Brundage 2019).

Not all studies have shown improved wound healing with PBM. Both Kurach et al. (2015) and Gammel et al. (2018) found the application of LLLT (using 635 and 980 nm, respectively) had no benefit on the healing of surgically created wounds in dogs.

Safety

There are multiple safety components to consider when operating a Class IIIb or Class IV laser, including operator, client, and patient safety, cautions and contraindications, and side effects.

Occupational Safety and Health Administration

The Occupational Safety and Health Administration (OSHA) is a division of the United States Department of Labor (OSHA 2014). OSHA was created by congress with the Occupational Safety and Health Act of 1970 "to ensure safe and healthful working conditions for workers by setting and enforcing standards and by providing training, outreach, education, and assistance. . .OSHA standards are rules that describe the methods employers are legally required to follow to protect their workers from hazards" (OSHA 2014). Figure 6.25 summarizes the employer requirements and employee rights outlined in the Occupational Safety and Health Act of 1970. A free downloadable copy of the "OSHA At-A-Glance" handout is available on the companion website.

As summarized in Table 6.3 all lasers have potential hazards associated with their use.

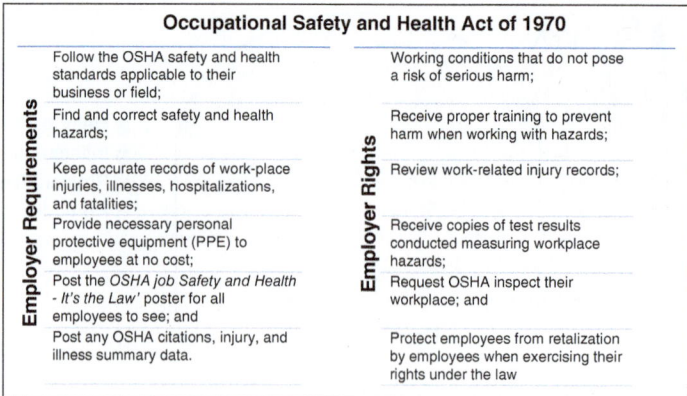

Figure 6.25 The Occupational Safety and Health Act of 1970 created the Occupational Safety and Health Administration (OSHA). The Act set out requirements for all employers and rights ensured for all employees. Source: Lisa P. McFaddin.

A Laser Safety Program (LSP) Must Contain the Following Information

1) A description of the class or classes of lasers used in the hospital.
2) Documents describing the safe use of lasers.
3) A designated Laser Safety Officer (LSO).
4) A written laser safety program including standard operating procedures (SOPs).
5) Approved locations for storage and use of lasers.
6) Description of the required personal protective equipment (PPE).
7) Employee training program.
(OSHA 2021)

OSHA has specific standards regarding the safe use of therapeutic lasers (OSHA 2021). Specifically, OSHA requires employers have an adequate Laser Safety Program (OSHA 2021).

Laser Classes

Class IIIb and IV are the most used lasers in veterinary hospitals.

Laser Safety Documents

OSHA lists the American National Standards Institute (ANSI) Z136 series (Safe Use of Lasers) as a good resource for consensus laser safety standards. The documents, written and produced by the Laser Institute of America (LIA), are frequently used as the foundation of laser safety programs and SOPs for multiple industries, including medical, military, industrial, and educational (LIA 2017). The ANSI Z136.1 describes the responsibilities of the

LSO, defines a laser hazard classification system, and establishes the educational and training requirements of the facility.

Laser Safety Officer

The ANSI Z136.1 requires facilities using a Class III or IV laser have a designated LSO who oversees the safety of all operational, maintenance, and servicing issues associated with the laser (LIA 2017). The LSO is responsible for monitoring and enforcing the control of laser hazards, establishing and updating laser SOPs, employee safety training, and maintenance and purchasing of personal protective equipment (PPE) (LIA 2017).

Laser Locations

SOPs should be established describing the proper storage location for the laser and PPE, as well as approved locations when using the laser.

Personal Protective Equipment

SOPs should be written outlining required PPE and warning signs used when operating a laser, as well as appropriate storage locations for these items.

Training Programs

SOPs outlining training requirements, as well as the training materials, should be created. OSHA offers additional laser safety resources, including training and safety materials, available for download on the companion website.

1) *Introduction to Laser Safety Training*: A free downloadable PowerPoint presentation created by Bob Curtis and OSHA covering laser basics, bioeffects on the skin and eyes, classifications, and administrative control measures and safety practices.
2) *Introduction to Laser Safety*: A free downloadable handout, produced by Alliance (an OSHA Cooperative Program) and LIA, briefly defining lasers and their potential hazards.
3) *Laser Effects on the Human Eye*: A free downloadable handout, produced by Alliance and LIA, discussing the potential negative effects of lasers on the human eye when directly exposed to laser beams.
4) *Questions That an OSHA Inspector May Ask You About Laser Safety*: A question and answer handout, produced by Alliance and LIA, covering questions commonly asked by OSHA inspectors evaluating workplaces in which lasers are used.

A training video or presentation should be created, downloaded, or purchased outlining the proper use of the hospital's laser. It should also discuss how to properly program the laser and the most common techniques used for different situations (i.e. skin wound vs. muscle injury).

Operator, Client, and Patient Safety

The primary safety concerns associated with laser PBM involve potential damage to the eyes and overheating of the tissues. Simple measures and methods can be used to minimize and avoid these issues. Knowledge regarding cautions, contraindications, and potential adverse effects is also important.

Personal Protective Equipment

Visible light, when shone directly into the eyes, will elicit a blink reflex protecting the eyes from damage. Infrared light cannot be seen by the eye and will not elicit a blink reflex (FDA 2021). The eye is designed to collect and focus light onto the retina which intensifies the energy of the light reaching the eye. Eyes can focus laser beams (already a narrow light source) into even smaller, more intense (by up to 100 000 times) spots on the retina potentially causing retinal damage (burns) or blind spots (FDA 2021). Class IIIb lasers are classified as having a high risk of immediate damage to the eye upon exposure to a direct beam, while Class IV are high risk for the eyes with direct and reflected (indirect) exposure (FDA 2021).

Special laser eye protection can protect the eyes from direct and indirect exposure to laser beams. Laser glasses or goggles are not the same as run of the mill laboratory glasses. This eyewear is designed to filter specific wavelengths of light and is often based on the output parameters of a specific laser. Proper PPE is required for anyone operating a laser or in the room with an active laser. The patient's eye protection should also be considered. Figure 6.26 shows an example of human and canine laser PPE.

All persons in the same room as a running therapeutic laser should wear protective eyewear. This should include hospital employees, clients, and ideally patients (if they tolerate doggles or a towel over their eyes). Patients requiring treatment around the face *must* have their eyes covered.

> **Remember: The eyes of the operator, patient, and anyone else in the room with a laser actively emitting beams must be protected at all times.**

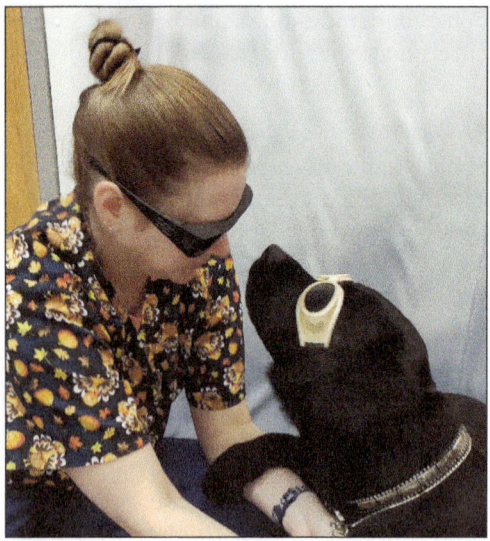

Figure 6.26 Both the operator and patient are wearing appropriate PPE designed to protect the eyes from potential exposure to the wavelengths of light emitted by the laser. Keep in mind this image does not depict appropriate patient restraint during PBM therapy. The dog in the picture is a friend of the clinic. Source: Lisa P. McFaddin.

Safety Signs

Signs warning employees and clients a therapeutic laser is or will be used in a specific area should be posted. Signs should also be posted in the area where the laser is stored. The signs should provide a warning about the presence or use of a laser, ideally specifying the type of laser to be used and reminding users to wear proper eye protection. A note recommending people avoid direct eye exposure may also be included. Figure 6.27 provides an example laser safety sign.

Cautions and Contraindications

When used correctly by trained personnel, PBM is a very safe, effective, and practical treatment modality. As with any therapy there

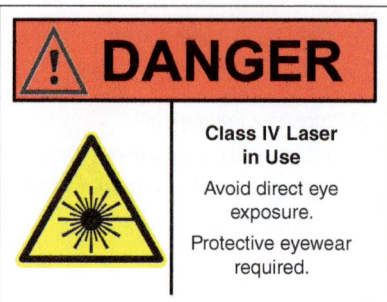

Figure 6.27 Example of a laser safety sign for a Class IV therapeutic laser. This sign should be posted in the room with an operational laser and where the laser is stored. Source: Lisa P. McFaddin.

are several precautions but only one true contraindication for which the entire hospital team should be aware. This information is outlined in Table 6.6 and described in more detail in the Veterinarians section.

Adverse Effects

Side effects are uncommon but may include a rise in skin or hair temperature, mild skin redness, or skin irritation. If noted these effects are temporary and self-resolving. Adverse effects may include overheating of treated tissues, sedation for 24–48 hours following treatment (rare), or transient pain following treatment (rare) (Niebaum 2013; Hagler 2019).

Cautions and Contraindications for Veterinarians

Darker Skin and Coat

Darker skin and coat pigmentation absorbs laser photons more easily, increasing the risk of overheating the tissue (Souza-Barros et al. 2017; Luna et al. 2020; Shah and Alster 2010). To avoid excess heat a faster scanning technique may be needed, and the person performing the PBMT should use their fingers or hand to check the fur and skin for excess warmth throughout the treatment (Godbold 2014).

Melanin has a wide absorption spectrum (250–1200 nm), but the absorption of laser energy decreases as the wavelength increases

Table 6.6 An overview of the most common areas of cautions and the single contraindication, as well as potential corrective measures, seen with veterinary PBM).

PBM cautions	Potential negative effects	Corrective measures
Darker skin and coat	Overheating of the skin and fur	Adjust scanning technique; periodically check skin and fur temperature
	Decreased laser penetration	Use longer wavelength lasers
Photosensitive skin	Overheating of the skin and fur	Adjust scanning technique; periodically check skin and fur temperature
Wet fur	None	Not applicable
Injection sites	Affect absorption of the injection; decrease penetration of the laser beam	Perform PBM before the injection; wait to perform PBM after the injection has absorbed
Bleeding	Vasodilation which could increase bleeding	Perform PBM after hemorrhage is stopped
Growth plates	± Effects on bone growth or premature growth plate closure (conflicting data)	Limited use for short periods of time, such as a maximum of six to eight treatments or over three to four days
Fontanel	Potential negative effects and corrective measures are grouped with active growth plates	
Thyroid gland	Potential changes to thyroid tissue and function	Avoid prolonged exposure of the thyroid gland to laser photons; treatment of the tissue around the thyroid gland is appropriate
Testicles	Low-dose exposure may improve sperm production, motility, and viability	No adjustments required
	High-dose prolonged exposure may negatively affect sperm viability	Avoid high-dose prolonged exposure
Implants	Non-superficial implants: little to none in practice	No adjustments required
	Implants reflect light which could increase skin temperature for superficial implants	Adjust scanning technique and/or reduce dosage (and treatment time) for superficial implants
Pregnancy	None	No adjustment required
Cancer	± Increase tumor size	Avoid PBM directly over tumors, distant sites of tumor spread (metastasis), and postsurgical incisions (even if "clean margins" are obtained)
		Safe to use as treatment for cancer therapy-related conditions and palliative (hospice) care (even directly over the cancer)
PBM contraindication	**Potential negative effects**	**Corrective measures**
Ocular exposure	Retinal damage; blindness	Wear protective eyewear; avoid direct treatment of the eye and immediate surrounding tissue

Source: Lisa P. McFaddin.

(Shah and Alster 2010; Gaffey and Johnson 2022). When possible, lasers with longer wavelength are used to ensure the laser photons reach the target tissue.

Photosensitive Skin

A sensitivity of the skin to light (photosensitivity) can occur focally or be generalized. Focal photosensitivity in the dog and cat is usually noted on areas of the body which lack fur and/ or are color dilute, such as eyelids, ears, muzzle, axilla, inner forelimbs and pelvic limbs, and the groin (Barrington 2022). These areas may be normal or develop due to concurrent illness. Generalized photosensitivity of the skin is rare and typically occurs as a side effect of another illness (such as immune-mediated skin disease or Cushing's disease) (Barrington 2022). Overheating of tissues is the primary concern associated with PBM and photosensitive skin. As for darker skin and fur, a faster scanning technique and repeated checking of the skin and fur is recommended.

Drug-induced photosensitivity is relatively common in people but rare in dogs and cats. There are quite a few medications (both topical and oral) causing photosensitive reactions at certain wavelengths which preclude the use of PBM while taking or applying these pharmaceuticals (Kerstein et al. 2014). This does not appear to be a concern in veterinary medicine.

Wet Fur

Anecdotally some practitioners are concerned about using therapeutic lasers on wet fur, with the fear that the moisture could increase the risk of thermal injury. There are no data to support this idea. Theoretically, an air–water interface could increase the risk of laser beam reflection, but again there are no data to support this concern. Currently there is no need to use caution when treating wet or damp fur or skin.

Injection Sites

PBM should not be performed directly over a subcutaneous or intramuscular injection site immediately following administration (Godbold 2017). PBM may affect absorption (increasing or decreasing) of the vaccine or medication and/or penetration of the laser beam may be negatively affected. Practitioners can either perform PBM before giving the injection or wait until the injectable has been absorbed.

Bleeding

PBM should not be performed during active bleeding (hemorrhage) due to its vasodilatory (widens blood vessels) properties (Maegawa et al. 2000; Chung et al. 2012). PBM can safely be performed, and accelerates wound healing, once the bleeding is stopped (hemostasis) (Godbold 2017).

Growth Plates

PBM of an active epiphysis was initially considered a contraindication in veterinary and human medicine. Class III lasers are now considered safe when treating the skin overlying active epiphyses and should be used with caution when treating an active epiphysis (Houghton et al. 2010; de Andrade et al. 2012; Jenkins 2022). Caution is still recommended when treating the bone itself because studies on rats have shown conflicting data, with some studies demonstrating a negative effect (de Oliveira et al. 2012) and others demonstrating a positive effect on longitudinal bone growth (Choi et al. 2015). Some practitioners anecdotally recommend a maximum of six to eight treatments on epiphyses (Rivera 2022). To date no studies have investigated the use of Class IV lasers on epiphyses, and the recommendation is typically to use caution or avoid (Dycus 2014). More than likely acute use of a therapeutic laser over an active growth plate for three to four days should not have negative effects (Godbold 2017).

Open Fontanel

To date there is no research investigating the effects (positive or negative) associated with PBM of an open fontanel. Most academics and clinicians lump open fontanels into the same category as active epiphyses, suggesting acute use should be safe but long-term (repeated) applications are not recommended (Edge-Hughes 2020). Further research is clearly needed to draw specific conclusions.

Thyroid Gland

Initial animal studies suggested laser treatment of the thyroid gland caused cellular changes within the gland but the functional significance was unclear (Parrado et al. 1990, 1999). Later studies found no change in thyroid function following PBM with a potential application for chronic autoimmune thyroiditis (hypothyroidism) in humans (Azevedo et al. 2005; Höfling et al. 2013). Currently there is no documented beneficial effect for the direct treatment of the thyroid glands in veterinary medicine. It is unlikely that limited exposure of the thyroid glands to laser photons would cause a problem, i.e. if treating the soft tissue around the thyroid glands, but direct treatment is not advised at this time (Godbold 2017).

Testicles

Direct exposure of the testes and scrotum to low-dose PBM is considered safe but may cause increased spermatogenesis and sperm motility (Firestone et al. 2012; Siqueira et al. 2016). Prolonged exposure to high-dose PBM may reduce sperm viability (Firestone et al. 2012).

Implants

Historical concerns regarding overheating of implants and surrounding tissue is unfounded. The implants will reflect light back into the surrounding tissue which may be beneficial to its therapeutic effect. In cases with a thin layer of tissue covering the implant, the operator can move the probe faster and/or reduce the dose (and thus treatment time) to prevent overheating (Godbold 2017).

Class IIIb and IV lasers do not have documented negative effects on implants (metal or synthetic), suture, or tissue adhesives used in veterinary medicine (Godbold 2017). PBM has been shown to improve soft tissue and bone health around dental implants in humans and animals, thus improving implant success (Tang and Arany 2013; Razaghi et al. 2022).

Pregnancy

The use of laser therapy over a gravid uterus was initially considered a contraindication due to presumed negative effects on the fetus. The wavelengths typically used in veterinary PBM have not been shown to posses mutagenic or teratogenic effects (Godbold 2017). Current literature suggests a fetus (animal or human) will not be harmed by exposure (direct or indirect) to a Class IIIb or Class IV laser (Godbold 2017). There are no indications to specifically treat a gravid uterus, but PBM can be performed safely on surrounding tissues (such as or lower back pain).

Malignancies

The use of PBM on malignant neoplasia is controversial and initial recommendations relied heavily on data obtained from *in vitro* studies (Godbold 2017). There are several *in vitro* studies, using human malignant cell lines, which found PBM increased the growth rate of cancer cells in cell culture (Hamblin et al. 2018).

In vivo studies using animal models have yielded conflicting results. Depending on the wavelength and treatment protocol, as well as the type of cancer, PBM was shown to increase tumor cell growth (Frigo et al. 2009), elicit no change (Barasch et al. 2020), or decrease tumor cell growth (Petrellis et al. 2017). A recent systematic review conducted by Bensadoun et al. and the WALT concluded PBMT is safe to use over neoplasms, is safe and effective in treating cancer treatment-related conditions and may benefit overall patient survival (Bensadoun et al. 2020).

There are three potential means by which PBM can have a beneficial effect on cancer: a direct effect on tumor cell death, an indirect effect on tumor cell death, and stimulation of antitumor immunity (Hamblin et al. 2018). High-dose PBM can be used to kill tumor cells through the deliberate use of the biphasic dose–response curve. This can be thought of as an "overdose" for the cancer cells (Kiro et al. 2017). Wu et al. (2014), through *in vitro* and *in vivo* testing, determined PBM can damage and even kill cancer cells by triggering fatal mitochondrial burst through the increased production of ROS. This approach is often called "high fluence low-power laser irradiation, HF-LPLI" (Wu et al. 2014).

The indirect effect of PBM on tumor cells relies on the Warburg effect: "the propensity of cancer cells under aerobic conditions to metabolize glucose to lactate (aerobic glycolysis)" (Kalyanaraman 2017). This occurs because the rapidly dividing tumor cells outgrow their blood supply forcing the cells to tolerate chronic hypoxia (low oxygen). As a result, the mitochondria of normal cells behave differently compared to those of cancer cells, and PBM mitochondrial stimulation will produce different results in both cell types. Cancer cells, which typically have a limited ATP supply, will experience an ATP boost following PBM, increasing their responsivity to pro-apoptotic cytotoxic stimuli from adjunct cancer therapies (Hamblin et al. 2018). Conversely, normal cells typically experience an increase in the production of ROS following PBM which can protect healthy cells and tissue from the damaging effects of adjunct cancer therapies (Hamblin et al. 2018).

Finally, PBM has been shown, in mostly animal models, to positively affect the host's immune system through the recruitment of immune cells (T lymphocytes and dendritic cells), reduction of angiogenic macrophages within tumors, and by increasing the expression of certain inflammatory mediators (IL-1β, IL-6, IL-10, and TNF-α) (Ottaviani et al. 2016; Petrellis et al. 2017; Hamblin et al. 2018).

Currently, there are no *in vivo* studies investigating the effects of PBM on malignancies in companion animals. Until such studies exist the recommendation is to avoid the use of PBMT directly over malignant tumors, sites of potential metastasis, and surgical sites (even when "clean margins" are achieved) (Godbold 2017). Be aware with time (and further studies) these recommendations will likely change.

In people, PBM is recommended to reduce the negative effects of cancer treatment. Multiple studies have demonstrated the safety and efficacy of PBMT in the treatment of chemotherapy-induced and chemoradiotherapy-induced oral mucositis (Legouté et al. 2019; Al-Rudayni et al. 2021), radiation-induced dermatitis (Rocha et al. 2022), and chemotherapy-induced peripheral neuropathy (Lodewijckx et al. 2022; Teng et al. 2022). These studies also support the use of PBM in areas away from the initial malignancy.

To date there are no veterinary studies investigating PBMT as a means for alleviating the negative effects of cancer treatment or at sites distant to the original malignancy. Extrapolating from the human research applications of PBM under these circumstances should be considered safe (Godbold 2017).

Due to its profound analgesic and anti-inflammatory properties, PBM can also be used as a palliative treatment for patients with terminal cancers, even if a malignant neoplasm is located in the treatment area (Godbold 2017). An open discussion and agreement with the client, regarding the pros and cons of incorporating PBM, must occur before initiating therapy.

Contraindication

As discussed in the section on PPE, direct and indirect retinal exposure, depending on the class of laser, can have deleterious effects on the eye including retinal burns and blindness. This can be avoided by having the patient wear protective eyewear. Additionally, PBM should not be performed on the eye itself and the tissue immediately surrounding it (periocular).

The Why

Applications in Human Medicine

As of 2019 more than 3500 scientific articles had been published on PBM, and 85–90% of the research involved lasers as the light source

(Heiskanen and Hamblin 2018). Both laser and LED PBM are most used to control and reduce pain, accelerate wound healing (skin, tendons, ligaments, and nerves), reduce inflammation, and treat a variety of dermatologic conditions (Desmet et al. 2006; Kim and Calderhead 2011; de Freitas and Hamblin 2016; Ablon 2018).

One of the first medical applications of PBM involved the use of HeNe lasers on the treatment of skin ulcers (Mester et al. 1968). Since then PBM has proven effective for the treatment of acute and chronic wounds caused by trauma, burns, venous ulcers, pressure sores, and diabetic foot ulcers (Chung et al. 2012; Mosca et al. 2019).

The analgesic and anti-inflammatory effects of PBM are well studied. PBM is effective in reducing neck pain, dental pain, muscle pain and injury, chronic joint pain, and postoperative pain (Bjordal et al. 2006; Chung et al. 2012; Ferraresi et al. 2016; Chow et al. 2019; Ezzati et al. 2019; Cronshaw et al. 2020). The anti-inflammatory properties undoubtedly contribute to the analgesic effects.

PBM has also been shown to improve cognition and memory and restore blood flow in damaged areas of the brain (Hamblin 2016, 2018; Cardoso et al. 2021). PBM is also being studied as an adjunct therapy in the treatment of Alzheimer's disease, Parkinson's disease, and psychiatric disorders (Hamblin 2016; Tsai and Hamblin 2017; Cardoso et al. 2021).

Historically, the application of light therapy directly over a tumor was considered contraindicated. Several flawed animal studies suggested PBM increased tumor growth or changed tumor pathology (Frigo et al. 2009; Monteiro et al. 2011; Ree et al. 2016). Since that time multiple animal and human studies have shown the beneficial effects of PBM in cancer treatment through the direct damage of tumors, potentiation of adjunct cancer therapies, and stimulation of the host's immune system (Hamblin et al. 2018; Legouté et al. 2019; Al-Rudayni et al. 2021; Lodewijckx et al. 2022; Rocha et al. 2022; Teng et al. 2022). A few clinical trials have suggested the use of PBM may improve quality of life and survival time in patients with certain cancers (Santana-Blank et al. 2002; Antunes et al. 2017). Further research is needed to solidify PBMT's place in cancer management.

PBM in people is considered very safe. Side effects are uncommon, often self-resolving, and dose-dependent including skin irritation, itching and redness (Dompe et al. 2020).

Applications in Veterinary Medicine

PBM is most used in veterinary medicine to aid in the treatment of skin wounds, dermatologic infections, acral lick granulomas, musculoskeletal injuries (tendon, ligament, muscle, and bone), osteoarthritis, neurologic injuries, postoperative pain and healing, and other sources of pain (Downing 2017; Brunke 2018; Fessehav 2020). Refer to Table 6.7 for a list of conditions and studies for which PBM has demonstrated a positive effect. PBM can also be used in a more targeted fashion for laser acupuncture and laser trigger point therapy (see Chapters 1 and 9 for additional information).

Veterinary Research

While still a relatively new modality, veterinary PBMT has a moderate amount of research. As of February 2023 a quick search on PubMed.gov yielded over 100 articles using the criteria "photobiomodulation canine/feline/veterinary," "low level light therapy canine/feline/veterinary," and "cold laser canine/feline/veterinary." Presented in the following boxes are the summaries of three veterinary PBM studies.

Not all research has yielded positive results. Studies by Kennedy et al. (2018) and Bennaim et al. (2017) found no beneficial effects on pain or function following TPLO and hemilaminectomy surgeries, respectively. Additionally, studies by Kurach et al. (2015) and Gammel et al. (2018) found the application of LLLT (using 635 and 980 nm, respectively) had no benefit on the surgical wound healing in dogs.

The use of PBM to treat certain cancers in veterinary patients is controversial. Historically the application of light therapy directly over a tumor was considered contraindicated. Several flawed animal studies suggested PBM increased tumor growth or changed tumor pathology (Frigo et al. 2009; Monteiro et al. 2011; Ree et al. 2016). Since that time multiple animal and human studies have shown the beneficial effects of PBM in cancer treatment through the direct damage of tumors, potentiation of adjunct cancer therapies, and stimulation of the host's immune system (Hamblin et al. 2018; Legouté et al. 2019; Al-Rudayni et al. 2021; Lodewijckx et al. 2022; Rocha et al. 2022; Teng et al. 2022). A few clinical trials have suggested the use PBM may improve quality of life and survival time in patients with certain cancers (Santana-Blank et al. 2002; Antunes et al. 2017). The use of PBM for the direct treatment of

---

A Randomized Blind Placebo-Controlled Trial Investigating the Effects of Photobiomodulation Therapy (PBMT) on Canine Elbow Osteoarthritis

Authors: Andrea L. Looney, Janice L. Huntingford, Lauren L. Blaeser, and Sabine Mann

Journal: *Canadian Veterinary Journal*

Date: 2018

Study design: Randomized blind placebo-controlled clinical trial

Study hypothesis: The use of photobiomodulation therapy (PBMT) would improve pain and lameness in dogs with naturally occurring elbow joint osteoarthritis.

Sample size: 20 client-owned dogs.

Materials and methods: All participants have clinical exam and radiographic or computed technology confirmation of unilateral or bilateral elbow degenerative joint disease. Baseline complete blood count, serum chemistry, electrolytes, thyroid status, and tick serology was performed prior to their inclusion. Dogs were on nonsteroidal anti-inflammatory dugs (NSAIDs) for more than one week before the trial and could be on other pain medications and nutraceuticals provided they had been taking them for more than one week before the trial and dose did not change throughout the study. A baseline blinded clinician lameness score and owner-assigned Helskinki Chronic Pain Index Score was assigned to each dog. Dogs were randomly placed in the active PMBT group or the sham group using a coin toss. The treatment laser used was a Class IV emitting NIR 980 nm at 12 W and visible red light 650 nm at 3.5 mW. The sham laser emitted only the 650 nm light. Both groups received twice weekly treatments by blinded technicians. The PBMT group used a fluence of $10-20 J/cm^2$ $(5-10 W)$. The sham group used a fluence of $0 J/cm^2$. After three weeks clients were instructed to reduce the NSAID dose by 50%. Laser treatments then continued weekly for another three weeks. NSAID dose was adjusted as needed based on client perception of discomfort. The blinded clinician lameness score and client Helsinki chronic pain score, as well as the final NSAID dose, was obtained at the end of the study and 7–10 days after the last treatment.

Results

1) Dogs in the PBMT group had a significant reduction in their NSAID dose compared to the sham group.

2) Dogs in the PBMT group had a significant improvement in their lameness scores compared to the sham group.

3) There was a marked, though not statistically significant, improvement in the pain scores of the dogs receiving PBMT compared to the sham group.

Study conclusions: Six weeks of regular PBMT $(10-20 J/cm^2)$ improved the pain and lameness scores, as well as reduced the required NSAID dose, in dogs with elbow osteoarthritis.

Study limitations

1) Small sample size.
2) NSAID use and type was not standardized.
3) Concurrent drug administration was not standardized.
4) Nutraceutical use was not standardized.
5) No true control group (i.e. group receiving no PBMT or sham treatment).
6) The sham laser may still have had a beneficial effect.

L.P.M. conclusion: This study supports the use of PBMT as an effective adjunct therapy in the short-term management of canine elbow arthritis. Further studies are necessary to determine if other wavelengths, fluences, and treatment regimens are equally effective. As arthritis is a chronic condition, long-term studies are needed to determine the length of improvement following PBMT and if repeated (maintenance) PBMT is necessary.

Retrospective Observational Study and Analysis of Two Different Photobiomodulation Therapy Protocols Combined with Rehabilitation Therapy as Therapeutic Interventions for Canine Degenerative Myelopathy

Authors: Lisa A. Miller, DVM, CCRT, CVA; Debbie (Gross) Torraca, DPT, MSPT, OCS, CCRP; and Luis De Taboada, MSEE
Journal: *Photobiomodulation, Photomedicine, and Laser Surgery*
Date: 2020
Study design: Retrospective observational study
Study hypothesis: Determine the effects of two photobiomodulation therapy (PBMT) protocols on the progression of degenerative myelopathy (DM) in dogs from the onset of clinical signs to either nonambulatory paresis (NAP), paralysis, or euthanasia.
Sample size: 20 client-owned dogs with presumed DM taken to a specialty physical rehabilitation facility between 2003 and 2012.
Materials and methods: Inclusion criteria included referral or consultation with a board-certified veterinary neurologist before referral to the rehabilitation facility; history of slowly progressive clinical signs; body weight over 33 lbs (15 kg); neurologic examination consistent with stage 1 DM (upper motor neuron paraparesis, general pelvic limb proprioceptive ataxia, absence of spinal hyperesthesia); lack of other orthopedic or neurologic comorbidities; consistent PBMT (same laser and treatment parameters) throughout the treatment. Almost all dogs received twice-weekly in-clinic rehabilitation therapy (including PBMT) and at-home exercises. In-clinic and at-home therapies were similar, if not the same, for all dogs. For all PBMT the probe was in direct contact with the fur and skin. The treatment area was along the dorsal midline from approximately the third thoracic vertebrae (T3) to the lumbosacral junction (LS) and extending 5–7 cm laterally on both sides. Two PBMT treatment protocols were evaluated: Protocol A (PTCL-A), n = 6, 904 nm, 0.5 W, 8 J/cm^2 per point (total of 20 points used), with a treatment time of approximately five minutes; Protocol B (PTCL-B) n = 14, 980 nm, 6–12 W, 14–21 J/cm^2 continuous grid pattern at a speed of 1–3 inches per second, with a treatment time of 25–26 minutes.

Results

1) The length of time between onset of clinical signs and euthanasia was significantly longer in PTCL-B (38.2 ± 14.67 months) compared to PTCL-A (11.09 ± 2.68 months).
2) The length of time between onset of clinical signs and NAP or paralysis was significantly longer in the PTCL-B (31.76 ± 12.53 months) versus PTCL-A (8.79 ± 1.6 months).

Study conclusions: A specific PBMT protocol significantly slows disease progression and lengthens survival time for dogs with degenerative myelopathy.

(Continued)

Study limitations

1) Retrospective study.
2) Small sample size.
3) Only compared two protocols (wavelengths, fluences, doses).

L.P.M. conclusion: The use of a Class IV laser with 980 nm at 6–12 W, 14–21 J/cm^2 continuous grid pattern at a speed of 1–3 inches per second, with a treatment time of 25–26 minutes significantly improved quality of life, survival time, and delayed symptom onset in dogs with DM. Prospective clinical trials (randomized and blinded) are necessary to confirm these findings. Additional studies evaluating other wavelengths and dosages is warranted as well, as having a technician perform PBMT for almost 30 minutes straight one to two times a week is a large time commitment on the part of the hospital, client, and patient.

Effect of Low-Level Laser Therapy on Bacterial Counts of Contaminated Traumatic Wounds in Dogs

Authors: Samuel Rico-Holgado, Gustavo Ortiz-Díez, María C Martín-Espada, Cristina Fernández-Pérez, María R Baquero-Artigao, and María Suárez-Redondo
Journal: *Journal of Lasers in Medical Science*
Date: 2021
Study design: Randomized blinded placebo-controlled pilot clinical trial
Study hypothesis: The application of low-level light therapy (LLLT) to contaminated wounds will reduce the bacterial load.
Sample size: 14 client-owned dogs with naturally occurring wounds
Materials and methods: Inclusion criteria included dogs presenting with contaminated traumatic wounds with signs of infection or contamination and no history of prior treatment. Microbial analysis was performed on each wound before starting LLLT and on day 2. Dogs were randomly divided into three groups: Group A (n = 4, 6 J/cm^2), Group B (n = 5; 2 J/cm^2), and Group C (n = 5, 0 J/cm^2). The laser used for Groups A and B was a Class IV using four wavelengths simultaneously (660, 800, 905, and 970 nm) with continuous wave and pulsed wave and power range 2–4 W. A noncontact mode was used. The "placebo" laser was 5 mW using a 660 nm wavelength. The area treated included the wound itself plus a 2–4 cm margin of healthy tissue around the wound. Pre-cut sterile silicone templates were used to ensure consistent treatment area for each wound. Following LLLT the wounds were cleaned with lactated Ringer's solution. The laser and irritation treatments were performed on Day 0 and 1. Antibiotics were used as deemed appropriate. All dogs were placed in an Elizabethan collar for 72 hours. Photographs of the wounds were taken on Days 0, 1, and 2.

Results

1) Statistically significant reduction in the colony-forming units noted between Group B and Group C.

Study conclusions: LLLT with these specified parameters decreases bacterial contamination of wounds.

Study limitations

1) Small sample size.
2) Clinician administering the LLLT was not blinded to the treatment group.
3) Different types of wounds with varying degrees of severity and contamination.
4) No true control.
5) Only received two LLLT treatments.
6) Use of antibiotics may confound the results.

L.P.M. conclusion: This is a good pilot study examining the clinical efficacy of LLLT in wound management. Further studies with more standardization, an actual control group, and longer follow-up are necessary to prove LLLT's efficacy for this application.

Table 6.7 Canine studies demonstrating the efficacy of PBMT in companion animals as of February 2023.

Category	Condition	Light specifics	Studies
Anti-inflammatory	Post-dental prophylaxis	LLLT; 650 nm	Watson and Brundage (2019)
		LLLT; Class IV	Alves et al. (2023)
Dermatology	Hair growth	LLLT; 470 nm + 685 nm + 830 nm	Olivieri et al. (2014)
		LLLT + LED	Schnedeker et al. (2021)
	Interdigital	Fluorescence	Marchegiani et al. (2019, 2022)
	Otitis externa	LED-illuminated gel	Tambella et al. (2020)
Gastrointestinal	Large bowel diarrhea	LLLT; Class IV	Alves et al. (2022a)
Osteoarthritis	Elbow	LLLT; 980 nm	Looney et al. (2018)
	Hip joint	LLLT; 980 ± 808 nm	Alves et al. (2022b)
	Multiple joints	LLLT; 808 nm	Barale et al. (2020)
Rehabilitation	Degenerative myelopathy	LLLT; 904 and 908 nm	Miller et al. (2020)
	Postoperative hemilaminectomy	LLLT; 810 nm	Draper et al. (2012), Bruno et al. (2020)
	Postoperative TPLO	LLLT; 650 nm, 800 + 905 + 970 nm	Renwick et al. (2018)
		LLLT; 800–900 nm	Rogatko et al. (2017)
Wound healing	Dental extractions	980 nm	Hamid et al. (2021)
	Postsurgical	LLLT; 850 nm LED; 670 nm	Wardlaw et al. (2019)
	Acute traumatic	Fluorescence; LED	Marchegiani et al. (2020)
		LLLT; 660 + 800 + 905 + 970 nm	Rico-Holgado et al. (2021)
	Chronic wounds	LLLT; 830 nm and 660 + 875 + 905 nm	Hoisang et al. (2021)

LLLT, low-level laser therapy; LED, light emitting diode; TPLO, tibial plateau leveling osteotomy. Source: Lisa P. McFaddin.

cancer in companion animals has promise but further studies are needed before this technique can be recommended.

Table 6.7 specifies many of the diseases and conditions for which canine PBM has shown a scientifically beneficial effect. This list is not all inclusive, as new studies documenting the beneficial effects of PBM in veterinary research are being continually published.

The How

Team Members

This section reviews the potential return on investment (ROI), how to effectively train the entire team, how to promote, and how to integrate the integrative therapy.

Return on Investment

ROI can be determined by evaluating client interest, veterinarian demand, hospital costs, applicability of the service, appointment scheduling, and pricing.

Client Interest

Currently there are no studies documenting client interest or the popularity of veterinary PBMT. By evaluating trends in client opinion and pet health insurance, interest in PBMT may be judged.

Client Opinion   Table 6.8 summarizes the pet owner demographics and statistics mentioned in the My Lessons section of the Introduction. If even half of those owners are open to PBMT, that is still 53.1 million potential patients.

Pet Health Insurance   Many pet insurance plans include coverage for integrative therapies, especially acupuncture (Woodley 2018). The presence of this type of coverage re-emphasizes the mainstream incorporation of these treatment modalities, as well as reflecting client demand.

Veterinarian Demand

As of February 2023 a census of the number of veterinary hospitals offering PBMT has not

Table 6.8   Summary of the 2022 pet ownership and pet health insurance demographics in the United States discussed in the Introduction of the book (Burns 2018; MFAF 2018; APPA 2022; Burns 2022; Nolen 2022; NAPHIA 2023).

• 83% of pets are owned by millennials (32%), generation X (24%), and baby boomers (27%)
• 69 million households owned dogs
• 45.3 million households owned cats
• Estimated over 81.1 million owned dogs
• Estimated over 60.7 million owned cats
• 68% of owners are interested in alternative treatment modalities for their pets
• 4.41 million pets have pet health insurance
• 82% of insurance pets are dogs

Source: Lisa P. McFaddin.

been performed. Unlike other integrative modalities veterinarian demand is less of a concern for a few reasons. First, support team members can be trained to perform PBMT, making the treatment dependent safely and effectively on hospital demand not veterinarian demand. Secondly, the wide diversity of conditions and situations for which PBMT can be used means market saturation is not a concern. The limiting factor is usually veterinarians "remembering" to utilize PBM, not lack of client interest. Finally, PBMT is often thought of as an add-on treatment not a sole therapeutic modality. The number of patients suitable for receiving PBM is again limited by the number of recommendations made for its use, not the number of new or referred patients.

Hospital Costs

Let's start by reviewing the potential costs associated with introducing and offering PBMT: veterinarian training, staff training, supplies and equipment, staffing, facilities, and advertising. Tables 6.9 and 6.10 demonstrate varying start-up costs, depending on the hospital's contribution toward the veterinarian's training and prior utilization of regular all-staff meetings. For more information on potential hospital costs, refer to the Introduction at the beginning of this book.

Veterinarian Training

Course   As of February 2023, there are no accredited certification courses in veterinary PBMT. Attending formal training in PBMT is not required but is encouraged, ensuring PBM is performed safely and effectively. Many national and state veterinary conferences have American Association of Veterinary State Boards (AAVSB) Registry of Approved Continuing Education (RACE) approved lectures on PBM which can be a great introduction to the modality. There are several online laser training courses, for which additional information can be found in the Veterinarians section of this chapter (cost range, $189–799).

Textbooks Textbooks are not required but may come in handy as a quick reference for point-of care. As of February 2023 there are two well-known veterinary laser books. Here we assume purchase of at least one of the books (total, $150).

Travel Expenses As all of the courses are offered online, there will be no travel expenses (cost, $0).

Time Off Veterinarian paid time-off (PTO) for on-site courses only factors in as an added expense if additional PTO is provided outside of their contractual annual PTO. Clinics offer an average of 4.1 paid continuing education (CE) days per year (AAHA 2019). As all of the CE options are online, it is assumed there will be no additional cost for the hospital (cost, $0).

Staff Training Team training expenses are highly variable and dependent on the preexistence staff meetings and use of a staff meeting for training (compared to self-study). Refer to the Introduction for a breakdown of these variables (cost range, $230–1295).

Another factor to consider is the cost of additional training materials. If the clinic elects to purchase training videos for PBM and laser safety, this would need to be added to the tangible costs.

Supplies Supplies break down to the laser unit itself, laser accessories (probe attachments, carrying case or stand) and PPE (human and animal goggles). Refer to Table 6.9 for a breakdown of the costs (cost range, $9300–41 900).

Staffing PBMT appointments are typically scheduled as assistant or technician appointments ranging from 10 to 45 minutes in length, depending on the treatment time and number of treatment sites. The staffing requirements for PBMT should not exceed those required for a normal day, assuming the clinic usually has assistant or technician appointments (cost, $0).

Table 6.9 Total potential hospital start-up costs for PBMT as of February 2023.

Category	Subcategories	Projected cost	
Veterinarian training	Course	$185–799	Average $528
	Textbooks	$150	
	Travel expenses	$0	
	Time-off	$0	
Staff training	Variable	$230–1295	
Supplies	Laser unit	$9000–40 000	Estimate average $25 000
	Case or stand	$100–1000	± Included
	PPE people	$200–500	Average $350; ± Included
	PPE pets	$0–400	Average $200
Staffing	Variable	≥$0	
Facilities	Overhead	$2–5 per minute for 10–45 minute appointment	$20–225 per patient
Advertising	Variable	≤$420	

PPE, personal protective equipment. Source: Lisa P. McFaddin.

Facilities Facilities expenses represent the costs needed to keep the doors open (aka overhead). Overhead includes rent or mortgage, utilities, administrative costs, and often employee costs divided by the minutes the practice is open (Stevenson 2016). The price per minute equals the amount of revenue needed just to break even. Overhead is extremely hospital specific, but the range tends to be $2–5/minute.

While a specific area does not need to be designated for PBM, OSHA requires a list of places in the hospital where PBMT will be performed and where the laser will be stored. Having set areas can help with appointment flow, especially when performing a number of PBMTs each day. No additional expense will be needed to design or decorate a PBM-specific room.

Advertising There are numerous ways to advertise a new service. On average veterinary hospitals spend 0.7% of revenue on promotion and advertisement (AVMA 2019). Most of the advertisement can be done with little to no additional expenditure. The national median gross revenue for companion animal practices was $1.2 million in 2022 (AVMA 2023). Advertising costs are calculated assuming no more than 5% of the current advertising budget would be used for promotion of the new service (estimated maximal cost, $420).

Start-Up Costs Table 6.9 summarizes projected start-up costs for PBMT. Table 6.10 calculates potential start-up costs based on the price of the laser unit and degree of hospital contribution toward veterinarian and staff training.

Table 6.10 Projected PBMT start-up costs for six hospital scenarios, with varying hospital contributions toward training and staff training as of February 2023. The course and textbook costs are based on averages. Staff training costs assumes a 1.5-hour-long all-staff meeting, using national averages for employee numbers: eight non-veterinarians and two veterinarians (AVMA 2019). The overhead is based on an average of $3.5/minute. Missed revenue is calculated using $250 as the veterinarian revenue per hour. Examples 1–3 assume the laser unit cost $9000, no accessories or pet personal protective equipment (PPE) were purchased, and two human goggles (PPE) were purchased. Examples 4–6 assume the laser unit cost $40 000, accessories cost $1000, human PPE cost $500, and pet PPE cost $400. Advertising costs include printed materials, digital advertisement, and community engagement.

Category	Projected expenses	Ex. 1	Ex. 2	Ex. 3	Ex. 4	Ex. 5	Ex. 6	Ex. 7	Ex. 8
Training	Course cost	$528	n/a	$528	n/a	$528	$528	$528	$528
	Textbooks	$150	n/a	$150	n/a	$150	n/a	$150	n/a
Staff training	Office supplies	$30	$30	$30	$30	$30	$30	$30	$30
	Lunch	$200	$200	$200	$200	$200	$200	$200	$200
	Overhead	$315	$315	n/a	n/a	$315	$315	n/a	n/a
	Missed revenue	$851	$851	n/a	n/a	$851	$851	n/a	n/a
Supplies	Laser unit	$9000	$9000	$9000	$9000	$40 000	$40 000	$40 000	$40 000
	Accessories	$0	$0	$0	$0	$1000	$1000	$1000	$1000
	Human PPE	$200	$200	$200	$200	$500	$500	$500	$500
	Pet PPE	$0	$0	$0	$0	$400	$400	$400	$400
Advertising		$420	$420	$420	$420	$420	$420	$420	$420
Total		**$11 694**	**$11 016**	**$10 528**	**$9850**	**$44 394**	**$44 244**	**$43 228**	**$43 078**

Source: Lisa P. McFaddin.

Applicability

As stated earlier PBM is a versatile treatment modality useful for a variety of conditions. A conservative estimate will be used to calculate potential PBM patients on a weekly and annual basis. Most PBMT protocols have a finite number of applications. This is not to say PBM cannot be used long term, but most of the conditions for which PBM is recommended are acute. For example, postoperative PBM for spays and neuters or dental extractions is typically performed one time immediately after wound closure. PBM for wounds, acute pain, dermatologic conditions, and acute inflammation or pain often have a set number of treatments followed by reassessment of the problem. Chronic conditions, like osteoarthritis, often start with a set of PBM sessions; one common protocol is two to three treatments weekly for a total of six treatments, then reassess.

The average companion animal practice employees 2.1 full-time veterinarians (AVMA 2023). If each veterinarian has one surgery and averages three spays or neuters a week, that is at least six potential PBM treatments a week on post-alteration surgeries alone. The average companion animal veterinarian receives 21 paid days of vacation and holiday pay annually and 4.1 paid days off for CE (AAHA 2019; iVet360 2023). Over a one-year period this example would yield 290 post-surgery PBM treatments alone.

There are no studies documenting the average weekly or annual number of wounds seen, but a conservative estimate would be 5%, and this would include acute and chronic wounds caused by a variety of conditions. Most small animal clinics are open for appointments 5.6 days/week (AVMA 2023). Veterinarians works on average 45 hours a week, spending 78% of their time in appointments (35 hours/week), and see on average 2.1 patients per hour (AVMA 2023). This equals approximately 74 patients a week. In this scenario the clinic would treat eight wounds a week and 387 annually. Keep in mind each wound would receive roughly six treatments for a total of 2322 PBM sessions in one year.

Depending on the study, osteoarthritis affects at least 2.5–6.6% of dogs of all ages and breeds (O'Neill et al. 2014; Anderson et al. 2018) and over 20% of dogs over the age of one year (Johnston 1997; Clements et al. 2006). Using the lower end of 6.6%, and assuming 70% of the patient base is canine, that is 3.4 canine osteoarthritis patients who could benefit from PBMT weekly, per doctor. That is a total of 329 annually, and assuming each receives at least six treatments, that is a total of 1074 PBM sessions in one year.

The feline statistics are even more varied, with one study finding 40% of cats of all ages have clinical signs consistent with osteoarthritis (Kerwin 2010), while up to 90% of cats 12 years and older had radiographic findings of osteoarthritis (Hardie et al. 2002). Using the low end, that equals 860 feline patients with osteoarthritis who could benefit from PBMT annually, and with six sessions each the total is 5160.

Adding all of these "ideal" situations together, the total annual PBM sessions for a two-doctor practice could be as high as 8846. There are obviously more applications for PBMT, but this exercise at least allows visualization of the practicalities. In the end the limits of PBMT are only limited by the veterinarian's imagination and effectiveness of the hospital's promotion.

Appointment Scheduling

Scheduling PBMT is different from other modalities where the veterinarian must perform the procedure. When the treatment can be performed by veterinary assistants and licensed technicians (VA/LT) scheduling is primarily limited by support staff availability. Once the hospital knows there will be an available and properly trained VA/LT, the customer service representatives (CSRs) can schedule based on appointment length and follow-up recommendations. Unlike other therapies, exam room availability should be less of an issue, especially if multiple areas within the hospital are designated as acceptable laser treatment zones.

Most PBM is performed to address acute or chronic pain. The goal is for the treatment to be relaxing. Scheduling potentially stressful adjunct procedures, such as nail trims, anal gland expressions, ear cleaning, blood draws, and vaccinations, is discouraged.

Pricing

An in-depth look into appointment pricing can be found in the Introduction of this book. Here we discuss two pricing methods: current market fees and hospital cost-based pricing.

Current Market Fees   There are no studies documenting the average price of PBMT. A quick internet search of veterinary clinics with posted PBMT pricing in February 2023 revealed prices ranging from $25 to $150 per treatment depending on the region of the country, type of laser used, and target area or areas (i.e. length of the treatment).

Hospital Cost-Based Pricing   The practice needs to consider how it will charge for PBMT. One approach is to charge solely by the number of areas treated. This approach ignores the treatment time, as some target tissues and/or areas take longer than others, but instead relies on making more profit on shorter treatment times and less on longer ones. Keep in mind if multiple areas are treated, each site would be one charge. This approach is also dependent on the class of laser purchased, as Class IV treatment times are generally shorter compared to Class III. Having one set price does make it easier for the staff to provide estimated costs.

Another pricing method charges by the number of treatments and the treatment area. For example, a relatively small wound or otitis treatment would cost less than treating the entire lumbar spine. This approach accounts more for support staff time but is a little more complicated when providing estimated costs to clients.

A final consideration is the inclusion of "packages." Some practices and clients like the idea of having one charge for a single treatment ($\pm$ per area as well) and a bundle price for multiple treatments that typically offers a slight discount to the client. In the case of "packages" the clients pay up front. This can be a lucrative approach but does have a few drawbacks. First, the management team needs to have clear definitions regarding an appropriate length of time in which the treatments must be completed (i.e. three to four weeks, depending on the number of treatments). Secondly, the management team must decide if they will refund unused treatments. Finally, keep in mind the end-of-day will be much higher the day the client purchases the package and lower when the client returns for the prepaid service.

Unlike other modalities, most of the cost comes from the equipment (laser and PPE), so instead of calculating the hospital cost per patient we calculate the hospital cost per treatment. To more easily demonstrate hospital cost and potential pricing, the following examples use the approach of charging per treatment, i.e. the same charge regardless of the target tissue.

Table 6.11 outlines the hospital cost per treatment using roughly one-quarter of the projected number of annual treatments calculated in the Applicability section, rounded down to 2000 for ease of calculations. This was done because when calculating the realistic daily number of treatments, the schedule of the persons predominantly performing the PBMT, the VAs and LTs, must be taken into consideration. Assuming a VA/LT has her or his own appointments, during an eight-hour shift if they have appointments every 15–30 minutes that is 16–32 patients per day; 2000 annual PBM treatments would equate to almost seven sessions daily, accounting for 22–44% of their appointment load.

Overhead includes rent or mortgage, utilities, administrative costs, and often employee costs divided by the minutes the practice is

Table 6.11 Estimated hospital cost per PBM treatment based on one- and two-year amortization periods. The total start-up costs are taken from Table 6.10. The amortization per treatment is based on an estimated 2000 PBM treatments annually. Overhead was calculated using 20% of $3.5/minute for 15 minutes.

	$9000 Laser unit				$40 000 Laser unit			
	Ex. 1	Ex. 2	Ex. 3	Ex. 4	Ex. 5	Ex. 6	Ex. 7	Ex. 8
Amortization period of 1 year								
Table 6.10 totals	$11 694	$11 016	$10 528	$9850	$44 394	$44 244	$43 228	$43 078
Amortization	$5.85	$5.51	$5.26	$4.93	$22.20	$22.12	$21.61	$21.54
Overhead	$10.50	$10.50	$10.50	$10.50	$10.50	$10.50	$10.50	$10.50
Total	**$16**	**$16**	**$16**	**$15**	**$33**	**$33**	**$32**	**$32**
Amortization period of 2 years								
Table 6.10 totals	$11 694	$11 016	$10 528	$9850	$44 394	$44 244	$43 228	$43 078
Amortization	$2.92	$2.75	$2.63	$2.46	$11.10	$11.06	$10.81	$10.77
Overhead	$10.50	$10.50	$10.50	$10.50	$10.50	$10.50	$10.50	$10.50
Total	**$13**	**$13**	**$13**	**$13**	**$22**	**$22**	**$21**	**$21**

Source: Lisa P. McFaddin.

open (Stevenson 2016). Total overhead was calculated using the following assumptions:

1) Hospital overhead is $3.5/minute.
2) Each chargeable treatment would take no more than 15 minutes.
3) At any given hour there are three employees seeing appointments and generating revenue: two veterinarians and one VA/LT (AAHA 2019; AVMA 2023).
4) Non-veterinarian income accounts for 40% of mean hourly revenue (AVMA 2023).
5) Assume half of the hourly non-veterinarian revenue is from medications (prescription and over-the-counter) and food.

With these assumptions, VA/LT overhead would be 20% of the $3.5/minute for 15 minutes (i.e. $10.5). Table 6.12 lists potential PBM treatment prices based on hospital costs.

Team Training

The concept of phase training is used when introducing PBM to the hospital team. A multimedia approach is used to assist with the training program and is outlined Table 6.13.

Practice Manager's Role in Training

To conquer this task the practice manager needs his or her own checklist which includes the following information:

- Create the hospital's Laser Safety Program (LSP) with the medical director. The LSP must include:
  - A description of the class or classes of lasers used in the hospital.
  - Documents describing the safe use of lasers (refer to the Safety section of this chapter and the companion website for resources).
  - A designated LSO.
  - A written LSP including SOPs.
  - Approved locations for storage and use of lasers.
  - Description of the required PPE.
  - Employee training program (refer to the Safety section of this chapter and the companion website for resources).
- Schedule a date and time for the team training.
- Ensure all information pertaining to the new service is reviewed with the staff.

Table 6.12 Potential PBM treatment pricing using hospital costs from Table 6.11 at varying percentage markups as of February 2023.

		$9000 Laser unit				$40 000 Laser unit			
		Ex. 1	Ex. 2	Ex. 3	Ex. 4	Ex. 5	Ex. 6	Ex. 7	Ex. 8
Amortization period of 1 year									
Total hospital cost		$16	$16	$16	$15	$33	$33	$32	$32
Potential appointment price	40% Markup	$22	$22	$22	$21	$46	$46	$45	$45
	50% Markup	$24	$24	$24	$23	$50	$50	$48	$48
	60% Markup	$26	$112	$107	$94	$118	$111	$105	$93
	70% Markup	$27	$27	$27	$26	$56	$56	$54	$54
	80% Markup	$29	$29	$29	$27	$59	$59	$58	$58
	90% Markup	$30	$30	$30	$29	$63	$63	$61	$61
	100% Markup	$32	$32	$32	$30	$66	$66	$64	$64
Amortization period of 2 years									
Total hospital cost		$13	$13	$13	$13	$22	$22	$21	$21
Potential appointment price	40% Markup	$18	$18	$18	$18	$31	$31	$29	$29
	50% Markup	$20	$20	$20	$20	$33	$33	$32	$32
	60% Markup	$21	$112	$107	$94	$118	$111	$105	$93
	70% Markup	$22	$22	$22	$22	$37	$37	$36	$36
	80% Markup	$23	$23	$23	$23	$40	$40	$38	$38
	90% Markup	$25	$25	$25	$25	$42	$42	$40	$40
	100% Markup	$26	$26	$26	$26	$44	$44	$42	$42

Source: Lisa P. McFaddin.

Table 6.13 The breakdown of phase training steps and resources for the entire hospital team.

Phase 1: Background information	
Team training guide	The handout walks the practice manager and/or veterinarian through Phase 1 of the training
	A downloadable and editable copy of the handout is located on the companion website
Training presentation	The video covers background information on the modality
	PowerPoints can be downloaded, edited, and personalized from the companion website
	The document can be used as a PowerPoint or saved as an mp4 creating a personalized movie
Team training handout	The handout provides additional background information for the CSRs, VAs, and LTs to complement the knowledge gained from watching the training presentation
	A downloadable and editable copy of the handout is located on the companion website

Phase 2: Knowledge proficiency	
Quiz	A short quiz to ensure all team members have a good understanding of the service being offered
	A downloadable and editable copy of the handout is located on the companion website
	A key is provided
Phase 3: Expectations	
Training worksheets	A training checklist is provided for CSRs and VA/LTs with role-specific expectations and tasks for each staff member
	A recommended completion time is provided
	A downloadable and editable copy of the handout is located on the companion website
Phase 4: Client education	
Client scripts	Bullet point information and scripted examples used when discussing the therapy with clients
	A downloadable and editable copy of the handout is located on the companion website
Client education presentation	A short (5–7 minute) client educational video about the therapeutic modality
	PowerPoints can be downloaded, edited, and personalized from the companion website
	The document can be used as a PowerPoint or saved as an mp4 creating a personalized movie
Client education handout	An informational handout about the therapeutic modality written specifically for clients
	A downloadable and editable copy of the handout is located on the companion website

CSR, customer service representative; VA, veterinary assistant; LT, licensed technician. Source: Lisa P. McFaddin.

- Confirm all team members have completed the training.
- Certify all team members understand the information and can successfully educate clients.

Promotion

There are six common avenues of promotion for a VIM service: hospital website, social media, email blasts, mailers, in-hospital promotions, and client education.

Hospital Website

Advertise "Photobiomodulation Therapy" or "Cold Laser Therapy" or "Low Level Light Therapy" in several locations on the website. Checkout AAHA's Publicity Toolbox, available free of charge to AAHA accredited hospitals, for client consent forms when discussing specific patients and using their photographs.

On the made page insert "Now offering veterinary photobiomodulation" with a link to success stories or client testimonials. Utilize the hospital website to advertise the VIM treatment under the "Services" section. Create a blog page discussing patient success stories.

Social Media

Utilize Facebook, Instagram, and/or Twitter to post facts, photographs, hashtags, and patient success stories. Include fun and intriguing facts about PBM. Clients love patient photographs, especially when receiving PBM. Create or utilize PBM specific hashtags.

Email Blasts

Send fun mass emails to your clients introducing PBM. Consider monthly case presentations illustrating how the service has benefited patients. Almost everyone has at least one email address these days. CSRs should be amassing client emails at the same rate as phone numbers.

Mailers

Mailers can be expensive and are largely unnecessary in this digital age. Mailers can be used to announce the introduction of PBM to existing clients. The mailer should include the name of the new service, a brief description of how PBM can help pet patients, the name of the doctor performing PBM, possibly a brief description of the training the team has received, and possibly a photograph of a pet receiving PBM.

In-Hospital Promotions

Advertise PBM within the hospital using small promotional signs, informational signs, invoice teasers, and staff buttons. Small promotional signs can be placed in the waiting room and exam rooms. Include photographs of pets receiving PBM. Buttons can be made for the staff to wear with kitchy phrases reminding owners, in a fun way, of the new VIM service. Consider catchphrases such as "Need a Light?" or "Let It Shine" or "Ask me about my laser beams?"

Informational signs should include a brief description of how PBM can help pet patients, photographs of pets receiving PBM, and a brief description of the training the team received.

Invoice teasers should consist of short phrases reminding and enticing owners regarding a new service offered at the practice. Examples include "Now offering Veterinary Photobiomodulation," "Curious if PBM can help your pet?," "Introducing Veterinary Photobiomodulation" and "Would your pet benefit from Veterinary Photobiomodulation?" (Note that the terms "Cold Laser" or "Low Level Light Therapy" can be substituted for the term "Photobiomodulation".)

Client Education

Education is crucial to understanding the purpose and importance of any given treatment. The client handouts and videos solidify pet owner knowledge base, reducing concerns and conveying value.

Integration

The key components for proper integration include availability of the service to the right patients; appropriate patient scheduling; appropriate support staff scheduling; and staff buy-in (understanding the benefits of the offered service).

Veterinarians

There are several factors to contemplate when veterinarians are considering, and preparing to incorporate, a VIM in their clinical repertoire: state requirements and restrictions, return on investment, course availability, supplies and equipment, veterinary organizations, and continuing education.

State Requirements and Restrictions

Is PBM Considered the Practice of Veterinary Medicine?

While most states do not specifically reference PBM in their definition of the "practice of veterinary medicine," the use of PBM is likely categorized as such for two reasons. First, Class IIIb and Class IV lasers are classified as medical equipment by the FDA. Secondly, these units are used to treat specific conditions in our veterinary patients. Appropriately trained veterinary assistants and technicians should be allowed to perform the laser treatments when under the direct supervision of a veterinarian. Consultation with each state board is the best way to ensure all veterinarians and hospitals are complying with state law.

Does PBM Continuing Education Count Toward Licensure Continuing Education Requirements?

All veterinary establishments using a Class IIIb or Class IV laser are required to provide laser safety training for all employees. Ideally this training should be completed annually, ensuring continued safe use of the equipment. Currently no states require specific CE hours for veterinarians offering PBMT nor do they specifically reference PBM CE.

Are Your Assets Covered?

The research supporting the efficacy of PBM combined with its ubiquitous use in general practice suggest it should be considered standard of care for certain conditions. As such, the practice of PBMT should be covered under veterinary liability insurance policies. To be safe check with your liability insurance to determine if you are covered when practicing PBM. Refer to the Introduction at the beginning of this book for additional information.

Return on Investment

Specifics are discussed in the Team Members section of this chapter.

Course Availability

At this time there are no accredited certification courses in veterinary PBMT. Training is still vital, providing the foundation for understanding how PBMT can best help your veterinary patients. Completion of formal training also helps legitimize the modality. The following initial certification course offerings and pricing are current as of February 2023.

Most veterinarians learn about PBM attending lectures at the state or national conferences. There are also a variety of online veterinary organizations, such as Veterinary Information Network (VIN), Vetfolio, DVM360 Flex, and Vet Girl on the Run, which offer AAVSB RACE-approved CE on PBM. Additionally, the College of Integrative Veterinary Therapies (CIVT, https://civtedu.org) and the Canine Rehabilitation Institute (CRI, https://www.caninerehabinstitute.com) will occasionally have webinars discussing PBM.

American Institute of Medical Laser Applications (AIMLA)

- **Course name**: Introduction to Companion Animal Laser Therapy
- **Prerequisites**: None specified
- **Description**
  - Three-hour AAVSB RACE-approved CE.
  - Covers the following information:
    - Medical laser safety.

- Biological effects of lasers for treating common companion animal conditions.
- Practical applications for laser therapy.
- Treatment of conditions in the oral cavity, ear, cervical region, elbow, lumbar spine, hip, stifle, tarsus, and more.
- Quiz following completion each module.
- Provides certificate of completion.

- **Online**: Three modules
- **On-site**: Not applicable
- **Cost**: $189
- **Contact information**
  - Phone: 888-566-7244
  - Website: https://aimla.org
  - Email: support@aimla.info

American Institute of Medical Laser Applications (AIMLA)

- **Course name**: Introduction to Laser Therapy for the Veterinary Technician, Veterinary Assistant, and Veterinary Nurse
- **Prerequisites**: None specified
- **Description**
  - Four-hour AAVSB RACE-approved CE.
  - Covers material presented in the other course but geared toward non-veterinarian team members.
  - Quiz following completion each module.
  - Provides certificate of completion.

- **Online**: Five modules
- **On-site**: Not applicable
- **Completion time**: Not applicable
- **Cost**: $199.95
- **Contact information**
  - Phone: 888-566-7244
  - Website: https://aimla.org
  - Email: support@aimla.info

American Institute of Medical Laser Applications (AIMLA)

- **Course name**: Veterinary Medical Laser Safety Officer
- **Prerequisites**: None specified
- **Description**
  - Two-hour AAVSB RACE-approved CE.
  - Discusses laser basics, safety controls and eye protection, additional safety

precautions, and the responsibilities of the veterinary medical laser safety officer.
– Quiz.
– Provides certificate of completion.

- **Online**: One module
- **On-site**: Not applicable
- **Cost**: $169.85
- **Contact information**
  – Phone: 888-566-7244
  – Website: https://aimla.org
  – Email: support@aimla.info

American Institute of Medical Laser Applications (AIMLA)
- **Course name**: Laser Therapy Principles in the Companion Animal Practice
- **Prerequisites**: None specified
- **Description**
  – 1.5-hour AAVSB RACE-approved CE.
  – Discusses the biological effects of medical lasers in the treatment of common veterinary conditions.
  – Quiz.
  – Provides certificate of completion.

- **Online**: One module
- **On-site**: Not applicable
- **Completion time**: Not applicable
- **Cost:** $109.95
- **Contact Information**
  – Phone: 888-566-7244
  – Website: https://aimla.org
  – Email: support@aimla.info

American Institute of Medical Laser Applications (AIMLA)
- **Course name**: The Scientific Basis of Medical Lasers
- **Prerequisites**: None specified
- **Description**
  – One-hour AAVSB RACE-approved CE.
  – Discusses the scientific principles of medical lasers.
  – Quiz.
  – Provides certificate of completion.

- **Online**: One module
- **On-site**: Not applicable

- **Completion time**: Not applicable
- **Cost**: $84.95
- **Contact information**
  – Phone: 888-566-7244
  – Website: https://aimla.org
  – Email: support@aimla.info

Companion Animal Laser
- **Course name**: Introduction to Laser Therapy
- **Prerequisites**: Licensed veterinarians, veterinary technicians, and clinics
- **Description**
  – Four-hour AAVSB RACE-approved CE.
  – Covers the following topics:
    o Laser physics
    o Mechanisms of action
    o Safety
    o Practical applications
    o Optimizing use.
  – Covers many other web series and webinars on various topics pertaining to PBM, pain management, diagnostics, and business.

- **On-site training**: Not applicable
- **Online training**: Nine modules of varying length
- **Completion time**: Not applicable
- **Cost**: Unclear. Website did not allow pricing, but it does appear a coupon code allows free access.
- **Contact information**: https://www.companionanimalhealth.com

CuraCore
- **Course name**: Photomedicine for Veterinarians
- **Prerequisites**: License, in good standing, to practice veterinary medicine, third or fourth year veterinary student, or animal rehabilitation practitioner
- **Description**
  – 40-hours of CE, does not specify if AAVSB RACE-approved.
  – Course covers
    o Medical application of light using laser and LEDs
    o Tissue–light interactions

o PBM for various conditions in veterinary patients

o Pros and cons of various LED units.

- **On-site training**: Not applicable
- **Online training**: 12 modules
- **Completion time**: One year
- **Cost**: $799
- **Contact information**
  - Address: 4007 Automation Way, Fort Collins, CO 80525
  - Phone: (970) 818-0851
  - Website: www.curacore.org
  - Email: info@curacore.org

NC State Veterinary Medicine and Northwest Seminars

- **Course name**: Introduction to Companion Animal Laser Therapy
- **Prerequisites**: Licensed veterinarians and veterinary technicians
- **Description**
  - An introductory course discussing the biological effects of medical lasers used to treat common conditions in veterinary patients.
  - Provides access to the Companion Animal Therapy Certification Course.
  - AAVSB RACE-approved CE credit.

- **Online training**: Three hours
- **On-site training**: Not applicable
- **Cost**: $149
- **Contact information**: https://www.ncsu-vetce.com

Optimum Pet Vitality

- **Course name**: Optimum Laser Therapy Course and Community
- **Prerequisites**: Licensed veterinarians, veterinary technicians, physical therapists, and clinics
- **Description**
  - 20-hours AAVSB RACE-approved CE.
  - Covers the following topics:
    o Laser fundamentals
    o Instructions for treating over 25 conditions and areas
    o Technique and protocol recommendations

o Information on different laser manufacturers.
  - Includes
    o Printable indication charts
    o Customizable patient record templates.

- **Online training**: Yes
- **On-site training**: Not applicable
- **Completion time**: One year
- **Cost**: $597
- **Contact information**: https://www.optimumpetvitality.com

Supplies and Equipment

The necessary supplies are a laser unit and PPE. There are several companies marketing Class IIIb and Class IV veterinary lasers and each have pros and cons. The practitioner and hospital should look at as many options before purchase as possible to determine which unit will best fit their needs. As of February 2023 the most used companies include Companion Animal Laser (https://www.companionanimal-health.com), Cutting Edge Laser (https://cela-sers.com), Diowave Laser System (https://diowavelaser.com), Erchonia (https://www.erchonia.com), EvoLaser (http://www.evolaser.net), K Laser (https://k-laser.com), Multi Radiance Medical (https://www.multiradiance.com), Pegasus Therapy (https://www.pegasus-therapy.com), Respond Systems (https://respondsystems.com), and Thor Laser (https://www.thorlaser.com). The price range is huge and depends on the laser class, wavelength(s), pulse structure, and probe attachments. As of February 2023 the range is between $9000 and $40 000. Purchasing a stand or carrying case for the laser typically adds an additional $100–1000 depending on the product and company.

At bare minimum the PPE should consist of goggles for people, at least two pairs. Ideally the clinic would purchase pet goggles as well, generally in two to three sizes. As of February 2023, the people and pet goggles run approximately $100–150 a pair. Some companies will include ocular PPE as part of the package when purchasing a laser.

Veterinary Organizations

A description of the most common veterinary organizations with a special interest in PBMT are provided below. Table 6.14 summarizes organization names, contact information, and membership dues as of February 2023.

There are two laser-specific organizations which offer CE for both human and veterinary medical professions: the AIMLA (https://aimla.org) and the ASLMS (https://www.aslms.org). AIMLA, mentioned in the course section, appears to offer free registration, requiring the veterinarian only pay as needed for online courses. Since the AIMLA functions more as a CE distributor, specifics regarding the membership are not discussed further.

The ASLMS does discuss veterinary medicine, but all of the references appear to end in 2016. There is no mention of current CE events for veterinarians. Membership, $350/year, may be required to purchase online course and webinar information. Given the confusing relevance in veterinary medicine this organization is not discussed further.

American Holistic Veterinary Medical Association (AHVMA)

- **Description**: The AHVMA was founded in 1982 at the Western States Veterinary Conference with the goal of advancing integrative medicine through the education of integrative and non-integrative veterinarians, the introduction of integrative medicine

to veterinary students, the promotion of research, and representation in the AVMA House of Delegates. There is no annual CE requirement to maintain membership.

- **Membership benefits**

  - Free subscription to the *AHVMA Journal*, a peer-reviewed journal.
  - Online resources for client education.
  - Searchable member directory.
  - Discounted vaccination titers through Kansas State University (KSU) Diagnostic Lab.
  - Free access to the Natural Medicines Database, an online resource for supplements, natural medicines, and integrative therapies.
  - Reduced cost for the AHVMA annual conference.

College of Integrative Veterinary Therapies (CIVT)

- **Description**: An online organization open to all licensed animal health providers interested in integrative medicine. There are two membership options: full membership for veterinarians and associate membership for registered animal health professionals. CIVT strives to promote all aspects of evidence-based integrative medicine through online education and discussion forums. CIVT provides financial support to veterinary students interested in studying integrative

Table 6.14 Veterinary associations and organizations with a special interest in PBM as of February 2023.

Organization	Contact information	Membership dues
American Holistic Veterinary Medical Association (AHVMA)	PO Box 630, Abingdon, MD 21009 (410) 569-0795 office@ahvma.org	$300/year
College of Integrative Veterinary Therapies (CIVT)	PO Box 352, Yeppoon, 4703 QLD, Australia (303) 800-5460 membership@civtedu.org	$185/year
International Veterinary Academy of Pain Management (IVAPM)	PO Box 1868, Mt Juliet, TN 371211 info@ivapm.org	$150/year

Source: Lisa P. McFaddin.

medicine. CIVT also helps fund integrative medicine research. There is no annual CE requirement to maintain membership.

- **Membership benefits**

  - Access to the online electronic library.
  - Access to the electronic *Journal of Integrative Veterinary Therapies*.
  - Three free CE webinars annually.
  - 20% discount on all webinars.
  - Discounts on specific CIVT courses.
  - Searchable member directory.
  - Access to the Natural Medicines Databases and the American Botanical Council Library.

International Veterinary Academy of Pain Management (IVAPM)

- **Description**: Originally known as the Companion Animal Pain Management Consortium, then the Academy of Pain Management Interest Group, and finally IVAPM. Founded in 2001 to provide pain management education and certification programs. The organization's goal is to provide acute and chronic pain relief for veterinary patients. Both traditional and alternative therapies are embraced, including acupuncture and rehabilitation and physical therapy.
- **Membership benefits**

  - Members can become Certified Veterinary Pain Practitioners (CVPP).
  - Access to member's-only Facebook group offering case consultations and questions.
  - Reduced subscription rate for IVAPM's journal *Veterinary Anaesthesia and Analgesia*.
  - Reduced registration fee for the International Veterinary Emergency and Critical Care (IVECCS) conference.
  - Reduced registration for all IVAPM continuing education events (online and on-site).
  - Complementary World Small Animal Veterinary Association (WSAVA) membership.

Reference Books

The following is a list of my recommended references pertaining to PBM and other forms of light therapy as of February 2023. A summary of each book is provided.

Canine Rehabilitation and Physical Therapy
- Author: Darryl Mills, DVM, DACVS, DACVSMT, CCRP and David Levine, PhD, PT
- Summary: A comprehensive reference book covering canine rehabilitation protocols for a variety of conditions, printable medical record forms, canine exercises, therapeutic modality options available, physical examination specifics, and a companion website. A must-have for veterinarians interested in manual therapy, orthopedics, and rehabilitation.

Canine Sports Medicine and Rehabilitation
- Authors: M. Christine Zink, DVM, PhD, DACVP, DACVSMR and Janet D. Van Dyke, DVM, DACVSMR
- Summary: A comprehensive reference book discussing common canine musculoskeletal conditions and ailments, with particular interest in the canine athlete. The book covers gait analysis and physiology, various therapeutic approaches (including nutrition, rehabilitation, manual therapy, acupuncture, chiropractic, therapeutic exercise, aquatic therapy, conditioning and retraining, and assistive devices), and specific diagnoses and treatment recommendations for disorders of the forelimbs and pelvic limbs. A must-have for veterinarians interested in manual therapy, orthopedics, and rehabilitation.

Laser Therapy in Veterinary Medicine: Photobiomodulation
- Authors: Ronald J. Riegel, DVM and Hohn C. Godbold, Jr., DVM
- Summary: An in-depth review of the science behind photobiomodulation as well as a practical reference for the clinical applications of laser therapy in veterinary medicine.

Integrating Complementary Medicine into Veterinary Practice
- Authors: Robert S. Goldstein, VMD, Paula Jo Broadfoot, DVM, Richard E. Plamquist, DVM, Karen Johnstons, DVM, Jiu Jia Wen, DVM, Barbara Fougère, BSc, BVMs (Hons), BHSc (comp Med), MODT, MHSc (Herb Med), CVA (IVAs), CVBM, CVCP, and Margo Roman, DVM
- Summary: A comprehensive review of multiple integrative therapies including Chinese herbal medicine, acupuncture, homotoxicology, nanopharmacology, homotoxicology, and therapeutic nutrition. The book aims to educate veterinary practitioners on the validity, effectiveness, and incorporation of each modality within daily practice.

Manual of Natural Veterinary Medicine: Science and Tradition
- Authors: Susan G. Wynn, DVM and Steve Marsden, DVM, ND, MSOM, Lac, Dipl. CH., RH(AHG)
- Summary: A quick reference book discussing the integrative therapy options for numerous diseases in veterinary medicine. The book is organized by Western conditions. For each category the potential TCVM diagnoses and treatment options are reviewed in succinct detail. A must-have for all integrative veterinarians.

Veterinary Laser Therapy in Small Animal Practice
- Authors: Maria Suárez Rendondo, DVM, PhD, CVA and Bryan J. Stephens, PhD

- Summary: Practical guide to laser therapy for the clinician discussing the fundamentals of light therapy and clinical applications. Case studies are included to demonstrate how laser therapy can be incorporated into everyday practice.

Promotion

Information regarding the hospital's promotion of PBM can be found in the Team Members section.

Integration

Key components for proper integration include availability, scheduling, and staff buy-in. Availability means offering the service to the right patient. Scheduling refers to appropriate patient and support staff scheduling. Staff buy-in ensures all team members understand the benefits of the offered service.

Conclusion

PBMT is a relatively new but thriving therapeutic modality in veterinary medicine. The therapeutic benefits center on reducing pain and inflammation, modulating the immune system, and stimulating tissue healing and regeneration. This chapter and online resources describe in detail how veterinary PBMT can be successfully introduced into daily practice, as well as provide practical tools for implementation.

References

AAHA (American Animal Hospital Association) (2019). *Compensation and Benefits*, 9e. Denver, CO: AAHA Press.

Ablon, G. (2018). Phototherapy with light emitting diodes: treating a broad range of medical and aesthetic conditions in dermatology. *Journal of Clinical and Aesthetic Dermatology* 11 (2): 21–27.

Abrahamse, H. (2012). Regenerative medicine, stem cells, and low-level laser therapy: future directives. *Photomedicine and Laser Surgery* 30 (12): 681–682.

Acin-Perez, R., Salazar, E., Kamenetsky, M. et al. (2009). Cyclic AMP produced inside mitochondria regulates oxidative phosphorylation. *Cell Metabolism* 9 (3): 265–276.

Adcock, I. and Caramori, G. (2009). Transcription factors. In: *Asthma and COPD: Basic Mechanisms and Clinical Management*, 2e (ed. P. Barnes, J. Drazen, S. Rennard, and N. Thomson), 373–380. San Diego, CA: Academic Press.

Alayat, M.S.M., Battecha, K.H., Elsodany, A.M. et al. (2022). Effectiveness of photobiomodulation therapy in the treatment of myofascial pain syndrome of the upper trapezius muscle: a systematic review and meta-analysis. *Photobiomodulation, Photomedicine, and Laser Surgery* 40 (10): 661–674.

AlGhamdi, K.M., Kumar, A., Ashour, A.E., and AlGhamdi, A.A. (2015). A comparative study of the effects of different low-level lasers on the proliferation, viability, and migration of human melanocytes in vitro. *Lasers in Medical Science* 30 (5): 1541–1551.

Aliodoust, M., Bayat, M., Jalili, M.R. et al. (2014). Evaluating the effect of low-level laser therapy on healing of tentomized Achilles tendon in streptozotocin-induced diabetic rats by light microscopical and gene expression examinations. *Lasers in Medical Science* 29: 1495–1503.

Al-Rudayni, A.H.M., Gopinath, D., Maharajan, M.K. et al. (2021). Efficacy of photobiomodulation in the treatment of cancer chemotherapy-induced oral mucositis: a meta-analysis with trial sequential analysis. *International Journal of Environmental Research and Public Health* 18 (14): 7418.

Alves, A., Vieira, R., Leal-Junior, E. et al. (2013). Effect of low-level laser therapy on the expression of inflammatory mediators and on neutrophils and macrophages in acute joint inflammation. *Arthritis Research and Therapy* 15 (5): R116.

Alves, J., Jorge, P., and Santos, A. (2022a). The effect of photobiomodulation therapy on the management of chronic idiopathic large-bowel diarrhea in dogs. *Lasers in Medical Science* 37 (3): 2045–2051.

Alves, J., Santos, A., Jorge, P., and Carreira, L.M. (2022b). Randomized double-blinded controlled trial on the effects of photobiomodulation therapy in dogs with osteoarthritis. *American Journal of Veterinary Research* 83 (8): ajvr.22.03.0036.

Alves, J.C., Jorge, P., and Santos, A. (2023). The effect of photobiomodulation therapy on inflammation following dental prophylaxis. *Journal of Veterinary Dentistry* https://doi.org/10.1177/08987564221150525.

Amid, R., Kadkhodazadeh, M., Ahsaie, M.G., and Hakakzadeh, A. (2014). Effect of low level laser therapy on proliferation and differentiation of the cells contributing in bone regeneration. *Journal of Lasers in Medical Sciences* 5 (4): 163–170.

Anders, J., Lanzadame, R., and Arany, P. (2015). Low-level light/laser therapy versus photobiomodulation therapy. *Photomedicine and Laser Surgery* 33 (4): 183–184.

Anderson, K.L., O'Neill, D.G., Brodbelt, D.C. et al. (2018). Prevalence, duration and risk factors for appendicular osteoarthritis in a UK dog population under primary veterinary care. *Scientific Reports* 8 (1): 5641.

de Andrade, A.R., Meireles, A., Artifon, E.L. et al. (2012). The effects of low-level laser therapy, 670 nm, on epiphyseal growth in rats. *Scientific World Journal* 2012: 231723.

Antunes, H., Herchenhorn, D., Small, I.A. et al. (2017). Long-term survival of a randomized phase III trial of head and neck cancer patients receiving concurrent chemoradiation therapy with or without low-level laser therapy (LLLT) to prevent oral mucositis. *Oral Oncology* 71: 11–15.

APPA (American Pet Products Association) (2022). Pet industry market size and ownership statistics. https://www.americanpetproducts.org/research-insights/industry-trends-and-stats (accessed 23 February 2023).

Arany, P. (2016). Craniofacial wound healing with photobiomodulation therapy: new insights and current challenges. *Journal of Dental Research* 95 (9): 977–984.

Aras, M., Omezli, M., and Güngörmüs, M. (2010). Does low-level laser therapy have an antoanesthetic effect? A review. *Photomedicine and Laser Surgery* 28 (6): 719–722.

Araújo, T., de Oliveira, A.G., Tobar, N. et al. (2013). Liver regeneration following partial hepatectomy is improved by enhancing the HGF/Met axis and Akt and Erk pathways after low-power laser irradiation in rats. *Lasers in Medical Science* 28: 1511–1517.

ASLMS (American Society for Laser Medicine and Surgery) (2021). ASLMS history. https://www.aslms.org/about-aslms/history (accessed 8 April 2021).

AVMA (American Veterinary Medical Association) (2019). Economic state of the veterinary profession. https://www.avma.org/news/press-release/AVMA-2019-Economic-State-of-the-Veterinary-Profession-Report-now-available (accessed 26 July 2021).

AVMA (American Veterinary Medical Association) (2023). *2023 AVMA Report on the Economic State of the Veterinary Profession.* Schaumburg, IL: AVMA.

Azevedo, L.H., Aranha, A.C.C., Stolf, S.F. et al. (2005). Evaluation of low intensity laser effects on the thyroid gland of male mice. *Photomedicine and Laser Surgery* 23 (6): 567–570.

Barale, L., Monticelli, P., Raviola, M., and Adami, C. (2020). Preliminary clinical experience of low-level laser therapy for the treatment of canine osteoarthritis-associated pain: a retrospective investigation on 17 dogs. *Open Veterinary Journal* 10 (1): 116–119.

Barasch, A., Li, H., Rajasekhar, V.K. et al. (2020). Photobiomodulation effects on head and neck squamous cell carcinoma (HNSCC) in an orthotopic animal model. *Support Care Cancer* 28 (6): 2721–2727.

Barrington, G. (2022). Photosensitization in Dogs: Pet Owner Version. https://www.merckvetmanual.com/dog-owners/skin-disorders-of-dogs/photosensitization-in-dogs#:~:text=Photosensitive%20dogs%20squirm%20in%20apparent,is%20soon%20followed%20by%20swelling (accessed 13 February 2023).

Bennaim, M., Porato, M., Jarleton, A. et al. (2017). Preliminary evaluation of the effects of photobiomodulation therapy and physical rehabilitation on early postoperative recovery of dogs undergoing hemilaminectomy for treatment of thoracolumbar intervertebral disk disease. *American Journal of Veterinary Research* 78 (2): 195–206.

Bensadoun, R.-J., Epstein, J.B., Nair, R.G. et al. (2020). Safety and efficacy of photobiomodulation therapy in oncology: a systematic review. *Cancer Medicine* 9 (22): 8279–8300.

Biophysical Society (2023). What is Biophysics? https://www.biophysics.org/what-is-biophysics (accessed 5 February 2023).

Bjordal, J., Johnson, M.I., Iversen, V. et al. (2006). Low-level laser therapy in acute pain: a systematic review of possible mechanisms of action and clinical effects in randomized placebo-controlled trials. *Photomedicine and Laser Surgery* 24 (2): 158–168.

van den Bosch, M., van Lent, P., and van der Kraan, P. (2020). Identifying effector molecules, cells, and cytokines of innate immunity in OA. *Osteoarthritis and Cartilage* 28 (5): 532–543.

Britannica Editors (2020). Joule. https://www.britannica.com/science/joule (accessed 7 January 2023).

Brunke, M. (2018). Photobiomodulation facts and function in veterinary rehab. https://www.dvm360.com/view/photobiomodulation-facts-and-functions-veterinary-rehab (accessed 12 April 2021).

Bruno, E., Canal, S., Antonucci, M. et al. (2020). Perilesional photobiomodulation therapy and physical rehabilitation in post-operative recovery of dogs surgically treated for thoracolumbar disk extrusion. *BMC Veterinary Research* 16 (1): 120.

Burns, K. (2018). Pet ownership stable, veterinary care variable. https://www.avma.org/javma-news/2019-01-15/pet-ownership-stable-veterinary-care-variable (accessed 11 August 2021).

Burns, K. (2022). New report takes a deep dive into pet ownership. https://www.avma.org/

news/new-report-takes-deep-dive-pet-ownership (accessed 6 November 2022).

Butow, R. and Avadhani, N. (2004). Mitochondrial signaling. *Molecular Cell* 14 (1): 1–15.

Cardoso, F.D.S., Gonzalez-Lima, F., and da Silva, S.G. (2021). Photobiomodulation for the aging brain. *Aging Research Review* 70: 101415.

Caterina, M. and Pang, Z. (2016). TRP channels in skin biology and pathophysiology. *Pharmaceuticals* 9 (4): 77.

Chen, C.-H., Wang, C.-Z., Wang, Y.-H. et al. (2014). Effects of low-level laser therapy on M1-related cytokine expression in monocytes via histone modification. *Mediators of Inflammation* 2014: 625048.

Chen, N.-F., Sung, C.-S., Wen, Z.-H. et al. (2018). Therapeutic effect of platelet-rich plasma in rat spinal cord injuries. *Frontiers in Neuroscience* 12: 252.

Cheng, K., Martin, L.F., Slepian, M.J. et al. (2021). Mechanisms and pathways of pain photobiomodulation: a narrative review. *Journal of Pain* 22 (7): 763–777.

Choi, J.W., Jang, I.S., and Jeong, M.J. (2015). Review of low level laser therapy on the growth of epiphyseal plate. *Journal of Pediatrics of Korean Medicine* 29 (4): 29–38.

Chow, R., Johnson, M., Lopes-Martin, R., and Bjordal, J. (2019). Efficacy of low-level laser therapy in the management of neck pain: a systematic review of meta-analysis of randomized placebo or active-treatment controlled trials. *Lancet* 374 (9705): 1897–1908.

Chung, H., Dai, T., Sharma, S.K. et al. (2012). The nuts and bolts of low-level laser (light) therapy. *Annals of Biomedical Engineering* 40 (2): 516–533.

Ciolek, J. (1985). Cryotherapy: review of physiologic effects and clinical application. *Cleveland Clinic Quarterly* 52 (2): 193–201.

Clements, D.N., Carter, S.D., Innes, J.F., and Ollier, W.E. (2006). Genetic basis of secondary osteoarthritis in dogs with joint dysplasia. *American Journal of Veterinary Research* 67 (5): 909–918.

ColdLasers.org (2021). The 2021 cold laser guide. https://www.coldlasers.org/coldlaserguide (accessed 11 May 2021).

Cooper, G. (2000). Signaling molecules and their receptors. In: *The Cell: A Molecular Approach*, 2e. Sunderland, MA: Sinauer Associates.

Cronshaw, M., Parker, S., Anagnostaki, E. et al. (2020). Photobiomodulation and oral mucositis: a systematic review. *Denistry Journal* 8 (3): 87.

Cury, V., Moretti, A.I.S., Assis, L. et al. (2013). Low level laser therapy increases angiogenesis in a model of ischemic skin flap in rats mediated by VEGF, HIF-1α and MMP-2. *Journal of Photochemistry and Photobiology B: Biology* 125: 164–170.

Damante, C., De Micheli, G., Miyagi, S.P.H. et al. (2009). Effect of laser phototherapy on the release of fibroblast growth factors by human gingival fibroblasts. *Lasers in Medical Science* 24: 885–891.

Dederich, D. (1991). Laser/tissue interaction. *The Alpha Omegan* 84 (4): 33–36.

Desmet, K., Paz, D.A., Corry, J.J. et al. (2006). Clinical and experimental applications of NIR-LED photobiomodulation. *Photobiomodulation and Laser Surgery* 24 (2): 121–128.

Dompe, C., Moncrieff, L., Matys, J. et al. (2020). Photobiomodulation: underlying mechanism and clinical applications. *Journal of Clinical Medicine* 9 (6): 1724.

Dos Anjos, L., da Fonseca, A., Gameiro, J., and de Paoli, F. (2017). Apoptosis induced by low-level laser in polymorphonuclear cells of acute joint inflammation: comparative analysis of two energy densities. *Lasers in Medical Science* 32: 975–983.

Dos Santos, S.A., Sampaio, L.M., Caires, J.R. et al. (2019). Parameters and effects of photobiomodulation in plantar fasciitis: a meta-analysis and systematic review. *Photobiomodulation, Photomedicine, and Laser Surgery* 37 (6): 327–335.

Downing, R. (2017). Laser therapy in veterinary medicine. https://ivcjournal.com/laser-therapy-veterinary-medicine (accessed 10 April 2021).

Draper, W., Schubert, T., Clemmons, R., and Mile, S. (2012). Low-level laser therapy reduces time to ambulation in dogs after hemilaminectomy: a preliminary study. *Journal of Small Animal Practice* 53 (8): 465–469.

Dycus, D. (2014). Laser therapy in companion animals. https://todaysveterinarypractice.com/wp-content/uploads/sites/4/2016/06/T1405C05.pdf. (accessed 11 May 2021).

Edge-Hughes, L. (2020). Safety of Laser Therapy. https://physiotherapy.ca/app/uploads/2022/07/safety_of_laser_therapy.pdf (accessed 14 February 2023).

Edwards, K.D. (2005). Light emitting diodes. https://web.archive.org/web/20190214175634/http://faculty.sites.uci.edu/chem11/files/2013/11/RDGLED.pdf (accessed 10 January 2023).

Eells, J.T., Henry, M.M., Summerfelt, P. et al. (2003). Therapeutic photobiomodulation for methanol-induced retinal toxicity. *Proceedings of the National Academy of Sciences of the United States of America* 100 (6): 3429–3444.

Esmaeelinejad, M., Bayat, M., Darbandi, H. et al. (2014). The effects of low-level laser irradiation on cellular viability and proliferation of human skin fibroblasts cultured in high glucose mediums. *Lasers in Medical Sciences* 29 (1): 121–129.

Ezzati, K., Fekrazad, R., and Raoufi, Z. (2019). The effects of photobiomodulation therapy on post-surgical pain. *Journal of Lasers in Medical Sciences* 10 (2): 79–85.

Farivar, S., Malekshahabi, T., and Shiari, R. (2014). Biological effects of low level laser therapy. *Journal of Lasers in Medicine and Science* 5 (2): 58–62.

FDA (Food and Drug Administration) (2020). Device Advice: Comprehensive Regulatory Assistance. https://www.fda.gov/medical-devices/device-advice-comprehensive-regulatory-assistance/overview-device-regulation (accessed 7 January 2022).

FDA (Food and Drug Administration) (2021). Laser Products and Instruments. https://www.fda.gov/radiation-emitting-products/home-business-and-entertainment-products/laser-products-and-instruments (accessed 22 January 2023).

FDA (Food and Drug Administration) (2022). Center for Devices and Radiological Health. https://www.fda.gov/about-fda/fda-organization/center-devices-and-radiological-health (accessed 22 January 2023).

FDA (Food and Drug Administration) (2023). Title 21: Chapter 1, Subchapter J, Radiological Health. https://www.ecfr.gov/current/title-21/chapter-I/subchapter-J (accessed 22 January 2023).

Fekrazad, R., Katayoun, K., Farzaneh, A., and Nikoo, T. (2011). Laser in orthodontics. In: *Principles in Contemporary Orthodontics* (ed. S. Naretto), 129–180. Tehran: ResearchGate.

Ferlito, J.V., Ferlito, M.V., Leal-Junior, E.C.P. et al. (2022). Comparison between cryotherapy and photobiomodulation in muscle recovery: a systematic review and meta-analysis. *Lasers in Medical Science* 37 (3): 1375–1388.

Ferraresi, C., Huang, Y.-Y., and Hamblin, M. (2016). Photobiomodulation in human muscle tissue: an advantage in sports performance? *Journal of Biophotonics* 9 (11–12): 1273–1299.

Fessehav, H. (2020). Laser therapy and its potential application in veterinary practice: a review. *Journal of Light and Laser: Current Trends* 3: 007.

Firestone, R.S., Esfandiari, N., Moskovtsev, S.I. et al. (2012). The effects of low-level laser light exposure on sperm motion characteristics and DNA damage. *Journal of Andrology* 33 (3): 469–473.

de Freitas, L. and Hamblin, M. (2016). Proposed mechanisms of photobiomodulation or low-level light therapy. *IEEE Journal of Selected Topics in Quantum Electronics* 22 (3): 7000417.

Frigo, L., Luppi, J.S.S., Favero, G.M. et al. (2009). The effect of low-level laser irradiation (In-Ga-Al-AsP - 660 nm) on melanoma in vitro and in vivo. *BMC Cancer* 9: 404.

Gaffey, M. and Johnson, A. (2022). *Laser Treatment of Pigmented Lesions*. Treasure Island, FL: StatPearls https://www.ncbi.nlm.nih.gov/books/NBK560613.

Gammel, J., Biskup, J.J., Drum, M.G. et al. (2018). Effects of low-level laser therapy on the healing of surgically closed incisions and surgically created open wounds in dogs. *Veterinary Surgery* 47 (4): 499–506.

Ganju, L., Salhan, A., Karan, D. et al. (1999). Immunomodulatory effect of laser on whole body exposure. *Indian Journal of Experimental Biology* 37 (5): 444–449.

Gaynor, J.S. (2015). Energy modalities: therapeutic laser and pulsed electromagnetic field therapy. In: *Handbook of Veterinary Pain Management*, 3e (ed. J.S. Gaynor and W.W. Muir), 356–357. St. Louis, MO: Elsevier.

Ginani, F., Soares, D., Barreto, M., and Barboza, C. (2015). Effect of low-level laser therapy on mesenchymal stem cell proliferation: a systematic review. *Lasers in Medical Science* 30 (8): 2189–2194.

Godbold, J. (2014). Laser therapy: lighting the way to improved patient care.

Godbold, J. (2017). The Science of Laser Therapy and Photobiomodulation. *Pacific Veterinary Conference* (29 June to 2 July 2017) Long Beach, CA. https://www.vin.com/members/cms/project/defaultadv1.aspx?pid=18559&catId=&id=8026136&said=&meta=&authorid=&preview=

Gross, D. (2014). Practical applications of laser therapy in practicw. *Western Veterinary Conference*.

Hagler, K. (2019). *Lights, Camera, Action: Using and Understanding Therapeutic Lasers for Pain Management*. Bridgewater, NJ: American Association of Feline Practitioners.

Hamblin, M.R. (2016). Shining light on the head: photobiomodulation for brain disorders. *BBA Clinical* 6: 113–124.

Hamblin, M. (2017). Mechanisms and applications of the anti-inflammatory effects of photobiomodulation. *AIMS Biophysics* 4 (3): 337–361.

Hamblin, M. (2018). Photobiomodulation for traumatic brain injury and stroke. *Journal of Neuroscience Research* 96 (4): 731–743.

Hamblin, M., Nelson, S., and Strahan, J. (2018). Photobiomodulation and cancer: what is the truth? *Photomedicine and Laser Surgery* 36 (5): 241–245.

Hamid, M., Zaied, A.A., Zayet, M.K. et al. (2021). Efficacy of flat-top hand-piece using 980 nm diode laser photobiomodulation on socket healing after extraction: split-mouth experimental model in dogs. *Photochemistry and Photobiology* 97 (3): 627–633.

Hardie, E., Roe, S.C., and Martin, F. (2002). Radiographic evidence of degenerative joint disease in geriatric cats: 100 cases (1994–1997). *Journal of the American Veterinary Medical Association* 220 (5): 628–632.

Harvard (2018). Laser Hazard Classification. https://www.ehs.harvard.edu/sites/default/files/laser_hazard_classification.pdf (accessed 22 January 2023).

Hashmi, J., Huang, Y.-Y., Sharma, S.K. et al. (2010). Effect of pulsing on low-level light therapy. *Lasers in Surgery and Medicine* 42 (6): 450–466.

Haslerud, S., Naterstad, I.F., Bjordal, J.M. et al. (2017). Achilles tendon penetration for continuous 810 nm and superpulsed 904 nm lasers before and after ice application: an in situ study on healthy young adults. *Photomedicine and Laser Surgery* 35 (10): 567–575.

Hawkins, D., Houreld, N., and Abrahamse, H. (2005). Low level laser therapy (LLLT) as an effective therapeutic modality for delayed wound healing. *Annals of the New York Academy of Sciences* 1056: 486–493.

Heiskanen, V. and Hamblin, M. (2018). Photobiomodulation: lasers and light emitting diodes? *Photochehmical and Photobiological Sciences* 17 (8): 1003–1017.

Hochman-Elam, L., Heidel, R.E., and Shmalberg, J.W. (2020). Effects of laser power, wavelength, coat length, and coat color on tissue penetration using photobiomodulation in healthy dogs. *Canadian Journal of Veterinary Research* 84 (2): 131–137.

Höfling, D.B., Chavantes, M.C., Juliano, A.G. et al. (2013). Low-level laser in the treatment of patients with hypothyroidism induced by chronic autoimmune thyroiditis: a randomized, placebo-controlled clinical trial. *Lasers in Medicine and Science* 28 (3): 743–753.

Hoisang, S., Kampa, N., Seesupa, S., and Jitpean, S. (2021). Assessment of wound area reduction on chronic wounds in dogs with photobiomodulation therapy: a randomized controlled clinical trial. *Veterinary World* 14 (8): 2251–2259.

Houghton, P.E., Nussbaum, E.L., and Hoens, A.M. (2010). Electrophysical agents: contraindications and precautions: an evidence-based approach to clinical decision making in physical therapy. *Physiotherapy Canada* 62 (5): 1–80.

Huang, Y.-Y., Sharma, S., Carroll, J., and Hamblin, M. (2011). Biphasic dose response in low level light therapy: an update. *Dose Response* 9 (4): 602–618.

iVet360 (2023). Benefits Matter. https://ivet360.com/recruiting-tool-kit/wages-benefits/benefits-matter/#:~:text=Most%20companies%20provide%20a%20minimum,and%20holidays%2C%20plus%20sick%20time (accessed 23 February 2023).

JEDEC (2023). Dictionary: JESD88. https://www.jedec.org/standards-documents/dictionary (accessed 7 January 2023).

Jenkins, P. (2022). Is LLLT over active epiphyses contraindicated? https://www.veterinarypracticenews.ca/lasers-june-2022/ (accessed 13 February 2023).

Johnson, J. (2016). An introduction to laser therapy in veterinary practice. *Pacific Veterinary Conference* (June 23–26), San Francisco. https://www.vin.com/members/cms/project/defaultadv1.aspx?pid=15054&catId=&id=7351637&said=&meta=&authorid=&preview=

Johnson, J. and Kellogg, D.L. Jr. (2010). Local thermal control of the human cutaneous circulation. *Journal of Applied Physiology* 109 (4): 1229–1238.

Johnston, S. (1997). Osteoarthritis. Joint anatomy, physiology, and pathobiology. *Veterinary Clinics of North America Small Animal Practice* 27 (4): 699–723.

Kalyanaraman, B. (2017). Teaching the basics of cancer metabolism: developing antitumor strategies by exploiting the differences between normal and cancer cell metabolism. *Redox Biology* 12: 833–842.

Kampa, N., Jitpean, S., Seesupa, S., and Hoisang, S. (2020). Penetration depth study of 830 nm low-intensity laser therapy on living dog tissue. *Veterinary World* 13 (7): 1417–1422.

Karu, T. (2008). Mitochondrial signaling in mammalian cells activated by red and near-IR radiation. *Photochemistry and Photobiology* 84 (5): 1091–1099.

Karu, T. (2010). Multiple roles of cytochrome c oxidase in mammalian cells under action of red and IR-A radiation. *IUBMB Life* 62 (8): 207–210.

Karu, T., Pyatibrat, L., Kolyakov, S., and Afanasyeva, N. (2005). Absorption measurements of a cell monolayer relevant to phototherapy: reduction of cytochrome C oxidase under near IR radiation. *Journal of Photochemistry and Photobiology B: Biology* 81 (2): 98–106.

Kennedy, K., Martinez, S.A., Martinez, S.E. et al. (2018). Effects of low-level laser therapy on bone healing and signs of pain in dogs following tibial plateau leveling osteotomy. *American Journal of Veterinary Research* 79 (8): 898–904.

Kerstein, R., Lister, T., and Cole, R. (2014). Laser therapy and photosensitive medication: a review of the evidence. *Lasers in Medicine and Science* 29 (4): 1449–1452.

Kerwin, S.C. (2010). Osteoarthritis in cats. *Top Companion Animal Medicine* 25 (4): 218–223.

Kim, W.-S. and Calderhead, R.G. (2011). Is light-emitting diode phototherapy (LED-LLLT) really effective? *Laser Therapy* 20 (3): 205–215.

Kiro, N., Hamblin, M., and Abrahamse, H. (2017). Photobiomodulation of breast and cervical cancer stem cells using low-intensity laser irradiation. *Tumour Biology* 39 (6): 1010428317706913.

Kneebone, W. (2011). Immune-modulating effects of therapeutic laser. *MeCentral, Practical Pain Management* 10 (9): https://www.medcentral.com/pain/chronic/immune-modulating-effects-therapeutic-laser.

Kurach, L.M., Stanley, B.J., Gazzola, K.M. et al. (2015). The effect of low-level laser therapy on the healing of open wounds in dogs. *Veterinary Surgery* 44 (8): 988–996.

Landén, N., Li, D., and Ståhle, M. (2016). Transition from inflammation to proliferation: a critical step during wound healing. *Cellular and Molecular Life Sciences* 73: 3861–3885.

Legouté, F., Bensadoun, R.-J., Seegers, V. et al. (2019). Low-level laser therapy in treatment of chemoradiotherapy-induced mucositis in head and neck cancer: results of a randomised, triple blind, multicentre phase III trial. *Radiation Oncology* 14 (1): 83.

Li, X., Fang, P., Mai, J. et al. (2013). Targeting mitochondrial reactive oxygen species as novel therapy for inflammatory diseases and cancers. *Journal of Hematology and Oncology* 6: 19.

LIA (Laser Institute of America) (2017). ANSI Z136.1. https://www.lia.org/resources/laser-safety-information/laser-safety-standards/ansi-z136-standards/z136-1 (accessed 19 May 2021).

Liang, H., Whelan, H.J., Eells, J.T. et al. (2006). Photobiomodulation partially rescues visual cortical neurons from cyanide-induced apoptosis. *Neuroscience* 139 (2): 639–649.

Liao, X., Xie, G.H., Liou, H.-W. et al. (2014). Helium-neon laser irradiation promotes the proliferation and migration of human epidermal stem cells in vitro: proposed mechanism for enhanced wound re-epithelialization. *Photomedicine and Laser Surgery* 32 (4): 219–225.

Lim, W., Kim, J., Kim, S. et al. (2013). Modulation of lipopolysaccharide-induced NF-κB signaling pathway by 635 nm irradiation via heat shock protein 27 in human gingival fibroblast cells.

Photochemistry and Photobiology 89 (1): 199–207.

de Lima, F., Vitoretti, L., Coelho, F. et al. (2012). Suppressive effect of low-level laser therapy on tracheal hyperresponsiveness and lung inflammation in rat subjected to intestinal ischemia and reperfusion. *Lasers in Medical Science* 28: 551–564.

Lindgård, A., Hultén, L., Svensson, L., and Soussi, B. (2006). Irradiation at 634 nm releases nitric oxide from human monocytes. *Lasers in Medical Science* 22: 30–37.

Lodewijckx, J., Robijns, J., Claes, M. et al. (2022). The use of photobiomodulation therapy for the prevention of chemotherapy-induced peripheral neuropathy: a randomized, placebo-controlled pilot trial (NEUROLASER trial). *Supportive Care in Cancer* 30 (6): 5509–5517.

Looney, A., Huntingfod, J., Blaeser, L., and Mann, S. (2018). A randomized blind placebo-controlled trial investigating the effects of photobiomodulation therapy (PBMT) on canine elbow osteoarthritis. *Canadian Veterinary Journal* 59 (9): 989–966.

Lopez, A. and Brundage, C. (2019). Wound photobiomodulation treatment outcomes in animal models. *Journal of Veterinary Medicine* 2019: 6320515.

Luna, S.P.L., Schoen, A., Trindade, P.H.E., and da Rocha, P.B. (2020). Penetration profiles of a class IV therapeutic laser and a photobiomodulation therapy device in equine skin. *Journal of Equine Veterinary Science* 85: 102846.

Maegawa, Y., Itoh, T., Hosokawa, T. et al. (2000). Effects of near-infrared low-level laser irradiation on microcirculation. *Lasers in Surgery and Medicine* 27 (5): 427–437.

MAGLAB (2021). Magnet Academy from the National High Magnetic Field Laboratory. https://nationalmaglab.org/education/magnet-academy/history-of-electricity-magnetism/pioneers/theodore-maiman (accessed 8 April 2021).

Marchegiani, A., Spaterna, A., and Cerquetella, M. (2019). Fluorescence biomodulation in the management of canine interdigital pyoderma cases: a prospective, single-blinded, randomized and controlled clinical trial. *Veterinary Dermatology* 30 (5): 371.

Marchegiani, A., Spaterna, A., Piccionello, A.P. et al. (2020). Fluorescence biomodulation in the management of acute traumatic wounds in two aged dogs. *Veterinární Medicína* 65 (5): 215–220.

Marchegiani, A., Fruganti, A., Gavazza, A. et al. (2022). Fluorescence biomodulation for canine interdigital furunculosis: updates for once-weekly schedule. *Frontiers in Veterinary Science* 9: 880349.

Mehani, H. (2017). Immunomodulatory effects of two different physical therapy modalities in patients with chronic obstructive pulmonary disease. *Journal of Physical Science* 29 (9): 1527–1533.

Meng, C. and Xing, Z.D. (2013). Low-level laser therapy rescues dendrite atrophy via upregulating BDNF expression: implications for Alzheimer's disease. *Journal of Neuroscience* 33 (33): 13505–13517.

Merriam-Webster (2021). Light. https://www.merriam-webster.com/dictionary/light (accessed 8 August 2021).

Mester, E., Szende, B., and Gärtner, P. (1968). The effect of laser beams on the growth of hair in mice. *Radiobiology and Radiotherapy (Berlin)* 9 (5): 621–626.

Mester, E., Nagylucskay, S., Döklen, A., and Tisza, S. (1976). Laser stimulation of wound healing. *Acta Chirurgica Academiae Scientiarum Hungaricae* 17 (1): 49–55.

MFAF (Michelson Found Animals Foundation) (2018). Furred lines: Pet trends. https://www.prnewswire.com/news-releases/furred-lines-pet-trends-2019-300741947.html. (accessed 26 July 2021).

Miller, L., Torraca, D.G., and Taboada, L.D. (2020). Retrospective observational study and analysis of two different photobiomodulation therapy protocols combined with rehabilitation therapy as therapeutic interventions for canine degenerative myelopathy. *Photobiomodulation,* *Photomedicine, and Laser Surgery* 38 (4): 195–205.

Millis, D., Francis, D., and Adamson, C. (2005). Emerging modalities in veterinary rehabilitation. *Veterinary Clinics of North America: Small Animal Practice* 35 (6): 1335–1355.

Mills, D. and Gross, S. (2014). Laser therapy in canine rehabilitation. In: *Canine Rehabilitation and Physical Therapy* (ed. D. Mills and D. Levine), 359–372. Philadelphia, PA: Elsevier.

Mizutani, K., Musya, Y., Wakae, K. et al. (2004). A clinical study on serum prostaglandin E2 with low-level laser therapy. *Photomedicine and Laser Surgery* 22 (6): 537–539.

Monteiro, J., Pinheiro, A.N.L.B., de Oliveira, S.C.P.S. et al. (2011). Influence of laser phototherapy (λ660 nm) on the outcome of oral chemical carcinogenesis on the hamster cheek pouch model: histological study. *Photomedicine and Laser Surgery* 29 (11): 741–745.

Moriyama, Y., Moriyama, E.H., Blackmore, K. et al. (2005). In vivo study of the inflammatory modulating effects of low-level laser therapy on iNOS expression using bioluminescence imaging. *Photochemistry and Photobiology* 81: 1351–1355.

Mosca, R., Ong, A.A., Albasha, O. et al. (2019). Photobiomodulation therapy for wound care: a potent, noninvasive, photoceutical approach. *Advances in Skin and Wound Care* 32 (4): 157–167.

Nagaraja, M. (2021). Visible light. https://science.nasa.gov/ems/09_visiblelight (accessed 10 January 2023).

NAPHIA (North American Pet Health Insurance Association) (2023). Industry Data. https://naphia.org/industry-data/#my-menu (accessed 18 February 2023).

NASA (National Aeronautics and Space Administration) (2013). The electromagnetic spectrum. https://imagine.gsfc.nasa.gov/science/toolbox/emspectrum1.html (accessed 8 April 2021).

NASA (National Aeronautics and Space Administration) (2021). What is a laser?

https://spaceplace.nasa.gov/laser/en (accessed 22 January 2023).

Niebaum, K. (2013). Rehabilitation physical modalities. In: *Canine Sports Medicine and Rehabilitation* (ed. M.C. Zink and J.V. Dyke), 115–131. Oxford: Wiley-Blackwell.

Nobel, M. (1967). *Nobel Lectures, Physiology or Medicine 1901–1921: Niels Ryberg Finsen Biographical.* Amsterdam: Elsevier.

Nolen, R.S. (2022). Pet owner ship rate stabilizes as spending increases. https://www.avma.org/news/pet-ownership-rate-stabilizes-spending-increases (accessed 22 February 2023).

Nolfi-Donegan, D., Braganza, A., and Shiva, S. (2020). Mitochondrial electron transport chain: oxidative phosphorylation, oxidant production, and methods of measurement. *Redox Biology* 37: 101674.

de Oliveira, S.P., Rahal, S.C., Pereira, E.J. et al. (2012). Low-level laser on femoral growth plates in rats. *Acta Cirurgica Brasiliera* 27 (2): 117–122.

Olivieri, L., Cavina, D., Radicchi, G. et al. (2014). Efficacy of low-level laser therapy on hair regrowth in dogs with noninflammatory alopecia: a pilot study. *Veterinary Dermatology* 26 (1): 35–e11.

O'Neill, D.G., Church, D.B., McGreevy, P.D. et al. (2014). Prevalence of disorders recorded in dogs attending primary-care veterinary practices in England. *PLoS One* 9 (3): e90501.

OSHA (Occupational Safety and Health Administration) (2014). OSHA At-A-Glance. https://www.osha.gov/sites/default/files/publications/3439at-a-glance.pdf (accessed 19 May 2021).

OSHA (Occupational Safety and Health Administration) (2021). Laser Hazards - Standards. https://www.osha.gov/laser-hazards/standards (accessed 19 May 2021).

Ottaviani, G., Martinelli, V., Rupel, K. et al. (2016). Laser therapy inhibits tumor growth in mice by promoting immune surveillance and vessel normalization. *eBioMedicine* 11: 165–172.

Parrado, C., Peláez, A., Vidal, L., and Vargas, I.P.D. (1990). Quantitative study of the morphological changes in the thyroid gland following IR laser radiation. *Lasers in Medicine and Science* 5: 77–80.

Parrado, C., de Albornoz, F.C., Vidal, L., and de Vargas, I.P. (1999). A quantitative investigation of microvascular changes in the thyroid gland after infrared (IR) laser radiation. *Histology and Histopathology* 14 (4): 1067–1071.

Patil, U. and Dhami, L. (2008). Overview of lasers. *Indian Journal of Plastic Surgery* 41 (Suppl): S101–S113.

Petrellis, M.C., Frigo, L., Marcos, R.L. et al. (2017). Laser photobiomodulation of pro-inflammatory mediators on Walker Tumor 256 induced rats. *Journal of Photochemistry and Photobiology B* 177: 69–75.

Poyton, R. and Ball, K. (2011). Therapeutic photobiomodulation: nitric oxide and a novel function of mitochondrial cytochrome c oxidase. *Discovery Medicine* 11 (57): 154–159.

Prohaska, J. and Hohman, M. (2022). *Laser Complications.* Treasure Island, FL: StatPearls https://www.ncbi.nlm.nih.gov/books/NBK532248.

Ramezani, F., Razmgir, M., Tanha, K. et al. (2020). Photobiomodulation for spinal cord injury: a systematic review and meta-analysis. *Physiology and Behavior* 224: 112977.

Razaghi, P., Haghgou, J.M., Khazaei, S. et al. (2022). The effect of photobiomodulation therapy on the stability of orthodontic mini-implants in human and animal studies: a systematic review and meta-analysis. *Journal of Lasers in Medicine and Science* 23: e27.

Ree, Y.-H., Moon, J.-H., Choi, S.-H., and Ahn, J.-C. (2016). Low-level laser therapy promoted aggressive proliferation and angiogenesis through decreasing of transforming growth factor-β1 and increasing of Akt/hypoxia inducible factor-1α in anaplastic thyroid cancer. *Photomedicine and Laser Surgery* 36 (6): 229–235.

Reis, V.P., Rego, C.M.A., Setubal, S.S. et al. (2021). Effect of light emitting diode photobiomodulation on murine macrophage function after Bothrops envenomation. *Chemico-Biological Interactions* 333: 109347.

Renwick, S.M., Renwick, A.I., Brodbelt, D.C. et al. (2018). Influence of class IV laser therapy on the outcomes of tibial plateau leveling osteotomy in dogs. *Veterinary Surgery* 47 (4): 507–515.

Reusch, W. (2013). Photochemistry. https://www2.chemistry.msu.edu/faculty/reusch/VirtTxtJml/photchem.htm (accessed 10 January 2023).

Ribeiro, M.A.G., Albuquerque, R.L.C. Jr., Ramalho, L.M.P. et al. (2009). Immunohistochemical assessment of myofibroblasts and lymphoid cells during wound healing in rats subjected to laser photobiomodulation at 660 nm. *Photomedicine and Laser Surgery* 27 (1): 49–55.

Rico-Holgado, S., Ortiz-Díez, G., Martín-Espada, M.C. et al. (2021). Effect of low-level laser therapy on bacterial counts of contaminated traumatic wounds in dogs. *Journal of Lasers in Medical Science* 12: e78.

Rivera, P. (2022). Thermal Therapy and Photobiomodulation - Course Notes. Veterinary Massage and Rehabilitation Therapy Postgraduate Certification Program. The Healing Oasis Center, Sturtevant, WI.

Rocha, S.R., de Ferreira, S.A.C., Ramalho, A. et al. (2022). Photobiomodulation therapy in the prevention and treatment of radiodermatitis in breast cancer patients: systematic review. *Journal of Lasers in Medicine and Science* 13: e42.

Rochkind, S., El-Ani, D., Nevo, Z., and Shahar, A. (2009). Increase of neuronal sprouting and migration using 780 nm laser phototherapy as procedure for cell therapy. *Lasers in Surgery and Medicine* 41 (4): 277–281.

Rogatko, C., Baltzer, W., and Tennant, R. (2017). Preoperative low-level laser therapy in dogs undergoing tibial plateau levelling osteotomy: a blinded, prospective, randomized clinical trial. *Veterinary and Comparative Orthopaedics and Traumatology* 30 (1): 46–53.

Santana-Blank, L., Rodríguez-Santana, E., Vargas, F. et al. (2002). Phase I trial of an infrared pulsed laser device in patients with advanced neoplasia. *Clinical Cancer Research* 8 (10): 3082–3091.

Schnedeker, A.H., Cole, L.K., Diaz, S.F. et al. (2021). Is low-level laser therapy useful as an adjunctive treatment for canine acral lick dermatitis? A randomized, double-blinded, sham-controlled study. *Veterinary Dermatology* 32 (2): 148–e35.

Schultz, G., Chin, G., Moldawer, L., and Diegelmann, R. (2015). Principles of wound healing. In: *Mechanisms of Vascular Disease: A Reference Book for Vascular Speciliasts* (ed. R. Fitridge and M. Thompson), 423–450. Adelaide: University of Adelaide Press.

Shah, S. and Alster, T. (2010). Laser treatment of dark skin: an updated review. *American Journal of Clinical Dermatology* 11 (6): 389–397.

Shields, H., Traa, A., and Raamsdonk, K.V. (2021). Beneficial and detrimental effects of reactive oxygen species on lifespan: a comprehensive review of comparative and experimental studies. *Frontiers in Cell and Developmental Biology* 9: 628157.

Siekevitz, P. (1957). Powerhouse of the cell. *Scientific American* 197 (1): 131–144.

Silva, R.S.D.L., Pessoa, D.R., Mariano, R.R. et al. (2020). Systematic review of photobiomodulation therapy (PBMT) on the experimental calcaneal tendon injury in rats. *Photochemistry and Photobiology* 96 (5): 981–997.

Sineshchekov, V. (1995). Photobiophysics and photobiochemistry of the heterogeneous phytochrome system. *Biochimica et Biophysica Acta, Bioenergetics* 1228 (2–3): 125–164.

Siqueira, A.F.P., Maria, F.S., Mendes, C.M. et al. (2016). Effects of photobiomodulation therapy (PBMT) on bovine sperm function. *Lasers in Medicine and Science* 31 (6): 1245–1250.

de Souza Costa, M., Teles, R.H.G., Dutra, Y.M. et al. (2018). Photobiomodulation reduces neutrophil migration and oxidative stress in mice with carrageenan-induced peritonitis. *Lasers in Medical Science* 33 (9): 1983–1990.

Souza-Barros, L., Dhaidan, G., Maunula, M. et al. (2017). Skin color and tissue thickness effects on transmittance, reflectance, and skin temperature when using 635 and 808 nm lasers in low intensity therapeutics. *Lasers in Surgery and Medicine* 50 (4): 291–301.

Sperandio, F.F., Simoes, A., Correa, L. et al. (2015). Low-level laser irradiation promotes the proliferation and maturation of keratinocytes during epithelial wound repair. *Journal of Biophotonics* 8 (10): 795–803.

Stevenson, P. (2016). How to set practice service fees. https://cliniciansbrief.com/article/how-set-practice-service-fees. (accessed 10 June 2020).

Stitch, A., Rosenkrantz, W., and Griffin, C. (2014). Clinical efficacy of low-level laser therapy on localized canine atopic dermatitis severity score and localized pruritic visual analog score in pedal pruritus due to canine atopic dermatitis. *Veterinary Dermatology* 25 (5): 464–474.

Sutherland, J. (2002). Biological effects of polychromatic light. *Photochemistry and Photobiology* 76 (2): 164–170.

Szymanska, J., Goralczyk, K., Klawe, J.J. et al. (2013). Phototherapy with low-level laser influences the proliferation of endothelial cells and vascular endothelial growth factor and transforming growth factor-beta secretion. *Journal of Physiology and Pharmacology* 64 (3): 387–397.

Tambella, A.M., Attili, A.R., Beribe, F. et al. (2020). Management of otitis externa with an led-illuminated gel: a randomized controlled clinical trial in dogs. *BMC Veterinary Research* 16 (1): 91.

Tang, E. and Arany, P. (2013). Photobiomodulation and implants: implications for dentistry. *Journal of Periodontal and Implant Sicence* 43 (6): 262–268.

Teng, C., Egger, S., Blinman, P.L., and Vardy, J.L. (2022). Evaluating laser

photobiomodulation for chemotherapy-induced peripheral neuropathy: a randomised phase II trial. *Supportive Care in Cancer* 31 (1): 52.

Tsai, S.-R. and Hamblin, M. (2017). Biological effects and medical applications of infrared radiation. *Journal of Photochemistry and Photobiology B: Biology* 170: 197–207.

Tsai, W.-C., Hsu, C.-C., Pang, J.-H.S. et al. (2012). Low-level laser irradiation stimulates tenocyte migration with up-regulation of dynamin II expression. *PLoS One* 7 (5): e38235.

Wang, L., Jacques, S., and Zheng, L. (1995). MCML: Monte Carlo modeling of light transport in multi-layered tissues. *Computer Methods and Programs in Biomedicine* 47 (2): 131–146.

Wardlaw, J., Gazzola, K.M., Wagoner, A. et al. (2019). Laser therapy for incision healing in 9 dogs. *Frontiers in Veterinary Science* 5: 349.

Watson, A. and Brundage, C. (2019). Photobiomodulation as an inflammatory therapeutic following dental prophylaxis in canines. *Photobiomodulation, Photomedicine, and Laser Surgery* 37 (5): 276–278.

Whitley, D., Goldberg, S., and Jordan, W. (1999). Heat shock proteins: a review of the molecular chaperones. *Journal of Vascular Surgery* 29 (4): 748–751.

Wong-Riley, M.T., Liang, H.L., Eells, J.T. et al. (2005). Photobiomodulation directly benefits primary neurons functionally inactivated by toxins: role of cytochrome c oxidase. *Journal of Biological Chemistry* 280 (6): 4761–4771.

Woodley, K. (2018). Pet insurance for holistic and integrative practice. https://ivcjournal.com/pet-insurance-integrative-practices. (accessed 11 August 2021).

Wu, Z.-H., Zhou, Y., Chen, J.-Y., and Zhou, L.-W. (2010). Mitochondrial signaling for histamine releases in laser-irradiated RBL-2H3 mast cells. *Lasers in Surgery and Medicine* 42 (6): 503–509.

Wu, S., Zhou, F., Wei, Y. et al. (2014). Cancer phototherapy via selective photoinactivation of respiratory chain oxidase to trigger a fatal superoxide anion burst. *Antioxidants and Redox Signaling* 20 (5): 733–746.

Xiang, A., Deng, H., Cheng, K. et al. (2020). Laser photobiomodulation for cartilage defect in animal models of knee osteoarthritis: a systematic review and meta-analysis. *Lasers in Medical Science* 35 (4): 789–796.

Zein, R., Selting, W., and Hamblin, M. (2018). Review of light parameters and photobiomodulation efficacy: dive into complexity. *Journal of Biomedical Optics* 23 (12): 190901.

Zhang, H., Wu, S., and Xing, D. (2012). Inhibition of Aβ(25–35)-induced cell apoptosis by low-power-laser-irradiation (LPLI) through promoting Akt-dependent YAP cytoplasmic translocation. *Cell Signaling* 24 (1): 224–232.

Zhao, R.-Z., Jian, S., Zhang, L., and Yu, Z.-B. (2019). Mitochondrial electron transport chain, ROS generation and uncoupling (Review). *International Journal of Molecular Medicine* 44 (1): 3–15.

Zorov, D., Juhaszova, M., and Sollott, S. (2014). Mitochondrial reactive oxygen species (ROS) and ROS-induced ROS release. *Physiological Reviews* 94 (3): 909–950.

7

Prolotherapy

Introduction

Prolotherapy can aid in the management of chronic musculoskeletal pain in veterinary patients. Prolotherapy offers a nonsurgical option for chronic pain due to a variety of joint, tendon, and ligament diseases. Small volumes of irritating solutions, primarily dextrose, are injected directly into these areas stimulating the body's natural ability to heal itself.

The introduction of prolotherapy into a veterinary practice may be beneficial for both the patient and the health of the practice. The successful incorporation and utilization of prolotherapy does not end with the veterinarian's training. Support staff training and client education are crucial. This chapter discusses the what, why, and how for effective integration of prolotherapy within your practice.

The What

Word Origin

Prolotherapy is derived from the words "proliferate," meaning to multiply, and "therapy," meaning a treatment used to heal a disorder.

Definition

Prolotherapy, also known as Proliferation Therapy, is the injection of a small volume of a sterile irritant into a painful joint, tendon, or ligament (Hauser et al. 2016; AOAPRM 2020). The irritating solution induces a local inflammatory response, stimulating the body's natural healing ability, stabilizing the weakened tissues, and reducing pain (Hauser et al. 2016; AOAPRM 2020). The most common substances used include dextrose and ozone. The inclusion of orthobiologics, such as platelet-rich plasma and stem cells, within the

Integrative Medicine in Veterinary Practice, First Edition. Lisa P. McFaddin.
© 2024 John Wiley & Sons, Inc. Published 2024 by John Wiley & Sons, Inc.
Companion website: www.wiley.com/go/mcfaddin/integrativemedicine

umbrella of prolotherapy is controversial. For the purposes of this book, prolotherapy and regenerative medicine are classified separately but share similar mechanisms of action and beneficial effects.

Human History

Dr. Earl Gedney, an osteopathic surgeon, is considered the father of modern day prolotherapy (Alderman 2009). In 1936, a mishap with a surgical suite door irreparably injured the ligaments in his thumb. Faced with the possibility of never performing surgery again Dr. Gedney turned to herniologists for help. Physicians practicing herniology injected irritating solutions into the muscles around abdominal hernias, creating scar tissue, and non-surgically sealing the hernias (Alderman 2009).

Dr. Gedney surmised the same solutions could be injected into tendons, ligaments, and joints with a similar healing effect. Using himself as the first test subject, he injected his own damaged thumb with sclerosing (scaring) solutions. The treatment was successful, and Dr. Gedney was able to continue his surgical practice. Dr. Gedney published his findings in June 1937 and continued to research and practice prolotherapy for the rest of his career. The technique exploded in popularity throughout the 1940s and 1950s (Alderman 2009; Andersen 2015).

Originally called "sclerotherapy," the procedure included the injection of joints and veins (Alderman 2009; Andersen 2015). In the 1950s Dr. George Hackett focused the treatment on joints, tendons, and ligaments calling it prolotherapy because of the proliferation of new tissue at the site of injection (Andersen 2015). Today sclerotherapy is used when describing the injection of vascular abnormalities, including varicose veins, spider veins, and hemorrhoids (Andersen 2015).

The usefulness of prolotherapy in the management of chronic musculoskeletal pain continued to expand. In 1996, the American Osteopathic College of Sclerotherapy renamed themselves the American College of Osteopathic Sclerotherapeutic Pain Management (ACOSPM) to reflect the importance of prolotherapy in the management of musculoskeletal pain (Alderman 2009).

Throughout the 2000s research demonstrated prolotherapy did not create scar tissue, but instead led to the proliferation of normal ligament and tendon tissues. Without the formation of scar tissue the term "sclerotherapy" was incorrect, and the organization changed its name to the American Osteopathic Association of Prolotherapy Regenerative Medicine (AOAPRM). The AOAPRM continues to educate and train physicians in regenerative medicine through annual conferences and specialized training courses (AOAPRM 2020).

Veterinary History

Veterinary prolotherapy dates back as far as 1350 BCE where Egyptians used hot iron cautery to treat equine lameness (Andersen 2015). The first published use of veterinary prolotherapy was in 1979. In the article Dr. Lambert described the use of electrosurgery to heal cruciate ligament rupture in dogs (Lambert 1979); 20–24 holes were created in the bones above and below the knee causing acute inflammation which, when resolved, improved stability in the knees of 94 dogs. The procedure was repeated in only six of the cases. No dog required surgical correction following prolotherapy.

Prolotherapy is still considered a niche market in veterinary medicine. Prolotherapy has been divided into two categories: traditional prolotherapy and prolozone. The injection of dextrose and other irritants fall under the traditional prolotherapy grouping. Prolozone uses ozone as the injectable substance (Tiekert 2013). Currently there are no prolotherapy-specific veterinary organizations.

Terminology

There a lot of terms used when discussing prolotherapy. A basic understanding of these terms is crucial, allowing effective communication amongst professionals and with clients.

Anterior (aka ventral): Closer to the front of the body.

Arthritis (aka osteoarthritis): Degeneration of the cartilage (smooth covering) within a joint. Over time physical changes occur to the underlying bone (CDC 2020).

Articular cartilage (aka hyaline cartilage): The translucent, blue-hued cartilage covering the joint end of bones, comprising synovial joints. The tissue serves to reduce concussive forces and friction within the joint (Pasquini et al. 2003). Cartilage thickness is dependent on the joint location and function.

Bioregulatory medicine: The use of non-pharmaceutical agents to stimulate the body's natural healing abilities (Reinders and Haghighat 2019).

Bursa: A fluid-filled sac located between bone and other tissues (muscles, tendons, ligaments, and skin) which reduces friction during movement (Pasquini et al. 2003).

Bursitis: Inflammation of the small fluid-filled cushions, called bursa, found between bone and other tissues, such as muscles, tendons, ligaments, and skin (MedlinePlus 2016).

Caudal: Located farther from the head.

Collagen: The most abundant protein in the body found within all types of connective tissue, including skin, cartilage, tendon, ligaments, and bone (Bliss 2013).

Contralateral: Opposite side.

Cranial: Located closer to the head.

Dextrose (aka d-glucose): A natural sugar, or more specifically a D-isomer of glucose (Hauser et al. 2016).

Distal: Away from the body.

Dorsal: Closer to the back of the body.

Elastin: A highly elastic protein found in connective tissue, tendons, ligaments, joint capsules, and cartilage (Frantz et al. 2010).

Enthesis: The fibrocartilaginous junction where tendon attaches to bone (Tresoldi et al. 2013).

Extracellular matrix (ECM): A three-dimensional network of big non-cellular molecules, including collagen, elastin, and proteoglycans, outside of the cells found within all tissues and organs (Frantz et al. 2010). The ECM functions as a physical framework for cells and is intimately involved in numerous biochemical and biomechanical processes crucial for tissue health and growth (Frantz et al. 2010).

Fibrocartilage: A tough and strong avascular connective tissue found at the insertion sites of ligaments and tendons, as well as intervertebral discs (Benjamin and Evans 1990).

Inferior (aka caudal): Located farther from the head.

In Vitro (latin for "within the glass"): Studies performed outside of a living organism. Most commonly microorganisms, tissue cultures, and cells are studied in petri dishes and/or test tubes.

In Vivo (latin for "in glass"): Studies performed within living organisms, not tissue extracts or cells.

Ipsilateral: Same side.

Joint (aka articulations): Area where two or more bones meet covered by a fibrous, elastic, cartilaginous, or combination of connective tissue types (Evans and De Lahunta 2013).

Joint capsule: Tissue covering a joint comprised of two layers: an outer fibrous layer and an inner synovial membrane (Pasquini et al. 2003).

Joint cavity: The space within a synovial joint containing synovial fluid (Pasquini et al. 2003).

Lateral: Farther away from the median plane or midline of the body or organ.

Ligament: Bands of fibrous connective tissue connecting bone to bone.

Intracapsular ligaments are located within a joint, while extracapsular ligaments are found outside of the joint or function as part of the joint capsule (Pasquini et al. 2003).

Ligament laxity: A ligament which is too loose to properly stabilize the joint and prevent misalignment during movement.

Luxation: Dislocation of a joint.

Medial: Closer to the median plane or midline of the body or organ.

Orthobiologics: The use of biological materials to treat musculoskeletal injuries.

Periosteum: The fibrous tissue covering the non-articulating surfaces of a bone. The periosteum nourishes and repairs bone and functions as the attachment site for tendons and ligaments (Pasquini et al. 2003).

Posterior (aka dorsal): Closer to the back of the body.

Prolotherapy (aka nonsurgical ligament and tendon reconstruction and regenerative joint injection): The injection of a small volume of a sterile irritant into a painful joint, tendon, or ligament with the goal of stimulating the body's natural healing ability, stabilizing the weakened tissues, and reducing pain (Hauser et al. 2016; AOAPRM 2020).

Prolozone: The injection of ozone or a combination of ozone plus an irritant or pharmaceutical into a joint, tendon, or ligament for the purposes of relieving pain and improving dysfunction (Shallenberger 2011b).

Proteoglycans Glycosylated proteins present in all connective tissues which form hydrogel matrices allowing tissues to withstand intense compressive forces (Frantz et al. **2010).**

Proximal: Closer to the body.

Regenerative medicine: The use of biological materials, including stem cells and platelet-rich plasma, to treat disease and injury through the restoration of the body's natural healing abilities (Barrett 2016).

Repetitive motion disorder (RMD): A category of muscular conditions caused by repeated motions performed during routine work or daily activities (NINDS 2019).

Sclerotherapy: The injection of an irritating solution into a vein or lymphatics causing transient swelling of the area, followed by collapse of the abnormal vein or lymph vessel. Most commonly used to treat varicose veins (aka chronic venous insufficiency), hemorrhoids, and malformed lymph vessels in people (Villines 2017).

Sprain: Injury to one or more ligaments. Ligaments are either stretched or torn (NIAMSD 2015).

Strain: Injury to a muscle or tendon because of stretching or tearing of the tissue (NIAMSD 2015).

Synovial fluid: The thick gelatinous liquid produced by the synovial membrane used to lubricate and nourish a synovial joint (Pasquini et al. 2003).

Tendon: Fibrous connective tissue attaching muscle to bone (Pasquini et al. 2003).

Tendonitis: Inflammation of a tendon.

Veterinary regenerative medicine: The injection of a substance derived from animal cells or tissues into a joint, tendon, or ligament with the intent of reducing pain and inflammation and promoting the body's natural healing abilities.

Anatomy Fundamentals

Anatomy and physiology are crucial to successfully and safely performing prolotherapy. Anatomy is a branch of science focusing on the bodily structure of living organisms. A thorough understanding of anatomy is crucial to safely and effectively perform prolotherapy (Tiekert 2013; Osborn 2018). Without this foundation, the patient response may be unfavorable and there is a higher risk of injury. An in-depth discussion of anatomy is beyond the scope of this book, but more detail is provided in the veterinarian subsection. Further information can also be found in the recommended references.

Anatomy for Veterinarians

The anatomy used during prolotherapy and regenerative medicine focuses on injured tendons, ligaments, and joints. As a review the anatomy of the shoulder, elbow, hip, and stifle joints are provided in Tables 7.1 and 7.2. (Tables 9.1 and 9.2 in Chapter 9 provide the origin, insertion, innervation, and primary function of the major muscles associated with these thoracic and pelvic limb joints, respectively.) Refer to anatomy textbooks for more in-depth information on these and other joints, muscles, tendons, and ligaments.

Physiology Fundamentals

Physiology is the branch of science focusing on the function of living organisms and their parts. The veterinarian must understand prolotherapy directly affects the cellular makeup of the musculoskeletal system and the body as w hole. Figure 7.1 illustrates the complexities of the anatomy and physiology within a joint. The veterinarian subsection provides a brief glimpse into the physiology of the tendons, ligaments, and joints.

Physiology for Veterinarians

Musculoskeletal physiology can be categorized into a molecular, cellular, and tissue levels. For the purposes of this chapter the most important molecular and cellular components are the ECM, collagen, elastin, and proteoglycans. The

Table 7.1 The primary bones, muscles, tendons, and ligaments comprising the shoulder (glenohumeral) and elbow (cubital) in the canine (Pasquini et al. 2003; Marcellin-Little et al. 2007; Evans and De Lahunta 2013).

Glenohumeral joint		
Bones	Scapula, humerus	
Primary muscles	Brachiocephalicus, omotransversarius, trapezius, latissimus dorsi, supraspinatus, infraspinatus, subscapularis, deltoideus, teres major, teres minor, biceps brachii	
Primary tendons	Supraspinatus[a]	Inserts onto the greater and lesser tubercles of the humerus
	Infraspinatus[a]	Inserts onto the greater tubercle of the humerus
	Biceps brachii	Originates on the supraglenoid tubercle of the scapula
	Subscapularis[a]	Inserts on the lesser tubercle of the humerus
Ligaments	Medial glenohumeral ligament, lateral glenohumeral ligament	
Cubital joint		
Bones	Humerus, radius, ulna	
Muscles	Biceps brachii, brachialis, triceps, anconeus	
Primary tendons	Biceps brachii	Inserts on the radial tuberosity
	Triceps brachii	Inserts (all heads) on the olecranon
Ligaments	Medial collateral ligament, lateral collateral ligament, cranial crura, caudal crura, annular ligament, oblique ligament, olecranon ligament	

[a] These tendons cross the joint and function as ligaments. Source: Lisa P. McFaddin.

Table 7.2 The primary bones, muscles, tendons, and ligaments comprising the hip (coxofemoral) and knee (stifle) joints in the canine (Pasquini et al. 2003; Marcellin-Little et al. 2007; Evans and De Lahunta 2013).

Coxofemoral joint		
Bones	Os coxae (ilium, ischium, pubis, and acetabulum), femur	
Primary muscles	Superficial gluteal, middle gluteal, deep gluteal, tensor fascia latae, piriformis, biceps femoris, semitendinosus, semimembranosus, rectus femoris, vastus (lateralis, intermedius, and medialis), sartorius, iliopsoas group, external obturator, pectineus, adductor, gracilis, internal obturator	
Primary tendons	Psoas major	Inserts on the lesser trochanter of the femur
	Iliacus	Inserts on the lesser trochanter of the femur
	External obturator	Inserts onto the trochanteric fossa of the femur
	Internal obturator	Inserts onto the trochanteric fossa of the femur
Ligaments	Ligament of the head of the femur (formerly the round ligament), transverse acetabular ligament, sacrotuberous ligament	
Stifle joint		
Bones	Femur, tibia, fibula	
Primary muscles	Biceps femoris, semitendinosus, semimembranosus, rectus femoris, vastus group, gastrocnemius, popliteus	
Tendons	Quadriceps group	Inserts onto the patella and tibial tuberosity
	Popliteus	Inserts onto the sesamoid bone (caudal to the tibia)
	Long digital extensor	Originates from the extensor fascia of the femur
Ligaments	Femoropatellar ligament, patellar ligament, medial collateral ligament, lateral collateral ligament, cranial cruciate ligament, caudal cruciate ligament, meniscofemoral ligament, cranial tibial ligament of medial meniscus, caudal tibial ligament of medial meniscus, cranial tibial ligament of lateral meniscus, caudal tibial ligament of lateral meniscus, transverse ligament, cranial ligament of femoral head, caudal ligament of femoral head	

Source: Lisa P. McFaddin.

tissues of primary concern are tendons, ligaments, and joints.

Musculoskeletal Molecular and Cellular Physiology
Extracellular Matrix The ECM is a three-dimensional network of non-cellular macromolecules outside of the cells. The ECM, found within all tissues and organs, functions as a physical framework for cells and is intimately involved in numerous biochemical and biomechanical processes crucial for tissue health and growth (Frantz et al. 2010).

The macromolecules within the ECM can be divided into two categories: proteoglycans and fibrous proteins (Frantz et al. 2010). With respect to the musculoskeletal system the fibrous proteins collagen and elastin are the most important.

Collagen As the main structural protein in connective tissue, collagens are one of the most plentiful and important proteins in the body, comprising approximately 30% of the total protein mass in mammals (Ricard-Blum 2011). All collagen is composed of amino acids linked together to form polypeptides, called α-chains (Bliss 2013). Three α-chains are bound together forming a triple helix or tropocollagen, as shown in Figure 7.2.

Within the α-chains every third amino acid is glycine. The most common collagen sequences are glycine-proline-X or glycine-X-hydroxyproline, where X can be any one of 17 different amino acids (Wu et al. 2022).

Collagen synthesis primarily occurs within fibroblasts, but extracellular synthesis can also occur (Wu et al. 2022). Transcription and

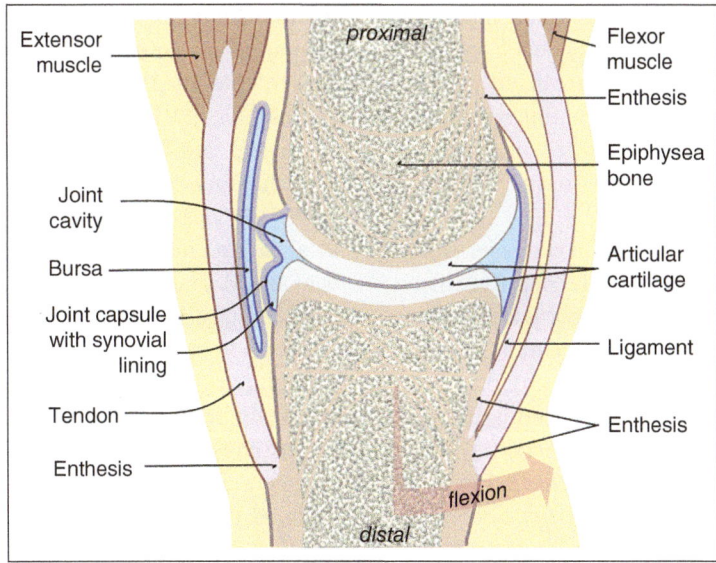

Figure 7.1 A schematic representation of a synovial joint and the surrounding structures. The joint is located between two bones, proximal (close to the body) and distal (away from the body). The joint consists of a joint capsule with a synovial membrane lining, articular cartilage, and a resulting joint cavity. The joint is flanked by collateral ligaments providing stability. The joint is moved through the contraction and relaxation of the surrounding musculature. Contraction of the extensor muscles straighten the joint; while contraction of the flexor muscles cause compression of the joint and bending (flexion) of the bones. The tendons connecting muscle to bone, as well as the entheses, are also pictured. Source: Jmarchn, August 17, 2015; https://en.wikipedia.org/wiki/File:Joint.svg.

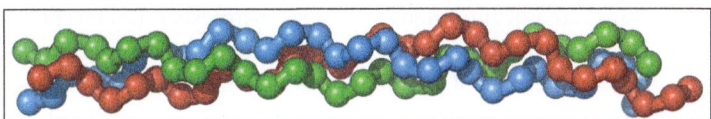

Figure 7.2 A cartoon model of the collagen triple helix or tropocollagen. Each colored strand represents one of the polypeptide chains called α-chains. Source: JWSchmidt, October 20, 2005, https://en.wikipedia.org/wiki/File:Collagentriplehelix.png.

translation of the α-chain genes within the cell create a pre-pro-polypeptide. The pre-pro-polypeptide becomes a procollagen following post-translational modifications within the endoplasmic reticulum (Wu et al. 2022). The procollagen is excreted from the cell in secretory vesicles following additional modifications within the Golgi apparatus. Once in the extracellular space, collagen peptidase enzymes cleave the ends of the procollagen creating a tropocollagen (Wu et al. 2022).

The three α-chains maybe identical, creating a homotrimer, or different, forming a heterotrimer. Mammals have 34 α-chain varieties, creating 28 distinct collagen types (Ricard-Blum 2011; Bliss 2013). The individual α-chains are numbered with Roman numerals.

Collagens contain at least one triple helix and represent a diverse group of ECM glycoproteins with a tendency to form supramolecular systems (Exposito et al. 2010). Collagens are classified into several groups. Within the musculoskeletal system the fibrillar collagens are the most important. Type I, II, III, V, XI, XXIV, and XXVII collagens constitute the fibrillar collagen family (Exposito et al. 2010; Bliss 2013).

Type I and II are by far the most common collagen proteins found within the musculoskeletal system (Bliss 2013). Type I collagen is found within skin, tendon, ligaments, blood vessels, organs, and bone. Type I collagen are heterotrimers arranged in long, thin cross-linked fibrils, creating a structural and mechanical matrix which increases the tensile strength of the tissue (Exposito et al. 2010; Bliss 2013).

Type II collagen is found in cartilage, particularly hyaline cartilage. Type II collagen are homotrimers forming cross-linked fibrils arranged in a three-dimensional matrix which traps proteoglycan aggregates (Exposito et al. 2010; Bliss 2013). Type II collagen increases the cartilage's resistance to deformation and increases tensile strength (Exposito et al. 2010; Bliss 2013).

Elastin Elastin is a highly elastic protein found in connective tissue, tendons, ligaments, joint capsules, and articular cartilage. Elastin fibers allow tissues to recoil and return to normal when exposed to repeated stretch and deformation (Frantz et al. 2010). Tissue elasticity is directly related to its elastin content. The associated collagen fibrils affect elastin's stretching ability (Bliss 2013).

Transcription and translation of the tropoelastin gene within the cell creates a soluble elastin subunit called tropoelastin (Frantz et al. 2010). Tropoelastin and specific elastin-binding proteins are excreted from the cell. Within the ECM tropoelastin is assembled into fibers, cross-linked together by lysine residues. These fibers are covered by fibrillins (glycoprotein microfibrils) which enhance the integrity of the elastin (Frantz et al. 2010; Bliss 2013). The result is a high molecular weight insoluble biopolymer.

Elastin fibers are strong, resilient, and durable. Fibers can sustain and recover from a 200% increase in length (Bliss 2013). Elastin fibers are primarily produced during the growth, repair, and remodeling phases of tissue healing, and once produced can persist for years (Bliss 2013).

Proteoglycans Proteoglycans (PGs) are one of the primary components of the ECM and found in all types of connective tissue. PGs are composed of a core protein with variable numbers of attached glycosaminoglycan (GAG) chains (Bliss 2013). All GAGs, except in hyaluronic acid, are covalently bonded to the core proteins (Frantz et al. 2010).

PGs are classified by the core protein type, localization, and GAG composition (Frantz et al. 2010). The core protein length and amino acid composition vary. Categorization of PG localization includes intracellular, cell surface, pericellular and basement membrane, and extracellular (Iozzo and Schaefer 2015). GAG chains consist of unbranched polysaccharide chains made up of repeating disaccharide units. GAGs are either sulfated (chondroitin sulfate, heparan sulfate, and keratan sulfate) or non-sulfated (hyaluronic acid) (Iozzo and Schaefer 2015).

PGs are extremely hydrophilic and tend to create large aggregates forming a hydrogel matrix which can withstand strong compressive forces (Frantz et al. 2010; Bliss 2013). PG aggregates may be firm, solidified, and reinforced by associated collagen fibrils.

PG synthesis relies on the transcription and translation of the core protein followed by attachment of the GAG chains, and finally extracellular secretion of the mature PG (Bliss 2013). PG synthesis is a highly regulated process which can be altered by exposure to biochemical, both biological and pharmaceutical, stimuli.

There are numerous PGs associated with tendons, ligaments, and articular cartilage. Table 7.3 summarizes the key PGs found within these tissues.

Tissue Physiology

Tendons

Tendons are composed of fibrous connective tissue which connects muscle to bone. Tendons are designed to transfer forces from muscles to the bone and must withstand the force of muscle contraction. The "non-linear, viscous-elastic, anisotropic, and heterogeneous mechanical properties" of the tendon provide its rigidity and

Table 7.3 The name, classification, and primary functions of common proteoglycans (PG) found in tendons, ligaments, and articular cartilage (Knudson and Knudson 2001; Kiani et al. 2002; Yoon and Halper 2005; Fox et al. 2009; Gupta et al. 2019).

Name	Classification	Functions
Aggrecan	Lectican	Major PG in articular cartilage
		90% of the GAG chains are chondroitin sulfate
		Non-covalently bound to hyaluronic acid
		Provides resiliency
		Assists with load-bearing
Biglycan	SLRP	Binds to fibrillar collagen
		Inhibits collagen fibrillogenesis
		Plays a role in bone mineralization
Decorin	SLRP	Binds to fibrillar collagen
		Binds growth factors
		Improves tensile strength
Fibromodulin	SLRP	Binds to type I collagen
		Regulates collagen fibril diameter
		Modulates tendon strength
Hyaluronan (hyaluronic acid)	Non-sulfated	Non-covalently binds with aggrecan and versican
		Maintains viscoelasticity
		Maintains lubrication
		Regulates metabolism of fibroblasts
Lumican	SLRP	Binds to type I collagen
		Limits collagen fibril size
		Modulates tendon strength
Versican	Lectican	Non-covalently binds to hyaluronic acid
		Contains many chondroitin sulfate chains
		Increases viscoelasticity
		Maintains cell shape

GAG, glycosaminoglycans; SLRP, small leucine-rich repeat proteoglycan. Source: Lisa P. McFaddin.

flexibility (Tresoldi et al. 2013). There are multiple types of tendons, the most common being summarized in Table 7.4. Figure 7.3 depicts an example of an ossified tendon from a dinosaur.

Tendons are composed of 70% water and 30% dry mass, with 60–80% of the dry mass consisting of type I collagen and 2% elastin (Tresoldi et al. 2013). The primary cell type are specialized fibroblasts called tenocytes which are responsible for generating the tendon's ECM.

Tendons are covered by a loose sheath of connective tissue, the epitenon, which contains blood vessels, lymphatic vessels, and nerves (Tresoldi et al. 2013). The attachment site of the tendon to the bone, called the enthesis, is composed of either fibrous or fibrocartilaginous tissue (Tresoldi et al. 2013).

Ligaments Ligaments are strong, dense, inelastic bands of white fibrous connective tissue which originate and insert on bone (Pasquini et al. 2003).

Table 7.4 Classification of the most common tendon types with description of their features, primary function, and examples (Bliss 2013).

Energy-storing tendons	Description:	Pronounced tissue recoil due to their high concentration of elastin
	Function:	Maintain weight-bearing and posture
	Example:	Tarsal extensor tendon
Positional tendons	Description:	Solid and rope-like, specific sites of bony attachment, and may be encased in a fluid-filled sheath reducing friction during movement
	Function:	Control joint position
	Example:	Biceps brachii tendon of origin
Wrap-around tendons	Description:	A form of positional tendon; changes direction when crossing a joint
	Function:	Control joint position
	Example:	Digital extensor tendon

Source: Lisa P. McFaddin.

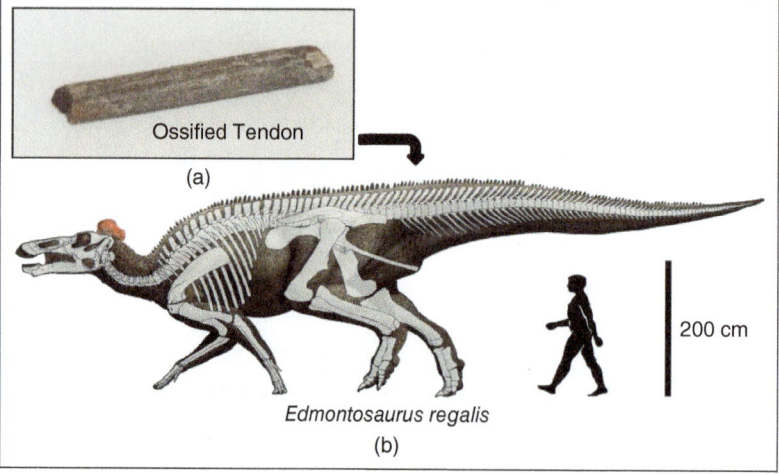

Ossified Tendon

(a)

Edmontosaurus regalis

(b)

200 cm

Figure 7.3 (a) An ossified tendon from an *Edmontosaurus* found in Wyoming. (b) *Edmontosaurus* were a herbivorous dinosaur, weighing approximately 3400 kg, living during the Late Cretaceous Period (76–65 million years ago). Source: (a) HCA/Wikimedia Commons/CC BY-SA 4.0. (b) Xiang et al. (2017); Epstein et al. (2015), Figure 2, doi: 10.1371/journal.pone.0175253.

Ligaments typically attach two different bones together but can originate and insert on the same bone, as in the transverse acetabular ligament (Pasquini et al. 2003). Ligaments serve to stabilize joints by keeping joint surfaces in correct apposition, while ensuring appropriate joint movement (Pasquini et al. 2003; Bliss 2013).

Ligaments are divided into two categories: extracapsular and intracapsular. Extracapsular (aka capsular) ligaments are found on the outside of or contained within the joint capsule. Extracapsular ligaments, such as collateral ligaments, are collagen-rich and function to stabilize the joint and limit side-to-side movement (Pasquini et al. 2003; Bliss 2013).

Intracapsular (aka intra-articular) ligaments are found within the joint capsule but are not considered within the joint space because they are covered by the synovial membrane (Pasquini et al. 2003). Intra-articular ligaments have a vascular outer layer, called the epiligament, which is grossly indistinguishable from the ligament itself (Frank 2004). The epiligament fuses with the periosteum at the site of origin and insertion.

Histologically and biochemically tendons and ligaments are very similar. Ligaments are composed of approximately 67% water and 33% dry mass, with 85% of the dry mass consisting of type I collagen and less than 1% elastin (Frank 2004). Fibroblasts are the primary cell population responsible for creating the ligament's ECM (Frank 2004). The collagen bundles comprising the ligament are aligned along its long axis and have a wavy appearance microscopically. The waviness or crimping provides extra slack when the ligament is under tension (loaded), reducing the risk of damage (Frank 2004).

Joints There are three primary classification systems for joints: clinical, structural, and functional (outlined in Table 7.5). Clinical classifications are defined by the number of articulating bones (Pasquini et al. 2003). Structural classifications are broken down by the type of tissue used to connect bone to bone (Pasquini et al. 2003). Functional classifications are defined by their type and degree of movement (Pasquini et al. 2003).

When performing prolotherapy synovial joints are the most important. The primary components of a joint are the joint cavity and the joint capsule.

Table 7.5 Summary of the three joint classification systems including the name and description of joint types, as well as an example of each (Pasquini et al. 2003; Evans and De Lahunta 2013).

Clinical joint classification system		
Simple joints	Description:	Contains two articulating bones
	Example:	Glenohumeral (hip) joint
Compound joints	Description:	Involves more than two articulating bones
	Example:	Stifle joint
Structural joint classification system		
Fibrous joints	Description:	Joints united by fibrous connective tissue with limited to no movement; joint may ossify as in the case of cranial sutures
	Example:	Hyoid apparatus to the temporal bone
Cartilaginous joints	Description:	(aka synchondroses) Slightly mobile to immobile joints united by hyaline cartilage, fibrocartilage, or a combination
	Example:	Hyaline cartilage joints, fibrocartilaginous joints
	Hyaline cartilage joints	
	Description:	(aka primary joints) Temporary cartilaginous joints in fetal skeletons and growing bone; often ossify with time
	Example:	Cartilaginous physeal plate between the epiphysis and diaphysis of an immature long bone
	Fibrocartilaginous joints	
	Description:	(aka secondary joints) Restricted movement; generally found along the midline of the body; fibrocartilage tightly connects bones together in areas where limited movement is needed
	Example:	Vertebral bodies
Synovial joints	Description:	(aka diarthrosis) Freely moveable joints found in the extremities; all contain a joint capsule, joint cavity, synovial fluid, and articular cartilage
	Example:	Stifle joint

(Continued)

Table 7.5 (Continued)

Functional joint classification system		
Synarthrosis	Description:	Immobile joint often comprising fibrous tissue
	Example:	Cranial sutures
Amphiarthrosis	Description:	Joint with limited movement usually containing fibrocartilage or other connective tissue
	Example:	Pubic symphysis
Diarthrosis	Description:	(aka synovial joint) Freely mobile joint
	Example:	Elbow joint

Source: Lisa P. McFaddin.

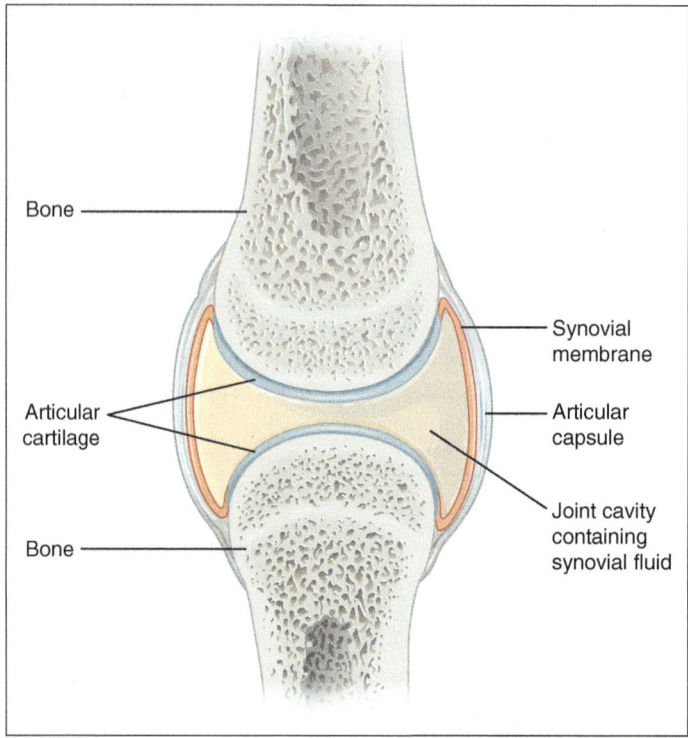

Figure 7.4 A schematic drawing of primary components within a synovial joint: joint (articular) capsule, joint cavity, articular cartilage, and synovial fluid. Source: OpenStax College Anatomy & Physiology, Connexions web site. June 19, 2013, http://cnx.org/content/col11496/1.6.

Joint Cavity The space between the articulating bones, surrounded by joint capsule, and filled with synovial fluid.

Joint Capsule As shown in Figure 7.4 the joint capsule is composed of an outer fibrous layer and an inner synovial membrane (SM). The outer fibrous membrane (FM), the membrane fibrosa, consists of avascular dense white fibrous tissue with yellow elastic fibers (Evans and De Lahunta 2013). The FM covers the entire circumference of the joint attaching to the articular end of each associated bone. The capsular ligament is an extension of the FM in some joints, as with collateral ligaments. In other joints the capsular ligament is a separate structure, such as the patellar ligament (Evans and De Lahunta 2013).

The SM is composed of an avascular connective tissue and covers everything within the joint except, when present, the articular cartilage and fibrocartilaginous plates (Evans and De Lahunta 2013). Instead of coating the articular cartilage, the SM blends with the periosteum. SM also forms sleeves around intra-articular ligaments, blood vessels, nerves, muscles, and tendons found within the joint (Evans and De Lahunta 2013).

The SM generally consists of two layers: subintima and intima. The subintima is the thicker fibrous outer layer. The inner synovial intima is one to three cell layers deep, depending on the joint, and comprises synoviocytes (Iwanaga et al. 2000). There are two types of synoviocytes: type A (macrophagic) and type B (fibroblastic). Type A synoviocytes remove waste substances from the synovial fluid (Iwanaga et al. 2000). Type B synoviocytes produce hyaluronan, proteoglycans, surfactants, and matrix metalloproteinases which, when combined with lubricin, create the synovial fluid within the joint cavity (Iwanaga et al. 2000).

Synovial Fluid   Synovial fluid is a clear, straw-colored viscous fluid found within the joint cavities of all synovial joints. Synovial fluid is composed of hyaluronan, lubricin, and plasma proteins (primarily albumin and globulin) (Hui et al. 2011).

Hyaluronan and lubricin are the primary lubricating macromolecules within synovial fluid. Hyaluronan, or hyaluronic acid, is a non-sulfated proteoglycan produced by type B synoviocytes within the SM's intima layer (Gupta et al. 2019). Hyaluronan helps maintain viscoelasticity and lubrication within the joint.

Lubricin is a mucinous glycoprotein secreted by synovial fibroblasts. Lubricin coats the surface of the articular cartilage providing lubrication and preventing cell and protein adhesion to the cartilage surface (Hui et al. 2011).

The primary role of synovial fluid is to keep joints well lubricated. Synovial fluid also serves to reduce friction and absorb shock within the joint, transport nutrients and waste products out of the joint, and mediate communication between cells within the joint (Iwanaga et al. 2000; Hui et al. 2011). Normally there is a very small amount of synovial fluid within the joint cavity, but the quantity and quality of synovial fluid changes with age and pathology.

Joint inflammation causes changes in the composition, volume, and function of synovial fluid. During inflammation the protein content increases, the hyaluronan and lubricin concentrations decrease, and the volume of joint fluid increases (Hui et al. 2011). The altered synovial fluid composition and volume inhibit its natural lubricating properties causing the joints to become swollen, stiff, and painful (Hui et al. 2011).

Articular Cartilage   Articular cartilage, or hyaline cartilage, is a smooth, translucent, and blue-hued specialized connective tissue covering the articulating bones of diarthrodial joints (Fox et al. 2009). Articular cartilage serves as a surface for low friction articulation and transfers weight to the underlying subchondral bone during normal joint movement and dynamic loading (Fox et al. 2009).

Articular cartilage is primarily composed of a dense ECM and chondrocytes. The ECM consists of water, collagen (primarily type II), proteoglycans (primarily aggrecan), noncollagenous proteins, and glycoproteins (Fox et al. 2009). Articular cartilage has a high water content, accounting for approximately 60–85% of the total weight (Fox et al. 2009). On a dry-matter basis 50% of the weight is from collagen, while proteoglycans account for 35% (Fox et al. 2009; Bliss 2013; Evans and De Lahunta 2013). The remaining 10% is made up of proteins, lipids, and minerals.

Chondrocytes are the primary cell found within articular cartilage comprising approximately 2% of the total volume (Fox et al. 2009). These highly specialized cells play a huge role in the development, maintenance, and repair of the ECM. Chondrocytes differ in size and appearance and primary function throughout the articular cartilage.

Articular cartilage is organized into four zones: superficial zone, middle zone, deep zone, and calcified zone (Bautista et al. 2016). Figure 7.5 illustrates the histologic appearance of articular cartilage the first three zones.

The superficial zone, or Zone I, accounts for 10–20% of the articular cartilage's thickness (Fox et al. 2009). Being in direct contact with the synovial fluid, Zone I helps resist compressive forces and protect the deeper layers. Type II and IX collagen are arranged closely together parallel to the articular surface (Fox et al. 2009). Zone I also contains many flat chondrocytes.

The middle zone, or Zone II, provides resistance to compressive forces and acts as a transition between the superficial and deep layers (Fox et al. 2009). Zone II accounts for 40–60% of the articular cartilage's total volume and is composed of thick obliquely organized collagen fibrils, proteoglycans, and spherical chondrocytes (Fox et al. 2009).

The deep zone, or Zone III, accounts for 30% of the articular cartilage's total volume. It plays the biggest role in resisting compressive forces

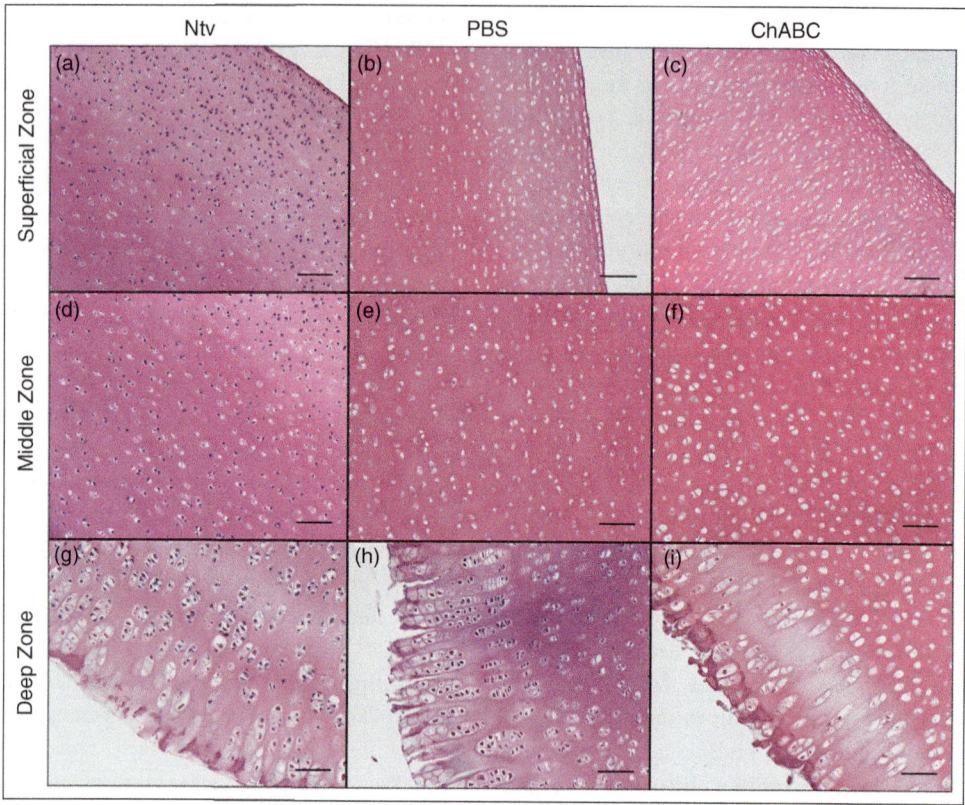

Figure 7.5 A cross-section of decellularized articular cartilage stained with hematoxylin and eosin. The superficial (Zone I), middle (Zone II), and deep (Zone III) zones are shown. Zone I comprises 10–20% of the articular cartilage thickness, contains primarily types II and IX collagen, is in direct contact with the synovial fluid, helps resist compressive forces, and protects the deeper layers. Zone II comprises 40–60% of the total volume, contains thick obliquely organized collagen fibrils, proteoglycans, and spherical chondrocytes, provides resistance to compressive forces, and acts as a transition between the superficial and deep layers. Zone III comprises 30% of the total volume, contains large-diameter collagen fibrils and chondrocytes arranged parallel to the collagen, and contains the largest concentration of proteoglycans, with the least amount of water. Zone IV comprises a few large chondrocytes and serves to firmly attach the articular cartilage to the subchondral bone (the calcified Zone IV is not pictured). Source: Catherine A. Bautista et al. 2016/PLOS ONE/CC0 1.0.

through the special perpendicular arrangement of its large diameter collagen fibrils (Fox et al. 2009). Zone III also contains chondrocytes arranged parallel to the collagen and the largest concentration of proteoglycans, with the least amount of water (Fox et al. 2009). The calcified zone, or Zone IV, comprises a few large chondrocytes and serves to firmly attach the articular cartilage to the subchondral bone (Fox et al. 2009).

The collagen and proteoglycans help retain water within the ECM contributing to the articular cartilage's ability to withstand high cyclic loads (Fox et al. 2009). Articular cartilage undergoes significant elastic and reversible deformation during normal joint loading. The initial compressive forces increase interstitial fluid pressure causing fluid to move out of the ECM (Fox et al. 2009). When the pressure is removed the fluid returns.

Articular cartilage thickness is dependent on the joint, location within the joint, age of the animal, and health of the joint (Bliss 2013; Fox et al. 2009). Joints expected to undergo heavy and repetitive loading contain thicker articular cartilage. With age, and repetitive stress, the quantity and distribution of chondrocytes changes within the different zones of the articular cartilage (Fox et al. 2009). The number of chondrocytes in the superficial layer decreases, while chondrocytes in the deep layers increase. The ECM also loses hydration, reducing its compliance and ability to effectively absorb loading forces. As a result, the subchondral bone is exposed to higher forces and undergoes physical changes. Additionally, the articular cartilage's lack of vascular and lymphatic supply, as well as innervation, hinders the capacity for healing.

Wound Healing Fundamentals

Wound healing is divided into four overlapping phases: hemostasis, inflammation, proliferation, and remodeling. Figure 7.6 illustrates the coinciding nature and approximate timing for each phase.

- **Hemostasis**: Before healing can start hemostasis must be achieved. Bleeding is generally halted within seconds to hours following injury (Wallace et al. 2022). Initially vessels constrict reducing blood flow, followed by platelets plugging the hole by attaching to the lining (subendothelium) of the disrupted blood vessel (Guo and DiPietro 2010).

- **Inflammatory phase**: The inflammatory phase generally lasts one to five days, occurring with hemostasis (Landén et al. 2016). This phase, summarized in Figure 7.7, causes increases in the size of blood vessels (vasodilation), leakage of fluids, proteins, and cells from the blood vessels (increased vascular permeability), movement of cells to the site of injury (chemotaxis), and the recruitment of more white blood cells to the area (Patil et al. 2019; Chen et al. 2018). This cascade of events results in the classic signs of inflammation: redness, swelling, heat, pain, and loss of function (Punchard et al. 2004).

- **Proliferative phase**: The primary goal of the proliferative phase is to create the initial scar tissue by laying the groundwork for new tissue formation. This starts with a disorganized matrix of connective tissue and blood vessels. The proliferative phase typically lasts 4–21 days (Landén et al. 2016).

- **Remodeling phase**: The final phase of wound healing can last 21 days to over one year

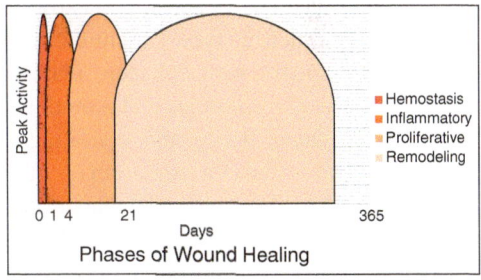

Figure 7.6 The timeline for the phases of wound healing (Landén et al. 2016). Hemostasis occurs within seconds to hours. The inflammatory phase lasts one to five days. The proliferative phase lasts 4–21 days. The remodeling phase lasts 21 days to over one year. Source: Lisa P. McFaddin.

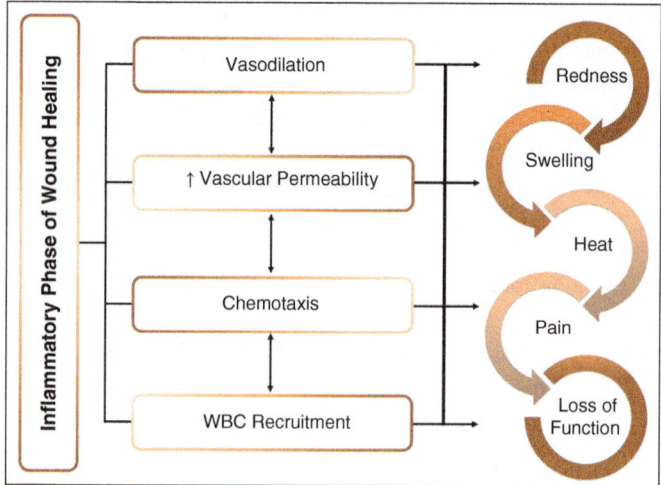

Figure 7.7 Schematic summary of the inflammatory phase of wound healing which comprises four primary interconnected physiologic changes (vasodilation, increased vascular permeability, chemotaxis, and the recruitment of more white blood cells) and leads to the five cardinal signs of inflammation (redness, swelling, heat, pain, and loss of function). WBC, white blood cells. Source: Lisa P. McFaddin.

(Landén et al. 2016). The remodeling phase focuses on replacing the proliferative (granulation) tissue with tissue like that before the injury (aka a functional scar). Keep in mind the repaired tendons, ligaments, and joints are never as strong as undamaged tissues.

> **The end goal of wound healing is a functional scar.**

Wound Healing for Veterinarians

Hemostasis

Platelets are triggered by exposure to extravascular collagen, such as type I (Schultz et al. 2015). Upon contact with collagen, platelets release adhesive glycoproteins and growth factors, making them sticky and encouraging aggregation and initial clot formation (Schultz et al. 2015). The fibrin plug also encourages activation of the clotting cascade. Platelet released growth factors aid in wound healing (see Table 8.2 in Chapter 8 for additional information).

Inflammatory Phase

Tissue injury causes a cascade of chemical signaling, summarized in Figure 7.8. Damaged endothelial cells release inflammatory mediators and other proteins which attract white blood cells and platelets (Chen et al. 2018; Patil et al. 2019). Proinflammatory proteins include cytokines, chemokines, arachidonic acid metabolites, adhesion molecules, and platelet-activating factors (PAF) (Chen et al. 2018; Patil et al. 2019). Neutrophils are the first to arrive, followed by monocytes, lymphocytes, and mast cells (Chen et al. 2018; Patil et al. 2019). Each cell contributes to the propagation of inflammation.

The inflammatory phase is essential to hemostasis and recruitment of the immune system, and without these processes wound healing would not occur. Exaggerated or prolonged inflammation within the musculoskeletal system can be detrimental, leading to pain and loss of function.

Proliferative Phase

Approximately three days after injury monocytes recruited to the site differentiate into macrophages (Landén et al. 2016). Macrophages are critical to the transition from the inflammatory to proliferative phases of wound healing. The proliferative phase generally takes 4–21 days (Landén et al. 2016).

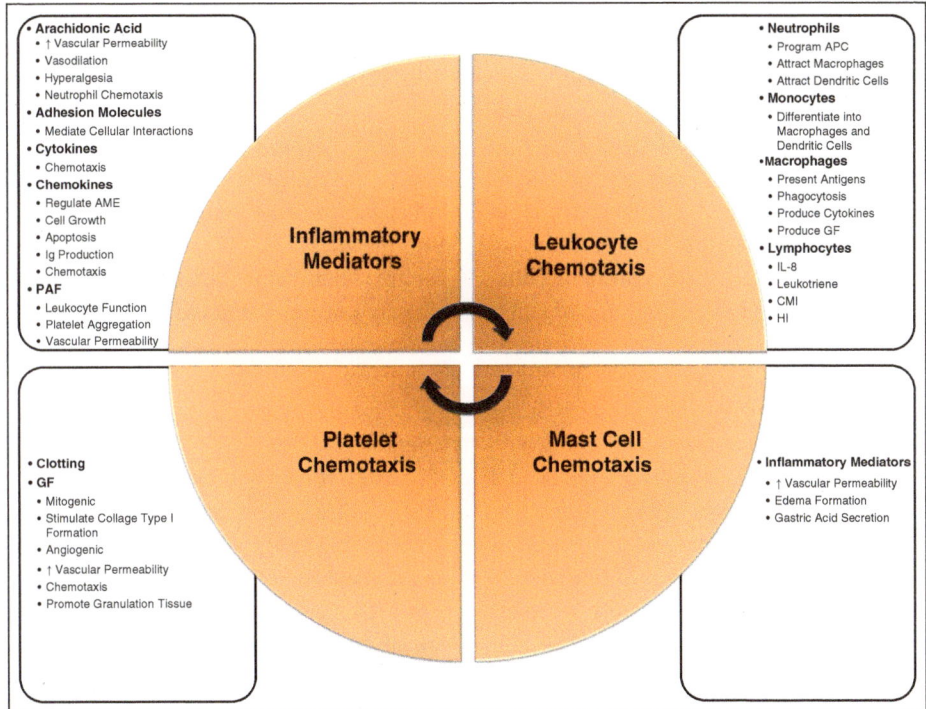

Figure 7.8 An overview of the inflammatory cascade. Most inflammatory mediators are arachidonic acid (prostaglandins and leukotrienes), adhesion molecules (immunoglobulin-like, integrins, cadherins, and selectins), cytokines (interleukin-1, interleukin-6, tumor necrosis factor alpha, and lipopolysaccharide), chemokines (interleukin-8 or IL-8), and platelet-activating factor (PAF). The most common leukocytes are neutrophils, monocytes, macrophages, and lymphocytes (natural killer cells, T cells, and B cells). The predominant inflammatory mediators released by mast cells include cytokines, chemokines, histamine, protease, prostaglandin, leukotrienes, serglycin proteoglycans, and complement activation. The primary growth factors (GF) involved are platelet-derived growth factor, transforming growth factor, vascular endothelial growth factor, basic fibroblast growth factor, platelet-derived epidermal growth factor, insulin-like growth factor, and mesenchymal stem cells (Yates 2014; Tambella et al. 2018; Chen et al. 2018; Patil et al. 2019;). Source: Lisa P. McFaddin.

The primary goals of the proliferative phase are to establish a new connective tissue matrix, lay down vasculature, and form granulation tissue (Schultz et al. 2015). The connective tissue matrix is composed of disorganized collagen fibers, proteoglycans, and fibronectin (Schultz et al. 2015).

Platelets and macrophages initially bind to matrix proteins, migrate along the fibrils within the ECM, and recruit fibroblasts to the site of injury (Schultz et al. 2015). Fibroblasts are responsible for synthesizing and depositing the collagen, proteoglycans, elastin, and other proteins found within granulation tissue (Schultz et al. 2015).

Angiogenesis is necessary to sustain tissue viability. The tissue oxygen saturation, pH, and lactate levels help stimulate angiogenesis along with soluble mediators produced by endothelial cells, fibroblasts, vascular endothelial cells, and macrophages (Schultz et al. 2015). Angiogenic factors trigger adjacent capillary endothelial cells to migrate and proliferate (Schultz et al. 2015).

Remodeling Phase

The established transitional granulation tissue remodels and matures over 21 days to one year forming functional scar tissue (Landén et al. 2016). The initial scar tissue is replaced by an ECM resembling the pre-injury tissue (Schultz et al. 2015). The remodeling process relies heavily on ECM proteins and proteolytic enzymes, specifically metalloproteinases and serine proteases (Schultz et al. 2015). The ECM composition is ultimately dependent on the tissue type, i.e. tendon, ligament, or joint.

Maturation of granulation tissue involves formation of larger blood vessels (aggregation of capillaries), decreased concentrations of fibroblast, GAGs, and proteoglycans, and reduction of cellular metabolism and density (Schultz et al. 2015). The predominant collagen type, concentration, and organization (from random deposition to orderly covalent cross-linking) changes (Schultz et al. 2015). Collagen reorganization is the primary factor affecting tissue tensile strength.

During typical wound healing, the healed tissue has greater tensile strength, mobility, and shock absorption compared to the granulation tissue. The new tissue over time develops a tensile strength approximately 80% that of the uninjured tissue (Landén et al. 2016).

Administration Techniques

The most common sterile injectable irritants used in veterinary medicine are dextrose and ozone.

Dextrose Prolotherapy
Description
A simple sugar, whose molecular structure is pictured in Figure 7.9, typically produced from corn (PubChem 2023). Dextrose is identical to glucose, the primary sugar found in the blood (PubChem 2023). Sterile dextrose solution typically comes as a 50% solution (500 mg/ml). The solution must be diluted with sterile water prior to administration.

Dextrose is the most common prolotherapy irritant used in human medicine. Typically, 12.5–25% sterile solutions are used in human and veterinary medicine (Hauser et al. 2016). In veterinary medicine a 15% dextrose solution is often used for ligaments, while a 25% solution is used for joint injections (Tiekert 2013); 50% dextrose is diluted with sterile water to create the desired concentration. Often lidocaine is added, in varying quantities, to the mixture (Tiekert 2013). Injectable dextrose is approved

by the Food and Drug Administration (FDA) but its use for prolotherapy is considered off-label (DHHS 2020).

Required Supplies
Sterile 50% dextrose for injection, sterile 2% lidocaine for injection, sterile water, syringes, and needles (25, 27, or 30g; 1.5 inches in length) (Ben-Yakir 2020). The procedure may or may not require anesthesia, but sedation is often recommended depending on the area being injected (Tiekert 2013).

Injection Locations
The most common injection locations in veterinary medicine are (Tiekert 2013; Osborn 2018) patellar tendon in the stifle (knee); biceps tendon in the shoulder and elbow; brachiocephalicus tendon in the neck and shoulder; cruciate ligament in the stifle; collateral ligaments in the stifle; and cervical, thoracolumbar, and lumbar spine.

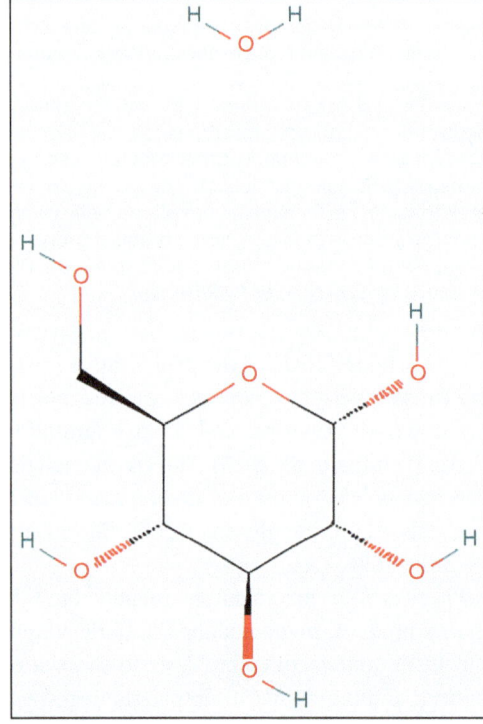

Figure 7.9 The molecular structure of dextrose, $C_6H_{14}O_7$. Source: PubChem, created August 8, 2005, https://pubchem.ncbi.nlm.nih.gov/compound/66370.

Injection Techniques

Multiple areas are injected with small volumes of liquid instead of injecting one area with a large volume of fluid (Tiekert 2013). The smallest gauge needle, 25–30g, is recommended. Light sedation or anesthesia may be needed depending on the location being treated. Always pull back on the syringe to ensure the needle is not placed in a blood vessel (Osborn 2018).

When injecting irritants the needle should contact, or peck, the bone. Stimulation of the periosteum (covering of the bone) activates the vascular covering of the bone facilitating the healing process (Gladstein 2012). Both the presence of the needle and the solution being injected trigger inflammation followed by healing.

Treatment Frequency

Prolotherapy sessions are generally administered every two to six weeks for three to five sessions (Ben-Yakir 2020; Tiekert 2013). The patient should be re-evaluated to determine if further prolotherapy sessions are necessary. The intervals between treatments are gradually lengthened until they are repeated every few years or may no longer be needed (Ben-Yakir 2020; Tiekert 2013).

Post-Treatment Recommendations

Patients may need to be placed on nonsteroidal anti-inflammatory drugs (NSAIDs) for a few weeks following the injection (Ben-Yakir 2020). Steroids are not recommended immediately following prolotherapy (Ben-Yakir 2020). Improvement is generally seen within a month following injection (Ben-Yakir 2020). Post-treatment movement is crucial to healing, especially for the first 48 hours after injection (Osborn 2018). Short, controlled walks should be encouraged, but jumping should be prohibited.

Ozone

Description

Ozone, depicted in Figure 7.10, is an inorganic molecule composed of three oxygen atoms, O_3

(PubChem 2022). Ozone is a colorless to pale blue explosive gas with a characteristic odor (PubChem 2022). Ozone occurs naturally (atmospheric) and can be synthesized.

An ozone generator (ozonator) is a device designed to create ozone from room air or pure oxygen gas using either an electrical discharge (corona), UV light, plasma, or electrolysis (Rodriguez 2016). Only pure oxygen gas should be used for medical applications of ozone therapy in people and animals (Shallenberger 2011a). The machine can be set to generate a specific concentration of ozone, typically 1–3% (Shallenberger 2011a).

The instability of ozone causes the O_3 molecules to interact and break down into more stable O_2 molecules relatively quickly in a process called dismutation, as shown in Figure 7.11 (Shallenberger 2011a). In a glass container 50% of the ozone will dismutate every 45 minutes; while plastic containers result in 50% dismutation every 30 minutes (Elvis and Ekta 2011; Shallenberger 2011a). This means ozone must be generated and used as needed (see Chapter 5 for further information).

Required Supplies

An ozone generator and oxygen tank are required to create ozone. Refer to Chapter 5 for a more detailed list of supplies required for ozone therapy. Syringes and needles are needed to inject the ozone.

Injection Locations

Common injection locations include neck, back, hips, stifles, carpi (wrists), and hocks (ankles) (Shallenberger 2011a,b).

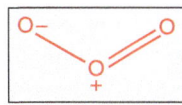

Figure 7.10 Molecular structure of ozone or triatomic oxygen, O_3. Source: Pubchem, https://pubchem.ncbi.nlm.nih.gov/compound/24823, August 1, 2005.

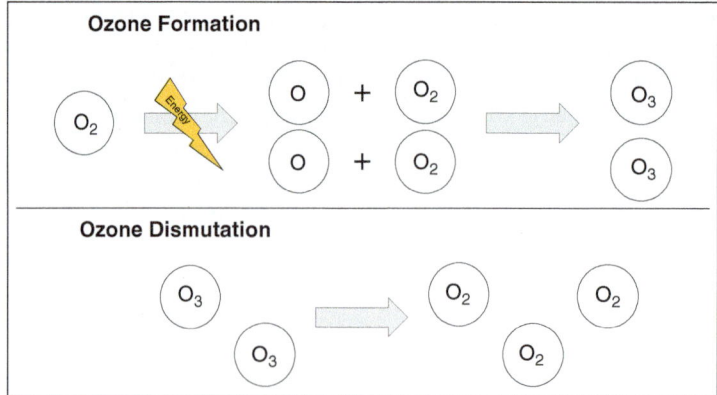

Figure 7.11 A schematic representation of the formation and dismutation of ozone. As oxygen gas is exposed to an energy source some of the oxygen (O_2) molecules dissociate into oxygen (O) atoms. The oxygen atoms recombine with non-dissociated oxygen molecules forming ozone (O_3). Ozone molecules are unstable and break down into more stable oxygen (O_2) molecules quickly. Source: Lisa P. McFaddin.

Injection Technique

Larger volumes of gas are injected, compared to solution-based prolotherapy. Because the gas will diffuse and expand once injected, a single injection location is used (Shallenberger 2011b).

Treatment Frequency

Three to six treatments every three to four weeks are recommended initially (Tiekert 2013). Long-term frequency is assessed on a case-by-case basis. Some patients require treatments every three to four months for chronic pain conditions.

Post-Treatment Recommendations

No special aftercare instructions are needed.

Mechanisms of Action

Like many therapies the mechanisms of action are complex and not fully understood. The injection of a substance into a tendon, ligament, or joint causes a controlled injury or insult which incites a predictable response by the body leading to inflammation followed by healing (Osborn 2018). The result is improved stability, strength, and pain reduction (Gladstein 2012). The repair and reinforcement of stability and strength within the joint, tendon, or ligament contributes to prolotherapy's ability to reduce pain (Gladstein 2012).

Tendons, ligaments, and articular cartilage have relatively poor blood supply compared to muscles and skin which slows their healing times following injury (Steilen et al. 2014). Muscles typically require two to four weeks to heal; while tendons, ligaments, and cartilage take 4–6, 10–12, and 12 weeks, respectively (Woo and Buckwalter 1988; Henderson and Millis 2014).

The goal of prolotherapy is to cause local inflammation which triggers the innate healing abilities of the body (Hauser et al. 2016). Regardless of the location, the post-prolotherapy healing process takes six to eight weeks (Osborn 2018). After injecting the solution, the tissue undergoes several overlapping phases of healing, as shown in Figure 7.12 (Steilen et al. 2014).

Mechanisms of Action for Veterinarians

Ben-Yakir (2020) describes six steps in the mechanism of action for prolotherapy (Figure 7.13). The healing process incited by prolotherapy, like that of normal wound healing, consists of four overlapping phases or cascades: hemostasis, inflammation, proliferation, and remodeling (Steilen et al. 2014). Using Ben-Yakir's model, steps 1 and 2 represent the initial tissue insult resulting in bleeding followed by hemostasis and the initiation of the inflammatory cascade. Steps 3–5 are predominantly the proliferation

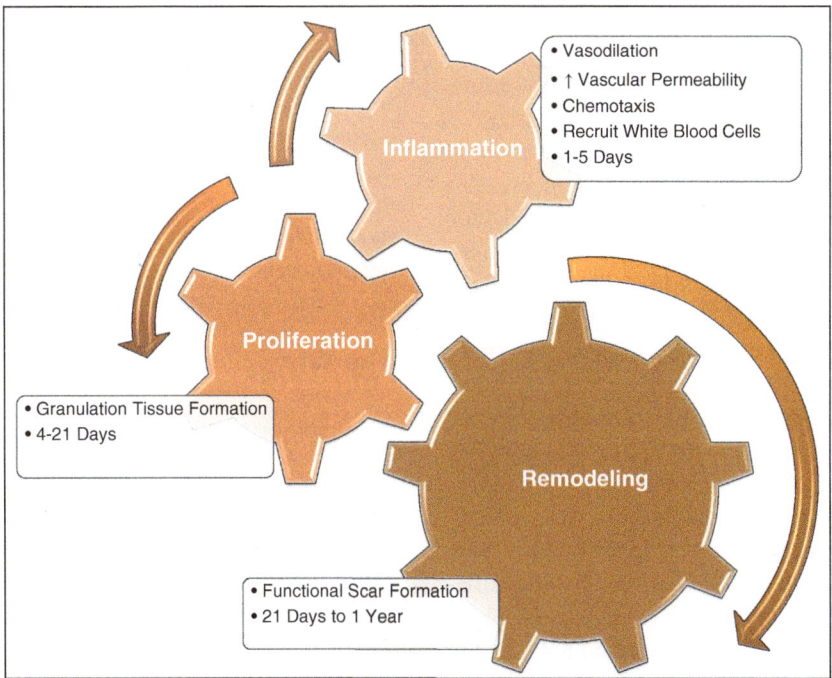

Figure 7.12   The overlapping phases of healing, primary beneficial effects, and approximate timeline associated with prolotherapy. Source: Lisa P. McFaddin.

phase but also involve tissue remodeling. Step 6 is the end result of tissue remodeling.

Initially localized tissue injury occurs due to the mechanical presence of the needle and solution. Disrupted tissue and blood vessels trigger the release of proinflammatory substances and

the recruitment of platelets and white blood cells to the area (see Figure 7.8) (Yates 2014; Chen et al. 2018; Patil et al. 2019). This causes increased vascular permeability, vasodilation, and recruitment of cells including white blood cells and fibroblasts (chemotaxis) leading to the

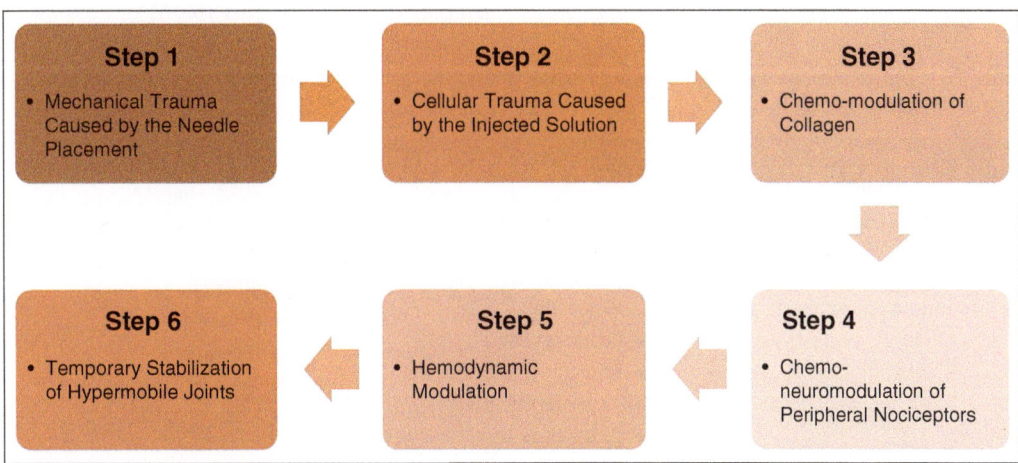

Figure 7.13   An algorithmic depiction of Ben-Yakir's (2020) proposed mechanism of action for prolotherapy. Source: Lisa P. McFaddin.

hallmarks of inflammation: redness, swelling, heat, pain, and loss of function.

While inflammation is the body's initial response to injury, the proliferation phase is the beginning of the body's healing process. Collagen and ECM are laid down creating the scaffolding upon which additional connective tissue and microscopic blood vessels (i.e. granulation tissue) are built (Schultz et al. 2015).

Over time granulation tissue is remodeled into functional scar tissue (Landén et al. 2016). The healed tissue is stronger and has greater mobility and shock absorption compared to granulation tissue. Prolotherapy is used to trigger wound healing and improve the proliferative and remodeling responses improving tendon, ligament, and joint stability and relieving pain. A positive outcome is generally defined as improved mobility and reduction of pain (Tiekert 2013).

Dextrose is water soluble, dispersing easily within the tissues surrounding the injection site. The hypertonic solution causes dehydration of local cells inciting an inflammatory response which leads to proliferation and tissue remodeling (Hauser et al. 2016). The peritendinous injection of dextrose has been shown to cause the production and proliferation of growth factors, the proliferation of fibroblast and chondrocytes, and the deposition of collagen (Sit et al. 2016).

Safety

As with any therapeutic modality there are potential cautions, contraindications, and adverse effects associated with prolotherapy, as outlined in Table 7.6. The most common adverse effect following prolotherapy is pain, which is generally mild and resolves within two to seven days following the injection (Gladstein 2012).

The Why

Applications in Human Medicine

Opinions on the use of prolotherapy are mixed in human medicine. Dextrose and other sterile injectables are not FDA-approved for use in prolotherapy. These injectables are used in an off-label manner and most insurance policies will not cover prolotherapy.

In the 2019 the American College of Rheumatology/Arthritis Foundation Guideline for the Management of Osteoarthritis of the Hand, Hip, and Knee stated prolotherapy is "conditionally recommended against in patients with knee and/or hip [osteoarthritis]" due to "a limited number of trials involving small number of participants" (Kolasinski et al. 2020). The National Center for Complementary and Integrative Health (NCCIH) states the use of prolotherapy for lower back pain has shown inconsistent results in their handout *Chronic Pain* (NCCIH 2015).

Table 7.6 The conditions under which prolotherapy should not be used or should be used with caution (Ben-Yakir 2020; Gladstein 2012).

Cautions	Contraindications	Adverse effects
• Senior pets (dogs older than 12 years of age and cats older than 15 years of age) • Immuno-compromised	• Cancer (affecting local muscle, connective tissue, and bone) • Acute non-reduced luxations or dislocations • Septic arthritis • Post-traumatic arthritis • Acute tendonitis • Acute bursitis • Allergy to the injectable solution	• Infection • Pain • Stiffness • Bruising • Bleeding • Transient nerve damage • Therapy failure

Source: Lisa P. McFaddin.

There are several studies demonstrating the efficacy of prolotherapy in the treatment of lower back pain and osteoarthritis (Rabago et al. 2010, 2013). In a systematic review of 32 dextrose prolotherapy studies, Hauser et al. (2016) concluded the therapy was efficacious in the treatment of tendinopathies, osteoarthritis of the knee and fingers, and spinal and pelvic pain in patients who failed to respond to conservative treatments. Sit et al. (2016) reviewed two randomized clinical trials utilizing peri- and intra-articular knee injections of dextrose. Both studies demonstrated statistically significant improvement in pain and joint function after three to five sessions of prolotherapy. Sit et al. (2016) also noted the use of prolotherapy was safe with rare adverse effects.

Prolotherapy when performed correctly is relatively safe. However, anytime anything is injected into or around a joint there is risk of pain and stiffness, bleeding, bruising, swelling, infection, and allergic reactions. Rare side effects may include spinal headache, spinal cord or disk injury, damage to a nerve, ligament, or tendon, and pneumothorax (Gossett 2020).

Applications in Veterinary Medicine

"Soft-tissue injury" is a name given to any painful stimuli affecting the musculoskeletal system whose cause is either not immediately identified or for which an obvious bony abnormality has been ruled out. This catch-all term can refer to anything from bruised muscles, sprained muscles, trigger points, tendon strain, or ligament sprain. In the case of tendinous strains and ligamentous sprains, damage to the connective tissue causes hypermobility, weakness, and pain. Complete tendon or ligament tears often require surgical correction. But partial tears and connective tissue laxity are still a major source of pain and can benefit from prolotherapy (Gladstein 2012; Tiekert 2013; Sherebrin 2014).

Specific conditions for which prolotherapy may be of benefit include (Gladstein 2012; Ben-Yakir 2020):

- Ankylosing spondylosis
- Carpal and tarsal ligament laxity
- Cervical vertebral instability (CVI) or wobbler's
- Chronic ligament or tendon sprains or strains
- Cruciate laxity or partial tear
- Elbow dysplasia
- Hip dysplasia
- Intervertebral disk disease (IVDD)
- Intolerance of traditional medications (NSAIDs, steroids, opioids, etc.)
- Myofascial pain syndromes
- Osteochondrosis dissecans (OCD)
- Pain from repetitive motion disorder
- Patellar luxation
- Sacroiliac laxity
- Shoulder, elbow, and carpal joint laxity
- Spinal stenosis
- Stifle collateral ligament injury
- Tarsocrural luxations
- Temporomandibular joint (TMJ) laxity.

Between 75 and 90% of veterinary patients show significant improvement following prolotherapy (Ben-Yakir 2020), though it should be noted that not all data is positive when discussing prolotherapy. There is an estimated 10–20% failure rate associated with prolotherapy (Gladstein 2012). Possible causes include insufficient number of treatments; weak injectable solution (i.e. dextrose concentration is too low); inappropriate injection technique; additional unidentified source of compensatory pain; concurrent administration of NSAIDs preventing an appropriate inflammatory response; early return to normal activity without a proper resting and rehabilitation period; senior pets (dogs >12 years of age, cats >15 years of age); and immunocompromised patients (Gladstein 2012). There is also questionable efficacy for large to giant breed dogs and/or those with complete cruciate ligament tears (Tiekert 2013).

Veterinary Research

As of February 2023, a search on PubMed and GoogleScholar for clinical trials of "prolotherapy veterinary medicine" and "prolotherapy canine" yielded one article; while a search for "prolotherapy feline" produced no results.

The lone prolotherapy article, published by Sherwood et al. (2017), was a randomized, double-blind, placebo-controlled prospective pilot study investigating the effect of dextrose prolotherapy in the treatment of elbow and stifle arthritis in dogs. The results did not show a significant improvement in lameness, range of motion, and radiographic improvement of arthritic changes in the treatment group. There was improvement in weight-bearing in the prolotherapy group compared to the placebo group, but the difference was not statistically significant. The sample size was extremely limited, 10 dogs in total, which likely affected the results. The authors commented on the limited sample size, suggesting 26–106 dogs per group would be necessary to demonstrate significant improvement in weight-bearing following prolotherapy (Sherwood et al. 2017).

These results, and lack of additional studies, highlight the need for more research investigating the use of procedures in veterinary medicine. There are several studies showing significant improvement in the healing of ligament and muscle damage using dextrose prolotherapy in rodents (Jensen et al. 2008; Tsai et al. 2018). Anecdotal evidence and case studies suggest dextrose prolotherapy shows promise in canine arthritis management, but currently there is not enough evidence to support the modality's efficacy. Presented below are the summaries of two prolotherapy studies using rodent models.

Response of Knee Ligaments to Prolotherapy in a Rat Injury Model

Authors: Kristina Jensen, PhD; David Rabago, MD; Thormas Best, MD, PhD, FACSM; Jeffrey Patterson, DO; and Ray Vanderby Jr., PhD
Journal: *American Journal of Sport Medicine*
Date: 2008
Study design: Controlled laboratory study
Study hypothesis: Dextrose prolotherapy will help heal injured medial collateral ligaments (MCLs)
Sample size: 24 rats
Materials and methods: The MCL of 24 rats were injured through stretching, and the resulting laxity was measured. Two weeks later 32 of the MCLs were injected with either saline or dextrose solution into the tibial and femoral insertion sites twice one week apart. There were 16 negative MCL controls (i.e. no stretch injury and no injections). Two weeks after the last injection all animals were humanely euthanized and the MCL laxity, mechanical properties, and collagen fibril diameter and density were measured. Statistical analysis was performed using analysis of variance (ANOVA) and Fisher protected least significant difference tests.

Results

1) There was no significant difference in ligament laxity between the dextrose and saline groups.
2) The cross-sectional area of the MCL increased significantly in the dextrose compared to saline and negative control groups.
3) Collagen fibril diameter and density was significantly reduced in the injured compared to non-injured animals, but no significant difference was found between the dextrose and saline groups.

Study conclusions: Dextrose prolotherapy increased the MCL thickness but did not alter the other measured properties. The authors suggest the clinical improvement seen with "prolotherapy may not result from direct effects on ligament biomechanics."

Study limitations:

1) Saline can be irritating by itself suggesting the saline placebo group may have been more of a treatment group. Sterile water may have been a better choice for a placebo effect.
2) The experimentally induced MCL trauma may have been more severe compared to real-life trauma.
3) The experimentally induced trauma is more consistent with acute injury compared to the chronic ligament injury more commonly seen in veterinary patients.
4) Weight-bearing and range of motion pre and post injections were not evaluated.
5) The animal's pain levels were not scored.

L.P.M. conclusions: No beneficial effects of prolotherapy can be drawn from this study. This study opens doors for further evaluations and demonstrates what factors must be considered when designing prolotherapy studies: how best to replicate acute and chronic ligament injury in the lab. Is saline an appropriate placebo? Does ligament laxity and collagen fibril diameter and density reflect weight-bearing ability, range of motion, and pain levels?

Effects of Dextrose Prolotherapy on Contusion-Induced Muscle Injuries in Mice

Authors: Sen-Wei Tsai, Yi-Ju Hsu, Mon-Chien Lee, Hao-En Huang, Chi-Chang Huang, and Yu-Tang Tung
Journal: *International Journal of Medical Science*
Date: 2018
Study design: Randomized controlled study
Study hypothesis: Dextrose prolotherapy will help heal injured muscles in mice.
Sample size: 48 laboratory mice
Materials and methods: Mice were randomly divided into six groups: control, no injury with saline injections, mass-drop injury (MDI) to the gastrocnemius muscle with saline injection two hours post injury, MDI with 10% dextrose injection two hours post injury, MDI with 20% dextrose injection two hours post injury, MDI with 30% dextrose injection two hours post injury, and MDI with diclofenac (an NSAID) injection two hours post injury. Seven days after treatment all mice were humanely euthanized. Serum samples, organ (liver, lung, kidney, heart, and epididymal fat pad) tissues, and gastrocnemius muscle samples were obtained. Muscle was frozen and stored. Histology and immunohistochemistry (IHC) was performed on all tissue samples. One-way analysis of variance with Duncan's post-hoc test were used for statistical analysis.

Results

1) The serum creatine kinase (CK), blood urea nitrogen (BUN), creatinine (CREA), and low-density lipoprotein (LDL) was significantly higher in the MDI-alone group compared to the control.
2) Serum levels of CK, BUN, CREA, and lactate dehydrogenase (LDH) were significantly lower in all dextrose treatment groups compared to the control group.
3) Based on histology and IHC, macrophage response was suppressed in the dextrose groups compared to the control group.
4) Muscle satellite cell regeneration (defined by desmin protein levels) was higher in the dextrose groups compared to the control group.
5) Desmin protein levels were lower in the NSAID group compared to the dextrose groups.

Study conclusions: Dextrose prolotherapy aided in the repair of injured muscles.

Study limitations

1) Validity of the MDI compared to real-life muscle injury.
2) Relatively small individual group sample sizes.

(Continued)

Effects of Dextrose Prolotherapy on Contusion-Induced Muscle Injuries in Mice (Continued)	
3) Lack of statistical analysis of the histology and IHC results. 4) Use of saline as a control compared to sterile water. **L.P.M. conclusions**: This study suggests dextrose prolotherapy may aid in the healing of	muscle injury by stimulating local muscle inflammation. Additional studies, especially ones investigating natural muscle trauma in canine and feline patients, are necessary to solidify the use of this therapy in veterinary patients.

The How

Team Members

This section reviews the potential return on investment (ROI), how to effectively train the entire team, how to promote, and how to integrate the integrative therapy.

Return on Investment

ROI can be determined by evaluating client interest, veterinarian demand, hospital costs, applicability of the service, appointment scheduling, and pricing.

Client Interest

Currently there are no studies documenting client interest or the popularity of prolotherapy. By evaluating trends in client opinion and pet health insurance, interest in prolotherapy can be inferred.

Client Opinion Table 7.7 summarizes the pet owner demographics and statistics mentioned the My Lessons section of the Introduction. Even if 1% of the owners are open to prolotherapy, that is still 1.4 million potential patients.

The treatment of pain in veterinary patients is a hot button issue amongst both owners and practitioners. The existence of the International Veterinary Academy of Pain Management (IVAPM), Certified Veterinary Pain Practitioners (CVPP), 2015 and 2022 American Animal Hospital Association (AAHA) and American Association of Feline Practitioners (AAFP) Pain Management for Dogs and Cats consensus statement, and Animal Pain Awareness Month

in September highlights the importance and community awareness of this issue (Epstein et al. 2015; Grant et al. 2022). As such, any treatment which effectively reduces companion animal pain should and will spark the interest of clients and veterinarians.

Pet Health Insurance Many pet insurance plans include coverage for integrative therapies (Woodley 2018). While most do not specify prolotherapy, the presence of this type of coverage re-emphasizes the mainstream incorporation of these treatment modalities, as well as reflecting client demand.

Veterinarian Demand

Currently, prolotherapy is a niche market with few veterinarians offering the service. Over-saturation

Table 7.7 Summary of the 2022 pet ownership and pet health insurance demographics in the United Sates discussed in the Introduction of the book (Burns 2018, 2022; MFAF 2018; APPA 2022; Nolen 2022; NAPHIA 2023).

• 83% of pets are owned by millennials (32%), generation X (24%), and baby boomers (27%)
• 69 million households owned dogs
• 45.3 million households owned cats
• Estimated over 81.1 million owned dogs
• Estimated over 60.7 million owned cats
• 68% of owners are interested in alternative treatment modalities for their pets
• 4.41 million pets have pet health insurance
• 82% of insurance pets are dogs

Source: Lisa P. McFaddin.

of the market is unlikely. Erring on the side of cation, the pratice manager could compare the number of general practitioners within a 5-, 10-, or 20-mile radius to the number of veterinarians advertising prolotherapy. The search radius is dependent on your hospital's demographics. Most comparisons follow the 5% trend. In other words, you want to ensure less than 5% of the surrounding hospitals are offering the service.

Hospital Costs

Let us start by reviewing the potential costs associated with introducing and offering prolotherapy: veterinarian training, staff training, supplies and equipment, staffing, facilities, and advertising. For more information on potential hospital costs refer to the Introduction chapter of this book.

Veterinarian Training   For most modalities this includes the course cost, cost of reference material, travel expenses, and time off. The American Holistic Veterinary Medical Association's (AHVMA) annual conference often has lectures discussing prolotherapy. As there are no available courses these costs are not applicable (estimated cost, $0).

Staff Training   Team training expenses are highly variable and dependent on the preexistence staff meetings and use of a staff meeting for training (compared to self-study). Refer to the Introduction of the book for a breakdown of these variables (cost range, $230–1295).

Supplies   There are no additional supply costs for prolotherapy, discounting prolozone. The veterinarians can perform the procedure with supplies readily available within the hospital including sedatives, syringes, needles, 50% dextrose, sterile saline, sterile water, chlorhexidine scrub, and isopropyl alcohol (estimated cost, $0).

Staffing   As sedation is often required, prolotherapy is typically scheduled as a procedure, not a regular appointment. Following the American Animal Hospital Association (AAHA) recommendations a veterinary assistant or licensed technician (VA/LT) should be present to monitor the patient while under sedation. Assuming the hospital has preexisting procedure hours for the veterinarians, there would be no additional staffing costs (estimated cost, $0).

Facilities   Facility expenses represent the costs needed to keep the doors open (aka overhead). Overhead includes rent or mortgage, utilities, administrative costs, and often employee costs divided by the minutes the practice is open (Stevenson 2016). The price per minute equals the amount of revenue needed just to break even. Overhead is extremely hospital specific, but the range tends to be $2–5/minute. With prolotherapy overhead is determined by the length of the procedure performed as this will affect doctor and support staff time. Presumably each procedure would take 30–60 minutes from the start of sedation to recovery.

Advertising   There are numerous ways to advertise a new service. On average veterinary hospitals spend 0.7% of revenue on promotion and advertisement (AVMA 2019). Most of the advertisement can be done with little to no additional expenditure. The Promotion section discusses advertising ideas in further detail. The national median gross revenue for companion animal practices was $1.2 million in 2022 (AVMA 2023). Advertising costs are calculated assuming no more than 5% of the current advertising budget would be used for promotion of the new service (estimated maximum cost, $420).

Start-Up Costs   The cost of prolotherapy is largely dependent on the hospital's preexisting cost for sedation, surgeon's time or procedural time, and supplies. Given the highly variable nature of these expenses, potential start-up costs are not calculated in this chapter. Refer to other chapters for examples of start-up cost calculations.

Applicability

According to the Healthy Paws Pet Insurance and Foundation 2019 Cost of Pet Health Care Report, 18.8% of canine vet visits were related to pain and musculoskeletal injuries, while 6.8% of feline visits were related to painful conditions (HPPIF 2019). As stated previously, prolotherapy is very useful in the management and prevention of pain. This treatment modality can be a valuable addition to any practitioner's toolbox when it comes to treating the third most common reason for taking a dog, and seventh most common reason for taking a cat, to the veterinarian (HPPIF 2019).

Appointment Scheduling

Factors to consider when planning prolotherapy appointments include the type of procedure performed (dextrose or prolozone), the level of sedation required for the procedure, the length of time needed for the procedure, the support staff availability, and room availability.

Pricing

An in-depth look into appointment pricing can be found in the Introduction at the beginning of this book. There are two primary pricing methods: current market fees and hospital cost-based pricing.

Current Market Fees There are no current studies evaluating the average cost or price range for prolotherapy. Hospitals can survey client pricing for said services from practices in the area to get an idea of market fees.

Hospital Cost-Based Pricing The hospital cost per patient is calculated using the initial start-up cost. Service fee is then calculated using the formula: Service Fee = Hospital Cost + Profit. The service fee can be obtained by marking up the start-up cost per patient, usually between 40 and 100%. Refer to other chapters for specific examples as to how this is calculated.

Team Training

The concept of phase training is used when introducing acupuncture to the hospital team. A multi-media approach is used to assist with the training program and is outlined in Table 7.8.

Practice Manager's Role in Training

To conquer this task the pratice manager needs his or her own checklist which includes the following information:

- Schedule a date and time for the team training.
- Ensure all information pertaining to the new service is reviewed with the staff.
- Confirm all team members have completed the training.
- Certify all team members understand the information and can successfully educate clients.

Promotion

There are six common avenues of promotion for a veterinary integrative medicine (VIM) service: hospital website, social media, email blasts, mailers, in-hospital promotions, and client education.

Hospital Website

Advertise "Veterinary Prolotherapy" in several locations on the website. On the made page insert "Now offering veterinary prolotherapy" with a link to success stories or client testimonials. Utilize the hospital website to advertise the VIM treatment under the "Services" section. Under Veterinarian Biograph include a description of the specialized training. Create a Prolotherapy blog page discussing patient success stories.

Social Media

Utilize Facebook, Instagram, and/or Twitter to post facts, photographs, hashtags, and patient success stories. Include fun and intriguing facts about prolotherapy. Clients love pet photographs, especially receiving prolotherapy

Table 7.8 The breakdown of phase training steps and resources for the entire hospital team.

Phase 1: Background information	
Team training guide	The handout walks the practice manager and/or veterinarian through Phase 1 of the training
	A downloadable and editable copy of the handout is located on the companion website
Training presentation	The video covers background information on the modality
	PowerPoints can be downloaded, edited, and personalized from the companion website
	The document can be used as a PowerPoint or saved as an mp4 creating a personalized movie
Team training handout	The handout provides additional background information for the CSRs, VAs, and LTs to complement the knowledge gained from watching the training presentation
	A downloadable and editable copy of the handout is located on the companion website
Phase 2: Knowledge proficiency	
Quiz	A short quiz to ensure all team members have a good understanding of the service being offered
	A downloadable and editable copy of the handout is located on the companion website
	A key is provided
Phase 3: Expectations	
Training worksheets	A training checklist is provided for CSRs and VA/LTs with role-specific expectations and tasks for each staff member
	A recommended completion time is provided
	A downloadable and editable copy of the handout is located on the companion website
Phase 4: Client education	
Client scripts	Bullet point information and scripted examples used when discussing prolotherapy with clients
	A downloadable and editable copy of the handout is located on the companion website
Client education presentation	A short (five to seven minute) client educational video about the therapeutic modality
	PowerPoints can be downloaded, edited, and personalized from the companion website
	The document can be used as a PowerPoint or saved as an mp4 creating a personalized movie
Client education handout	An informational handout about the therapeutic modality written specifically for clients
	A downloadable and editable copy of the handout is located on the companion website

CSR, customer service representative; VA, veterinary assistant; LT, licensed technician. Source: Lisa P. McFaddin.

treatments. Create or utilize prolotherapy specific hashtags. Provide posts with patient success stories.

Email Blasts

Send fun mass emails to your clients introducing prolotherapy. Consider monthly case presentations illustrating how the service has benefited patients. Almost everyone has at least one email address these days. Customer service representatives should be amassing client emails at the same rate as phone numbers.

Mailers

Mailers can be expensive and are largely unnecessary in this digital age. Mailers can be used to announce the introduction of prolotheray to existing clients. The mailer should include the name of the new service, a brief description of how veterinary prolotherapy can help pet patients, the name of the doctor performing the procedure, possibly a brief description of the training the doctor received, and possibly a photograph of a pet receiving prolotherapy or after having received the treatment.

In-Hospital Promotions

Advertise veterinary prolotherapy within the hospital using small promotional signs, informational signs, invoice teasers, and staff buttons. Small promotional signs can be placed in the waiting room and exam rooms. Include photographs of pets receiving or having received prolotherapy. Informational signs should include a brief description of how veterinary prolotherapy can help pet patients, photographs of pets, and name of the doctor performing the procedure.

Invoice teasers should consist of short phrases reminding and enticing owners regarding a new service offered at the practice. Examples include "Now offering Veterinary Prolotherap"; "Curious if Veterinary Prolotherapy could help your pet?"; "Introducing Veterinary Prolotherapy"; and "Would your pet benefit from Veterinary Prolotherapy?"

Buttons can be made for the staff to wear with kitchy phrases reminding owners, in a fun way, of the new VIM service. Examples include "Got Prolotherapy?" and "Want to learn more about Prolotherapy?"

Client Education

Education is crucial to understanding the purpose and importance of any given treatment. The client handouts and videos solidify pet owner knowledge base, reducing concerns and conveying value.

Integration

The key components for proper integration include availability of the service to the right patients; appropriate patient scheduling; appropriate support staff scheduling; and staff buy-in (understanding the benefits of the offered service).

Veterinarians

There are several factors to contemplate when veterinarians are considering, and preparing to incorporate, a VIM in their clinical repertoire: state requirements and restrictions, return on investment, course availability, supplies and equipment, veterinary organizations, and continuing education.

State Requirements and Restrictions

Is Prolotherapy Considered the Practice of Veterinary Medicine?

Each state has its own veterinary provisions outlining what is and is not considered the practice of veterinary medicine. While at present no state specifically defines prolotherapy as the practice of veterinary medicine, joint injections (regardless of the material used) is considered the practice of veterinary medicine. Refer to the companion website for links to each state's veterinary rules and regulations.

Does Prolotherapy Continuing Education Count Toward Licensure Continuing Education Requirements?

Currently no states require specific continuing education (CE) hours for veterinarians offering prolotherapy nor do they specifically reference prolotherapy CE. Some states limit the use of integrative medicine CE hours toward the annual CE requirement for license renewal. Most states permit the use of integrative CE if the lectures or webinars are performed by an approved provider. Table 1.16 in Chapter 1 provides a list of each states CE allotments as it pertains to certain forms of integrative medicine. Refer to the companion website for links to each state's veterinary rules and regulations.

Are Your Assets Covered?

Check with your liability insurance to determine if you are covered when practicing veterinary prolotherapy. Refer to the Introduction of this book for additional information.

Return on Investment

Specifics are discussed in the Team Members section of this chapter.

Course Availability

Currently, there are no online or onsite veterinary prolotherapy courses. The AHVMA often has lectures on prolotherapy at their annual conference.

Supplies and Equipment

The necessary supplies are dependent on the procedure performed. For example, dextrose prolotherapy requires 50% dextrose, sterile water or sterile saline, syringes, needles, and surgical preparation materials. All materials can be purchased from your hospital's typical vendor(s).

Hospital remodeling is generally not required when offering prolotherapy. Prolotherapy is usually performed in the treatment room with easy access to anesthesia machines.

Veterinary Organizations

A description of the most common veterinary organizations with a special interest in acupuncture are provided below. Table 7.9 summarizes the organizations' names, contact information, and membership dues as of February 2023.

American Holistic Veterinary Medical Association (AHVMA)

- **Description**: The AHVMA was founded in 1982 at the Western States Veterinary Conference with the goal of advancing integrative medicine through the education of integrative and non-integrative veterinarians, the introduction of integrative medicine to veterinary students, the promotion of research, and representation in the AVMA House of Delegates. There is no annual CE requirement to maintain membership.
- **Membership benefits**
  - Free subscription to the *AHVMA Journal*, a peer-reviewed journal.
  - Online resources for client education.
  - Searchable member directory.
  - Discounted vaccination titers through Kansas State University (KSU) Diagnostic Lab.
  - Free access to the Natural Medicines Database, an online resource for supplements, natural medicines, and integrative therapies.
  - Reduced cost for the AHVMA annual conference.

Table 7.9 Veterinary associations and organizations with a special interest in veterinary integrative medicine and prolotherapy as of February 2023.

Organization	Contact information	Membership dues
American Holistic Veterinary Medical Association (AHVMA)	PO Box 630, Abingdon, MD 21009 (410) 569-0795 office@ahvma.org	$300/year
College of Integrative Veterinary Therapies (CIVT)	PO Box 352, Yeppoon, 4703 QLD, Australia (303) 800-5460 membership@civtedu.org	$185/year
International Veterinary Academy of Pain Management (IVAPM)	PO Box 1868, Mt. Juliet, TN 371211 info@ivapm.org	$250/year
North American Veterinary Regenerative Medicine Association (NAVRMA)	conference@narvma.org	Conference cost/year

Source: Lisa P. McFaddin.

College of Integrative Veterinary Therapies (CIVT)

- **Description**: An online organization open to all licensed animal health providers interested in integrative medicine. There are two membership options: full membership for veterinarians and associate membership for registered animal health professionals. CIVT strives to promote all aspects of evidence-based integrative medicine through online education and discussion forums. CIVT provides financial support to veterinary students interested in studying integrative medicine. CIVT also helps fund integrative medicine research. There is no annual CE requirement to maintain membership.
- **Membership benefits**
  - Access to the online electronic library.
  - Access to the electronic *Journal of Integrative Veterinary Therapies.*
  - Three free CE webinars annually.
  - 20% discount on all webinars.
  - Discounts on specific CIVT courses.
  - Searchable member directory.
  - Access to the Natural Medicines Databases and the American Botanical Council Library.

International Veterinary Academy of Pain Management (IVAPM)

- **Description**: Originally known as the Companion Animal Pain Management Consortium, then the Academy of Pain Management Interest Group, and finally IVAPM. Founded in 2001 to provide pain management education and certification programs. The organization's goal is to provide acute and chronic pain relief for veterinary patients. Both traditional and alternative therapies are embraced, including acupuncture and rehabilitation and physical therapy.
- **Membership benefits**
  - Members can become Certified Veterinary Pain Practitioners (CVPP).
  - Access to member's only Facebook group offering case consultations and questions.
  - Reduced subscription rate for IVAPM's journal *Veterinary Anaesthesia and Analgesia.*
  - Reduced registration fee for the International Veterinary Emergency and Critical Care (IVECCS) conference.
  - Reduced registration for all IVAPM continuing education events (online and onsite).
  - Complementary World Small Animal Veterinary Association (WSAVA) membership.

Reference Books

As of February 2023, there are no veterinary prolotherapy-specific books. There are a number of human prolotherapy books which may contain useful information for the veterinarian practicing this modality. The recommended list of reference books is based on the importance of knowing the patient's anatomy and additional therapeutic modalities which may complement the use of prolotherapy. A summary of each book is provided.

Anatomy of Domestic Animals: Systemic and Regional Approach
- Authors: Chris Pasquini, DVM, MS; Tom Spurgeon, PhD; and Susan Pasquini, DVM
- Summary: Most veterinarians already own a copy from vet school. This in-depth, thorough, and entertaining anatomy book provides tons of information on the anatomy of most domestic animals.

Canine Sports Medicine and Rehabilitation
- Authors: M. Christine Zink, DVM, PhD, DACVP, DACVSMR and Janet D. Van Dyke, DVM, DACVSMR
- Summary: A comprehensive reference book discussing common canine musculoskeletal conditions and ailments, with particular interest in the canine athlete. The book covers gait analysis and physiology, various therapeutic approaches (including nutrition, rehabilitation, manual therapy, acupuncture, chiropractic, therapeutic

exercise, aquatic therapy, conditioning and retraining, and assistive devices), and specific diagnoses and treatment recommendations for disorders of the forelimbs and pelvic limbs. A must-have for veterinarians interested in manual therapy, orthopedics, and rehabilitation.

Integrating Complementary Medicine into Veterinary Practice

- Authors: Robert S. Goldstein, VMD; Paula Jo Broadfoot, DVM; Richard E. Plamquist, DVM; Karen Johnstons, DVM; Jiu Jia Wen, DVM; Barbara Fougère, BSc, BVMs (Hons), BHSc (comp Med), MODT, MHSc (Herb Med), CVA (IVAs), CVBM, CVCP; and Margo Roman, DVM
- Summary: A comprehensive review of multiple integrative therapies including: Chinese herbal medicine, acupuncture, homotoxicology, nanopharmacology, homotoxicology, and therapeutic nutrition. The book aims to educate veterinary practitioners on the validity, effectiveness, and incorporation of each modality within daily practice.

Miller's Anatomy of the Dog

- Authors: Howard Evans, PhD and Alexander de Lahunta, DVM, PhD
- Summary: Most veterinarians already own a copy from vet school. This is a comprehensive guide to the canine anatomy.

Promotion

Information regarding the hospital's promotion of acupuncture can be found in the Team Members section.

Integration

Key components for proper integration include availability, scheduling, and staff buy-in. Availability means offering the service to the right patient. Scheduling refers to appropriate patient and support staff scheduling. Staff buy-in ensures all team members understand the benefits of the offered service.

Conclusion

Prolotherapy is a relatively new therapeutic modality. The effects and benefits for veterinary patients center on the facilitation of self-healing, restoration of mobility, and reduction of pain. This chapter and companion website describe in detail how prolotherapy can be successfully introduced into practice, as well as provide practical tools for implementation.

References

Alderman, D. (2009). A history of the American College of Osteopathic Sclerotherapeutic Pain Management, the oldest prolotherapy Organization. *Journal of Prolotherapy* 1 (4): 200–204.

Andersen, A. (2015). The history of prolotherapy. *Practical Pain Management* 15 (4): https://www.medcentral.com/pain/chronic/history-prolotherapy.

AOAPRM (American Osteopathic Association of Prolotherapy Regenerative Medicine) (2020). What is Prolotherapy. https://prolotherapycollege.org/ (accessed 29 October 2020).

APPA (American Pet Products Association) (2022). Pet industry market size and ownership statistics. https://www.americanpetproducts.org/research-insights/industry-trends-and-stats (accessed 23 February 2023).

AVMA (American Veterinary Medical Association) (2019). Economic state of the veterinary profession. https://www.avma.org/news/press-release/AVMA-2019-Economic-State-of-the-Veterinary-Profession-Report-now-available (accessed 26 July 2021).

AVMA (American Veterinary Medical Association) (2023). *2023 AVMA Report on the Economic State of the Veterinary Profession.* Schaumburg, IL: AVMA.

Barrett, J. (2016). A set of grand challenges for veterinary regenerative medicine. *Frontiers in Veterinary Science* 3: 20.

Bautista, C.A., Park, H.J., Mazur, C.M. et al. (2016). Effects of chondroitinase ABC-mediated proteoglycan digestion on decellularization and recellularization of articular cartilage. *PLoS One* 11 (7): e0158976.

Benjamin, M. and Evans, E. (1990). Fibrocartilage. *Journal of Anatomy* 171: 1–15.

Ben-Yakir, S. (2020). Prolotherapy in Animals. https://www.med-vetacupuncture.org/english/articles/prolovet.html (accessed 29 October 2020).

Bliss, S. (2013). Musculoskeletal structure and physiology. In: *Canine Sports Medicine and Rehabilitation* (ed. M.C. Zink and J.B. Van Dyke), 32–59. Oxford: Wiley-Blackwell.

Burns, K. (2018). Pet ownership stable, veterinary care variable. https://www.avma.org/javma-news/2019-01-15/pet-ownership-stable-veterinary-care-variable (accessed 11 August 2021).

Burns, K. (2022). New report takes a deep dive into pet ownership. https://www.avma.org/news/new-report-takes-deep-dive-pet-ownership (accessed 6 November 2022).

CDC (Centers for Disease Control and Prevention) (2020). Arthritis: Osteoarthritis. http://www.cdc.gov/arthritis/basics/osteoarthritis.htm (accessed August 2020).

Chen, L., Deng, H., Cui, H. et al. (2018). Inflammatory responses and inflammation-associated diseases in organs. *Oncotarget* 9: 7204–7218.

DHHS (Department of Health and Human Services) (2020). Approved Drug Products with Therapeutic Equivalence Evaluations. https://www.fda.gov/media/136324/download (accessed 4 May 2021).

Elvis, A. and Ekta, J. (2011). Ozone therapy: a clinical review. *Journal of Natural Sicence, Biology and Medicine* 21 (1): 66–70.

Epstein, M., Rodan, I., Griffenhagen, G. et al. (2015). 2015 AAHA/AAFP pain management guidelines for dogs and cats. *Journal of the American Animal Hospital Association* 51 (2): 67–84.

Evans, H. and De Lahunta, A. (2013). *Miller's Anatomy of the Dog*, 4e. St. Louis, MO: Elsevier.

Exposito, J.-Y., Valcourt, U., Cluzel, C., and Lethias, C. (2010). The fribrillar collagen family. *International Journal of Molecular Sciences* 11 (2): 407–426.

Fox, A., Bedi, A., and Rodeo, S. (2009). The basic science of articular cartilage: structure, composition, and function. *Sports Health: A Multidisciplinary Approach* 1 (6): 461–468.

Frank, C.B. (2004). Ligament structure, physiology, and function. *Journal of Musculoskeletal and Neuronal Interactions* 4 (2): 199–201.

Frantz, C., Stewart, K., and Weaver, V. (2010). The extracellular matrix at a glance. *Journal of Cell Science* 123: 4195–4200.

Gladstein, B. (2012). A case for prolotherapy and its place in veterinary medicine. *Journal of Prolotherapy* 2012 (4): e870–e885.

Gossett, T. (2020). How does prolotherapy work? https://www.healthline.com/health/prolotherapy (accessed 4 May 2021).

Grant, M., Lascelles, B.D.X., Colleran, E. et al. (2022). 2022 AAHA pain management guidelines for dogs and cats. *Journal of the American Animal Hospital Association* 58: 55–76.

Guo, S. and DiPietro, L.A. (2010). Factors affecting wound healing. *Journal of Dental Research* 89 (3): 219–229.

Gupta, R., Lall, R., Srivastava, A., and Sinha, A. (2019). Hyaluronic acid: molecular mechanisms and therapeutic trajectory. *Frontiers in Veterinary Science* 192.

Hauser, R., Lackner, J., Steilen-Matias, D., and Harris, D. (2016). A systematic review of dextrose prolotherapy for chronic musculoskeletal pain. *Clinical Medicine Insights. Arthritis and Musculoskeletal Disorders* 9: 139–159.

Henderson, A. and Millis, D. (2014). Tissue healing: tendons, ligaments, bone, muscles, and cartilage. In: *Canine Rehabilitation and*

Physical Therapy, 2e (ed. D. Millis and D. Levine), 79–91. Elsevier https://veteriankey.com/tissue-healing-tendons-ligaments-bone-muscles-and-cartilage/.

HPPIF (Healthy Paws Pet Insurance and Foundation) (2019). 2019 Cost of Pet Health Care Report. https://www.healthypaw spetinsurance.com/content/costofcare/pet-care-costs-health-conditions_2019.pdf (accessed 2 September 2020).

Hui, A., McCarty, W.J., Masuda, K. et al. (2011). A systems biology approach to synovial joint lubrication in health, injury and disease. *Wiley Interdisciplinary Reviews. Systems Biology and Medicine* 4 (1): 15–37.

Iozzo, R. and Schaefer, L. (2015). Proteoglycan form and function: a comprehensive nomenclature of proteoglycans. *Matrix Biology* 42: 11–55.

Iwanaga, T., Shikichi, M., Kitamura, H. et al. (2000). Morphology and functional roles of synoviocytes in the joint. *Archives of Histology and Cytology* 63 (1): 17–31.

Jensen, K., Rabago, D.P., Best, T.M. et al. (2008). Early inflammatory response of knee ligaments to prolotherapy in a rat model. *American Journal of Sports Medicine* 36 (7): 1347–1357.

Kiani, C., Chen, L., Wu, Y.J. et al. (2002). Structure and function of aggrecan. *Cell Research* 12: 19–32.

Knudson, C. and Knudson, W. (2001). Cartilage proteoglycans. *Cell and Development Biology* 12: 69–78.

Kolasinski, S., Neogi, T., Hochberg, M.C. et al. (2020). 2019 American College of Rheumatology/Arthritis Foundation guideline for the management of osteoarthritis of the hand, hip, and knee. *Arthritis and Rheumatology* 72 (2): 220–233.

Lambert, R. (1979). Electrosurgical treatment of cranial cruciate ligament rupture. *Modern Veterinary Practice* 60 (7): 557.

Landén, N., Li, D., and Ståhle, M. (2016). Transition from inflammation to proliferation: a critical step during wound healing. *Cellular and Molecular Life Sciences* 73: 3861–3885.

Marcellin-Little, D., Levine, D., and Canapp, S. (2007). The canine shoulder: selected disorders and their management with physical therapy. *Clinical Techniques in Small Animal Practice* 22 (4): 171–182.

MedlinePlus (2016). Bursitis. https://medlineplus.gov/bursitis.html (accessed 1 May 2020).

MFAF (Michelson Found Animals Foundation) (2018). Furred lines: Pet trends. https://www.prnewswire.com/news-releases/furred-lines-pet-trends-2019-300741947.html (accessed 26 July 2021).

NAPHIA (North American Pet Health Insurance Assocition) (2023). Industry Data. https://naphia.org/industry-data/#my-menu (accessed 18 February 2023).

NCCIH (National Center for Complemetary and Integrated Health) (2015). Chronic Pain. https://files.nccih.nih.gov/s3fs-public/Chronic_Pain_08-11-2015.pdf (accessed 5 May 2020).

NIAMSD (National Institute of Arthritis and Musculoskeletal and Skin Diseases) (2015). Sprains and Strains. http://niams.nih.gov/health-topics/sprains-and-strains (accessed 3 May 2020).

NINDS (National Institute of Neurological Disorders and Stroke) (2019). Repetitive Motion Disorders. https://www.ninds.nih.gov/health-information/disorders/repetitive-motion-disorders#:~:text=Definition,%2C%20 tenosynovitis%2C%20and%20trigger%20finger (accessed 2 May 2020).

Nolen, R.S. (2022). Pet ownership rate stabilizes as spending increases. https://www.avma.org/news/pet-ownership-rate-stabilizes-spending-increases (accessed 22 February 2023).

Osborn, J. (2018). Prolotherapy in practice. https://ivcjournal.com/prolotherapy-practice (accessed 5 May 2023).

Pasquini, C., Spurgeon, T., and Pasquini, S. (2003). *Anatomy of Domestic Animals: Systemic and Regional Approach*, 10e. Pilot Point: Sudz Publishing.

Patil, K., Mahajan, U.B., Unger, B.S. et al. (2019). Animal models of inflammation for screening of anti-inflammatory drugs: implications for the discovery and development of phytopharmaceuticals. *International Journal of Molecular Sciences* 20: 4367.

PubChem (2022). Ozone. https://pubchem.ncbi. nlm.nih.gov/compound/24823 (accessed 5 September 2022).

PubChem (2023). Dextrose. https://pubchem. ncbi.nlm.nih.gov/compound/66370 (accessed 4 March 2023).

Punchard, N.A., Whelan, C.J., and Adcock, I. (2004). The Journal of Inflammation. *Journal of Inflammation* 1: 1. https:// journal-inflammation.biomedcentral.com/arti cles/10.1186/1476-9255-1-1#citeas.

Rabago, D., Slattengren, A., and Zgierska, A. (2010). Prolotherapy in primary care practice. *Primary Care: Clinics in Office Practice* 37 (1): 65–80.

Rabago, D., Patterson, J.J., Mundt, M. et al. (2013). Dextrose prolotherapy for knee osteoarthritis: a randomized controlled trial. *Annals of Family Medicine* 11 (3): 229–237.

Reinders, M. and Haghighat, S. (2019). Modified platelet rich plasma (PRP) for cruciate ligament injuries in dogs. https://ivcjournal. com/prp-cruciate-ligament-injuries/ (accessed 5 May 2020).

Ricard-Blum, S. (2011). The collagen family. *Cold Spring Harbor Perspectives in Biology* 3 (1): a004978.

Rodriguez, Z.B.Z. (2016). Ozone therapy. In: *Veterinary Medicine*. La Habana, Cuba: @ Collective of Authors.

Schultz, G., Chin, G., Moldawer, L., and Diegelmann, R. (2015). Principles of wound healing. In: *Mechanisms of Vascular Disease: A Reference Book for Vascular Speciliasts* (ed. R. Fitridge and M. Thompson), 423–450. Adelaide: University of Adelaide Press.

Shallenberger, F. (2011a). *Principles and Applications of Ozone Therapy: A Practical Guideline for Physicians*. CreateSpace Independent Publishing Platform.

Shallenberger, F. (2011b). Prolozone™: regenerating joints and eliminating pain. *Journal of Prolotherapy* 3 (2): 630–638.

Sherebrin, R. (2014). Prolotherapy for canine joint pain. https://animalwellnessmagazine. com/prolotherapy-for-joint-pain/ (accessed 5 May 2021).

Sherwood, J., Roush, J., Armbrust, L., and Renberg, W. (2017). Prospective evaluation of intra-articular dextrose prolotherapy for treatment of osteoarthritis in dogs. *Journal of the American Animal Hospital Association* 53 (3): 135–142.

Sit, R., Chung, V.C., Reeves, K.D. et al. (2016). Hypertonic dextrose injections (prolotherapy) in the treatment of symptomatic knee osteoarthritis: a systematic review and meta-analysis. *Scientific Reports* 6: 25247.

Steilen, D., Hauser, R., Woldin, B., and Sawye, S. (2014). Chronic neck pain: making the connection between capsular ligament laxity and cervical instability. *The Open Orthopaedics Journal* 8: 326–345.

Stevenson, P. (2016). How to set practice service fees. https://cliniciansbrief.com/article/ how-set-practice-service-fees (accessed 10 June 2020).

Tambella, A., Martin, S., Cantalamessa, A. et al. (2018). Platelet-rich plasma and other hemocomponents in veterinary regenerative medicine. *Wounds* 30 (11): 329–336.

Tiekert, C.G. (2013). Prolotherapy 2013: a simple, natural technique that stimulates the body to repair damaged/loose ligaments. North American Veterinary Conference, January 19–23, Orlando, FL. Vetfolio.

Tresoldi, I., Oliva, F., Benvenuto, M. et al. (2013). Tendon's ultrastructure. *Muscles, Ligaments and Tendons Journal* 3 (1): 2–6.

Tsai, S.-W., Hsu, Y.J., Lee, M.C. et al. (2018). Effects of dextrose prolotherapy on contusion-induced muscle injuries in mice. *International Journal of Medical Sciences* 15 (11): 1251–1259.

Villines, Z. (2017). What is sclerotherapy? https://www.medicalnewstoday.com/ articles/320282 (accessed 2 May 2020).

Wallace, H.A., Basehore, B.M., and Zito, P.M. (2022). Wound Healing Phases. Treasure Island, FL: StatPearls. https://www.ncbi.nlm.nih.gov/books/NBK470443/ (accessed 27 February 2023).

Woo, S.L.-Y. and Buckwalter, J.A. (1988). Injury and repair of the musculoskeletal soft tissues. *Journal of Orthopaedic Research* 6 (6): 907–931.

Woodley, K. (2018). Pet insurance for holistic and integrative practice. https://ivcjournal.com/pet-insurance-integrative-practices/. (accessed 11 August 2021).

Wu, M., Cronin, K., and Crane, J. (2022). *Biochemistry, Collagen Synthesis*. Treasure Island, FL: StatPearls https://www.ncbi.nlm.nih.gov/books/NBK507709/.

Xiang, H., Mallon, J., and Currie, M. (2017). Supplementary cranial description of the types of *Edmontosaurus regalis* (Ornithischia: Hadrosauridae), with comments on the phylogenetics and biogeogreograph of Hadrosaurinae. *PLoS One* 12 (4): e0175253.

Yates, R. (2014). Initiators and mediators of acute inflammation. In: *Basic Veterinary Immunology*. Boulder, CO: University Press of Colorado https://www.vin.com/members/cms/project/defaultadv1.aspx?pid=8449&id=6262076&f5=1.

Yoon, J. and Halper, J. (2005). Tendon proteoglycans: biochemistry and function. *Journal of Musculoskeletal and Neuronal Interactions* 5 (1): 22–34.

8

Veterinary Regenerative Medicine

Introduction

Veterinary regenerative medicine (VRM) can aid in the management of chronic musculoskeletal pain in veterinary patients. VRM offers a nonsurgical option for chronic pain due to a variety of joint, tendon, and ligament diseases. Small volumes of platelet-rich plasma (PRP) or stem cells are injected directly into these areas, stimulating the body's natural ability to regenerate and heal itself.

The introduction of VRM into a veterinary practice can be beneficial for both the patient and the health of the practice. The successful incorporation and utilization of VRM does not end with the veterinarian's training. Support staff training and client education are crucial. This chapter discusses the what, why, and how for effective integration of regenerative medicine within your practice.

The What

Definition

The Association for the Advancement of Blood and Biotherapies (AABB) defines regenerative medicine (RM) "as the process of replacing or 'regenerating' human cells, tissues or organs to restore or establish normal function" (AABB 2023). The Food and Drug Administration (FDA) defines regenerative medicine therapies (RMT) in section 506(g)8 of the Food Drug and Cosmetic Act "as including cell therapies, therapeutic tissue engineering products, human cell and tissue products, and combination products using any such therapies or products" (FDA 2020). The FDA defined VRM as the use of "material from cells and tissues – such as living cells, serum, or bone – . . . in animals with the hope of repairing diseased or damaged tissues or organs" (FDA 2022a).

Integrative Medicine in Veterinary Practice, First Edition. Lisa P. McFaddin.
© 2024 John Wiley & Sons, Inc. Published 2024 by John Wiley & Sons, Inc.
Companion website: www.wiley.com/go/mcfaddin/integrativemedicine

For the purposes of this chapter VRM is defined as the injection of a substance derived from animal cells or tissues into a joint, tendon, or ligament with the intent of reducing pain and inflammation by promoting the body's natural healing abilities. VRM is frequently used as an adjunct to surgery or as part of a multimodal approach to rehabilitation (Carr and Canapp 2016). The two primary biologicals used in regenerative medicine are PRP and stem cells. In this book, prolotherapy is not included within the umbrella of VRM as it does not use biological substances.

Human History

The history of RM started long before the name was coined, as outlined in Table 8.1. The term "regenerative medicine" was first used in an editorial article in 1992 by Dr. Leland Kaiser about the future of technology in medicine (Kaiser 1992). Dr. William Haseltine popularized

Table 8.1 A brief review of the history of research leading to the establishment of regenerative medicine.

Date	Study purpose	Reference
1968	First bone marrow transplantation	Starzl (2000)
1978	Human stem cells discovered in umbilical cord blood	Prindull et al. (1978)
1981	First *in vitro* stem cell line from mice	Evan and Kaufman (1981)
1981	First artificial skin transplant on burn victims	Burke et al. (1981)
1996	First cloned animal, a sheep named Dolly	Campbell et al. (1996)
1998	Isolation of human embryonic stem cells	Thomson et al. (1998)
1999	First artificial laboratory-grown bladder transplant	Atala et al. (2006)

Source: Lisa P. McFaddin.

the term at a conference in 1999 when describing a new field of medicine blending tissue engineering, cell transplantation, stem cell biology, biomechanics prosthetics, nanotechnology, and biochemistry (Sampogna et al. 2015). In 1998, the FDA began establishing regulations regarding the use of animal and human cells, tissues, and cell- and tissue-based products.

Over the past 20 years RM has evolved into three primary disciplines: tissue engineering and biomaterials; cellular therapies; and medical devices and artificial organs (Sampogna et al. 2015; MIRM 2022). Research in each field has exploded (and continues to thrive) as have the number of professional organizations associated with each field of study. The study of cellular biologics has also been fraught with controversy, especially involving the procurement, storage, and use of stem cells (Lo and Parham 2009).

Veterinary History

Much of VRM's history mirrors that of human RM, given the use of laboratory animals in research, VRM predominantly focusing on orthobiologics, substances derived from animal cells or tissues used to aid the healing of musculoskeletal injuries, such as the injection of PRP or stem cells into joints and around ligaments and tendons.

The North American Veterinary Regenerative Medicine Association (NAVRMA) was established in 2010 highlighting the profession's interest in VRM. NARVMA is a nonprofit organization dedicated to the promotion, clinical application, and education of VRM.

The FDA began regulating veterinary cell therapy in 2015. A more detailed account of this regulatory process is discussed later in this chapter. The American Veterinary Medical Association (AVMA) "supports the continued scientific development of these modalities while at the same time encouraging its members to employ caution with respect to their use" (AVMA 2020).

Terminology

A lot of terms are used when discussing RM. A basic understanding of these terms is crucial, allowing effective communication amongst professionals and with clients.

Allogeneic transplant: Cells or tissue obtained from a donor are transplanted into a different patient.

Anterior (AKA ventral): Closer to the front of the body.

Arthritis (aka osteoarthritis): Degeneration of the cartilage (smooth covering) within a joint. Over time physical changes occur to the underlying bone (CDC 2020).

Articular cartilage (aka hyaline cartilage): The translucent, blue-hued cartilage covering the joint end of bones, comprising synovial joints. The tissue serves to reduce concussive forces and friction within the joint (Pasquini et al. 2003). Cartilage thickness is dependent on the joint location and function.

Autologous transplant: Cells or tissue obtained from and transplanted into the same patient.

Bioregulatory medicine: The use of non-pharmaceutical agents to stimulate the body's natural healing abilities (Reinders and Haghighat 2019).

Bursa: A fluid-filled sac located between bone and other tissues (muscles, tendons, ligaments, and skin) which reduces friction during movement (Pasquini et al. 2003).

Bursitis: Inflammation of the small fluid-filled cushions, called bursa, found between bone and other tissues, such as muscles, tendons, ligaments, and skin (MedlinePlus 2016).

Caudal: Located farther from the head.

Collagen: The most abundant protein in the body found within all types of connective tissue, including skin, cartilage, tendon, ligaments, and bone (Bliss 2013).

Contralateral: Opposite side.

Cranial: Located closer to the head.

Distal: Away from the body.

Dorsal: Closer to the back of the body.

Elastin: A highly elastic protein found in connective tissue, tendons, ligaments, joint capsules, and cartilage (Frantz et al. 2010).

Enthesis: The fibrocartilaginous junction where tendon attaches to bone (Tresoldi et al. 2013).

extracellular matrix (ECM): A three-dimensional network of big non-cellular molecules, including collagen, elastin, and proteoglycans, outside of the cells found within all tissues and organs (Frantz et al. 2010). The ECM functions as a physical framework for cells and is intimately involved in numerous biochemical and biomechanical processes crucial for tissue health and growth (Frantz et al. 2010).

Fibrocartilage: A tough and strong avascular connective tissue found at the insertion sites of ligaments and tendons, as well as intervertebral disks (Benjamin and Evans 1990).

Inferior (aka caudal): Located farther from the head.

In Vitro (latin for "within the glass"): Studies performed outside of a living organism. Most commonly microorganisms, tissue cultures, and cells are studied in petri dishes and/or test tubes.

In Vivo (latin for "in glass"): Studies performed within living organisms, not tissue extracts or cells.

Ipsilateral: Same side.

Joint (aka articulations): Area where two or more bones meet covered by a fibrous, elastic, cartilaginous, or combination of connective tissue types (Evans and Lahunta 2013).

Joint capsule: Tissue covering a joint comprised of two layers: an outer fibrous layer and an inner synovial membrane (SM) (Pasquini et al. 2003).

Joint cavity: The space within a synovial joint containing synovial fluid (Pasquini et al. 2003).

Lateral: Farther away from the median plane or midline of the body or organ.

Ligament: Bands of fibrous connective tissue connecting bone to bone. Intracapsular ligaments are located within a joint, while extracapsular ligaments are found outside of the joint or function as part of the joint capsule (Pasquini et al. 2003).

Ligament laxity: A ligament which is too loose to properly stabilize the joint and prevent misalignment during movement.

Luxation: Dislocation of a joint.

Medial: Closer to the median plane or midline of the body or organ.

Orthobiologics: The use of biological materials to treat musculoskeletal injuries.

Periosteum: The fibrous tissue covering the non-articulating surfaces of a bone. The periosteum nourishes and repairs bone and functions as the attachment site for tendons and ligaments (Pasquini et al. 2003).

Platelet: Small cell fragments found in large numbers in whole blood involved in clotting.

Platelet-rich plasma (PRP): Blood that has been processed, generally spun down using a centrifuge, to separate and concentrate the platelets from the blood. PRP has a higher concentration of platelets than that found in whole blood (Reinders and Haghighat 2019).

Platelet-rich therapy: The injection of PRP into damaged and painful areas of the musculoskeletal system with the goal of stimulating the body's natural healing ability, stabilizing the weakened

tissues, and reducing pain (Reinders and Haghighat 2019).

Posterior (aka dorsal): Closer to the back of the body.

Prolotherapy (aka nonsurgical ligament and tendon reconstruction and regenerative joint injection): The injection of a small volume of a sterile irritant into a painful joint, tendon, or ligament with the goal of stimulating the body's natural healing ability, stabilizing the weakened tissues, and reducing pain (Hauser et al. 2016; AOAPRM 2020).

Proteoglycans (PGs): Glycosylated proteins present in all connective tissues which form hydrogel matrices allowing tissues to withstand intense compressive forces (Frantz et al. 2010).

Proximal: Closer to the body.

Regenerative medicine: The use of biological materials, including stem cells and PRP, to treat disease and injury through the restoration of the body's natural healing abilities (Barrett 2016).

Repetitive motion disorder (RMD): A category of muscular conditions caused by repeated motions performed during routine work or daily activities (NINDS 2019).

Sprain: Injury to one or more ligaments. Ligaments are either stretched or torn (NIAMSD 2015).

Stem cells: Cells which can self-renew and develop into specific cells. Self-renewal involves the unlimited production of daughter cells identical to the original cell (Biehl and Russell 2009).

Stem cell therapy: The injection of prepared stem cells into the body with the goal of stimulating the body's natural healing ability.

Strain: Injury to a muscle or tendon because of stretching or tearing of the tissue (NIAMSD 2015).

Synovial fluid: The thick gelatinous liquid produced by the synovial membrane used to lubricate and nourish a synovial joint (Pasquini et al. 2003).

Tendon: Fibrous connective tissue attaching muscle to bone (Pasquini et al. 2003).

Tendonitis: Inflammation of a tendon.

Veterinary regenerative medicine: The injection of a substance derived from animal cells or tissues into a joint, tendon, or ligament with the intent of reducing pain and inflammation and promoting the body's natural healing abilities.

Human RM Regulation

The FDA defines RM as "a general approach to restore, replace, or recreate cells, tissues, or organs to treat or mitigate disease" (FDA 2022b).

> "Regenerative medicine therapies (RMTs) are defined in section 506(g)(8) of the Food Drug & Cosmetic Act as including cell therapies, therapeutic tissue engineering products, human cell and tissue products, and combination products using any such therapies or products, except for those regulated solely under section 361 of the Public Health Service Act (42 U.S.C. 264) and Title 21 of the Code of Federal Regulations Part 1271 (21 CFR Part 1271)" (FDA 2020).

For the purposes of this chapter, the focus will be on the regulation of autologous (from oneself) PRP and stem cell injections. PRP is considered a blood product and falls outside of 21 CFR Part 1271 (FDA 2020). As a result, the FDA does not directly regulate the injection of autologous PRP. The FDA does provide guidelines for how the PRP is obtained (i.e. blood draw), processed, and stored (CFR 2023). The FDA also governs the devices used to prepare PRP (FDA 2020). Only FDA-approved devices should be used to prepare PRP for human administration.

Stem cells do fall within the definition of RMT, and the FDA has the authority to regulate stem cell products in the United States (FDA 2019). Currently, the only FDA-approved stem cell-based products consist of blood-forming stem cells derived from cord blood (FDA 2019). Additionally, the FDA has only approved the use of stem cells to treat certain hematopoietic (blood production) conditions and disorders (FDA 2019). The use of stem cells to treat musculoskeletal conditions has not been FDA-approved and is illegally marketed.

VRM Regulation

Food and Drug Administration

The FDA labels animal cells, tissues, and cell- and tissue-based products as ACTPs, which includes PRP and stem cells (FDA 2022a).

> "ACTPs are intended to be implanted, transplanted, infused, or transferred from a donor into an animal recipient. Sometimes the donor and recipient are the same animal. Sometimes the donor and recipient are different animals of the same species. And other times, the donor and recipient are different species" (FDA 2022a).

According to the FDA "most of the cell-based products meet the legal definition of 'drug' because they are intended to treat, control, or prevent a disease or other condition" (FDA 2022a). ACTPs are required to adhere to the laws and regulations applied to other animal drugs. Prior to release the FDA reviews the safety and efficacy data, as well as the labeling and packaging, for drugs. Approved ACTPs are approved only for the purposes listed on the label. Unapproved ACTPs are illegal to market without FDA pre-market review and approval (FDA 2022a). Currently there are no FDA-approved animal cell-based drugs.

The FDA Center for Veterinary Medicine (CVM) is aware of some unapproved ACTP products which have a low risk to human and animal safety. In response to these products the FDA

> "intends to prioritize use of its resources for certain ACTPs in a manner that is

protective of human and animal health, based on risk, and informed by available science and data. FDA provides a publicly available list of those ACTPs that the agency has determined are lower risk following a review of product-specific information" (FDA 2022a).

American Veterinary Medical Association

As of 2020, the AVMA provided recommendations for veterinarians considering VRM (AVMA 2020):

1) Animal-based cell products must follow FDA Guidance for Industry #218 (GFI #218).
2) Evidence-based medicine should be used to create regenerative medicine protocols.
3) Protocols should pertain to the sample collection, preparation, and administration.
4) Regenerative medicine should be recommended for conditions in which studies have demonstrated efficacy.
5) Sample production must be validated prior to administration.
6) Outside laboratories should comply with laws and regulations governing cell-based products.
7) Veterinarians who process cell-based products within their hospitals are considered a manufacturer by the FDA and must adhere to good manufacturing practices.
8) Veterinarians who process cell-based products assume any and all liability associated with adverse effects from the products.
9) Only minimally manipulated autologous stem cells (Type II) can be used.
10) Advertising the use of regenerative medicine through any means (client communication, handouts, websites, etc.) can only make claims for which there are published studies documenting a beneficial effect of the therapy.
11) Liability insurance may not cover the practice of regenerative medicine.

Anatomy Fundamentals

As with prolotherapy, anatomy, and physiology are crucial to successfully and safely performing VRM. Anatomy is a branch of science focusing on the bodily structure of living organisms (see Chapter 7 for further information).

Anatomy for Veterinarians

Refer to Tables 7.1 and 7.2 for the primary bones, muscles, tendons, and ligaments comprising the proximal joints of the thoracic and pelvic limbs, respectively. Tables 9.1 and 9.2 in Chapter 9 provide the origin, insertion, innervation, and primary function of the major muscles associated with these thoracic and pelvic limb joints, respectively.

Physiology Fundamentals

Physiology is the branch of science focusing on the function of living organisms and their parts. Refer to Chapter 9 for further information.

Physiology for Veterinarians

A summary of the key physiology information from the previous chapter is provided below.

Molecular and Cellular Physiology

Extracellular Matrix The macromolecules within the ECM can be divided into two categories: proteoglycans and fibrous proteins (Frantz et al. 2010). The primary fibrous proteins are collagen and elastin.

Collagen Type I and II are the most common within the musculoskeletal system (Bliss 2013). Type I collagen is arranged in long, thin cross-linked fibrils, creating a structural and mechanical matrix which increases the tensile strength of the tissue (Exposito et al. 2010; Bliss 2013). Type II collagen is found in cartilage, especially hyaline cartilage. Type II collagen is formed from cross-linked fibrils arranged in a three-dimensional matrix which traps proteoglycan aggregates, increasing its tensile strength and resistance to deformation (Exposito et al. 2010; Bliss 2013).

Elastin Elastin fibers allow tissues to recoil and return to normal when exposed to repeated stretch and deformation (Frantz et al. 2010). Tissue elasticity is directly related to its elastin content.

Proteoglycans PGs are classified by the core protein type, localization, and glycosaminoglycan (GAG) composition (Frantz et al. 2010). GAG chains consist of unbranched polysaccharide chains made up of repeating disaccharide units and are either sulfated (chondroitin sulfate, heparan sulfate, and keratan sulfate) or non-sulfated (hyaluronic acid) (Iozzo and Schaefer 2015). PGs are extremely hydrophilic and tend to create large aggregates forming a hydrogel matrix which can withstand strong compressive forces (Frantz et al. 2010; Bliss 2013). The most common musculoskeletal proteoglycans are aggrecan, biglycan, decorin, fibromodulin, hyaluronan (hyaluronic acid), lumican, and versican (see Table 7.3).

Tissue Physiology

Tendons Comprised of fibrous connective tissue connecting muscle to bone. The "non-linear, viscous-elastic, anisotropic and heterogeneous mechanical properties" of the tendon provide its rigidity and flexibility (Tresoldi et al. 2013). Tendons are covered by a loose sheath of connective tissue (epitenon) which contains blood vessels, lymphatic vessels, and nerves (Tresoldi et al. 2013).

The attachment site of the tendon to the bone, called the enthesis, comprises either fibrous or fibrocartilaginous tissue (Tresoldi et al. 2013). The three most common tendon types are energy-storing, positional, and wrap-around tendons (see Table 7.4).

Ligaments Ligaments are strong, dense, inelastic bands of white fibrous connective tissue which originate and insert on bone (Pasquini et al. 2003). Ligaments serve to stabilize joints by keeping joint surfaces in correct apposition, while ensuring appropriate joint movement (Pasquini et al. 2003;

Bliss 2013). Extracapsular (aka capsular) ligaments are found on the outside of or contained within the joint capsule, rich in collagen, and function to stabilize the joint (especially limiting side-to-side movement) (Pasquini et al. 2003; Bliss 2013). Intracapsular (aka intra-articular) ligaments are found within the joint capsule but not considered within the joint space, and have a vascular outer layer (epiligament) which fuses with the periosteum at the site of origin and insertion (Pasquini et al. 2003; Frank 2004).

Joints Refer to Table 7.5 for information on the three classification systems for joints: clinical, structural, and functional. The synovial joint, depicted in Figure 8.1, is the most important joint in VRM.

Synovial fluid (SF) is a clear, straw-colored viscous fluid found within the joint cavities of all synovial joints, and is composed of hyaluronan, lubricin, and plasma proteins (Hui et al. 2011). SF keeps joints well lubricated, reduces friction, absorbs shock, transports nutrients and waste products out of the joint, and mediates communication between cells within the joint (Iwanaga et al. 2000; Hui et al. 2011).

Articular cartilage, or hyaline cartilage, is a smooth, translucent, and blue-hued specialized connective tissue covering the articulating bones of diarthrodial joints (Fox et al. 2009). Articular cartilage serves as a surface for low friction articulation and transfers weight to the underlying subchondral bone during normal joint movement and dynamic loading (Fox et al. 2009).

Wound Healing Fundamentals

Wound healing is described in more detail in Chapter 7. Figure 8.2 provides a recap of the four phases of wound healing: hemostasis, inflammation, proliferation, and remodeling. Remember the primary goal of wound healing is a functional scar.

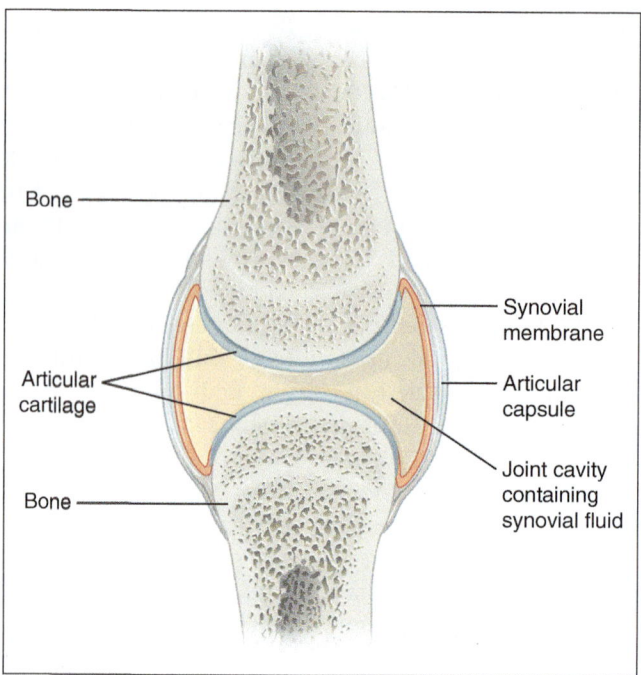

Figure 8.1   A schematic drawing of primary components within a synovial joint: joint (articular) capsule, joint cavity, articular cartilage, and synovial fluid. The joint capsule is composed of an outer fibrous layer and an inner synovial membrane (SM). The fibrous membrane (FM) consists of avascular dense white fibrous tissue with yellow elastic fibers, covering the entire circumference of the joint attaching to the articular end of each associated bone. The SM comprises an avascular connective tissue, covering everything within the joint except the articular cartilage and fibrocartilaginous plates, when present (Evans and Lahunta 2013). The SM instead blends with the periosteum and forms sleeves around the intra-articular ligaments, blood vessels, nerves, muscles, and tendons found within the joint. The SM generally consists of two layers: subintima and intima. The subintima is the thicker fibrous outer layer. The intima is one to three cell layers deep, depending on the joint, and comprises synoviocytes (Iwanaga et al. 2000; Evans and Lahunta 2013). Source: OpenStax College Anatomy & Physiology, Connexions website. June 19, 2013, http://cnx.org/content/col11496/1.6.

Administration Techniques

PRP, bone marrow, and adipose tissue are the most common regenerative agents used (Hauser et al. 2016). All injectables are sterile. Administration of a combination of PRP and stem cells, as well as PRP and hyaluronic acid, is also being used (Canapp et al. 2016a,b; Lee et al. 2019).

PRP

Required Supplies

Between 10 and 60 ml of blood is obtained from the patient (Carr and Canapp 2016). Following phlebotomy, blood is placed in a specialized tube and spun down in a PRP centrifuge. Centrifugation separates substances based on their particle size and density (Apakupakul et al. 2020). A specialized syringe is used to isolate the platelet-rich plasma from the red blood cells (RBCs) and white blood cells (WBCs) (Hakhamian and Schulman 2012). There are multiple commercially available PRP kits requiring one or two step centrifugation. The patient may need to be sedated for both blood draw and PRP injection.

Injection Locations

PRP is commonly used for tendon and ligament strains in the shoulders, elbows, and knees (Carr and Canapp 2016). PRP has also been used to heal muscle and other soft tissue injuries (Osborn 2018). Investigation into the use of

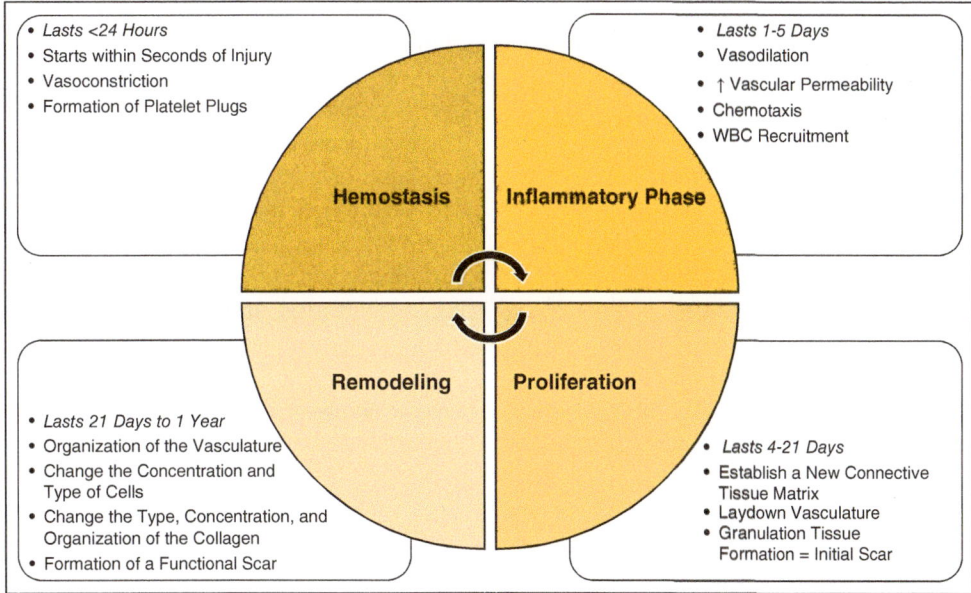

Figure 8.2 An overview of the phases of wound healing. The first step is cessation of bleeding (hemostasis) which starts within seconds, can last for several hours and up to one day (Wallace et al. 2022). Blood vessels initially constrict followed by an influx of platelets to plug the leak (Guo and DiPietro 2010). The inflammatory phase starts during hemostasis and lasts one to five days. During this phase the size of the blood vessels increases (vasodilation), fluid and cells leak from blood vessels (increases vascular permeability), cells move to the site of injury (chemotaxis), and more white blood cells are recruited to the area (Chen et al. 2018a; Patil et al. 2019). This cascade of events results in the classic signs of inflammation: redness, swelling, heat, pain, and loss of function (Punchard et al. 2004). The primary goal of the proliferative phase is to create the initial scar tissue by laying the groundwork for new tissue formation starting with a disorganized matrix of connective tissue and blood vessels. The proliferative phase typically lasts 4–21 days (Landén et al. 2016). The remodeling phase focuses on replacing the proliferative (granulation) with pre-injury tissue. Formation of the functional scar takes at a minimum 21 day but can occur over a one-year period. This tissue is never as strong as undamaged tissues. Source: Lisa P. McFaddin.

topical PRP for wound healing is a current area of scientific interest (Tambella et al. 2018).

Injection Technique

Local anesthesia, sedation or general anesthesia is required for PRP injections (Hakhamian and Schulman 2012). The degree of sedation is dependent on the area being treated. The area is clipped and surgically prepared prior to injection. For tendon and ligament injuries PRP is injected directly into the affected tissue. Ultrasound guidance may be required, especially when used for the treatment of muscle injuries. PRP can also be combined with dextrose to create a greater inflammatory reaction (Osborn 2018).

Treatment Frequency

The need to repeat the treatment is patient and injury specific.

Post-Treatment Recommendations

The patient may be uncomfortable for 12–24 hours following injection (Carr and Canapp 2016). Pain medication can be used if needed. Concurrent administration of nonsteroidal anti-inflammatory drugs (NSAIDs) or steroids is not recommended two weeks before or following PRP therapy (Hakhamian and Schulman 2012). These medications are meant to reduce inflammation, and NSAIDs alter platelet function, which may lessen the effects of the treatment.

Concurrent rehabilitation therapy is recommended along with PRP therapy. The use of therapeutic ultrasound, electrostimulation, class IV low-level laser therapy, and hydrotherapy should be avoided for four to eight weeks after PRP therapy (Carr and Canapp 2016).

Stem Cells

Description

Stem cell therapy relies on the use of autologous or allogeneic materials. Autologous stem cells are extracted from and transplanted into the same patient; while allogeneic stem cells are taken from a donor and transplanted into the patient. The risks and benefits of both approaches are a point of contention at present. The use of allogeneic materials requires specific regulations and raises potential safety concerns but also allows for standardization and banking of cells for future use (Mocchi et al. 2020).

Autologous adult-derived mesenchymal stem cells (MSC) are obtained from the patient's bone marrow or fat (adipose tissue). There are no current studies suggesting one MSC source is more effective than the other (Carr and Canapp 2016).

To ensure the continued development and proper application of VRM, all biological agents used should adhere to the following criteria (Barrett 2016): validate reagents used in sample preparation; standardize protocols for cell culturing, sample preparation, and sample storage; standardize nomenclature; and focus on evidence-based medicine.

Required Supplies

The necessary supplies depend on the stem cell source. Sedation or general anesthesia is required for sample collection. Specialized needles and syringes, as well as imaging equipment, are needed for bone marrow collection. Surgical supplies are required for fat tissue collection. Once the sample is collected it is either processed in-house or sent to a laboratory for processing (Carr and Canapp 2016). An in-depth description of the multitude of materials needed for the various collection and administration techniques is beyond the scope of this book.

Injection Location

The size of the needles, location of injection, and injection technique all affect cell viability and must be taken into consideration (Mocchi et al. 2020). Intra-articular injections can be performed for any type of joint issues, including osteoarthritis. Intra-lesion injections are used for tendon and ligament problems.

Injection Technique

Refer to the PRP section.

Treatment Frequency

The need to repeat the treatment is patient and injury specific.

Post-Treatment Recommendations

Refer to the PRP section.

Mechanisms of Action

PRP

PRP stimulates, supports, and fortifies the body's natural healing ability reducing inflammation and pain, as well as restoring function. PRP is a small volume of concentrated platelets created from blood. PRP is generally created from the patient's own blood (autologous). There are a few commercially available PRP products made from donor dogs (autogeneic) but none have received FDA approval at this time. There are multiple techniques for the generation of PRP. Currently there are no standard protocols in veterinary medicine. PRP can differ in the concentration of platelets, WBCs, and RBCs depending on the isolation technique utilized and variations in the patient's own blood (Carr and Canapp 2016).

Platelets have three jobs: initiate clot formation, bring WBCs to areas of injury, and release growth factors (Hakhamian and Schulman 2012). Injured tissue releases multiple proteins causing inflammation and recruitment of other cells for help, especially platelets. Platelets help "plug the hole" and provide scaffolding for additional clotting proteins. Platelets also guide WBCs to the site of injury helping clean up the area by combating infection and cleaning up the area. Growth factors are crucial to the repair and regeneration of damaged tissue (Hakhamian and Schulman 2012).

PRP for Veterinarians

PRP is defined as a hemoconcentrate in which the proportions of platelets are higher than those of whole blood. The platelet concentration must be over $1000\,K/\mu l$ or two to five times that of the baseline WBC concentration (Ferrari and Schwartz 2020).

PRP does contain some RBCs and WBCs. Currently, there is no standardization regarding the recommended concentration for RBCs and WBCs. The beneficial effects of WBCs is a hotly debated topic, with some practitioners claiming leukocytes improve PRP therapy results while others state the presence of neutrophils can increase tissue inflammation and damage (Ferrari and Schwartz 2020).

PRP contains more than 1500 bioactive proteins which reduce inflammation and encourage cellular healing (Reinders and Haghighat 2019). Growth factors are one of the most important proteins involved in tissue healing and contribute greatly to the beneficial effects associated with PRP therapy.

During coagulation platelets release α-granules which stimulate the release of multiple growth factors (Tambella et al. 2018). Growth factors curb the inflammatory cascade and aid in proliferation and tissue remodeling. A description of the most important growth factors involved in tissue healing is provided in Table 8.2.

Commercially available PRP preparation systems create PRP substrate with inconsistent concentrations of platelets, WBCs, and RBCs (Ferrari and Schwartz 2020). This highlights the importance of sample validation prior to use. Ferrari and Schwartz (2020) evaluated the use of two commercial systems in the preparation of feline PRP. Neither preparation method resulted in PRP solutions with a platelet concentration two to five times that of baseline. Feline tendency toward platelet aggregation immediately following phlebotomy presented a unique challenge in the preparation of PRP. While PRP therapy in felines has potential, the logistics surrounding autologous sample preparation still need to be hammered out.

Stem Cell

Stem cells have been shown to aid tissue healing, reduce inflammation, improve blood supply, function as a framework for new cell growth, protect cells, and break down scar tissue (Carr and Canapp 2016). Once injected into the affected tissue, stem cells can develop into multiple cell types. Each cell type can secrete proteins which either directly or indirectly (by attracting other cells to the area) reduce inflammation and promote healing (Mocchi et al. 2020).

Stem Cell for Veterinarians

MSC are multipotent progenitor cells. MSC can be isolated from all tissues within the body, but the source has been shown to affect cell development and efficacy (Mocchi et al. 2020). Bone marrow and adipose tissue are the primary sources used in veterinary medicine (Carr and Canapp 2016). Peripheral blood is being investigated as another source for MSC (Mocchi et al. 2020). Adipose tissue is often the preferred tissue for dogs because sample collection is relatively simple, there is limited pain associated with sample collection, and the produced MSC counts are high, especially from the falciform fat pad (Carr and Canapp 2016; Mocchi et al. 2020).

Cost is the primary limitation in the use of MSC. MSC production requires strict procedures regarding tissue sampling, MSC culturing, expansion, and cryopreservation. Inconsistences or errors in the production of MSC negatively affect the viability of the cells and case outcome.

Adipose tissue contains MSC, endothelial progenitor cells, pericytes, immune cells, fibroblasts, and growth factors (Carr and Canapp 2016). Isolation and harvesting of these cells is called the stromal vascular fraction (SVF) and can be used in VRM (Carr and Canapp 2016). Stem cells can also be isolated, cultured, and expanded from adipose tissue. This procedure creates a large quantity of adipose-derived cultured progenitor cells (ADPC) (Carr and Canapp 2016). Studies have not proven the efficacy of one cell-based therapy over the other.

There are two techniques for processing bone-marrow derived MSC (BM-MSC): bone marrow aspirate concentrate (BMAC) and culture-expanded (Carr and Canapp 2016). BMAC concentrates the nucleated cells of the aspirate, and the concentrate is injected into the desired site. BMAC processing takes less than two hours and there is less cellular altering. Culture-expanded BM-MSC generate a more homogeneous cell population, but the process takes three to four weeks and cell phenotypes can be altered. There are no studies proving the efficacy of one technique over the other.

MSC possess several beneficial properties which aid in the repair and regeneration of damaged tissues including the ability to differentiate into multiple cell types; secrete trophic factors (therapeutic proteins); secrete cytokines (inflammatory compounds) which inhibit certain immune cells (natural killer cells, helper T cells, and cytotoxic T cells) and activate regulatory T cells; and migrate to the site of cell injury and inflammation (homing) (Mocchi et al. 2020).

MSC efficacy is due, in large part, to the release of paracrine factors (diffusible proteins, also called secretomes) (Voga et al. 2020). Secretomes consists of cytokines, chemokines, growth factors, and extracellular vesicles (EVs) (Wangler et al. 2021). Studies are investigating the therapeutic properties of EVs alone as a potentially safer and less immunogenic alternative to stem cell therapy (Voga et al. 2020).

Table 8.2 Common growth factors released by platelets during coagulation and crucial for proper tissue healing. These growth factors are present in platelet-rich plasma (PRP), contributing to its beneficial effects.

Name	Therapeutic effects
PDGF	Mitogenic for fibroblasts, osteoblasts, and adipocytes
	Stimulates formation of collagen type I
TGF	Promotes proliferation and differentiation of MSC
	Stimulates production of collagen type I
	Angiogenic
	Inhibits osteoclast formation
	Inhibits epithelial cell production
VEGF	Promotes angiogenesis
	Increased blood vessel permeability
	Mitogenic for fibroblasts, epithelial, renal, and glial cells
bFGF	Aids in MSC mitogenesis
	Enhances angiogenesis
PDEGF	Chemotactic for fibroblasts and epithelial cells
	Mitogenic for fibroblasts and epithelial cells
	Induces cell migration
	Promotes granulation tissue formation
IGF	Promotes pre-osteoblast formation
	Stimulates the production of osteocalcin, alkaline phosphatase, and collagen type I from osteoblasts
	Stimulates MSC proliferation and differentiation
	Promotes neuronal differentiation
	Chemotactic effect on vascular endothelial cells

PDGF, platelet-derived growth factor; TGF, transforming growth factor; VEGF, vascular endothelial growth factor; bFGF, basic fibroblast growth factor; PDEGF, platelet-derived epidermal growth factor; IGF, insulin-like growth factor; MSC, mesenchymal stem cells. Source: adapted from Tambella et al. (2018).

Table 8.3 The conditions under which VRM should not be used or should be used with caution.

Cautions	Contraindications	Adverse effects
• Immunocompromised	• Cancer (affecting local muscle, connective tissue, and bone) • Acute non-reduced luxations or dislocations • Septic arthritis • Post-traumatic arthritis • Acute tendonitis • Acute bursitis • Bleeding disorders • Clotting disorders	• Infection • Pain • Stiffness • Bruising • Bleeding • Transient nerve damage • Therapy failure

Source: adapted from Gladstein (2012).

Safety

As with any therapeutic modality there are potential cautions, contraindications, and adverse effects associated with VRM, as outlined in Table 8.3. The potential risks and adverse effects associated with sedation or general anesthesia must be considered as well. Caution is necessary when sedating or anesthetizing patients with comorbidities (illnesses) which may increase their anesthetic risk, such as patients with heart disease or brachycephalic (short-nosed) dogs. As mentioned earlier the use of therapeutic ultrasound, electrostimulation, class IV low-level laser therapy, and hydrotherapy should be avoided for four to eight weeks after PRP therapy (Carr and Canapp 2016).

The Why

Applications in Human Medicine

As mentioned in the Humn RM Regulation section, PRP is not classified as a drug but a blood product by the FDA. The FDA does not approve PRP but does govern the methods by which PRP is prepared and thus the PRP kits (FDA 2020). Currently, there are several FDA-approved PRP kits.

Alternatively, stem cells are classified as a drug. The use of stem cells to treat musculoskeletal conditions has not been FDA-approved and any advertised product is considered illegally marketed (FDA 2020). The limited available research dose show promising results for applications in the treatment of heart failure, wound healing, and tooth regeneration (Rajabzadeh et al. 2019).

In the 2019 the American College of Rheumatology/Arthritis Foundation Guideline for the Management of Osteoarthritis of the Hand, Hip, and Knee stated PRP and stem cell injections are "strongly recommended against in patients with knee and/or hip [osteoarthritis]" due "concern(s) regarding the heterogeneity and lack of standardization in available preparations" (Kolasinski et al. 2020).

Chen et al. (2018b) reviewed 21 studies investigating the use of PRP in the treatment of primarily rotator cuff injuries and lateral epicondylitis. Results of the systematic review suggest PRP may reduce pain associated with these injuries. In contrast, a meta-analysis of 36 randomized controlled trials by Franchini et al. (2018) determined PRP was only marginally effective when compared to control groups and did not support the use of the treatment.

In a systematic review of five studies, Rhatomy et al. (2020) found there is evidence of improved tendon and ligament healing following stem-cell therapy in preclinical studies. Conversely, a review of eight trials by van den Boom et al. (2020) concluded there was a high risk of bias and lack of evidence to support the use of stem cell therapy for tendon disorders.

PRP, when performed correctly following FDA guidelines, is considered relatively safe. However, anytime anything is injected into or around a joint there is risk of pain and stiffness, bleeding, bruising, swelling, infection, and allergic reactions.

Applications in Veterinary Medicine

"Soft-tissue injury" is a name given to basically any painful stimuli affecting the musculoskeletal system whose cause is either not immediately identified or for which an obvious bony abnormality has been ruled out. This catch-all term can refer to anything from bruised muscles, sprained muscles, trigger points, tendon strain, to ligament sprain. In the case of tendinous strains and ligamentous sprains damage to the connective tissue causes hypermobility, weakness, and pain. Complete tendon or ligament tears often require surgical correction. Partial tears, connective tissue laxity, and sprained muscles are still a major source of pain and can benefit from VRM.

Specific conditions for which VRM may be of benefit include ankylosing spondylosis, carpal and tarsal ligament laxity, cervical vertebral instability (CVI) or wobbler's, chronic ligament or tendon sprains or strains, cruciate laxity or partial tear, elbow dysplasia, hip dysplasia, intervertebral disk disease (IVDD), intolerance of traditional medications (NSAIDs, steroids, opioids, etc.), myofascial pain syndromes,

osteochondrosis dissecans (OCD), pain from repetitive motion disorder, patellar luxation, sacroiliac laxity, shoulder, elbow, and carpal joint laxity, spinal stenosis, stifle collateral ligament injury, tarsocrural luxations, and temporomandibular joint (TMJ) laxity (Mocchi et al. 2020; Sharun et al. 2021).

While this chapter focuses on the use of PRP and stem cells in the treatment of musculoskeletal conditions, Table 8.4 outlines studies investigating the use of VRM for the treatment of a multitude of conditions in animals.

Both PRP and stem cell therapy are considered safe and effective in veterinary medicine (Carr and Canapp 2016; Sharun et al. 2021; Armitage et al. 2023). As mentioned earlier the primary concern with PRP is the lack of standardization regarding sample preparation. Further research is necessary to determine the best preparation protocols to ensure safety and efficacy.

Veterinary Research

As of February 2023, a quick search on PubMed. gov for "regenerative medicine canine" and "regenerative medicine feline" yielded 1157 results, while a search for "platelet rich plasma canine," "platelet rich plasma feline," "stem cell therapy canine," and "stem cell therapy feline" yielded 1488 results. Even assuming there is some overlap between the two search categories, that is still an appreciable amount of research in the field of VRM. Presented below are the summaries of three VRM studies in canines.

Multiple Injections of Leukoreduced Platelet Rich Plasma Reduce Pain and Functional Impairment in a Canine Model of CCL and Meniscal Deficiency

Authors: James Cook, Patrick Smith, Chantelle Bozynski, Keiichi Kuroki, Cristi Cook, Aaron Stoker, and Ferris Pfeiffer **Journal**: *Journal of Orthopaedic Research* **Date**: 2016 **Study design**: Controlled trial **Study hypothesis**: Multiple intra-articular injections of leukoreduced platelet-rich plasma	following cranial cruciate ligament (CCL) damage will improve CCL and meniscal repair compared to saline injections. **Sample size**: 12 dogs **Materials and methods**: 12 dogs received a surgical partial CCL transection and meniscal release in one stifle joint. At one, two, three, six, and eight weeks after CCL trauma dogs

were either treated with intra-articular injections of 2 ml of leukoreduced platelet-rich plasma (ACP) or saline. The following parameters were measured over six months: comfortable range of motion (CROM), lameness, pain, effusion, kinetics, and radiographic and arthroscopic assessments. After six months the CCLs of all dogs were evaluated visually and using histopathology. Practitioners involved in the monitoring parameters were blinded to the dog's treatment group. A one-way analysis of variance (ANOVA) and Tukey's post hoc test were used for statistical analysis.

Results

1) Lameness was significantly higher in the saline-treated dogs compared to the dextrose-treated group.
2) CROM was significantly lower in the saline-treated dogs compared to the ACP-treated group.
3) Limb function was significantly lower in the saline-treated dogs compared to the ACP-treated group.
4) Pain was significantly higher in the saline-treated dogs compared to the ACP-treated group.
5) Radiographic evidence of arthritis increased significantly in both groups.
6) Arthroscopic evaluation of the ACP-treated group more closely resembled normal stifle joints compared to the saline-treated groups, but the result was not statistically significant.

7) Histopathologic changes were significantly lower in the ACP-treated dogs compared to the saline-treated group.

Study conclusions: Five intra-articular injections of ACP improved pelvic limb function and reduced pain following CCL injury.

Study limitations

1) Small sample size.
2) There was no true negative control group, i.e. no normal dogs or dogs undergoing sham surgery.
3) How closed does surgical damage to the CCL resemble real-life chronic degradative changes?
4) Did meniscal release reduce pain levels because in normal CCL injury with meniscal tears the torn meniscus represents its own source of significant pain.
5) Study did not address the effects of ACP on the meniscus directly.
6) Did not evaluate the effect of different numbers of ACP treatments.
7) This study was designed to use canines as a human model and not specifically to investigate methods for CCL repair in veterinary patients.

L.P.M. conclusion: This study does show promise for the use of platelet-rich plasma in the treatment of CCL injury in canines. Additional studies addressing the outlined study limitations would go a long way to solidifying the effectiveness of this therapeutic modality.

Partial Cranial Cruciate Ligament Tears Treated with Stem Cell and Platelet-Rich Plasma Combination Therapy in 36 Dogs: A Retrospective Study

Authors: Sherman Canapp Jr., Christopher Leasure, Catherine Cox, Victor Ibrahim, and Brittany Carr
Journal: *Frontiers in Veterinary Science*
Date: 2016
Study design: Retrospective analysis

Study hypothesis: The use of autologous bone marrow aspirate concentrate (BMAC) and adipose-derived progenitor cells (ADPC) with platelet-rich plasma (PRP) will improve recovery in dogs with partial cranial cruciate ligament (CCL) tears.

(Continued)

Partial Cranial Cruciate Ligament Tears Treated with Stem Cell and Platelet-Rich Plasma Combination Therapy in 36 Dogs: A Retrospective Study (Continued)

Sample size: 36 client-owned dogs

Materials and methods: Medical records of client-owned dogs with early partial (<50%) CCL tear treated with BMAC-PRP or ADPC-PRP between 2010 and 2015. The following parameters were evaluated: signalment, medical history, physical and orthopedic examination findings, objective temporospatial gait analysis, radiographs, arthroscopy findings on days 0 and 90, treatment, and outcome. Owners were sent a questionnaire with a validated Helsinki chronic pain index (HCPI). Data was analyzed using paired *t*-test, chi-square test, and Fisher's exact test.

Results

1) Stifle arthroscopy 90 days post-treatment was available in 13 dogs, nine of whom had neovascularization and normal ligament in previously damaged areas. Three of the dogs received surgery (tibial plateau leveling osteotomy, TPLO), and one dog received one additional treatment.
2) Baseline and 90-day post-treatment gait analysis was available for 11 dogs. A significant improvement was noted in the treated limb on day 90 compared to day 0.

There was no significant difference between the treated and untreated limbs on day 90.

3) 12 owners returned questionnaires. Eight of the dogs were sporting dogs, and seven of the dogs returned to sport. All owners reported improved quality following injections rating the outcome as excellent or good.

Study conclusions: BMAC + PRP and ADPC + PRP improved patient outcome and shows promise for the treatment of partial CCL tears.

Study limitations

1) Retrospective study.
2) Lack of continuity of treatment types given the retrospective nature of the study.
3) Did not compare recovery of dogs without injections.
4) Owner compliance may have been biased.

L.P.M. conclusion: This study supports the use of BMAC, ADPC, and PRP as viable treatment options for partial CCL tears. Further studies are needed to determine the efficacy of these treatments for CCL tears and other musculoskeletal conditions. Ideally double-blinded randomized clinical trials are needed.

Adipose-Derived Mesenchymal Stem Cells and Platelet-Rich Plasma Synergistically Ameliorate the Surgical-Induced Osteoarthritis in Beagle Dogs

Authors: Sungho Yun, Sae-Kwang Ku, and Young-Sam Kwon

Journal: *Journal of Orthopaedic Surgery and Research*

Date: 2016

Study design: Controlled trial

Study hypothesis: The use of platelet-rich plasma (PRP) with mesenchymal stem cells (MSC) will improve cartilage regeneration in surgically induced arthritis in the canine knee.

Sample size: 24 laboratory dogs

Materials and methods: The CCL of the right stifle was surgically excised in all dogs. Dogs were divided into four groups based on the type of intra-articular injections received: control (phosphate-buffered saline), PRP, MSC, and PRP+MSC. The PRP and MSC were autologous, with the MSC derived from fat tissue collected from the dog's flank. Injections were given weekly for one month starting one week after surgery.

Dogs were humanely euthanized after another two months. Dogs received the following evaluations: lameness scoring before surgery and every month after surgery, post-mortem focal compressive strength measurement of the femoral and tibial articular surfaces, post-mortem histopathology of the articular cartilage of the lateral femoral and tibial condyles, post-mortem analysis of the extracellular matrix (ECM) of the femoral and tibial articular cartilage, and measurement of ECM-related chondrogenic gene mRNA expression. Multiple statistical analyses were used to evaluate the data.

Results

1) Results of the lameness scoring, focal compression strength, articular ECM composition, histopathology, and gene expression were significantly improved in all treatment groups compared to the control group.
2) Histopathologic changes were significantly improved in the PRP and/or MSC group.

Study conclusions: PRP and MSC treatments have beneficial effects on arthritis.

Study limitations

1) The stifle joints of dogs with no arthritis and surgically excised CCL do not have the same level of chronic inflammation or degenerative changes as those seen in dogs with naturally ruptured CCLs.
2) The study's focus was using canines as a model for human arthritis, and not performed as a means to improve veterinary medicine.
3) There was no negative control, i.e. dogs who had surgery but no injections.
4) The sample size of each treatment group was small.

L.P.M. conclusion: The study demonstrated PRP and MSC improved patient outcome following surgical removal of the CCL. The study did not prove PRP+MSC was a superior therapy. Further studies are needed investigating the use of PRP and MSC in naturally occurring arthritis and CCL injury, especially as compared to surgery alone, without surgery, or compared to other supportive treatments for arthritis (pharmaceuticals, photobiomodulation, acupuncture, etc.).

There are numerous studies supporting the safety and efficacy of PRP and stem cell therapy. A number of these are summarized in Table 8.4. Not every study has yielded positive results. Several studies found administration of PRP did not improve bone healing following implant placement (Garcia et al. 2010; Streckbein et al. 2014; Franklin et al. 2017). Use of adipose-derived allogeneic MSC in the treatment of feline chronic renal disease did not prove effective (Quimby et al. 2016). Intravenously administered autogenous adipose-derived MSC did not improve the clinical signs associated with canine atopic dermatitis (Hall et al. 2010). Edelmann et al. (2018) found no difference in wound healing of the cornea following diamond-burr epithelial debridement when autologous PRP was used compared to tradiotional therapies.

Table 8.4 specifies many of the diseases and conditions for which VRM has shown a scientifically beneficial effect. This list is not all inclusive, as new studies are continually published.

The How

Team Members

This section reviews the potential return on investment (ROI), how to effectively train the entire team, how to promote, and how to integrate the integrative therapy.

Table 8.4 Examples of studies demonstrating the efficacy of VRM in the treatment of multiple diseases and conditions as of 2023.

Condition studied	Technique	Study examples
Allergic asthma	ADMSC	Trzil et al. (2016)
Aural hematomas	L-PRP	Perego et al. (2021)
Chronic degenerative musculoskeletal conditions	PRP	Armitage et al. (2023)
Cruciate ligament repair	PRP + ADPC; PRP + BMAC	Canapp et al. (2016b)
	PRP	Cook et al. (2016), Vilar et al. (2018), Venator et al. (2020)
	PRP; PRP + HA	Lee et al. (2019)
	PRP; MSC; PRP + MSC	Yun et al. (2016)
Hip dysplasia	PRGF	Cuervo et al. (2020)
Inflammatory bowel disease	MSC	Pérez-Merino et al. (2015)
Fracture repair	PRP	López et al. (2019)
	PRP + TCP	Szponder et al. (2018)*
Fragmented MCP	PRP	Cruz and Mason (2022)
Lumbosacral stenosis	PRP	Hernández-Guerra et al. (2021)
Osteoarthritis	PRP	Catarino et al. (2020)
	PRP + ADMSC	Sanghani-Kerai et al. (2021)
	ADMSC	Black et al. (2007), Vilar et al. (2013)
Periodontal disease	PRP	Chung et al. (2023)
Prostatic cysts	PRP	Bigliardi et al. (2018)
Spinal cord repair	PRP	Chen et al. (2018b)**
	ADMSC	Ryu et al. (2009)
Supraspinatus tendinopathy	PRP	Ho et al. (2015)
	PRP + ADPC	Canapp et al. (2016a,b)
	PRP + BMAC	McDougall et al. (2018)
Wound healing	PRP	Karayannopoulou et al. (2014), Tambella et al. (2014), Farghali et al. (2017), Jee et al. (2016), Iacopetti et al. (2020)
	MSC	Kim et al. (2013)

ADPC, adipose-derived progenitor cells; ADMSC, adipose-derived mesenchymal stem cells; BMAC, bone marrow aspirate concentrate; HA, hyaluronic acid; L-PRP, leukocyte- and platelet-rich plasma; MCP, medial coronoid process; MSC, mesenchymal stem cell; PRGF, plasma rich in growth factors (a PRP derivative); PRP, platelet-rich plasma; TCP, tricalcium phosphate.
All studies used canine subjects unless otherwise indicated (*, rabbit; **, rat). Source: Lisa P. McFaddin.

Return on Investment

ROI can be determined by evaluating client interest, veterinarian demand, hospital costs, applicability of the service, appointment scheduling, and pricing.

Client Interest

Currently there are no studies documenting client interest or the popularity of VRM. By evaluating trends in client opinion and pet health insurance, interest in VRM can be inferred.

Client Opinion   Table 8.5 summarizes the pet owner demographics and statistics mentioned in the My Lessons section of the Introduction. Even if 5% of the owners are open to VRM, that is still 4.8 million potential patients.

The treatment of pain in veterinary patients is a hot button issue amongst both owners and practitioners. The existence of the International Veterinary Academy of Pain Management (IVAPM), Certified Veterinary Pain Practitioners (CVPP), 2015 and 2022 American Animal Hospital Association (AAHA) and American Association of Feline Practitioners (AAFP) Pain Management for Dogs and Cats consensus statement, and Animal Pain Awareness Month in September highlights the importance and community awareness of this issue (Epstein et al. 2015; Grant et al. 2022). As such, any treatment which effectively reduces companion animal pain should and will spark the interest of clients and veterinarians.

Pet Health Insurance   Many pet insurance plans include coverage for integrative therapies, including VRM (Woodley 2018). The presence of this type of coverage re-emphasizes the mainstream incorporation of these treatment modalities, as well as reflecting client demand.

Veterinarian Demand

Currently, VRM is a niche market with few veterinarians offering the service. Over-saturation of the market is unlikely. Erring on the side of

Table 8.5   Summary of the 2022 pet ownership and pet health insurance demographics in the United States discussed in the Introduction of the book (Burns 2018, 2022; MFAF 2018; Nolen 2022; APPA 2022; NAPHIA 2023).

• 83% of pets are owned by millennials (32%), generation X (24%), and baby boomers (27%)
• 69 million households owned dogs
• 45.3 million households owned cats
• Estimated over 81.1 million owned dogs
• Estimated over 60.7 million owned cats
• 68% of owners are interested in alternative treatment modalities for their pets.
• 4.41 million pets have pet health insurance
• 82% of insurance pets are dogs.

Source: Lisa P. McFaddin.

cation, the pratice manager could compare the number of general practitioners within a 5-, 10-, or 20-mile radius to the number of veterinarians advertising VRM. The search radius is dependent on your hospital's demographics. Most comparisons follow the 5% trend. In other words, you want to ensure less than 5% of the surrounding hospitals are offering the service.

Hospital Costs

Let us start by reviewing the potential costs associated with introducing and offering acupuncture: veterinarian training, staff training, supplies and equipment, staffing, facilities, and advertising. For more information on potential hospital costs refer to the Introduction of this book.

Veterinarian Training

Course   There are a few online course options. Veterinarians can also learn about VRM by attending national conferences and through traditional online veterinary continuing education (CE) sources (approximate cost, $100).

Textbooks   Textbooks are not required but are often highly recommended. Cost depends on the quantity and type of book purchased (estimated cost, $100).

Travel Expenses Not applicable. Veterinarians attending national conferences would not be attending solely to learn about VRM, so there would be no additional travel costs (estimated cost, $0).

Time Off Veterinarian paid time-off (PTO) expenses are not projected because the online courses could be completed on the veterinarian's own time. Additionally, if a veterinarian attended a major veterinary conference, it is assumed he or she would use their allotted PTO for CE (estimated cost, $0).

Staff Training Team training expenses are highly variable and dependent on the preexistence staff meetings and use of a staff meeting for training (compared to self-study). Refer to the Introduction of the book for a breakdown of these variables (cost range, $230–1295).

Supplies The necessary supplies are dependent on the procedure performed. PRP requires specialized collection, preparation, and administration materials, as well as a specific type of centrifuge. For stem cell therapy costs include the specialized collection and sample preparation materials, stem cell production through an outside facility, and shipping the materials to and from the facility. Given the wide range of potential supplies and costs, it is not feasible to provide specific information on these costs.

Staffing As sedation is often required, VRM is typically scheduled as a procedure, not a regular appointment. Following the AAHA recommendations a veterinary assistant or licensed technician (VA/LT) should be present to monitor the patient while under sedation. Assuming the hospital has preexisting procedure hours for the veterinarians, there would be no additional staffing costs (estimated costs, $0).

Facilities Facility expenses represent the costs needed to keep the doors open (aka overhead). Overhead includes rent or mortgage, utilities, administrative costs, and often employee costs divided by the minutes the practice is open (Stevenson 2016). The price per minute equals the amount of revenue needed just to break even. Overhead is extremely hospital specific, but the range tends to be $2–5/minute. With VRM, overhead is determined by the length of the procedure performed as this will affect doctor and support staff time. Presumably each procedure would take 30–90 minutes from the start of sedation to recovery.

Advertising There are numerous ways to advertise a new service. On average veterinary hospitals spend 0.7% of revenue on promotion and advertisement (AVMA 2019). Most of the advertisement can be done with little to no additional expenditure. The Promotion section discusses advertising ideas in further detail. The national median gross revenue for companion animal practices was $1.2 million in 2022 (AVMA 2023). Advertising costs are calculated assuming no more than 5% of the current advertising budget would be used for promotion of the new service (estimated maximum cost, $420).

Start-Up Costs The cost of VRM is not only dependent on the supply costs but the hospital's preexisting cost for sedation, surgeon's time or procedural time, and supplies. Given the highly variable nature of these expenses, potential start-up costs are not calculated in this chapter. Refer to other chapters for examples of start-up cost calculations.

Applicability

According to the Healthy Paws Pet Insurance and Foundation 2019 Cost of Pet Health Care Report 18.8% of canine vet visits were related to pain and musculoskeletal injuries; while 6.8% of feline visits were related to painful conditions (HPPIF 2019). As stated previously, VRM is very useful in the management and prevention of pain. This treatment modality can be a valuable addition to any practitioner's toolbox when it comes to treating the third most common reason for taking a dog, and seventh most common reason for taking a cat, to the veterinarian (HPPIF 2019).

Appointment Scheduling

Factors to consider when planning VRM appointments include the type of procedure performed (PRP or stem cell); the level of sedation required for the procedure; the length of time needed for the procedure; the support staff availability; and room availability.

Pricing

An in-depth look into appointment pricing can be found in the Introduction of this book. There are two primary pricing methods: current market fees and hospital cost-based pricing.

Current Market Fees   There are no current studies evaluating the average cost or price range for VRM. Hospitals can survey client pricing for said services from practices in the area to get an idea of market fees.

Hospital Cost-Based Pricing   The hospital cost per patient is calculated using the initial start-up cost. Service fee is then calculated using the formula: Service Fee = Hospital Cost + Profit. The service fee can be obtained by marking up the start-up cost per patient, usually between 40 and 100%. Refer to other chapters for specific examples as to how this is calculated.

Team Training

The concept of phase training is used when introducing acupuncture to the hospital team. A multi-media approach is used to assist with the training program and is outlined in Table 8.6.

Practice Manager's Role in Training

To conquer this task the pratice manager needs his or her own checklist which includes the following information:

- Schedule a date and time for the team training.
- Ensure all information pertaining to the new service is reviewed with the staff.
- Confirm all team members have completed the training.
- Certify all team members understand the information and can successfully educate clients.

Promotion

There are six common avenues of promotion for a veterinary integrative medicine (VIM) service: hospital website, social media, email blasts, mailers, in-hospital promotions, and client education.

Hospital Website

Advertise "Veterinary Regenerative Medicine" or "Veterinary Stem Cell Therapy" in several locations on the website. On the made page insert "Now offering veterinary regenerative medicine" or "Now offering veterinary stem cell therapy" with a link to success stories or client testimonials. Utilize the hospital website to advertise the VIM treatment under the "Services" section. Under Veterinarian Biograph include a description of the specialized training. Create a regenerative medicine blog page discussing patient success stories.

Social Media

Utilize Facebook, Instagram, and/or Twitter to post facts, photographs, hashtags, and patient success stories. Include fun and intriguing facts about VRM. Clients love photographs, especially of the preparation procedure and pets receiving VRM treatments. Create or utilize VRM specific hashtags. Provide posts with patient success stories.

Table 8.6 The breakdown of phase training steps and resources for the entire hospital team.

Phase 1: Background information	
Team training guide	The handout walks the practice manager and/or veterinarian through Phase 1 of the training
	A downloadable and editable copy of the handout is located on the companion website
Training presentation	The video covers background information on the modality
	PowerPoints can be downloaded, edited, and personalized from the companion website
	The document can be used as a PowerPoint or saved as an mp4 creating a personalized movie
Team training handout	The handout provides additional background information for the CSRs, VAs, and LTs to complement the knowledge gained from watching the training presentation
	A downloadable and editable copy of the handout is located on the companion website
Phase 2: Knowledge proficiency	
Quiz	A short quiz to ensure all team members have a good understanding of the service being offered
	A downloadable and editable copy of the handout is located on the companion website
	A key is provided
Phase 3: Expectations	
Training worksheets	A training checklist is provided for CSRs and VA/LTs with role-specific expectations and tasks for each staff member
	A recommended completion time is provided.
	A downloadable and editable copy of the handout is located on the companion website
Phase 4: Client education	
Client scripts	Bullet point information and scripted examples used when discussing acupuncture with clients
	A downloadable and editable copy of the handout is located on the companion website
Client education presentation	A short (five to seven minute) client educational video about the therapeutic modality
	PowerPoints can be downloaded, edited, and personalized from the companion website
	The document can be used as a PowerPoint or saved as an mp4 creating a personalized movie
Client education handout	An informational handout about the therapeutic modality written specifically for clients
	A downloadable and editable copy of the handout is located on the companion website

CSR, customer service representative; VA, veterinary assistant; LT, licensed technician. Source: Lisa P. McFaddin.

Email Blasts

Send fun mass emails to your clients introducing VRM. Consider monthly case presentations illustrating how the service has benefited patients. Almost everyone has at least one email address these days. Customer service representatives should be amassing client emails at the same rate as phone numbers.

Mailers

Mailers can be expensive and are largely unnecessary in this digital age. Mailers can be used to announce the introduction of VRM to existing clients. The mailer should include the name of the new service, a brief description of how VRM can help pet patients, the name of the doctor performing the procedure, possibly a brief description of the training the doctor received, and possibly a photograph of a pet receiving VRM or after having received the treatment.

In-Hospital Promotions

Advertise VRM within the hospital using small promotional signs, informational signs, invoice teasers, and staff buttons. Small promotional signs can be placed in the waiting room and exam rooms. Include photographs of pets receiving or having received VRM. Informational signs should include a brief description of how VRM can help pet patients, photographs of pets, and name of the doctor performing the procedure.

Invoice teasers should consist of short phrases reminding and enticing owners regarding a new service offered at the practice. Examples include "Now offering Veterinary Regenerative Medicine/Stem Cell Therapy"; "Curious if Veterinary Regenerative Medicine/Stem Cell Therapy could help your pet?"; "Introducing Veterinary Regenerative Medicine/Stem Cell Therapy"; and "Would your pet benefit from Veterinary Regenerative Medicine/Stem Cell Therapy?"

Buttons can be made for the staff to wear with kitchy phrases reminding owners, in a fun way, of the new VRM service. Examples include "Got PRP?" and "Want to learn more about PRP/Stem Cell Therapy?"

Client Education

Education is crucial to understanding the purpose and importance of any given treatment. The client handouts and videos solidify pet owner knowledge base reducing concerns and conveying value.

Integration

The key components for proper integration include availability of the service to the right patients; appropriate patient scheduling; appropriate support staff scheduling; and staff buy-in (understanding the benefits of the offered service).

Veterinarians

There are several factors to contemplate when veterinarians are considering and preparing to incorporate VRM in their clinical repertoire: state requirements and restrictions, return on investment, course availability, supplies and equipment, veterinary organizations, and continuing education.

State Requirements and Restrictions
Is VRM Considered the Practice of Veterinary Medicine?

Each state has its own veterinary provisions outlining what is and is not considered the practice of veterinary medicine. All states would consider the methods used to obtain samples for VRM and joint injections the practice of veterinary medicine. Refer to the companion website for links to each state's veterinary rules and regulations.

Does VRM Continuing Education Count Toward Licensure Continuing Education Requirements?

Currently no states require specific CE hours for veterinarians offering VRM nor do they specifically reference VRM CE. Some states limit the use of integrative medicine CE hours toward the annual CE requirement for license renewal. Most states permit the use of integrative CE if the lectures or webinars are performed by an approved provider. Table 1.16 in Chapter 1 provides a list of each states CE allotments as it pertains to certain forms of integrative medicine. Refer to the companion website for links to each state's veterinary rules and regulations.

Are Your Assets Covered?

Check with your liability insurance to determine if you are covered when practicing all forms of VRM. Refer to the Introduction of this book for additional information.

Return on Investment

Specifics are discussed in the Team Members section of this chapter.

Course Availability

Formal training for VRM is very limited. There are several online introductory courses available. Pricing is accurate as of February 2023.

Many of the major veterinary conferences have lectures discussing regenerative medicine, but wet labs are uncommon. The North American Veterinary Regenerative Medicine Association (NAVRMA) annual conference is dedicated to advancing VRM knowledge and practical applications. The American Holistic Veterinary Medical Association (AHVMA) annual conference often has lectures discussing regenerative medicine. There also a variety of online veterinary organizations, such as Veterinary Information Network (VIN), Vetfolio, DVM360 Flex, and Vet Girl on the Run, which offer American Association of Veterinary State Boards (AAVSB) Registry of Approved Continuing Education (RACE)-approved CE on VRM.

NC State Veterinary Medicine and Northwest Seminars

- **Course name**: Introduction to Veterinary Stem Cell and Regenerative Medicine
- **Prerequisites**: Licensed veterinarians and veterinary technicians
- **Description**
  - An introductory course discussing regenerative medicine in veterinary science.
  - Covers the application of adipose-derived stem cells and platelet-rich plasma.
  - No mention of RACE-approved CE credit.
- **Online training**: Three hours
- **On-site training**: Not applicable
- **Cost**: $195
- **Contact information**: https://www.ncsu-vetce.com

Rocky Mountain School of Animal Acupressure and Massage

- **Course name**: Evidence-Based Small Animal Regenerative Medicine Course
- **Prerequisites**: Licensed veterinarians, veterinary technicians, and physical therapists
- **Description**

- Described as the VetStem Credentialing Course for small animal and equine veterinarians.
- Four modules in the course.
- Up to four hours of RACE-approved CE hours.
- Limited information available about the courses without applying and/or creating an account.
- As of February 2023 it appears this course may no longer be offered.

- **Online training**: Up to four hours
- **On-site training**: Not applicable
- **Cost**: Free
- **Contact information**
  - Address: 12860 Danielson Court, Suite B, Poway, CA 92064
  - Website: www.vetstem.com
  - Email: info@vetstem.com

VetStem

- **Course name**: VetStem Credentialing Course and/or Regenerative Medicine and the Feline Patient Course
- **Prerequisites**: Veterinarian
- **Description**: CE provided by a company which offers adipose tissue processing, dose banking, banked dose processing, cell culturing, and client referral. No real information on the course found.
- **Online training**: Yes, length unknown
- **On-site training**: Not applicable
- **Cost**: $0 if working in the US or Canada
- **Contact information**: https://vetstem.com

Veterinary Teaching Academy

- **Course name**: Regenerative Medicine
- **Prerequisites**: Veterinarian, veterinary technician, rehabilitation profession, industry profession, administrative staff
- **Description**
  - Three-part series covering the basics of regenerative medicine, PRP, and preventing and slowing progression of arthritis in a young dog.
  - Includes:
    - Video
    - Time-stamped index

- ○ Key points summary
- ○ Transcript PDF
- ○ Slide workbook
- ○ Downloadable audio
- ○ 24/7 lifetime access
  - – No mention of AAVSB RACE-approval.
- **Online training**: Unknown
- **On-site training**: Not applicable
- **Cost**: Purchase options include one-time fee of $97 or a membership for access to all their online CE ($297/year or $37/month).
- **Contact information**: https://vetstem.com

Supplies and Equipment

PRP requires specialized equipment for collection, preparation, and administration. The effectiveness of PRP preparation is dependent on the supplies used and protocols followed. Factors to consider include patient's starting blood sample (volume of whole blood collected and starting platelet count) and the type of centrifuge and settings used (speed, number of spins, and separation time) (Apakupakul et al. 2020).

A detailed list of the manufacturers and necessary supplies for regenerative medicine procedures is beyond the scope of this book.

Veterinarians are encouraged to research manufacturers meeting FDA standards and discuss preferences with other regenerative medicine practitioners prior to purchasing equipment.

Hospital remodeling is generally not required when offering VRM as it is usually performed in the treatment room with easy access to anesthesia machines.

Veterinary Organizations

A description of the most common veterinary organizations with a special interest in integrative medicine, pain, and VRM are provided below. Table 8.7 summarizes the organizations' names, contact information, and membership dues as of February 2023.

American Holistic Veterinary Medical Association (AHVMA)

- **Description**: The AHVMA was founded in 1982 at the Western States Veterinary Conference with the goal of advancing integrative medicine through the education of integrative and non-integrative veterinarians, the introduction of integrative medicine to veterinary students, the promotion of research, and representation in the AVMA

Table 8.7 Veterinary associations and organizations with a special interest in veterinary integrative medicine and VRM as of February 2023.

Organization	Contact information	Membership dues
American Holistic Veterinary Medical Association (AHVMA)	PO Box 630, Abingdon, MD 21009 (410) 569-0795 office@ahvma.org	$300/year
College of Integrative Veterinary Therapies (CIVT)	PO Box 352, Yeppoon, 4703 QLD, Australia (303) 800-5460 membership@civtedu.org	$185/year
International Veterinary Academy of Pain Management (IVAPM)	PO Box 1868, Mt Juliet, TN 371211 info@ivapm.org	$250/year
North American Veterinary Regenerative Medicine Association (NAVRMA)	conference@narvma.org	Conference cost/year

Source: Lisa P. McFaddin.

House of Delegates. There is no annual CE requirement to maintain membership.

- **Membership benefits**
  - Free subscription to the *AHVMA Journal*, a peer-reviewed journal.
  - Online resources for client education.
  - Searchable member directory.
  - Discounted vaccination titers through Kansas State University (KSU) Diagnostic Lab.
  - Free access to the Natural Medicines Database, an online resource for supplements, natural medicines, and integrative therapies.
  - Reduced cost for the AHVMA annual conference.

College of Integrative Veterinary Therapies (CIVT)

- **Description**: An online organization open to all licensed animal health providers interested in integrative medicine. There are two membership options: full membership for veterinarians and associate membership for registered animal health professionals. CIVT strives to promote all aspects of evidence-based integrative medicine through online education and discussion forums. CIVT provides financial support to veterinary students interested in studying integrative medicine. CIVT also helps fund integrative medicine research. There is no annual CE requirement to maintain membership.
- **Membership benefits**
  - Access to the online electronic library.
  - Access to the electronic *Journal of Integrative Veterinary Therapies*.
  - Three free CE webinars annually.
  - 20% discount on all webinars.
  - Discounts on specific CIVT courses.
  - Searchable member directory.
  - Access to the Natural Medicines Databases and the American Botanical Council Library.

International Veterinary Academy of Pain Management (IVAPM)

- **Description**: Originally known as the Companion Animal Pain Management

Consortium, then the Academy of Pain Management Interest Group, and finally IVAPM. Founded in 2001 to provide pain management education and certification programs. The organization's goal is to provide acute and chronic pain relief for veterinary patients. Both traditional and alternative therapies are embraced, including acupuncture and rehabilitation and physical therapy.

- **Membership benefits**
  - Members can become Certified Veterinary Pain Practitioners (CVPP).
  - Access to members-only Facebook group offering case consultations and questions.
  - Reduced subscription rate for IVAPM's journal *Veterinary Anaesthesia and Analgesia*.
  - Reduced registration fee for the International Veterinary Emergency and Critical Care (IVECCS) conference.
  - Reduced registration for all IVAPM CE events (online and on-site).
  - Complementary World Small Animal Veterinary Association (WSAVA) membership.

North American Veterinary Regenerative Medicine Association

- **Description**: Founded by speakers and attendees of the North American Veterinary Regenerative Medicine Conference in 2010. The organization's goals are to educate veterinarians about regenerative medicine, improve techniques and expertise, encourage and facilitate clinical trials, support veterinarian training, discuss policies and regulations pertaining to VRM, and collaborate with other organizations as needed.
- **Membership benefits**
  - The organization sponsors an annual meeting and publishes the proceedings.
  - Cost of the membership includes the price of the annual conference.

Reference Books

The following is a list of my recommended books pertaining to VRM as of February 2023. A summary of each book is provided.

Anatomy of Domestic Animals: Systemic and Regional Approach

- Authors: Chris Pasquini, DVM, MS; Tom Spurgeon, PhD; and Susan Pasquini, DVM
- Summary: Most veterinarians already own a copy from vet school. This in-depth, thorough, and entertaining anatomy book provides tons of information on the anatomy of most domestic animals.

Canine Sports Medicine and Rehabilitation

- Authors: M. Christine Zink, DVM, PhD, DACVP, DACVSMR and Janet D. Van Dyke, DVM, DACVSMR
- Summary: A comprehensive reference book discussing common canine musculoskeletal conditions and ailments, with particular interest in the canine athlete. The book covers gait analysis and physiology, various therapeutic approaches (including nutrition, rehabilitation, manual therapy, acupuncture, chiropractic, therapeutic exercise, aquatic therapy, conditioning and retraining, and assistive devices), and specific diagnoses and treatment recommendations for disorders of the forelimbs and pelvic limbs. A must-have for veterinarians interested in manual therapy, orthopedics, and rehabilitation.

Frontiers in Stem Cell and Regenerative Medicine Research

- Editors: Atta-ur-Rahman, FRS and Shazia Anjum
- Summary: A review of the use of stem cell therapy through retrodifferentiation, mesodermal regeneration, hematopoiesis, and mesenchymal stem cells.

Integrating Complementary Medicine into Veterinary Practice

- Authors: Robert S. Goldstein, VMD, Paula Jo Broadfoot, DVM, Richard E. Plamquist, DVM, Karen Johnstons, DVM, Jiu Jia Wen, DVM, Barbara Fougère, BSc, BVMs (Hons), BHSc (comp Med), MODT, MHSc (Herb Med), CVA (IVAs), CVBM, CVCP, and Margo Roman, DVM

- Summary: A comprehensive review of multiple integrative therapies including: Chinese herbal medicine, acupuncture, homotoxicology, nanopharmacology, homotoxicology, and therapeutic nutrition. The book aims to educate veterinary practitioners on the validity, effectiveness, and incorporation of each modality within daily practice.

Mesenchymal Stem Cell in Veterinary Services

- Editors: Mudasir Bashir Gugjoo, PhD and Amar Pal
- Summary: Discusses the production, properties, clinical applications, and mechanisms of action for MSC in regenerative medicine.

Miller's Anatomy of the Dog

- Authors: Howard Evans, PhD and Alexander de Lahunta, DVM, PhD
- Summary: Most veterinarians already own a copy from vet school. This is a comprehensive guide to canine anatomy.

Stem Cells in Veterinary Science

- Authors: Ratan Kumar Choudhary, PhD, MS and Shant Choudhary, PhD
- Summary: An overview of the use of stem cell therapy in veterinary medicine focusing on the mechanisms of action, preclinical evidence, safety, and therapeutic efficacy. The book covers a variety of stem cell types and practical applications.

Therapeutic Applications of Mesenchymal Stem Cells in Veterinary Medicine

- Author: Mudasir Bashir Gugjoo, PhD
- Summary: An in-depth review of the application of MSC in veterinary regenerative and reproductive medicine. The book discusses applications for the musculoskeletal, nervous, gastrointestinal, cardiovascular, urogenital, respiratory, and integumentary systems.

Promotion

Information regarding the hospital's promotion of VRM can be found in the Team Members section.

Integration

The key components for proper integration include availability of the service to the right patients; appropriate patient scheduling; appropriate support staff scheduling; and staff buy-in.

Conclusion

VRM is a rapidly advancing therapeutic modality. The effects and benefits for veterinary patients center on the facilitation of self-healing, restoration of mobility, and reduction of pain. The practical applications in veterinary patients beyond the musculoskeletal are still being explored. This chapter and companion website describe in detail how VRM can be successfully introduced into practice, as well as provide practical tools for implementation.

References

AABB (Association for the Advancement of Blood and Biotherapies) (2023). Regenerative Medicine. https://www.aabb.org/news-resources/resources/cellular-therapies/facts-about-cellular-therapies/regenerative-medicine (accessed 25 February 2023).

AOAPRM (American Osteopathic Association of Prolotherapy Regenerative Meicine) (2020). What is Prolotherapy. https://prolotherapycollege.org/ (accessed 29 October 2020).

Apakupakul, J., Sattasatchuchana, P., Chanloinapha, P., and Thengachaisri, N. (2020). Optimization of a rapid one-step platelet-rich plasma preparation method using syringe centrifugation with and without carprofen. *BMC Veterinary Research* 16 (1): 124.

APPA (American Pet Products Association) (2022). Pet industry market size and ownership statistics. https://www.americanpetproducts.org/press_

industrytrends.asp (accessed 23 February 2023).

Armitage, A.J., Miller, J.M., Sparks, T.H. et al. (2023). Efficacy of autologous mesenchymal stromal cell treatment for chronic degenerative musculoskeletal conditions in dogs: a retrospective study. *Frontiers in Veterinary Science* 13 (9): 1014687.

Atala, A., Bauer, S.B., Soker, S. et al. (2006). Tissue-engineered autologous bladders for patients needing cystoplasty. *Lancet* 367 (9518): 1241–1246.

AVMA (American Veterinary Medical Association) (2019). Economic state of the veterinary profession. https://www.avma.org/news/press-release/AVMA-2019-Economic-State-of-the-Veterinary-Profession-Report-now-available (accessed 26 July 2021).

AVMA (American Veterinary Medical Association) (2020). Therapeutic use of stem cells and regenerative medicine. https://www.avma.org/resources-tools/avma-policies/therapeutic-use-stem-cells-and-regenerative-medicine (accessed 7 December 2020).

AVMA (American Veterinary Medical Association) (2023). *2023 AVMA Report on the Economic State of the Veterinary Profession*. Schaumburg, IL: AVMA.

Barrett, J. (2016). A set of grand challenges for veterinary regenerative medicine. *Frontiers in Veterinary Science* 3: 20.

Benjamin, M. and Evans, E. (1990). Fibrocartilage. *Journal of Anatomy* 171: 1–15.

Biehl, J. and Russell, B. (2009). Introduction to stem cell therapy. *Journal of Cardiovascular Nursing* 24 (2): 98–103.

Bigliardi, E., Cantoni, A.M., De Cesaris, V. et al. (2018). Use of platelet-rich plasma for the treatment of prostatic cysts in dogs. *Canadian Journal of Veterinary Research* 82 (4): 264–270.

Black, L.L., Gaynor, J., Gahring, D. et al. (2007). Effect of adipose-derived mesenchymal stem and regenerative cells on lameness in dogs with chronic osteoarthritis of the coxofemoral joints: a randomized, double-blinded, multicenter, controlled trial. *Veterinary Therapeutics* 8 (4): 272–284.

Bliss, S. (2013). Musculoskeletal structure and physiology. In: *Canine Sports Medicine and Rehabilitation* (ed. M.C. Zink and J.B. Van Dyke), 32–59. Oxford: Wiley-Blackwell.

van den Boom, N., Winters, M., Haisma, H., and Moen, M. (2020). Efficacy of stem cell therapy for tendon disorders: a systematic review. *Orthopaedic Journal of Sports Medicine* 8 (4): 2325967120915857.

Burke, J.F., Yannas, I.V., Quinby, W.C. Jr. et al. (1981). Successful use of a physiologically acceptable artificial skin in the treatment of extensive burn injury. *Annals of Surgery* 194 (4): 413.

Burns, K. (2018). Pet ownership stable, veterinary care variable. https://www.avma.org/javma-news/2019-01-15/pet-ownership-stable-veterinary-care-variable (accessed 11 August 2021).

Burns, K. (2022). New report takes a deep dive into pet ownership. https://www.avma.org/news/new-report-takes-a-deep-dive-pet-ownership (accessed 6 November 2022).

Campbell, K.H., McWhir, J., Ritchie, W.A., and Wilmut, I. (1996). Sheep cloned by nuclear transfer from a cultured cell line. *Nature* 380 (6569): 64–66.

Canapp, S., Canapp, D.A., Ibrahim, V. et al. (2016a). The use of adipose-derived progenitor cells and platelet-rich plasma combination for the treatment of supraspinatous tendinopathy in 55 dogs: a retrospective. *Frontiers in Veterinary Science* 3: 61.

Canapp, S., Leasure, C.S., Cox, C. et al. (2016b). Partial cranial cruciate ligament tears treated with stem cell and platelet-rich plasma combination therapy in 36 dogs: a retrospective study. *Frontiers in Veterinary Science* 3: 112.

Carr, B. and Canapp, S. (2016). Regenerative medicine for soft tissue injury and osteoarthritis. https://todaysveterinarypractice.com/wp-content/uploads/sites/4/2016/07/TVP_2016-0708_NavcInst-Regenerative_WEB.pdf (accessed 3 May 2020).

Catarino, J., Carvalho, P., Santos, S. et al. (2020). Treatment of canine osteoarthritis with allogenic platelet-rich plasma: review of five cases. *Open Veterinary Journal* 10 (2): 226–231.

CDC (Centers for Disease Control) (2020). Arthritis: Osteoarthritis. http://www.cdc.gov/arthritis/basics/osteoarthritis.htm (accessed August 2020).

CFR (Code of Federal Regulations) (2023). Title 21 - Food and Drugs, Chapter 1, Subchapter F, Part 640, Subpart D - Plasma, Sec 640.34 Processing. https://www.accessdata.fda.gov/scripts/cdrh/cfdocs/cfcfr/CFRSearch.cfm?fr=640.34 (accessed 4 March 2023).

Chen, L., Deng, H., Cui, H. et al. (2018a). Inflammatory responses and inflammation-associated diseases in organs. *Oncotarget* 9: 7204–7218.

Chen, N.-F., Sung, C.S., Wen, Z.H. et al. (2018b). Therapeutic effect of platelet-rich plasma in rat spinal cord injuries. *Frontiers in Neuroscience* 12: 252.

Chung, C.-S., Wi, Y.-F., and Lin, L.-S. (2023). Submucosal injection of activated platelet-rich plasma for treatment of periodontal disease in dogs. *Journal of Veterinary Dentistry* 40 (1): 19–27.

Cook, J., Smith, P.A., Bozynski, C.C. et al. (2016). Multiple injections of leukoreduced platelet rich plasma reduce pain and functional impairment in a canine model of ACL and meniscal deficiency. *Journal of Orthopaedic Research* 34 (4): 607–615.

Cruz, A.M.M. and Mason, D.R. (2022). Owner assessed outcomes following elbow arthroscopy with or without platelet rich plasma for fragmented medial coronoid process. *Fronteirs in Veterinary Science* 9: 938706.

Cuervo, B., Rubio, M., Chicharro, D. et al. (2020). Objective comparison between platelet rich plasma alone and in combination with physical therapy in dogs with osteoarthritis caused by hip dysplasia. *Animals* 10 (2): 175.

Edelmann, M.L., Mohammed, H.O., Wakshlag, J.J., and Ledbetter, E.C. (2018). Clinical trial of adjunctive autologous platelet-rich plasma treatment following diamond-burr debridement for spontaneous chronic corneal epithelial defects in dogs. *Journal of the American Veterinary Medical Association* 253 (8): 1012–1021.

Epstein, M., Rodan, I., Griffenhagen, G. et al. (2015). 2015 AAHA/AAFP pain management guidelines for dogs and cats. *Journal of the American Animal Hospital Association* 51 (2): 67–84.

Evan, M. and Kaufman, M. (1981). Establishment in culture of pluripotential cells from mouse embryos. *Nature* 292 (5819): 154–156.

Evans, H. and De Lahunta, A. (2013). *Miller's Anatomy of the Dog*, 4e. St. Louis, MO: Elsevier.

Exposito, J.-Y., Valcourt, U., Cluzel, C., and Lethias, C. (2010). The fribrillar collagen family. *International Journal of Molecular Sciences* 11 (2): 407–426.

Farghali, H., AbdElKader, N., Khattab, M., and AbuBakr, H. (2017). Evaluation of subcutaneous infiltration of autologous platelet-rich plasma on skin-wound healing in dogs. *Bioscience Reports* 37 (2): BSR20160503.

FDA (Food and Drug Administration) (2022b). Focus Area: Regenerative Medicine. https://www.fda.gov/science-research/focus-areas-regulatory-science-report/focus-area-regenerative-medicine (accessed 4 March 2023).

FDA (Food and Drug Administration) (2019). FDA Warns About Stem Cell Therapies. https://www.fda.gov/consumers/consumer-updates/fda-warns-about-stem-cell-therapies (accessed 4 March 2023).

FDA (Food and Drug Administration) (2020). Resources Related to Regenerative Medicine Therapies. https://www.fda.gov/vaccines-blood-biologics/cellular-gene-therapy-products/resources-related-regenerative-medicine-therapies (accessed 25 February 2023).

FDA (Food and Drug Administration) (2022a). FDA's Role in Veterinary Regenerative Medicine. https://www.fda.gov/animal-veterinary/cell-and-tissue-products-animals/fdas-role-veterinary-regenerative-medicine (accessed 25 February 2023).

Ferrari, J. and Schwartz, P. (2020). Prospective evaluation of feline sourced platelet-rich plasma using centrifuge-based systems. *Frontiers in Veterinary Science* 7: 322.

Fox, A., Bedi, A., and Rodeo, S. (2009). The basic science of articular cartilage: structure, composition, and function. *Sports Health: A Multidisciplinary Approach* 1 (6): 461–468.

Franchini, M., Cruciani, M., Mengoli, C. et al. (2018). Efficacy of platelet-rich plasma as conservative treatment in orthopaedics: a systematic review and meta-analysis. *Blood Transfusion* 16 (6): 502–513.

Frank, C.B. (2004). Ligament structure, physiology, and function. *Journal of Musculoskeletal and Neuronal Interactions* 4 (2): 199–201.

Franklin, S., Burke, E., and Holmes, S. (2017). The effect of platelet-rich plasma on osseous healing in dogs undergoing high tibial osteotomy. *PLoS One* 12 (5): e0177597.

Frantz, C., Stewart, K., and Weaver, V. (2010). The extracellular matrix at a glance. *Journal of Cell Science* 123: 4195–4200.

Garcia, R.V., Gabrielli, M.A.C., Hochuli-Vieira, E. et al. (2010). Effect of platelet-rich plasma on peri-implant bone repair: a histologic study in dogs. *Journal of Oral Implantology* 36 (4): 281–290.

Gladstein, B. (2012). A case for prolotherapy and its place in veterinary medicine. *Journal of Prolotherapy* 2012 (4): e870–e885.

Grant, M., Lascelles, B.D.X., Colleran, E. et al. (2022). 2022 AAHA pain management guidelines for dogs and cats. *Journal of the American Animal Hospital Association* 58: 55–76.

Guo, S. and DiPietro, L.A. (2010). Factors affecting wound healing. *Journal of Dental Research* 89 (3): 219–229.

Hakhamian, A. and Schulman, A. (2012). Platelet rich plasma: its place in cranial cruciate ligament repair. *Today's Veterinary Practice* 2: 42–45.

Hall, M.N., Rosenkrantz, W.S., Hong, J.H. et al. (2010). Evaluation of the potential use of adipose-derived mesenchymal stromal cells in the treatment of canine atopic dermatitis: a pilot study. *Veterinary Therapeutics* 11 (2): E1–E14.

Hauser, R., Lackner, J., Steilen-Matias, D., and Harris, D. (2016). A systematic review of dextrose prolotherapy for chronic musculoskeletal pain. *Clinical Medicine Insights. Arthritis and Musculoskeletal Disorders* 9: 139–159.

Hernández-Guerra, Á.M., Carrillo, J.M., Sopena, J.J. et al. (2021). Platelet-rich plasma for the treatment of degenerative lumbosacral stenosis: a study with retired working dogs. *Animals* 11 (10): 2965.

Ho, L., Baltzer, W., Nemanic, S., and Stieger-Vanegas, S. (2015). Single ultrasound-guided platelet-rich plasma injection for treatment of supraspinatus tendinopathy in dogs. *Canadian Veterinary Journal* 56 (8): 845–849.

HPPIF (Healthy Paws Pet Insurance and Foundation) (2019). 2019 Cost of Pet Health Care Report. https://www.healthypawspetinsurance.com/content/costofcare/pet-care-costs-health-conditions_2019.pdf (accessed 2 September 2020).

Hui, A., McCarty, W.J., Masuda, K. et al. (2011). A systems biology approach to synovial joint lubrication in health, injury and disease. *Wiley Interdisciplinary Reviews. Systems Biology and Medicine* 4 (1): 15–37.

Iacopetti, I., Patruno, M., Melotti, L. et al. (2020). Autologous platelet-rich plasma enhances the healing of large cutaneous wounds in dogs. *Frontiers in Veterinary Science* 7: 575449.

Iozzo, R. and Schaefer, L. (2015). Proteoglycan form and function: a comprehensive nomenclature of proteoglycans. *Matrix Biology* 42: 11–55.

Iwanaga, T., Shikichi, M., Kitamura, H. et al. (2000). Morphology and functional roles of synoviocytes in the joint. *Archives of Histology and Cytology* 63 (1): 17–31.

Jee, C.-H., Eom, N.Y., Jang, H.M. et al. (2016). Effect of autologous platelet-rich plasma application on cutaneous wound healing in dogs. *Journal of Veterinary Science* 17 (1): 79–87.

Kaiser, L. (1992). The future of multihospital systems. *Topics in Health Care Financing* 18 (4): 32–45.

Karayannopoulou, M., Papazoglou, L.G., Loukopoulos, P. et al. (2014). Locally injected autologous platelet-rich plasma enhanced tissue perfusion and improved survival of long subdermal plexus skin flaps in dogs. *Veterinary and Comparative Orthopaedics and Traumatology* 27 (5): 379–386.

Kim, J.-W., Lee, J.H., Lyoo, Y.S. et al. (2013). The effects of topical mesenchymal stem cell transplantation in canine experimental cutaneous wounds. *Veterinary Dermatology* 24 (2): 242–e53.

Kolasinski, S., Neogi, T., Hochberg, M.C. et al. (2020). 2019 American College of Rheumatology/Arthritis Foundation guideline for the management of osteoarthritis of the hand, hip, and knee. *Arthritis and Rheumatology* 72 (2): 220–233.

Landén, N., Li, D., and Ståhle, M. (2016). Transition from inflammation to proliferation: a critical step during wound healing. *Cellular and Molecular Life Sciences* 73: 3861–3885.

Lee, M.-I., Kim, J.H., Kwak, H.H. et al. (2019). A placebo-controlled study comparing the efficacy of intra-articular injections of hyaluronic acid and a novel hyaluronic acid-platelet-rich plasma conjugate in a canine model of osteoarthritis. *Journal of Orthopaedic Surgery and Research* 14 (1): 314.

Lo, B. and Parham, L. (2009). Ethical issues in stem cell research. *Endocrine News* 30 (3): 204–213.

López, S., Vilar, J.M., Sopena, J.J. et al. (2019). Assessment of the efficacy of platelet-rich plasma in the treatment of traumatic canine fractures. *International Journal of Molecular Sciences* 20 (5): 1075.

McDougall, R., Canapp, S., and Canapp, D. (2018). Ultrasonographic findings in

41 dogs treated with bone marrow aspirate concentrate and platelet-rich plasma for a supraspinatus tendinopathy: a retrospective study. *Frontiers in Veterinary Science* 5: 98.

MedlinePlus (2016). Bursitis. https://medlineplus.gov/bursitis.html (accessed 1 May 2020).

MFAF (Michelson Found Animals Foundation) (2018). Furred lines: Pet trends. https://www.prnewswire.com/news-releases/furred-lines-pet-trends-2019-300741947.html. (accessed 26 July 2021).

MIRM (McGowan Institute for Regenerative Medicine) (2022). What is Regenerative Medicine? https://mirm-pitt.net/about-us/what-is-regenerative-medicine/ (accessed 25 February 2023).

Mocchi, M., Dotti, S., Del Bue, M. et al. (2020). Veterinary regenerative medicine for musculoskeletal disorders: can mesenchymal stem/stromal cells and their secretome be the new frontier? *Cells* 9 (6): 1453.

NAPHIA (North American Pet Health Insurance Association) (2023). Industry Data. https://naphia.org/industry-data/#my-menu (accessed 18 February 2023).

NIAMSD (National Institute of Arthritis and Musculoskeletal and Skin Diseases) (2015). Sprains and Strains. niams.nih.gov/health-topics/sprains-and-strains (accessed 3 May 2020).

NINDS (National Institute of Neurological Disorders and Stroke) (2019). Repetitive Motion DIsorders. https://www.ninds.nih.gov/health-information/disorders/repetitive-motion-disorders#:~:text=Definition,%2C%20tenosynovitis%2C%20and%20trigger%20finger (accessed 2 May 2020).

Nolen, R.S. (2022). Pet ownership rate stabilizes as spending increases. https://www.avma.org/news/pet-ownership-rate-stabilizes-spending-increases (accessed 22 February 2023).

Osborn, J. (2018). Prolotherapy in practice. https://ivcjournal.com/prolotherapy-practice (accessed 5 May 2023).

Pasquini, C., Spurgeon, T., and Pasquini, S. (2003). *Anatomy of Domestic Animals: Systemic and Regional Approach*, 10e. Pilot Point, TX: Sudz Publishing.

Patil, K., Mahajan, U.B., Unger, B.S. et al. (2019). Animal models of inflammation for screening of anti-inflammatory drugs: implications for the discovery and development of phytopharmaceuticals. *International Journal of Molecular Sciences* 20: 4367.

Perego, R., Spada, E., Moneta, E. et al. (2021). Use of autologous leucocyte- and platelet-rich plasma (L-PRP) in the treatment of aural hematoma in dogs. *Veterinary Science* 8 (9): 172.

Pérez-Merino, E.M., Usón-Casaús, J.M., Zaragoza-Bayle, C. et al. (2015). Safety and efficacy of allogeneic adipose tissue-derived mesenchymal stem cells for treatment of dogs with inflammatory bowel disease: clinical and laboratory outcomes. *Veterinary Journal* 206 (3): 385–390.

Prindull, G., Prindull, B., and Meulen, N. (1978). Haematopoietic stem cells (CFUc) in human cord blood. *Acta Paediatrica Scandinavica* 67 (4): 413–416.

Punchard, N.A., Whelan, C.J., and Adcock, I. (2004). The Journal of inflammation. *Journal of Inflammation* 1 (1): 1–4.

Quimby, J.M., Webb, T.L., Randall, E. et al. (2016). Assessment of intravenous adipose-derived allogeneic mesenchymal stem cells for the treatment of feline chronic kidney disease: a randomized, placebo-controlled clinical trial in eight cats. *Journal of Feline Medicine and Surgery* 18 (2): 165–171.

Rajabzadeh, N., Fathi, E., and Farahzadi, R. (2019). Stem cell-based regenerative medicine. *Stem Cell Investigation* 6: 19.

Reinders, M. and Haghighat, S. (2019). Modified platelet rich plasma (PRP) for cruciate ligament injuries in dogs. https://ivcjournal.com/prp-cruciate-ligament-injuries/ (accessed 5 May 2020).

Rhatomy, S., Prasetyo, T.E., Setyawan, R. et al. (2020). Prospect of stem conditioned medium (secretome) in ligament and tendon healing: a systematic review. *Stem Cells Translational Medicine* 9 (8): 895–902.

Ryu, H.H., Lim, J.H., Byeon, Y.E. et al. (2009). Functional recovery and neural differentiation after transplantation of allogenic adipose-derived stem cells in a canine model of acute spinal cord injury. *Journal of Veterinary Science* 10 (4): 273–284.

Sampogna, G., Guraya, S.Y., and Forgionea, A. (2015). Regenerative medicine: historical roots and potential strategies in modern medicine. *Journal of Microscopy and Ultrastructure* 3 (3): 101–107.

Sanghani-Kerai, A., Black, C., Cheng, S.O. et al. (2021). Clinical outcomes following intra-articular injection of autologous adipose-derived mesenchymal stem cells for the treatment of osteoarthritis in dogs characterized by weight-bearing asymmetry. *Bone and Joint Research* 10 (10): 650–658.

Sharun, K., Jambagi, K., Dhama, K. et al. (2021). Therapeutic potential of platelet-rich plasma in canine medicine. *Archives of Razi Institute* 76 (4): 721–730.

Starzl, T.E. (2000). History of clinical transplantation. *World Journal of Surgery* 24 (7): 759–782.

Stevenson, P. (2016). How to set practice service fees. https://cliniciansbrief.com/article/how-set-practice-service-fees. (accessed 10 June 2020).

Streckbein, P., Kleis, W., Buch, R.S. et al. (2014). Bone healing with or without platelet-rich plasma around four different dental implant surfaces in beagle dogs. *Clinical Implant and Dental Related Research* 16 (4): 479–486.

Szponder, T., Wessely-Szponder, J., Sobczyńska-Rak, A. et al. (2018). Application of platelet-rich plasma and tricalcium phosphate in the treatment of comminuted fractures in animals. *In Vivo* 32 (6): 1449–1455.

Tambella, A.M., Attili, A.R., Dini, F. et al. (2014). Autologous platelet gel to treat chronic decubital ulcers: a randomized, blind controlled clinical trial in dogs. *Veterinary Surgery* 43 (6): 726–733.

Tambella, A., Martin, S., Cantalamessa, A. et al. (2018). Platelet-rich plasma and other hemocomponents in veterinary regenerative medicine. *Wounds* 30 (11): 329–336.

Thomson, J.A., Itskovitz-Eldor, J., Shapiro, S.S. et al. (1998). Embryonic stem cell lines derived from human blastocysts. *Science* 282 (5391): 1145–1147.

Tresoldi, I., Oliva, F., Benvenuto, M. et al. (2013). Tendon's ultrastructure. *Muscles, Ligaments and Tendons Journal* 3 (1): 2–6.

Trzil, J.E., Masseau, I., Webb, T.L. et al. (2016). Intravenous adipose-derived mesenchymal stem cell therapy for the treatment of feline asthma: a pilot study. *Journal of Feline Medicine and Surgery* 18 (12): 981–990.

Venator, K., Frye, C., Gamble, L.-J., and Wakshlag, J. (2020). Assessment of a single intra-articular stifle injection of pure platelet rich plasma on symmetry indices in dogs with unilateral or bilateral stifle osteoarthritis from long-term medically managed cranial cruciate ligament disease. *Veterinary Medicine* 11: 31–38.

Vilar, J.M., Morales, M., Santana, A. et al. (2013). Controlled, blinded force platform analysis of the effect of intraarticular injection of autologous adipose-derived mesenchymal stem cells associated to PRGF-Endoret in osteoarthritic dogs. *BMC Veterinary Research* 9: 131.

Vilar, J., Manera, M.E., Santana, A. et al. (2018). Effect of leukocyte-reduced platelet-rich plasma on osteoarthritis caused by cranial cruciate ligament rupture: a ccanine gait analysis model. *PLoS One* 13 (3): e0194752.

Voga, M., Adamic, N., Vengust, M., and Majdic, G. (2020). Stem cells in veterinary medicine: current state and treatment options. *Frontiers in Veterinary Science* 7: 278.

Wallace, H.A., Basehore, B.M., and Zito, P.M. (2022). *Wound Healing Phases*. Treasure Island, FL: StatPearls https://www.ncbi.nlm.nih.gov/books/NBK470443/.

Wangler, S., Kamali, A., Wapp, C. et al. (2021). Uncovering the secretome of mesenchymal stromal cells exposed to healthy, traumatic, and degenerative intervertebral discs: a proteomic analysis. *Stem Cell Research and Therapy* 12 (11): 1–7.

Woodley, K. (2018). Pet insurance for holistic and integrative practice. https://ivcjournal.com/pet-insurance-integrative-practices. (accessed 11 August 2021).

Yun, S., Ku, S.-K., and Kwon, Y.-S. (2016). Adipose-derived mesenchymal stem cells and platelet-rich plasma synergistically ameliorate the surgical-induced osteoarthritis in beagle dogs. *Journal of Orthopaedic Surgery and Research* 11: 9.

9

Trigger Point Therapy

CHAPTER MENU

Introduction

Trigger point therapy (TrPT) is an emerging and effective treatment modality for musculo-skeletal pain in veterinary patients. TrPT focuses on reducing, and ideally resolving, myofascial trigger points through manual techniques, therapeutic ultrasound, photobio-modulation, thermal techniques, dry needling, and trigger point injections.

The introduction of TrPT into a veterinary practice can be beneficial for both the patient and the health of the practice. The successful incorporation and utilization of TrPT does not end with the veterinarian's training. Support staff training and client education are crucial. This chapter discusses the what, why, how for effective integration of TrPT within your practice.

The What

Definition

TrPT refers to a group of treatment modalities used to reduce, and ideally resolve, the pain associated with myofascial trigger points. Therapeutic techniques include physical ther-apy (massage, stretching, ischemic compres-sion technique, taping, and neuromuscular techniques), therapeutic ultrasound, photobio-modulation, thermal techniques (hot and cold packs), dry needling, and trigger point injec-tion (Physiopedia 2016).

Human History

Guillaume de Baillou, a sixteenth-century French physician, was the first to write about

Integrative Medicine in Veterinary Practice, First Edition. Lisa P. McFaddin.
© 2024 John Wiley & Sons, Inc. Published 2024 by John Wiley & Sons, Inc.
Companion website: www.wiley.com/go/mcfaddin/integrativemedicine

disorders involving muscle pain (Shah et al. 2016). In 1816, Balfour, a British physician, described "thickenings" and "nodular tumors" within the muscle as a source of local and regional pain. In 1843, Robert Froriep, a German anatomist, described callouses within the muscle ("muskelshwiele") of people with rheumatic diseases (Shah et al. 2016). This condition was later defined as fibromyalgia.

In the mid-1900s, three physicians (Michael Gutstein of Germany, Michael Kelly of Australia, and J.H. Kellgren of Britain) working independently charted the areas of referred pain when hypertonic saline was injected into various fascia, tendons, and muscles (Shah et al. 2016). Janet G. Travell, an American physician, applied this information to the treatment of myofascial pain and trigger points. In the 1950s, Drs. Travell and Rinzler devised the term "myofascial trigger point" (Shah et al. 2016).

In 1955, Dr. Travell used her skills to dramatically reduce then-Senator John F. Kennedy's debilitating back pain following two failed back surgeries (McPartland 2004). Dr. Travell published over 40 papers on myofascial trigger points and co-wrote a two-volume book with Dr. David Simons, *Myofascial Pain and Dysfunction: The Trigger Point Manual* (McPartland 2004). This information serves as the foundation for future clinical applications and research pertaining to myofascial pain syndromes (MPS) and trigger points.

Fast forward 40–50 years the National Association of Myofascial Trigger Point Therapists (NAMTPT) was established. This is a nonprofit organization "dedicated to increasing public awareness of and access to myofascial pain treatment" (NAMTPT 2020). The NAMTPT offers continuing education (CE) for its members.

TrPT is well known among osteopathic physicians, chiropractors, physical therapists, and massage therapists. The diagnosis of MPS and trigger points are gaining traction in mainstream human medicine, especially as research demonstrates significant reduction of pain through the application of TrPT.

Veterinary History

Dr. LA Janssens (1991) was the first veterinarian to describe MPS in a retrospective study of 48 dogs (Janssens 1991). Dr. Janssens observed the palpation of trigger points in various muscles elicited pain responses and needling or injection of local anesthetic into the trigger points improved pain in 60% of the dogs (Janssens 1991).

Unfortunately, there have been limited studies assessing the efficacy of TrPT in veterinary medicine. That being said TrPT is well known by veterinarians practicing rehabilitation and integrative therapies. TrPT is discussed in most acupuncture and spinal manipulation certification programs. Additionally, the International Veterinary Academy of Pain Management (IVAPM) considers the identification and appropriate treatment of trigger points a valuable skill in the management of pain (IVAPM 2020).

Mirroring human medicine, TrPT is an up and coming field of study and practical pain management in veterinary patients. Interest in these techniques continues to grow as benefits are continually demonstrated in all species.

Terminology

There are a lot of terms used when discussing muscle conditions and treatments. A basic understanding of these terms is crucial, allowing effective communication amongst veterinary professionals and with clients.

Afferent: Signals or nerve cells (neurons) sending information <u>toward</u> the central nervous system.

Autonomic nervous system (ANS): Contains components of the central nervous system (CNS) and peripheral nervous system (PNS) which function to control involuntary activity, maintain homeostasis, and react to stress (Darby 2014). The ANS is divided into the sympathetic and parasympathetic nervous systems.

Concentric muscle contraction: A type of isotonic (normal) contraction in which muscle tension increases as the muscle shortens (Padulo et al. 2013).

Eccentric muscle contraction: A type of isotonic (normal) contraction in which muscle elongates under tension (Padulo et al. 2013).

Efferent: Signals or nerve cells (neurons) sending information away from the central nervous system.

Facilitation: Increased nerve cell (neuronal) stimulation causing hyperactive responses.

Fascia: A band of connective tissue composed primarily of collagen, covering and separating muscles, tendons, ligaments, joint capsules, blood vessels, nerves, and internal organs (Evans and Lahunta 2013). The terms deep fascia or myofascia are used when referring to the connective tissue surrounding individual muscle groups.

Isometric muscle contraction: There is no change in muscle length as tension (aka contraction) increases (Padulo et al. 2013).

Isotonic muscle contraction: There is change in muscle length as tension (aka contraction) increases (Padulo et al. 2013).

Jump sign: A behavioral response involving an involuntary movement or jerk of the head or limb, and often vocalization, after digital palpation of a trigger point (Al-Shenqiti and Oldham 2005). The reaction represents a disproportionate pain response when pressure is applied to a trigger point (Al-Shenqiti and Oldham 2005).

Local twitch response: Mechanical stimulation of the trigger point, most commonly needling, results in a visible or palpable contraction of the muscle and skin. This is most often observed when needling the trigger point (Perreault et al. 2017).

Motor neurons: Nerve cells transmitting information from the brain and spinal cord to muscles and some glands (Purves et al. 2012a).

Myalgia: Muscle pain.

Myofascia (aka deep fascia): The connective tissue sheath surrounding and passing between muscles. The myofascia is particularly thick in the limbs. For some muscles the myofascia takes the place of a tendon (aponeurosis) attaching to the outside of the bone (periosteum) at the origin or insertion of the muscle (Evans and Lahunta 2013).

Myofascial pain: Pain associated with one or multiple muscles and surrounding fascia.

Myofascial pain syndrome (MPS): A chronic condition in people affecting a specific area or areas of muscle and the surrounding fascia (Akamatsu et al. 2015; Shah et al. 2016). Associated clinical signs include the presence of one or more trigger point(s), regional pain, ± referred pain, increased tension, and reduced flexibility (Akamatsu et al. 2015; Shah et al. 2016). MPS is classified as a separate disorder from fribromyalgia, tendonitis, and bursitis.

Neuron (aka nerve cell): A cell capable of electrical excitability which sends signals to other cells over long distances (Purves et al. 2012c).

Neuropathic pain: Pathologic pain caused by damage or injury to nerves responsible for transferring information from the body (peripheral nervous system) to the spinal cord or brain (central nervous system).

Neuroplasticity: Ability of the nervous system to reorganize and create new synaptic connections within the central nervous system (Jackman and Regehr 2017; Maltese et al. 2019). Typically used to describe the brain's ability to learn and heal following injury, but the concept can also be applied to the spinal cord (Maltese et al. 2019).

Neurotransmitters: A chemical released at the end of a neuron whose release is triggered by an action potential (Nolte 2009). Neurotransmitters serve to stimulate other cells (nerve, muscle) or structures.

Nociception: Detection and communication of noxious stimuli by the nervous system.

Nociceptors (aka free nerve endings): Sensory nerves stimulated by damaging or noxious stimuli which send information to the central nervous system where the information is interpreted as pain (Purves et al. 2012b).

Nociceptive pain: Physiologic pain caused by damage to the body and is typically well localized and temporary.

Noxious stimulus: A signal which is damaging or threatening to normal tissue.

Parasympathetic nervous system ("rest and digest"): Sends signals from the brain and spinal cord to the internal organs ensuring normal day-to-day function.

Proprioception: Perception or awareness of the body and limb positions in space (Purves et al. 2012c).

Referred pain: Pain perceived in site distant from the painful stimulus or origin of the pain (Physiopedia 2016).

Referred pain maps have been created for human trigger points and visceral pain.

Sensory neuron: Nerve cells which respond to stimuli (touch, sound, light, and temperature changes) and send information to the spinal cord or brain (Purves et al. 2012b).

Stretch and hold: The application of a sustained stretch to a tight muscle with the intent of passively inducing muscle relaxation.

Sympathetic nervous system ("fight or flight"): Sends signals from the brain and spinal cord to the internal organs in times of stress.

Trigger point (TrP, aka myofascial trigger point): A hyperirritable palpable nodule or taut band within the skeletal muscle or associated fascia (Finando 2005). Direct manipulation of the nodule or band will elicit a disproportionately painful response locally and often distantly (referred pain) (Finando 2005).

Muscular Anatomy Fundamentals

Anatomy, physiology, and neurology lay the groundwork for understanding and applying veterinary TrPT. Anatomy is a branch of science focusing on the bodily structure of living organisms. The veterinarian must have a deep understanding of anatomy and functional physiology to effectively identify TrPs and potential areas of referred pain. Without this foundation the patient may not respond favorably and there is potential risk of injury. Tables 9.1 and 9.2 provides a list of the common muscles in which TrPs are found, as well as information regarding the muscle's origin, insertion, innervation, and function. More detailed information on the anatomy and physiology of TrPT can be found in the following sections.

Muscle Anatomy for Veterinarians

Table 9.1 lists the primary muscles affecting the canine head, neck, and thoracic limbs. Table 9.2 lists the primary muscles affecting the canine pelvic limbs. Additional information can be found in the recommended reference books.

Muscle Physiology Fundamentals

Physiology is the branch of science focusing on the function of living organisms and their parts. The veterinarian must understand how TrPT directly affects the patient's body as whole down to the cellular level. TrPT has direct effects on nerves, muscles, connective tissue, blood flow, hormones, and the immune system.

Muscle Physiology for Veterinarians

Skeletal muscle is the muscle of interest when discussing myofascial pain and TrPs. While in-depth discussion of muscle physiology is beyond the scope of this book, a summary of the cellular components, blood supply, and innervation of muscles is provided.

Cellular Components

Skeletal (aka striated, voluntary, or somatic) muscles are the primary contractile organs responsible for movement within the body and account for 33–50% of the total body weight of mammals (Evans and Lahunta 2013). Each muscle is composed of long, cylindrical multinucleated muscle fibers (myofibers) housed in connective tissue sheaths (Pasquini et al. 2003). Within each myofiber there are hundreds to thousands of parallel myofibrils which attach to each other through cross-striations. Myofibrils are composed of hundreds of thick (myosin) and thin (actin) myofilaments mixed with other proteins (Evans and Lahunta 2013).

Actin and myosin group together in longitudinally repeating units, bordered by anchors (Z-line), called sarcomeres (McCuller et al. 2022). The specific arrangement of actin and myosin creates the microscopic, striated appearance of muscle. During muscle contraction the H-band and I-band shorten, but the A-band maintains its length (McCuller et al. 2022). Figure 9.1 illustrates the arrangement of sarcomeres within myofibrils.

Connective tissue or fascia is interwoven and surrounds all skeletal muscle. Connective tissue attachments are either cord-like (tendon) or flat sheet-like (aponeurosis) and anchor skeletal muscles to bone and cartilage at their origin and insertion (Evans and Lahunta 2013). Figure 9.2 illustrates the organization and nomenclature of the various fascia associated with skeletal muscle.

Blood Supply

Skeletal muscle vasculature is quite impressive and extensive due to the high metabolic rate of muscle cells. Arteries enter the muscles at specific locations and frequently anastomose within the muscle (Evans and Lahunta 2013). As a result, there are abundant capillaries within each muscle fiber, ensuring adequate oxygen distribution throughout the entire muscle. Both lymphatics and veins follow a similar course as the arteries. Muscle contractions are responsible for pushing blood through venules and into larger veins (Evans and Lahunta 2013).

Innervation

The nervous supply of skeletal muscles accompanies the blood vessels and lymphatics. Both sensory and motor neurons are present in approximately equal proportions within muscles (Evans and Lahunta 2013).

Efferent motor neurons terminate at motor endplates on muscle fibers, called the neuromuscular junction (Purves et al. 2012a). A single alpha motor neuron innervates the extrafusal fibers within a muscle, called a

Table 9.1 The primary muscles affecting the canine head, neck, and thoracic limbs. The origin, insertion, innervation, and primary function(s) are provided (Pasquini et al. 2003; Marcellin-Little et al. 2007; Evans and Lahunta 2013).

Temporalis	Origin:	Temporal fossa
	Insertion:	Coronoid process of the mandible
	Innervation:	Cranial nerve V3 (third branch of the trigeminal nerve)
	Function:	Close the jaw (flex the temporomandibular joint)
Masseter	Origin:	Zygomatic arch
	Insertion:	Masseteric fossa and angular process of the mandible
	Innervation:	Cranial nerve V3 (third branch of the trigeminal nerve)
	Function:	Close the jaw (flex the temporomandibular joint)
Splenius	Origin:	Median raphe of the first/second thoracic vertebrae
	Insertion:	Nuchal crest and mastoid part of the temporal bone
	Innervation:	Segmental nerves
	Function:	Support the head; cervical dorsiflexion
Scalenus	Origin:	Ventral vertebral bodies of the third/fourth through seventh cervical vertebrae
	Insertion:	Transverse process of the fifth through seventh cervical vertebrae and the first four to five ribs
	Innervation:	Segmental nerves
	Function:	Cervical ventroflexion and ventrolateral flexion
Rhomboideus	Origin:	Median fibrous raphe fifth cervical through eighth thoracic vertebrae
	Insertion:	Dorsomedial border of the scapula
	Innervation:	Segmental nerves
	Function:	Elevate the scapula dorsomedially
Brachiocephalicus	Origin:	Occiput and first cervical vertebrae (atlas)
	Insertion:	Distal one-third of the humerus
	Innervation:	Cranial nerve XI (spinal accessory nerve)
	Function:	Extend the shoulder joint; cervical ventroflexion

Omotransversarius	Origin:	Acromion
	Insertion:	Transverse process of the atlas
	Innervation:	Cranial nerve XI (spinal accessory nerve)
	Function:	Move the shoulder blade forward
Cervical trapezius	Origin:	Median raphe of the third cervical vertebrae to the first/second thoracic vertebrae
	Insertion:	Scapular spine and acromion
	Innervation:	Cranial nerve XI (spinal accessory nerve)
	Function:	Elevate the scapula dorsomedially
Sternocephalicus	Origin:	Cephalic region of the head
	Insertion:	Manubrium
	Innervation:	Cranial nerve XI (spinal accessory nerve)
	Function:	Cervical ventroflexion and ventrolateral flexion
Serratus ventralis	Origin:	Transverse processes of the last four cervical vertebrae through the ninth/tenth ribs
	Insertion:	Dorsomedial third of the scapula
	Innervation:	Long thoracic nerve
	Function:	Suspends the thorax between the forelimbs
Cranial pectorals	Origin:	Cranial third of the sternum
	Insertion:	Lateral proximal humerus
	Innervation:	Cranial pectoral nerve
	Function:	Adduct the forelimb
Caudal pectorals	Origin:	Ventrocaudal sternum
	Insertion:	Lateral proximal humerus
	Innervation:	Caudal pectoral nerve
	Function:	Adduct the forelimb
Latissimus dorsi	Origin:	Median raphe of the dorsal spinous process of the fifth/sixth thoracic vertebrae caudal to the fourth lumbar vertebrae
	Insertion:	Teres major tuberosity
	Innervation:	Thoracodorsal nerve
	Function:	Flex the shoulder joint
Supraspinatus	Origin:	Supraspinous fossa
	Insertion:	Greater tubercle of the humerus
	Innervation:	Suprascapular nerve
	Function:	Stabilize the shoulder joint; extend the shoulder joint

(Continued)

Table 9.1 (Continued)

Infraspinatus	Origin:	Infraspinous fossa
	Insertion:	Lesser tubercle of the humerus
	Innervation:	Suprascapular nerve
	Function:	Stabilize the shoulder joint; extend or flex the shoulder joint
Subscapularis	Origin:	Subscapular fossa
	Insertion:	Lesser tubercle of the humerus
	Innervation:	Subscapular nerve
	Function:	Stabilize the shoulder joint; adduct the shoulder
Deltoideus	Origin:	Scapular spine and acromion
	Insertion:	Deltoid tuberosity
	Innervation:	Axillary nerve
	Function:	Flex the shoulder joint; stabilize the shoulder joint; abducts the forelimb
Teres major	Origin:	Dorsocaudal border of the scapula
	Insertion:	Teres major tuberosity
	Innervation:	Axillary nerve
	Function:	Flex the shoulder joint; stabilize the shoulder joint; shoulder joint rotation
Teres minor	Origin:	Infraglenoid tubercle and distal third of the caudal scapular border
	Insertion:	Teres minor tuberosity
	Innervation:	Axillary nerve
	Function:	Flex the shoulder joint; stabilize the shoulder joint; shoulder joint rotation
Biceps brachii	Origin:	Supraglenoid tubercle
	Insertion:	Ulnar and radial tuberosities
	Innervation:	Musculocutaneous nerve
	Function:	Flex the elbow joint; extend the shoulder joint
Brachialis	Origin:	Proximal third of the lateral surface of the humerus
	Insertion:	Ulnar and radial tuberosities
	Innervation:	Musculocutaneous nerve
	Function:	Flex the elbow joint
Triceps	Origin:	Caudal edge of the scapula and humerus
	Insertion:	Olecranon tuber
	Innervation:	Radial nerve
	Function:	Extend the elbow joint

Anconeus	Origin:	Distal half of the caudal humerus
	Insertion:	Lateral surface of the proximal ulna
	Innervation:	Radialis nerve
	Function:	Extends the elbow joint; helps tense the antebrachial fascia
Extensor carpi radialis	Origin:	Lateral epicondyle of the humerus
	Insertion:	Dorsal surface of the base of the second and third metacarpals
	Innervation:	Radial nerve
	Function:	Extend the carpal joint
Common digital extensor	Origin:	Lateral epicondyle of the humerus
	Insertion:	Extensor process of the second through fifth distal phalanges
	Innervation:	Radial nerve
	Function:	Extend the carpal joint; extend the digits
Lateral digital extensor	Origin:	Lateral epicondyle of the humerus
	Insertion:	Proximal ends of the third through fifth phalanges
	Innervation:	Radial nerve
	Function:	Extend the carpal joint; extend the digits
Extensor carpi ulnaris	Origin:	Lateral epicondyle of the humerus
	Insertion:	Lateral aspect of the proximal end of the fifth metacarpal and accessory carpal bones
	Innervation:	Radial nerve
	Function:	Extend the carpal joint; extend the digits; abduct the paw
Flexor carpi radialis	Origin:	Medial epicondyle of the humerus and medial border of the radius
	Insertion:	Palmar side of the second and third metacarpals
	Innervation:	Medial nerve
	Function:	Flex the carpal joint
Superficial digital flexor	Origin:	Medial epicondyle of the humerus
	Insertion:	Palmar surfaces of the middle phalanges of the second through the fifth digits
	Innervation:	Median nerve
	Function:	Flex the carpal joint; flex the digits

(Continued)

Table 9.1 (Continued)

Deep digital flexor	Origin:	Medial epicondyle of the humerus
	Insertion:	Distal phalanx of the third through fifth digits
	Innervation:	Ulnar nerve
	Function:	Flex the carpal joint; flex the digits
Flexor carpi ulnaris	Origin:	Medial epicondyle of the humerus
	Insertion:	Accessory carpal bone
	Innervation:	Ulnar nerve
	Function:	Flex the carpal joint

Source: Lisa P. McFaddin.

Table 9.2 The primary muscles affecting the canine pelvic limbs. The origin, insertion, innervation, and primary function(s) are provided (Pasquini et al. 2003; Marcellin-Little et al. 2007; Evans and Lahunta 2013).

Superficial gluteal	Origin:	Fascia of the sacrococcygeal region
	Insertion:	Third trochanter of the femur
	Innervation:	Caudal gluteal nerve
	Function:	Extend the hip joint; abduct the pelvic limb
Middle gluteal	Origin:	Iliac crest
	Insertion:	Greater trochanter of the femur
	Innervation:	Cranial gluteal nerve
	Function:	Extend the hip joint
Deep gluteal	Origin:	Body of the ilium
	Insertion:	Greater trochanter of the femur
	Innervation:	Cranial gluteal nerve
	Function:	Extend the hip joint; abduct the pelvic limb
Tensor fascia latae	Origin:	Tuber coxae
	Insertion:	Fascia of the lateral femur and tibial crest
	Innervation:	Cranial gluteal nerve
	Function:	Flex the hip joint; stabilize the hip; abduct the hip
Piriformis	Origin:	Sacrum and first coccygeal vertebrae
	Insertion:	Greater trochanter of the femur
	Innervation:	Cranial gluteal nerve
	Function:	Extend the hip joint

Biceps femoris	Origin:	Sacrotuberous ligament
	Insertion:	Cranial one-third of the tibia and calcaneus
	Innervation:	Sciatic nerve
	Function:	Extend the hip joint; flex the stifle joint; extend the tibiotarsal joint
Semitendinosus	Origin:	Ischiatic tuberosity
	Insertion:	Craniomedial tibia and calcaneus
	Innervation:	Sciatic nerve
	Function:	Extend the hip joint; flex the stifle joint; extend the tibiotarsal joint
Semimembranosus	Origin:	Ischiatic tuberosity and medial aspect of the ischium
	Insertion:	Mediodistal femurs and proximal tibia
	Innervation:	Sciatic nerve
	Function:	Extend the hip joint; flex the stifle joint
Rectus femoris	Origin:	Cranial acetabulum
	Insertion:	Patellar tendon
	Innervation:	Femoral nerve
	Function:	Extend the stifle joint; flex the hip joint
Vastus group (lateralis, intermedius, and medialis)	Origin:	Proximal femur
	Insertion:	Patellar tendon
	Innervation:	Femoral nerve
	Function:	Extend the stifle joint
Sartorius	Origin:	Tuber coxae and ventral iliac crest
	Insertion:	Medial proximal aspect of the stifle and fascia of the cranial tibia
	Innervation:	Femoral nerve
	Function:	Flex the hip joint; adduct the pelvic limb; cranial belly extend the stifle joint; caudal belly flex the stifle joint
Iliopsoas group	Origin:	Eleventh through 13th thoracic vertebrae; interdigitates with the diaphragm
	Insertion:	Lesser trochanter of the femur
	Innervation:	Femoral nerve
	Function:	Flex the hip joint; assist flexion of the lumbar spine

(Continued)

Table 9.2 (Continued)

Pectineus		
	Origin:	Pubic symphysis
	Insertion:	Distal medial femur
	Innervation:	Obturator nerve
	Function:	Adduct the pelvic limb; stabilize the hip
Adductor	Origin:	Pubic symphysis
	Insertion:	Lateral and caudal femur
	Innervation:	Obturator nerve
	Function:	Adduct the pelvic limb
Gracilis	Origin:	Pubic symphysis
	Insertion:	Cranial border of the tibia; calcaneus
	Innervation:	Obturator nerve
	Function:	Adduct the pelvic limb; stabilize the stifle joint; flex the stifle joint; extend the hock joint; extend the hip joint
Gastrocnemius	Origin:	Distal medial and lateral caudal femur
	Insertion:	Calcaneus
	Innervation:	Tibial nerve
	Function:	Extend the hock joint; flex the stifle joint
Popliteus	Origin:	Caudolateral femoral condyle
	Insertion:	Proximal quarter of the tibia
	Innervation:	Tibial nerve
	Function:	Stabilize the stifle joint; internally rotate the tibia
Superficial digital flexor	Origin:	Distal femur
	Insertion:	Calcaneus; middle second through fifth phalanges
	Innervation:	Tibial nerve
	Function:	Flex the digits; extend the hock joint
Deep digital flexor	Origin:	Proximal caudal tibia and fibula
	Insertion:	Plantar surface of P3 on the second through fifth digits
	Innervation:	Tibial nerve
	Function:	Flex the digits

Cranial tibialis	Origin:	Proximal craniolateral tibia
	Insertion:	Plantar surface of the base of the first and second metatarsus
	Innervation:	Fibular nerve
	Function:	Flex the hock joint; rotate the paw laterally
Long digital extensor	Origin:	Extensor fossa of the ventral aspect of the lateral femoral condyle
	Insertion:	Extensor process of P3 on the second through fifth digits
	Innervation:	Fibular nerve
	Function:	Extend the digits
Peroneus longus	Origin:	Lateral femoral condyle and tibial condyle; proximal fibula
	Insertion:	Proximal plantar aspect and proximal aspect of the metatarsals
	Innervation:	Fibular nerve
	Function:	Flex the hock joint; rotate the paw laterally
Lateral digital extensor	Origin:	Proximal caudal tibia
	Insertion:	Extensor process of P3 on the second through fifth digits
	Innervation:	Fibular nerve
	Function:	Extend the digits

Source: Lisa P. McFaddin.

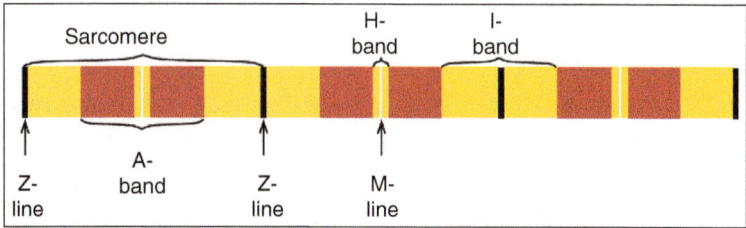

Figure 9.1 A schematic representation of the organization of sarcomeres within a myofibril. Z-lines (the terminal boundary of the sarcomere) function to anchor the actin filaments. M-lines (the central line within the sarcomere) anchor the myosin filaments. H-bands comprise myosin only, are in the center of the sarcomere, and contain the M-line. A-bands consist of myosin filaments, are the largest portion of the sarcomere, and include areas of actin–myosin overlap. I-bands cover the terminal region of each sarcomere and contain only actin myofilaments (McCuller et al. 2022). Source: *Richfield, David (2014)*. "Medical gallery of David Richfield." *WikiJournal of Medicine 1(2)*. DOI:10.15347/wjm/2014.009. ISSN 2002-4436.

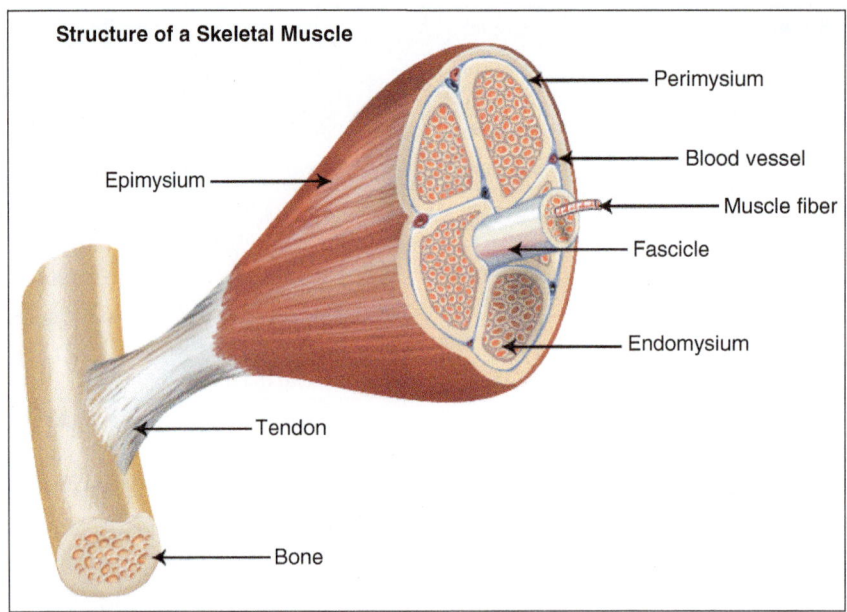

Figure 9.2 An illustration of the structure of skeletal muscle. The outermost connective tissue layer covering the whole muscle is called the epimysium. The perimysium covers a group of muscle fibers called fascicles. The endomysium is a thin sheath of connective tissue covering each individual muscle fiber. Source U.S. Department of Health and Human Services, https://training.seer.cancer.gov/images/anatomy/muscular/muscle_structure.jpg/ last accessed June 14, 2023/Public Domian CC BY 4.0.

motor unit. Each alpha motor neuron sends numerous branches to synapse on multiple extrafusal fibers throughout the muscle (Purves et al. 2012a). This redundancy ensures adequate contractile force throughout the muscle and protects the muscle if some of the motor branches are damaged (Purves et al. 2012a).

Physiologically there are three types of motor units slow motor units, fast fatigable motor units, and fast fatigue-resistant motor units. Slow motor units are small, slow to contract, generate little force during contraction, are resistant to fatigue, used for sustained muscle contraction, and associated with "red" muscle fibers due to their high myoglobin content and extensive capillary beds (Purves et al. 2012a). Fast fatigable motor units are innervated by larger diameter alpha motor neurons, associated with larger paler muscles, contract quickly,

generate a lot of force during contraction, and fatigue within a few seconds (Purves et al. 2012a). Fast fatigue-resistant motor units are intermediate in size, speed of contraction, force of contraction, and resistance to fatigue (Purves et al. 2012a).

The primary afferent sensory receptors found within muscles include free nerve endings, muscle spindle cells (MSC), and Golgi tendon organs (GTO). Table 9.3 summarizes the classification and primary function of these receptors.

Nociceptors are classified as either A-delta (Aδ) group (lightly myelinated axons with conduction velocities of 5–30 m/s) or C fiber group (unmyelinated axons with conduction velocities of 2 m/s) (Purves et al. 2012b). Aδ nociceptors are further divided into type I Aδ (respond to truly noxious chemical and mechanical stimuli) and type II Aδ (respond to exposure to heat) (Purves et al. 2012b). C fiber nociceptors

Table 9.3 The classification and primary function of the main afferent sensory receptors within muscles (Purves et al. 2012; Purves et al. 2012b,c; Zhu 2014).

Receptor type	Classification	Primary function
Free sensory nerve endings	Nociceptors	Respond to damaging stimuli and their activation results in pain
Muscle spindle cells	Mechanoreceptors	Stretch receptors within muscles assessing muscle length
Golgi tendon organs	Mechanoreceptors	Measure muscle tension at the origin and insertion during concentric contraction

Source: Lisa P. McFaddin.

are considered polymodal, responding to all forms of noxious stimuli.

Nociceptor cell bodies are primarily located in the dorsal horn of the spinal cord. C nerve fiber first order neurons terminate in the laminae I (marginal zone) and II (substantia gelatinosa) of the dorsal horn of the spinal cord (Yam et al. 2018). Aδ first-order neurons from the periphery enter the spinal cord through Lissauer's tract, travel cranial or caudally for three to four spinal segments then enter laminae II (substantia gelatinous) connecting to a second-order neuron (Purves et al. 2012b).

Once in the substantia gelatinosa a portion of the sensory information crosses midline below the central canal entering the spinothalamic tract, a set of sensory tracts located in the ventral funiculus of the spinal cord white matter (Purves et al. 2012b). Within the substantia gelatinosa inhibitory interneurons are also stimulated blocking the transmission of nociceptive information to the higher centers of the brain (Purves et al. 2012b; Mittleman and

Gaynor 2000). This local inhibition of pain is known as Melzack and Wall's Gate Theory.

Most of the sensory information then travels to the ipsilateral thalamus. The thalamus is a gate through which all sensory information travels, except olfaction. The spinothalamic tract terminates at a third-order neuron where most information travels to the somatosensory region of the ipsilateral cortex, parietal lobe (Purves et al. 2012b). On the way to the thalamus branches are sent to several connections in the midbrain, especially the periaqueductal gray matter (PAG) and rostral ventral medulla (RVM) (Yam et al. 2018).

The PAG helps regulate the response to nociceptive input integrating information from the higher brain centers, including the cortex, and the dorsal horn of the spinal cord. The RVM downregulates excitatory information from the dorsal horn of the spinal cord. Both the PAG and RVM express a variety of neurotransmitters (endogenous opioids and cannabinoids, 5-hydroxytryptamine, and norepinephrine) heavily involved in the regulation and recognition of pain (Yam et al. 2018).

Trigger Point Physiology

TrP Characteristics

A trigger point (also called myofascial trigger point) is a hyperirritable palpable nodule or taut band within the skeletal muscle or associated fascia (Finando 2005). Direct manipulation of the nodule or band will elicit a disproportionately painful response locally and often distantly (referred pain) (Finando 2005).

Wall (2010, 2019) described the classic characteristics of TrPs in veterinary patients as having the following characteristics (summarized in Figure 9.3): a tight band or nodule within the muscle which causes marked pain upon palpation; visible or palpable contraction of the muscle during TrP palpation (local twitch response, LTR); weakness of the affected

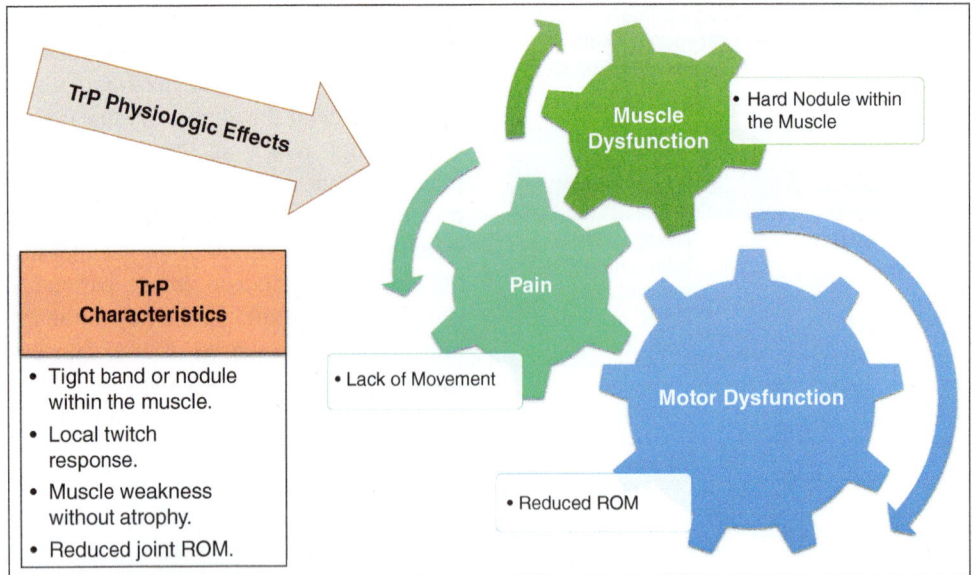

Figure 9.3 The common characteristics and physiologic effects of trigger points (TrPs). ROM, range of motion. Source: Lisa P. McFaddin.

muscle, without atrophy; and reduced range of motion of the associated joint.

A "jump sign" is commonly seen after palpation of a TrP in both humans and dogs. Common responses associated with a "jump sign" in dogs include a quick turn of the head toward the painful stimuli, attempting to move away from the stimuli, attempting to bite, and vocalization (crying, whining, barking, growling, and yelping) (Wall 2010).

Referred pain is a common characteristic of TrP in people but cannot be easily assessed in veterinary patients (Wall 2010). Abnormal behaviors such as licking, biting, scratching, and chewing at a specific area of the body or limbs may represent referred pain in canine and feline patients.

TrP Formation

Microscopic changes to the intricate systems involved in muscle contraction lead to TrP formation. These alterations are outlined in Figure 9.4. Specifically, changes in areas where the nerve and muscle fibers meet (the neuromuscular junction) lead to improper communication between the nerves and muscles, causing excessive contraction of certain muscle fibers (Bron and Dommerholt 2012). If enough neighboring fibers become dysfunctional, a taut band can develop within the muscle belly (Bron and Dommerholt 2012). Figure 9.5 illustrates an example of the gross location and microscopic changes associated with TrPs.

Once formed, the presence of the TrP itself causes mechanical stress within the muscle and to other muscles serving similar functions. TrPs also cause pain and reduce range of motion which can lead to postural changes and chronic lameness reinforcing the presence of the TrP (Bron and Dommerholt 2012). Overuse and trauma are the primary causes of TrP formation in both people and animals (Simons 1983). Additional propagating factors for TrP in people include postural changes, chronic lameness, postoperative pain, postoperative trauma, neuropathy, degenerative joint disease, osteoarthritis, joint dysfunction, other

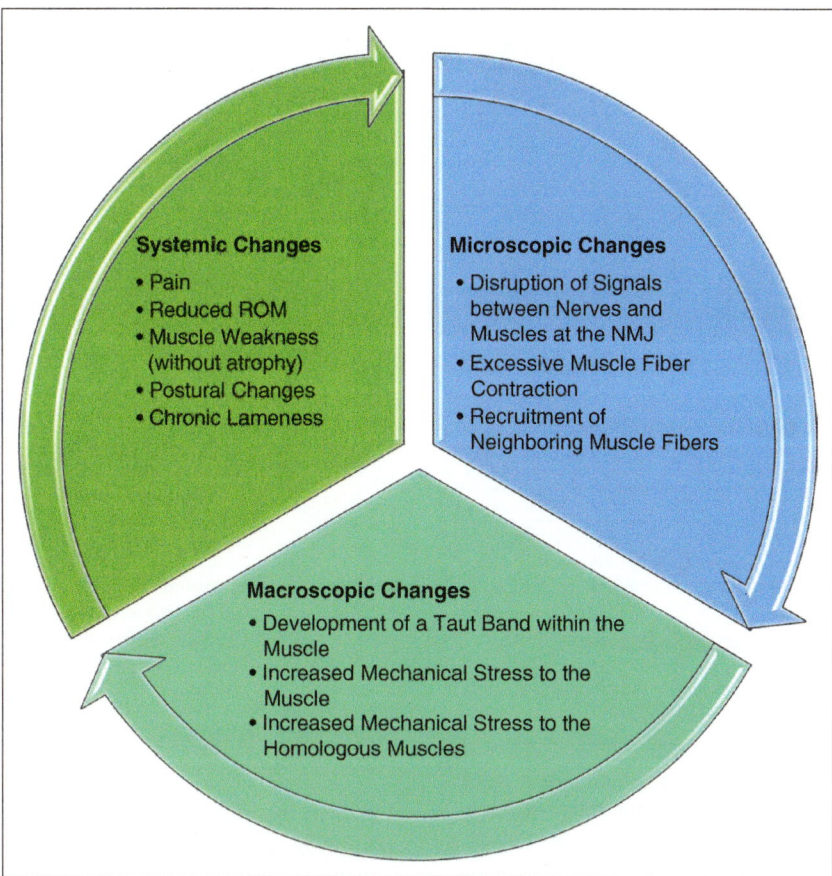

Figure 9.4 The multifactor process of trigger point (TrP) formation divided into microscopic and macroscopic muscular changes, as well as systemic changes. The process of TrP formation is self-driving and cyclical. NMJ, neuromuscular junction; ROM, range of motion. Source: Lisa P. McFaddin.

causes of chronic pain, nutritional deficiencies, endocrine disorders, metabolic derangements, nerve impingement, and visceral-somatic pain (McPartland 2004; Dommerholt 2011). Table 9.4 lists many of the conditions leading to the development of TrPs in veterinary patients (Wall 2019).

Muscle weakness is associated with TrPs without accompanying muscle atrophy or loss (Bron and Dommerholt 2012). TrP are believed to interfere with muscle activation, as demonstrated by the restoration of muscle strength with resolution or inactivation of the TrP (Bron and Dommerholt 2012). The presence of TrP within one muscle can also affect the contractile forces (function and strength) of other muscles (Jafri 2014).

TrP Classification

TrPs are classified as either active or latent. Active TrPs cause spontaneous pain even when not directly manipulated; latent TrPs only cause pain when direct pressure is applied (Bron and Dommerholt 2012; Shah et al. 2016). Both active and latent TrPs cause muscle dysfunction (stiffness and reduced range of motion), and both appear anatomically similar (Bron and Dommerholt 2012). It remains unclear why some TrPs are active while others are latent, and why some TrPs change between

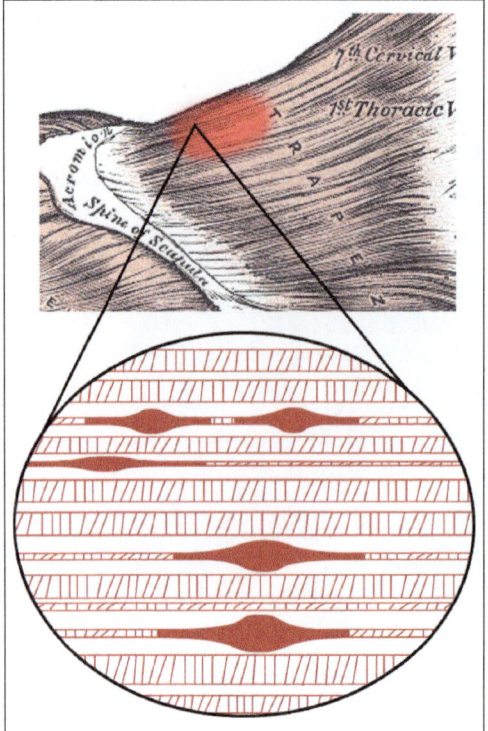

Figure 9.5 Schematic diagram of a trigger point in a human trapezius muscle. The solid red areas represent trigger points within the muscle fibers. Source: Davidparmenter. https://commons. wikimedia.org/wiki/File:Trigger_Point_Complex. jpg#globalusage February 17 2014.

Table 9.4 A list of many of the conditions responsible for the development of trigger points in veterinary patients (Wall 2010, 2019; Shah et al. 2016; Kitchens 2016).

Category	Examples
Trauma	Blunt-force; falling; slipping; sprain; strain
Overuse	Poorly conditioned athletes; repetitive stress injury; weekend warrior
Neurologic	Ataxia; intervertebral disk disease; myopathies
Orthopedic	Any orthopedic surgery; cruciate ligament ligament injury; developmental orthopedic diseases; fractures; lameness; osteoarthritis
Other	Hormone disorders; overweight or obesity; viscero-somatic pain (intestinal disorders, bladder stones, feline lower urinary tract disorder)

Source: Lisa P. McFaddin.

the two states. Distinguishing between active and latent TrPs is almost impossible in veterinary medicine because trigger point diagnosis depends, in large part, on palpating a band within the muscle. Once the TrP is palpated, pain is elicited regardless of whether the TrP caused pain without being touched.

TrP Diagnosis

Veterinarians are not routinely taught how to properly assess for TrPs or myalgia, in general. Careful palpation with an intimate knowledge of anatomy is required. There are two fundamental palpation techniques: flat palpation and pincer palpation. Both techniques utilize the sensitive sensory nerve endings and receptors within the fingertips to detect the taut bands in the muscle fibers. Figures 9.6 and 9.7 demonstrate these techniques.

Palpation can be performed with patients standing or gently restrained in a recumbent (non-weight-bearing) position. Most anti-gravity muscles are tense while standing, making the taut bands within TrP difficult to find. Muscle tension can be reduced by lifting the limb during palpation or laying the patient on their side. Muscle spasms are often more easily appreciated while patients are standing.

Client education is critical. The goal is to identify areas of discomfort so they can be treated. Unfortunately, our veterinary patients do not understand they may experience some pain to help them. If palpation elicits a jump sign an uneducated and unwarned client may assume their pet is being harmed.

Interestingly, in human medicine "there is no accepted reference standard for the diagnosis of trigger points, and data on the reliability of physical examination for trigger points is

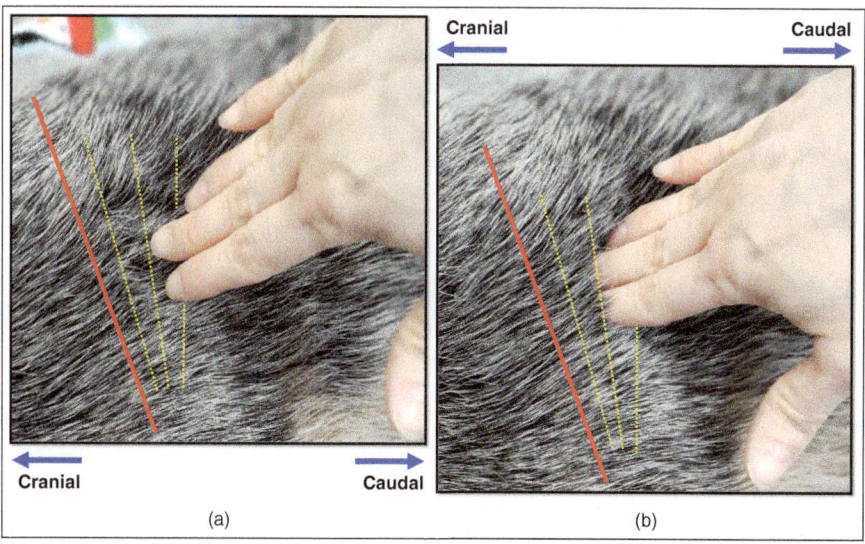

Figure 9.6 Demonstration of the flat palpation technique for myalgia and trigger points. (a) The alignment of the fingers prior to contact with the fur and skin. (b) The application of steady downward digital pressure onto the muscle fibers of the infraspinatus. The muscle is supported medially (underneath) by the scapula or shoulder blade. The red line represents the approximate location of the scapular spine, while the dotted yellow lines represent the direction of the infraspinatus muscle fibers. The patient is laying on their right side (right lateral recumbency), and the blue arrows mark the direction toward the head (cranial) and tail (caudal). Source: Lisa P. McFaddin.

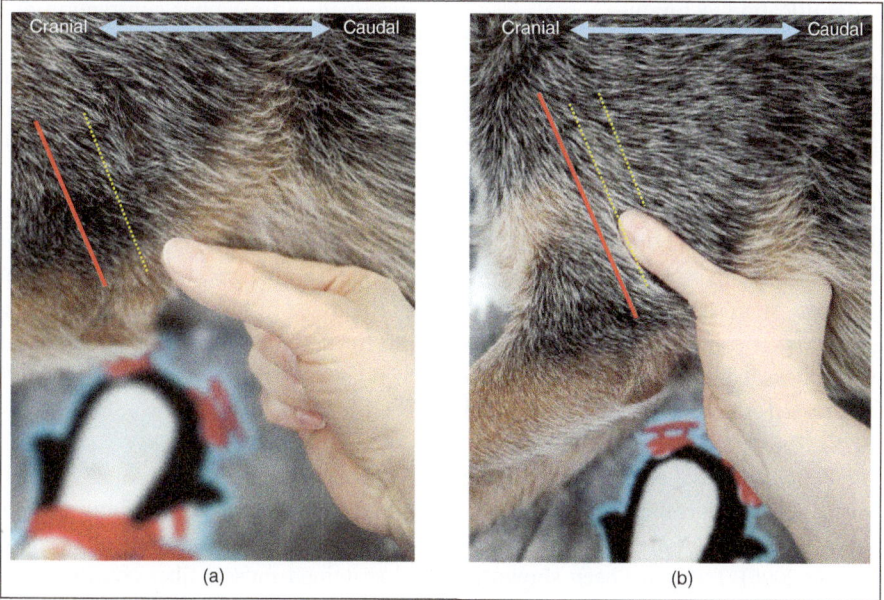

Figure 9.7 Demonstration of the pincer palpation technique for myalgia and trigger points. (a) The proper positioning of the thumb and index finger. (b) How the pincer grasp can be used to palpate part of the triceps muscle, with the thumb on the outside (lateral) and the index finger on the inside (medial) of the left front limb. The red line represents the approximate location of the humerus bone. The dotted yellow lines represent the direction of the triceps muscle fibers. The patient is laying on their right side (right lateral recumbency), and the blue arrows mark the direction toward the head (cranial) and tail (caudal). Source: Lisa P. McFaddin.

conflicting" (Lucas et al. 2009). Studies have shown large discrepancies in inter-examiner detection of TrPs, with Lew et al. (1997) finding only 21% of examiners agreed on the presence and location of specific TrPs (Dunning et al. 2014). Other studies suggest experienced practitioners can reliably agree on the presence of TrPs but not the exact location (Myburgh et al. 2011). Sciotti et al. (2001) found an identification error rate of 3.3–66 cm (or 1.2–26 inches).

As of February 2023, there are no studies documenting the accuracy of TrP detection in veterinary patients. It is reasonable to assume the veterinary agreement and error rate is comparable, especially given the absence of verbal communication between patient and clinician (though an error rate of 26 inches in a Chihuahua would be near impossible). This is not to say TrPs cannot be identified or effectively treated in veterinary medicine. This does highlight the need for practitioners to hone their palpation skills and the need for standardized identification techniques.

TrP Physiology for Veterinarians

TrPs are anatomically defined as a taut linear band or stiff tender nodule of hardened muscle fibers within normal muscle which can produce local and referred pain, as well as potential stimulation of the ANS (Bron and Dommerholt 2012). The TrP itself is composed of numerous contraction knots. Microscopically, an individual contraction knot is composed of muscle fibers with hypercontracted sarcomeres with abnormally increased diameters (Simons and Stolov 1976).

The taut band runs parallel to normal muscle fibers. Formation of the contracted muscle fibers occurs without activation of the motor unit (Dommerholt 2006). TrPs have been shown to exhibit spontaneous electrical activity and affect the peripheral nervous system (sensory and motor) and ANS (Dommerholt 2006; Kitchens 2016).

Conversely, muscle spasms are muscle fibers which repeatedly contract due to increased neuromuscular tone (Mense 2008). Both TrPs and muscle spasms can occur with or without associated pain (Gerwin et al. 2004).

As mentioned previously, overuse and trauma are the primary causes of TrP development (McPartland 2004). These conditions lead to several myopathologic changes including low-level muscle contractions, uneven pressure within muscles, and inappropriate eccentric muscle contractions (Bron and Dommerholt 2012; Shah et al. 2016).

The underlying mechanisms responsible for TrP formation are complex and center around variations of Simon's integrative trigger point hypothesis (ITPH), also called the "energy crisis theory" (Simons 1983). Roughly, the expanded ITPH suggests muscle injury leads to vascular changes causing muscular ischemia and cell damage which acidifies the tissue, triggers the release of inflammatory mediators, and activates muscle nociceptors (Gerwin et al. 2004). The lowered pH causes increased and persistent acetylcholine (ACh), causing sustained muscle fiber contraction and eventual formation of a taut band or nodule. ACh and inflammatory mediators change the activity and sensitivity of the motor endplates and nociceptors resulting in potentiation and neuroplasticity (Gerwin et al. 2004).

Delving deeper, the ITPH can be broken down into three components: biochemical changes, circulatory changes, and neurologic changes, summarized in Figure 9.8. All the changes are interrelated causing both feed-forward and feed-back systems leading to the formation and persistence of TrPs.

Biochemical Changes

Muscle injury causes calcium accumulation outside of the sarcoplasmic reticulum resulting in sustained muscle fiber contraction (Simons and Stolov 1976). Additionally, excessive ACh release from dysfunctional motor endplates causes disproportionate muscle fiber contraction (Bron and Dommerholt 2012). Unlike normal skeletal muscle contractions, TrP formation and persistence do not rely on stimulation of

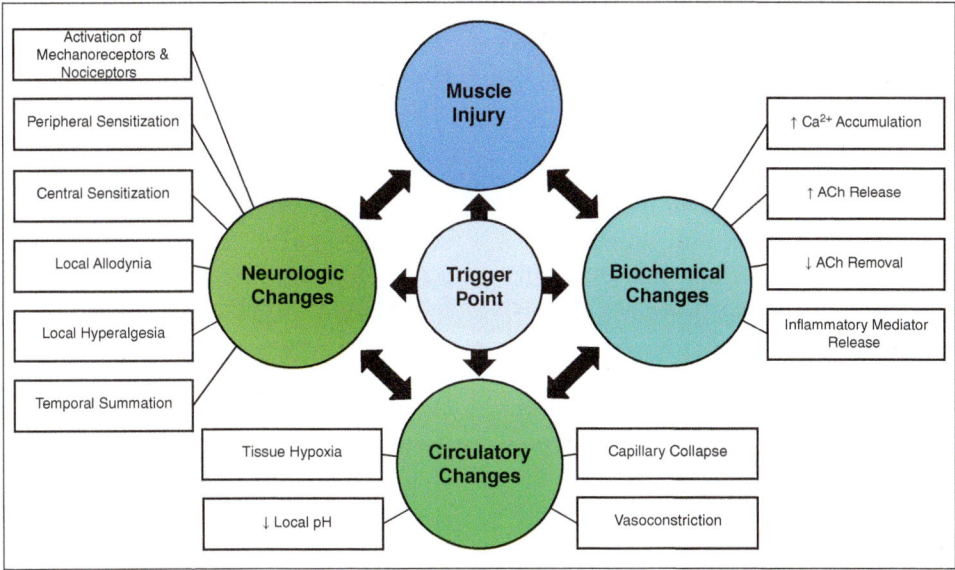

Figure 9.8 An overview of the complex and interwoven etiology of trigger point formation and continuation. This schematic is based on the expanded integrative trigger point hypothesis. Ca^{2+}, calcium; ACh, acetylcholine; ATP, adenosine triphosphate. Source: Lisa P. McFaddin.

alpha motor neurons, unlike normal skeletal muscle contractions (Dommerholt 2011).

Hypercontractility increases the muscle's metabolic demand and reduces the available energy sources, in the form of adenosine triphosphate (ATP) (McPartland 2004). The ATP-dependent calcium pump on the sarcoplasmic reticulum cannot restore calcium homeostasis perpetuating high local calcium concentrations and sustained muscle fiber contractions. Muscle injury also inhibits the removal of ACh from the postsynaptic ACh receptors by ACh (McPartland 2004). Inflammatory mediators (calcitonin gene related peptide [CGRP], substance P, bradykinins, cytokines, histamine, prostaglandins, and leukotrienes) released during muscle injury increase ACh release, prevent ACh breakdown, prime ACh receptors, and chemically activate and sensitize nociceptors (Gerwin et al. 2004).

Circulatory Changes

The mechanical stress of the TrP itself causes chronic muscle overload while also triggering capillary collapse and activation of nociceptors (Gerwin et al. 2004). Reduced oxygen supply further depletes available ATP and leads to the release of more inflammatory mediators and neuroreactive substances from oxygen-deprived tissues (Bron and Dommerholt 2012).

Under anaerobic conditions pyruvic acid, a breakdown product of glucose, is converted to lactic acid (Gerwin et al. 2004; McPartland 2004). Vasoconstriction prevents the dispersal of lactic acid lowering the pH. Acidic environments excite muscle nociceptors, downregulate acetylcholinesterase, increase ACh efficacy, and encourage sustained sarcomere contraction (Gerwin et al. 2004).

Neurologic Changes

The local tissue injury and subsequent release of inflammatory mediators and neuroactive substances causes sensitization of nociceptors (Gerwin et al. 2004). This peripheral sensitization is perpetuated by concomitant neurogenic inflammation, caused by retrograde neurotransmitter release by small-fiber unmyelinated afferents (Shah et al. 2016). Additionally, constant nociception bombardment of the dorsal horn leads to the release of more inflammatory mediators within the peripheral tissues (Gerwin et al. 2004).

Neurogenic inflammation creates a self-perpetuating cycle. The inflammatory mediators and neurotransmitters cause further inflammation and pain which, in turn, stimulates the production of even more inflammatory mediators and neurotransmitters (Gerwin et al. 2004). This cycle creates local allodynia and hyperalgesia worsening the pain associated with a TrP. Sustained afferent stimulation disrupts the normal function and response of the dorsal horn (aka central sensitization), leading to worsening hyperalgesia and temporal summation of pain (Shah et al. 2016).

Latent TrPs

The exact nature of latent TrPs is not well understood. Currently, the presence of subthreshold afferent signaling and ineffective synapses are thought to explain the lack of spontaneous pain, despite the presence of a physical trigger point, associated with latent TrPs (Dommerholt 2006; Shah et al. 2016).

Latent TrPs are constantly sending afferent information to the dorsal horn but, unlike active TrP, the excitatory information does not trigger an action potential within the dorsal horn allowing sensitization without eliciting pain (Mense 2010). Once the threshold of nociceptive information increases, for example with direct palpation of the latent TrP, pain is experienced.

The presence of ineffective or damaged synapses within the dorsal horn further reduces the chances nociceptive information is conveyed to the central nervous system. Palpation of a latent TrP increases the nociceptive signals basically overpowering the ineffective synapses resulting in the perception of pain (Mense 2010; Shah et al. 2016).

Similar to active TrPs, latent TrPs have the potential to induce referred pain. The constant barrage of afferent information, subsequent sensitization, and abnormal synapses contributes to

the sensation of pain at distant unrelated muscle sites, i.e. referred pain (Jafri 2014; Shah et al. 2016).

Unfortunately, our veterinary patients cannot tell us if a palpable TrP is active or latent. Ultimately this distinction is not as important in veterinary medicine given the fluidity of active–latent TrPs. Latent TrPs can become active TrPs when repeatedly exposed to detrimental stimuli, such as overuse or trauma (Celik and Mutlu 2013). Active TrPs can be inactivated, or converted back to latent TrPs, but many never fully disappear regardless of the therapy used (Celik and Mutlu 2013).

TrPT Techniques

TrPT techniques can be classified as noninvasive or invasive. Noninvasive procedures include medications, thermal techniques, photobiomodulation, transcutaneous electrical nerve stimulation (TENS), therapeutic ultrasound, and physical or manual therapies. Alternatively, dry needling and TrP injections are classified invasive therapies.

Regardless of the technique chosen, most patients will require multiple treatments. The number and frequency of treatments is dependent on the cause and chronicity of the TrPs. Specific client educational information and homework (typically involving passive stretching, massage, and home exercises) are based on the TrPTs chosen.

Noninvasive TrPTs
Pharmaceuticals

Prescription medications are used to reduce the pain and inflammation associated with TrPs. The most common medications chosen include nonsteroidal anti-inflammatory drugs (NSAIDs), muscle relaxers, opioids, gabapentin, and amantadine. Unfortunately, these medications cannot fix the TrPs but, instead, mask the pain making the patient more comfortable. Depending on the chronicity of the TrPs and the patient, additional treatment may be necessary.

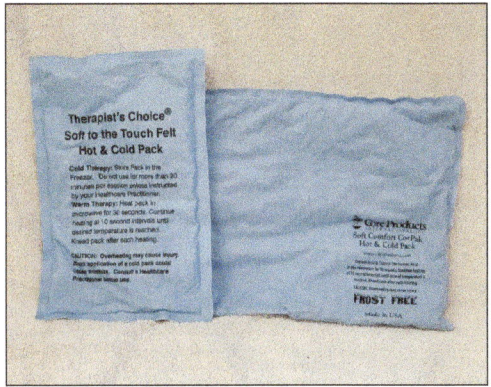

Figure 9.9 One type of warm and cold packs/devices used in veterinary medicine. Source: Lisa P. McFaddin.

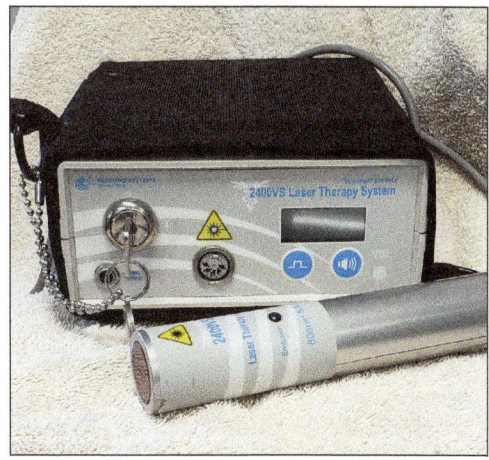

Figure 9.10 One type of veterinary Class IIIb therapeutic laser. Source: Lisa P. McFaddin.

Thermal Techniques

Superficial thermal techniques include the application of cold (cryotherapy) or heat to the skin and fur. In cryotherapy a cold pack or ice pack is wrapped in a thin towel and applied to the fur or skin for no more than 20 minutes. Cryotherapy is often administered in 20 minutes on, 20 minutes off cycle.

In heat therapy various heat packs are wrapped in a thin towel and applied to the fur or skin for 15–30 minutes (Niebaum 2013). Veterinary hot packs and warming pads wrapped in a towel are the most used resources. Human heating pads can be used but with extreme caution. The device should only be used on a low setting, with a towel between the pad and the animal, for less than 20 minutes, and under direct supervision. Pets can be, and have been, burned when a heating pad is used improperly. Figure 9.9 depicts an example of multipurpose thermal packs which can be used for both cold and heat.

Photobiomodulation

Photobiomodulation (PBM, aka cold laser or low-level light therapy, LLLT) involves the application of a Class IIIb or IV therapeutic laser directly over the TrP (Wall 2019). The recommended therapeutic dose (J/cm^2) depends on the muscle involved and is often practitioner dependent (Wall 2019). Figure 9.10 shows one type of Class IIIb therapeutic laser. Refer to Chapter 6 for further information on veterinary PBM.

Transcutaneous Electrical Nerve Stimulation

TENS is a form of electrical stimulation in which electrodes are placed directly onto the skin over areas of pain or over the peripheral nerves innervating the painful areas (Niebaum 2013). The frequency, pulse duration, amplitude, and treatment duration are dependent on the area being treated. The fur must be shaved before applying the pads. Figure 9.11 shows one type of TENS unit used in veterinary medicine.

Therapeutic Ultrasound

Therapeutic ultrasound uses sound waves (frequencies greater than 20000 Hz) to heat deep tissues (3–5 cm) without causing thermal damage. The frequency, intensity, and mode (continuous or pulsed) are based on the target tissues (Niebaum 2013). For therapeutic ultrasound to work the fur must be shaved and special ultrasound gel applied before placing the probe on the skin. Figure 9.12 shows one type of therapeutic ultrasound used in veterinary medicine.

Physical or Manual Therapies

Manual therapy options in people include ischemic compression, massage, passive

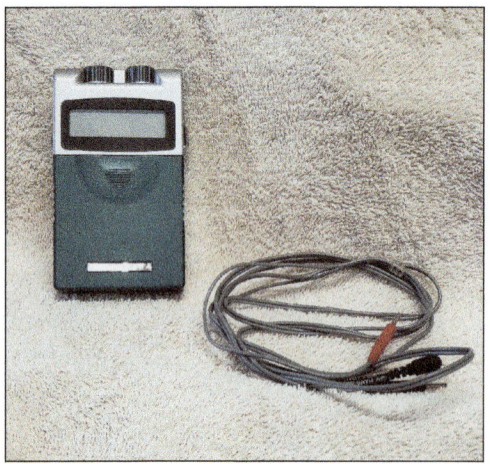

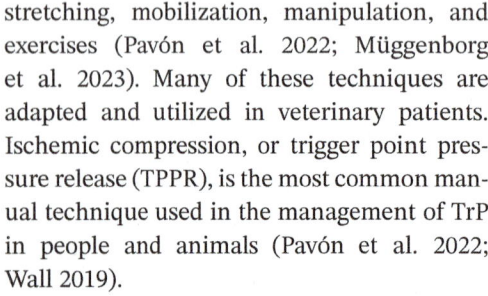

Figure 9.11 One type of transcutaneous electrical nerve stimulation (TENS) unit used in veterinary medicine. Source: Lisa P. McFaddin.

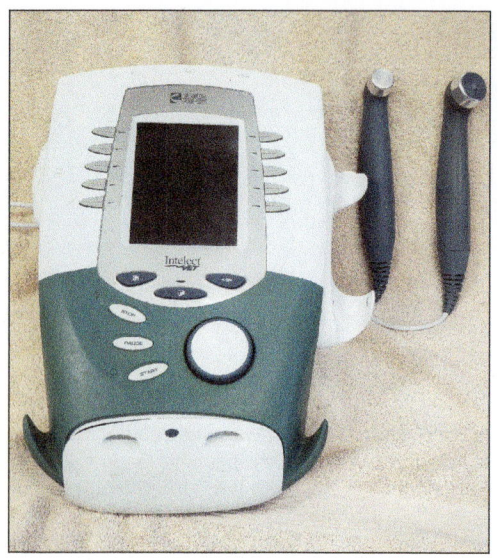

Figure 9.12 One type of therapeutic ultrasound used in veterinary medicine. Source: Lisa P. McFaddin.

stretching, mobilization, manipulation, and exercises (Pavón et al. 2022; Müggenborg et al. 2023). Many of these techniques are adapted and utilized in veterinary patients. Ischemic compression, or trigger point pressure release (TPPR), is the most common manual technique used in the management of TrP in people and animals (Pavón et al. 2022; Wall 2019).

In TPPR digital compression is applied to the palpable TrP for 60–120 seconds until relaxation of the taut band or nodule is appreciated (Coates 2013; Boyles et al. 2015). Initially digital pressure is gentle, but every 10–15 seconds, as the band or nodule relaxes, the tension increases (Coates 2013). The amount of pressure applied is based on the patient's pain tolerance. The hand positioning used for the pincher palpation technique, depicted in Figure 9.7, can be used to perform TPPR.

Invasive TrPTs
Dry Needling
Dry needling (DN) is the placement of a thin solid acupuncture needle through the skin directly into a TrP. DN is uncomfortable and

sometimes painful. Veterinary patients may need to be sedated for patient and practitioner/staff safety. Explaining the need to cause pain to stop pain is not feasible with our patients. Pain can make even the most docile animal bite. Sedation prevents the hair-trigger response of teeth on flesh. Additionally, stress makes patients tense their muscles. TrPs are very difficult to palpate and accurately place a needle into when muscles are actively contracting.

DN has many of the same physiologic effects as acupuncture, but theory and application differ greatly. As with acupuncture, DN causes local and systemic effects through stimulation of the nervous, circulatory, and immune systems. DN placement does use preset points on the body. Instead, needle placement is dependent on the location of the TrP.

Once the TrP is identified the non-dominant hand stabilizes the muscle, while the dominant hand places the acupuncture needle through the skin into the TrP, as shown in Figure 9.13. The abnormal muscle fibers within a TrP create a different texture compared to the surrounding normal muscle tissue

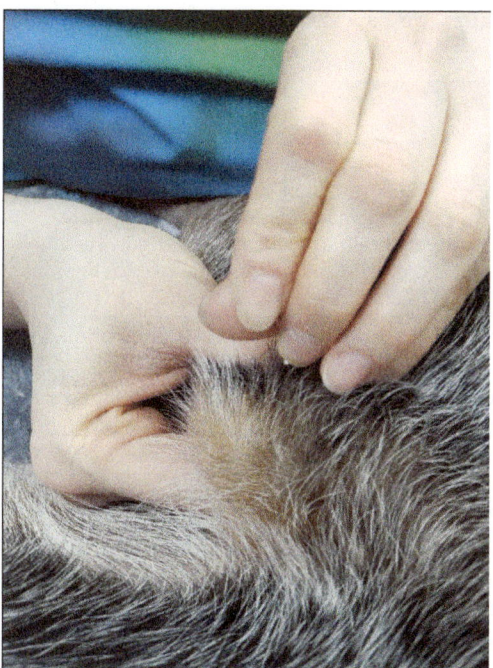

Figure 9.13 An example of trigger point dry needling. A 28g 1-inch sterile acupuncture needle is placed through the skin into a trigger point within the triceps muscle of a dog. Source: Lisa P. McFaddin.

(Wall 2010, 2019). TrPs often feel like trying to place a needle through sand or leather.

Placement of the needle within the TrP often results in an LTR. The LTR is a visible or palpable muscle twitch immediately following needle placement (Hong 1994; Shah et al. 2016). The necessity of eliciting an LTR during DN, as it pertains to therapeutic efficacy, is currently being debated. The presence of an LTR was originally believed to correlate with clinical improvement (both short and long term), but recent human clinical trials and meta-analyses suggest an LTR may not be necessary (Hakim et al. 2019; Fernández-de-Las-Peñas et al. 2022).

Following needle placement there are several recommended techniques including pistoning, needle winding, and in situ placement (Dunning et al. 2014; Perreault et al. 2017; Butts et al. 2021). During the pistoning technique (aka sparrow pecking or fast-in fast-out) the needle is moved back and forth (in and out

of the TrP while staying within the muscle) until an LTR is no longer appreciated or the TrP is subjectively less defined (Dunning et al. 2014; Wall 2019).

Needle winding involves the twisting of the needle following placement within the TrP, regardless of the presence of an LTR (Perreault et al. 2017). The needle may be removed quickly after winding or left in place, a form of in situ placement, for a period (Perreault et al. 2017).

The in situ technique involves leaving one or more needles in place for 5–40 minutes (Dunning et al. 2014). Currently, there are no standards regarding the number of needles, retention time (length of time needles remain in the muscle), and level of stimulation (digital manipulation or electric stimulation) in human or veterinary medicine (Dunning et al. 2014).

Most veterinary practitioners recommend the pistoning technique, though data supporting the superiority of this technique is lacking (Kitchens 2016; Wall 2019). There is a decisive lack of veterinary (and human) DN protocol standardization. At present the technique used, number of needles placed, and frequency of DN appointments is primarily based on evidence extrapolated from human studies, practitioner bias, and patient condition.

As an aside there is a connection between DN and acupuncture. TrPs are often identified as A-shi points in acupuncture. A-shi points represent painful areas on the skin or connective tissue not associated with acupuncture points found on the major meridians or classical points. A-shi points often correlate with active and latent TrPs (Dunning et al. 2014). Electroacupuncture (the use of an electric current between at least two acupuncture needles) is like the application of electric stimulation to in situ DN techniques. To learn more about veterinary acupuncture, see Chapter 1.

Trigger Point Injections

TrP injections (TrPI or wet needling) involve the injection of a small amount of a sterile

Table 9.5 Most common pharmaceutical agents used to treat the pain associated with trigger points in veterinary patients.

Drug category	Examples	Mechanism of action
NSAIDS	Carprofen Deracoxib Firocoxib Meloxicam Robenacoxib	Selective or nonselective cyclooxygenase-2 (COX-2) inhibitors, a substance produced by inflamed muscles and tissues. These medications reduce pain centrally (within the CNS) and peripherally (within the affected tissues outside the CNS)
Opioids	Codeine Hydromorphone Tramadol	Centrally acting pain medication primarily interacting with mu (μ) receptors. All opioids are chemical derivatives of compounds from opium
Muscle relaxant	Methocarbamol	Centrally acting skeletal muscle relaxant
Other analgesics	Gabapentin	Centrally acting to reduce nerve pain
	Amantadine Ketamine	Centrally acting pain medication by inhibiting NMDA receptors

CNS, central nervous system; NSAIDs, nonsteroidal anti-inflammatory drugs; NMDA, *N*-methyl-D-aspartate.
Source: Lisa P. McFaddin.

solution into a TrP. The most used solutions include local anesthetics (lidocaine or bupivacaine, with or without sodium bicarbonate), corticosteroids, sterile saline, or dextrose (Tantanatip et al. 2021; Hammi et al. 2022). The use of sterile saline or dextrose is technically considered a form of prolotherapy (see Chapter 7 for further information). TrPIs are not commonly utilized in veterinary medicine.

Mechanisms of Action

Pharmaceuticals
The mechanisms of action are dependent on the class of medication selected. The most common class of drugs used help reduce inflammation (NSAIDS), reduce pain (opioids, gabapentin, and amantadine), or relax muscles (muscle relaxants) are shown in Table 9.5.

Thermal Techniques
Cryotherapy is used to reduce pain, inflammation, and swelling primarily through the constriction of blood vessels (vasoconstriction) and reduction of inflammatory proteins within the skin and underlying tissues, reduction of tissue metabolism, and dampening the transmission of pain signals from superficial nerves (Ciolek 1985; Niebaum 2013). Cryotherapy will penetrate tissues 2–4 cm deep (Niebaum 2013).

Superficial heat is used to reduce pain, promote tissue and muscle relaxation, increase blood flow, and improve tissue and joint mobility (Niebaum 2013; Nanneman 1991). Heat therapy penetrates 1–2 cm deep (Niebaum 2013).

Photobiomodulation
PBM relies on the absorption of monochromatic, coherent, and collimated electromagnetic radiation by light-absorbing molecules within the mitochondria of local tissues (Hamblin 2017). The energy absorption causes a host of cellular changes resulting in a reduction of pain and inflammation, modulation of the immune system, and improved tissue healing and regeneration (Arany 2016). See Chapter 6 for further information.

Transcutaneous Electrical Nerve Stimulation

TENS is a noninvasive technique using pulsed electric currents (delivered across intact skin) to reduce pain through the stimulation of peripheral nerves (Johnson 2007). TENS requires direct contact between the electrode pads and the skin, necessitating shaving of the fur.

Therapeutic Ultrasound

Therapeutic ultrasound increases blood flow, promotes muscle relaxation, reduces pain, and improves muscle and joint mobility by thermal (heating tissues) and nonthermal effects (increase cellular chemical and biological reactions, as well as tissue mechanical changes) (Niebaum 2013).

Manual Therapy

There are many effective manual therapies used to manage TrPs (Pavón et al. 2022). As TPPR is the most common manual therapy used to treat veterinary TrPs, this section focuses solely on TPPR. There are several excellent veterinary rehabilitation books and online resources available discussing the other manual therapies in detail.

TPPR directly affects the circulatory, biochemical and neurologic changes caused by TrP (Dommerholt 2006). When digital pressure is applied to the TrP, blood flow decreases. The degree to which blood flow decreases is proportional to the amount of applied compression (Simons 1983). Once pressure is released local blood flow returns restoring circulation, facilitating muscle fiber relaxation, reducing local inflammation, and promoting healing (Coates 2013).

Dry Needling

Placement of the needle punctures the skin causing counter-irritation within the epidermis, dermis, subcutaneous tissues, and muscle leading to microtrauma (Clemmons 2007). This tissue disruption directly affects local nerves, muscle fibers, blood vessels, and immune cells improving blood flow, immune response, and relaxation of tissues and muscles (Dommerholt 2011). Signals carried by the nerve cells spread from the point of impact to the spinal cord and eventually the brain, propagating the beneficial effects throughout the body (Chiu et al. 2001).

Trigger Point Injections

The injection of a sterile liquid into or near a TrP has similar effects to that of DN (Hammi et al. 2022). TrPIs also improve the movement of myofascial tissues helping to normalize muscle function and reduce pain (Tantanatip et al. 2021). Additionally, TrPIs incite a predictable response by the body: controlled inflammation followed by healing (Osborn 2018).

Mechanisms of Action for Veterinarians

This section provides more detailed information on the pathophysiology of thermal therapy.

Thermal Techniques

Limited studies have shown both cryotherapy and heat therapy can have beneficial effects on the management of active and latent TrPs, typically when combined with other therapeutic modalities (Gutiérrez-Rojas et al. 2015; Petrofsky et al. 2020). The physiologic effects of cryotherapy include local vasoconstriction, local analgesia, reduction of tissue edema and hypoxia, reduction of muscle spasms, reduces lymphatic and venous drainage, reduces nerve conduction velocity, and reduces the metabolic rate of injured tissue (Ciolek 1985; Nanneman 1991). The primary therapeutic effects are vasoconstriction and reduction of the concentration of inflammatory mediators (inflammatory soup). Cryotherapy decreases the nerve conduction velocity of thermoreceptors (Aδ and C fibers), blocks pain centers at the dorsal horn, and affects MSC and GTO (Niebaum 2013). The reduction of nerve conduction velocity, while important, plays a smaller role than original theorized.

The physiologic effects of heat therapy include release of histamine and prostaglandin, local vasodilation, increased local cellular metabolism, increased capillary permeability, increased lymphatic and venous drainage, local analgesia, increased motor and sensory nerve conduction velocity, increased axon reflex activity, increased muscle contractility, decreasing muscle spasms, and increasing connective tissue elasticity (Nanneman 1991; Kim et al. 2020). The analgesic effects are caused by decreased firing of type II afferents and gamma efferents, increased firing of type Ib and GTOs, decreased firing of the alpha motor neurons, and muscle relaxation (Malanga et al. 2015).

Photobiomodulation

PBM has shown promising effects when used as monotherapy or part of a multimodal treatment of TrPs (Simunovic 1996; Shiryan et al. 2022). Specifics regarding the mechanisms of action of PBM are discussed in detail Chapter 6.

Transcutaneous Electrical Nerve Stimulation

Limited, yet promising, studies have demonstrated improved myofascial pain, from trigger points, following TENS treatments in humans (Dissanayaka et al. 2016; Ebadi et al. 2021). TENS can be used to elicit excitatory (stimulating peripheral nerves through depolarization), non-excitatory (cellular changes including increased cell membrane permeability, promotion of protein synthesis, and tissue growth and repair), and noxious (tissue irritation, typically undesired) effects (Johnson 2007). The electrical current causes muscle contraction through depolarization of the motor nerve and subsequent activation of muscle fibers. TENS reduces pain by stimulating sensory nerves through the Gate Theory of pain inhibition (Niebaum 2013).

Therapeutic Ultrasound

Limited randomized controlled studies suggest therapeutic ultrasound is effective in the management of active TrPs (Yildirim et al. 2018). Therapeutic ultrasound is dependent on the conversion of electrical energy into mechanical energy in the form of sound waves. An electrical current is passed through a crystal (typically lead-zirconium-titanate) causing it to vibrate and produce sound waves (Niebaum 2013). Ultrasound waves have an affinity for tissues that are highly organized and contain a high water content (Yadollahpour and Rashidi 2017).

The thermal mechanisms are like those seen with superficial heat therapy (improve blood flow, decrease muscle spasms, increase collagen fiber extensibility, and proinflammatory) but applicable to deeper tissues (Yadollahpour and Rashidi 2017). The nonthermal effects are caused by sound waves creating pressure changes in the cellular fluid (microstreaming) and the compression/expansion of gas bubbles within body fluids (cavitation) (Miller et al. 2012). The nonthermal effects have a greater therapeutic effect increasing the rate of cellular chemical reactions, increasing the permeability of cell membranes, decreasing muscle spasms, increasing range of motion, decreasing adhesions, and breaking up calcified deposits.

TPPR

Several human studies have shown TPPR effectively reduces pain (both directly and by increasing the pressure pain threshold, or PPT) and muscle tension (Moraska et al. 2017; Kashyap et al. 2018; Pecos-Martin et al. 2019; Nikam and Varadharajulu 2021; Lu et al. 2022). Further examples are provided in The Why section of this chapter.

TPPR was initially referred to as ischemic compression by Travell and Simons because digital pressure caused blanching of the skin followed by a reactive hyperemia once the pressure was released (Simons 1983). After determining the therapeutic benefits affected more than local circulation, the name was changed to TPPR.

TPPR dilates the sarcomere within the TrP, improves local circulation, and facilitates the removal of inflammatory mediators and lactic acid (Esparza et al. 2019; Moraska et al. 2013). These focal changes help to normalize muscle

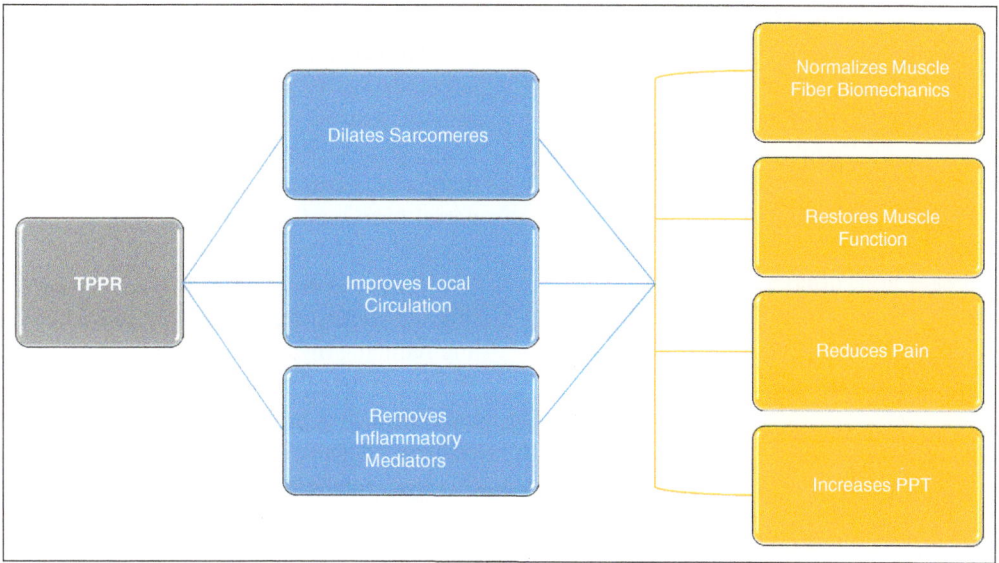

Figure 9.14 A summary of the mechanisms of action and physiologic effects of trigger point pressure release (TPPR). PPT, pressure pain threshold. Source: Lisa P. McFaddin.

fiber biomechanics, restore muscle function, and reduce pain (Álvarez et al. 2022). Pain is reduced through removal of inflammatory mediators within the TrP; stimulation and attenuation of nociceptors and mechanoreceptors within the skin, connective tissue and muscles; increasing PPT; and modulation of the prefrontal cortical activity affecting the way pain is interpreted (Kostopoulos et al. 2008; Kodama et al. 2019; Lu et al. 2022). Figure 9.14 summarizes the mechanisms of action and therapeutic effects of TPPR.

In cases of hyperalgesia, due to active or latent TrPs, TPPR may be more effective than DN (Álvarez et al. 2022). In some cases, TPPR may not be enough to improve muscle contraction, motor control, convert an active TrP to a latent TrP, or fully resolve the TrP (Mauntel et al. 2014; Esparza et al. 2019).

Dry Needling

Multiple studies have demonstrated the efficacy of DN on the reduction of pain intensity, increases in the PPT, and quality of life of people suffering from both myalgia due to active and latent TrPs (Álvarez et al. 2022; Cagnie et al. 2015; Shah et al. 2016). Additional detail and examples are provided in "The Why" section of this chapter.

DN has been shown to improve range of motion, muscle activation, and reduce pain through multiple mechanisms, listed in Table 9.6 and outlined in Figure 9.15.

Occurrence of an LTR following needle placement is still considered important to the efficacy of DN, especially in veterinary medicine (Wall 2019; Cruz-Montecinos et al. 2021), despite recent research suggesting the LTR may not be necessary (Hakim et al. 2019; Fernández-de-Las-Peñas et al. 2022). The LTR is an involuntary local spinal cord reflex causing rapid contraction of the abnormal muscle band immediately following stimulation, either with palpation or through insertion of a needle (Cruz-Montecinos et al. 2021). The LTR represents a rapid depolarization of muscle fibers within the TrP. Previous research suggests once the muscle twitching stops the preexisting spontaneous electrical activity within the TrP ceases, motor-endplate dysfunction resolves, and pain is reduced (Kalichman and Vulfsons 2010).

Table 9.6 A list of many of the mechanisms through which trigger point dry needling exerts its beneficial therapeutic effects. Studies supporting the mechanisms are provided.

Mechanisms of action	Supporting research
Relaxes sarcomeres within the TrP	Castro-Sánchez et al. (2017)
Decreases spontaneous motor endplate activity	Abbaszadeh-Amirdehi et al. (2016)
Reduces acetylcholine (ACh) release from the motor endplate	Dommerholt (2011)
Improves local circulation	Dunning et al. (2014), Abbaszadeh-Amirdehi et al. (2016), and Castro-Sánchez et al. (2017)
Reduces and removes the chemical soup of inflammatory mediators	Boyles et al. (2015) and Abbaszadeh-Amirdehi et al. (2016)
Overstimulates nociceptors which normalizes sensory input	Dommerholt (2011)
Stimulates inhibitory interneurons within the dorsal horn, blocking afferent pain information to the cortex	Boyles et al. (2015)
Increases the release of endogenous opioids (β-endorphins and enkephalins) through the stimulation of Aδ nerve fibers	Boyles et al. (2015), Abbaszadeh-Amirdehi et al. (2016), and Castro-Sánchez et al. (2017)
Induces short-term segmental neuromodulation	Srbely et al. (2010)

Source: Lisa P. McFaddin.

Trigger Point Injections

Multiple studies have shown TrPI effectively reduces the pain associated with TrPs and improves function (Tantanatip et al. 2021; Cho et al. 2022). The exact mechanism(s) of TrPI is unknown. Many of the mechanical and neurologic effects associated with DN are also seen with TrPI, including relaxation of the sarcomeres within the TrP, improvement in local circulation, decreased spontaneous motor endplate activity, reduced ACh release from the motor endplate, normalization of sensory input, stimulation of inhibitory interneurons within the dorsal horn, and short-term segmental neuromodulation (Wong and Wong 2012).

TrPIs also loosen tightened fascial tissue surrounding TrPs, normalizing muscle function, and reducing myalgia (Tantanatip et al. 2021). The injection of a sterile liquid also causes a controlled wound with predictable wound healing responses (hemostasis → inflammation → proliferation → remodeling). See Chapter 7 for further information on wound healing.

Safety

All TrPTs are considered safe and effective. Potential risks and specific cautions/contraindications are dependent on the TrPT being utilized.

Pharmaceutical

Pharmaceutical selection is dependent on the species being treated, preexisting conditions, and concurrent medications. Specific medications are contraindicated in patients allergic to ingredients or medications. Adverse effects (AEs) are also dependent on the medication prescribed.

Thermal Therapy

Cryotherapy should be used with caution in patients hypersensitive to the cold, around areas of vascular compromise, open wounds, and very young or old patients (Niebaum 2013). When used appropriately cryotherapy has very few, and typically self-resolving, side effects including numbness and reddening of the skin. If used incorrectly severe skin or soft tissue damage can occur.

Heat therapy should be avoided in cases of acute inflammation, loss of sensation, skin or subcutaneous hemorrhage, over neoplasms of

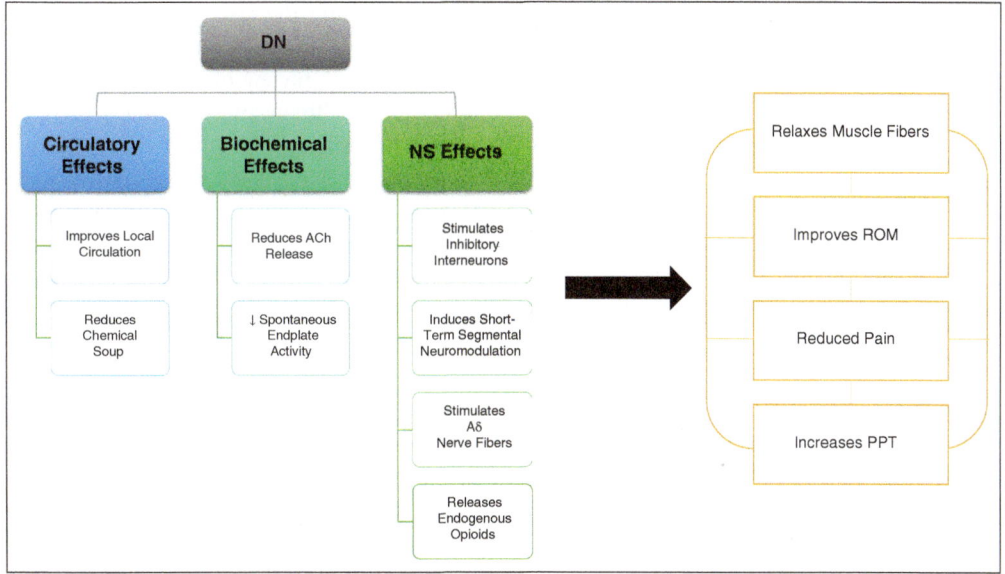

Figure 9.15 A summary of the mechanisms of action and physiologic effects of trigger point dry needling (DN). NS, nervous system; ACh, acetylcholine; ROM, range of motion. Source: Lisa P. McFaddin.

the skin or subcutaneous tissue, and open wounds (Niebaum 2013). Caution should be used in obese patients, as subcutaneous fat insulates against rewarming. The potential AEs are like those seen with cryotherapy.

Photobiomodulation

PBM should be used with caution over photosensitive skin, darker skin and coats, injection sites, areas with active bleeding, growth plates, and malignancies (Shah and Alster 2010; Godbold 2017; Maegawa et al. 2000; Barrington 2022). See Chapter 6 for additional information, including potential AE.

Transcutaneous Electoral Nerve Stimulation

TENS is contraindicated in animals with pacemakers. Caution should be taken when using TENS over the heart, in animals with seizure disorders, areas of blood clots (thrombosis), areas of infection, neoplasia, the carotid sinus, areas with impaired sensation, irritated or damaged skin, and electronic sensing devices (Johnson 2007).

Therapeutic Ultrasound

Therapeutic ultrasound should not be used over a gravid (pregnant) uterus, malignancies, metal implants, electronic devices, and infected or damaged skin (Mathews and Stretanski 2023). Caution should be taken when using over bony prominences, growth plates, or non-metal implants (Mathews and Stretanski 2023). When used appropriately the patient may experience mild heating of the skin, which is self-resolving, following treatment. Inappropriate use could lead to irreversible tissue damage (Mathews and Stretanski 2023).

TPPR

TPPR is contraindicated in patients with fractures, bone infections (osteomyelitis), muscle or bone cancer, and active bleeding (especially internally) (Wall 2010, 2019). Caution is required when treating patients with cancer or immune-mediated diseases. Pain and bruising are the most likely AEs (Wall 2010, 2019).

Invasive Techniques

The contraindications, cautions, and adverse effects for DN and TrPI are similar to those seen with TPPR. Invasive TrPTs are also contraindicated in areas with skin infections and patients with a high anesthetic or sedation risk, if required (Wall 2010, 2019). Pain, bruising, bleeding, hematoma formation, and an adverse reaction to the sedation/anesthetic are the most likely AEs (Wall 2010, 2019).

The Why

Applications in Human Medicine

MPS is a common source of musculoskeletal pain in people, comprising 30–85% of patients with musculoskeletal pain (Tantanatip and Chang 2022). MPS is a chronic condition affecting a specific area or areas of muscle and the surrounding fascia (Akamatsu et al. 2015; Shah et al. 2016). Associated clinical signs include the presence of one or more trigger point(s), regional pain, ± referred pain, increased tension, and reduced flexibility (Akamatsu et al. 2015; Shah et al. 2016). MPS is classified as a separate disorder from fribromyalgia, tendonitis, and bursitis. A variety of therapeutic modalities are routinely used to manage and treat MPS, as well as other conditions involving TrPs. This section focuses on the use of TPPR, DN, and wet needling or TrPI.

The use of TPPR is very common among human massage therapists, physical therapists, and chiropractors. In a randomized placebo-controlled study by Moraska et al. (2017), TPPR was shown to reduce the pain associated tension headaches caused by TrPs. Affected muscles included the trapezius and suboccipital muscles. Moraska et al. (2017) discovered multiple TPPR sessions are often necessary to fully resolve TrPs. Dissolution of the TrPs may not be possible, but pain reduction and/or transition of the TrPs from active to latent is feasible.

DN is becoming more common in the treatment of TrPs and MPS and show promising results (Dommerholt 2011; Castro-Sánchez et al. 2017; Álvarez et al. 2022). Unfortunately, double-bind placebo-controlled studies are very hard to perform because placement of a needle anywhere in the body, even in a non-TrP, can induce an effect on the nervous system, making the use of sham or placebo controls very difficult (Dommerholt 2011).

A systematic review of randomized clinical trials by Kalichman and Vulfsons (2010) supported the efficacy of DN in the successful treatment of pain caused by TrP. Another systematic review by Morihisa et al. (2016) concluded DN was effective in reducing the pain associated with lower limb TrPs, but the studies did not demonstrate a positive effect on range of motion or strength. In a third systematic review of randomized controlled trials, Boyles et al. (2015) revealed DN of TrP was effective in reducing pain and local tenderness (especially in the head, trunk, upper extremities, and lower extremities). The authors did report a lack of consistency among studies with respect to patient selection, needle placement location, and methodology. Additionally, several systematic reviews revealed there is low-to-moderate quality of evidence (Fernández-De-Las-Peñas et al. 2021; Jiménez-Del-Barrio et al. 2022) or inconclusive evidence supporting the use of DN in the treatment of TrPs (Lucena-Anton et al. 2022).

To better understand and standardize TrPT, the National Center for Complementary and Integrative Health (NCCIH), a branch of the National Institutes of Health (NIH), announced their intentions to investigate myofascial pain disorders in the beginning of 2020 (Chen and Sabri 2020). The goal of the study will be to standardize myofascial pain diagnoses (Phase 1) and test nonpharmacological treatment options (Phase 2) (Chen and Sabri 2020). DN and TPPR are two of the main therapies that will be investigated.

Another factor to consider is the legality of DN, which is highly state dependent. Some states permit physical therapists and chiropractors to perform DN, while other states only permit medical doctors or acupuncturists.

The AEs associated with TPPR and DN are uncommon and considered mild and self-resolving. The most common AE is transient pain and bruising. The most common AEs seen with DN include bruising, bleeding, and pain. Uncommon DN AEs include hematoma formation, infection, and temporary nerve damage (Kalichman and Vulfsons 2010). Extremely rare DN AEs involve fainting and pneumothorax (accumulation of air within the chest cavity around the lungs due to a puncture of the lung with a needle) (Kalichman and Vulfsons 2010; Boyles et al. 2015).

Applications in Veterinary Medicine

TrPT is used for the treatment of musculoskeletal pain caused by TrPs; 85% of pain from injury is due to muscle pain, myalgia (Wall 2019). The list of conditions in Table 9.4 which can lead to TrP formation would also benefit from TrPT.

Myalgia, in people, is defined as an aching or cramping pain within the muscles that is difficult to isolate. The source of the pain may originate from the muscle or radiate from the viscera. Myalgia does occur in our veterinary patients, though its description in the literature is limited. The most common causes of myalgia in dogs and cats include muscle injury (overuse or trauma), inflammatory myopathies, metabolic conditions, endocrine disorders, nutritional deficiencies, and myofascial pain (Wall 2010). Another cause of myalgia is the formation of TrPs within the muscles.

Veterinary Research

As of February 2023, there are no studies validating the efficacy of the most common TrPT techniques used in veterinary medicine (Wall 2019). Therapeutic recommendations are extrapolated from the human literature, for which there are numerous studies documenting efficacy. Many of the human studies use animal subjects, but these studies are not often performed by veterinarians.

As of February 2023, a quick search on PubMed for "trigger point veterinary," "trigger point canine," and "trigger point feline" yielded only 14 articles. The number of articles increased by almost 30 when the search parameters included "trigger point rodent" and "trigger point rabbit." Presented below are the summaries of three veterinary TrPT studies.

Not all research promotes the use of TrPT. A systematic review of soft tissue mobilization techniques, which included TrPTs, in veterinary sport and companion animals revealed a moderate to high risk of bias and lack of standardization among the studies (Bergh et al. 2022). The authors concluded there was not sufficient evidence to support the clinical efficacy of stretching, massage, and other manual therapies in horses, dogs, and cats (Bergh et al. 2022).

Neuromuscular Damage and Repair After Dry Needling in Mice

Authors: Ares Domingo, Orlando Mayoral, Sonia Monterde, and Manel Santafé
Journal: *Evidence Based Complementary and Alternative Medicine*
Date: 2013
Study design: Controlled trial
Study hypothesis: Dry needling (DN) causes scar tissue formation within the muscle and damages nerve fibers through repetitive needle insertion.
Sample size: 23 male Swiss mice
Materials and methods: Mice were anesthetized and 15 repeated punctures were performed on the levator auris longus (LAL) muscle using an acupuncture needle (0.16 mm thick and 25 mm long). Tissue samples were obtained at 3 hours and one, three, five, and seven days after DN. The right LAL muscles were used for immunohistochemistry and the left LAL muscles were used for methylene blue staining. Electron microscopy evaluation was performed on either the right or left LAL muscles. All samples were prepared in formalin or paraformaldehyde prior to evaluation.

(Continued)

Neuromuscular Damage and Repair After Dry Needling in Mice   (Continued)

Results

1) Evidence of inflammation was present 3 and 24 hours post DN.
2) Inflammatory cells were still seen seven days post DN.
3) Muscle regeneration was almost complete seven days post DN.
4) Changes in receptor distribution in the denervated postsynaptic nerve fibers was seen one day after DN.
5) Reinnervation started three hours post and was complete three days after DN.

Study conclusions: Repeated needle placement through the muscle during DN causes initial muscle and nerve fiber damage but does not inhibit muscle and nerve fiber regeneration.

Study limitations

1) No statistical analysis of the data.
2) Needle size to muscle size is different in a mouse compared to a cat, dog, and human.
3) The possibility of sample collection causing muscle and nerve damage was not addressed.
4) Healthy tissue, non-trigger points, were used.
5) Does not address repeated DN sessions used in the management of trigger points, i.e. does fibrosis play a role in trigger point healing?

L.P.M. conclusion: This study supports to concept of counter-irritation as a source of healing in TrPT. Counter-irritation is one of the main methods through which acupuncture exerts its beneficial effects. More studies are needed to further understand the mechanisms through which DN exerts its positive effects.

(Domingo et al. 2013)

Acupotomy Alleviates Energy Crisis at Rat Myofascial Trigger Points

Authors: Zhang, Yi, Ning-Yu Du, Chen Chen, Tong Wang, Li-Juan Wang, Xiao-Lu Shi, Shu-Ming Li, and Chang-Qing Guo
Journal: *Evidence Based Complementary and Alternative Medicine*
Date: 2020
Study design: Randomized controlled trial
Study hypothesis: Acupotomy is an effective method of treatment for trigger points (TrP). Acupotomy is the use of surgical incisions and acupuncture needle placement.
Sample size: 32 male Sprague Dawley rats
Materials and methods: Rats were randomly divided into four groups (control, TrP, acupotomy, and lidocaine injection). All rats, except the control group, were subjected to trauma to the middle of the left vastus medialis muscle. Non-control rats were then exercised the

next day using a treadmill. The presence of TrP was confirmed using electromyography in rats in all groups. The TrP group received model preparation but no therapeutic treatment. Enzyme-linked immunosorbent assays were used to measure acetylcholinesterase (AChE) and free sarcoplasmic calcium concentrations. High-performance liquid chromatography was used to measure adenosine triphosphate (ATP), adenosine monophosphate (AMP), substance P (SP), and calcitonin gene-related peptide (CGRP). Analysis of variance (ANOVA) was used for statistical analysis.

Results

1) Sarcoplasmic calcium, SP, and CGRP were reduced in the acupotomy and lidocaine injection groups.

2) AChE and ATP were lower in the acupotomy and lidocaine injection groups.
3) Compared to the TrP group the acupotomy group decreased AMP and increased ATP levels.

Study conclusions: Acupotomy helps reduce ACh levels dampening the chemical noise associated with trigger points. ACh reduction is a key requirement in resolving trigger points suggesting acupotomy could be useful in the management of trigger points.

Study limitations

1) Trigger points were experimentally created which may affect their biochemical, circulatory, and neurologic responses.
2) Only was method was used to test each variable limiting experimental verification.
3) Multiple anesthetic events may have affected muscle response.

L.P.M. conclusions: Acupotomy is an interesting and novel treatment approach for trigger point management. Further studies are needed to determine the validity and efficacy of this therapeutic approach in veterinary medicine.

(Zhang et al. 2020)

Experimental Myofascial Trigger Point Creation in Rodents

Authors: Ramon Margalef, March Sisquella, Marc Bosque, Clara Romeu, Orlando Mayoral, Sonia Monterde, Mercedes Priego, Rafael Guerra-Perez, Nicolau Ortiz, Josep Tomás, and Manel Santafe
Journal: *Journal of Applied Physiology*
Date: 2020
Study design: Controlled trial
Study hypothesis: The use of electrical stimulation at trigger points (TrP) will increase the number and speed of LTR compared to dry needling (DN).
Sample size: 35 young male Swiss mice
Materials and methods: Neostigmine methyl sulfate was injected subcutaneously into the mice to create a model for TrP. 30 minutes after injecting the neostigmine electric current was applied to the gastrocnemius muscle and LAL muscles. The electric current was applied at 0.4, 1.5, and 3 mA for three to five seconds with three to four repetitions. A lower intensity protocol was used for 10 minutes as well. Electromyography (EMG) and intracellular (spontaneous miniature endplate potentials or mEPPs) recordings were taken 3 and 24 hours after current application. Muscular ultrasound was used to measure the number

and strength of LTR. A two-tailed Welch's *t*-test was used for statistical analysis.

Results

1) An increase in the frequency of mEPPs was measured in the LAL muscle 30 minutes after neostigmine injection. The 3 mA (three seconds with three repetitions) reversed the frequency of mEPPs to control values after 3 hours, and the change was sustained at 24 hours. The other pulsed frequencies slightly reduced the mEPPs, but no real change was observed with the low intensity protocol.
2) An increase in endplate noise was noted in the gastrocnemius muscle following neostigmine injection. The 3 and 1.5 mA (five seconds, three repetitions) completely reverse the endplate noise after three hours, and the change was sustained after 24 hours. A slight reduction was noted with the 0.4 mA (five second, three repetitions), but no appreciable change was noted with the low intensity protocol.
3) The 1.5 mA electrical current increased the LTR by 144% compared to DN, and the speed of the LTR was 230% faster.

(Continued)

Experimental Myofascial Trigger Point Creation in Rodents (Continued)	
Study conclusions: Higher intensity electrical current is effective in reducing the mEPP and endplate noise associated with TrP. Higher intensity electrical currents also increase the number and speed of LTRs.	2) mEPP and EMG results were compared to a control but not the DN technique.
	L.P.M. conclusions: The use of electrical current, coupled with dry needling, may be an effective TrPT for veterinary patients. Further studies are needed to confirm the efficacy and practicality of this methodology.
Study limitations	(Margalef et al. 2019)
1) TrP were experimentally induced which may affect their biochemical, circulatory, and neurologic responses.	

Table 9.7 Examples of studies demonstrating the efficacy of trigger point therapy in laboratory animals in the treatment of multiple diseases and conditions as of 2023.

Condition studied	Therapeutic technique	Species studied	Studies
Biochemical changes	DN	Rat	Li et al. (2019), Zhang et al. (2020), Felber et al. (2022)
Cessation of spontaneous electrical activity	DN	Rat	Huang et al. (2015), Meng et al. (2015)
Neuromuscular damage	DN	Mice	Domingo et al. (2013)
Reduction of substance P levels	DN	Rabbit	Hsieh et al. (2014)
Trigger point creation	n/a	Mice	Margalef et al. (2019)
		Rat	Lv et al. (2018), Zhang et al. (2017)
Trigger point reversal	DN with current	Mice	Margalef et al. (2020)

DN, dry needle. Source: Lisa P. McFaddin.

Almost all the available research in companion animals is extrapolated from human and laboratory animal studies, and/or based on case studies. Table 9.7 lists the most common conditions, and their studies, for which TrPT in laboratory animals has shown a scientifically beneficial effect. This list is not all inclusive as new research is continually published.

The How

Team Members

This section reviews the potential return on investment (ROI), how to effectively train the entire team, how to promote, and how to integrate the integrative therapy.

Return on Investment

ROI can be determined by evaluating client interest, veterinarian demand, hospital costs, applicability of the service, appointment scheduling, and pricing.

Client Interest

Currently there are no studies documenting client interest or the popularity of TrPTs. By evaluating trends in client opinion and pet health insurance, interest in TrPTs can be inferred.

Table 9.8 Summary of the 2022 pet ownership and pet health insurance demographics in the United States discussed in the Introduction of the book (Burns 2018, 2022; MFAF 2018; APPA 2022; Nolen 2022; NAPHIA 2023).

- 83% of pets are owned by millennials (32%), generation X (24%), and baby boomers (27%)
- 69 million households owned dogs
- 45.3 million households owned cats
- Estimated over 81.1 million owned dogs
- Estimated over 60.7 million owned cats
- 68% of owners are interested in alternative treatment modalities for their pets
- 4.41 million pets have pet health insurance
- 82% of insurance pets are dogs

Source: Lisa P. McFaddin.

Client Opinion   Table 9.8 summarizes the pet owner demographics and statistics mentioned in the My Lessons section of the Introduction. Even if 25% of those owners are open to TrPTs, that is still 26.6 million potential patients.

The treatment of pain in veterinary patients is a hot button issue amongst both owners and practitioners. The existence of the International Veterinary Academy of Pain Management (IVAPM), Certified Veterinary Pain Practitioners (CVPP), 2015 and 2022 American Animal Hospital Association (AAHA) and American Association of Feline Practitioners (AAFP) Pain Management for Dogs and Cats consensus statement, and Animal Pain Awareness Month in September highlights the importance and community awareness of this issue (Epstein et al. 2015; Grant et al. 2022). As such, any treatment which effectively reduces companion animal pain should and will spark the interest of clients and veterinarians.

Pet Health Insurance   Many pet insurance plans include coverage for integrative therapies, including manual therapies such as TrPTs (Woodley 2018). The presence of this type of coverage re-emphasizes the mainstream incorporation of these treatment modalities, as well as reflecting client demand.

Veterinarian Demand

The best way to determine veterinarian demand is to compare the number of general practitioners to the number of veterinarians advertising trigger point therapy, massage, acupuncture, and rehabilitation within a 5-, 10-, or 20-mile radius of the hospital. Less than 10% of the practices should offer TrPT to avoid oversaturation of the market and the introduction of a redundant service.

Hospital Costs

Let us start by reviewing the potential costs associated with introducing and offering TrPTs: veterinarian training, staff training, supplies and equipment, staffing, facilities, and advertising. Tables 9.9 and 9.10 demonstrate varying start-up costs, dependent on the hospital's contribution toward the veterinarian's training and prior utilization of regular all-staff meetings. For more information on potential hospital costs refer to the Introduction of this book.

Veterinarian Training

Course Costs   There are currently three courses on TrPT in the United States. The programs focus on on-site only or hybrid on-site/online training. The hands-on portion lasts two to four days, depending on the program. Only one of the courses offers a certification program. Additional information can be found in the Veterinarians section of this chapter (cost range, $1195–1347).

Textbooks   Textbooks are typically required. The price range for two to three books is $200–500 (average cost, $350).

Travel Expenses   Travel costs include airfare, lodging, car rental, and meals. The estimated pricing is based on one on-site session with two to four full days of training.

- *Airfare:* The average roundtrip domestic flight within the United States was $398 in June 2022 and has continued to rise by at least 3.4% in the last eight months to

Table 9.9 Total potential hospital start-up costs and per patient expenses for trigger point therapy as of 2023.

Category	Sub-categories	Projected cost	
Veterinarian training	Course costs	$1195–1347	Average $1281
	Textbooks	$200–500	Average $250
	Travel expenses	$1475	
	Time-off	$0–386	Average $193
Staff training	Variable	$230–1295	
Supplies	Acupuncture needles	$12 per box	$2.50 per patient
	Electroacupuncture unit	$400 per unit	$0.76–4.02 per patient
Staffing	Variable	≥$0	
Facilities	Overhead	$2–5/minute per 30–60-minute appointment	$60–300 per patient
Advertising	Variable	≤$420	

Source: Lisa P. McFaddin.

approximately $412 (BLS 2023; Trcek 2023). The $412 value was used when calculating the cost of airfare for one roundtrip flights (total cost, $412).

- *Lodging:* As of February 2023 the federal per diem rate for lodging on business trips is $98 per night (FederalPay.org 2023). The cost range for three to five nights of lodging is $294–490 (average cost, $392).
- *Car rental:* As of January 2023, the average weekly car rental price was $551 (French and Kemmis 2023). Rideshare and cabbing are extremely popular, but the variability in travel distances makes calculating an average cost impractical. It is suspected this cost would be comparable, if not lower, than that of a rental car. The total was based on one five-day rental (total cost, $551).
- *Meals:* The federal per diem rate for business trip meals from October 2022 through September 2023 is $59 a day (FederalPay. org 2023). Most training programs provide at least one meal, as well as snacks. Meal expenditure is estimated to be $40/day for two to four days (average cost, $120).
- *Time Off:* Veterinarian paid time-off (PTO) for on-site courses only factors in as an added expense if additional PTO is provided outside of the veterinarian's contractual annual PTO. Clinics offer an average of 4.1 paid CE days per year according to the last AAHA Compensation and Benefits Guide (AAHA 2019). If the total number of CE days exceeds the allotted CE days per year, the hospital can either require the veterinarian use PTO or pay the veterinarian for some or all the remaining CE days. Requiring the use of PTO would not "cost" the hospital anything additional.

The clinic accrues an added expense if they agree to pay for the additional CE days. The price range provided represents a clinic offering 5–12 days of additional paid CE leave. The median pay for a full-time veterinarian, calculated by the United States Bureau of Labor Statistics in 2022, was $100 370 or $48.26/hour

Table 9.10 Projected trigger point therapy (TrPT) start-up costs for eight hospital scenarios, with varying hospital contributions toward veterinary certification and staff training as of February 2023. The cost of veterinarian training is based on the averages presented in Table 9.9. Staff training costs assume a 1.5-hourlong all-staff meeting, using national averages for employee numbers: eight non-DVMs and two DVMs (AVMA 2019, 2023). The cost of office supplies and lunch as estimated based on 10 employees attending the meeting. The overhead is based on an average of $3.5/minute. Missed revenue is calculated using the 2022 national mean revenue per hour for companion animal practices ($567/hour) (AVMA 2023). All examples assume dry needling (DN), with the potential for electric current, will be an offered service. If an electroacupuncture unit is not required, the total start-up cost would be $400 less. Advertising includes printed materials, digital advertisement, and community engagement.

Category	Projected expenses	Ex. 1	Ex. 2	Ex. 3	Ex. 4	Ex. 5	Ex. 6	Ex. 7	Ex. 8
Veterinarian training	Average course cost	$1281	$1281	$1281	n/a	$1281	$1281	$1281	n/a
	Average textbooks	$250	n/a	n/a	n/a	$250	n/a	n/a	n/a
	Travel expenses	$1475	n/a	n/a	n/a	$1475	n/a	n/a	n/a
	Average time-off	$193	$193	n/a	n/a	$193	$193	n/a	n/a
Staff training	Office supplies	$30	$30	$30	$30	$30	$30	$30	$30
	Lunch	$200	$200	$200	$200	$200	$200	$200	$200
	Overhead	$315	$315	$315	$315	n/a	n/a	n/a	n/a
	Missed revenue	$851	$851	$851	$851	n/a	n/a	n/a	n/a
Supplies	Five boxes acupuncture needles	$50	$50	$50	$50	$50	$50	$50	$50
	Electroacupuncture unit	$400	$400	$400	$400	$400	$400	$400	$400
Advertising		$420	$420	$420	$420	$420	$420	$420	$420
Total		**$5465**	**$3740**	**$3547**	**$2266**	**$4299**	**$2574**	**$2381**	**$1100**

Source: Lisa P. McFaddin.

(BLS 2022). Each paid CE day was counted as eight hours. The total does not include potential lost revenue due to the veterinarian's absence, nor does it include relief veterinarian expenses. The number of additional paid CE days was estimated to be zero to one day (average cost, $193).

Staff Training Team training expenses are highly variable and dependent on the preexistence of staff meetings and use of a staff meeting for training (compared to self-study). Refer to the Introduction of the book for a breakdown of these variables (cost range, $230–1295).

Supplies Supplies are only needed if DN is performed. TPPR can be performed without sedation during an integrative appointment.

The specific type and quantity of needles kept on-hand is dependent on practitioner preference and the hospital's goal for consumables on-hand. Given this variability the expected expenditure for acupuncture needles is based on the cost per patient. The range assumes a cost of $12 for a box of 100 needles with 10–30 needles used per patient (total per patient, $2.50).

If electric current is used during the DN session, an electroacupuncture unit can be used. The average cost is $400 per unit. The price range per patient is based on the frequency of use and the assumptions and calculations presented by a 2015 paper discussing the profitability of veterinary acupuncture, which is being applied to DN for TrPs (Marks and Shmalberg 2015) (total per patient, $0.76–4.02).

Additional supplies for DN include various medications used for sedation, anesthetic monitoring, an oxygen source, and crash cart (just in case). The price of these materials is not included because the majority of hospitals already have these items on hand, the medications and quantities used for sedation are practitioner dependent, and not all practitioners will sedate patients for DN.

Staffing TrPT appointments range from 30 to 60 minutes depending on the treatment method and number of TrPs being treated. Following the American Animal Hospital Association (AAHA) recommendations a veterinary assistant or licensed technician (VA/LT) should restrain patients for physical examinations and procedures. A VA/LT should also be used to monitor patients while under sedation.

Facilities Facility expenses represent the costs needed to keep the doors open (aka overhead). Overhead includes rent or mortgage, utilities, administrative costs, and often employee costs divided by the minutes the practice is open (Stevenson 2016). The price per minute equals the amount of revenue needed just to break even. Overhead is extremely hospital specific, but the range tends to be $2–5/minute. The low end of the range in Table 9.9 represents the cost for a 30-minute appointment at a clinic with a $2/minute overhead, while the high end represents the cost for a 60-minute appointment at a clinic with a $5/minute overhead.

Designating a specific room for integrative appointments minimizes the chances other associates will need the room for their appointments. However, there is then an added expense for designing the room and potential lost revenue if the room is not used regularly. The absence of a designated room theoretically reduces redecoration costs, but this can be disruptive for appointment flow if the treatment takes longer than the allotted time.

Procedures requiring sedation are typically performed in the treatment room, often without the owner present. Hospitals can use their current treatment area eliminating the need for further renovations.

Advertising There are numerous ways to advertise a new service. On average veterinary hospitals spend 0.7% of revenue on promotion and advertisement (AVMA 2019). Most of the advertising can be done with little to no additional expenditure. The Promotion section discusses advertising ideas in further detail. The national median gross revenue for companion animal practices was $1.2 million in 2022 (AVMA 2023). Advertising costs are calculated assuming no more than 5% of the current advertising budget would be used for promotion of the new service (estimated maximal cost, $420).

Start-Up Costs Table 9.9 summarizes projected start-up costs for TrPT. Table 9.10 calculates potential start-up costs based on the degree of hospital contribution toward veterinarian and staff training. Different scenarios are presented in which the hospital covers all, some, or none of the expenses.

Applicability

According to the Healthy Paws Pet Insurance and Foundation 2019 Cost of Pet Health Care Report 18.8% of canine vet visits were related to pain and musculoskeletal injuries, while 6.8% of feline visits were related to painful conditions (HPPIF 2019). As stated previously TrPT is useful in the management and prevention of pain. This treatment modality is an invaluable addition to any practitioner's toolbox when it comes to treating the third most common reason for taking a dog, and seventh most common reason for taking a cat, to the veterinarian (HPPIF 2019).

Appointment Scheduling

There are four main factors to consider when planning TrPTs appointment protocols: appointment length; support staff availability; exam room availability; and follow-up appointment scheduling. There are several additional issues to consider when scheduling TrPT appointments. First, TPPR and DN should be scheduled separately from traditional Western appointments. Secondly, the initial TPPR appointment is longer compared to follow-up appointments, often 60 minutes. Follow-up appointments should be scheduled for 30–60 minutes depending on the patient and if additional treatments are performed.

Third, DN appointments should always be scheduled separately if sedation is required. On average these procedures take 60 minutes from the time of the pre-sedation exam to recovery. Finally, keep the appointment positive. You want to pet to enjoy the experience. A relaxed pet is more easily treated. Avoid ancillary procedures which may cause stress: nail trims, anal gland expression, sanitary trims, anything with the ears, etc. Additional information on appointment scheduling can be found in the Introduction of this book.

Pricing

An in-depth look into appointment pricing can be found in the Introduction of this book. Here we discuss two pricing methods: current market fees and hospital cost-based pricing.

Current Market Fees There are no average current market fees available for TPPR and/or DN. The average cost of veterinary massage and/or rehabilitation services could be used to infer the cost of TPPR, while the average cost of veterinary acupuncture ± the cost of sedation can be used to surmise the cost of DN. See Chapter 1 for specific acupuncture pricing information.

Hospital Cost-Based Pricing Table 9.11 outlines the hospital cost per patient for 30- and 60-minute TrPT appointments, assuming sedation is not performed. Hospitals will need to review their current pricing structure for sedation and anesthesia monitoring to adjust treatment prices accordingly.

The veterinarian training amortization per patient was calculated using the following assumptions:

1. The average companion animal practice employees 2.1 full-time veterinarians (AVMA 2023).

Table 9.11 Estimated hospital costs per patient for 30- and 60-minute trigger point therapy (TrPT) appointments as of February 2023. Start-up costs are taken from the totals in Table 9.10. Amortization is per patient and is based on the veterinarian seeing 952 acupuncture patients in two years. Overhead is calculated using $3.5/minute in a practice with two veterinarians. Multiple examples are provided with the variance determined by the total cost within each category. The total is rounded to the nearest whole number.

	Ex. 1	Ex. 2	Ex. 3	Ex. 4	Ex. 5	Ex. 6	Ex. 7	Ex. 8
30-Minute appointments								
Table 9.10 totals	$5465	$3740	$3547	$2266	$4299	$2574	$2381	$1100
Amortization	$5.74	$3.93	$3.73	$2.38	$4.52	$2.70	$2.50	$1.16
Overhead	$52.50	$52.50	$52.50	$52.50	$52.50	$52.50	$52.50	$52.50
Total	**$58**	**$56**	**$56**	**$55**	**$57**	**$55**	**$55**	**$54**
60-Minute appointments								
Table 1.9 totals	$5465	$3740	$3547	$2266	$4299	$2574	$2381	$1100
Amortization	$5.74	$3.93	$3.73	$2.38	$4.52	$2.70	$2.50	$1.16
Overhead	$105	$105	$105	$105	$105	$105	$105	$105
Total	**$111**	**$109**	**$109**	**$107**	**$110**	**$108**	**$108**	**$106**

Source: Lisa P. McFaddin.

2. The average companion animal practice is open for appointments 5.6 days per week (AVMA 2023).
3. The average companion animal veterinarian sees two patients per hour (AVMA 2023).
4. The average companion animal veterinarian works 45 hours a week (AVMA 2023).
5. The average companion animal veterinarian spends 78% of their work week seeing appointments (AVMA 2023).
6. The average companion animal veterinarian receives 21 paid days of vacation and holiday pay annually (iVet360 2023).
7. The average companion animal veterinarian receives 4.1 paid days off for CE per year (AAHA 2019).
8. Using the percentages established for veterinary acupuncture appointments, TrPT treatments were presumed to account for 14% of a veterinarian's appointments (Marks and Shmalberg 2015).
9. The amortization is calculated over a two-year period.

Using the above information, the typical companion animal veterinarian sees 3398 patients a year (70 patients a week, working 48.4 weeks a year); 476 of these patients would receive TrPT, for a total of 952 patients in two years.

Supply assumptions were based on the average cost per patient for each supply listed in Table 9.9. Appointments without DN would cost the hospital $2.5–5 less per patient, depending on the use of an electroacupuncture unit.

Overhead includes rent or mortgage, utilities, administrative costs, and often employee costs divided by the minutes the practice is open (Stevenson 2016). A $3.5/minute overhead was used. The national average of two DVMs per hospital was used, rounded down from 2.1 (AAHA 2019; AVMA 2023).

The formula to determine service fees is quite simple: Service Fee = Hospital Cost + Profit. The big question becomes how much profit? Table 9.12 illustrates the potential fee for 30- and 60-minute TrPT appointments, based on hospital cost and variable markup percentages. It becomes readily apparent that the lower the hospital contribution, the higher the

Table 9.12 Potential 30- and 60-minute trigger point therapy (TrPT) appointment prices using hospital costs from Table 1.11 at varying percentage markups as of February 2023.

		Ex. 1	Ex. 2	Ex. 3	Ex. 4	Ex. 5	Ex. 6	Ex. 7	Ex. 8
30-Minute appointments									
Total hospital cost		**$58**	**$56**	**$56**	**$55**	**$57**	**$55**	**$55**	**$54**
Potential appointment price	40% Markup	$81	$78	$78	$77	$80	$77	$77	$76
	50% Markup	$87	$84	$84	$83	$86	$83	$83	$81
	60% Markup	$93	$112	$107	$94	$118	$111	$105	$93
	70% Markup	$99	$95	$95	$94	$97	$94	$94	$92
	80% Markup	$104	$101	$101	$99	$103	$99	$99	$97
	90% Markup	$110	$106	$106	$105	$108	$105	$105	$103
	100% Markup	$116	$112	$112	$110	$114	$110	$110	$108
60-Minute appointments									
Total hospital cost		**$111**	**$109**	**$109**	**$107**	**$110**	**$108**	**$108**	**$106**
Potential appointment price	40% Markup	$155	$153	$153	$150	$154	$151	$151	$148
	50% Markup	$167	$164	$164	$161	$165	$162	$162	$159
	60% Markup	$178	$112	$107	$94	$118	$111	$105	$93
	70% Markup	$189	$185	$185	$182	$187	$184	$184	$180
	80% Markup	$200	$196	$196	$193	$198	$194	$194	$191
	90% Markup	$211	$207	$207	$203	$209	$205	$205	$201
	100% Markup	$222	$218	$218	$214	$220	$216	$216	$212

Source: Lisa P. McFaddin.

comparative profit. Keep in mind for sedated procedures the hospital's cost for sedation and/or current pricing for sedation must be factored into the final appointment price.

Additional Considerations   Most of my patients receive other treatments or diagnostics when they come in for their treatments. Frequently we adjust current medication regimens, run diagnostics (blood work, urinalysis, radiographs, etc.), discuss dietary and environmental modifications, and discuss nutrition and nutraceuticals, all of which increases revenue, average transaction charge (ATC), and DVM revenue per hour. Offering TrPT also helps improve current client retention and drive new client acquisition.

Team Training
The concept of phase training is used when introducing TrPT to the hospital team. A multimedia approach is used to assist with the training program and is outlined in Table 9.13.

Practice Manager's Role in Training
To conquer this task the pratice manager needs his or her own checklist which includes the following information:

- Schedule a date and time for the team training.
- Ensure all information pertaining to the new service is reviewed with the staff.
- Confirm all team members have completed the training.
- Certify all team members understand the information and can successfully educate clients.

Table 9.13 The breakdown of phase training steps and resources for the entire hospital team.

Phase 1: Background information	
Team training guide	The handout walks the practice manager and/or veterinarian through Phase 1 of the training
	A downloadable and editable copy of the handout is located on the companion website
Training presentation	The video covers background information on the modality
	PowerPoints can be downloaded, edited, and personalized from the companion website
	The document can be used as a PowerPoint or saved as an mp4 creating a personalized movie
Team training handout	The handout provides additional background information for the CSRs, VAs, and LTs to complement the knowledge gained from watching the training presentation
	A downloadable and editable copy of the handout is located on the companion website
Phase 2: Knowledge proficiency	
Quiz	A short quiz to ensure all team members have a good understanding of the service being offered
	A downloadable and editable copy of the handout is located on the companion website
	A key is provided
Phase 3: Expectations	
Training worksheets	A training checklist is provided for CSRs and VA/LTs with role-specific expectations and tasks for each staff member
	A recommended completion time is provided
	A downloadable and editable copy of the handout is located on the companion website
Phase 4: Client education	
Client scripts	Bullet point information and scripted examples used when discussing acupuncture with clients
	A downloadable and editable copy of the handout is located on the companion website
Client education presentation	A short (five to seven minute) client educational video about the therapeutic modality
	PowerPoints can be downloaded, edited, and personalized from the companion website
	The document can be used as a PowerPoint or saved as an mp4 creating a personalized movie
Client education handout	An informational handout about the therapeutic modality written specifically for clients
	A downloadable and editable copy of the handout is located on the companion website

CSR, customer service representative; VA, veterinary assistant; LT, licensed technician. Source: Lisa P. McFaddin.

Promotion

There are six common avenues of promotion for a veterinary integrative medicine (VIM) service: hospital website, social media, email blasts, mailers, in-hospital promotions, and client education.

Hospital Website

Advertise "Trigger Point Therapy" or "Dry Needling" in several locations on the website. On the made page insert "Now offering veterinary trigger point therapy" or "Now offering veterinary dry needling" with a link to success stories or client testimonials. Utilize the hospital website to advertise the VIM treatment under the "Services" section. Under Veterinarian Biograph include a description of the specialized training. Create a TrPT blog page discussing patient success stories.

Social Media

Utilize Facebook, Instagram, and/or Twitter to post facts, photographs, hashtags, and patient success stories. Include fun and intriguing facts about TrPT. Clients love patient photographs, especially when receiving TrPT treatments. Create or utilize veterinary TrPT specific hashtags.

Email Blasts

Send fun mass emails to your clients introducing TrPT. Consider monthly case presentations illustrating how the service has benefited patients. Almost everyone has at least one email address these days. Customer service representatives should be amassing client emails at the same rate as phone numbers.

Mailers

Mailers can be expensive and are largely unnecessary in this digital age. Mailers can be used to announce the introduction of a new service to existing clients. The mailer should include the name of the new service, a brief description of how TrPT can help pet patients, the name of the doctor performing the treatments, possibly a brief description of the training the doctor received, and possibly a photograph of a pet receiving TrPT.

In-Hospital Promotions

Advertise TrPT within the hospital sing promotional signs, invoice teasers, and wearable pieces of flare. Small promotional signs can be placed in the waiting room and exam rooms. Include photographs of pets receiving TrPT.

Informational signs should include a brief description of how TrPT can help pet patients, photographs of pets receiving TrPT, name of the doctor performing the treatment, and possibly a brief description of the training the doctor received.

Invoice teasers should consist of short phrases reminding and enticing owners regarding a new service offered at the practice. Examples include "Now offering Veterinary Trigger Point Therapy"; "Now offering Veterinary Dry Needling"; "Curious if trigger point therapy can help your pet?"; "Curious if dry needling can help your pet?"; "Introducing Veterinary Trigger Point Therapy"; "Introducing Veterinary Dry Needling"; "Would your pet benefit from Veterinary Trigger Point Therapy?"; "Would your pet benefit from Veterinary Dry Needling?"

Buttons can be made for the staff to wear reminding owners of the new VIM service. Examples include "What's TrPT?"; "Want to learn more about Veterinary Trigger Point Therapy?"; "Want to learn more about Veterinary Dry Needling?"

Client Education

Education is crucial to understanding the purpose and importance of any given treatment. The client handouts and videos solidify pet owner knowledge base, reducing concerns and conveying value.

Integration

The key components for proper integration include availability of the service to the right patients; appropriate patient scheduling; appropriate support staff scheduling; and staff buy-in (understanding the benefits of the offered service).

Veterinarians

There are several factors to contemplate when veterinarians are considering, and preparing to incorporate, a VIM in their clinical repertoire: state requirements and restrictions, return on investment, course availability, supplies and equipment, veterinary organizations, and continuing education.

State Requirements and Restrictions
Is TrPT Considered the Practice of Veterinary Medicine?
Each state has its own veterinary provisions outlining what is and is not considered the practice of veterinary medicine. Currently no state specifically defines veterinary TrPT as the

Table 9.14 The most used veterinary acupuncture suppliers.

Jing Tang Herbal	A Time to Heal	Lhasa Oms
9700 West Hwy 318, Reddick, FL 32686	140 Webster Road, Shelburne, VT 05482	230 Libbey Parkway, Weymouth, MA 02189
(352) 591-2141 (800) 891-1986	(802) 497-2375	(800) 722-8775
https://store.tcvmherbal.com	https://atimetohealherbs.com	https://www.lhasaoms.com

Source: Lisa P. McFaddin.

practice of veterinary medicine. Although many states do consider acupuncture the practice of veterinary medicine and these states may consider dry needling TrPs akin to acupuncture (see Table 1.14 in Chapter 1). Keep in mind these rules can change, and careful review of your specific state requirements is recommended.

Does TrPT Continuing Education Count toward Licensure Continuing Education Requirements?
Currently no states require specific CE hours for veterinarians offering TrPT nor do they specifically reference TrPT CE. Some states limit the use of integrative medicine CE hours toward the annual CE requirement for license renewal. Most states permit the use of integrative CE if the lectures or webinars are performed by an approved provider. Review your specific state's requirements for further details. Table 1.14 in Chapter 1 lists each state's CE requirements and provides links for their Board of Veterinary Medicine on the companion website.

Are Your Assets Covered?
Check with your liability insurance to determine if you are covered when practicing TrPT. Refer to the Introduction of this book for additional information.

Return on Investment
Specifics are discussed in the Team Members section of this chapter.

Course Availability
While certification is not required, formal training is highly recommended. Training

and certification provide the foundation for understanding how TrPT can best help your veterinary patients. Completion of formal training also helps legitimize the modality. While the current training options are limited, major conferences may offer RACE-approved lectures on TrPT. Unfortunately, wet labs at these conferences is almost unheard of. Some veterinary organizations, such as the College of Integrative Veterinary Therapies (CIVT), offer paid webinars. These introductory lectures can provide a basic understanding regarding the mechanisms of action and practical applications of TrPT, hopefully priming interested veterinarians to undergo more extensive training. Additionally, most acupuncture certification and training courses briefly discuss TrPT. Course pricing is accurate as of February 2023.

Myopain Seminar
- **Course name**: Canine Trigger Point Management
- **Prerequisite**: Licensed veterinarians, veterinary technicians, and physical therapists
- **Description**
  - Approximately 16 hours of American Association of Veterinary State Boards (AAVSB) Registry of Approved Continuing Education (RACE)-approved CE hours.
  - Introductory course on canine trigger point diagnosis and management including anatomy, trigger point pressure release, and dry needling.
  - Small class sizes (maximum 20 people).
  - Lectures and wet labs.

- **Online training**: Not applicable
- **On-site training**: Two days with varying locations.
- **Cost**: $1195
- **Contact information**

  – Address: 4405 East-West Highway, Suite 401, Bethesda, MD 20814
  – Website: www.myopainseminars.com
  – Email: info@myopainseminars.com
  – Telephone: 855-209-1832

NC State Veterinary Medicine and Northwest Seminars

- **Course name**: Small Animal Myofascial Practitioner Program (CSMP)
- **Prerequisites**: Licensed veterinarians, veterinary technicians, and physical therapists
- **Description**

  – A 24-hour (pending AAVSB RACE approval) certification course affording the post-nominal initials CSMP (Certified Small Animal Myofascial Practitioner) upon completion.
  – Provides foundational information on the diagnosis and treatment of MPS and TrPs in the canine and feline patient.
  – Covers manual therapies and dry needling for 25 major muscle groups including the most common TrP locations, referral patterns, and treatment protocols.
  – Combination online and on-site.
  – Online portion covers myofascial pain, TrPs, anatomy, and a multimodal treatment approach.
  – On-site portions involve hands-on labs focusing on TrP identification and treatment options, as well as reviewing gait analysis, movement patterns, and compensatory mechanisms.
  – Completion of the course requires passing an online final exam and three case studies within 90 days of completion of the hands-on portion of the course.
- **Online training**: 10 hours and final exam
- **On-site training**: Two days in Colchester, CT
- **Cost**: $1347
- **Contact information**: https://www.ncsu-vetce.com

Rocky Mountain School of Animal Acupressure and Massage

- **Course name**: Canine TrPT
- **Prerequisites**: Licensed veterinarians, veterinary technicians, massage therapists, and physical therapists
- **Description**

  – No information provided on the number of CE hours, and no mention of AAVSB RACE approval.
  – Online portion covers neuromuscular physiology, muscular anatomy, and functional anatomy.
  – Hands-on portion covers trigger point identification and manual therapies.
  – Dry needling is not covered in this course.
- **Online training**: Not specified
- **On-site training**: Four days in Littleton, CO.
- **Cost**: $1300
- **Contact information**:

  – Address: 7745 N Moore Rd., Littleton, CO 80125
  – Website: www.rmsaam.com
  – Email: information@rmsaam.com
  – Telephone: 303-660-9390

Supplies and Equipment

TPPR does not require additional supplies. DN requires acupuncture needles and possibly an electroacupuncture unit. DN may also require the use of syringes, needles, and sedation materials, but these supplies are generally already used in a veterinary practice for other sedated or anesthetized procedures.

Acupuncture needles (28, 30, and 32g) of varying lengths (1, 1.5, and 2 inches) are used. Acupuncture needles typically cost $12 for a box of 100. Table 9.14 lists commonly used suppliers.

Hospital remodeling and/or redecorating is generally not required when offering TrPT. DN is usually performed in the treatment room with easy access to anesthesia machines in the unlikely event of an adverse drug reaction.

TPPR can be performed in traditional exam rooms. Some practitioners prefer to have a dedicated manual therapy room while others use existing spaces. Having comfy places for the patient to lie down is highly recommended. This can be accomplished with yoga mats or puzzle floor mats and towels or blankets. Creating a relaxing environment with soft music and diffusors (lavender or pheromones) is also beneficial.

Veterinary Organizations

A description of the most common veterinary organizations with a special interest in acupuncture are provided below. Table 9.15 summarizes the organizations' names, contact information, and membership dues as of February 2023.

American Academy of Veterinary Acupuncture (AAVA)

- **Description**: The AAVA was founded in 1998 and is affiliated with IVAS. The goals of the AAVA are to promote the education, understanding, and professional development of veterinarians practicing veterinary acupuncture, TCVM, and other Eastern medicine practices. There is no annual CE requirement to maintain membership.
- **Membership benefits**

  – Free subscription to the *American Journal of Traditional Chinese Veterinary Medicine*, a peer-reviewed journal.
  – Searchable member directory.
  – Help advance integrative medicine through the AAVA's seat on the AVMA House of Delegates.
  – Access to the career center with open positions and potential candidates.
  – Option to advance the veterinarian's acupuncture development through completion

Table 9.15 Veterinary associations and organizations with a special interest in trigger point therapy (TrPT) as of February 2023.

Organization	Contact information	Membership dues
American Academy of Veterinary Acupuncture (AAVA)	PO Box 803, Fayetteville, TN 37334 (931) 438-0238 office@aava.org	$150/year
American Holistic Veterinary Medical Association (AHVMA)	PO Box 630, Abingdon, MD 21009 (410) 569-0795 office@ahvma.org	$300/year
College of Integrative Veterinary Therapies (CIVT)	PO Box 352, Yeppoon, 4703 QLD, Australia (303) 800-5460 membership@civtedu.org	$185/year
International Veterinary Academy of Pain Management (IVAPM)	PO Box 1868, Mt. Juliet, TN 371211 info@ivapm.org	$150/year
International Veterinary Acupuncture Society (IVAS)	PO Box 271 458, Fort Collins, CO 80527 (970) 266-0666 office@ivas.org	$110/year
World Association of Traditional Chinese Veterinary Medicine (WATCVM)	WATCVM and AATCVM PO Box 141 324, Gainesville, FL 32614 (844) 422-8286 support@aatcvm.org	$85/year

Source: Lisa P. McFaddin.

of the Fellows of American Academy of Veterinary Acupuncturists (FAAVA) certification process.
- The AAVA hosts an annual CE.

American Holistic Veterinary Medical Association (AHVMA)
- **Description**: The AHVMA was founded in 1982 at the Western States Veterinary Conference with the goal of advancing integrative medicine through the education of integrative and non-integrative veterinarians, the introduction of integrative medicine to veterinary students, the promotion of research, and representation in the AVMA House of Delegates. There is no annual CE requirement to maintain membership.
- **Membership benefits**

  - Free subscription to the *AHVMA Journal*, a peer-reviewed journal.
  - Online resources for client education.
  - Searchable member directory.
  - Discounted vaccination titers through Kansas State University (KSU) Diagnostic Lab.
  - Free access to the Natural Medicines Database, an online resource for supplements, natural medicines, and integrative therapies.
  - Reduced cost for the AHVMA annual conference.

College of Integrative Veterinary Therapies (CIVT)
- **Description**: An online organization open to all licensed animal health providers interested in integrative medicine. There are two membership options: full membership for veterinarians and associate membership for registered animal health professionals. CIVT strives to promote all aspects of evidence-based integrative medicine through online education and discussion forums. CIVT provides financial support to veterinary students interested in studying integrative medicine. CIVT also helps fund integrative medicine research. There is no annual CE requirement to maintain membership.

- **Membership benefits**

  - Access to the online electronic library.
  - Access to the electronic *Journal of Integrative Veterinary Therapies*.
  - Three free CE webinars annually.
  - 20% discount on all webinars.
  - Discounts on specific CIVT courses.
  - Searchable member directory.
  - Access to the Natural Medicines Databases and the American Botanical Council Library.

International Veterinary Academy of Pain Management (IVAPM)
- **Description**: Originally known as the Companion Animal Pain Management Consortium, then the Academy of Pain Management Interest Group, and finally IVAPM. Founded in 2001 to provide pain management education and certification programs. The organization's goal is to provide acute and chronic pain relief for veterinary patients. Both traditional and alternative therapies are embraced, including acupuncture and rehabilitation and physical therapy.
- **Membership benefits**

  - Members can become Certified Veterinary Pain Practitioners (CVPP).
  - Access to member's only Facebook group offering case consultations and questions.
  - Reduced subscription rate for IVAPM's journal *Veterinary Anesthesia and Analgesia*.
  - Reduced registration fee for the International Veterinary Emergency and Critical Care (IVECCS) conference.
  - Reduced registration for all IVAPM CE events (online and on-site).
  - Complementary World Small Animal Veterinary Association (WSAVA) membership.

International Veterinary Acupuncture Society (IVAS)
- **Description**: IVAS was founded in 1974 to promote and educate veterinary acupuncture.

IVAS held the first veterinary acupuncture course in 1974 in Cincinnati, Ohio. Current membership numbers are over 1800 veterinarians. Helps promote, educate, and set the global standards for veterinary acupuncture. Certified Veterinary Acupuncturists (CVA) are required to have 10 hours of acupuncture CE every two years.

- **Membership benefits**

  - Searchable member directory.
  - Access to IVAS member-only publications *The Point* published quarterly and *The Flashpoint* published monthly.
  - Discounted IVAS events and seminars.
  - Online access to IVAS Congress Proceedings.
  - Free digital subscription to the *American Journal of Traditional Chinese Veterinary Medicine*, a peer-reviewed journal.
  - Access to the in-print and online IVAS classifieds.
  - Access to online forums with other IVAS members.
  - Access to veterinary acupuncture templates for in-hospital promotion.
  - Access to veterinary acupuncture educational materials.
  - IVAS has multiple CE events annually.

World Association of Traditional Chinese Veterinary Medicine (WATCVM)

- **Description**: The WATCVM promotes the education, research, and practice of TCVM throughout the world. The WATCVM provides financial support to veterinary students interested in studying TCVM as well as establishing student organizations within veterinary schools. The WATCVM funds TCVM research programs. There is no annual CE requirement to maintain membership.
- **Membership benefits**
  - Access to online case discussion forums.
  - Free subscription to the *American Journal of Traditional Chinese Veterinary Medicine*, a peer-reviewed journal.
  - Access to the quarterly online TCVM newsletter.
  - Access to the online TCVM library.

  - Discounted TCVM conferences.
  - Access to the online classified ads.
  - Assistance with scientific writing as well as research design of grant proposals.
  - Dual membership in WATCVM and American Association of TCVM (AATCVM).
  - The WATCVM and AATCVM offer an annual International Conference on TCVM

Reference Books

The following is a list of my recommended reference books as of February 2023. A summary of each book is provided.

Acu-Cat: A Guide to Feline Acupressure
- Authors: Nancy Zidonis and Amy Snow
- Summary: An introduction to traditional Chinese veterinary medicine (TCVM) theory, the location of feline acupuncture points (acupoints), practical tips for performing acupressure, and suggested acupressure acupoints by disease condition. This book can be utilized by veterinarians, others working in the animal health field, and owners.

Acu-Dog: A Guide to Canine Acupressure
- Authors: Amy Snow and Nancy Zidonis
- Summary: A introduction to TCVM theory, the location of canine acupoints, practical tips for performing acupressure, and suggested acupressure acupoints by disease condition. This book can be utilized by veterinarians, others working in the animal health field, and owners.

Acupuncture for Dogs and Cats: A Pocket Atlas
- Author: Christina Matern, DVM
- Summary: A quick reference pocket guide introducing the basic concepts of TCVM and veterinary acupuncture. A brief outline of the location, indication, systemic effect, and technique for each canine acupoint is discussed.

Anatomy of Domestic Animals: Systemic and Regional Approach
- Authors: Chris Pasquini, DVM, MS; Tom Spurgeon, PhD; and Susan Pasquini, DVM

- Summary: Most veterinarians already own a copy from vet school. This in-depth, thorough, and entertaining anatomy book provides tons of information on the anatomy of most domestic animals.

Canine Ergonomics: The Science of Working Dogs
- Author: William S. Helton
- Summary: A comprehensive review of the physiology, cognition, and ergonomics of working dogs. There is also a discussion on training service dogs.

Canine Lameness
- Author: Felix Duerr, DVM
- Summary: An in-depth reference book covering the diagnosis and treatment of musculoskeletal diseases in dogs. There is a companion website with videos of examination techniques and lameness conditions.

Canine Rehabilitation and Physical Therapy
- Author: Darryl Mills, DVM, DACVS, DACVSMT, CCRP and David Levine, PhD, PT
- Summary: A comprehensive reference book covering canine rehabilitation protocols for a variety of conditions, printable medical record forms, canine exercises, therapeutic modality options available, physical examination specifics, and a companion website.

Canine Sports Medicine and Rehabilitation
- Authors: M. Christine Zink, DVM, PhD, DACVP, DACVSMR and Janet D. Van Dyke, DVM, DACVSMR
- Summary: A comprehensive reference book discussing common canine musculoskeletal conditions and ailments, with particular interest in the canine athlete. The book covers gait analysis and physiology, various therapeutic approaches (including nutrition, rehabilitation, manual therapy, acupuncture, chiropractic, therapeutic exercise, aquatic therapy, conditioning and retraining, and assistive devices), and specific diagnoses and treatment recommendations for disorders of the forelimbs and pelvic limbs. A must-have for veterinarians interested in manual therapy, orthopedics, and rehabilitation.

Clinician's Guide to Canine Acupuncture
- Author: Curtis Wells Dewey, DVM, MS, DACVIM (Neurology), DACVS and Huisheng Xie, DVM, MS, PhD
- Summary: An in-depth discussion of canine acupuncture focusing on the anatomic location of acupoints. A summary of the Western and Eastern indications for each acupoint is provided.

Dogs in Motion
- Authors: Martin S. Fischer and Karin E. Lije
- Summary: An in-depth look into the anatomy of canine locomotion across 32 different breeds. There is a companion DVD with over 400 movies, X-rays, and 3D animations.

Essentials of Western Veterinary Acupuncture
- Authors: Samantha Lindley, BVSc, MRCVS and Mike Cummings, DVM
- Summary: A discussion of the history, mechanisms of action, safety, and practical uses of veterinary acupuncture from a Western medicine perspective.

The Human Brain: An Introduction to its Functional Anatomy
- Author: John Notle
- Summary: A comprehensive look into the anatomy and functional neurology of the brain. While geared toward the study of the human brain, the information is applicable to veterinary patients.

Interactive Medical Acupuncture Anatomy
- Author: Narda G. Robinson, DO, DVM, MS, FAAMA
- Summary: A combination book and CD set providing detailed anatomic locations for human acupoints.

Manual of Natural Veterinary Medicine: Science and Tradition
- Authors: Susan G. Wynn, DVM and Steve Marsden, DVM, ND, MSOM, Lac, Dipl. CH., RH(AHG)

- Summary: A quick reference book discussing the integrative therapy options for numerous diseases in veterinary medicine. The book is organized by Western conditions. For each category the potential TCVM diagnoses and treatment options are then discussed in succinct detail. Chiropractic recommendations are provided for most musculoskeletal and neurologic conditions. A must-have for all integrative veterinarians.

Miller's Anatomy of the Dog
- Authors: Howard Evans, PhD and Alexander de Lahunta, DVM, PhD
- Summary: Most veterinarians already own a copy from vet school. This is a comprehensive guide to canine anatomy.

Myofascial Pain and Dysfunction: The Trigger Point Manual, Volumes 1 and 2
- Authors: David Simons, MD, Janet Travell MD, and Lois Simons PT
- Summary: A comprehensive look into the etiology, diagnosis, and treatment of human trigger points.

Trigger Point Dry Needling: An Evidence and Clinical-Based Approach
- Authors: Jan Dommerholt, PT, DPT, MPS and Cesar Fernandez de las Penas, PT, PhD Dr. SciMed
- Summary: The neurophysiology of trigger points and dry needling in people. Contains detailed descriptions and images of dry needling techniques.

Trigger Point Therapy for Myofascial Pain: The Practice of Informed Touch
- Authors: Donna Finando, Lac, LMT and Steven Finando, PhD, Lac
- Summary: Human reference book for the evaluation, common locations, and treatment of trigger-points. The book is organized by muscle grouping.

Veterinary Acupuncture
- Author: Allen M. Schoen, DVM, MS
- Summary: A detailed discussion of the history, anatomy, neurophysiologic mechanisms of action, scientific research, techniques, and practical application of veterinary acupuncture for small and large animals.

Promotion
Information regarding the hospital's promotion of TrPT can be found in the Team Members section.

Integration
Key components for proper integration include availability, scheduling, and staff buy-in. Availability means offering the service to the right patient. Scheduling refers to appropriate patient and support staff scheduling. Staff buy-in ensures all team members understand the benefits of the offered service.

Conclusion

TrPT is rapidly advancing therapeutic modality. The effects and benefits for veterinary patients center on the cessation or reduction of pain through the inactivation or dissolution of trigger points. This chapter and companion website describe in detail how TrPT can be successfully introduced into daily practice, as well as provide practical tools for implementation.

Acknowledgments

I would like to thank Dr. Matt Brunke for reviewing this chapter for content. Matt Brunke, DVM, Diplomate ACVSMR, CCRP, CVPP, CVA, CCMT is a sports medicine and rehabilitation specialist sports medicine and rehabilitation specialist at Veterinary Referral Associated in Maryland. He is an instructor through Northeast Seminars for the UT CCRP (Certified Canine Rehabilitation Practitioner) course and the small animal myofascial practitioner program. He also lectures domestically and internationally on veterinary rehabilitation and pain management. Additionally, he has authored numerous articles and several research papers on these topics.

References

AAHA (American Animal Hospital Association) (2019). *Compensation and Benefits*, 9e. Denver, CO: AAHA Press.

Abbaszadeh-Amirdehi, M., Ansari, N.N., Naghdi, S. et al. (2016). Therapeutic effects of dry needling in patients with upper trapexius myofascial trigger points. *Acupuncture in Medicine* 35 (2): 85–92.

Akamatsu, F., Ayres, B.R., Saleh, S.O. et al. (2015). Trigger points: an anatomical substratum. *BioMed Research Internation* 2015: 623287.

Al-Shenqiti, A. and Oldham, J. (2005). Test–retest reliability of myofascial trigger point detection in patients with rotator cuff tendonitis. *Clinical Rehabilitation* 19 (5): 482–487.

Álvarez, S.D., Velázquez Saornil, J., Sánchez Milá, Z. et al. (2022). Effectiveness of dry needling and ischemic trigger point compression in the gluteus medius in patients with non-specific low back pain: a randomized short-term clinical trial. *International Journal of Environmental Research and Public Health* 19 (19): 12468.

APPA (American Pet Products Association) (2022). Pet industry market size and ownership statistics. https://www.americanpetproducts.org/press_industrytrends.asp (accessed 23 February 2023).

Arany, P. (2016). Craniofacial wound healing with photobiomodulation therapy: new insights and current challenges. *Journal of Dental Research* 95 (9): 977–984.

AVMA (American Veterinary Medical Association) (2019). Economic state of the veterinary profession. https://www.avma.org/news/press-release/AVMA-2019-Economic-State-of-the-Veterinary-Profession-Report-now-available (accessed 26 July 2021).

AVMA (American Veterinary Medical Association) (2023). *2023 AVMA Report on the Economic State of the Veterinary Profession*. Schaumburg, IL: AVMA.

Barrington, G. (2022). Photosensitization in Dogs: Pet Owner Version. https://www.merckvetmanual.com/dog-owners/skin-disorders-of-dogs/photosensitization-in-dogs#:~:text=Photosensitive%20dogs%20squirm%20in%20apparent,is%20soon%20followed%20by%20swelling. (accessed 13 February 2023).

Bergh, A., Asplund, K., Lund, I. et al. (2022). A systematic review of complementary and alternative veterinary medicine in sport and companion animals: soft tissue mobilization. *Animals* 12 (11): 1440.

BLS (Bureau of Labor Statistics) (2022). Occupational outlook handbook: veterinarians 2022 median pay. https://www.bls.gov/ooh/healthcare/veterinarians.htm (accessed 18 February 2023).

BLS (Bureau of Labor Statistics) (2023). News Release: Consumer Price Index January 2023. https://www.bls.gov/news.release/pdf/cpi.pdf (accessed 18 February 2023).

Boyles, R., Fowler, R., Ramsey, D., and Burrows, E. (2015). Effectiveness of trigger point dry needling for multiple body regions: a systematic review. *Journal of Manual and Manipulative Therapy* 23 (5): 276–293.

Bron, C. and Dommerholt, J. (2012). Etiology of myofascial trigger points. *Current Pain and Headache Reports* 16 (5): 439–444.

Burns, K. (2018). Pet ownership stable, veterinary care variable. https://www.avma.org/javma-news/2019-01-15/pet-ownership-stable-veterinary-care-variable (accessed 11 August 2021).

Burns, K. (2022). New report takes a deep dive into pet ownership. https://www.avma.org/news/new-report-takes-deep-dive-pet-ownership (accessed 6 November 2022).

Butts, R., Dunning, J., and Serafino, C. (2021). Dry needling strategies for musculoskeletal conditions: do the number of needles and needle retention time matter? A narrative literature review. *Journal of Bodywork and Movement Therapies* 26: 353–363.

Cagnie, B., Castelein, B., Pollie, F. et al. (2015). Evidence for the use of ischemic compression and dry needling in the management of trigger points of the upper trapezius in patients with neck pain: a systematic review. *American Journal of Physical Medicine and Rehabilitation* 94 (7): 573–583.

Castro-Sánchez, A., García-López, H., Matarán-Peñarrocha, G.A. et al. (2017). Effects of dry needling on spinal mobility and trigger points in patients with fibromyalgia syndrome. *Pain Physician* 20 (2): 37–52.

Celik, D. and Mutlu, E.K. (2013). Clinical implication of latent myofascial trigger point. *Current Pain and Headache Reports* 17 (8): 353.

Chen, W. and Sabri, M. (2020). Concept: Quantitative evaluations of myofascial tissues: potential impact on musculoskeletal pain research. https://www.nccih.nih.gov/grants/concepts/quantitative-evaluations-of-myofascial-tissues-potential-impact-on-musculoskeletal-pain-research (accessed 5 May 2021).

Chiu, J.-H., Cheng, H.C., Tai, C.H. et al. (2001). Electroacupuncture-induced neural activation detected by use of manganese-enhanced functional magnetic resonance imaging in rabbits. *American Journal of Veterinary Research* 62 (2): 178–184.

Cho, S.-C., Kwon, D.R., Seong, J.W. et al. (2022). A pilot analysis on the efficacy of multiple trigger-point saline injections in chronic tension-type headache: a retrospective observational study. *Journal of Clinical Medicine* 11 (18): 5423.

Ciolek, J. (1985). Cryotherapy: review of physiologic effects and clinical application. *Cleveland Clinic Quarterly* 52 (2): 193–201.

Clemmons, R.M. (2007). Functional neuroanatomical physiology of acupuncture. In: *Xie's Veterinary Acupuncture* (ed. H. Xie and V. Preast), 341–347. Ames, IA: Blackwell Publishing.

Coates, J. (2013). Manual therapy. In: *Canine Sports Medicine and Rehabilitation* (ed. M.C. Zink and J.B. van Dyke), 100–114. Oxford: Wiley-Blackwell.

Cruz-Montecinos, C., Cerda, M., Becerra, P. et al. (2021). Qualitative ultrasonography scale of the intensity of local twitch response during dry needling and its association with modified joint range of motion: a cross-sectional study. *BMC Musculoskeletal Disorders* 22: 790.

Darby, S.A. (2014). Neuroanatomy of the autonomic nervous system. In: *Clinical Anatomy of the Spine, Spinal Cord, and ANS*, 3e (ed. G.D. Cramer and S.A. Darby), 413–507. St. Louis, MO: Elsevier.

Dissanayaka, T.D., Pallegama, R.W., Suraweera, H.J. et al. (2016). Comparison of the effectiveness of transcutaneous electrical nerve stimulation and interferential therapy on the upper trapezius in myofascial pain syndrome: a randomized controlled study. *American Journal of Physical Medicine and Rehabilitation* 95 (9): 663–672.

Domingo, A., Mayoral, O., Monterde, S., and Santafé, M. (2013). Neuromuscular damage and repair after dry needling in mice. *Evidence Based Complementary and Alternative Medicine* 2013: 260806.

Dommerholt, J. (2006). Trigger point dry needling. *Journal of Manual and Manipulative Therapy* 14 (4): E70–E87.

Dommerholt, J. (2011). Dry needling: peripheral and central considerations. *Journal of Manual and Manipulative Therapy* 19 (4): 223–227.

Dunning, J., Butts, R., Mourad, F. et al. (2014). Dry needling: a literature review with implications for clinical practice guidelines. *Physical Therapy Reviews* 19 (4): 252–265.

Ebadi, S., Alishahi, V., Ahadi, T. et al. (2021). Acupuncture-like versus conventional transcutaneous electrical nerve stimulation in the management of active myofascial trigger points: a randomized controlled trial. *Journal of Bodyworks and Movement Therapy* 28: 483–488.

Epstein, M., Rodan, I., Griffenhagen, G. et al. (2015). 2015 AAHA/AAFP pain management guidelines for dogs and cats. *Journal of the American Animal Hospital Association* 51 (2): 67–84.

Esparza, D., Aladro-Gonzalvo, A., and Rybarczyk, Y. (2019). Effects of local ischemic compression on upper limb latent myofascial trigger points: a study of subjective pain and linear motor performance. *Rehabilitation Research and Practice* 2019: 5360924.

Evans, H. and De Lahunta, A. (2013). *Miller's Anatomy of the Dog*, 4e. St. Louis, MO: Elsevier.

FederalPay.org (2023). FY 2023 Federal Per Diem Rates October 2022-September 2023. https://www.federalpay.org/perdiem/2023 (accessed 18 February 2023).

Felber, D.T., Malheiros, R.T., Tentardini, V.N. et al. (2022). Dry needling increases antioxidant activity and grip force in a rat model of muscle pain. *Acupuncture in Medicine* 40 (3): 241–248.

Fernández-De-Las-Peñas, C., Plaza-Manzano, G., Sanchez-Infante, J. et al. (2021). Is dry needling effective when combined with other therapies for myofascial trigger points associated with neck pain symptoms? A systematic review and meta-analysis. *Pain Research Management* 2021: 8836427.

Fernández-de-Las-Peñas, C., Plaza-Manzano, G., Sanchez-Infante, J. et al. (2022). The importance of the local twitch response during needling interventions in spinal pain associated with myofascial trigger points: a systematic review and meta-analysis. *Acupuncture Medicine* 40 (4): 299–311.

Finando, D.S.F. (2005). *Trigger Point Therapy for Myofascial Pain*. Rochester, VT: Healing Art Press.

French, S. and Kemmis, S. (2023). Rental Car Pricing Statistics:2023. https://www.nerdwallet.com/article/travel/car-rental-pricing-statistics#:~:text=The%20average%20weekly%20rental%20price,in%20advance%2C%20it%20was%20%24513 (accessed 18 February 2023).

Gerwin, R., Dommerholt, J., and Shah, J. (2004). An expansion of Simons' integrated hypothesis of trigger point formation. *Current Pain and Headache Reports* 8: 468–475.

Godbold, J. (2017). The Science of Laser Therapy and Photobiomodulation. Pacific Veterinary Conference, 29 June to 2 July 2017, Long Beach, CA. https://www.vin.com/members/cms/project/defaultadv1.aspx?pid=18559&catId=&id=8026136&said=&meta=&authorid=&preview=

Gruen, M.E., Lascelles, B.D.X., Colleran, E. et al. (2022). 2022 AAHA pain management guidelines for dogs and cats. *Journal of the American Animal Hospital Association* 58: 55–76.

Gutiérrez-Rojas, C., González, I., Navarrete, E. et al. (2015). The effect of combining myofascial release with ice application on a latent trigger point in the forearm of young adults: a randomized clinical trial. *Journal of Myofascial Pain and Fibromyalgia* 23 (3–4): 201–208.

Hakim, I.K., Takamjani, I.E., Sarrafzadeh, J. et al. (2019). The effect of dry needling on the active trigger point of upper trapezius muscle: eliciting local twitch response on long-term clinical outcomes. *Journal of Back and Musculoskeletal Rehabilitation* 32 (5): 717–724.

Hamblin, M. (2017). Mechanisms and applications of the anti-inflammatory effects of photobiomodulation. *AIMS Biophysics* 4 (3): 337–361.

Hammi, C., Schroeder, J. and Yeung, B. (2022). Trigger Point Injection. Treasure Island, FL: StatPearls. https://www.ncbi.nlm.nih.gov/books/NBK542196 (accessed 26 March 2023).

Hong, C. (1994). Lidocaine injection versus dry needling to myofascial trigger point. The importance of the local twitch response. *American Journal of Physical Medicine and Rehabilitation* 73 (4): 256–263.

HPPIF (Healthy Paws Pet Insurance and Foundation) (2019). 2019 Cost of Pet Health Care Report. https://www.healthypawspetinsurance.com/content/costofcare/pet-care-costs-health-conditions_2019.pdf (accessed 2 September 2020).

Hsieh, Y.-L., Yang, C.C., Liu, S.Y. et al. (2014). Remote dose-dependent effects of dry needling at distant myofascial trigger spots of rabbit skeletal muscles on reduction of substance P levels of proximal muscles and spinal cords. *BioMed Research International* 2014: 982121.

Huang, Q.-M., Lv, J.-J., Ruanshi, Q.-M., and Liu, L. (2015). Spontaneous electrical activities at myofascial trigger points at different stages of recovery from injury in a rat model. *Acupuncture in Medicine* 33 (4): 319–324.

IVAPM (International Veterinary Academy of Pain Management) (2020). Advocating for best practices in the prevention, detection and management of animals in pain. https://ivapm.org (accessed 22 September 2020).

iVet360 (2023). Benefits matter. https://ivet360.com/recruiting-tool-kit/wages-benefits/benefits-matter/#:~:text=Most%20companies%20provide%20a%20minimum,and%20holidays%2C%20plus%20sick%20time (accessed 23 February 2023).

Jackman, S. and Regehr, W. (2017). The mechanisms and functions of synaptic facilitation. *Neuron* 94 (3): 447–464.

Jafri, M.S. (2014). Mechanisms of myofascial pain. *International Scholarly Research Notices* 2014: 523924.

Janssens, L.A.A. (1991). Trigger points in 48 dogs with myofascial pain syndromes. *Veterinary Surgery* 20 (4): 274–278.

Jiménez-Del-Barrio, S., Medrano-de-la-Fuente, R., Hernando-Garijo, I. et al. (2022). The effectiveness of dry needling in patients with hip or knee osteoarthritis: a systematic review and meta-analysis. *Life* 12 (10): 1575.

Johnson, M. (2007). Transcutaneous electrical nerve stimulation: mechanisms, clinical application and evidence. *Reviews in Pain* 1 (1): 7–11.

Kalichman, L. and Vulfsons, S. (2010). Dry needling in the management of musculoskeletal pain. *Journal of the American Board of Family Medicine* 23 (5): 640–646.

Kashyap, R., Iqbal, A., and Alghadir, A. (2018). Controlled intervention to compare the efficacies of manual pressure release and the muscle energy technique for treating mechanical neck pain due to upper trapezius trigger points. *Journal of Pain Research* 11: 3151–3160.

Kim, K., Reid, B.A., Casey, C.A. et al. (2020). Effects of repeated local heat therapy on skeletal muscle structure and function in humans. *Journal of Applied Physiology* 128: 483–492.

Kitchens, A. (2016). Trigger points: definitions, identification, and therapeutic options. Southwest Veterinary Symposium, 21–24 September, Dallas, TX. https://www.vin.com/members/cms/project/defaultadv1.aspx?pid=16700&catId=&id=7671959&said=&meta=&authorid=&preview=

Kodama, K., Takamoto, K., Nishimaru, H. et al. (2019). Analgesic effects of compression at trigger points are associated with reduction of frontal polar cortical activity as well as functional connectivity between the frontal polar area and insula in patients with chronic low back pain: a randomized trial. *Frontiers in Systems Neuroscience* 13: 68.

Kostopoulos, D., Nelson, A., Ingber, R.S., and Larkin, R.W. (2008). Reduction of spontaneous electrical activity and pain perception of trigger points in the upper trapezius muscle through trigger point compression and passive stretching. *Journal of Musculoskeletal Pain* 16 (4): 266–278.

Lew, P., Lewis, J., and Story, I. (1997). Inter-therapist reliability in locating latent myofascial trigger points using palpation. *Manual Therapy* 2 (2): 87–90.

Li, L.-H., Huang, Q.M., Barbero, M. et al. (2019). Quantitative proteomic analysis to identify biomarkers of chronic myofascial pain and therapeutic targets of dry needling in a rat model of myofascial trigger points. *Journal of Pain Research* 12: 283–298.

Lu, W., Li, J., Tian, Y., and Lu, X. (2022). Effect of ischemic compression on myofascial pain syndrome: a systematic review and meta-analysis. *Chiropractic and Manual Therapies* 30: 34.

Lucas, N., Macaskill, P., Irwig, L. et al. (2009). Reliability of physical examination for diagnosis of myofascial trigger points: a systematic review of the literature. *Clinical Journal of Pain* 25 (1): 80–89.

Lucena-Anton, D., Luque-Moreno, C., Valencia-Medero, J. et al. (2022). Effectiveness of dry needling of myofascial trigger points in the triceps surae muscles: systematic review. *Healthcare* 10 (10): 1862.

Lv, H., Li, Z., Hu, T. et al. (2018). The shear wave elastic modulus and the increased nuclear factor kappa B (NF-kB/p65) and cyclooxygenase-2 (COX-2) expression in the area of myofascial trigger points activated in a rat model by blunt trauma to the vastus medialis. *Journal of Biomechanics* 66 (3): 44–50.

Maegawa, Y., Itoh, T., Hosokawa, T. et al. (2000). Effects of near-infrared low-level laser irradiation on microcirculation. *Lasers in Surgery and Medicine* 27 (5): 427–437.

Malanga, G.A., Yan, N., and Stark, J. (2015). Mechanisms and efficacy of heat and cold therapies for musculoskeletal injury. *Postgraduate Medical Journal* 127 (1): 57–65.

Maltese, P., Michelini, S., Baronio, M., and Bertelli, M. (2019). Molecular foundations of chiropractic therapy. *Acta Biomedica* 90 (Suppl. 10): 93–102.

Marcellin-Little, D., Levine, D., and Canapp, S. (2007). The canine shoulder: selected disorders and their management with physical therapy. *Clinical Techniques in Small Animal Practice* 22 (4): 171–182.

Margalef, R., Sisquella, M., Bosque, M. et al. (2019). Experimental myofascial trigger point creation in rodents. *Journal of Applied Physiology* 126 (1): 160–169.

Margalef, R., Bosque, M., Monclús, P. et al. (2020). Percutaneous application of galvanic current in rodents reverses signs of myofascial trigger points. *Evidence-Based Complementary and Alternative Medicine* 2020: 4173218.

Marks, D. and Shmalberg, J. (2015). Profitability and financial benefits of acupuncture in small animal private practice. *American Journal of Traditional Chinese Veterinary Medicine* 10 (1): 43–48.

Mathews, M. and Stretanski, M. (2023). *Ultrasound Therapy*. Treasure Island, FL: StatPearls https://www.ncbi.nlm.nih.gov/books/NBK547717.

Mauntel, T., Clark, M.A., and Padua, D.A. (2014). Effectiveness of myofascial release therapies on physical performance measurements: a systematic review. *Athletic Training and Sports Health Care* 6 (4): 189–196.

McCuller, C., Jessu, R., and Callahan, A. (2022). *Physiology, Skeletal Muscle*. Treasure Island, FL: StatPearls https://www.ncbi.nlm.nih.gov/books/NBK537139.

McPartland, J.M. (2004). Travell trigger points: molecular and osteopathic perspectives. *Journal of Osteopathic Medicine* 104 (6): 244–249.

Meng, F., Ge, H.-Y., Wang, Y.-H., and Yue, S.-W. (2015). Myelinated afferents are involved in pathology of the spontaneous electrical activity and mechanical hyperalgesia of myofascial trigger spots in rats. *Evidence-based Complementary and Alternative Medicine* 2015: 404971.

Mense, S. (2008). Muscle pain: mechanisms and clinical significance. *Deutsches Ärzteblatt International* 105 (12): 214–219.

Mense, S. (2010). How do muscle lesions such as latent and active trigger points influence central nociceptive neurons? *Journal of Musculoskeletal Pain* 18 (4): 348–353.

MFAF (Michelson Found Animals Foundation) (2018). Furred lines: Pet trends. https://www.prnewswire.com/news-releases/furred-lines-pet-trends-2019-300741947.html. (accessed 26 July 2021).

Miller, D., Smith, N.B., Bailey, M.R. et al. (2012). Overview of therapeutic ultrasound applications and safety considerations. *Journal of Ultrasound Medicine* 31 (4): 626–634.

Mittleman, E. and Gaynor, J. (2000). A brief overview of the analgesic and immunologic effects of acupuncture in domestic animals. *Journal of the American Veterinary Medical Association* 217 (8): 1201–1205.

Moraska, A.F., Hickner, R.C., Kohrt, W.M., and Brewer, A. (2013). Changes in blood flow and cellular metabolism at a myofascial trigger point with trigger point release (ischemic compression): a proof-of-principle pilot study. *Archives of Physical Medicine and Rehabilitation* 94 (1): 196–200.

Moraska, A., Schmiege, S.J., Mann, J.D. et al. (2017). Responsiveness of myofascial trigger points to single and multiple trigger point release massages: a randomized, placebo controlled trial. *Journal of Physical Medicine and Rehabilitation* 96 (9): 639–645.

Morihisa, R., Eskew, J., McNamara, A., and Young, J. (2016). Dry needling in subjects with muscular trigger points in the lower quarter: a systematic review. *International Journal of Sports Physical Therapy* 11 (1): 1–14.

Müggenborg, F., de Castro Carletti, E.M., Dennett, L. et al. (2023). Effectiveness of manual trigger point therapy in patients with myofascial trigger points in the orofacial region: a systematic review. *Life (Basel)* 13 (2): 336.

Myburgh, C., Lauridsen, H.H., Larsen, A.H., and Hartvigsen, J. (2011). Standardized manual palpation of myofascial trigger points in relation to neck/shoulder pain; the influence of clinical experience on inter-examiner reproducibility. *Manual Therapy* 16 (2): 136–140.

NAMTPT (National Association of Myofascial Trigger Point Therapists) (2020). About Us. https://www.myofascialtherapy.org/about-us (accessed 22 September 2020).

Nanneman, D. (1991). Thermal modalities: heat and cold. A review of physiologic effects with clinical applications. *American Association of Occupational Health Nurses Journal* 39 (2): 70–75.

NAPHIA (North American Pet Health Insurance Association) (2023). Industry data. https://naphia.org/industry-data/#my-menu (accessed 18 February 2023).

Niebaum, K. (2013). Rehabilitation physical modalities. In: *Canine Sports Medicine and Rehabilitation* (ed. M.C. Zink and J.B. van Dyke), 115–131. Oxford: Wiley-Blackwell.

Nikam, P.P. and Varadharajulu, G. (2021). Effect of variants of positional release technique vs. ischemic compression technique on trigger point in myofascial pain syndrome: a randomized controlled trial. *International Journal of Life Science and Pharma Research* 11 (2): L54–L57.

Nolen, R.S. (2022). Pet ownership rate stabilizes as spending increases. https://www.avma.org/news/pet-ownership-rate-stabilizes-spending-increases (accessed 22 February 2023).

Nolte, J. (2009). Synaptic transmission between neurons. In: *The Human Brain: An Introduction to its Functional Anatomy*, 6e, 177–200. Philadelphia, PA: Mosby Elsevier.

Osborn, J. (2018). Prolotherapy in practice. https://ivcjournal.com/prolotherapy-practice (accessed 5 May 2021).

Padulo, J., Laffaye, G., Chamari, K., and Concu, A. (2013). Concentric and eccentric: muscle contraction or exercise? *Sports Healths: A Multidisciplinary Approach* 5 (4): 306.

Pasquini, C., Spurgeon, T., and Pasquini, S. (2003). *Anatomy of Domestic Animals: Systemic and Regional Approach*, 10e. Pilot Point, TX: Sudz Publishing.

Pavón, M.J.G., Redondo, I.C., Vizcaíno, V.M. et al. (2022). Comparative effectiveness of manual therapy interventions on pain and pressure pain threshold in patients with myofascial trigger points: a network meta-analysis. *Clinical Journal of Pain* 38 (12): 749–760.

Pecos-Martin, D., Ponce-Castro, M.J., Jiménez-Rejano, J.J. et al. (2019). Immediate effects of variable durations of pressure release technique on latent myofascial trigger points of the levator scapulae: a double-blinded randomised clinical trial. *Acupuncture in Medicine* 37 (3): 141–150.

Perreault, T., Dunning, J., and Butts, R. (2017). The local twitch response during trigger point dry needling: is it necessary for successful outcomes? *Journal of Bodywork and Movement Therapies* 21 (4): 940–947.

Petrofsky, J., Laymon, M., and Lee, H. (2020). Local heating of trigger points reduces neck and plantar fascia pain. *Journal of Back and Musculoskeletal Rehabilitation* 33 (1): 21–28.

Physiopedia (2016). Trigger points. https://www.physio-pedia.com/Trigger_Points?utm_source=physiopedia&utm_medium=search&utm_campaign=ongoing_internal (accessed 20 September 2020).

Purves, D., Augustine, G., FitzPatrick, D. et al. (2012a). Lower motor neuron circuits and motor control. In: *Neuroscience*, 5e, 343–374. Sunderland, MA: Sinauer Associates.

Purves, D., Augustine, G., FitzPatrick, D. et al. (2012b). Pain. In: *Neuroscience*, 5e, 209–227. Sunderland, MA: Sinauer Associates.

Purves, D., Augustine, G., FitzPatrick, D. et al. (2012c). The somatic sensory system: touch and proprioception. In: *Neuroscience*, 5e, 189–227. Sunderland, MA: Sinauer Associates.

Sciotti, V.M., Mittak, V.L., DiMarco, L. et al. (2001). Clinical precision of myofascial trigger point location in the trapezius muscle. *Pain* 93 (3): 259–266.

Shah, S. and Alster, T. (2010). Laser treatment of dark skin: an updated review. *American Journal of Clinical Dermatology* 11 (6): 389–397.

Shah, J., Thaker, N., Heimur, J. et al. (2016). Myofascial trigger points then and now: a historical and scientific perscpective. *Physical Medicine and Rehabilitation* 7 (7): 746–761.

Shiryan, G.T., Amin, F.S., and Embaby, E.A. (2022). Effectiveness of polarized polychromatic light therapy on myofascial trigger points in chronic non-specific low back pain: a single blinded randomized controlled trial. *Bulletin of Faculty of Physical Therapy* 27: 33.

Simons, D.J.T. (1983). *Myofascial Pain and Dysfunction: The Trigger Point Manual*. Baltimore, MD: Williams and Wilkins.

Simons, D. and Stolov, W. (1976). Microscopic features and transient contraction of palpable bands in canine muscle. *American Journal of Physical Medicine and Rehabilitation* 55 (2): 65–88.

Simunovic, Z. (1996). Low level laser therapy with trigger points technique: a clinical study on 243 patients. *Journal of Clinical Laser Medicine and Surgery* 14 (4): 163–167.

Srbely, J., Dickey, J., Lee, D., and Lowerison, M. (2010). Dry needle stimulation of myofascial trigger points evokes segmental anti-nociceptive effects. *Journal of Rehabilitation Medicine* 42 (5): 463–468.

Stevenson, P. (2016). How to set practice service fees. https://cliniciansbrief.com/article/how-set-practice-service-fees. (accessed 10 June 2020).

Tantanatip, A. and Chang, K.-V. (2022). *Myofascial Pain Syndrome*. Treasure Island, FL: StatPearls https://www.ncbi.nlm.nih.gov/books/NBK499882.

Tantanatip, A., Patisumpitawong, W., and Lee, S. (2021). Comparison of the effects of physiologic saline Interfascial and lidocaine trigger point injections in treatment of myofascial pain syndrome: a double-blind randomized controlled trial. *Archives of Rehabilitation Research and Clinical Translation* 3 (2): 100119.

Trcek, L. (2023). This is how much flight prices increase in 2023 (+FAQs). https://www.travelinglifestyle.net/this-is-how-much-flight-prices-increase-in-2023 (accessed 18 February 2023).

Wall, R. (2010). Myofascial pain in dogs. https://www.dvm360.com/view/myofascial-pain-dogs-proceedings (accessed 22 September 2020).

Wall, R. (2019). Myofascial pain and dysfunction: trigger points (part 1 and 2). Pacific Veterinary Conference, 21–23 June, Long Beach, CA. https://www.vin.com/members/cms/project/defaultadv1.aspx?pid=23140&catId=&id=9111958&said=&meta=&authorid=&preview=

Wong, C.S. and Wong, S.H. (2012). A new look at trigger point injections. *Anesthesiology Research and Practice* 2012: 492452.

Woodley, K. (2018). Pet insurance for holistic and integrative practice. https://ivcjournal.com/pet-insurance-integrative-practices. (accessed 11 August 2021).

Yadollahpour, A. and Rashidi, S. (2017). A review of mechanism of actions of ultrasound waves for treatment of soft tissue injuries. *International Journal of Green Pharmacy* 11 (1): S13–S20.

Yam, M.F., Loh, Y.C., Tan, C.S. et al. (2018). General pathways of pain sensation and the major neurotransmitters involved in pain regulation. *International Journal of Molecular Sciences* 19 (8): 2164.

Yildirim, M.A., Öneş, K., and Gökşenoğlu, G. (2018). Effectiveness of ultrasound therapy on myofascial pain syndrome of the upper trapezius: randomized, single-blind, placebo-controlled study. *Archives of Rheumatology* 33 (4): 418–423.

Zhang, H., Lü, J.J., Huang, Q.M. et al. (2017). Histopathological nature of myofascial trigger points at different stages of recovery from injury in a rat model. *Acupuncture in Medicine* 35 (6): 445–451.

Zhang, Y., Du, N.Y., Chen, C. et al. (2020). Acupotomy alleviates energy crisis at rat myofascial trigger points. *Evidence Based Complementary and Alternative Medicine* 2020: 5129562.

Zhu, H. (2014). Acupoints initiate the healing process. *Medical Acupuncture* 26 (5): 264–270.

10

Veterinary Spinal Manipulation Therapy

Introduction

Veterinary spinal manipulation therapy (VSMT) was officially included as a valid therapeutic modality in the 1980s. VSMT focuses on the correction of poorly mobile (hypomobile) joints, especially within the spine. Restoration of joint mobility improves nerve and muscle function locally and throughout the body. VSMT is primarily used to treat disorders of the musculoskeletal and nervous system.

The introduction of VSMT into a veterinary practice can be beneficial for both the patient and the health of the practice. The successful incorporation and utilization of VSMT does not end with the veterinarian's training. Support staff training and client education are crucial. This chapter discusses the what, why, and how for effective integration of VSMT within your practice.

The What

Word Origin

Chiropractic is derived from the Greek words *cheir*, meaning hand, and *praktos*, meaning done (ACA 2020).

Definition

VSMT is also known as veterinary chiropractic or animal chiropractic. VSMT is an integrative medical system rooted in the diagnosis and treatment of hypomobile joints, especially those within the spinal column, which cause local and systemic dysfunction of nerves, muscles, and organs. Improvement in joint mobility, generally through manual therapy, allows the body's innate forces to heal itself, achieving homeostasis (WFC 2001; Cooperstein and Gleberzon 2004; Rivera 2015).

Integrative Medicine in Veterinary Practice, First Edition. Lisa P. McFaddin.
© 2024 John Wiley & Sons, Inc. Published 2024 by John Wiley & Sons, Inc.
Companion website: www.wiley.com/go/mcfaddin/integrativemedicine

September 18, 1895

D.D. Palmer performed the first "chiropractic adjustment" on a deaf janitor. The man lost his hearing 17 years earlier after he felt "something give in his back" (ACA 2020). Palmer palpated what he believed to be a misaligned vertebra. After performing a "forceful thrust" the misalignment resolved, and the janitor's hearing improved (Rivera 2015).

Human History

Dr. Daniel David Palmer is considered the first true practitioner of chiropractic therapy in 1895. While manual therapy had been used to treat physical ailments for thousands of years, Palmer was the first to develop a scientific explanation, using anatomy and physiology, for the benefits of manual therapy, specifically spinal manipulation (ACA 2020).

Palmer founded the first chiropractic school, now known as the Palmer College of Chiropractic, in Davenport, Iowa in 1897 (ACA 2020). Bartlett Joshua Palmer, D.D. Palmer's son, continued his father's teachings.

In 1913, Kansas became the first American state to officially recognize and license chiropractic therapy as a medical practice (ACA 2020). The United States Council of State Chiropractic Examining Boards, now known as the Federation of Chiropractic Licensing Boards, was established in 1933 standardizing state licensure requirements. The United States National Board of Chiropractic Examiners was established in 1963 to standardize the various state boards. The United States Council on Chiropractic Education was federally recognized in 1974 as the official accreditation body for chiropractic schools (WFC 2009; ACA 2020).

Until 1983 the American Medical Association (AMA) considered chiropractic an unscientific practice and decreed it unethical for physicians to professionally associate with anyone practicing unscientific medicine. In 1987 the Wilk v. AMA trial declared the AMA's actions unlawful. The trial resulted in revision of the AMA's position on the referral of patients to chiropractors (WFC 2009).

In 1994 government-sponsored panels included chiropractic as a valid treatment modality in their evidence-based guidelines for the treatment of back pain. Two years later the United States began funding chiropractic research through the National Institutes of Health (NIH). In 2005 the World Health Organization (WHO) published their recommendations regarding chiropractic educational standards in the Guidelines on Basic Training and Safety in Chiropractic (WFC 2009).

Veterinary History

Dr. Sharon Willoughby was the first veterinarian to practice chiropractic manipulations on her patients in the 1980s. Dr. Willoughby received her veterinary degree from Michigan State University College of Veterinary Medicine and went on to graduate from the Palmer School and obtain a Doctor of Chiropractic (DC). With the help of Dr. Tom Offen DC, the pair adapted chiropractic techniques to animals. Drs. Willoughby and Offen are considered the "mother" and "father" of veterinary chiropractic. Dr. Willoughby created the first veterinary chiropractic course and founded the American Veterinary Chiropractic Association (AVCA) in 1989 (Jurek 2013; Rivera 2015).

VSMT is becoming more popular in veterinary medicine, especially among equine and small animal rehabilitation practitioners. To date there are multiple certification programs for VSMT (aka animal chiropractic) available to both veterinarians and human chiropractors. The ability to practice veterinary chiropractic as a non-veterinarian is state dependent (see Table 10.24 for state-specific information).

Terminology

Like any medical system chiropractors have their own vocabulary. A basic understanding of these terms is crucial, allowing effective communication amongst professionals and with clients. Below are common terms used in veterinary and human spinal manipulation, anatomy, physiology, and neurology.

Action potential (aka nerve spike or nerve impulse): Electrical signals generated by neruons which travel along their axons (Purves et al. 2012a).

Adjustment: The application of any chiropractic technique on a specific motion segment or anatomic region resulting in the improvement, and ideally restoration, of neurologic and physiologic function to that area (Cooperstein and Gleberzon 2004; Gatterman 2005).

Afferent: Signals or nerve cells (neurons) sending information toward the central nervous system.

Anterior (aka ventral): Closer to the front of the body.

Autonomic nervous system (ANS): Contains components of the central nervous system (CNS) and peripheral nervous system (PNS) which function to control involuntary activity, maintain homeostasis, and react to stress (Darby 2014). The ANS is divided into the sympathetic and parasympathetic nervous systems.

Biomechanics: The study of the structure, function, and mechanical motion of biological systems.

Caudal: Located farther from the head.

Central nervous system: Brain and spinal cord.

Chiropractic (aka spinal manipulation): An integrative medical system rooted in the diagnosis and treatment of hypomobile joints, especially those within the spinal column, which cause local and systemic dysfunction of nerves, muscles, and organs. Improvement in joint mobility, generally through manual therapy, allows the body's innate forces to heal itself, achieving homeostasis (WFC 2001; Cooperstein and Gleberzon 2004; Rivera 2015).

Contralateral: Opposite side.

Cranial: Located closer to the head.

Distal: Away from the body.

Dorsal: Closer to the back of the body.

Efferent: Signals or nerve cells (neurons) sending information away from the central nervous system.

Facilitation: Increased nerve cell (neuronal) stimulation causing hyperactive responses.

Inferior (aka caudal): Located farther from the head.

Interneurons: Nerve cells transmitting information from one neuron to another within the brain or spinal cord (Purves et al. 2012a).

Intervertebral disk: A fibrocartilaginous joint located between the vertebral bodies helping hold the vertebrae together, as well as function as a shock absorber for the spine (Cramer and Darby 2005).

Intervertebral foramen: The hole (or foramen) between two vertebrae through which the spinal nerve exits (Evans and Lahunta 2013).

Ipsilateral: Same side.

Kinesiopathology: The abnormal movement or position of a spinal motion segment (Seaman and Faye 2005).

Lateral: Farther away from the median plane or midline of the body or organ.

Manipulation: Movement of a joint through passive range of motion to the paraphysiologic space without exceeding the joint's anatomical barrier (Gatterman 2005).

Medial: Closer to the median plane or midline of the body or organ.

Mobilization: Movement of a joint through normal range of motion to passive range of motion (Gatterman 2005).

Motion unit (spinal) (aka motion segment): The smallest unit of motion within the spine consisting of two articular facets and a disk (Rivera 2015).

Motor neurons: Nerve cells transmitting information from the brain and spinal cord to muscles and some glands (Purves et al. 2012b).

Myopathology: Abnormal muscle function.

Neuron (aka nerve cell): A cell capable of electrical excitability which sends signals to other cells over long distances (Purves et al. 2012a).

Neuropathic pain: Pathologic pain caused by damage or injury to nerves responsible for transferring information from the body (peripheral nervous system) to the spinal cord or brain (central nervous system).

Neuropathology: Abnormal nervous system function.

Neuroplasticity: Ability of the nervous system to reorganize and create new synaptic connections within the central nervous system (Jackman and Regehr 2017; Maltese et al. 2019). Typically used to describe the brain's ability to learn and heal following injury, but the concept can also be applied to the spinal cord (Maltese et al. 2019).

Neurotransmitters: A chemical released at the end of a neuron whose release is triggered by an action potential (Nolte 2009a). Neurotransmitters serve to stimulate other cells (nerve, muscle) or structures.

Nociceptor (aka free nerve endings): Sensory nerves stimulated by damaging or noxious stimuli which send information to the central nervous system where the information is interpreted as pain (Purves et al. 2012c).

Parasympathetic nervous system ("rest and digest"): Sends signals from the brain and spinal cord to the internal organs ensuring normal day-to-day function.

Pathoanatomy: Abnormal organ and tissue function.

Pathobiochemistry: Abnormal biochemical processes or reactions.

Pathophysiology: Abnormal physiologic function.

Peripheral nervous system: Cranial nerves and spinal nerves.

Posterior (aka dorsal): Closer to the back of the body.

Proprioception: Perception or awareness of the body and limb positions in space (Purves et al. 2012e).

Proximal: Closer to the body.

Sensory neurons: Nerve cells which respond to stimuli (touch, sound, light, and temperature changes) and send information to the spinal cord or brain (Purves et al. 2012e).

Spinal cord: A long column of nervous tissue, housed within the spinal canal of the vertebrae, extending from the level of the foramen magnum to the lumbosacral region (Pasquini et al. 2003).

Spinal manipulation: The use of manual therapy, most often a high-velocity low-amplitude thrust, to restore normal pain-free range of motion to a joint or motion unit (Gatterman 2005).

Subluxation: A joint with reduced mobility, also called hypomobility, restriction, fixation, or joint dysfunction (Gatterman 2005; Mai-Roecker and Roecker 2018).

Superior (aka cranial): Closer to the head.

Sympathetic nervous system ("fight or flight"): Sends signals from the brain and spinal cord to the internal organs in times of stress.

Thrust: The use of a specific contact point to deliver a deliberate, controlled, and unidirectional force to a particular motion segment (Gatterman 2005; Rivera 2015).

Vertebral subluxation complex (VSC): A model explaining the cascade of events resulting from and contributing to spinal segment hypomobility. The VSC comprises nine components which function individually and synergistically following the restriction of vertebral segments: kinesiology, neuropathology, myopathology, vascular pathology, connective tissue pathology, inflammatory response, pathoanatomy, pathophysiology, and pathobiochemistry (Seaman and Faye 2005).

Z-Joints (aka zygapophyseal joints): Joint between two articular facets.

Pain in Veterinary Patients

Simply put, pain is the worst. Pain is so awful our brains frequently try to shield us from the memories of pain. Unfortunately, people frequently anthropomorphize pain responses in animals. Clients often assume their pet is not in pain because they are not crying out loud or whimpering. Not many pets vocalize from pain, and if they do it is because the pain is severe.

Even though cats and dogs have been domesticated they still retain many "wild" characteristics. One of those traits is the concept of survival of the fittest. Animals that are visibly in pain are considered weak, and weak animals either get eaten or beaten up. As a result, pain signs in animals can be very subtle. The bottom line is animals in pain do not mirror people in pain. Table 10.1 compares pain responses between people, dogs, and cats.

Pain is considered the fifth vital sign (temperature, pulse [heart rate], respiratory rate, mucus membrane color, capillary refill time, and pain) (Epstein et al. 2015). A patient's pain status should be noted on every physical examination. One of the most used scales is the Colorado State University Veterinary Medicine Center Canine and Feline Acute Pain Scales. This is a 5-point scale where 0 is normal (no pain) and 5 is excruciating pain (CSU 2023).

The International Association for the Study of Pain (IASP) defines pain as "an unpleasant sensory and emotional experience associated with, or resembling that associated with, actual or potential tissue damage" (IASP 2021b). Pain is often categorized as acute or chronic. It was originally assumed both forms occurred through the same pathway with the duration being the only distinction. A more

Table 10.1 A comparison of the common pain responses between people, dogs, and cats (Lamont et al. 2000; Epstein et al. 2015; Gruen et al. 2022).

Humans	Facial grimacing; frowning; moaning; groaning; whimpering or crying; complaining; yelling; anger or irritability; restlessness or agitation; grabbing/holding area in pain
Dogs	Antisocial behavior (hiding, wants to be alone); aggressive behavior; changes in eating habits; changes in drinking; changes in sleeping (more or less, fitfully); vocalization; excessive grooming; panting or abnormal breathing; mobility issues (limping, walking more slowly, slow to rise, reduced jumping); agitation or irritability; changes in body posture; holding tail down or tucked; holding ears back or pinned close to the head
Cats	Hiding; sitting still or hunched up; loss of interest in people, pets or activities; excessive grooming; decreased grooming; excessive purring or meowing; unusual vocalization (chitter, chirp, yowl, moan); inappropriate urination; inappropriate defecation; fast shallow breathing; reduced appetite

Source: Lisa P. McFaddin.

Nociception vs. Pain

Nociception is the process through which an organism detects potentially or actual damaging stimuli and the transmission of the that information to the brain (Purves et al. 2012c). Nociceptors are peripheral receptors which respond to triggers (chemical, thermal, mechanical, etc.) that induce cellular change. Nociceptors encode information and transform it into a pain signal (Purves et al. 2012c). Pain, on the other hand, always involves sensory and emotional components. Pain requires conscious recognition of the aversive stimulus and changes the animal's physiology and behavior to reduce or avoid further threat or damage of tissues.

---

thorough understanding of pain allowed for better understanding and changes in pain terminology.

"The IASP defines acute pain as happen[ing] suddenly, starts our sharp or intense, and serves as a warning sign of disease or threat to the body. It is caused by injury, surgery, illness, trauma, or painful medical procedures and generally lasts from a few minutes to less than six months. Acute pain usually disappears whenever the underlying cause is treated or healed" (IASP 2021a).

Acute pain (aka adaptive pain, physiologic pain, or nociceptive pain) is a normal physiologic response to actual or perceived tissue damage (Woolf 2010). Nociceptive pain has been described as "an adaptive alarm system" (Woolf and Ma 2007). This form requires a functioning nervous system and often occurs secondary to trauma, surgery, or medical issues, and the pain stops as soon as the underlying cause dissipates. Adaptive pain is necessary for survival. This response serves to protect individuals from repeated injury and prolonged tissue damage (Woolf 2010). A prime example of adaptive pain is why people avoid touching hot stoves.

Chronic pain is considered maladaptive pain, or "an ongoing false alarm," because there is no obvious protective or recovery advantages to its existence (Woolf and Ma 2007). During maladaptive pain the central nervous system becomes confused. The initial source of the pain has often resolved but the pain persists. Because maladaptive pain serves no purpose it can negatively affect survival (Costigan et al. 2009; Walters 2019).

Neuropathic pain, a form of maladaptive pain, can develop after nerve damage occurs (Costigan et al. 2009). Neuropathic pain can lead to wind-up pain. Wind-up pain is an unnecessarily complicated cascade of events that results in this never-ending cycle of pain causing more pain which causes more pain, and so on. Wind-up pain can be harder to treat and frequently requires multiple medications and manual therapy to relieve the symptoms.

In general, any uncontrolled chronic musculoskeletal, and many neurologic, conditions will eventually cause neuropathic pain. Even simpler still if a pet has arthritis, back pain, limps, has trouble getting up from a seated position, has trouble lying down, and/or refuses to jump up onto furniture he or she likely has chronic pain.

The logical question becomes, how do we treat chronic pain? Any pain management plan should have three parts: (i) control the acute pain and inflammation; (ii) plan for continuous pain control; and (iii) utilize a multimodal approach.

Patients with chronic pain have poorer quality of life, shorter lives, weaker immune systems, poorer gut motility, weaker muscles, water retention, increased stress hormone (cortisol) levels, reduced oxygen supply to the body, and slower healing (Epstein et al. 2015; Gruen et al. 2022). Lapses in pain control can allow wind-up pain to occur which makes stopping pain even harder.

The brain recognizes pain because of signals sent to it by various nerves throughout the body. Electrical, chemical, and/or thermal signals can be the inciting factors that trigger the nerves to fire. Each type of signal requires a different approach to treat and prevent it from causing pain. Because pain pathways are so complex, multiple treatment options are needed to stop and prevent pain. This includes supplements, herbs, pharmaceuticals, acupuncture, photobiomodulation, and manual therapy – in other words, integrative medicine. This chapter focuses on understanding VSMT in veterinary patients.

Anatomy Fundamentals

Anatomy, physiology, and neurology lay the groundwork for understanding and applying VSMT. Anatomy is a branch of science focusing on the bodily structure of living organisms. The veterinarian must have a deep understanding of anatomy and functional physiology to effectively identify problem areas and perform spinal manipulation therapy. Without this foundation the patient may not respond favorably and there is potential risk of injury.

VSMT anatomy focuses on the appendicular (limbs) and axial (head, neck, back, and chest) skeletons, muscles (specifically those under voluntary control), and the nervous system (both peripheral and central). The primary bones, muscles, tendons, and ligaments comprising the shoulder (glenohumeral) and elbow (humeroradial) joints and the hip (coxofemoral) and knee (stifle) joints are summarized in Tables 7.1 and 7.2 in Chapter 7. The primary muscles affecting the head, neck and thoracic limb, as well as the pelvic limb are listed in Tables 9.1 and 9.2 in the Chapter 9. The muscular anatomy tables provide the origin, insertion, primary functions, and innervation of each muscle.

The neuroanatomy of interest can be divided into the structures affecting the vertebral column, peripheral nervous system (PNS), and central nervous system (CNS).

Vertebral Column

The vertebral column of companion animals includes the bones, muscles, tendons, ligaments, joints, and other tissues from the base of the skull to the end of the coccygeal vertebrae. The primary components of interest within the vertebral column include the intervertebral disks (IVDs), intervertebral foramen (IVF), zygapophyseal joints, and vertebral ligaments.

Intervertebral Disk IVDs, depicted in Figure 10.1, are found between the vertebral bodies starting between the second and third cervical vertebrae and extending to the sacrum. IVDs are composed of water, proteoglycans, collagen, chondrocytes, and fribroblasts (Cramer and Darby 2005).

Intervertebral Foramen The IVF are paired "holes" on the lateral aspects of the spinal column. IVF start at the second cervical vertebrae (C2) and extend to the sacrum. The IVF boundaries are illustrated in Figure 10.2.

Ligaments VSMT has a direct effect on multiple ligaments throughout the vertebral column (see Table 10.2).

Zygapophyseal Joints (Z-joint) Z-joints are small synovial joints surrounding the cranial and caudal articular facets of the articular processes. Each coupled vertebrae have left and right Z-joints. The Z-joints guide and limit movement between the vertebrae (Cramer and Darby 2005).

Peripheral Nervous System

The PNS comprises nerves exiting (motor) and entering (sensory) the brain and spinal cord (cranial nerves + spinal nerves). Sensory nerves bring information from the entire body (cutaneous, subcutaneous, muscle, and viscera) to the CNS, while motor nerves send information from the CNS to muscles under voluntary and involuntary control (Purves et al. 2012d). See Tables 10.3 and 10.4 for more detailed information.

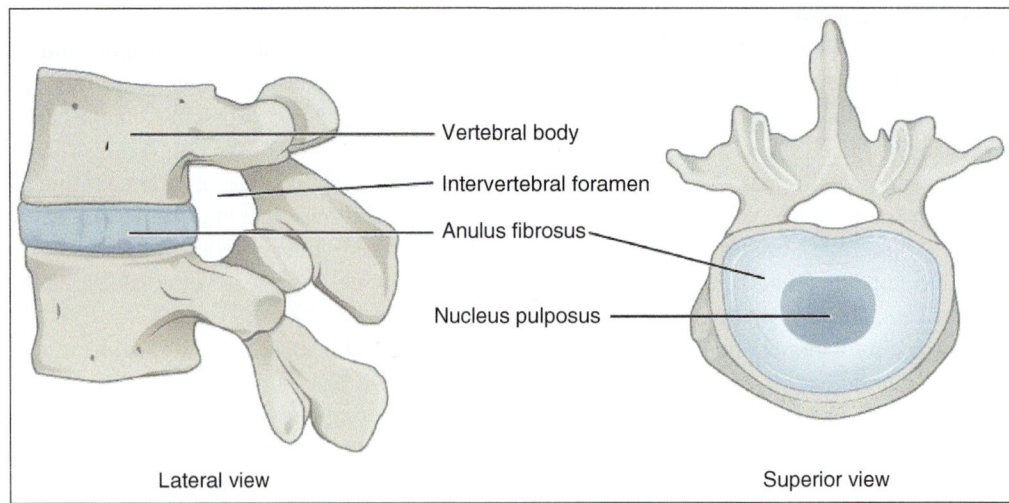

Figure 10.1   The location and anatomy of the intervertebral disk. The illustration is of a human lumbar vertebrae. The vertebral end plates are not depicted but would fall between the cranial (superior) and caudal (inferior) vertebral bodies and the annulus fibrosis. Source: Anatomy & Physiology/Rice University/ CC BY 4.0.

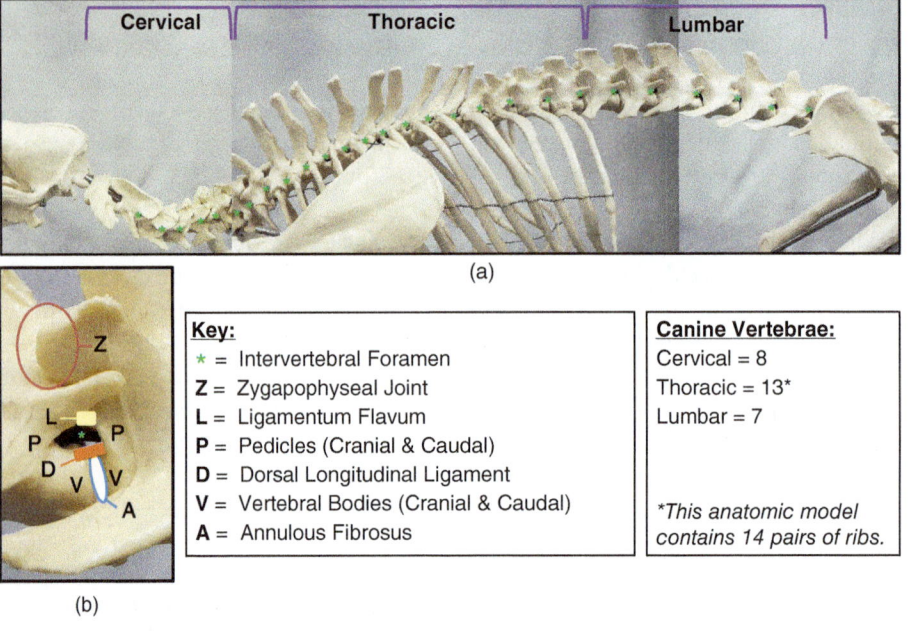

Figure 10.2   Intervertebral foramen (IVF) are paired holes between the vertebrae starting at the second cervical vertebrae and extending to the sacrum (Cramer and Darby 2005; Rivera 2015). (a) The anatomic model demonstrates the number of cervical (7), thoracic (13*), and lumbar (7) vertebrae. (*Note that this anatomic model contains 14 thoracic vertebrae.) (b) The IVF boundaries are shown. Z, zygapophyseal joint; L, ligamentum flavum; P, pedicle; D, dorsal longitudinal ligament; V, vertebral bodies; A, annulus fibrosus. Source: Lisa P. McFaddin.

Table 10.2 The ligaments affected by veterinary spinal manipulation therapy (Cramer and Darby 2005; Rivera 2015; Evans and Lahunta 2013; de Lahunta 1983).

Annulus fibrosis	Location	Outer portion of the intervertebral disk, specifically the convex
	Function	Transmits the stress and strain associated with lateral and dorsal–ventral movement
	Additional information	Convex fibrocartilaginous rings surrounding the nucleus pulposus; 1.5–3 times thicker ventrally compared to dorsally
Dorsal longitudinal ligament	Location	Ventral to the spinal cord and dorsal to the vertebral body
	Function	Limits spinal flexion
	Additional information	Aka posterior longitudinal ligament; location description depends on the reference point (i.e. vertebrae or cord); has an hourglass appearance (thicker over the intervertebral disk space, thinner and tapers when coursing over the vertebral body); thicker in the cervical spine; thinner in the thoracolumbar spine
Intercapital ligament	Location	Connects and stabilizes pairs of rib heads (left and right); runs over the annulus fibrosis but under the DLL
	Function	Stabilization
	Additional information	Joins rib heads (except T1, T12, and T13); inflammation of this ligament can mimic disk disease due to the high concentration of nociceptors
Interforamenal ligament	Location	Connect the periosteum of the vertebral pedicle and transforaminal ligament to the nerve root sleeves within the intervertebral foramen
	Function	Stabilizes the IVF
Interspinous ligament	Location	Connects adjacent dorsal spinous processes
	Function	Limits spinal flexion and axial rotation
	Additional information	Ligaments can become calcified and damaged (aka kissing spines)
Intertransverse ligament	Location	Connects transverse processes of adjacent vertebral bodies running from caudal aspect of one transverse process to the cranial aspect of the next transverse process
	Function	Limits spinal axial rotation and lateral bending
	Additional information	Runs from the cranial aspect of the transverse process of one vertebrae to the caudal transverse process of the vertebrae in front
Ligamentum flavum	Location	Dorsal boundary of the intervertebral foramen between the vertebral arches; ventromedial aspect of the joint capsule of the articular facet
	Function	Supports articular facets; slows down translation
	Additional information	Located between the vertebral arches; functions as the dorsal boundary of the IVF

(Continued)

Table 10.2 (Continued)

Nuchal ligament	Location	Caudal aspect of axis to dorsal aspect T10
	Function	Prevents overflexion of the neck and spine; helps with recoil
	Additional information	Funicular portion = thick strand; lamellar portion = elastic portion; canines only have the funicular portion; cats do not have a nuchal ligament
Sacrotuberous ligament	Location	Rope-like ligament running from the sacrum and first caudal vertebrae to the ischium
	Function	Prevents overflexion of the spine
	Additional information	Historically known as the ligamentum latum; not present in the feline
Supraspinous ligament	Location	Runs along the top of the dorsal spinous processes starting at the nuchal ligament's thoracic attachment and ending at the sacrum
	Function	Limits spinal flexion
	Additional information	Becomes vestigial at the lumbosacral region
Ventral longitudinal ligament	Location	Runs along the ventral aspect of the vertebral body
	Function	Limits spinal extension
	Additional information	Has a similar hourglass appearance to the DLL; in quadrupeds VLL becomes vestigial between C5/6 and T2; allows some overextension and lateral bending at the secondary curvature; cervical VLL is much thicker compared to the thoracic and lumbar spine; calcification (aka spondylosis) will affect the IVF by reducing joint and spinal mobility, decrease all afferent input, and with chronicity can develop into pseudo-joints

C, cervical vertebrae; DLL, dorsal longitudinal ligament; IVF, intervertebral foramen; T, thoracic vertebrae; VLL, ventral longitudinal ligament.
Source: Lisa P. McFaddin.

Central Nervous System

The CNS comprises seven parts: the spinal cord, medulla, pons, cerebellum, midbrain, thalamus, and cerebral hemispheres, as depicted in Figure 10.3 (Pasquini et al. 2003; Nolte 2009b; Evans and Lahunta 2013). The **spinal cord** receives and sends information from the brain and periphery. There are motor and sensory nerves (see the Spinal Cord section for further information).

The **medulla** and **pons** regulate blood pressure and respiration, with the former a part of the myelencephalon and the latter a part of the metencephalon. The **cerebellum** is responsible for coordinating voluntary movement, maintaining posture, and balance and is part of the metencephalon, with the pons. Sensory information is received from the spinal cord. Motor information is received from the cerebral cortex. Balance information is received from the vestibular organ.

Neuroanatomy for Veterinarians
Intervertebral Disks

IVDs have three distinct components: nucleus pulposus (NP), annulus fibrosus (AF), and the vertebral end plates (VEP). The VEP are fibrocartilaginous barriers connecting the AF and NP to the cranial and caudal vertebral bodies (Cramer and Darby 2005).

Table 10.3 The autonomic nervous system (ANS) is divided into the parasympathetic nervous system (PNS) and sympathetic nervous systems (SMS). This chart provides a brief overview of the defining characteristics of each division including primary function, control region, preganglionic length, neurotransmitter, and location of the ganglia. The intermedial lateral cell column (IML) is found within the spinal cord of all the thoracic segments and the first two to three lumbar segments. Acetylcholine (ACh) is a cholinergic neurotransmitter with a short duration of action because its enzyme, acetylcholinesterase, quickly inactivates it. Norepinephrine (NE) has different actions depending on the type of receptors in the responding cells. PNS ganglia within the brainstem include the Edinger Westphal nucleus (which is closely associated with the ganglia for cranial nerve III), nucleus ambiguus, and the superior and inferior salvatory nuclei, and the dorsal motor nucleus of the vagus nerve. The intermediate zone of the sacral segments innervates the kidneys, bladder, and colon. The cervical sympathetic ganglia actually comprise three divisions (superior, middle, and inferior) located between the first cervical through the eight cervical spinal segment (C1–C8). The sympathetic chain ganglia are found between the first thoracic through the fourth/fifth lumbar spinal segments (T1–L4/5). The celiac ganglia are located between the twelfth thoracic through the first lumbar spinal segments (T12–L1). The superior and inferior mesenteric ganglia innervate the gastrointestinal tract and urogenital systems. The pelvic–hypogastric ganglia are located caudal to the mesenteric ganglia (Purves et al. 2012d,e; Darby 2014; Rivera 2015).

	Parasympathetic	Sympathetic
Function	Rest and digest	Fight or flight
Control region	Brainstem	IML
Preganglionic length	Long	Short
Neurotransmitter	ACh: between preganglionic and postganglionic neurons and between postganglionic terminals and effector cells	ACh: between preganglionic and postganglionic neurons
		NE: between postganglionic terminals and effector cells and postganglionic neurons and enteric plexus
Ganglia	Brainstem; intermediate zone of the sacral segments	Cervical sympathetic ganglia; sympathetic chain ganglia; celiac ganglia, superior and inferior mesenteric ganglia; pelvic–hypogastric ganglia; adrenal medulla

Source: Lisa P. McFaddin.

Table 10.4 The name, function, location of the nucleus, reflexes, methods of assessment, signs of dysfunction, and additional information for the 12 paired cranial nerves (Pasquini et al. 2003; Evans and Lahunta 2013; Rivera 2015). CN, cranial nerves; LGN, lateral geniculate nucleus; C, cervical spinal segment; T, thoracic spinal segment; CNS, central nervous system; M, muscle; KCS, keratoconjunctivitis sicca. Reflexes often involve multiple CNs: pupilary light reflex (PLR) involves CN II and C III; menace reflex involves CN II and CN VII; dazzle reflex involves CN II, CN III, and CN VI (it does not check for cortical blindness); corneal reflex involves CN V1, CN VI, and CN VII; palpebral reflex involves slightly different nerves medially (CN V1 and CN VII) and laterally (CN V2 and CN VII); trigeminofacial reflex involves CN V and CN VII; tracking involves CN II, CN III, CN IV, and CN VI; gag involves CN IX and CN X; oculocardiac reflex involves CN V (sensory) and CN X (motor) (typically not very useful).

CN I (olfactory nerve)	
Function	Sensory = conscious perception of smell
Nucleus	Telencephalon (olfactory bulb of the frontal lobe)
Reflexes	None
Assessment	Hide treats; non-irritating aromatic substances
Dysfunction	Loss of smell

(Continued)

Table 10.4 (Continued)

Additional information	Smell can affect the frontal cortex and frontal lobe affecting behavior, emotions, movement, and memory
CN II (optic nerve)	
Function	Sensory = vision
Nucleus	Majority in the diencephalon (LGN of the thalamus); small portion in the midbrain (pretectal nucleus)
Reflexes	PLR; menace; dazzle
Assessment	Listed reflexes; sight avoidance (evaluates CN II and spinal nerves C1–T2); and tracking (evaluates CN II, CN III, CN IV, and CN VI)
Dysfunction	Blind
Additional information	Not a peripheral nerve but a specialized tract of CNS tissue
CN III (oculomotor nerve)	
Function	Motor = upper eyelid levator muscle; dorsal, medial, and ventral rectus muscle; ventral oblique muscle
Nucleus	CN III nuclei in the ventral mesencephalon
Reflexes	PLR; dazzle
Assessment	Listed reflexes; tracking (evaluates CN II, CN III, CNIV, and CN VI); anisocoria
Dysfunction	Lateral strabismus; sluggish, incomplete, or absent PLRs; anisocoria
Additional information	Closely associated with the Edinger–Westphal Nucleus (EWN). The preganglionic parasympathetic neurons from CN III originate in the EWN
	Miosis occurs due to stimulation of the parasympathetic nervous system
	Both eyes must move together (reflexogenic)
CN IV (trochlear nerve)	
Function	Motor = dorsal oblique muscle
Nuclei	CN IV nuclei in the mesencephalon
Reflexes	None
Assessment	Assessed with CN III, not individually
Dysfunction	If the pupil is round, the retinal vessels may appear tilted. If the pupil is not round, tilting of the pupil itself will be seen
CN V (trigeminal nerve)	
Branches	CN V1 (ophthalmic); CN V2 (maxillary); CN V3 (mandibular)
Function	**CN V1**: Sensory information from the cornea, dorsum of the nose, upper eyelid, and medial canthus
	CN V2: Sensory information from the lower lid, lateral head, maxillary region, nose, mucous membrane of maxillary sinus, nasopharynx, palate, medial nasal mucosa, maxillary teeth, and maxillary gingiva
	CN V3: Sensory information from mandibular and intermandibular skin, mandibular oral mucosa, taste rostral two-thirds of tongue (with CN VII), and proprioceptive information from ocular and masticatory muscles; motor to the muscles of mastication, mylohyoideus, soft palate, and middle ear
Nucleus	CN V nuclei in the pons
Reflexes	Corneal reflex; palpebral reflex; trigeminofacial reflex

Assessment	Listed reflexes; irritating nasal mucosa (CN V1 and CN VII); and muscles of mastication tone
Dysfunction	Loss of sensation to the listed areas of the head and neck; atrophy or loss of tone to the muscles of mastication; inability to close mouth; difficulty chewing
CN VI (abducens nerve)	
Function	Motor to the lateral rectus muscle, retractor bulbi, nictitating membrane
Nucleus	CN VI nuclei in the pons
Reflexes	Tracking; dazzle; corneal reflex
Assessment	Eye position; eye movements
Dysfunction	Medial strabismus; exophthalmos; third eyelid elevation
CN VII (facial nerve)	
Branches	Buccal; auriculopalpebral (or auricular); and lacrimal
Function	Motor to the muscles of facial expression, orbicularis oculi, stylohyoid, caudal portion of the digastricus, and stapedius of inner ear
	Sensory to the rostral two-thirds of the tongue (with CN V3 via the lingual nerve) and middle ear (with CN X via chordae tympani)
	Parasympathetic to the tear ducts, palatine, nasal glands, and mandibular and sublingual salivary glands
Nucleus	CN VII nuclei in the pons
Reflexes	Corneal reflex; palpebral reflex; trigeminofacial reflex
Assessment	Listed reflexes; irritating nasal mucosa; facial muscle tone; fascial symmetry; Schirmer tear test; atropine taste test
Dysfunction	Buccal: Drooping of the lip, cheek, drooling ipsilateral, and nose pulled to contralateral side
	Auriculopalpebral: Paresis of the ear and eyelid
	Lacrimal: No retraction of the lip with panting; no movement of the ipsilateral nares; loss of taste to rostral tongue, KCS
CN VIII (vestibulocochlea)	
Function	**Cochlear Nerve:** Sensory, hearing, and acoustic impulses from receptors in cochlea
	Vestibular Nerve: Sensory, proprioception, and head orientation
Nucleus	CN VIII in the pons and medulla
Reflexes	None
Assessment	Hearing; Balance
Dysfunction	Loss of hearing (complete or partial); Vestibular signs; and Nystagmus (CN VIII, Cerebellum)
CN IX (glossopharyngeal nerve)	
Function	Motor = pharyngeal muscles (with CN X) and stylo-pharyngoeus muscle of the palate
	Sensory = taste caudal one-third of the tongue, pharynx, and neck viscera
	Parasympathetic = parotid and zygomatic salivary glands
Nucleus	CN IX nuclei in the medulla
Reflexes	Gag reflex

(Continued)

Table 10.4 (Continued)

Assessment	Gag reflex; coughing (CN X [sensory], CN IX [motor], CN XI, CN II, and phrenic nerve); phonation; swallowing
Dysfunction	Trouble swallowing; change in bark/meow/voice
CN X (vagus nerve)	
Function	Motor = palate (with CN V), pharynx (with CN IX), esophagus, and larynx (with CN XI)
	Sensory = pharynx (with CN IX), larynx, palate, esophagus, epiglottis, thoracic, and abdominal viscera
	Parasympathetic = viscera of neck, thorax, and abdomen
Nucleus	CN X nuclei in the medulla
Reflexes	Gag reflex; oculocardiac reflex
Assessment	Gag reflex; coughing
Dysfunction	Soft stool; ulcers; malabsorption; maldigestion; parasympathetic issues
Additional information	Longest CN
CN XI (spinal accessory nerve)	
Function	Motor = trapezius, omotransversarius, part of sternocephalicus, brachiocephalicus, esophageal, and laryngeal muscles
Nucleus	CN XI nuclei in the medulla
Reflexes	None
Assessment	Muscle tone
Dysfunction	Atrophy of sternocephalicus, trapezius, omotransversarius, and/or brachiocephalicus
CN XII (hypoglossal nerve)	
Function	Motor = muscles of the tongue
Nucleus	CN XII nuclei in the caudal medulla
Reflexes	None
Assessment	Tongue position and tone
Dysfunction	Tongue atrophy; tongue deviation
Additional information	Shortest intracranial nerve

Source: Lisa P. McFaddin.

The NP is an avascular gelatinous remnant of the embryologic notochord (Evans and Lahunta 2013). The NP is the primary shock absorber for the vertebral column through the retention and loss of water (Cramer and Darby 2005). Protrusion and dehydration of the NP can result in IVD pathology.

The AF is primarily composed of convex fibrocartilaginous rings or lamellae. Only the outer layer is vascular. The outer one-third of the AF is heavily innervated, receiving sensory (nociceptive and proprioceptive) and vasomotor information. Tearing of the lamellae can also lead to IVD pathology (Cramer and Darby 2005).

Intervertebral Foramen

The boundaries of the IVF include zygapophyseal joint, ligamentum flavum, pedicles (cranial and caudal), dorsal longitudinal ligament, vertebral bodies (cranial and caudal), and AF (Cramer and Darby 2005). The IVF boundaries are illustrated in Figure 10.2.

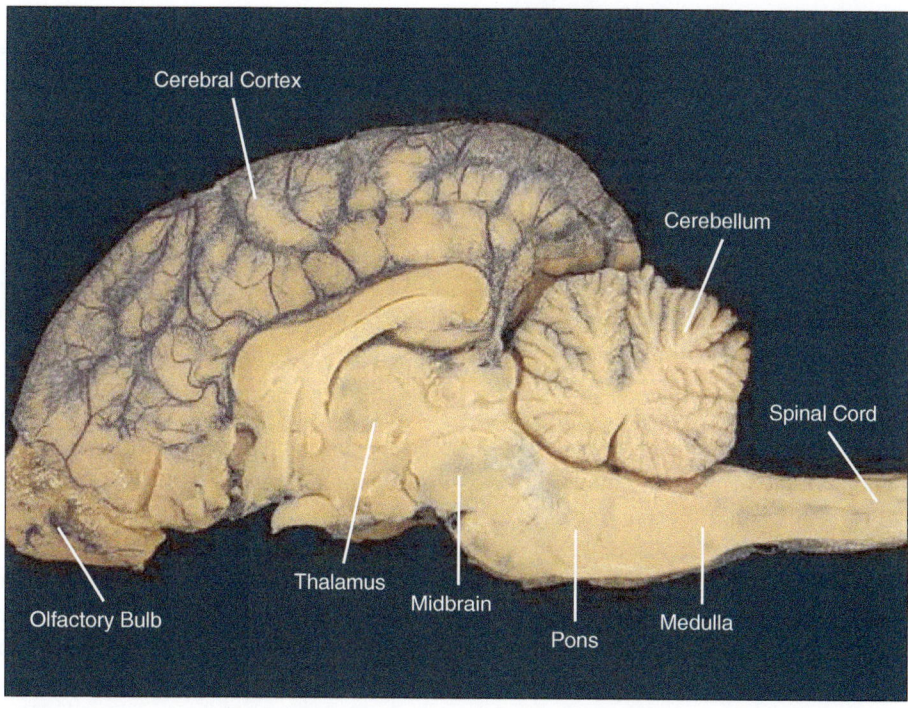

Figure 10.3 The anatomy of the canine brain. Source: PixCove, https://www.pixcove.com/brain-intelligence-medical-structure-health-dog-canine-anatomy-cerebellum-paerparat-veterinary-medicine-horse-biology-body-mount-dorsal/, last accessed June 09, 2023.

The IVF forms a boundary between the peripheral and central nervous systems (Cramer and Darby 2005). The structures exiting the IVF include the ventral horn, dorsal root ganglion (DRG), spinal nerve, dura (which transforms into the epineurium), cerebrospinal fluid (CSF), arteries, veins, lymphatics, fat, connective tissue, recurrent meningeal nerve, and transfo-raminal ligament (Rivera 2015). Disruption of these structures can result in pain, abnormal sensation (paresthesia), changes in muscle tone, and even changes to the autonomic nervous system (Henderson 2005).

Zygapophyseal Joints (Z-joint)
The outer articular capsule is made of fibroelastic connective tissue, while the inside lining contains a synovial membrane. The ventromedial capsule is lined by the ligamentum flavum (Cramer and Darby 2005). Damage to the Z-joint capsule is slow to heal given the area's limited blood supply.

The synovial lining of the articular capsule has extensions protruding into the Z-joint. Nociceptors have been found within the synovial folds (Cramer and Darby 2005). Trauma or inflammation affecting the Z-joint or IVF can contribute the development of hypomobilities and back pain (Cramer et al. 2007, 2010).

Peripheral Nervous System
The primary components of the PNS are ganglia, peripheral nerves, and nerve endings (Darby and Frysztak 2014). Ganglia are local groupings of nerve cell bodies and supporting cells. Peripheral nerves are composed of nerve fiber bundles, containing both myelinated and unmyelinated nerves, wrapped in connective tissue. The type of nerve ending is dependent on the nerve's function, i.e. sensory or motor,

and is discussed in more detail in the Physiology section of this chapter (Purves et al. 2012d).

Nerves innervating skeletal muscle (voluntary control) comprise the somatic nervous system, while nerves innervating smooth muscle, cardiac muscle, and glands (involuntary control) comprise the autonomic nervous system (ANS). The ANS is subdivided into the parasympathetic and sympathetic nervous systems, summarized in Table 10.3.

The PNS is also divided into cranial nerves and spinal nerves. The cranial nerves are 12 paired nerves arising from the brain and innervating specific regions within the head, neck, and body cavities, summarized in Table 10.4. The spinal nerves include all nerves emerging directly from spinal cord segments. Refer to textbooks referenced in the Veterinarian section for further detail on the PNS.

Central Nervous System

Spinal Cord   The spinal cord is a long column of nervous tissue, housed within the spinal canal of the vertebrae, extending from the level of the foramen magnum (large opening in the skull) to the lumbosacral region (where the last lumbar vertebrae meets the sacrum) (Evans and Lahunta 2013). The spinal cord is covered by the same meningeal layers as the brain. The cord can be divided into three portions: central canal, gray matter, and white matter.

The central canal contains CSF and is considered an extension of the ventricles within the brain. The gray matter surrounds the central canal and contains cell bodies, while the white matter contains ascending and descending axons (Nolte 2009a).

Spinal cord anatomy is complex and beyond the scope of this book. Refer to the neurology texts suggested in the Reference Books section towards the end of this chapter for detailed information and anatomical illustrations. The divisions within the white and gray matter are portrayed in Figures 10.4 and 10.5.

Brain   The **midbrain** regulates eye and skeletal muscle movement and is part of the mesencephalon. The **thalamus** integrates and redistributes almost all sensory and motor information destined to go to the cerebral cortex. It is part of the diencephalon with the hypothalamus, which regulates the autonomic nervous system. Finally, the **cerebral hemispheres**, separated by a groove (longitudinal fissure), are responsible for controlling muscle function and conscious thought, memory, and emotions.

Anatomically the brain is divided into the telencephalon, diencephalon, midbrain, metencephalon, and myelencephalon (Pasquini et al. 2003; Nolte 2009b; Evans and Lahunta 2013). The **telencephalon** contains the cerebral cortex and nuclei of cranial nerve (CN) I. The **diencephalon** contains the thalamus, hypothalamus, and CN II ganglia. The **midbrain** contains the ganglia of CN III and CN IV. The **metencephalon** comprises the pons, cerebellum, and ganglia of CN V, CN VI, CN VII, and CN VIII. The **myelencephalon** contains the medulla and ganglia of CN IX, CN X, CN XI, and CN XII. The area of the brain known as the brainstem comprises the midbrain, pons, and medulla.

Physiology Fundamentals

Physiology is the branch of science focusing on the function of living organisms and their parts. Physical manipulations have direct effects on nerves, muscles, connective tissue, blood flow, hormones, and the immune system. Neurophysiology is as complex as it is important. VSMT affects veterinary patients at a cellular level, and these cellular responses in turn affect nerves and muscles with the goal of improving mobility and reducing pain.

The neurophysiology of VSMT begins with understanding what makes a nerve cell (neurons), how the body receives and transmits information from external and internal sources, and how nerves and muscles respond to spinal manipulation.

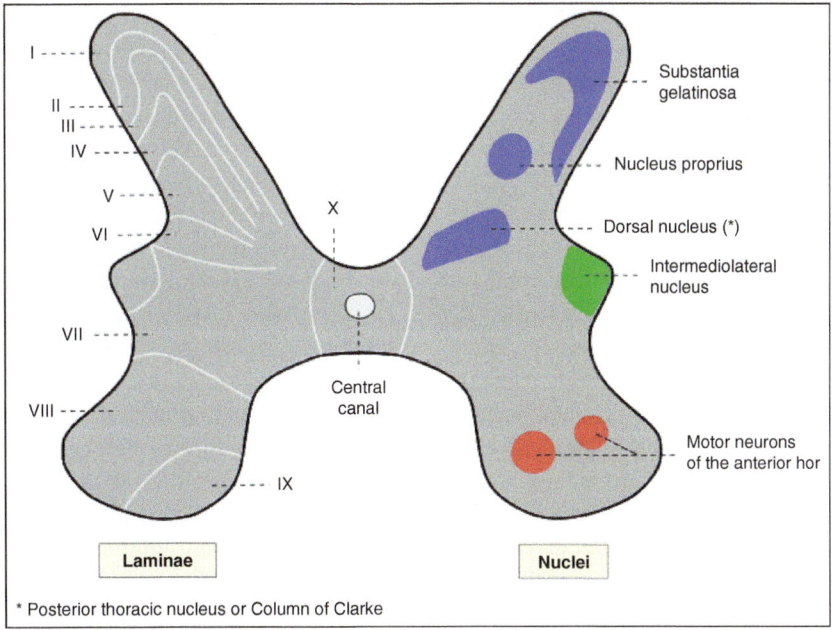

Figure 10.4 The nuclei and lamniae comprising the gray matter of the spinal cord. Source: Polarlys, June 3 2006, licensed by Creative Commons Attribution-Share Alike, https://en.wikipedia.org/wiki/File:Medulla_spinalis_-_Substantia_grisea_-_English.svg.

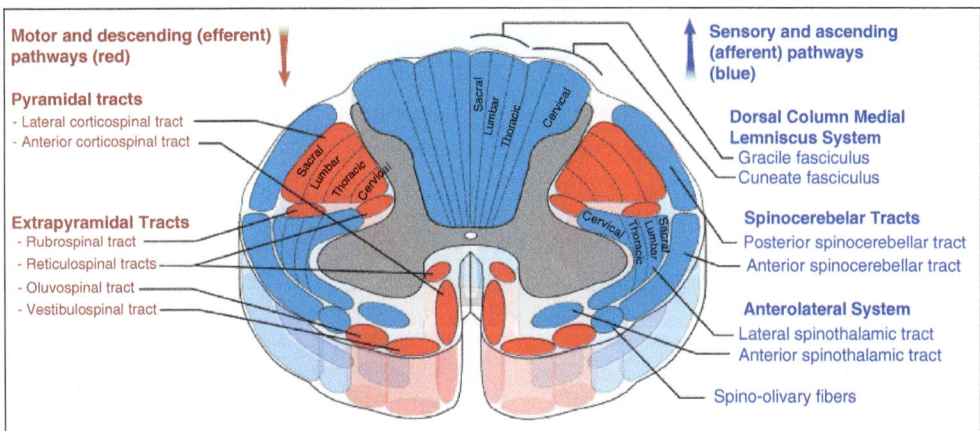

Figure 10.5 The tracts within the spinal cord white matter. Source: Polarlys and Mikael Häggström, July 17 2010, licensed by GNU Free Documentation License, https://en.wikipedia.org/wiki/File:Spinal_cord_tracts_-_English.svg.

VSMT Physiology Tidbit

Nerve cells need four things to maintain their health:

1) Oxygen
2) Energy (glucose)
3) Presynaptic stimulation
4) Specialized proteins which help nerve cells grow and mature (neurotrophic factors).

(Rivera 2015)

Neurons

Neurons are classified into two categories: nerve cells and glial cells. Nerve cells are specialized to carry electrical signals long distances. They can be further classified as sensory nerves, motor nerves, and interneurons (Purves et al. 2012d). **Sensory neurons** carry signals from the outside and inside of the body to the brain. **Motor neurons** carry information from the brain and spinal cord to muscles and some glands. The motor nervous system can be further divided into somatic and visceral efferents. Somatic efferents innervate striated skeletal muscle which is under voluntary control. Visceral efferents innervate involuntary smooth muscle associated with blood vessels, glands, cardiac muscles, and the viscera (Purves et al. 2012a-f). **Interneurons** transmit information from one neuron to another within the brain or spinal cord (Purves et al. 2012d).

Receptor Stimulation

Sensory afferent receptors can be stimulated by touch, pressure, temperature change, chemical exposure, noxious stimuli, and changes in body position. Tables 10.5–10.7 list the classification of sensory afferent receptors by their location, triggering stimulus, and structure, respectively.

All sensory receptors are important because *all* afferent fibers send information to the brain. Of particular interest are nociceptors and mechanoreceptors (specifically joint mechanoreceptors, muscle spindle cells, and Golgi tendon organs). Nociceptors are peripheral sensory neurons responding to damaging or noxious stimuli which terminate as unspecialized free nerve endings (Purves et al. 2012c). Pain is perceived by the brain from information transmitted by the nociceptors.

Mechanoreceptors send information to the CNS regarding the position (proprioception) of

Table 10.5 Sensory afferent receptors classified by their location (Mittleman and Gaynor 2000; Purves et al. 2012e; Zhu 2014; Rivera 2015).

Receptor type	Location	Function
Exteroceptors	Body surface	Receptors for touch, pressure, pain, and temperature
Interoceptors	Internal	(Aka visceroceptors); receptors on the viscera, blood vessels, glands, and other internal structures
Proprioceptors	Skeletal muscle, tendons, joints	(Aka mechanoreceptors); provide information from the musculoskeletal system about the position of the limbs and body in space

Source: Lisa P. McFaddin.

Table 10.6 Sensory afferent receptors classified by their triggering stimulus (Mittleman and Gaynor 2000; Purves et al. 2012e; Zhu 2014; Rivera 2015).

Receptor type	Location	Triggering stimulus
Mechanoreceptors	Throughout the body	Mechanical forces (directly or indirectly)
Thermoreceptors	Throughout the body	Temperature changes
Photoreceptors	Retina	Changes in light
Chemoreceptors	Tongue; nose; internal	Exposure to specific chemicals
Nociceptors	Throughout the body	Trauma or damage to tissues

Source: Lisa P. McFaddin.

Table 10.7 Sensory afferent receptors classified by their structure (Mittleman and Gaynor 2000; Purves, et al. 2012e; Zhu 2014; Rivera 2015).

Receptor type	Location	Function
Free sensory nerve endings	Epidermis Dermis	Nociceptors: respond to damaging stimuli and their activation results in pain
		Thermoreceptors: respond to temperature changes both hot and cold
Follicular nerve endings	Root hair plexus	Mechanoreceptors: respond to deformation of surrounding tissue including pressure and stretch
Merkel's complexes	Bottom epidermis	Mechanoreceptors: slow-adapting and respond to sustained pressure
Meissner's corpuscles	Top dermis	Mechanoreceptors: rapidly adapting and sensitive to fine or light texture and pressure
Ruffini's corpuscles	Middle dermis Joint	Thermoreceptors: triggered by heat
		Mechanoreceptors: slow-adapting and responsive to shearing stress and drag
Krause's end-bulbs	Dermis Conjunctiva Mouth and lips	Thermoreceptors: triggered by cold
Pacinian corpuscles	Deep dermis Subcutaneous Viscera	Mechanoreceptors: rapidly adapting and sensitive to strong pressure, jarring movements, and vibration
Muscle spindle cells	Skeletal muscle	Mechanoreceptors: stretch receptors within muscles assessing muscle length
Golgi tendon organs	Musculotendinous junction	Mechanoreceptors: measure muscle tension at the origin and insertion during concentric contraction
Joint kinesthetic receptors	Articular capsules	Mechanoreceptors: distinguish joint position and movement

Source: Lisa P. McFaddin.

and applied forces (stretch, compression, tension, acceleration, and rotation) to joints, ligaments, tendons, and muscles (Iheanacho and Vellipuram 2022). The primary mechanoreceptors of interest in VSMT are the muscle spindle cells (MSCs) and Golgi tendon organs (GTOs). MSCs monitor muscle length and speed of contraction. GTOs monitor muscle tone (especially tension at the origin and insertion).

Neurotransmitters

Neurotransmitters are endogenous chemicals (made within the body) which allow communication between neurons throughout the body. These chemical messages directly affect numerous bodily functions including heart rate, blood pressure, breathing rate and effort, muscle movements, thoughts, memory, learning, emotions, sleep, healing, aging, stress levels, hormone regulation, digestion, all five senses, and pain levels (Sheffler et al. 2022).

Nerurophysiology for Veterinarians
Neurons

All neurons have similar anatomy as depicted in Figure 10.6. The tree-like projections (dendrites) branch off the cell body (soma) and receive information from other neurons. A specialized portion of the cell body (axon

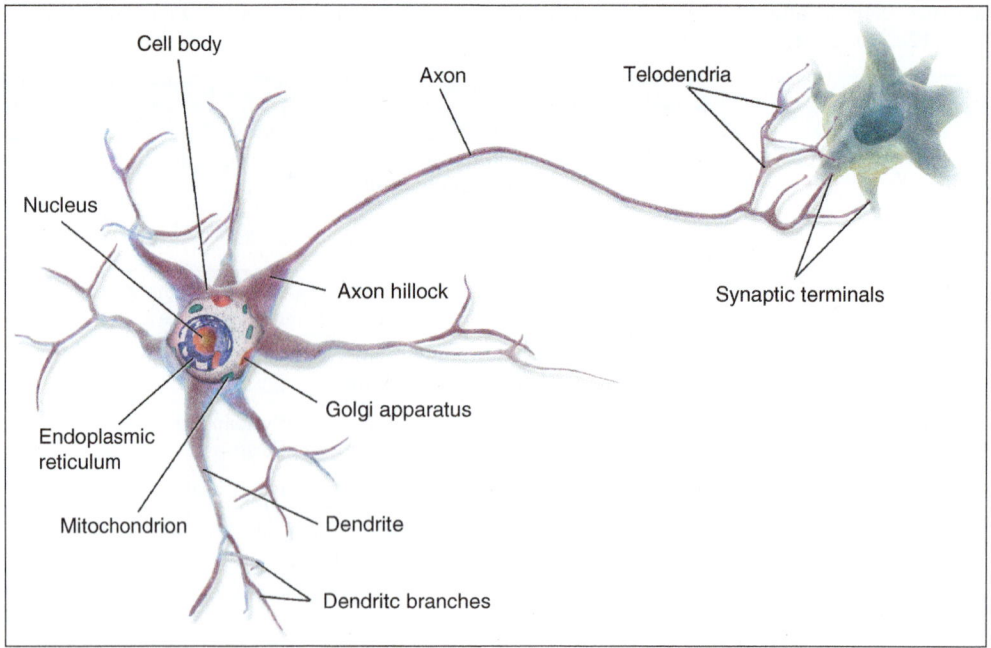

Figure 10.6 Anatomy of a multipolar neuron. Source: BruceBlaus/Wikimedia Commons/CC BY 3.0.

hillock) initiates the action potential. The electrical information is transmitted through the axon to the presynaptic terminals which propagate the information, either through chemical or electrical synapses, to the target cell (Purves et al. 2012d).

Some neurons have segments of fatty sheets (myelin) insulating the axon which serve to increase the rate at which the electrical impulses travel through the axon. The spaces between the myelin (nodes of Ranvier) are rich in ion channels allowing for the generation of action potentials. Myelinated neurons fire faster than unmyelinated neurons (Purves et al. 2012d).

Glial cells are primarily found within the CNS, outnumbering nerve cells three to one (Purves et al. 2012d). The anatomy of glial cells is similar that of nerve cells except glial cells do not produce electrical impulses. They serve to support the brain and PNS.

Astrocytes, ependymal cells, microglial cells, and oligodendrocytes are found within the CNS, while satellite cells and Schwann cells are in the

PNS (Purves et al. 2012d). Figure 10.7 depicts each cell type. Astrocytes maintain potassium concentrations within the intracellular space. Ependymal cells create and secrete CSF and create the blood–CSF barrier. Microglial cells act as scavengers removing debris associated with trauma and cell death, as well as modulating local inflammation through cytokine secretion. Oligodendrocytes generate and apply myelin sheets to axons. Satellite cells regulate the chemical environment of the intracellular space. Schwann cells generate and apply myelin sheets to axons (Purves et al. 2012d).

Action Potential

At rest neurons have a negative voltage, known as the resting membrane potential (RMP). The RMP of most neurons falls between −40 and −90 mV. The number of positive (cations = sodium and potassium) and negative (anions = chloride) ions within the fluid inside and outside of the nerve cell determines the RMP. The RMP is maintained through the passive diffusion and active transportation of

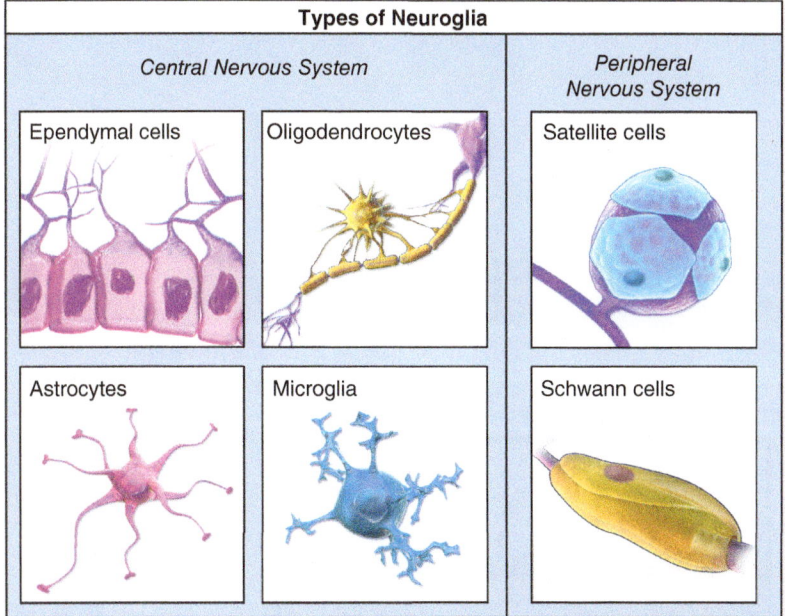

Types of Neuroglia

Central Nervous System

Peripheral Nervous System

Ependymal cells

Oligodendrocytes

Satellite cells

Astrocytes

Microglia

Schwann cells

Figure 10.7 Visual depiction of glial cells, also called neuroglia. Source: Blausen.com staff (2014)/CC BY SA 4.0.

electrolytes into and out of the cell (Purves et al. 2012a-f).

The electrical properties of the neuron are determined by the permeability of the cell membrane and the transport of electrolytes across the cell membrane. There are a variety of ion channels and pumps located in different parts of the neuron, making some portions of the cell more excitable than other (Purves et al. 2012a). The most well known are the voltage-gated ion channels and the sodium potassium pump. Voltage-gated ion channels, found at the nodes of Ranvier, open and close depending on the voltage difference between the inside and outside of the cell. The sodium/ potassium pump requires ATP to move three sodium ions into the cell while removing two potassium ions (Purves et al. 2012a-f). The complexity of voltage-gated ion channels is illustrated in Figure 10.8.

Currents or signals triggering the membrane potential to become more negative (hyperpolarization) cause a passive electrical response, meaning very little change occurs within the cell. Conversely, depolarization occurs when the membrane potential becomes more positive. Each neuron has a threshold potential or specific membrane voltage which triggers an active electrical response (action potential). Generation of an action potential (AP) takes approximately 1 ms (Purves et al. 2012a).

An AP, depicted in Figure 10.9, is considered an "all or none" response, meaning the strength of the stimulus does not affect the magnitude of the AP; however, the strength of the stimulus can affect the frequency. A stronger stimulus may incite multiple APs (Purves et al. 2012a).

Immediately following an AP the neuron experiences a refractory period during which the neuron's membrane potential dips below its normal RMP. Another AP cannot be triggered until the neuron's voltage returns to the RMP (Purves et al. 2012a).

The AP is one form of intercellular communication. Neurons can excite (depolarization) or inhibit (hyperpolarization) other nerve cells, stimulate muscle contraction, and regulate

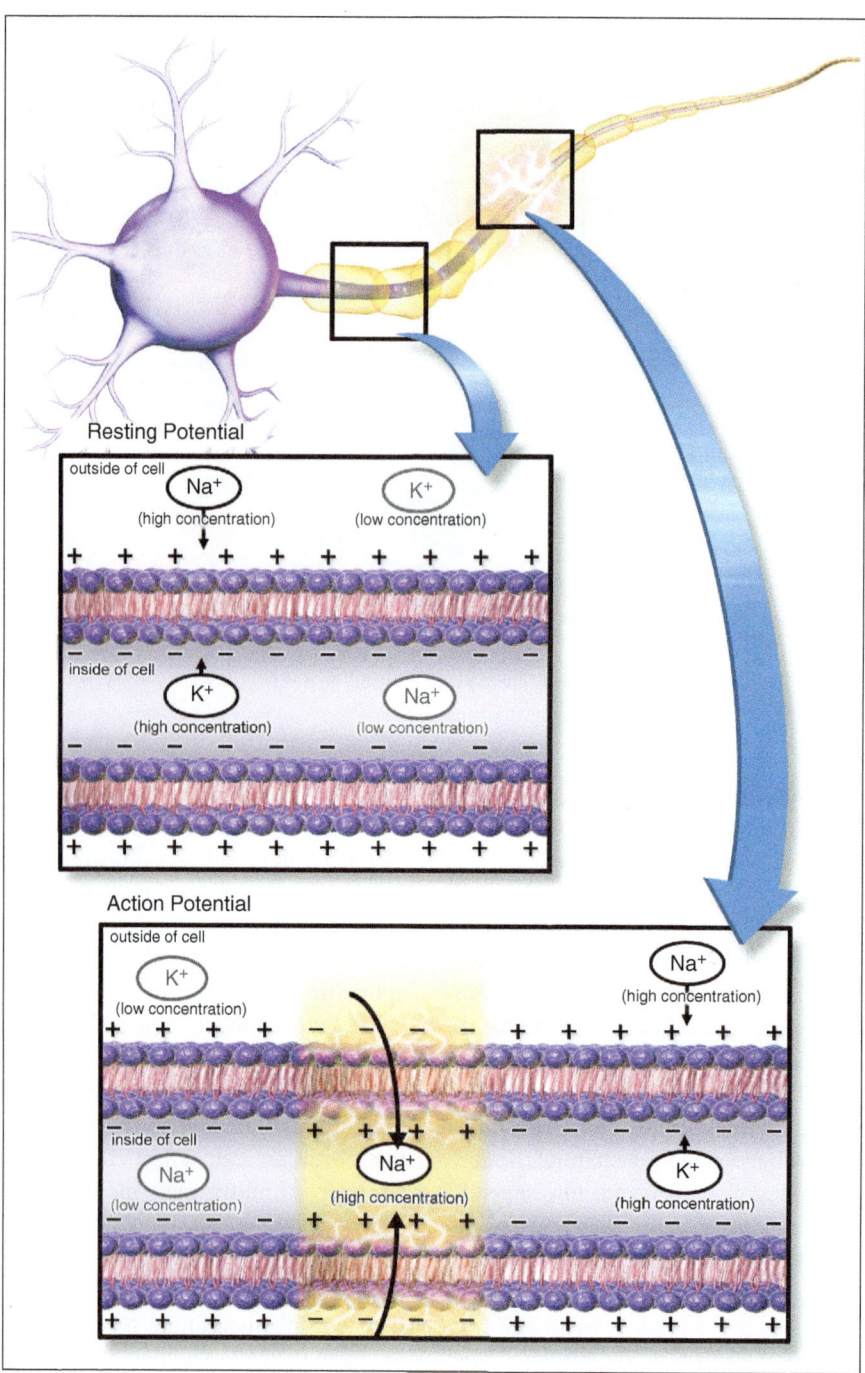

Figure 10.8 The function of voltage-gated ion channels during the propagation of an action potential along an axon. The voltage-gated ion channels are found along the axon between the myelin sheaths at the nodes of Ranvier. The influx of sodium (Na$^+$) depolarizes the region generating an action potential. Source: Blausen.com staff (2014)/CC BY SA 4.0.

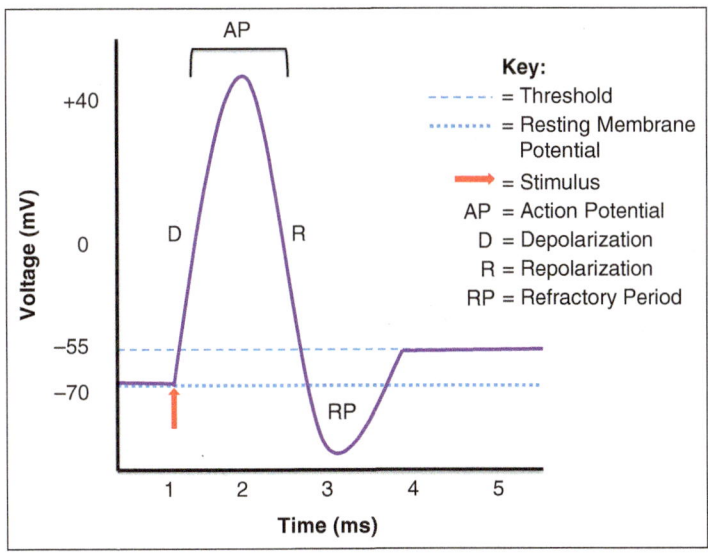

Figure 10.9   Approximation of an action potential. The nerve cell's resting membrane potential (RMP) is −70 mV. A stimulus initiates depolarization, making the inside of the nerve cell more positive. Once the threshold, defined as −55 mV, is reached an action potential occurs spiking the membrane potential to +40 mV within 1 ms. After reaching peak potential the voltage drops below the RMP over another millisecond. The membrane voltage then slowly rises back up to the RMP during the refractory period. Source: Lisa P. McFaddin.

hormone production and release (Purves et al. 2012d; Rivera 2015).

Sensory Receptors

Sensory receptors are classified by their location, triggering stimulus, and structure. As described in Tables 10.5–10.7, there is overlap between the classification systems. Figure 10.10 provides a schematic representation of various receptors within the skin.

Nociceptors

Nociceptors are thin small-diameter fibers classified as either A-delta (Aδ) group or C fiber group. Aδ nociceptors are lightly myelinated axons with conduction velocities of 5–30 m/s and divided into type I and type II. Type I Aδ respond to truly noxious chemical and mechanical stimuli (mechanosensitive), while type II Aδ respond to exposure to heat (mechanothermal). C fiber nociceptors are unmyelinated axons with conduction velocities of 2 m/s. They are considered polymodal,

responding to all forms of noxious stimuli (Purves et al. 2012c).

Nociceptor cell bodies are primarily located in the dorsal root of the spinal cord. C fiber first-order neurons terminate in the laminae I (marginal zone) and II (substantia gelatinosa) of the dorsal horn of the spinal cord (Yam et al. 2018). Aδ first-order neurons enter the spinal cord through Lissauer's tract, travel cranial or caudally for three to four spinal segments and then enter laminae II (substantia gelatinous) connecting to a second-order neuron (Purves et al. 2012c).

Once in the substantia gelatinosa, a portion of the sensory information crosses the midline below the central canal and enters the spinothalamic tract, a set of sensory tracts located in the ventral funiculus of the spinal cord white matter (Purves et al. 2012c). Within the substantia gelatinosa inhibitory interneurons are also stimulated, blocking the transmission of nociceptive information to the higher centers of the brain (Mittleman and Gaynor 2000; Purves

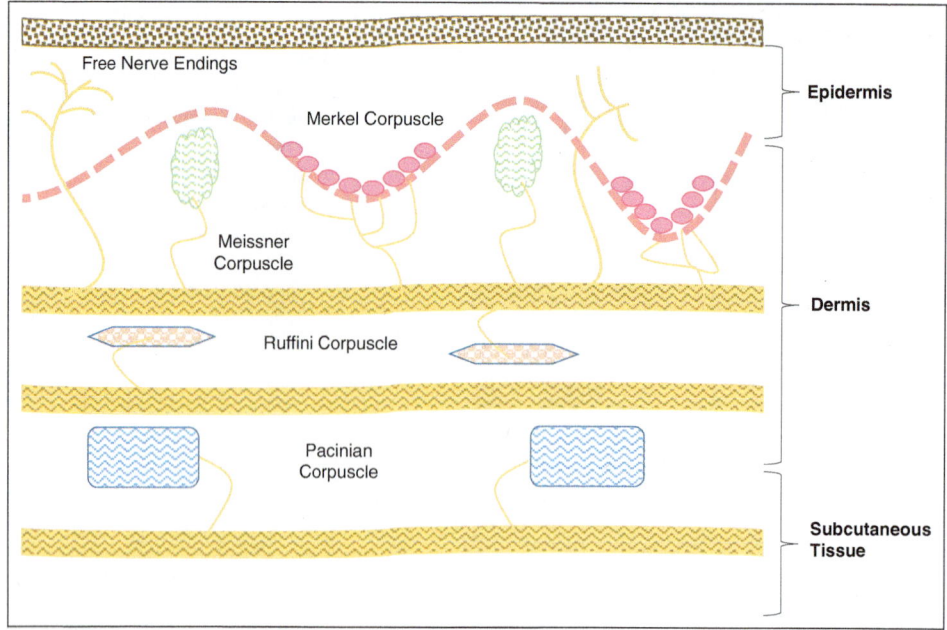

Figure 10.10 Schematic representation of common receptors found within the skin (Purves et al. 2012e). Source: Lisa P. McFaddin.

et al. 2012c).This local inhibition of pain is known as Melzack and Wall's Gate Theory.

Most of the sensory information then travels to the ipsilateral thalamus where it terminates at a third-order neuron. The thalamus is a gate through which all sensory information, except olfactory, travels. The third-order neuron sends information to the somatosensory region of the ipsilateral cortex, specifically the parietal lobe (Purves et al. 2012c). On the way to the thalamus, branches are sent to several connections in the midbrain, especially the periaqueductal gray matter (PAG) and rostral ventral medulla (RVM) (Yam et al. 2018).

The PAG helps regulate the response to nociceptive input, integrating information from the higher brain centers including the cortex and the dorsal horn of the spinal cord. The RVM downregulates excitatory information from the dorsal horn of the spinal cord. Both the PAG and RVM express a variety of neurotransmitters (endogenous opioids and cannabinoids, 5-hydroxytryptamine, and norepinephrine)

heavily involved in the regulation and recognition of pain (Yam et al. 2018).

Joint Mechanoreceptors
Mechanoreceptors are typically classified as types I–IV, as described in Table 10.8.

Muscle Spindle Cells
MSCs are specialized receptors found within striated muscles responsible for assessing muscle length and speed of contraction (Purves et al. 2012a-f; Purves et al. 2012b,e). Figure 10.11 is a schematic representation of a mammalian MSC.

The highest concentration of MSCs are found within the muscle belly (equatorial region). Each MSC consists of four to eight intrafusal muscle fibers housed within a connective tissue capsule capped by polar ends. The intrafusal fibers are arranged parallel to the extrafusal (force-producing) muscle fibers, and the MSC polar ends attach to the extrafusal fibers (Purves et al. 2012b,e).

Table 10.8 Classification of joint mechanoreceptors by their location and associated receptor types (Purves et al. 2012e; Rivera 2015).

Type	Location	Associated fiber types
I	Joint capsule; ligaments; tendons	Ruffini's corpuscles; Golgi tendon organs
II	Joint capsule	Pacinian corpuscles; Krause's end-bulbs
III	Ligaments; tendons	Golgi tendon organs; Golgi–Mazzoni
IV	Joint capsule; periosteum; ligaments; tendons; blood vessels	Free nerve endings

Source: Lisa P. McFaddin.

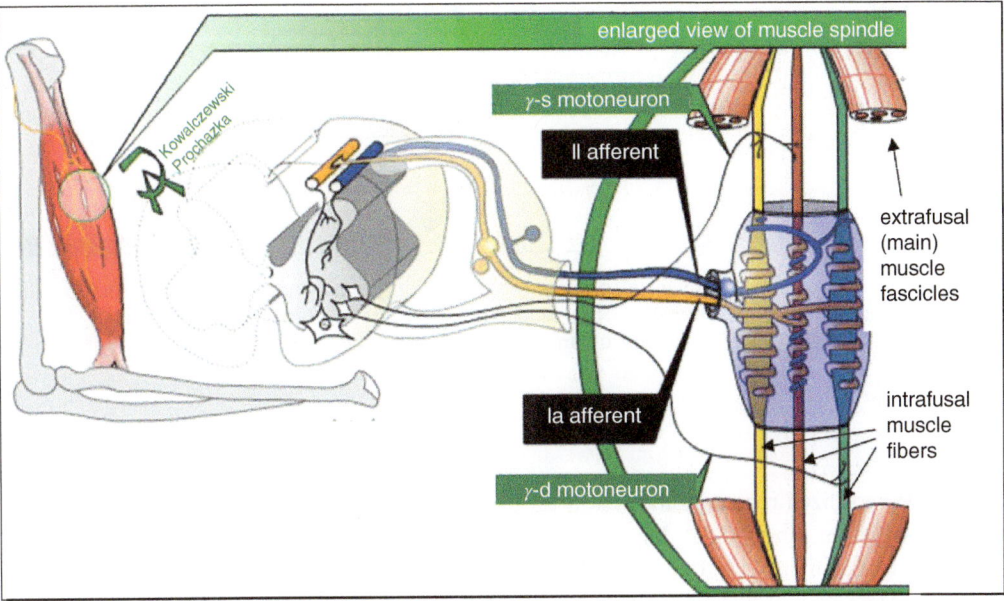

Figure 10.11 The location (left), sensory afferent receptors (right), motor innervation (right), and spinal cord connections (middle) of mammalian muscle spindle cells. Source: Neuromechanics, October 10 2005, https://commons.wikimedia.org/wiki/File:Muscle_spindle_model.jpg.

The primary sensory afferent innervations arise from Group Ia and Group II afferents. Group Ia afferents, large-diameter myelinated axons, respond to rapid changes in muscle length by transmitting information about limb movement and speed. Group II afferents, medium-diameter myelinated axons, respond to sustained muscle stretch by transmitting information about static limb position. Both sensory fibers send information to the dorsal horn of the spinal cord (Purves et al. 2012b,e).

Once in the dorsal horn both afferent fibers diverge causing a cascade of events, including inhibition of pain through the stimulation of interneurons within the dorsal horn; co-activation of alpha and gamma motor neurons in the ventral horn; stimulation of the contralateral cerebellum (Group Ia only); and inhibition of alpha and gamma motor neurons for the antagonistic and contralateral homologous muscles (Group Ia only) (Purves et al. 2012b,e; Rivera 2015).

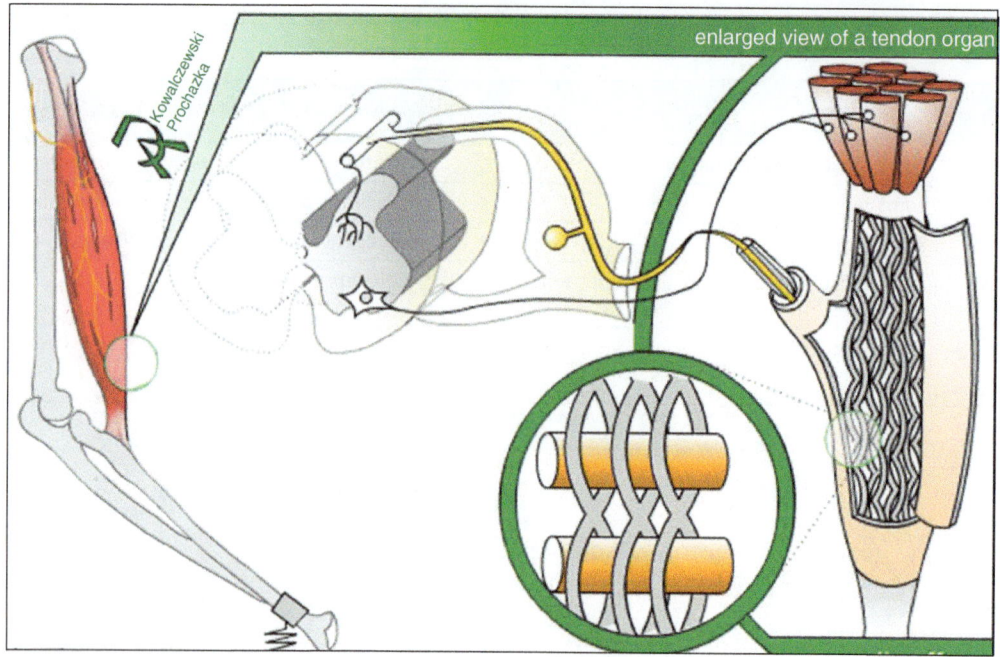

Figure 10.12 The location (left), sensory afferent receptors (right), motor innervation (right), and spinal cord connections (middle) of mammalian Golgi tendon organs. Source: Neuromechanics, January 5 2009, https://en.wikipedia.org/wiki/File:Tendon_organ_model.jpg.

Golgi Tendon Organs

GTOs are specialized receptors located in the musculotendinous junctions at the origin and insertion of striated muscles. GTOs are responsible for measuring muscle tension during concentric contraction (Purves et al. 2012b,e). Figure 10.12 is a schematic representation of a mammalian GTO.

GTOs are spindle shaped, slow-adapting receptors composed of interwoven collagen bundles surrounded by a thin capsule. GTOs are innervated by myelinated type Ib nerve fibers. Activation of Group Ib nerves inhibits alpha and gamma motor neurons innervating the muscle, as well inhibiting pain through stimulation of interneurons within the dorsal horn of the spinal cord (Purves et al. 2012b,e).

Alpha and Gamma Motor Neurons

MSC are innervated by efferent gamma motor neurons. Gamma motor neurons stimulate the polar ends of the MSC increasing their sensitivity to stretch. Alpha motor neurons stimulate the neuromuscular junction of the extrafusal muscle fibers causing muscle contraction (Purves et al. 2012b,e).

Each GTO will fire at its own tempo once stimulated. Together the receptors create spatial summation which can overwhelm type Ia afferent fibers and interneurons in the dorsal horn, hyperpolarizing alpha and gamma motor neurons resulting in muscle relaxation (Purves et al. 2012b,e; Rivera 2015).

The balance of alpha and gamma motor neuron stimulation (alpha–gamma gain) can be used to encourage muscle relaxation and pain reduction. There are four primary methods through which alpha–gamma gain is regulated: (i) decreasing the distance between MSC polar ends, often achieved by approximating muscles; (ii) stimulating GTOs; (iii) stretch and hold, fatiguing the muscles and stimulating GTOs; and (iv) pharmaceutical agents (Rivera 2015).

Neurotransmitters

Stimulation of nociceptors and mechanoreceptors cause the release of neurotransmitters
locally and within the CNS. These neurotransmitters function as biochemical mediators triggering inflammation, often modulating the
intensity and duration of the painful stimuli.
Table 10.9 lists some of the common neurotransmitters released by nociceptors. This is
not an exhaustive list.

Chiropractic Fundamentals

There are several terms and concepts fundamental to VSMT including range of motion,
planes of spinal movement, motion unit or
segment, and subluxation.

Range of Motion

There are four stages in the range of motion
within a joint, visualized in Figure 10.13: active

Table 10.9 Common neurotransmitters, and their primary functions, released by nociceptors and
associated with the modulation of pain. References are included in the body of the table.

Name	Function
Acetylcholine	Induces muscle contractions and modulates pain
Adenosine	Reduces pain through activation of Ia receptors on ascending afferent nerves from muscle spindle cells (Goldman et al. 2010)
β-Endorphin	Opioid peptide reducing pain through stimulation of μ-opiate receptors (Zhang et al. 2011)
Bradykinin	Inflammatory mediator of cardiovascular homeostasis, inflammation, and nociception through activation of bradykinin 1 and 2 receptors (Zhang et al. 2011)
Calcitonin gene-related peptide (CGRP)	Neuropeptide modulating pain sensation through interaction with an autoreceptor (Zhang et al. 2011)
Cytokines	Inflammatory proteins which augment afferent sensory nerve response reducing pain sensation and reducing production of additional inflammatory mediators from afferent terminals (Zhang et al. 2011)
GABA (γ-aminobutyeic acid)	Inhibitory neurotransmitter affecting autoreceptors within the CNS modulating the pain response (Zhao 2008)
Glutamate, aspartate	Excitatory amino acids modulating pain information peripherally and centrally through stimulation of autoreceptors, including NMDA receptors (Zhao 2008)
Histamine	Stimulation of H_1 receptors causes increased vascular permeability, relaxation of vascular smooth muscle, reduction in pain sensation, and increased concentration of β-endorphin in the cerebrospinal fluid (Huang et al. 2018)
Plasminogen	Precursor to plasmin involved in fibrinolysis
Prostaglandins	Proinflammatory factors affecting afferent sensory nerve excitability (Zhang et al. 2011)
Protease	Enzyme involved in proteolysis and functions as a proinflammatory mediator
Nitric oxide	Enhances acetylcholine and β-endorphin release while inhibiting release of substance P from primary afferent nerves (Zhang et al. 2011)
Norepinephrine	Modulates neuropathic pain through spinal α_2 receptors
Serotonin	Involved in the modulation of nociception through interactions with 5-HT_1 and 5-HT_3 receptors (Zhang et al. 2011)
Somatostatin	Endogenous non-opioid neuropeptide which modulates nociception (Zhao 2008)
Substance P	Tachykinin neuropeptide involved in peripheral and spinal nociception (Zhao 2008)

CNS, central nervous system; NMDA, *N*-methyl-D-aspartate; 5-HT, 5-hydroxytryptamine.Source: Lisa P. McFaddin.

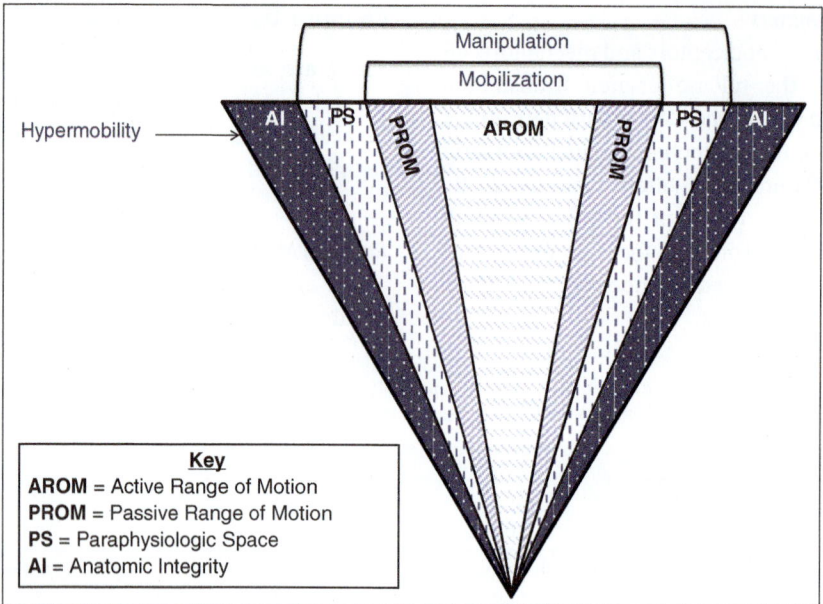

Figure 10.13 A schematic representation of joint movement from active range of motion (AROM), passive range of motion (PROM), mobilization, and manipulation. Adapted from (Evans and Breen 2006). Source: Lisa P. McFaddin.

range of motion (AROM), passive range of motion (PROM), manipulation, and joint sprain (Evans and Breen 2006).

1) AROM is achieved when opposing muscles contract and relax causing joint movement. AROM is typically less than that of PROM (Jurek 2013).
2) PROM occurs when an outside force is used to move a joint through AROM until it reaches paraphysiologic space (an elastic barrier of resistance representing the limit of anatomic integrity) (Sears 2023).
3) Manipulation occurs when a joint is brought through its normal range of motion into PROM without imparting a thrust (Rivera 2015). The goal is to restore joint mobility.
4) Manipulation occurs when a joint is taken abruptly through AROM, PROM, and the paraphysiologic space without exceeding the limit of anatomic integrity (Rivera 2015).

Joint sprain occurs when a joint is moved past the limit of anatomic integrity.

Table 10.10 The type of vertebral joint motion in bipeds and quadrupeds based on the axis of orientation (Inoue et al. 2020; Rivera 2015).

Axis	Biped	Quadruped
X	Flexion and extension	Flexion and extension
Y	Axial rotation	Lateral bending
Z	Lateral bending	Axial rotation

Source: Lisa P. McFaddin.

Spine Movement

Vertebral joint motion can occur in three primary axes: X, Y, and Z (Inoue et al. 2020). Regardless of the species, the Y-axis is always oriented vertically, the X-axis is always perpendicular to the Y-axis, and the Z-axis is perpendicular to the third dimension. The type of movement for each axis depends on the species (summarized in Table 10.10).

In our companion animal patients, the Y-axis runs parallel to the dorsal spinous process, and movement around this axis is considered lateral bending of the spine. The X-axis is perpendicular to the Y-axis, roughly parallel to the transverse processes. Movement around this axis would be spinal flexion and extension. The Z-axis is perpendicular to the Y-axis in the third dimension and runs through the spinal canal (hole in the vertebrae through which the spinal cord runs). Movement around the Z-axis would be considered axial rotation. Axial rotation and lateral bending are considered a coupled movement, as one does not occur without the other (Rivera 2015). Figures 10.14 and 10.15 allow visualization of these concepts using

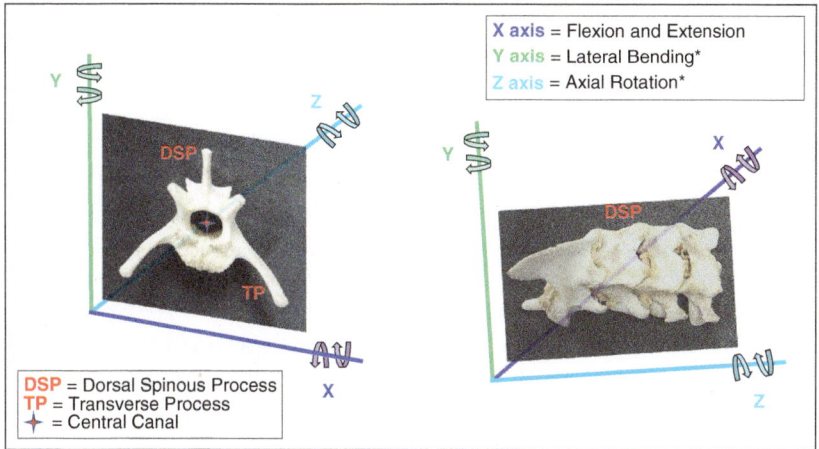

Figure 10.14 A schematic representation of the three-dimensional (3D) movement of the quadruped spine. Photographs taken by Lisa P. McFaddin using anatomical specimens provided by The Healing Oasis Wellness Center. Source: Lisa P. McFaddin.

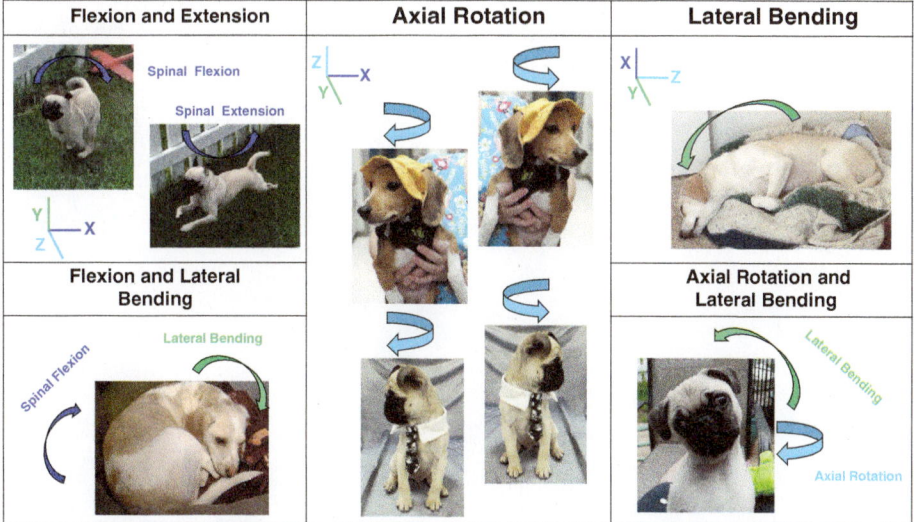

Figure 10.15 Real-life examples of three-dimensional (3D) spinal movements in canines. The Y-axis is always oriented parallel to the dorsal spinous process of the vertebrae. The X-axis is oriented perpendicular to the Y-axis (parallel to the transverse processes). The Z-axis is perpendicular to the Y-axis in the 3D plane, running parallel to the spinal canal. The example axis for flexion and extension, axial rotation, and lateral bending demonstrate the orientation of the axis moves with the dog as its position changes. Source: Lisa P. McFaddin.

anatomical vertebrae specimens and real-life canine examples.

Motion Unit or Segment

This is the smallest unit of motion within the spine consisting of two articular facets and a disk. Adjustment of the motion unit affects this three-joint complex and all of the surrounding structures, including the Z-joint, IVD, connective tissue, muscles, arteries, veins, and components of the IVF (Gatterman 2005; Jurek 2013; Rivera 2015). The motion unit in the canine lumbar spine is depicted in Figure 10.16.

Subluxation

The term "subluxation," while not a dirty word, elicits strong reactions from many human and veterinary chiropractors. D.D. Palmer initially used the term to describe a structural change between two adjacent vertebrae which causes

neurologic, musculoskeletal, and even metabolic changes throughout the body (Jurek 2013).

Over time the definition has evolved, with many practitioners steadfastly clinging to the original definition. Today "subluxation" typically refers to a joint with reduced mobility (Gatterman 2005). The resulting local and systemic effects caused by the subluxation, affecting everything from cellular function to the brain, are still implied (Mai-Roecker and Roecker 2018). To avoid confusion many chiropractors use terms like "hypomobility," "restriction," "fixation," or "joint dysfunction" when describing the affected joint or joints (Mai-Roecker and Roecker 2018).

Adjustment versus Mobilization versus Manipulation

There are several terms for techniques used in VSMT and chiropractic medicine which sound

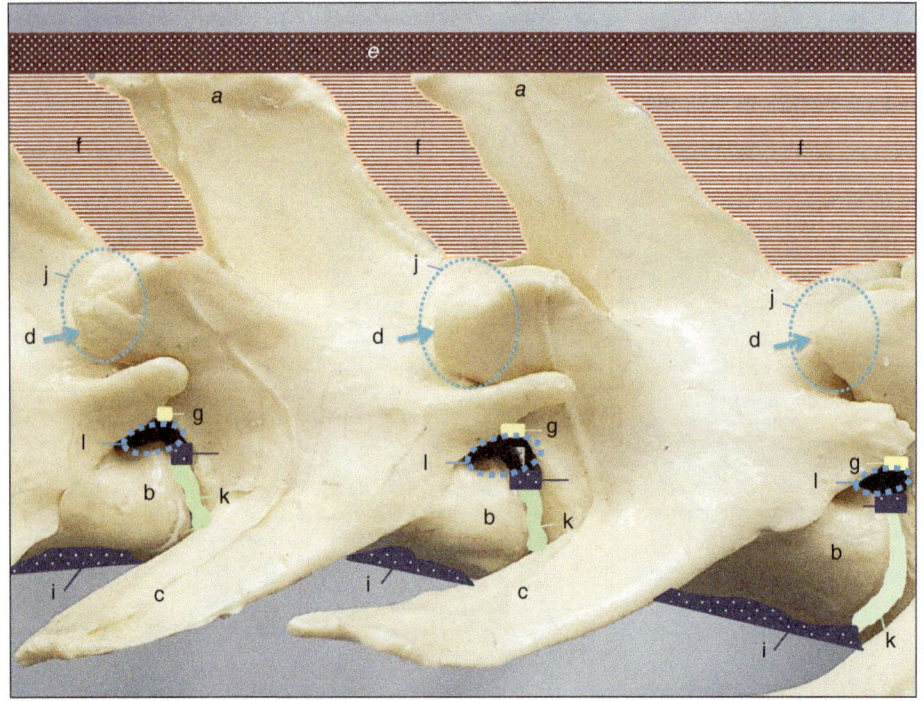

Figure 10.16 The canine lumbar motion unit. (a) Dorsal spinous process, (b) vertebral bodies, (c) transverse processes, (d) articular facets, (e) supraspinous ligament, (f) interspinous ligament, (g) ligamentum flavum, (h) dorsal longitudinal ligament, (i) ventral longitudinal ligament, (j) joint capsule, (k) intervertebral disk, (l) intervertebral foramen. Source: Lisa P. McFaddin.

similar but have different meanings including adjustment, manipulation, and mobilization. An **adjustment** is the application of any chiropractic technique on a specific motion segment or anatomic region resulting in the improvement, and ideally restoration, of neurologic and physiologic function to that area (Cooperstein and Gleberzon 2004). As stated earlier, a spinal motion segment or unit is the smallest unit of motion within the spine consisting of two articular facets (cranial and caudal) and an intervertebral disk (Gatterman 2005). **Mobilization** is the movement of a joint through normal range of motion to passive range of motion (Gatterman 2005). **Manipulation** is the movement of a joint through passive range of motion to the paraphysiologic space without exceeding the joint's anatomical barrier (Gatterman 2005). See Figure 10.13 for a visual depiction of these terms.

Motion Palpation

Prior to an adjustment the practitioner assesses the mobility of specific joints or areas of the body using digital and manual palpation, also known as motion palpation. The specific anatomic structures palpated on the patient are called segmental contacts.

The most common technique uses the practitioner's thumbs to assess the side-to-side and up-and-down movement of the dorsal spinous processes of the vertebrae. In the cervical spine the body of the vertebrae is also palpated, typically using the outside of the index finger. Figure 10.17 demonstrates the direction of motion palpation for the cervical, thoracic, and lumbar vertebrae. Motion palpation is used to identify poorly mobile (hypomobile) joints. VSMT is then used to correct the hypomobility.

Contact Point

A contact point is the area of the hand used to contact the patient. The most common points used in VSMT include pisiform, "V" trough, thenar, and calcaneal, as demonstrated in Figure 10.18 (Rivera 2015).

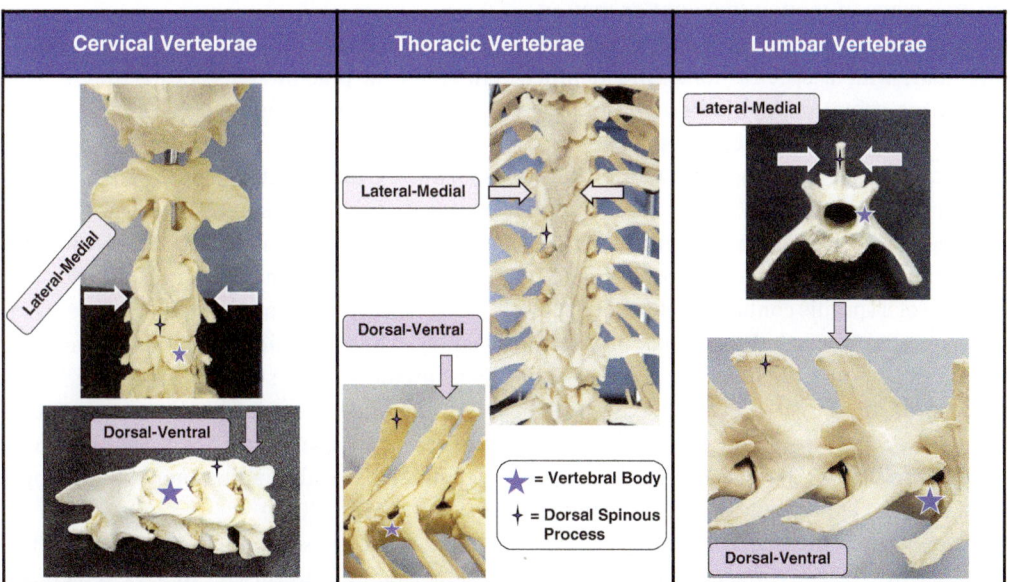

Figure 10.17 Examples of motion palpation landmarks for vertebrae in the cervical, thoracic, and lumbar spine. The dorsal spinous processes can be palpated up-and-down in the cervical, thoracic, and lumbar spine and side-to-side (lateral–medial) in the thoracic and lumbar spine. The vertebral body is used to palpate up-and-down (dorsal–ventral) in the cervical spine. Source: Lisa P. McFaddin.

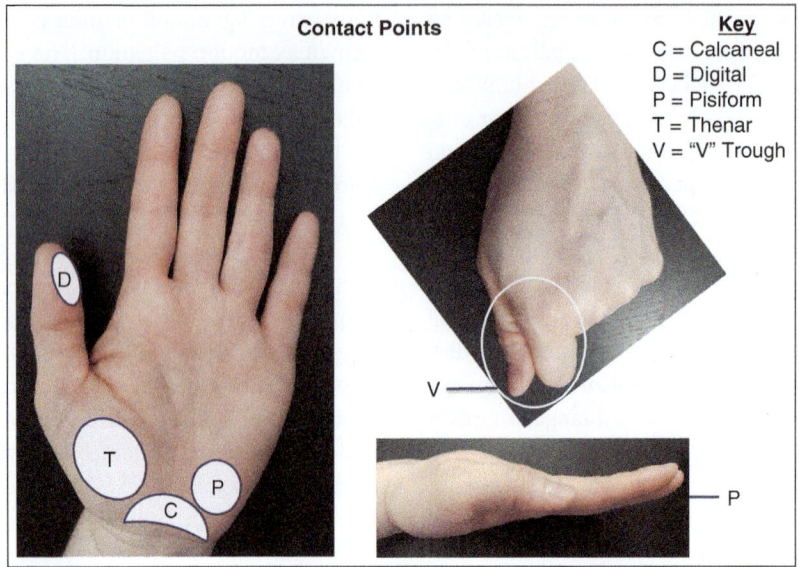

Figure 10.18 Common contact points used in veterinary spinal manipulation therapy. Source: Lisa P. McFaddin.

Thrust

Spinal manipulation refers to the use of manual therapy, most often a high-velocity low-amplitude (HVLA) thrust, to restore normal pain-free range of motion to a joint or motion unit (Gatterman 2005). An HVLA is a rapid movement, with a specific force and depth, used during spinal manipulation. The practitioner's contact point is placed on the patient's segmental contact over a specific motion segment (Jurek 2013; Rivera 2015).

While an HVLA is a type of thrust, not all thrusts are considered HVLA. Thrust is defined as the use of a specific contact point to deliver a deliberate, controlled, and unidirectional force to a particular motion segment (Gatterman 2005; Rivera 2015).

Line of Correction

Along with the appropriate segmental contact and contact point, the line of correction (LOC, or line of drive, LOD) is crucial. The alignment of the practitioner's body is necessary to deliver a proper thrust during spinal manipulation. The LOC starts at the practitioner's episternal notch (dip on the front of the chest between the clavicles) or shoulder, travels through the contact point, and through the segmental contact (Rivera 2015).

Body Mechanics

In VSMT the practitioner's body is their instrument. Proper positioning ensures their instrument stays healthy, free of injury, and maximizes the effectiveness of each adjustment. Proper form requires the practitioner's stance, upper body, and wrist positioning are correct before each manipulation.

The most common stance is a Fencer's stance. The practitioner stands with their legs greater than shoulder distance apart with the knees flexed. The distance between the legs and the degree of knee flexion is dependent on the adjustment being performed (Rivera 2015).

Upper body positioning is dependent on the contact point being used. Always remember the wrist should never be bent when performing an adjustment. A bent wrist is a sad wrist just waiting to get injured.

Chiropractic Fundamentals for Veterinarians

Additional key concepts in VSMT include vertebral subluxation complex, hypomobility pathogenesis, and neuroplasticity.

Vertebral Subluxation Complex

VSC is a model, depicted in Figure 10.19, explaining the cascade of events resulting from and contributing to spinal segment hypomobility. The VSC comprises nine components which function individually and synergistically following the restriction of vertebral segments: kinesiopathology, neuropathology, myopathology, vascular pathology, connective tissue pathology, inflammatory response, pathoanatomy, pathophysiology, and pathobiochemistry (Seaman and Faye 2005; Rivera 2015).

Kinesiopathology is the result of abnormal movement, position, or lack of normal movement of one or multiple spinal motion segments (Seaman and Faye 2005). Kinesiopathology is the principal condition in the VSC leading to pathobiochemistry, pathophysiology, pathoanatomy,

and inflammatory responses, as shown in Figure 10.20.

Movement (kinesiopathology) is influenced by the muscles (myopathology), connective tissue (connect tissue pathology), and nervous system (neuropathology); while the blood vessels (vascular pathology) feed and detoxify the tissues (Seaman and Faye 2005). The nervous system plays a central role mediating the effects of the VSC. Immobilized joints lead to disuse muscle atrophy. Like nerve roots, the vertebral vasculature is susceptible to impingement by osseous displacement, articular inflammation, and changes to surrounding connective tissue (Seaman and Faye 2005; Rivera 2015).

The connective tissues are negatively affected by immobilization. For example, synovial fluid can undergo fibro-fatty consolidation, develop fibrous connective tissue, and calcification of the matrix. This leads to loss of proteoglycans, inflammation, shrinkage of the articular cartilage, chondral calcification, adhesion formation between adjacent

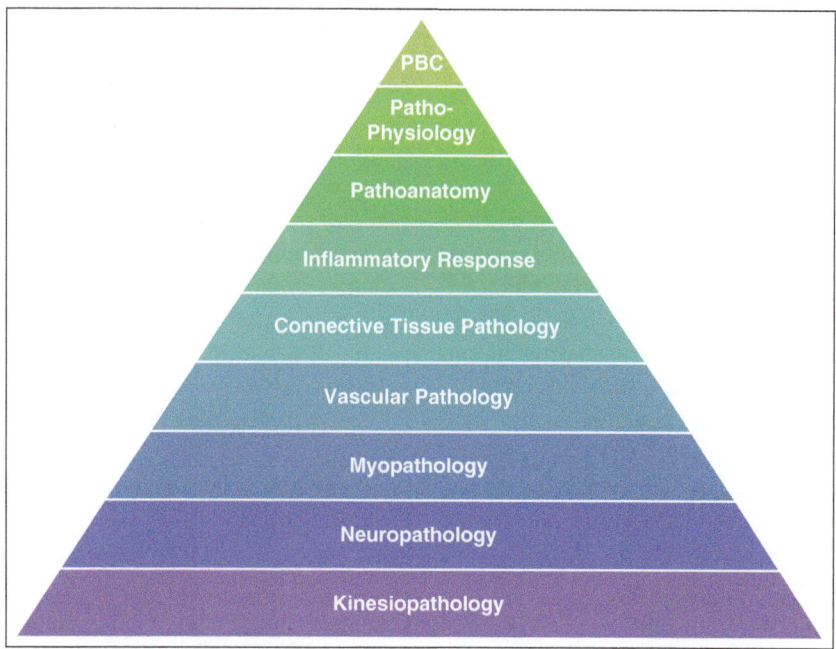

Figure 10.19 The components of the vertebral subluxation complex (VSC). PBC, Pathobiochemistry. Source: Lisa P. McFaddin.

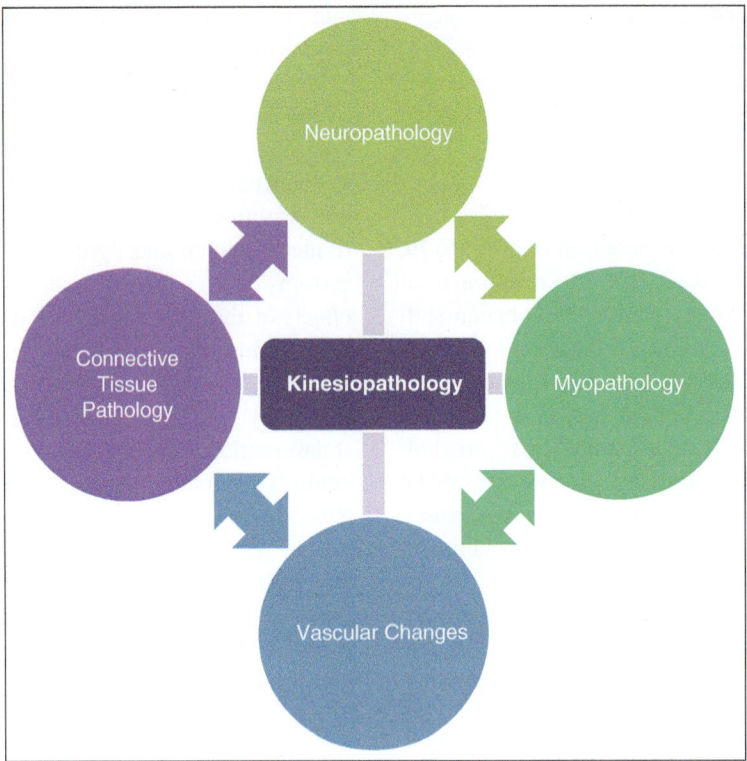

Figure 10.20 Kinesiopathology is the foundation of dysfunction within the VSC, and the most common causes of kinesiopahtology are listed. Source: Lisa P. McFaddin.

connective tissues, tendon contraction, and pain (Rivera 2015).

Hypomobility Pathogenesis

Changes within the VSC can lead to disease through one or more often a combination of six mechanisms: neurodystrophic changes, compressive myelopathologic changes, nerve compression changes, vertebrobasilar artery ischemia, facilitation changes, and secondary changes (Seaman and Faye 2005). The presence of hypomobilities causes a cascade of events, summarized in Figure 10.21, resulting in the development of pain and potentially loss of function.

- **Neurodystrophic changes**: Neuronal disruption can result in changes to the viscera, immune system, and endocrine system, which in turn causes further disturbance to the nervous system (Rivera 2015).

- **Compressive myelopathologic changes**: Chronic pressure on the spinal cord from masses, tumors, and hematomas can damage neuronal tissue leading to ischemia-induced myelopathy (Seaman and Faye 2005).

- **Nerve compression changes**: Motion segment hypomobility can result in inflammation and compression of nerve roots exiting the intervertebral foramen (Cramer and Darby 2005). Frequently, nerve compression results in pain but neuronal dysfunction can also occur.

- **Vertebrobasilar artery ischemia**: A segmental artery supplies each motion segment, transversing the intervertebral canal then splitting into the dorsal and ventral radicular arteries. Compression of the motion segment will adversely affect the nerves as well as the vascular supply. Within the cervical vertebrae these arteries can form loops, increasing their

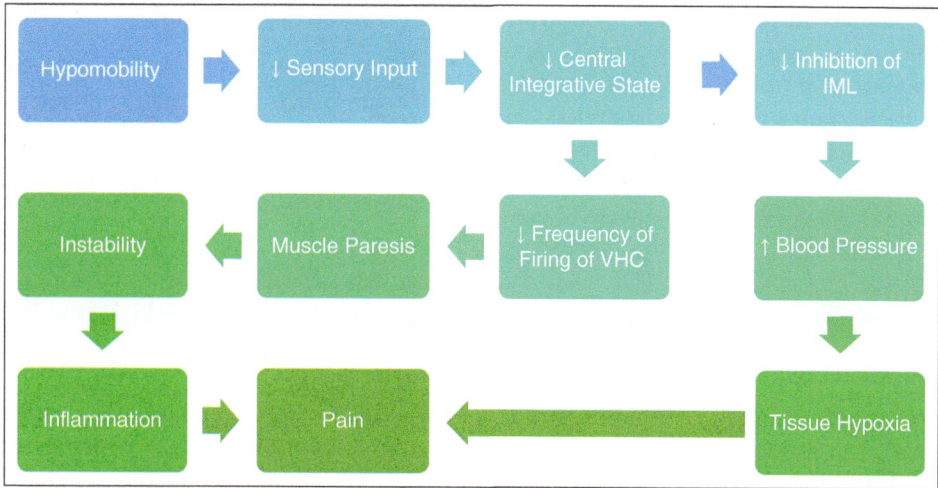

Figure 10.21 The complex sequelae of hypomobilities (Cramer et al. 2014; Rivera 2015). IML, intermedial lateral cell column; VHC, ventral horn cells. Source: Lisa P. McFaddin.

susceptibility to ischemic damage when exposed to sustained compression (Rivera 2015; Cramer and Darby 2005).

- **Facilitation changes**: Motion segment hypomobility or other spinal lesions cause excessive afferent signaling at the associated spinal cord segment, lowering the neuronal firing threshold (Bergman 2005). As a result, any stimuli, whether benign or pathologic, triggers neuronal firing leading to vasoconstriction, spinal muscle spasms, spinal muscle hypoxia, pain, trigger point formation, and accumulation of local inflammatory mediators (Jackman and Regehr 2017). This in turn leads to further stimulation of local pain receptors and afferent signaling, creating a self-perpetuating cycle of pain and inflammation (Rivera 2015).
- **Secondary changes**: Hypomobility can lead to a palpable reduction in spinal segment range of motion and paraspinal muscle tension. These changes are often what the chiropractor uses to identify areas of hypomobility.

Neuroplasticity

The reorganization and formation of new neuronal synapses and connections (i.e. neuroplasticity) within the CNS is typically described within the brain but can also occur within the spinal cord. Neuroplasticity can be defined as physiologic or pathologic (Maltese et al. 2019).

Physiologic neuroplasticity occurs during normal aging (development) and following CNS trauma or damage (adaptive). Adult hippocampal neurogenesis is a prime example of developmental neuroplasticity, in which the development of functional neurons within the adult hippocampus continues throughout life, contributing to a person's memory and behaviors (Kempermann et al. 2015). Adaptive neuroplasticity is commonly observed in people recovering from strokes, with physical therapy and rehabilitation consistently improving patient outcome (Pin-Barre and Laurin 2015).

Pathologic neuroplasticity results in the reorganization and adaptation of the CNS to noxious stimuli leading to the development of maladaptive pain. Repeated exposure to a painful stimulus continually stimulates nociceptors releasing inflammatory neurotransmitters that triggers the release of additional inflammatory mediators from non-neuronal cells. This is known as peripheral sensitization (Purves et al. 2012c).

These nociceptors bombard the dorsal horn of the spinal cord, lowering the firing threshold of second-order neurons making them hyper-excitable. As a result, they often fire without the presence of a truly painful stimulus. This central sensitization also causes stimulation of suprasegmental structures within the brainstem, thalamus, hypothalamus, cerebellum, and cortex leading to the development of more pain (Purves et al. 2012c; Boadas-Vaello et al. 2017).

Prolonged peripheral and central sensitization can lead to long-term potentiation (LTP) (Maltese et al. 2019). LTP represents the cellular mechanisms and changes occurring within the CNS because of hyperalgesia (Ruscheweyh et al. 2011).

Examination Fundamentals

Before an adjustment is performed the practitioner must perform a traditional and chiropractic examination. The chiropractic examination focuses on critically evaluating the musculoskeletal and neurologic systems.

Musculoskeletal Examination

The musculoskeletal (MS) examination involves visual observation of the animal in motion, at rest (standing, sitting, and laying down), and direct palpation. The key features of an MS exam are summarized in Table 10.11. Additionally, the patient's pain

Table 10.11 Overview of the canine musculoskeletal exam (Zink 2013; Duerr and Johnson 2015; Rivera 2015).

Gait	The patient is observed in motion. Abnormal movement patterns are identified. Lameness is identified			
	Walk	Four-beat symmetrical gait with three paws on the ground at one time		
	Trot	Diagonal two-beat symmetrical gait. Best gait for assessing lameness		
	Pace	Lateral two-beat symmetrical gait. Generally considered abnormal		
	Canter	Three-beat gait		
	Gallop	Four-beat gait with double suspension		
Lameness scoring	Allows quantification of the degree of lameness (scale 0–5)			
	0	No lameness	3	Moderate lameness
	1	Subtle lameness	4	Severe lameness
	2	Mild lameness	5	Broken bone
Standing	The patient is observed while standing. Limb placement and weight distribution is assessed			
Sitting	The patient is observed while seated. Limb placement and weight distribution is assessed			
Palpation	Long bone	Symmetry, swelling, heat, and pain		
	Muscle	Symmetry, swelling, atrophy, pain, and trigger points (muscle knots)		
	Joint	Flexion, extension, range of motion, swelling, crepitus (creaking), effusion (swelling), pain, and collateral ligament (cow-hocked, pigeon-toed, duck-footed)		
	Other	Cranial drawer, tibial thrust, etc.		

Source: Lisa P. McFaddin.

level is assessed and recorded using a pre-established pain scale.

Neurologic Examination

Neurology is the branch of science focusing on the nervous system. A comprehensive understanding of the nervous system is required to safely and effectively practice VSMT. The neurologic examination is used to assess the nervous system of the veterinary patient, identify potential deficits, and attempt to narrow down the potential problem area(s) (aka localization of the lesion). The primary objectives of the neurologic examination are listed in Table 10.12. The cranial nerve, postural reactions, and spinal reflex portions of the neurologic

Table 10.12 Key components of the veterinary neurologic examination. References are provided within the text of the table.

Exam components	Description
Mentation	Patient's attitude and level of consciousness are assessed. The attitude is considered appropriate or inappropriate based on the environment and systemic health. Any behavior changes, as observed by the owners, are noted (Bagley 2005)
Posture	Reflects the spine and limb positions with respect to gravity
Gait	Patient's ability to walk. Neurologic gait abnormalities are noted including incoordination (ataxia), scuffing of paws, dragging of limbs, exaggerated steps (hypermetric), leaning, falling, rolling, and circling. The affected limb(s) should be noted (Bagley 2005)
Muscles	Tone, symmetry, and distribution of muscle changes are identified
Cranial nerve	The 12 paired nerves arising from the brain and innervating specific regions within the head, neck, and body cavities. The nerves carry sensory information, motor, or a combination of both to the target organs (Pasquini et al. 2003; Evans and Lahunta 2013). Table 10.13 describes the techniques used for assessment
Postural reactions	Used to evaluate the patient's awareness of their body position in space. These responses require cerebral involvement to process the stimulus and are not reflexes. Examples of postural reaction assessments are detailed in Table 10.14
Spinal reflexes	Used to evaluate myotactic (proprioceptive response of muscles) reflexes of the thoracic and pelvic limbs. Abnormal spinal reflexes are only significant with abnormal postural reactions. Not all reflexes will elicit reliable results. Table 10.15 outlines the most common spinal reflexes evaluated in veterinary patients
Pain	*Superficial pain*: can be assessed by pinching the webbing between the digits of the thoracic and pelvic limbs. The patient should demonstrate a conscious response to the perception of the painful stimulus. Pulling away of the limb does not necessarily mean pain is perceived. Look for turning of the head toward the painful stimulus, trying to bite, vocalization, or even dilation of the pupils
	Deep pain: If the patient does not respond to superficial pain the presence of deep pain is assessed. The periosteum (outer covering of the bone) of the digits should be pinched. The patient should be observed for conscious response to the perception of the painful stimulus (Bagley 2005)
Spinal hyperpathia	Use to evaluate the presence of pain along the vertebrae from the neck to the sacrum
Panniculus	Also called cutaneous trunci, this is an involuntary movement of the skin along the top (dorsum). When lightly touched or pinched the skin will wriggle. Normally this response is not seen behind (caudal) the lower lumbar area. Absence of a panniculus in front of (cranial) the lower back is abnormal, and the approximate location should be noted (Bagley 2005)

Source: Lisa P. McFaddin.

examination requires specific assessments, as described in Tables 10.13–10.15, respectively.

Techniques

The primary techniques used in VSMT are manual adjustments, traction, mobilization, and stretch and hold. Less commonly utilized techniques include the activator method, Logan basic, and craniosacral therapy.

Manual Adjustments or Manipulation

Manual adjustments can be performed on the joints of the back of the head (occiput), jaw (temporomandibular joint), spine (cervical, thoracic, lumbar, and sacrum), pelvis, shoulders, elbows, knees (stifles), and ankles (hocks).

Figure 10.22 depicts the adjustment of several locations on a canine.

Manual adjustments involve the application of a unidirectional HVLA thrust to a specific motion segment (Rivera 2015). Pressure is applied to the hypomobile joint, taking the joint to the edge of its normal range of motion (end play). A rapid thrust is applied to the segmental contact, moving the joint through the paraphysiologic space and improving and ideally restoring range of motion (Jurek 2013). Figure 10.13 shows a graphic representation of the normal and pathologic movement within a joint.

Traction

Traction is the separation of joint surfaces through the application of gentle sustained

Table 10.13 Multiple techniques used to examine the cranial nerves during a veterinary neurologic examination (Bagley 2005; Rivera 2015). This is not an exhaustive list of potential assessments.

Assessment	Technique	CN(s)
Smell	Exposure to a pleasing aroma. Not often evaluated	CN I
Menace	Menacing gesture toward the face causing closing of the eyelids	CN II; CN VII
Pupillary light reflex	Shine a penlight or other bright light source directly into each eye. Observe the change in pupil diameter in both eyes	CN II; CN III
Eye position	Observe both eyes while at rest, lifting their head up, and with the patient on their side and back	CN III; CN IV; CN VI; CN VIII
Oculocephalic reflex	Move the head side to side watching for a normal compensatory movement of both eyes to the right/left interrupted by quick movements to the left/right	CN III; CN IV; CN VI; CN VII
Corneal reflex	Lightly touch cornea with cotton swab. Patient should blink and slightly retract the globe	CN V; CN VI; CN VII
Facial expression	Check for muscle tone and symmetry	CN V; CN VII
Facial sensation	Touch, pinch, or stroke hairs of the face on the nose, cheek, and ears	CN V; CN VII
Hearing	Make a loud noise to one side of the patient and watch for a response. Not always evaluated	CN VIII
Gag reflex	Put gloved hand near back of the throat and watch for swallowing and contraction of the soft palate	CN IX; CN X
Tongue	Examine tongue position and symmetry	CN XII

CN, cranial nerve; CN I, olfactory nerve; CN II, optic nerve; CN III, oculomotor nerve; CN IV, trochlear nerve; CN V, trigeminal nerve; CN VI, abducens nerve; CN VII, facial nerve; CN VIII, vestibulocochlear nerve; CN IX, glossopharyngeal nerve; CN X, vagus nerve; CN XI, spinal accessory nerve; CN XII, hypoglossal nerve.
Source: Lisa P. McFaddin.

Table 10.14 Multiple techniques used to examine the postural reactions during a veterinary neurologic examination (Bagley 2005; Rivera 2015). This is not an exhaustive list of potential assessments.

Assessment	Technique
Conscious proprioception	Flip the paw over onto the knuckles. Patient should either resist inappropriate paw placement or quickly correct the paw position
Hemistanding Hemihopping	Lift the front and rear limbs on the left or right half of the body and lean the patient away toward the ground. Patient should move their limbs once the center of gravity is crossed. This can also be performed on each individual limb
Wheelbarrowing	Lift both thoracic and pelvic limbs and walk the patient forward or backward. Patient should move their limbs once the center of gravity is crossed
Limb placement	(Small dogs and cats only.) Hold the patient in one arm, covering the eyes, and brush the top of their paws against the edge of a table or countertop. The pet should attempt to place their paws on the surface once contact is made with the limbs
Extensor postural thrust	(Small dogs and cats only) Similar to limb placement but with the pelvic limbs

Source: Lisa P. McFaddin.

Table 10.15 Multiple techniques used to examine the spinal reflexes during a veterinary neurologic examination (Bagley 2005; Rivera 2015). This is not an exhaustive list of potential assessments.

Reflex	Technique	Nerves assessed
Withdrawal reflex	Pinch the digits, and the entire limb should retract	Femoral nerve (TL) Sciatic nerve (PL)
Triceps reflex	Percuss the triceps tendon while the elbow is supported. The elbow joint should extend	Radial nerve
Biceps reflex	Percuss the biceps tendon, and the biceps muscle should contract slightly	Musculocutaneous nerve
Extensor carpi radialis	Percuss the extensor carpi radialis muscle, and the carpal (wrist) joint should extend	Radian nerve
Patellar reflex	Percuss the patellar tendon while the stifle (knee) is gently flexed and supported. The stifle joint should extend	Femoral nerve
Cranial tibial reflex	Percuss the cranial tibial muscle, and the tibiotarsal (hock) joint should flex	Peroneal nerve
Gastrocnemius reflex	Percuss the gastrocnemius tendon, and the tibiotarsal (hock) joint should extend	Tibial nerve
Sciatic reflex	Percuss your thumb covering the sciatic notch with the thigh supported. The entire pelvic limb should jerk	Sciatic nerve
Crossed extensor	Pinch the digits of the dependent pelvic limb. Extension of the opposite pelvic limb, while lying down, is a positive and abnormal response	N/A
Babinski	Apply moderate pressure to the bottom (plantar) surface of the metatarsals in a sweeping motion away from the digits. Extension (spreading out) of the digits is a positive and abnormal response	N/A
Perineal reflex	Touching or pinching of the perineal area should result in constriction of the anal sphincter	Pudendal nerve

TL, thoracic limb; PL, pelvic limb. Source: Lisa P. McFaddin.

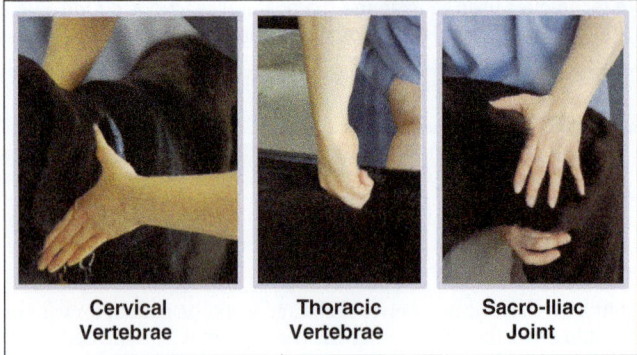

| Cervical Vertebrae | Thoracic Vertebrae | Sacro-Iliac Joint |

Figure 10.22 Examples of manual adjustments of the fifth cervical vertebrae, eleventh thoracic vertebrae, and left sacroiliac joint on a canine. Source: Lisa P. McFaddin.

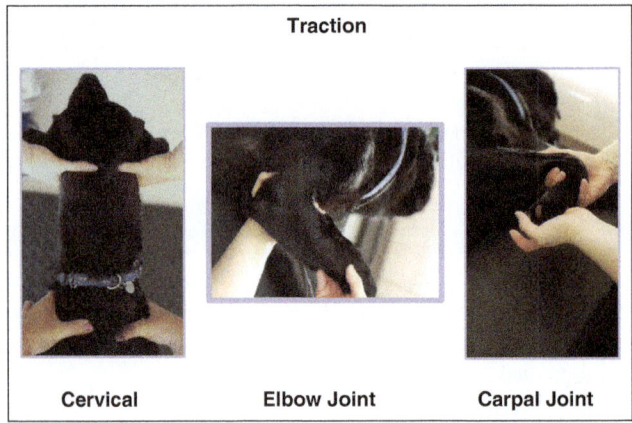

Traction

| Cervical | Elbow Joint | Carpal Joint |

Figure 10.23 Examples of cervical, right elbow joint, and right carpal joint traction on a canine. Source: Lisa P. McFaddin.

pressure (Bergman 2005). Traction is performed on the neck, elbow joints, wrist (carpal) joints, and tail. Figure 10.23 provides examples of performing traction on the neck, elbow joint, and carpal joint of a dog.

Gentle sustained pressure is used for 15–30 seconds, allowing separation of the joint surfaces, then slowly released (Bergman 2005). Traction should not start or stop abruptly as this can result in injury. Traction serves to rest the joint, open up the joint space encouraging the flow of synovial fluid, reduce joint compression and, in the case of cervical traction, open the intervertebral foramen reducing pressure on local vasculature, lymphatics, and nerves (Bergman 2005).

Mobilization

Mobilization is performed on the digits (thoracic and pelvic), metacarpals, metatarsals, wrist (carpus), accessory carpal bone, ankles (hocks), and tail vertebrae. During mobilization, the joint is passively moved through its range of motion multiple times. The goal of mobilization is to loosen areas and break up adhesions (Bergman 2005). The type of movement depends on the area of interest. For example, the accessory carpal bone is mobilized in a clockwise and counterclockwise fashion, while the metacarpals are isolated and moved forward and backward, as shown in Figure 10.24.

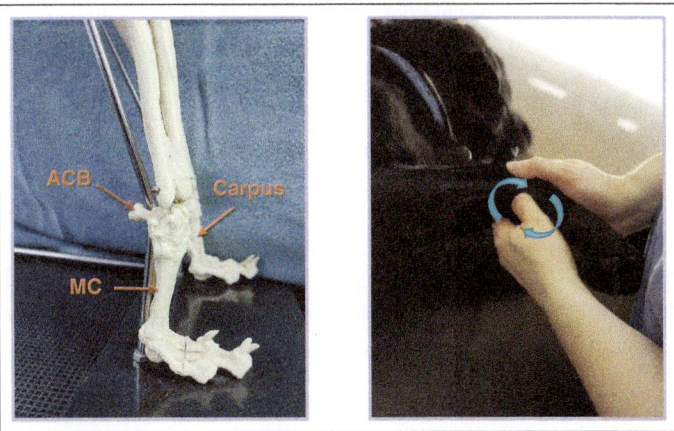

Figure 10.24 Example of mobilization of the right accessory carpal bone (ACB) on a canine. The picture on the left is a canine skeletal model with the labeled relevant anatomical landmarks. The picture on the right is the application of a clockwise mobilization of the right ACB. MC, metacarpals. Source: Lisa P. McFaddin.

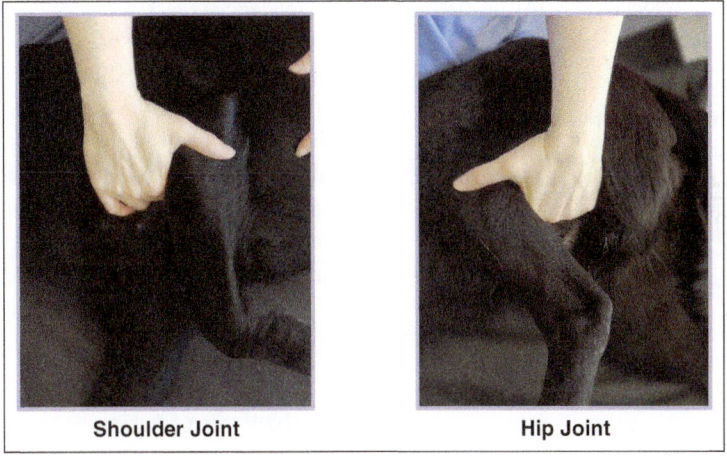

Figure 10.25 Examples of a stretch and hold on the right shoulder joint and right hip joint of a canine. The stretch and hold relaxes the respective joint extensor muscles. Source: Lisa P. McFaddin.

Stretch and Hold

The stretch and hold (SH) is the application of a sustained stretch to a tight muscle with the intent of passively inducing muscle relaxation. SH can be applied to the shoulder and hip joint flexors, as shown in Figure 10.25. The goal of the SH is to induce muscle relaxation through sustained elongation of the affected muscles (Bergman 2005). The SH tires muscles through the continuous stimulation of stretch receptors (MSCs). This technique also relaxes the surrounding connective tissue and fascia. The stretch is held for 60–90 seconds, or until palpable muscle relaxation is noted. Muscle relaxation prior to spinal manipulation improves patient response to the HVLA thrust.

Other Techniques

The **activator method** is a technique developed by W.C. Lee and A.W. Fuhr, centered on the concern that manual adjustments do not generate enough force to effect change

(Bergman 2005). A special device, called the activator adjusting instrument, produces a controlled repeatable percussive force on a specific area of the body.

Logan Basic is a technique developed by Hugh B. Logan based on the philosophy that the sacrum will rotate toward the least supported side (Bergman 2005). In veterinary medicine gentle pressure is applied to the sacrotuberous ligament until the ligament relaxes. This technique is used in both cats and dogs even though cats do not have the ligament.

Craniosacral therapy (aka cranial therapy or cranial osteopathy) is a form of manual therapy focusing on the application of light sustained pressure to the skull and sacrum (Bergman 2005). The timing and duration of pressure is often associated with the patient's respiratory pattern.

Post-Adjustment Recommendations

Common post-adjustment recommendations for clients, especially after a patient's first adjustment (Rivera 2015), include the following.

1) Encourage water intake for the first 24 hours.
2) If the patient seems sore, encourage gentle movement.
3) The first one to two bowel movements may be a little loose.
4) If the pet is still sore after 24 hours, call.

Water Consumption

Good hydration improves blood flow to all organs, including the musculoskeletal and nervous systems. Muscles with good blood flow are less likely to spasm. Increased water consumption following spinal manipulation reduces the risk of post-adjustment muscle stiffness and soreness.

Movement

Immobility causes muscle contraction and tightening which contributes to soreness. Gentle movement, especially short controlled leash walks, keeps muscles and the nervous system active, as well as encouraging blood flow to the muscles and joints. The administration of pain medication, without encouraging movement, may contribute to muscle disuse and stiffness.

Bowel Movements

Gut motility is regulated at the level of the brainstem, spinal cord, and locally within the small intestine and colon (Purves et al. 2012f). Spinal manipulation improves sensory input to the CNS and motor output to the intestines and colon. Subsequently, intestinal and colonic motility may transiently increase causing looser stools. The client should call if the loose stools persist for more than 24 hours.

Prolonged Soreness

If the patient is still sore or lethargic more than 24 hours after the adjustment, especially the initial treatment, the owner should inform the clinic. This may occur because of aggressive adjusting (too many sites or incorrect force) or there is another underlying condition not initially appreciated. Open communication improves client understanding and comfort levels regarding the therapy and guides future appointments improving efficacy.

Mechanisms of Action

VSMT causes physiologic changes to the nervous system (aka neurophysiology) and changes to the structure, function, and motion of the musculoskeletal system (biomechanics), summarized in Figure 10.26. The health of the nervous system is determined through the neurologic examination, described in Table 10.12. Biomechanics are assessed using the orthopedic examination, outlined in Table 10.11, and spinal motion palpation.

Spinal manipulation directly affects the structures comprising the IVF, IVD, zygapophyseal joints, muscles and connective tissue around the spine, blood flow, and nervous input and output (Cramer and Darby 2005). HVLA causes movement within the joints, breakdown of adhesions,

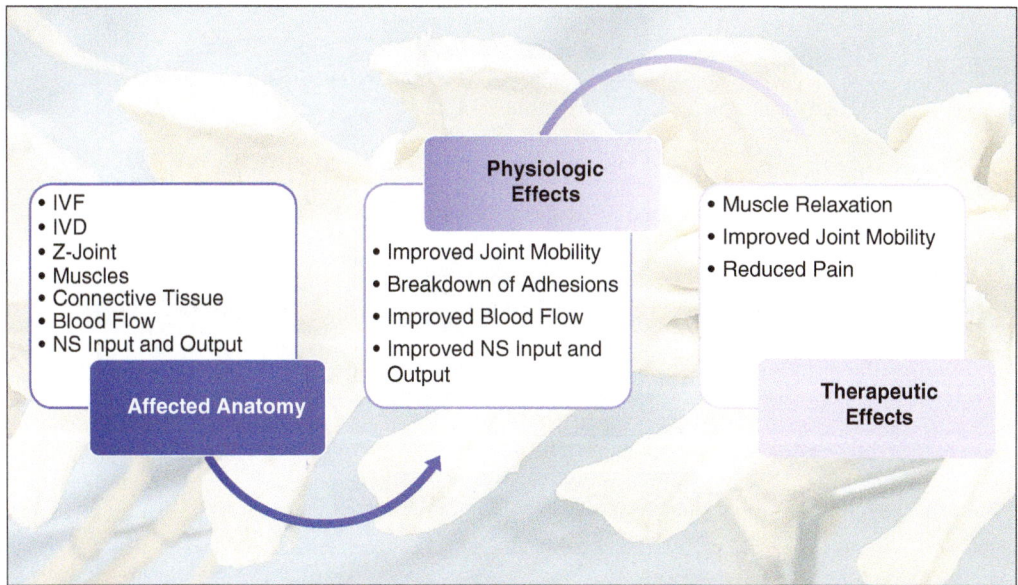

Figure 10.26 The affected anatomy, physiologic effects, and therapeutic benefits of veterinary spinal manipulation therapy. IVF, intervertebral foramen; IVD, intervertebral disk; Z-joint, zygapophyseal joint; NS, nervous system. Source: Lisa P. McFaddin.

improved blood flow, and improved nervous system function (Cramer 2015; Rivera 2015). The end result is muscle relaxation, improved joint mobility, and pain reduction.

Mechanisms of Action for Veterinarians

Pathologic changes in the anatomy, physiology, and biomechanics of the spine negatively affect the nervous system. Spinal manipulation helps correct these irregularities, restoring neurologic function. The mechanisms of action behind VSMT can be broken down into neurophysiologic and biomechanical effects, summarized in Figure 10.27.

Neurophysiologic Effects

VSMT stimulates sensory input to the CNS, stimulates and inhibits nociceptive input to the CNS, stimulates mechanoreceptors, in particular MSCs and GTOs, reduces central sensitization (facilitation) of pain, stimulates the neuroendocrine system, and promotes spinal cord neuroplasticity (Gillette 2005; Pickar et al. 2007; Rivera 2015; Maltese et al. 2019). The result is muscle relaxation, improved joint range of motion and mobility, and pain reduction.

Biomechanics of VSMT

Stimulation of the motion unit causes a host of biomechanical changes, including movement of the meniscus within the Z-joint, disruption of adhesions, stimulation of mechanoreceptors within the Z-joints, and restoration of IVD shape and pressure (Cramer 2015).

A fibro-adipose meniscus is attached to the Z-joint capsule by loose connective tissue. The meniscus can become entrapped between the articular cartilage causing pain (Panzer 2005). Extrapment of the synovial tissue within the Z-joint, between the joint capsule and articular cartilage, can also cause pain (Cramer 2015). Spinal manipulation effectively gaps the Z-joint releasing the trapped meniscus and synovial tissue. Once released these tissues return to their normal position within the Z-joint, stopping the painful stimuli caused by their misplacement (Panzer 2005; Cramer 2015).

Pain, inflammation, and disuse cause the development of fibro-adipose and collagen-like

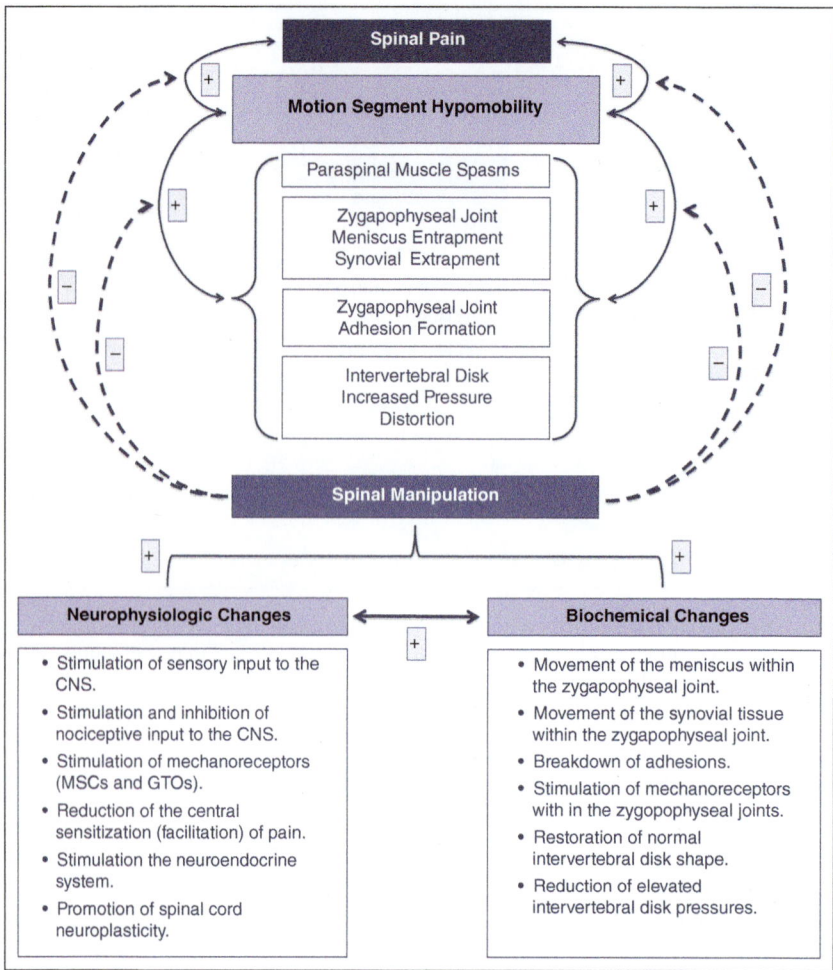

Figure 10.27 The primary causes of motion segment hypomobility, neurophysiologic and biochemical mechanisms involved in spinal manipulation, and the effects of both on pain (Mootz 2005; Pickar et al. 2007; Cramer 2015). (+) indicates promotion, (−) signifies inhibition. Source: Lisa P. McFaddin.

adhesions within the Z-joints and other affected synovial joints (Mootz 2005). The severity of adhesion formation is time dependent (Cramer et al. 2010). The presence of adhesions further limits mobility causing more pain and inflammation. The separation of the articular cartilage within the Z-joint (gapping) during spinal manipulation breaks up the adhesions, improving mobility of the Z-joint and the entire motion segment (Cramer 2015).

Z-joint capsules contain three types of mechanoreceptors: type I, type II, and type IV (Cramer 2015). Type I are very sensitive and

fire continuously, type II are stimulated by movement, and type IV are slow-conducting nociceptors (free nerve endings) (Cramer 2015). Pathologic changes to the Z-joints stimulate type IV receptors. Spinal manipulation will stimulate type I and II receptors (Cramer and Darby 2005). Type I and II inhibit pain through Melzack and Wall's Gate Theory (Mittleman and Gaynor 2000).

Prolonged hypomobility and inflammation within a motion segment can distort the AF and increase the pressure within the disk itself (Mootz 2005). Spinal manipulation and traction can improve mobility within the motion segment, reduce distortion of the AF, and reduce pressure within the IVD (Cramer 2015).

Safety

VSMT is a safe and well-tolerated medicinal practice. Like all therapies, there are conditions under which VSMT should be used with caution or avoided, summarized in Table 10.16. There are a few potential adverse effects including muscle stiffness, muscle pain (myalgia), and loose bowel movements. All adverse effects are mild and typically self-resolve within 24 hours.

The Why

Applications in Human Medicine

The 2017 National Health Interview Survey (NHIS), conducted by the National Center for Complementary and Integrative Health (NCCIH) and the National Center for Health Statistics (NCHS), revealed a 9.1% increase in chiropractic care in US adults, aged 18 years and older, between 2012 and 2017 (Clarke et al. 2018). The 2012 NHIS study revealed 67% of surveyed adults used chiropractic care for specific health problems; while 53% sought chiropractic care for general health and wellness and disease prevention (NHIS 2012). The NCCIH website (https://nccih.nih.gov) is an excellent resource to learn more about the effectiveness and usefulness of spinal manipulation for people.

NCCIH (2020) sites pain as the most common reason for which people seek chiropractic care specifically sciatica, lower-back pain, neck pain, headaches, and migraines. The NCCIH is currently funding studies investigating (NCCIH 2022):

- The impact of spinal manipulation of lower-back pain in U.S. veterans.
- How chiropractic care compares to the use of prescription drugs for the long-term management of chronic lower-back pain in older adults.
- The use of chiropractic care for chronic neck pain.

NCCIH (2022) considers spinal manipulation safe when performed by a trained and licensed practitioner. Adverse effects are uncommon with the majority being mild and temporary, resolving within 24–72 hours, including muscle soreness, stiffness, and a

Table 10.16 The conditions under which veterinary spinal manipulation therapy should be avoided or used with caution (Jurek 2013; Rivera 2015).

Cautions	Contraindications
<ul><li>Hypermobile joints</li><li>Spondylosis deformans</li><li>Cancer</li><li>Seizures</li><li>Immune-mediated diseases</li><li>Patient compliance (extremely aggressive or scared pets)</li></ul>	<ul><li>Severe acute pain</li><li>Fractures (spine, limb)</li><li>Vertebral abnormalities (hemivertebrae, block vertebrae)[a]</li><li>Intervertebral disk protrusion[a]</li><li>Bone infection (osteomyelitis)</li><li>Bone cancer</li><li>Splenic cancer</li><li>Active bleeding (especially internally)</li><li>Fever</li><li>Immediately postoperative</li><li>Heavily sedated or anesthetized patients</li></ul>

[a] Only adjustment of the affected vertebrae is contraindicated. Source: Lisa P. McFaddin.

transient increase in pain (Carnes et al. 2010; LeFebvre et al. 2012; NCCIH 2022).

Serious complications are rare but can occur. Cervical spinal manipulation has been linked to a potentially fatal tear in the walls of the arteries in the neck called cervical artery dissections (CAD) (NCCIH 2022). The risk of CAD increases in susceptible people with any sudden neck movement including playing sports, whiplash, extreme vomiting, and coughing (NCCIH 2022). CAD generally precedes a vertebrobasilar artery (VBA) stroke. A retrospective case analysis of 818 VBA stroke cases by Cassidy et al. (2008) revealed 4% of the cases had seen a chiropractor within seven days of hospitalization, while 53% of cases had seen their primary care physician. Headache and neck pain appeared to be the primary reason patients sought chiropractic care or physician evaluation. Another retrospective analysis of 1829 VBA stroke cases by Kosloff et al. (2015) demonstrated no statistical correlation between chiropractic visits and the development of a VBA stroke.

Applications in Veterinary Medicine

The primary application of VSMT is the treatment of pain, both adaptive and maladaptive. Realistically any disorder affecting the musculoskeletal and nervous systems can benefit from VSMT (Jurek 2013). Clients and referring veterinarians pursue VSMT when other treatments have failed, the client requests a more "holistic" approach, or as an adjunct to lessen the side effects of traditional medicine (Rivera 2015). VSMT may aid in the management of lameness, paresis (weakness), behavioral changes, sporting dog injuries, incontinence, temporomandibular joint (TMJ) issues, and as an adjunct to postoperative orthopedic rehabilitation (Rivera 2015; Haussler et al. 2021).

Veterinary Research

The 2015 American Animal Hospital Association (AAHA) and American Association of Feline Practitioners (AAFP) Pain Management Guidelines do not recommend animal chiropractic for pain control citing a lack of scientific evidence (Epstein et al. 2015). The paper does mention the evidence-based benefit of spinal manipulation in people. The 2022 AAHA Pain Management Guidelines for Dogs and Cats does not mention animal chiropractic or VSMT (Gruen et al. 2022).

Unfortunately, there is limited veterinarian-guided chiropractic research (Miscioscia and Repac 2022). As of February 2023, a quick search on PubMed for "veterinary chiropractic" and "veterinary spinal manipulation" yielded around 200 articles. There are numerous studies using animal models for human chiropractic research. As of February 2023, there are over 1000 articles involving searches for feline, canine, rat, murine, and rabbit chiropractic and spinal manipulation. While these studies are conducted to benefit the human population, the information is often still applicable to our veterinary patients. Presented below are the summaries of three VSMT studies.

Effect of Spinal Manipulation on the Development of History-Dependent Responsiveness of Lumbar Paraspinal Muscle Spindles in the Cat	
Authors: Dong-Yuan Cao and Joel G. Pickar	**Study hypothesis**: Spinal manipulation prevents muscle spindle cell (MSC) firing and improves MSC afferent input.
Journal: *Journal of the Canadian Chiropractic Association*	**Sample size**: 27 laboratory cats
Date: 2014	**Materials and methods**: Paraspinal tissue
Study design: Controlled study	dissection and bilateral L4, L5, and/or

L6 laminectomy was performed on 27 anesthetized cats. MSC action potentials were measured in the L6 dorsal root from the multifidus and longissimus muscles. Spinal manipulation was created using a feedback-controlled motor attached to the L6 spinous process. MSC action potentials were measured in relation to no change, static, and dynamic vertebral positioning. One-way analysis of variance (ANOVA) was used for data analysis.

Results

1) In the static test changes in MSC activity was significantly lower when spinal manipulation occurred after priming of the muscle but not before.
2) In the dynamic test there was no statistically significant difference in MSC activity when spinal manipulation was performed before or after muscle priming.

Study conclusions: Spinal manipulation improves abnormal muscle spindle cell activity negatively affected by changes in vertebral positioning.

Study limitations

1) Only the caudal lumbar spine was evaluated.
2) Anesthesia causes muscle relaxation which may impact muscle priming and response to spinal manipulation.

L.P.M. conclusions: Spinal manipulation improves muscle relaxation thus reducing pain from muscle tension and/or spasms.

(Cao and Pickar 2014)

Validation of the Cat as a Model for the Human Lumbar Spine During Simulated High-Velocity, Low-Amplitude Spinal Manipulation

Authors: Allyson Ianuzzi, Joel Pickar, and Partap Khalsa
Journal: *Journal of Biomechanical Engineering*
Date: 2010
Study design: Controlled study
Study hypothesis: Felines can be used as a model when studying the human lumbar spine, specifically facet joint capsule (FJC) strain and response to spinal manipulation.
Sample size: Six laboratory cats
Materials and methods: The cats were sacrificed and the lumbar spines (L2 to the sacrum) were removed. All tissues were then removed around the FJC surface exposing the capsular ligament. Specimens were arranged using an epoxy so the vertebral end-plates were parallel to the testing surface. All FJC were marked with infrared reflective markers. An apparatus was used to stimulate high-velocity low-amplitude (HVLA) thrusts. Cameras were used to capture movement of the spines following HVLA. Spinal manipulations were applied to the anterior surface of L5, L6, or L7. Optical measurements were taken of the vertebral kinematics, FJC (left and right) strain magnitudes, intervertebral angles, and plane of strain of the FJC. Results were compared to human FJC strain and kinematics data from a previously conducted study. One-way analysis of variance was used for data analysis.

Results

1) FJC strain was similar to that of human spines.
2) Joint motion and FJC strain was larger in the cat compared to human spine specimens.
3) HVLA thrust used and resultant FJC tensile strain was significantly correlated between feline and human specimens

(Continued)

Validation of the Cat as a Model for the Human Lumbar Spine During Simulated High-Velocity, Low-Amplitude Spinal Manipulation (Continued)

Study conclusions: The effect of HVLA thrusts on the feline lumbar spine can be used as a model for human responses to spinal manipulation.

Study limitations

1) Small sample size.
2) Spine models used in the study did not include superficial musculature which may affect FJC strain and biomechanics.

L.P.M. conclusions: Cats can be used to further research the physiologic effects of HVLA thrusts on the human lumbar spine. From a veterinary standpoint this means more research will be conducted on cats validating the applications of animal chiropractic. Research money can be hard to come by, especially in the veterinary field. This is a roundabout way of performing veterinary research while also furthering human medicine.

(Ianuzzi et al. 2010)

Paraspinal Muscle Spindle Response to Intervertebral Fixation and Segmental Thrust Level During Spinal Manipulation in an Animal Model

Authors: William Reed and Joel Pickar
Journal: *Spine*
Date: 2015
Study design: Controlled study
Study hypothesis: Unilateral facet joint fixations cause intervertebral fact joint dysfunction altering muscle spindle cell (MSC) response during high-velocity low-amplitude (HVLA) thrust.
Sample size: 23 laboratory cats
Materials and methods: A laminectomy was performed (exposing L5 and L6 dorsal rootlets) on anesthetized cats. The right sciatic nerves were cut to reduce afferent input from the pelvic limbs. L6 dorsal root filaments were dissected (in such a manner where they only responded to pressure applied to the multifidus and longissimus lumbar spinal muscles) and placed on monopolar electrodes. Electrodes also recorded information from left L4–L7 facet joints. MSC were identified using by measuring their response to succinylcholine. HVLA thrust was applied dorsoventrally at L4 or L6 spinous process under three spinal joint conditions: no fixation, two-level fixation (L5–6 and L6–7), or three-level fixation (L4–5, L5–6, and L6–7). HVLA thrust was generated using forceps attached to a feedback motor system. L6 MSC responses were measured. MSC neural discharge was measured as instantaneous frequency (IF) using the reciprocal time interval between action potentials. One-way analysis of variance (ANOVA) was used for data analysis.

Results

1) Fixation of the facets significantly increased lumbar spinal stiffness.
2) Fixation of the facets significantly decreased the L6 spindle response to HVLA thrusts.
3) L6 MSC response was significantly reduced when the HVLA thrust was applied at L4 compared to L6.

Study conclusions: Intervertebral facet fixation reduces paraspinal MSC response to HVLA thrusts. Targeted HVLA thrust have a greater effect than non-targeted spinal manipulation.

Table 10.17 specifies many conditions for which VSMT has shown a scientifically beneficial effect. This list is not all inclusive, as new studies documenting the beneficial effects of spinal manipulation in veterinary medicine are continually published.

The How

Team Members

This section reviews the potential return on investment (ROI), how to effectively train the entire team, how to promote, and how to integrate the integrative therapy.

Return on Investment

ROI can be determined by evaluating client interest, veterinarian demand, hospital costs, applicability of the service, appointment scheduling, and pricing.

Client Interest

Currently there are no studies documenting client interest or the popularity of VSMT. By evaluating trends in client opinion and pet health insurance client interest in VSMT can be inferred.

Client Opinion Table 10.18 summarizes the pet owner demographics and statistics mentioned in the My Lessons section of the Introduction. Even if one-quarter of those owners are open to VSMT, that is still 26.6 million potential patients.

Pet Health Insurance Many pet insurance plans include coverage for integrative therapies, including VSMT (Woodley 2018). The presence of this type of coverage re-emphasizes the mainstream incorporation of these treatment modalities, as well as reflecting client demand.

Veterinarian Demand

As of February 2023, there are no statistics on the number of veterinarians and human chiropractors practicing VSMT. The best way to determine veterinarian demand is to compare the number of general practitioners to the number of veterinarians and human chiropractors advertising VSMT or animal chiropractic within a 5-, 10-, or 20-mile radius of the hospital. Less than 10% of the practices should offer the service to avoid oversaturation of the market and the introduction of a redundant service.

Hospital Costs

Let's start by reviewing all the potential costs associated with introducing and offering VSMT: veterinarian training, staff training, supplies and equipment, staffing, facilities, and advertising. Tables 10.19 and 10.20 demonstrate the different potential start-up costs, dependent on the hospital's contribution toward the veterinarian's training and prior utilization of regular all-staff meetings. For more information on potential hospital costs refer to the Introduction of this book.

Table 10.17 Studies demonstrating the application and efficacy of spinal manipulation (SM) therapy in multiple animal species as of 2023.

Condition studied	Species	Studies
Back pain	Equine	Haussler et al. (2020)
Bone mobility	Feline	Adams et al. (1992)
Cervical vertebral mobilization	Equine	Ahern (1994)
	Canine	Verschooten (1991), Penning and Badoux (1987), Crisco et al. (1990)
Gait abnormalities	Equine	Vasseur et al. (1981)
Improved joint mobilization	Canine	Olson (1987)
IVD intradiscal pressure	Feline	Reed et al. (2022)
IVF innervation	Feline	Pickar and McLain (1995)
Kinematics	Equine	Alvarez et al. (2008)
Muscle relaxation	Equine	Acutt et al. (2019)
	Feline	Ge et al. (2005), Pickar et al. (2007), Pickar and Ge (2008), Cao et al. (2009), Ge et al. (2011), Ge and Pickar (2012), Cao et al. (2013), Cao and Pickar (2014), Reed et al. (2015), Reed et al. (2015), Reed and Pickar (2015), Reed et al. (2017), Lima et al. (2021) Studies focused on the effect of SM on MSC
Neuroendocrine connection	Canine	Brennan et al. (1991)
Neuropathic pain	Rat	Onifer et al. (2018)
Sciatic neuritis	Murine	Triano and Luttges (1980), Triano and Luttges (1982)
Spinal mobility	Equine	Haussler et al. (2007), Haussler et al. (2010)
Spinal nociceptive thresholds	Equine	Haussler and Erb (2003), Sullivan et al. (2008)
Spondylosis	Canine	Halle and Granhus (2021)
Stimulation of the GI NS	Rabbits	DeBoer et al. (1998)
Stimulation of the SNS	Canine	Dae et al. (1997)
	Rat	Sato and Swenson (1984)
Vertebral movement	Canine	Smith et al. (1989), Papakyriakou et al. (1991), Cao and Pickar (2011)
	Feline	Vaillant et al. (2012), Edgecombe et al. (2015)
Vertebral subluxation complex	Rat	Lin et al. (1978), Israel (1983)
Zygapophyseal joint changes	Rat	Cramer et al. (2004)

IVD, intervertebral disk; IVF, intervertebral facet; MSC, muscle spindle cells; GI, gastrointestinal tract; NS, nervous system; SNS, sympathetic nervous system.
Source: Lisa P. McFaddin.

Table 10.18 Summary of the 2022 pet ownership and pet health insurance demographics in the United States discussed in the Introduction of the book (Burns 2018; MFAF 2018; APPA 2022; Burns 2022; Nolen 2022; NAPHIA 2023).

• 83% of pets are owned by millennials (32%), generation X (24%), and baby boomers (27%)
• 69 million households owned dogs
• 45.3 million households owned cats
• Estimated over 81.1 million owned dogs
• Estimated over 60.7 million owned cats
• 68% of owners are interested in alternative treatment modalities for their pets
• 4.41 million pets have pet health insurance
• 82% of insurance pets are dogs

Source: Lisa P. McFaddin.

Table 10.19 Total potential hospital start-up costs for veterinary spinal manipulation therapy (VSMT) as of 2023.

Category	Subcategories	Projected cost	
Veterinarian training	Course costs	$7200–14 999.55	Average $8412
	Textbooks	$500	
	Travel expenses	$6060	
	Time-off	$0–4632.96	Average $2316.48
Staff training	Variable	$230–1295	
Supplies	Bale	$450	
Staffing	Variable	≥$0	
Facilities	Overhead	$2–5 per minute per 15–60-minute appointment	$30–300 per patient
Advertising	Variable	≤$420	

Source: Lisa P. McFaddin.

Veterinarian Training

Course Costs There are six main courses in the United States. Most programs are a hybrid of online and on-site training. On average there are four on-site modules lasting four days each. Typical completion time is five months, but many programs offer extended completion times of up to two years. Additional information can be found in the Veterinarians section of this chapter (cost range, $7200–14 999.55).

Textbooks

Textbooks may not be required for the courses but are often highly recommended. The price range for four to five books is $400–600 (average, $500).

Travel Expenses

Travel costs include airfare, lodging, car rental, and meals. The estimated pricing is based on four on-site sessions with four full days of training.

Table 10.20 Projected veterinary spinal manipulation therapy (VSMT) start-up costs for eight hospital scenarios, with varying hospital contributions toward veterinary certification and staff training as of February 2023. The cost of veterinarian training is based on the averages presented Table 10.19. Staff training costs assume a 1.5-hour-long all-staff meeting, using national averages for employee numbers: eight non-DVMs and two DVMs (AVMA 2019a, 2023). The cost of office supplies and lunch as estimated based on 10 employees attending the meeting. The overhead is based on an average of $3.5/minute. Missed revenue is calculated using the 2022 national mean revenue per hour for companion animal practices ($567/hour) (AVMA 2023). Advertising includes printed materials, digital advertisement, and community engagement.

Category	Projected expenses	Ex. 1	Ex. 2	Ex. 3	Ex. 4	Ex. 5	Ex. 6	Ex. 7	Ex. 8
Veterinarian training	Average course cost	$8412	$8412	$8412	n/a	$8412	$8412	$8412	n/a
	Average textbooks	$500	n/a	n/a	n/a	$500	n/a	n/a	n/a
	Travel expenses	$6060	n/a	n/a	n/a	$6060	n/a	n/a	n/a
	Average time-off	$2317	$2317	n/a	n/a	$2317	$2317	n/a	n/a
Staff training	Office supplies	$30	$30	$30	$30	$30	$30	$30	$30
	Lunch	$200	$200	$200	$200	$200	$200	$200	$200
	Overhead	$315	$315	$315	$315	n/a	n/a	n/a	n/a
	Missed DVM revenue	$851	$851	$851	$851	n/a	n/a	n/a	n/a
Supplies	Bale	$350	$350	$350	$350	$350	$350	$350	$350
Advertising		$420	$420	$420	$420	$420	$420	$420	$420
Total		**$19455**	**$12895**	**$10578**	**$2166**	**$18289**	**$11729**	**$9412**	**$1000**

Source: Lisa P. McFaddin.

- *Airfare*: Due to the global effects of the pandemic, the average roundtrip domestic flight within the United States was less expensive in 2021 compared to 2019, $293 vs. $359 (Damodaran 2021; Weir 2019). Airfare rose precipitously in June 2022 to an average of $398 for a roundtrip domestic flight and has continued to rise by at least 3.4% in the last eight months to approximately $412 (BLS 2023; Trcek 2023). The $412 value was used when calculating the cost of airfare for four roundtrip flights (total cost, $1648).
- *Lodging*: As of February 2023 the federal per diem rate for lodging on business trips is $98 per night (FederalPay.org 2023). The federal per diem rate was used for calculations, with four nights of lodging over four sessions (total cost, $1568).
- *Car rental*: As of January 2023, the average weekly car rental price is $551 (French and Kemmis 2023). Rideshare and cabbing are extremely popular, but the variability in travel distances makes calculating an average cost impractical. It is suspected this cost would be comparable, if not lower, than that of a rental car. The total was calculated using five-day car rentals for four sessions (total cost, $2204).
- *Meals*: The federal per diem rate for business trip meals from October 2022 through

September 2023 is $59 a day (FederalPay.org 2023). Most training programs provide at least one meal, as well as snacks. Meal expenditure is estimated to be $40/day for a total of 16 days (total cost, $640).

- *Time Off*: Veterinarian paid time-off (PTO) for on-site courses only factors in as an added expense if additional PTO is provided outside of the veterinarian's contractual annual PTO. Clinics offer an average of 4.1 paid continuing education (CE) days per year according to the last AAHA Compensation and Benefits Guide (AAHA 2019). If the total number of CE days exceeds the allotted CE days per year, the hospital can either require the veterinarian use PTO or pay the veterinarian for some or all the remaining CE days. Requiring the use of PTO, would not "cost" the hospital anything additional.

The clinic accrues an added expense if they agree to pay for the additional CE days. The price range provided represents a clinic offering 12 days of additional paid CE leave. The median pay for a full-time veterinarian, calculated by the United States Bureau of Labor Statistics in 2022, was $100 370 or $48.26/hour (BLS 2022). Each paid CE day was counted as eight hours. The total does not include potential lost revenue due to the veterinarian's absence, nor does it include relief veterinarian expenses. (total cost, $4632.96)

Staff Training

Team training expenses are highly variable and dependent on the preexistence of staff meetings and use of a staff meeting for training (compared to self-study). Refer to the Introduction of the book for a breakdown of these variables (cost range, $230–1295).

Supplies

No specific supplies are required to practice small animal VSMT. The use of floor mats or yoga mats allows better traction for larger dogs on slippery tile floors. Tables can be used when adjusting small dogs.

An equine spinal manipulation bale (basically a large compressed block of Styrofoam covered with heavy-duty nylon) is very helpful for medium sized dogs that are too small for the floor but too tall for a traditional exam room table (cost range, $400–500).

Staffing

VSMT appointments range from 15 to 60 minutes depending on the condition(s) being treated. Following the American Animal Hospital Association (AAHA) recommendations a veterinary assistant or licensed technician (VA/LT) should always restrain patients for physical examinations and procedures. A VA/LT is usually required for 15–30 minutes, so there is no difference in staffing cost for VSMT appointments compared to traditional appointments.

Facilities

Facility expenses represent the costs needed to keep the doors open (aka overhead). Overhead includes rent or mortgage, utilities, administrative costs, and often employee costs divided by the minutes the practice is open (Stevenson 2016). The price per minute equals the amount of revenue needed just to break even. Overhead is extremely hospital specific, but the range tends to be $2–5/minute. The low end of the range in Table 10.19 represents the cost for a 15-minute appointment at a clinic with a $2/minute overhead, while the high end represents the cost for a 60-minute appointment at a clinic with a $5/minute overhead.

Designating a specific room for VSMT minimizes the chances other associates will need the room for their appointments. However, there is then an added expense for designing the room and potential lost revenue if the room is not used regularly. The absence of a designated room theoretically reduces redecoration costs, but this can be disruptive for appointment flow if the treatment takes longer than the allotted time.

Advertising

There are numerous ways to advertise a new service. On average veterinary hospitals spend 0.7% of revenue on promotion and advertisement (AVMA 2019a). Most of the advertising can be done with little to no additional expenditure. The Promotion section discusses advertising ideas in further detail. The national median gross revenue for companion animal practices was $1.2 million in 2022 (AVMA 2023). Advertising costs are calculated assuming no more than 5% of the current advertising budget would be used for promotion of the new service (estimated maximal cost, $420).

Start-Up Costs Table 10.19 summarizes projected start-up costs for VSMT. Table 10.20 calculates potential start-up costs based on the degree of hospital contribution toward veterinarian and staff training. Different scenarios are presented in which the hospital covers all, some, or none of the expenses.

Applicability

According to the Healthy Paws Pet Insurance and Foundation 2019 Cost of Pet Health Care Report, 18.8% of canine vet visits were related to pain and musculoskeletal injuries, while 6.8% of feline visits were related to painful conditions. As stated previously, VSMT is very useful in the management and prevention of pain. This treatment modality is an invaluable addition to any practitioner's toolbox when it comes to treating the third most common reason for taking a dog, and seventh most common reason for taking a cat, to the veterinarian (HPPIF 2019).

Appointment Scheduling

here are four main factors to consider when planning VSMT appointment protocols: appointment length; support staff availability; exam room availability; and follow-up appointment scheduling.

There are other issues to consider as well. For example, will VSMT appointments be scheduled separately from traditional Western appointments, or will the appointment length be increased to allow time for the adjustment to be performed? Will wellness protocols be performed during the VSMT appointment?

Some practitioners prefer not to administer vaccines during the VSMT appointment while others do not mind.

The initial VSMT appointment is often longer compared to follow-up appointments. Follow-up appointments should be scheduled for 15–60 minutes depending on the patient and if additional treatments are performed.

Keep the appointment positive. You want to pet to enjoy the experience. A relaxed pet is more easily adjusted. Avoid ancillary procedures which may cause stress: nail trims, anal gland expression, sanitary trims, anything with the ears, etc. Ear problems should generally be addressed separately. Constant head shaking following an adjustment is often counterproductive. Additional information on appointment scheduling can be found in the Introduction of this book.

Pricing

An in-depth look into appointment pricing can be found in the Introduction of this book. Here we discuss two pricing methods: current market fees and hospital cost-based pricing.

Current Market Fees According to Wag! (2020) the cost of canine chiropractic treatments range from $50 to $200 per session.

Hospital Cost-Based Pricing Table 10.21 outlines the hospital cost per patient for 15-, 30-, and 60-minute VSMT appointments. The veterinarian training amortization per patient was calculated using the following assumptions:

1) The average companion animal practice employees 2.1 full-time veterinarians (AVMA 2023).
2) The average companion animal practice is open for appointments 5.6 days per week (AVMA 2023).
3) The average companion animal veterinarian sees two patients per hour (AVMA 2023).
4) The average companion animal veterinarian works 45 hours a week (AVMA 2023).

Table 10.21 Estimated hospital costs per patient for 15-, 30-, and 60-minute veterinary spinal manipulation therapy appointments as of February 2023. Start-up costs are taken from the totals in Table 10.20. Amortization is per patient and is based on the veterinarian seeing 952 integrative patients in two years. Overhead is calculated using $3.5/minute in a practice with two veterinarians. Multiple examples are provided with the variance determined by the total cost within each category. The total is rounded to the nearest whole number.

	Ex. 1	Ex. 2	Ex. 3	Ex. 4	Ex. 5	Ex. 6	Ex. 7	Ex. 8
15-Minute appointments								
Table 10.20 totals	$19 455	$12 895	$10 578	$2166	$18 289	$11 729	$9412	$1000
Amortization	$20.44	$13.55	$11.11	$2.28	$19.21	$12.32	$9.89	$1.05
Overhead	$26	$26	$26	$26	$26	$26	$26	$26
Total	**$46**	**$40**	**$37**	**$28**	**$45**	**$38**	**$36**	**$27**
30-Minute appointments								
Table 10.20 totals	$19 455	$12 895	$10 578	$2166	$18 289	$11 729	$9412	$1000
Amortization	$20.44	$13.55	$11.11	$2.28	$19.21	$12.32	$9.89	$1.05
Overhead	$52.50	$52.50	$52.50	$52.50	$52.50	$52.50	$52.50	$52.50
Total	**$73**	**$66**	**$64**	**$55**	**$72**	**$65**	**$62**	**$54**
60-Minute appointments								
Table 10.20 totals	$19 455	$12 895	$10 578	$2166	$18 289	$11 729	$9412	$1000
Amortization	$20.44	$13.55	$11.11	$2.28	$19.21	$12.32	$9.89	$1.05
Overhead	$105	$105	$105	$105	$105	$105	$105	$105
Total	**$125**	**$119**	**$116**	**$107**	**$124**	**$117**	**$115**	**$106**

Source: Lisa P. McFaddin.

5) The average companion animal veterinarian spends 78% of their work week seeing appointments (AVMA 2023).
6) The average companion animal veterinarian receives 21 paid days of vacation and holiday pay annually (iVet360 2023).
7) The average companion animal veterinarian receives 4.1 paid days off for continuing education per year (AAHA 2019).
8) Acupuncture appointments account for 14% of a veterinarian's appointments (Marks and Shmalberg 2015).
9) The amortization is calculated over a two-year period.

Using the above information, the typical companion animal veterinarian sees 3398 patients a year (70 patients a week, working 48.4 weeks a year). At least 476 of these patients would receive VSMT, for a total of 952 patients in two years.

Supply assumptions were considered negligible. Overhead includes rent or mortgage, utilities, administrative costs, and often employee costs divided by the minutes the practice is open (Stevenson 2016). A $3.5/minute overhead was used. The national average of two DVMs per hospital was used, rounded down from 2.1 (AAHA 2019; AVMA 2023).

The formula to determine service fees is quite simple: Service Fee = Hospital Cost + Profit. The big question becomes, how much profit? Table 10.22 illustrates the potential fee for 30- and 60-minute VSMT appointments, based on hospital cost and variable markup percentages. It becomes readily apparent that the lower the

Table 10.22 Potential 15-, 30-, and 60-minute veterinary spinal manipulation therapy appointment prices using hospital costs from Table 10.21 at varying percentage markups as of February 2023.

		Ex. 1	Ex. 2	Ex. 3	Ex. 4	Ex. 5	Ex. 6	Ex. 7	Ex. 8
15-Minute appointments									
Total hospital cost		$46	$40	$37	$28	$45	$38	$36	$27
Potential appointment price	40% Markup	$64	$56	$52	$39	$63	$53	$50	$38
	50% Markup	$69	$60	$56	$42	$68	$57	$54	$41
	60% Markup	$74	$64	$59	$45	$72	$61	$58	$43
	70% Markup	$78	$68	$63	$48	$77	$65	$61	$46
	80% Markup	$83	$72	$67	$50	$81	$68	$65	$49
	90% Markup	$87	$76	$70	$53	$86	$72	$68	$51
	100% Markup	$92	$80	$74	$56	$90	$76	$72	$54
30-Minute appointments									
Total hospital cost		**$73**	**$66**	**$64**	**$55**	**$72**	**$65**	**$62**	**$54**
Potential appointment price	40% Markup	$102	$92	$90	$77	$101	$91	$87	$76
	50% Markup	$110	$99	$96	$83	$108	$98	$93	$81
	60% Markup	$117	$106	$102	$88	$115	$104	$99	$86
	70% Markup	$124	$112	$109	$94	$122	$111	$105	$92
	80% Markup	$131	$119	$115	$99	$130	$117	$112	$97
	90% Markup	$139	$125	$122	$105	$137	$124	$118	$103
	100% Markup	$146	$132	$128	$110	$144	$130	$124	$108
60-Minute appointments									
Total hospital cost		**$125**	**$119**	**$116**	**$107**	**$124**	**$117**	**$115**	**$106**
Potential appointment price	40% Markup	$175	$167	$162	$150	$174	$164	$161	$148
	50% Markup	$188	$179	$174	$161	$186	$176	$173	$159
	60% Markup	$200	$190	$186	$171	$198	$187	$184	$170
	70% Markup	$213	$202	$197	$182	$211	$199	$196	$180
	80% Markup	$225	$214	$209	$193	$223	$211	$207	$191
	90% Markup	$238	$226	$220	$203	$236	$222	$219	$201
	100% Markup	$250	$238	$232	$214	$248	$234	$230	$212

Source: Lisa P. McFaddin.

hospital contribution, the higher the comparative profit.

Additional Considerations Scheduling integrative appointments presents a unique opportunity not afforded by traditional Western appointments. Most appointments in veterinary medicine are scheduled linearly: 8 a.m., 8:30 a.m., 9 a.m., etc. With VSMT appointments the veterinarian is really only in the exam room for the initial history, examination, and adjustment. If a hospital has enough exam rooms and personnel, integrative appointments could be staggered very easily. This would in essence double the DVM revenue. Staggered appointments should be considered once the veterinarian amasses enough demand. This tactic does require double the exam room capacity, support staff, and requires careful planning when scheduling appointments.

Team Training

The concept of phase training is used when introducing acupuncture to the hospital team. A multi-media approach is used to assist with the training program and is outlined in Table 10.23.

Practice Manager's Role in Training

To conquer this task the pratice manager needs his or her own checklist which includes the following information:

- Schedule a date and time for the team training.
- Ensure all information pertaining to the new service is reviewed with the staff.
- Confirm all team members have completed the training.

Table 10.23 The breakdown of phase training steps and resources for the entire hospital team.

Phase 1: Background information	
Team training guide	The handout walks the practice manager and/or veterinarian through Phase 1 of the training
	A downloadable and editable copy of the handout is located on the companion website
Training presentation	The video covers background information on the modality
	PowerPoints can be downloaded, edited, and personalized from the companion website
	The document can be used as a PowerPoint or saved as an mp4 creating a personalized movie
Team training handout	The handout provides additional background information for the CSRs, VAs, and LTs to complement the knowledge gained from watching the training presentation
	A downloadable and editable copy of the handout is located on the companion website
Phase 2: Knowledge proficiency	
Quiz	A short quiz to ensure all team members have a good understanding of the service being offered
	A downloadable and editable copy of the handout is located on the companion website
	A key is provided
Phase 3: Expectations	
Training worksheets	A training checklist is provided for CSRs and VA/LTs with role-specific expectations and tasks for each staff member
	A recommended completion time is provided
	A downloadable and editable copy of the handout is located on the companion website
Phase 4: Client education	
Client scripts	Bullet point information and scripted examples used when discussing acupuncture with clients
	A downloadable and editable copy of the handout is located on the companion website
Client education presentation	A short (5–7 minute) client educational video about the therapeutic modality
	PowerPoints can be downloaded, edited, and personalized from the companion website
	The document can be used as a PowerPoint or saved as an mp4 creating a personalized movie
Client education handout	An informational handout about the therapeutic modality written specifically for clients
	A downloadable and editable copy of the handout is located on the companion website

VSMT, veterinary spinal manipulation; CSR, customer service representative; VA, veterinary assistant; LT, licensed technician.
Source: Lisa P. McFaddin.

- Certify all team members understand the information and can successfully educate clients.

Promotion

There are six common avenues of promotion for a veterinary integrative medicine (VIM) service: hospital website, social media, email blasts, mailers, in-hospital promotions, and client education. Before enacting any promotions confirm what name is legally permissible in the state. The name "animal chiropractic" may not be legal. Some states only allow the term "chiropractor" or "chiropractic" to be used when referencing the treatment of people. For these states VSMT is the best option.

Hospital Website

Advertise "Veterinary Spinal Manipulation" or "Veterinary Chiropractic" or "Animal Chiropractic" in several locations on the website. On the made page insert "Now offering veterinary spinal manipulation" or "Now offering veterinary chiropractic treatments" with a link to success stories or client testimonials. Utilize the hospital website to advertise the VIM treatment under the "Services" section. Under Veterinarian Biograph include a description of the specialized training and professional initials. Create a VSMT blog page discussing patient success stories.

Social Media

Utilize Facebook, Instagram, and/or Twitter to post facts, photographs, hashtags, and patient success stories. Include fun and intriguing facts about VSMT. Clients love patient photographs, especially when receiving VSMT. Create or utilize VSMT specific hashtags.

Email Blasts

Send fun mass emails to your clients introducing VSMT. Consider monthly case presentations illustrating how the service has benefited patients. Almost everyone has at least one email address these days. Customer service representatives should be amassing client emails at the same rate as phone numbers.

Mailers

Mailers can be expensive, and are largely unnecessary in this digital age, but they can be used to announce the introduction of VSMT to existing clients. The mailer should include the following information: the name of the new service, a brief description of how VSMT can help pet patients, the name of the certified doctor, with their new initials, a brief description of the training the doctor received, and photograph of a pet receiving VSMT.

In-Hospital Promotions

Advertise VSMT within the hospital using promotional signs, invoice teasers, and wearable pieces of flare. Small promotional signs can be placed in the waiting room and exam rooms. Include photographs of pets receiving VSMT. Consider catchphrases such as "Got Chiro?"; "Veterinary Spinal Manipulation Therapy"; "Veterinary Chiropractic"; and "Animal Chiropractic."

Informational signs with photos of pets receiving VSMT should also include a brief description of how VSMT can help pet patients, the name of the doctor, with their new initials, performing VSMT, and a brief description of the training the doctor received.

Invoice teasers should consist of short phrases reminding and enticing owners regarding a new service offered at the practice. Examples include "Now offering Veterinary Spinal Manipulation"; "Now offering Veterinary Chiropractic"; "Now offering Animal Chiropractic"; "Curious if spinal manipulation can help your pet?"; "Curious if veterinary chiropractic can help your pet?"; "Curious if animal chiropractic can help your pet?"; "Introducing Veterinary Spinal Manipulation Therapy"; "Introducing Veterinary Chiropractic"; "Introducing Animal Chiropractic"; "Would your pet benefit from Veterinary Spinal Manipulation Therapy?"; "Would your pet benefit from Veterinary

Chiropractic?"; and "Would your pet benefit from Animal Chiropractic?".

Buttons can be made for the staff to wear with kitchy phrases reminding owners, in a fun way, of the new VIM service. Examples include "What's VSMT?"; "Want to learn more about Veterinary Chiropractic?"; and "Want to learn more about Animal Chiropractic?"

Client Education

Education is crucial to understanding the purpose and importance of any given treatment. The client handouts and videos solidify pet owner knowledge base, reducing concerns and conveying value.

Integration

The key components for proper integration include availability of the service to the right patients; appropriate patient scheduling; appropriate support staff scheduling; and staff buy-in (understanding the benefits of the offered service).

Veterinarians

There are several factors to contemplate when veterinarians are considering, and preparing to incorporate, a VIM in their clinical repertoire: state requirements and restrictions, return on investment, course availability, supplies and equipment, veterinary organizations, and continuing education.

State Requirements and Restrictions

Is VSMT Considered the Practice of Veterinary Medicine?

Table 10.24 details which states define VSMT as the practice of veterinary medicine. Some states permit non-veterinarians certified in VSMT to practice, usually under the supervision of a veterinarian. Table 10.24 also addresses which states allow human chiropractors to practice VSMT. These rules and regulations can change. Check your local state board for further information. Links to each

state's veterinary board can be found on the companion website.

Does VSMT Continuing Education Count toward Licensure Continuing Education Requirements?

Currently no states require specific CE hours for VSMT. Some states limit the use of integrative medicine CE hours toward the annual CE requirement for license renewal. Most states permit the use of VSMT CE if the lectures or webinars are performed by an approved provider.

Utilizing the AVMA (2019b) and each state's Board of Veterinary Medicine website, Table 10.24 addresses the following questions: Does the state define VSMT as the practice of veterinary medicine? Are licensed chiropractors certified in VSMT allowed to practice VSMT under the direct supervision of a veterinarian? Are VSMT CE hours applicable to the annual or biennial CE requirement? A link to each state's Board of Veterinary Medicine and Veterinary Laws or Statutes is available on the website.

Are Your Assets Covered?

Check with your liability insurance to determine if you are covered when practicing VSMT. Refer to the Introduction of this book for additional information.

Return on Investment

Specifics are discussed in the Team Members section of this chapter.

Course Availability

Formal training in VSMT should be considered a requirement. Training and certification provide the foundations for understanding how VSMT can best help your veterinary patients. Completion of formal training also helps legitimize the modality. Most training programs involve multiple online and on-site courses. Veterinarians can usually start practicing VSMT on their patients after the first on-site training session. The following initial certification course offerings and pricing are current as of February 2023.

Table 10.24 The legality of veterinary spinal manipulation therapy and applicability of continuing education (CE) hours by state as of 2023. A link to each state's veterinary board can be found on the companion website. PVM (practice of veterinary medicine): the state board considers VSMT to be the PVM. DC (Doctor of Chiropractic): a DC may perform VSMT under the direct supervision of a veterinarian with an active veterinary–client–patient relationship. DCE (DC exemption): a DC is not required to practice under direct veterinary supervision. ACE (applicable CE): VSMT CE is applicable to the state's mandated CE hours assuming approval by the American Association of Veterinary State Boards Registry (AAVSB) Register of Approved Continuing Education (RACE). NS: information not specified.

State	PVM	DC	DCE	ACE	References
Alabama	Yes	No	No	Yes	ASBVME (2021)
Alaska	No	Np	No	Yes	ADCBPL (2023)
Arizona	Yes	Yes	No	Yes	ASVMEB (2022)
Arkansas	Yes	Yes	No	≤5 hours per year	ADAVMEB (2008, 2019)
California	No	Yes	No	Yes	CDCAVMB (2022)
Colorado	No	Yes	No	Yes	CDRASBVM (2019)
Connecticut	No	No	No	Yes	CBVM (2023)
Delaware	No	NS	NS	Yes	DBVM (2023)
District of Columbia	Yes	NS	NS	Yes	DCVM (2023)
Florida	Yes	Yes	No	≤5 hours per year	FBVM (2022), eLaws.us (2020)
Georgia	No	NS	No	Yes	GSBVM (2022, 2023)
Hawaii	No	Yes	No	Yes	HDCCAPVLDBVM (2010)
Idaho	Yes	Yes	No	Yes	IBVM (2020)
Illinois	Yes	Yes	No	Yes	IGA (2004)
Indiana	No	Yes	No	Yes	IVMB (2019)
Iowa	Yes	NS	No	Yes	IBVM (2017)
Kansas	Yes	Yes	No	Yes	KBVE (2020)
Kentucky	Yes	No	No	Yes	KYBVE (2020)
Louisiana	No	Yes	No	Yes	LBVM (2022)
Maine	No	No	No	Yes	MSBVM (2022)
Maryland	No	Yes	No	Yes	MBVME (2019)
Massachusetts	Yes	Yes	No	Yes	MBRVM (2022)
Michigan	Yes	Yes	No	Yes	MBVM (2023)
Minnesota	Yes	Yes	No	Yes	MNBVM (2022)
Mississippi	Yes	Yes	No	Yes	MSBVM (2008)
Missouri	Yes	Yes	No	Yes	MOVMB (2022)
Montana	Yes	No	No	Yes	MCA (2021)
Nebraska	No	Yes	No	Yes	NLU (2019)
Nevada	Yes	Yes	Yes	Yes	NBVME (2023)
New Hampshire	Yes	No	No	Yes	NHBVM (2020, 2022)
New Jersey	Yes	Yes	No	Yes	NJSBVME (2021)
New Mexico	No	Yes	No	≤7 hours per year	NMBVM (2018), CaseText (2023)

State	PVM	DC	DCE	ACE	References
New York	Yes	No	No	Yes	NYSLPV (2023)
North Carolina	No	No	No	Yes	NCVMB (2014)
North Dakota	Yes	NS	No	Yes	NDVBME (2007)
Ohio	Yes	Yes	No	Yes	ORC (2006)
Oklahoma	Yes	Yes	No	Yes	OVB (2022)
Oregon	No	Yes	No	Yes	OL (2021)
Pennsylvania	No	Yes	No	Yes	CP (2022)
Rhode Island	No	No	No	Yes	RIDH (2006)
South Carolina	Yes	Yes	No	Yes	SCCL (2016)
South Dakota	No	no	No	Yes	SDL (2023)
Tennessee	Yes	Yes	No	Yes	TBVME (2014)
Texas	Yes	Yes	No	Yes	TAC (2012)
Utah	No	Yes	No	Yes	UC (2020)
Vermont	No	Yes	No	Yes	VGA (2023)
Virginia	Yes	No	No	Yes	DHP (2007)
Washington	No	No	No	Yes	WSL (2023)
West Virginia	No	No	No	Yes	WVBVM (2023)
Wisconsin	No	Yes	No	Yes	WVEB (2022)
Wyoming	Yes	No	No	Yes	WBVM (2018)

Source: Lisa P. McFaddin.

Many of the organizations offering the initial certification offer advanced training as well. Veterinarians who are on the fence about committing to a full training course are encouraged to attend introductory lectures first. Familiarizing yourself with the information is a great way to determine if pursuing this modality is right for you and your practice. State and national veterinary conferences, as well as many online veterinary educational platforms (Veterinary Information Network [VIN], Vetfolio, DVM360 Flex, Vet Girl on the Run, and CIVT) frequently offer AAVSB RACE-approved lectures on various integrative topics.

Animal Chiropractic Education Source (ACES)

- **Course name**: Animal Chiropractic 101
- **Prerequisites**: License, in good standing, to practice veterinary medicine or chiropractic

- **Description**
  - 240-hour introductory VSMT program covering:
    - Anatomy
    - Physiology
    - Neurology
    - Lameness examinations
    - Chiropractic philosophy and history
    - Chiropractic assessment
    - Case management
    - Marketing.
  - Completion of the course allows the student to sit for the:
    - American Veterinary Chiropractic Association (AVCA) examination for certification in Animal Chiropractic
    - Colorado DC licensing examination
    - Minnesota DC licensing examination
    - Oklahoma DC licensing examination.

- **Online training**:
  - 129 hours of online lectures.
  - Open book quizzes after each lecture (a passing score of 90% is required).
- **On-site training**:
  - 111 hours of on-site hands-on laboratory in Meridian, TX.
  - Each four-day module is available three times a year.
  - 5 : 1 student to teacher ratio.
  - Examinations at the end of each on-site laboratory module (a passing score of 75% is required).
- **Completion time**: Students are given up to two years to complete all online and on-site courses, as well as passing all examinations.
- **Cost**: $14 999.95
  - Downloadable noted for online lectures
  - Access to online lectures for two years after enrollment.
  - Bound notes for laboratory sessions
  - Adjustment bale
  - Canine spine model
  - Speeder board
  - Marketing materials
  - Access to doctor rounds
  - Access to private student Facebook account.
- **Contact information**:
  - Address: 10 771 Highway 6, Meridian, TX 76665
  - Phone: (843) 900-1502
  - Website: www.animalchiropracticeducation.com
  - Email: Admin@AnimalChiropracticEducation.com

Chi University

- **Course name**: Veterinary Medical Manipulation Certification Track
- **Prerequisites**: License, in good standing, to practice veterinary medicine or third or fourth year veterinary student
- **Description**
  - 107-hour AAVSB RACE-approved certification course training veterinarians in Small Animal Veterinary Medical Manipulation (SAVMM).
  - 32-hours of hands-on small group wet labs.
  - The course focuses on:
    - Anatomy
    - Physiology
    - Neurology
    - Lameness examinations
    - TMJ function and manipulation
    - Rehabilitation tools
    - Motion palpation
    - Lumbar manipulation.
  - Students who successfully complete the course are eligible for certification, Certified Veterinary Medical Manipulation Practitioner (CVMMP) endorsed by the IVMI. Certification requirements include:
    - Completion of all six modules
    - Pass 4 online homework assignments (score ≥75%)
    - Pass final written examination (score ≥75%)
    - Pass final practical examination (score ≥75%)
    - Submit 1 VMM case report.
  - Chi University is accredited by the Distance Education Accrediting Commission (DEAC).
  - Previously offered by the Integrative Veterinary Medical Institute (IVMI).
- **Online training**: Three online sessions
- **On-site training**: Three on-site sessions in Reddick, FL
- **Completion time**: The course takes approximately five months to complete.
- **Cost**: $7240
  - Free case consultation with faculty through email and online discussion
  - Digital class handouts and notes provided
  - Lunch and snacks provided
  - Printed binders available for an additional cost.
- **Contact information**:
  - Address: 9650 W Hwy 318, Reddick, FL 32686

- Phone: (800) 860-1543
- Website: www.chiu.edu
- Email: register@chiu.edu

Healing Oasis Wellness Center (HOWC)

- **Course name**: Veterinary Spinal Manipulative Therapy Certification Program
- **Prerequisites**: License, in good standing, to practice veterinary medicine or chiropractic
- **Description**
  - Minimum of 226-hour AAVSB RACE approved VSMT post-graduate, state-approved certification course covering:
    o Anatomy
    o Physiology
    o Neurology
    o Functional neurology
    o Lameness examinations
    o Chiropractic philosophy and history
    o Chiropractic assessment
    o Case management
    o Ethics and legality
    o Marketing.
  - Five modules in total which must be completed in order.
  - A total of four cases are presented by each student during Modules IV or V.
  - No external externships/internships are required.
  - Accredited by the Accrediting Council for Continuing Education and Training, an accrediting agency of the US Department of Education.
  - Approved by the Wisconsin Department of Safety and Professional Service – Educational Approval Program.
  - Approved for the GI Bill® by the Wisconsin State Approving Agency for Veteran's Education Benefits a Department of Veterans Affairs.
  - Cosponsored by the American Holistic Veterinary Medical Association.
  - An approved Basic Level Animal Chiropractic program by the College of Animal Chiropractors (CoAC).

- As a true school no third-party competency tests are required, and upon successful completion of the program a certificate of competency is awarded to graduates, CVSMT or Certificate of Competency Veterinary Spinal Manipulation Therapy.
- **Online training**:
  - Self-study at home averages a minimum of four to five hours per week.
  - One online module.
- **On-site training**:
  - Four modules of five days each in Sturtevant, WI.
  - On-site modules include didactic lecture and hands-on laboratories.
  - Closed-book examinations and/or practical assessments are completed at the end of each module.
  - Maximum of 20 students per class with maximum ratio of three to four students per teacher.
- **Completion time**: Five months
- **Cost**: $7310
  - Course notes
  - Unlimited access to consultations with the program director
  - Listed on the "Find a Graduate/Alumni" section
  - Access to the "Alumni" of the website which contains all videos of the explanations and techniques presented during the course.
- **Contact information**:
  - Address: 2555 Wisconsin St, Sturtevant, WI 53177
  - Phone: 262-898-1680
  - Website: www.healingoasis.edu
  - Email: contact@healingoasis.edu

Health Pioneers Institute (HPI)

- **Course name**: Animal Chiropractic Certification Program
- **Prerequisites**: License, in good standing, to practice veterinary medicine or chiropractic
Description
  - 210-hour VSMT course covering:
    o Anatomy

- ○ Physiology
- ○ Neurology
- ○ Lameness examinations
- ○ Chiropractic philosophy and history
- ○ Chiropractic assessment
- ○ Case management
- ○ Ethics and legality
- ○ Marketing
- ○ Introduction to Applied Kinesiology and Functional Neurology.
- – Completion of the course allows the student to sit for the:
  - ○ American Veterinary Chiropractic Association (AVCA) examination for certification in Animal Chiropractic
  - ○ International Veterinary Chiropractic Association examination for certification in Animal Chiropractic.
- **Online training**: 52 hours of online lectures, self-guided reading, and case studies.
- **On-site training**:
  - – 158 hours of on-site hands-on laboratory in Naperville, IL.
  - – Five modules of five to six days each.
- **Completion time**: Five months
- **Cost**: $7200
  - – Specific information regarding what is included with the cost of tuition is not provided.
- **Contact information**
  - – Address: 1120 E Diehl Rd, Naperville, IL 60563
  - – Phone: (630) 358-9644
  - – Website: www.healthpioneersinstitute.com
  - – Email: info@healthpioneersinstitute.com

Options for Animals College of Animal Chiropractic
- **Course name**: Post-Graduate Essentials in Animal Chiropractic Care
- **Prerequisites**: Licensed veterinarians, in good standing, a fourth year veterinary student, licensed chiropractor, in good standing, or a student in their last semester/trimester of chiropractor school
- **Description**
  - – 210-hour Essentials in Animal Chiropractic Course covering:

- ○ Anatomy
- ○ Physiology
- ○ Neurology
- ○ Lameness examinations
- ○ Chiropractic assessment
- ○ Case management.
- – Certificate of completion is provided at the completion of the course.
- – Completion of the course allows the student to sit for the:
  - ○ American Veterinary Chiropractic Association (AVCA) examination for certification in Animal Chiropractic
  - ○ International Veterinary Chiropractic Association examination for certification in Animal Chiropractic.
- – The program fulfills the requirements set by the College of Animal Chiropractors Certification Committee.
- **Online training**: Not applicable
- **On-site training**:
  - – Five on-site modules of 4.5 days each.
  - – Minimum of 135 hours of lecture and a minimum of 75 hours of hands-on laboratory.
- **Completion time**: Five to six months
- **Cost**: $7975
  - – Each student is assigned their own faculty advisor who will coach the student during the course and for three months after completion of the course.
  - – Specific information regarding what is included with the cost of tuition is not provided.
- **Contact information**:
  - – Address: 4267 Virginia Rd, Wellsville, KS 66092
  - – Phone: (309) 658-2920
  - – Website: www.optionsforanimals.com
  - – Email: Options4animals@aol.com

Parker University
- **Course name**: Animal Chiropractic Program
- **Prerequisites**: License, in good standing, to practice veterinary medicine or chiropractic
- **Description**
  - – 210-hour veterinary spinal manipulation course covering:

- o Anatomy
- o Physiology
- o Neurology
- o Lameness examinations
- o Chiropractic assessment
- o Ethics and Legality
- o Case management.
- – Completion of the course allows the student to sit for the American Veterinary Chiropractic Association (AVCA) examination for certification in Animal Chiropractic
- – Program fulfills the requirements set by the College of Animal Chiropractors Certification Committee.
- **Online training**: Not applicable
- **On-site training**: Five on-site modules of three days each in Dallas, TX.
- **Completion time**: Five months
- **Cost**: Current price not available
  - – Specific information regarding what is included with the cost of tuition is not provided.
- **Contact information**:
  - – Address: 2540 Walnut Hill Ln, Dallas, TX 75229
  - – Phone: (214) 902-2429
  - – Website: www.parker.edu
  - – Email: askadmissions@parker.edu

Supplies and Equipment

No specific supplies are required to practice small animal VSMT. The use of floor mats or yoga mats allows better traction for larger dogs on slippery tile floors. Tables can be used when adjusting small dogs.

An equine spinal manipulation bale (basically a large compressed block of Styrofoam covered with heavy-duty nylon) is very helpful for medium-sized dogs that are too small for the floor but too tall for a traditional exam room table. The bales typically run $400–$500 with shipping.

Hospital remodeling and/or redecorating is generally not required when offering VSMT. Most traditional exam rooms can be utilized. Some practitioners prefer to have a dedicated room while others use existing spaces. Creating a relaxing environment with soft music and diffusors (lavender or pheromones) is beneficial.

Veterinary Organizations

A description of the most common veterinary organizations with a special interest in VSMT is provided below. Table 10.25 lists the contact names, contact information, and membership dues for these organizations.

American Holistic Veterinary Medical Association (AHVMA)

- **Description**: The AHVMA was founded in 1982 at the Western States Veterinary Conference with the goal of advancing integrative medicine through the education of integrative and non-integrative veterinarians, the introduction of integrative medicine to veterinary students, the promotion of research, and representation in the AVMA House of Delegates. There is no annual CE requirement to maintain membership.
- **Membership benefits**
  - – Free subscription to the *AHVMA Journal*, a peer-reviewed journal.
  - – Online resources for client education.
  - – Searchable member directory.
  - – Discounted vaccination titers through Kansas State University (KSU) Diagnostic Lab.
  - – Free access to the Natural Medicines Database, an online resource for supplements, natural medicines, and integrative therapies.
  - – Reduced cost for the AHVMA annual conference.

American Veterinary Chiropractic Association (AVCA)

- **Description**
  - – A non-governmental organization which aims to develop standards of care for animal chiropractic in North America.
  - – ACCC has created a certification program and awards time-limited credentials to interested individuals meeting their criteria.
  - – ACVA created a voluntary, non-licensure, membership which issues certificates of

Table 10.25 Veterinary associations and organizations with a special interest in veterinary spinal manipulation therapy as of February 2023.

Organization	Contact information	Membership dues
American Holistic Veterinary Medical Association (AHVMA)	PO Box 630, Abingdon, MD 21009 (410) 569-0795 office@ahvma.org	$300/year
Animal Veterinary Chiropractic Association (ACVA)	442 236 E 140 Road, Bluejacket, OK 74333 (918) 784-2231 avcainfo@junct.com	$300/year
College of Animal Chiropractors (CoAC)	PO Box 262, Manistique, MI 49854 Info@coachiro.org	$325 initial fee $75/year
College of Integrative Veterinary Therapies (CIVT)	PO Box 352, Yeppoon, 4703 QLD, Australia (303) 800-5460 membership@civtedu.org	$185/year
International Veterinary Academy of Pain Management (IVAPM)	PO Box 1868, Mt Juliet, TN 371211 info@ivapm.org	$150/year
International Veterinary Chiropractic Association (IVCA)	Bahrenfelder Strasse 201a, 22765 Hamburg, Germany	€75 initial fee €85/year

competency to veterinarians and chiropractors meeting the standards outlined in the following section. Recertification is required to maintain the credentials.

- **Requirements**
  - Complete a postgraduate animal chiropractic program approved by the Education Committee of the ACVA.
  - Pass the AVCA exit examination.
  - Pass the ACCC written and practical examinations.
  - Hold a veterinary or chiropractic license in good standing.
  - Initial certification is granted for three years.
  - Recertification requires a minimum of 30 hours of AVCA approved continuing education every three years and pass the written and practice examinations.
- **Membership benefits**
  - Access to current articles and clinical information.
  - Network with other members through the "Community of Practice" forum.

- Name is listed on the "Find a Certified Doctor" directory.
- Information about upcoming CE seminars and conventions, including the annual meeting.
- Discounted prices on logo apparel and conferences.

College of Animal Chiropractors (CoAC)
- **Description**
  - An international nonprofit organization promoting the education and implementation of animal chiropractic care to the public.
  - Previously titled the American Canadian College of Animal Chiropractors
  - International nonprofit organization promoting animal chiropractic research, education, and practical applications.
  - CoAC created a voluntary, non-licensure, membership which issues certificates of competency to veterinarians and chiropractors meeting the standards outlined in the following section.

- **Requirements**
  - Complete a postgraduate animal chiropractic program approved by the ACVA, IVCA, or CoAC.
  - Pass the CoAC written certification examination.
  - Hold a veterinary or chiropractic license in good standing.
  - Recertification is required to maintain the credentials. A minimum of 20 hours of continuing education in animal chiropractic techniques, neurology, biomechanics, and anatomy is required.
- **Membership benefits**
  - Access to current articles and clinical information.
  - Network with other members through the "Community of Practice" forum.
  - Name is listed on the "Find a Certified Doctor" directory.
  - Information about upcoming CE seminars and conventions.
- **Cost**: $325 initial cost with $75 annual renewal fee.

College of Integrative Veterinary Therapies (CIVT)

- **Description**: An online organization open to all licensed animal health providers interested in integrative medicine. There are two membership options: full membership for veterinarians and associate membership for registered animal health professionals. CIVT strives to promote all aspects of evidence-based integrative medicine through online education and discussion forums. CIVT provides financial support to veterinary students interested in studying integrative medicine. CIVT also helps fund integrative medicine research. There is no annual CE requirement to maintain membership.
- **Membership benefits**
  - Access to the online electronic library.
  - Access to the electronic *Journal of Integrative Veterinary Therapies.*
  - Three free CE webinars annually.

- 20% discount on all webinars.
- Discounts on specific CIVT courses.
- Searchable member directory.
- Access to the Natural Medicines Databases and the American Botanical Council Library.

International Veterinary Academy of Pain Management (IVAPM)

- **Description**: Originally known as the Companion Animal Pain Management Consortium, then the Academy of Pain Management Interest Group, and finally IVAPM. Founded in 2001 to provide pain management education and certification programs. The organization's goal is to provide acute and chronic pain relief for veterinary patients. Both traditional and alternative therapies are embraced, including acupuncture and rehabilitation and physical therapy.
- **Membership benefits**
  - Members can become Certified Veterinary Pain Practitioners (CVPP).
  - Access to member's only Facebook group offering case consultations and questions.
  - Reduced subscription rate for IVAPM's journal *Veterinary Anaesthesia and Analgesia.*
  - Reduced registration fee for the International Veterinary Emergency and Critical Care (IVECCS) conference.
  - Reduced registration for all IVAPM continuing education events (online and on-site).
  - Complementary World Small Animal Veterinary Association (WSAVA) membership.

International Veterinary Chiropractic Association (IVCA)

- **Description**
  - An international nonprofit organization promoting veterinary chiropractic.
  - IVCA created a voluntary, non-licensure, membership which issues certificates of competency to veterinarians and chiropractors meeting the standards outlined in

the following section. Recertification is required to maintain the credentials.

- **Requirements**
  - Hold a veterinary or chiropractic license in good standing.
  - Complete an IVCA approved course.
  - Pass the IVCA certification examination.
  - Complete the IVCA requirements.
  - Annual membership fee.
  - Recertification is required every three years.
- **Membership benefits**
  - Source of patient referrals.
  - Case consultation with other IVCA members.
  - Free client education and promotional information.
  - Access to worldwide CE courses and seminars.
  - Access to research funding.

Reference Books

The following is a list of my recommended VSMT and neurology books. A brief summary of each book is provided.

Anatomy of Domestic Animals: Systemic and Regional Approach
- Authors: Chris Pasquini, DVM, MS; Tom Spurgeon, PhD; and Susan Pasquini, DVM
- Summary: Most veterinarians already own a copy from vet school. This in-depth, thorough, and entertaining anatomy book provides tons of information on the anatomy of most domestic animals.

Canine Ergonomics: The Science of Working Dogs
- Author: William S. Helton
- Summary: A comprehensive review of the physiology, cognition, and ergonomics of working dogs. There is also a discussion on training service dogs.

Canine Lameness
- Author: Felix Duerr, DVM
- Summary: An in-depth reference book covering the diagnosis and treatment of musculoskeletal diseases in dogs. There is a

companion website with videos of examination techniques and lameness conditions.

Canine Rehabilitation and Physical Therapy
- Authors: Darryl Mills, DVM, DACVS, DACVSMT, CCRP and David Levine, PhD PT
- Summary: A comprehensive reference book covering canine rehabilitation protocols for a variety of conditions, printable medical record forms, canine exercises, therapeutic modality options available, physical examination specifics, and a companion website.

Canine Sports Medicine and Rehabilitation
- Authors: M. Christine Zink, DVM, PhD, DACVP, DACVSMR and Janet D. Van Dyke, DVM, DACVSMR
- Summary: A comprehensive reference book discussing common canine musculoskeletal conditions and ailments, with particular interest in the canine athlete. The book covers gait analysis and physiology, various therapeutic approaches (including nutrition, rehabilitation, manual therapy, acupuncture, chiropractic, therapeutic exercise, aquatic therapy, conditioning and retraining, and assistive devices), and specific diagnoses and treatment recommendations for disorders of the forelimbs and pelvic limbs. A must-have for veterinarians interested in manual therapy, orthopedics, and rehabilitation.

Dogs in Motion
- Authors: Martin S Fischer and Karin E Lije
- Summary: An in-depth look into the anatomy of canine locomotion across 32 different breeds. There is a companion DVD with over 400 movies, X-rays, and 3D animations.

Foundations of Chiropractic: Subluxation
- Author: Meridel Gatterman, MA, DC, MED
- Summary: Evidence-based approach to the theories of joint dysfunction, common clinical syndromes, and practical application of chiropractic therapy in people.

The Human Brain: An Introduction to its Functional Anatomy
- Author: John Notle

- Summary: A comprehensive look into the anatomy and functional neurology of the brain. While geared toward the study of the human brain the information is applicable to veterinary patients.

Manual of Natural Veterinary Medicine: Science and Tradition

- Authors: Susan G. Wynn, DVM and Steve Marsden, DVM, ND, MSOM, Lac, Dipl. CH., RH(AHG)
- Summary: A quick reference book discussing the integrative therapy options for numerous diseases in veterinary medicine. The book is organized by Western conditions. For each category the potential TCVM diagnoses and treatment options are then discussed in succinct detail. Chiropractic recommendations are provided for most musculoskeletal and neurologic conditions. A must-have for all integrative veterinarians.

Miller's Anatomy of the Dog

- Authors: Howard Evans, PhD and Alexander de Lahunta, DVM, PhD
- Summary: Most veterinarians already own a copy from vet school. This is a comprehensive guide to the canine anatomy.

Veterinary Clinics of North America Small Animal Practice

- Authors: LoGiudice, R.J. & Rivera, P.L. Veterinary spinal manipulative therapy or animal chiropractic in veterinary rehabilitation. doi: 10.1016/j.cvsm.2023.02.008
- Summary: "Veterinary rehabilitation is a multimodal diagnostic and treatment approach that is recommended and provided to patients daily. One therapeutic modality that may be beneficial (diagnostically and therapeutically) is veterinary spinal manipulative therapy or animal chiropractic (AC). AC is a receptor-based health-care modality being provided more frequently in veterinary practices. All clinicians should strive to understand the mode of action, indications, contraindications, how it affects the patient from the neuro-anatomical and biomechanical point of view, and most importantly, when not to provide the requested modality, as further diagnostics may be indicated" (LoGiudice and Rivera 2023).

Promotion

Information regarding the hospital's promotion of VSMT can be found in the Team Members section.

Integration

Key components for proper integration include availability, scheduling, and staff buy-in. Availability means offering the service to the right patient. Scheduling refers to appropriate patient and support staff scheduling. Staff buy-in ensures all team members understand the benefits of the offered service.

Conclusion

VSMT is rapidly advancing therapeutic modality. The effects and benefits for veterinary patients center on the cessation or reduction of pain and restoration of musculoskeletal and neurologic function. This chapter and companion website describe in detail how VSMT can be successfully introduced into daily practice, as well as provide practical tools for implementation.

Acknowledgments

I would like to thank Dr. Pedro Rivera for reviewing this chapter for content. Pedro Luis Rivera, DVM, FACFN, DACVSMR, FCoAC graduated from Purdue University, School of Veterinary Medicine in 1986. He has been practicing integrative veterinary medicine and in particular veterinary spinal manipulative therapy and veterinary rehabilitation with emphasis in functional neurology for the last 35 years. Dr. Rivera is a proud Fellow of the

American College of Functional Neurology and a Diplomate of the American College of Veterinary Sport Medicine and Rehabilitation. Dr. Rivera and Michelle Rivera are the owners and main program directors of the Healing Oasis Wellness Center, a nationally accredited and recognized school (under the US Department of Education) providing state-approved postgraduate certifications (through the Educational Approval Programs of Wisconsin) and approved by the Veterans Affairs Office, among other national organization. The Healing Oasis has been providing postgraduate state-approved certification programs in VMRT (since 1998) and VSMT (since 1999) among providing many continuing education seminars and advanced programs with an emphasis in clinical applications in functional neurology to improve patient outcomes.

References

A. S. B. o. V. M. E.ASBVME (2021). Alabama Veterinary Practice Act. https://asbvme.alabama.gov/wp-content/uploads/2021/07/Alabama_Practice_Act_and_Administrative_Code_Updated_Working_Copy_2018_3_5_2019.pdf (accessed 19 February 2023).

AAHA (American Animal Hospital Association) (2019). *Compensation and Benefits*, 9e. Denver, CO: AAHA Press.

ACA (American Chiropractic Association) (2020). Origins and history of chiropractic care. https://www.acatoday.org/About/History-of-Chiropractic (accessed 8 July 2020).

Acutt, E.V., le Jeune, S.S., and Pypendop, B.H. (2019). Evaluation of the effects of chiropractic on static and dynamic muscle variables in sport horses. *Journal of Equine Veterinary Science* 73: 84–90.

Adams, M., Heisey, R., Smith, M., and Briner, B. (1992). Parietal bone mobility in the anesthetized cat. *Journal of the American Osteopathic Association* 92 (5): 599–622.

ADAVMEB (Arkansas Veterinary Medical Examining Board) (2008). 092.00.1–1 Rules and Regulations. https://arvetboard.statesolutions.us/wp-content/uploads/2019/01/Practice-Act-Rules-and-Regulations-2019.pdf (accessed 19 February 2023).

ADAVMEB (Arkansas Veterinary Medical Examining Board) (2019). Arkansas Veterinary Medical Practice Act. https://arvetboard.statesolutions.us/wp-content/uploads/2020/07/Practice-Act-2019.pdf (accessed 19 February 2023).

ADCBPL (Alaska Division of Corporations, Business and Professional Licensing) (2023). Veterinary Statutes and Regulations. https://www.commerce.alaska.gov/web/portals/5/pub/VeterinaryStatutes.pdf (accessed 19 February 2023).

Ahern, T. (1994). Cervical vertebral mobilization under anesthetic. *Journal of Equine Veterinary Science* 14 (10): 540–545.

Alvarez, C.B.G., L'ami, J.J., Moffat, D. et al. (2008). Effect of chiropractic manipulations on the kinematics of back and limbs in horses with clinically diagnosed back problems. *Equine Veterinary Journal* 40 (2): 153–159.

APPA (American Pet Products Association) (2022). Pet industry market size and ownership statistics. https://www.americanpetproducts.org/press_industrytrends.asp (accessed 23 February 2023).

ASVMEB (Arizona State Veterinary Medical Examining Board) (2022). AZ Revised Statues (Veterinary Practice Act). https://vetboard.az.gov/sites/default/files/AZ%20Revised%20Statutes%20Amended%20September%202022%20as%20of%209.24.22s.pdf (accessed 19 February 2023).

AVMA (American Veterinary Medical Association) (2019a). Economic state of the veterinary profession. https://www.avma.org/news/press-release/AVMA-2019-Economic-State-of-the-Veterinary-Profession-Report-now-available (accessed 26 July 2021).

AVMA (American Veterinary Medical Association) (2019b). Scope of practice: complementary and alternative veterinary medicine (CAVM) and other practice act exemptions. https://www.avma.org/advocacy/state-local-issues/scope-practice-complementary-and-alternative-veterinary-medicine-cavm-and-other-practice-act (accessed 11 August 2021).

AVMA (American Veterinary Medical Association) (2023). *2023 AVMA Report on the Economic State of the Veterinary Profession*. Schaumburg, IL: AVMA.

Bagley, R. (2005). *Veterinary Clinical Neurology*. Ames, IA: Wiley-Blackwell.

Bergman, T. (2005). Chiropractic technique. In: *Foundations of Chiropractic Subluxation*, 2e (ed. M.I. Gatterman), 133–167. St. Louis, MO: Elsevier Mosby.

BLS (Bureau of Labor Statistics) (2023). News Release: Consumer Price Index January 2023. https://www.bls.gov/news.release/pdf/cpi.pdf (accessed 18 February 2023).

BLS (Bureau of Labor Statistics) (2022). Occupational outlook handbook: veterinarians 2022 median pay. https://www.bls.gov/ooh/healthcare/veterinarians.htm (accessed 18 February 2023).

Boadas-Vaello, P., Homs, J., Reina, F. et al. (2017). Neuroplasticity of supraspinal structures associated with pathologic pain. *The Anatomical Record* 300 (8): 1481–1501.

Brennan, P., Kokjohn, K., Triano, J., et al. (1991). Immunologic correlates of reduced spinal mobility: preliminary observations in a dog model. *FCER's International Conference on Spinal Manipulation*, 118–121. https://chiro.org/Subluxation/Immunologic_Correlates.shtml

Burns, K. (2018). Pet ownership stable, veterinary care variable. https://www.avma.org/javma-news/2019-01-15/pet-ownership-stable-veterinary-care-variable (accessed 11 August 2021).

Burns, K. (2022). New report takes a deep dive into pet ownership. https://www.avma.org/news/new-report-takes-deep-dive-pet-ownership (accessed 6 November 2022).

Cao, D.-Y. and Pickar, J. (2011). Lengthening but no shortening history of paraspinal muscle spindles in the low back alters their dynamic sensitivity. *Journal of Neurophysiology* 105 (1): 434–441.

Cao, D.-Y. and Pickar, J. (2014). Effect of spinal manipulation on the development of history-dependent responsiveness of lumbar paraspinal muscle spindles in the cat. *Journal of the Canadian Chiropractic Association* 58 (2): 149–159.

Cao, D.-Y., Pickar, J.G., Ge, W. et al. (2009). Position sensitivity of feline paraspinal muscle spindles to vertebral movement in the lumbar spine. *Journal of Neurophysiology* 101 (4): 1722–1729.

Cao, D.-Y., Reed, W.R., Long, C.R. et al. (2013). Effects of thrust amplitude and duration of high velocity low amplitude spinal manipulation on lumbar muscle spindle responses to vertebral position and movement. *Journal of Manipulative and Physiological Therapeutics* 36 (2): 68–77.

Carnes, D., Mars, T.S., Mullinger, B. et al. (2010). Adverse events and manual therapy: a systematic review. *Manual Therapy* 15 (4): 355–363.

CaseText (2023). N.M. Code R. 16.25.4.8, Register Volume 34, No. 3. https://casetext.com/regulation/new-mexico-administrative-code/title-16-occupational-and-professional-licensing/chapter-25-veterinary-medicine-practitioners/part-4-continued-education-requirements-veterinarians/section-162548-general-requirements#:~:text= (accessed 19 February 2023).

Cassidy, J., Boyle, E., Cote, P. et al. (2008). Risk of vertebrobasilar stroke and chiropractic care. *European Spine Journal* 17 (Suppl. 1): 176–183.

CBVM (Connecticut Board of Veterinary Medicine) (2023). Chapter 384: Veterinary Medicine. https://www.cga.ct.gov/current/pub/chap_384.htm (accessed 19 February 2023).

CDCAVMB (California Veterinary Medical Board) (2022). California Veterinary Medicine Practice Act. www.vmb.ca.gov/laws_regs/vmb_act.pdf (accessed 19 February 2023).

CDRASBVM (Colorado State Board of Veterinary Medicine) (2019). Title 12: Division of Professions and Occupations, Articles 315: Veterinarians and Veterinary Technicians. https://drive.google.com/file/d/0B-K5DhxXxJZbTFdrR3FPZ0g0czg/view?resourcekey=0-Ub47Cye48cDfikSTtaciMg (accessed 19 February 2023).

Clarke, T., Barnes, P.M., Black, L.I., et al. (2018). The use of yoga, meditation, and chiropractors among U.S. adults aged 18 and over. NCHS Data Brief, No. 325. https://www.cdc.gov/nchs/data/databriefs/db325-h.pdf (accessed 20 May 2020).

Cooperstein, R. and Gleberzon, B. (2004). *Technique Systems in Chiropractic*. Philadelphia: Elsevier Science.

Costigan, M., Scholz, J., and Woolf, C.J. (2009). Neuropathic pain. *Annual Review of Neuroscience* 32: 1–32.

CP (Commonwealth of Pennsylvania) (2022). Chapter 31: State Board of Veterinary Medicine. http://www.pacodeandbulletin.gov/Display/pacode?file=/secure/pacode/data/049/chapter31/chap31toc.html&d=reduce (accessed 19 February 2023).

Cramer, G. (2015). *The Clinical Anatomy of Spinal Manipulative Therapy*. Sturtevant, WI: Healing Oasis Wellness Center.

Cramer, G. and Darby, S. (2005). Anatomy related to spinal subluxation. In: *Foundations of Chiropractic Subluxation*, 2e (ed. M.I. Gatterman), 30–46. St. Louis, MO: Elsevier Mosby.

Cramer, G., Fournier, J., Henderson, C., and Wolcott, C. (2004). Degenerative changes following spinal fixation in a small animal model. *Journal of Manipulative and Physiological Therapeutics* 27 (3): 141–154.

Cramer, G., Little, J., Henderson, C., and Daley, C. (2007). Zygapophyseal (Z) joint adhesions following induced segmental hypomobility in the rat. *FASEB Journal* 21: 777.8.

Cramer, G., Henderson, C.N.R., Little, J.W. et al. (2010). Zygapophyseal joint adhesion following induced segmental hypomobility. *Journal of Manipulative and Physiological Therapeutics* 33 (7): 508–518.

Cramer, G., Darby, S.A., and Frysztak, R. (2014). Pain of spinal origin. In: *Clinical Anatomy of the Spine, Spinal Cord, and ANS*, 3e, 508–539. St. Louis, MO: Elsevier.

Crisco, J., Panjabi, M.M., Wang, E. et al. (1990). The injured canine cervical spine after six months of healing. An in vitro three-dimensional study. *Spine* 11 (10): 1047–1052.

CSU (Colorado State University James L. Voss Veterinary Teaching Hospital) (2023). Animal Pain Scales. https://vetmedbiosci.colostate.edu/vth/services/anesthesia/animal-pain-scales (accessed 9 April 2023).

Dae, M., Lee, R.J., Ursell, P.C. et al. (1997). Heterogeneous sympathetic innervation in German shepherd dogs with inherited ventricular arrhythmia and sudden cardiac death. *Circulation* 96: 1337–1342.

Damodaran, A. (2021). Consumer airfare index report, May 2021. https://media.hopper.com/research/consumer-airfare-quarterly-index-report (accessed 8 August 2021).

Darby, S.A. (2014). Neuroanatomy of the autonomic nervous system. In: *Clinical Anatomy of the Spine, Spinal Cord, and ANS*, 3e, 413–507. St. Louis, MO: Elsevier.

Darby, S. and Frysztak, R. (2014). Neuroanatomy of the spinal cord. In: *Clinical Anatomy of hte Spine, Spinal Cord, and ANS*, 3e, 341–412. St Louis, MO: Elsevier Mosby.

DBVM (Delaware Board of Veterinary Medicine) (2023). Title 24: Progressions and Occupations, Chapter 33. Veterinarians, Subchapter I: General Terms. https://delcode.delaware.gov/title24/c033/sc01/index.html#:~:text=(9)%20%E2%80%9CVeterinary%20medicine%E2%80%9D,%2C%20%C2%A7%203302%3B%2057%20Del. (accessed 19 February 2023).

DCVM (District of Columbia Board of Veterinary Medicine) (2023). District of Columbia Municipal Regulations for Veterinarians. https://doh.dc.gov/sites/default/files/dc/sites/doh/publication/attachments/Veterinarian_DC_Municipal_Regulations_For_Veterinarians.pdf (accessed 19 February 2023).

DeBoer, K., Schut, M., and McKnight, M. (1998). Acute effects of spinal manipulation on gastrointestinal myoelectric activity in conscious rabbits. *Man and Medicine* 3: 85–94.

DHP (Department of Health Professions) (2007). Chapter 38 of Title 54.1 of the Code of Virginia Veterinary Medicine. https://www.dhp.virginia.gov/media/dhpweb/docs/vet/leg/Chapter38_VetMed.pdf (accessed 19 February 2023).

Duerr, F. and Johnson, T. (2015). Orthopedic Exam. www.vin.com (accessed 20 May 2020).

Edgecombe, T., Kawchuk, G., Long, C., and Pickar, J. (2015). The effect of application site of spinal manipulative therapy (SMT) on spinal stiffness. *Spine Journal* 15 (6): 1332–1338.

eLaws.us (2020). 61G18–16.002. Continuing Education Requirements for Active Status License Renewal. http://flrules.elaws.us/fac/61g18-16.002 (accessed 19 February 2023).

Epstein, M., Rodan, I., Griffenhagen, G. et al. (2015). 2015 AAHA/AAFP pain management guidelines for dogs and cats. *Journal of the American Animal Hospital Association* 51 (2): 67–84.

Evans, D. and Breen, A. (2006). A biomechanical model for mechanically efficient cavitation production during spinal manipulation: prethrust position and the neutral zone. *Journal of Manipulative and Physiological Therapeutics* 29 (1): 72–82.

Evans, H. and de Lahunta, A. (2013). *Miller's Anatomy of the Dog*, 4e. St. Louis, MO: Elsevier.

FBVM (Florida Board of Veterinary Medicine) (2022). The 2022 Florida Statues, Chapter 474, Veterinary Medical Practice. http://www.leg.state.fl.us/statutes/index.cfm?App_mode=Display_Statute&URL=0400-0499/0474/0474.html (accessed 19 February 2023).

FederalPay.org (2023). FY 2023 Federal Per Diem Rates October 2022–September 2023. https://www.federalpay.org/perdiem/2023 (accessed 18 February 2023).

French, S. and Kemmis, S. (2023). Rental Car Pricing Statistics:2023. https://www.nerdwallet.com/article/travel/car-rental-pricing-statistics#:~:text=The%20average%20weekly%20rental%20price,in%20advance%2C%20it%20was%20%24513. (accessed 18 February 2023).

Gatterman, M. (2005). What's in a word? In: *Foundations of Chiropractic Subluxation*, 2e (ed. M.I. Gatterman), 5–18. St. Louis, MO: Elsevier Mosby.

Ge, W. and Pickar, J. (2012). The decreased responsiveness of lumbar muscle spindles to a prior history of spinal muscle lengthening is graded with the magnitude of change in vertebral position. *Journal of Electromyography and Kinesiology* 22 (6): 814–820.

Ge, W., Long, C., and Pickar, J. (2005). Vertebral position alters paraspinal muscle spindle responsiveness in the feline spine: effect of positioning duration. *Journal of Physiology* 569 (2): 655–665.

Ge, W., Cao, D.-Y., Long, C., and Pickar, J. (2011). Plane of vertebral movement eliciting muscle lengthening history in the low back influences the decrease in muscle spindle responsiveness of the cat. *Journal of Applied Physiology* 111 (6): 1735–1743.

Gillette, R. (2005). Spinal cord mechanisms of referred pain and related neuroplasticity. In: *Foundations of Chiropractic Subluxation*, 2e (ed. M.I. Gatterman), 349–370. St. Louis, MO: Elsebier Mosby.

Goldman, N., Chen, M., Ujit, T. et al. (2010). Adenosine A1 receptors mediate local anti-nociceptive effects of acupuncture. *Nature Neuroscience* 13 (7): 883–888.

Gruen, M.E., Lascelles, B.D.X., Colleran, E. et al. (2022). 2022 AAHA pain management guidelines for dogs and cats. *Journal of the*

American Animal Hospital Association 58 (2): 55–76.

GSBVM (Georgia State Board of Veterinary Medicine) (2022). Georgia Veterinary Practice Act. https://sos.ga.gov/sites/default/files/2022-02/veterinary_minutes_20180116_vparc_subcommittee.pdf (accessed 19 February 2023).

GSBVM (Georgia State Board of Veterinary Medicine) (2023). Department 700. Rules of Georgia State Board of Veterinary Medicine. https://rules.sos.ga.gov/gac/700 (accessed 19 February 2023).

Halle, K.S. and Granhus, A. (2021). Veterinary chiropractic treatment as a measure to prevent the occurrence of spondylosis in boxers. *Veterinary Science* 8 (9): 199.

Haussler, K.K. and Erb, H.N. (2003). Pressure algometry: objective assessment of back pain and effects of chiropractic treatment. *AAEP Proceedings* 49: 66–70.

Haussler, K.K., Hill, A.E., Puttlitz, C.M., and McIlwraith, C.W. (2007). Effects of vertebral mobilization and manipulation on kinematics of the thoracolumbar region. *American Journal of Veterinary Research* 68 (5): 508–516.

Haussler, K., Martin, C., and Hill, A. (2010). Efficacy of spinal manipulation and mobilisation on trunk flexibility and stiffness in horses: a randomised clinical trial. *Equine Veterinary Journal* 38: 695–702.

Haussler, K.K., Manchon, P.T., Donnell, J.R., and Frisbie, D.D. (2020). Effects of low-level laser therapy and chiropractic care on back pain in quarter horses. *Journal of Equine Veterinary Science* 86: 102891.

Haussler, K.K., Hesbach, A.L., Romano, L. et al. (2021). A systematic review of musculoskeletal mobilization and manipulation techniques used in veterinary medicine. *Animals (Basel)* 11 (10): 2787.

HDCCAPVLDBVM (Hawaii Department of Commerce and Consumer Affairs, Professional and Vocational Licensing Division, Board of Veterinary Medicine) (2010). Chapter 471: Veterinary Medicine. https://files.hawaii.gov/dcca/pvl/pvl/hrs/hrs_pvl_471.pdf (accessed 19 February 2023).

Henderson, C. (2005). Three neurophysiologic theories on the chiropractic subluxation. In: *Foundations of Chiropractic Subluxation*, 2e (ed. M.I. Gatterman), 296–304. St. Louis. MO: Elsevier Mosby.

HPPIF (Healthy Paws Pet Insurance and Foundation) (2019). 2019 Cost of Pet Health Care Report. https://www.healthypawspetinsurance.com/content/costofcare/pet-care-costs-health-conditions_2019.pdf (accessed 2 September 2020).

Huang, M., Wang, X., Xing, B. et al. (2018). Critical roles of TRPV2 channels, histamine H1 and adenosine A1 receptors in the initiation of acupoint signals for acupuncture analgesia. *Scientific Reports* 8 (1): 6523.

Ianuzzi, A., Pickar, J., and Khalsa, P. (2010). Validation of the cat as a model for the human lumbar spine during simulated high-velocity, low-amplitude spinal manipulation. *Journal of Biomechanical Engineering* 132 (7): 071008.

IASP (International Association for the Study of Pain) (2021a). Acute Pain. https://www.iasp-pain.org/resources/topics/acute-pain (accessed 15 April 2023).

IASP (International Association for the Study of Pain) (2021b). Terminology: Pain. https://www.iasp-pain.org/resources/terminology/#pain (accessed 10 October 2022).

IBVM (Idaho Board of Veterinary Medicine) (2020). Veterinary Practice Act State of Idaho. https://elitepublic.bovm.idaho.gov/IBVMPortal/IBVM/VPA/Idaho%20Veterinary%20Practice%20Act.pdf (accessed 19 February 2023).

IBVM (Iowa Board of Veterianry Medicine) (2017). Chapter 169: Veterinary Practice. https://www.legis.iowa.gov/docs/ico/chapter/169.pdf (accessed 19 February 2023).

IGA (Illinois General Assembly) (2004). Professions, occupations, and business operations: (225 ILCS 115/) Veterinary Medicine and Surgery Practice Act of 2004.

https://www.ilga.gov/legislation/ilcs/ilcs3.asp?ActID=1326&ChapterID=24#:~:text=The%20practice%20of%20veterinary%20medicine,control%20in%20the%20public%20interest. (accessed 19 February 2023).

Iheanacho, F. and Vellipuram, A.R. (2022). *Physiology, Mechanoreceptors*. Treasure Island, FL: StatPearls https://www.ncbi.nlm.nih.gov/books/NBK541068.

Inoue, N., Orías, A.A.E., and Segami, K. (2020). Biomechanics of the lumbar facet joint. *Spine Surgery and Related Research* 4 (1): 1–7.

Israel, V. (1983). Changes in nerve physiology in the rat after induced subluxation. *Articulations* 1 (1): 9–10.

iVet360 (2023). Benefits Matter. https://ivet360.com/recruiting-tool-kit/wages-benefits/benefits-matter/#:~:text=Most%20companies%20provide%20a%20minimum,and%20holidays%2C%20plus%20sick%20time (accessed 23 February 2023).

IVMB (Indiana Veterinary Medical Board) (2019). Title 25: Professions and Occupations, Article 38.1 Veterinarians. https://iga.in.gov/legislative/laws/2022/ic/titles/025/#25-38.1 (accessed 19 February 2023).

Jackman, S. and Regehr, W. (2017). The mechanisms and functions of synaptic facilitation. *Neuron* 94 (3): 447–464.

Jurek, C. (2013). The role of physical manipulation (chiropratic) in canine rehabilitation. In: *Canine Sports Medicine and Rehabilitation* (ed. M.C. Zink and J.B. Van Dyke), 427–446. Oxford: Wiley-Blackwell.

KBVE (Kansas Board of Veterinary Examiners) (2020). State Board of Veterinary Examiners Statutes. https://kbve.kansas.gov/wp-content/uploads/2021/01/kbve-statutes-amp-regs-new-fees.pdf (accessed 19 February 2023).

Kempermann, G., Song, H., and Gage, F. (2015). Neurogenesis in the adult hippocampus. *Cold Spring Harbor Perspectives in Biology* 7 (9): 1–15.

Kosloff, T., Elton, D., Tao, J., and Bannister, W. (2015). Chiropractic care and the risk of vertebrobasilar stroke: results of a case-control study in U.S. commercial and Medicare advantage populations. *Chiropractic and Manual Therapies* 23: 19.

KYBVE (Kentucky Board of Veterinary Examiners) (2020). Kentucky Revised Statutes (KRS) Chapter 321. https://www.kybve.com/documents/laws-regulations-booklet.pdf (accessed 19 February 2023).

de Lahunta, A. (1983). *Veterinary Neuroanatomy and Clinical Neurology*, 2e. Philadelphia, PA: Elsevier Saunders.

Lamont, L., Tranquilli, W., and Grimm, K. (2000). Physiology of pain. *Veterinary Clinics of North America Small Animal Practice* 30 (4): 703–728.

LBVM (Louisiana Board of Veterinary Medicine) (2022). Louisiana Veterinary Practice Act. https://lsbvm.org/wp-content/uploads/LA-Veterinary-Practice-Act-CURRENT.pdf (accessed 19 February 2023).

LeFebvre, R., Peterson, D., and Haas, M. (2012). Evidence-based practice and chiropractic care. *Journal of Evidence Based Complementary and Alternative Medicine* 18 (1): 75–79.

Lima, C.R., Sozio, R.S., Lw, C. et al. (2021). Effects of thrust magnitude and duration on immediate postspinal manipulation trunk muscle spindle responses. *Journal of Manipulative and Physiologic Therapies* 44 (5): 363–371.

Lin, H.-L., Fujii, A., Rebechini-Zasadny, H., and Hartz, D. (1978). Experimental induction of vertebral subluxation in laboratory animals. *Journal of Manipulative and Physiological Therapeutics* 1 (1): 63–66.

LoGiudice, R. and Rivera, P.L. (2023). Veterinary spinal manipulative therapy or animal chiropractic in veterinary rehabilitation. *Veterinary Clinics of North America Small Animal Practice* 53 (4): 757–774.

Mai-Roecker, H. and Roecker, C. (2018). Improving interprofessional communication. https://www.acatoday.org/News-Publications/ACA-News-Archive/ArtMID/5721/ArticleID/347 (accessed 8 July 2020).

Maltese, P., Michelini, S., Baronio, M., and Bertelli, M. (2019). Molecular foundations of chiropractic therapy. *Acta Biomedica* 90 (Suppl. 10): 93–102.

Marks, D. and Shmalberg, J. (2015). Profitability and financial benefits of acupuncture in small animal private practice. *American Journal of Traditional Chinese Veterinary Medicine* 10 (1): 43–48.

MBRVM (Massachusetts Board of Registration in Veterinary Medicine) (2022). Massachusetts law about veterinary practice. https://www .mass.gov/info-details/massachusetts-law-about-veterinary-practice (accessed 19 February 2023).

MBVM (Michigan Board of Veterinary Medicine) (2023). Public Health Code Act 368 of 1978, Article 15 Occupations, Part 161 General Provisions. http://www.legislature.mi.gov/ (S(j2ynwbgd1j4kqisz4hw3osoq))/documents/ mcl/pdf/mcl-368-1978-15.pdf (accessed 19 February 2023).

MBVME (Maryland Board of Veterinary Medical Examiners) (2019). Agriculture Article, Title 2, Subtitltes 3 and 17; Code of Maryland Regulations 15.01.11 and 15.4, Board of Veterinary Medical Examiners. https://mda .maryland.gov/vetboard/Documents/Laws-Regs/Veterinary-Practice-Act-COMAR.pdf (accessed 19 February 2023).

MCA (Montana Code Annotated) (2021). Title 37. Professions and Occupations, Chapter 18. Veterinary Medicine, Part 1. General - Veterinary Medicine Defined. https://leg. mt.gov/bills/mca/title_0370/chapter_0180/ part_0010/section_0020/0370-0180-0010-0020 .html (accessed 19 February 2023).

MFAF (Michelson Found Animals Foundation) (2018). Furred lines: Pet trends. https://www .prnewswire.com/news-releases/furred-lines-pet-trends-2019-300741947.html. (accessed 26 July 2021).

Miscioscia, E. and Repac, J. (2022). Evidence-based complementary and alternative canine orthopedic medicine. *Veterinary Clinics of North America Small Animal Practice* 52 (4): 925–938.

Mittleman, E. and Gaynor, J. (2000). A brief overview of the analgesic and immunologic effects of acupuncture in domestic animals. *Journal of the American Veterinary Medical Association* 217 (8): 1201–1205.

MNBVM (Minnesota Board of Veterinary Medicine) (2022). Minnesota Statutes 2022, Chapter 156: Veterinarian. www.revisor. mn.gov/statutes/cite/156/pdf (accessed 19 February 2023).

Mootz, R. (2005). Theoretic models of subluxation. In: *Foundations of Chiropractic: Subluxation*, 2e (ed. M.I. Gatterman), 227–244. St. Louis, MO: Elsevier Mosby.

MOVMB (Missouri Veterinary Medical Board) (2022). Missouri Veterinary Medical Practice Act Chapter 340, RSMO Statutes. https:// pr.mo.gov/boards/veterinary/ RulesandRegulations.pdf (accessed 19 February 2023).

MSBVM (Maine State Board of Veterinary Medicine) (2022). Maine Veterinary Practice Act. https://www.mainelegislature.org/legis/ statutes/32/title32sec4853.html (accessed 19 February 2023).

MSBVM (Mississippi Board of Veterinary Medicine) (2008). The Mississippi Board of Veterinary Medicine Rules. www.sos.ms.gov/ ACCode/00000522c.pdf (accessed 19 February 2023).

NAPHIA (North American Pet Health Insurance Association) (2023). Industry Data. https:// naphia.org/industry-data/#my-menu (accessed 18 February 2023).

NBVME (Nevada Board of Veterinary Medical Examiners) (2023). Chapter 638 - Veterinary Medicine, Euthanasia Technicians. https:// www.leg.state.nv.us/NRS/NRS-638. html#NRS638Sec001 (accessed 19 February 2023).

NCCIH (National Center for Complementry and Integrated Health) (2022). Spinal Manipulation: What You Need to Know. https://www.nccih.nih.gov/health/spinal-manipulation-what-you-need-to-know (accessed 22 April 2023).

NCVMB (North Carolina Veterinary Medical Board) (2014). The North Carolina Veterinary

Practice Act. https://www.ncvmb.org/content/laws/documents/PRACTICE_ACT_PF.pdf (accessed 19 February 2023).

NDVBME (North Dakota Board of Veterinary Medical Examiners) (2007). Chapter 43–29 Veterinarians. https://www.ndbvme.org/image/cache/North_Dakota_Practice_Act.pdf (accessed 19 February 2023).

NHBVM (New Hampshire Board of Veterinary Medicine) (2020). Chapter Vet 100 Organizational Rules. https://www.gencourt.state.nh.us/rules/state_agencies/vet100-700.html (accessed 19 February 2023).

NHBVM (New Hampshire Board of Veterinary Medicine) (2022). Chapter Vet 600 Practice of Veterinary Medicine. https://www.oplc.nh.gov/sites/g/files/ehbemt441/files/inline-documents/sonh/vet-600-adopted-text.pdf (accessed 19 February 2023).

NHIS (National Health Interview Survey) (2012). National Health Interview Survey Series. https://www.icpsr.umich.edu/web/NACDA/studies/36146 (accessed 20 May 2020).

NJSBVME (New Jersey State Board of Veterinary Medical Examiners) (2021). New Jersey Administrative Coade Title 13, Law and Public Stafety, Chapter 44, State Board of Veterinary Medical Examiners. https://www.njconsumeraffairs.gov/regulations/Chapter-44-State-Board-of-Veterinary-Medical-Examiners.pdf (accessed 19 February 2023).

NLU (2019). Statutes relating to veterinary medicine and surgery practice act. https://dhhs.ne.gov/licensure/Documents/VeterinaryMedicineSurgery.pdf (accessed 19 February 2023).

NMBVM (New Mexico Board of Veterinary Medicine) (2018). 61–14-2 Definitions Veterinary Practice Act. https://www.nmbvm.org/wp-content/uploads/2021/07/Veterinary-Practice-Act-Turtle-image.pdf (accessed 19 February 2023).

Nolen, R.S. (2022). Pet ownership rate stabilizes as spending increases. https://www.avma.org/news/pet-ownership-rate-stabilizes-spending-increases (accessed 22 February 2023).

Nolte, J. (2009a). Synaptic transmission between neurons. In: *The Human Brain: An Introduction to Its Functional Anatomy*, 6e, 177–200. Philadelphia, PA: Mosby Elsevier.

Nolte, J. (2009b). *The Human Brain: An Introduction to Its Functional Anatomy*, 6e. Philadelphia, PA: Mosby Elsevier.

NYSLPV (New York State Licensed Professions Veterinarian) (2023). Article 135, Veterinarian. https://www.op.nysed.gov/professions/veterinarian/laws-rules-regulations/article-135 (accessed 19 February 2023).

OL (Oregon Legislature) (2021). Chapter 686 - Veterinarians; Veterinary Technicians. https://www.oregonlegislature.gov/bills_laws/ors/ors686.html (accessed 19 February 2023).

Olson, V. (1987). Evaluation of joint mobilization treatment: a method. *Physical Therapy* 67 (3): 351–356.

Onifer, S., Sozio, R.S., DiCarlo, M. et al. (2018). Long spinal manipulative therapy reduces peripheral neuropathic pain in the rat. *Neuroreport* 29 (3): 191–196.

ORC (Ohio Revised Code) (2006). Section 4741.01 Veterinarian Definitions. https://codes.ohio.gov/ohio-revised-code/section-4741.01 (accessed 19 February 2023).

OVB (Oklahoma Veterinary Board) (2022). Oklahoma Veterinary Practice Act. https://www.okvetboard.com/practice-act/388-practice-act-effective-2022/viewdocument/388 (accessed 19 February 2023).

Panzer, D. (2005). Facet subluxation syndrome. In: *Foundations of Chiropractic Subluxation*, 2e (ed. M.I. Gatterman), 509–521. St. Louis, MO: Elsevier Mosby.

Papakyriakou, M., Triano, J., and Brennan, P. (1991). Spine stiffness measures in a dog model of restricted joint motion. *International Conference on Spinal Manipulation* (12 April 1991), Arlington, VA.

Pasquini, C., Spurgeon, T., and Pasquini, S. (2003). *Anatomy of Domestic Animals: Systemic and Regional Approach*, 10e. Pilot Point, TX: Sudz Publishing.

Penning, L. and Badoux, D. (1987). Radiological study of the movements of the cervical spine in the dog compared with those in man. *Anatomia Histologia Embryologia* 16: 1–20.

Pickar, J. and Ge, W. (2008). Time course for the development of muscle history in lumbar paraspinal muscle spindles arising from changes in vertebral position. *Spine Journal* 8 (2): 320–328.

Pickar, J. and McLain, R. (1995). Responses of mechanosensitive afferents to manipulation of the lumbar facet in the cat. *Spine* 20 (22): 2379–2385.

Pickar, J.G., Sung, P.S., Kang, Y.-M., and Ge, W. (2007). Response of lumbar paraspinal muscles spindles is greater to spinal manipulative loading compared with slower loading under length control. *Spine Journal* 7 (5): 583–595.

Pin-Barre, C. and Laurin, J. (2015). Physical exercise as a diagnostic, rehabilitation, and preventative tool: influence on neuroplasticity and motor recovery after stroke. *Neural Plasticity* 2015: 608581.

Purves, D., Augustine, G., FitzPatrick, D. et al. (2012a). Electrical signals of nerve cells. In: *Neuroscience*, 5e, 25–40. Sunderland, MA: Sinauer Associates.

Purves, D., Augustine, G., FitzPatrick, D. et al. (2012b). Lower motor neuron circuits and motor control. In: *Neuroscience*, 5e, 343–374. Sunderland, MA: Sinauer Associates.

Purves, D., Augustine, G., FitzPatrick, D. et al. (2012c). Pain. In: *Neuroscience*, 5e, 209–227. Sunderland, MA: Sinauer Associates.

Purves, D., Augustine, G., FitzPatrick, D. et al. (2012d). Studying the nervous system. In: *Neuroscience*, 5e, 1–21. Sunderland, MA: Sinauer Associates.

Purves, D., Augustine, G., FitzPatrick, D. et al. (2012e). The somatic sensory system: touch and proprioception. In: *Neuroscience*, 5e, 189–227. Sunderland, MA: Sinauer Associates.

Purves, D., Augustine, G., FitzPatrick, D. et al. (2012f). The visceral motor system. In: *Neuroscience*, 5e, 2012. Sunderland, MA: Sinauer Associates.

Reed, W. and Pickar, J. (2015). Paraspinal muscle spindle response to intervertebral fixation and segmental thrust level during spinal manipulation in an animal model. *Spine* 40 (13): 752–759.

Reed, W., Long, C., Kawchuk, G., and Pickar, J. (2015). Neural responses to the mechanical parameters of a high velocity, low amplitude spinal manipulation: effect of preload parameters. *Manual Therapy* 20 (6): 797–804.

Reed, W., Pickar, J.G., Sozio, R.S. et al. (2017). Characteristics of paraspinal muscle spine response to mechanically-assisted spinal manipulation: a preliminary report. *Journal of Manipulative and Physiological Therapeutics* 40 (6): 371–380.

Reed, W.R., Lienschner, M.A.K., Lima, C.R. et al. (2022). In vivo measurement of intradiscal pressure changes related to thrust and non-thrust spinal manipulation in an animal model: a pilot study. *Chiropractic and Manual Therapies* 30 (1): 36.

RIDH (Rhode Island Department of Health) (2006). Rules and Regulations for the Licensure of Veterinarians. https://risos-apa-production-public.s3.amazonaws.com/DOH/DOH_3841.pdf (accessed 19 February 2023).

Rivera, P. (2015). *Introduction to Veterinary Spinal Manipulation: Lecture and Notes*. Sturtevant, WI: Healing Oasis Wellness Center.

Ruscheweyh, R., Wilder-Smith, O., Drdla, R. et al. (2011). Long-term potentiation in spinal nociceptive pathways as a novel target for pain therapy. *Molecular Pain* 7: 20.

Sato, A. and Swenson, R. (1984). Sympathetic nervous system response to mechanical stress of the spinal column in rats. *Journal of Manipulative and Physiological Therapeutics* 7: 141–147.

SCCL (South Carolina Code of Laws) (2016). Title 40 - Professions and Occupations, Chapter 69 Veterinarians, Article 1, General Provisions. https://www.scstatehouse.gov/code/t40c069.php (accessed 19 February 2023).

SDL (South Dakota Legislature) (2023). Codified Laws Chapter 36–12 Veterinarians. https://sdlegislature.gov/Statutes/Codified_Laws/2060135 (accessed 19 February 2023).

Seaman, D. and Faye, L.J. (2005). The vertebral subluxation complex. In: *Foundations in Chiropractic Subluxation*, 2e (ed. M.I. Gatterman), 195–226. St. Louis, MO: Elsevier Mosby.

Sears, B. (2023). What is range of motion? https://www.verywellhealth.com/overview-range-of-motion-2696650 (accessed 17 April 2023).

Sheffler, Z.M., Reddy, V. & Pillarisetty, L.S. (2022). Physiology, Neurotransmitters. Treasure Island, FL: SttPerls. https://www.ncbi.nlm.nih.gov/books/NBK539894 (accessed 16 April 2023).

Smith, D., Fuhr, A., and Davis, B. (1989). Skin accelerometer displacement and relative bone movement of adjacent vertebrae in response to chiropractic percussion thrusts. *Journal of Manipulative and Physiological Therapeutics* 12 (1): 26–37.

Stevenson, P. (2016). How to set practice service fees. https://cliniciansbrief.com/article/how-set-practice-service-fees. (accessed 10 June 2020).

Sullivan, K., Hill, A., and Haussler, K. (2008). The effects of chiropractic, massage and phenylbutazone on spinal mechanical nociceptive thresholds in horses without clinical signs. *Equine Veterinary Journal* 40 (1): 14–20.

TAC (Texas Admistrative Code) (2012). Title 22, Part 24 Texas Board of Veterinary Medical Examiners, Chapter 575 Practice and Procedure. https://texreg.sos.state.tx.us/public/readtac$ext.ViewTAC?tac_view=4&ti=22&pt=24&ch=575&rl=Y (accessed 19 February 2023).

TBVME (Tennessee Board of Veterinary Medical Examiners) (2014). Chapter 1730–1 General Rules Governing Veterinarians. https://publications.tnsosfiles.com/rules/1730/1730-01.20140821.pdf (accessed 19 February 2023).

Trcek, L. (2023). This is how much flight prices increase in 2023 (+FAQs). https://www.travelinglifestyle.net/this-is-how-much-flight-prices-increase-in-2023 (accessed 18 February 2023).

Triano, J. and Luttges, M. (1980). Subtle, intermittent mechanical irritation of sciatic nerves in mice. *Journal of Manipulative and Physiological Therapeutics* 3 (2): 75–80.

Triano, J. and Luttges, M. (1982). Nerve irritation: a possible model of sciatic neuritis. *Spine* 7 (2): 129–136.

UC (Utah Code) (2020). Chapter 28, Veterinary Practice Act, Part 1 General Provisions. https://le.utah.gov/xcode/Title58/Chapter28/C58-28_1800010118000101.pdf (accessed 19 February 2023).

Vaillant, M., Edgecombe, T., Long, C.R. et al. (2012). The effect of duration and amplitude of spinal manipulative therapy (SMT) on spinal stiffness. *Manual Therapy* 17 (6): 577–583.

Vasseur, P., Saunders, G., and Steinback, C. (1981). Anatomy and function of the ligaments of the lower cervical spine in the dog. *American Journal of Veterinary Research* 42 (6): 1002–1006.

Verschooten, F. (1991). Osteopathy in locomotion problems of the horse: a critical evaluation. *Swiss Veterinary Journal* 11: 115–116.

VGA (Vermont General Assembly) (2023). The Vermont Statutes Online, Title 26: Professions and Occupations, Chapter 44: Veterinary Medicine. https://legislature.vermont.gov/statutes/fullchapter/26/044 (accessed 19 February 2023).

Wag! (2020). Chiropractic Care in Dogs. https://wagwalking.com/treatment/chiropractic-care (accessed 2 September 2020).

Walters, E.T. (2019, 1785). Adaptive mechanisms driving maladaptive pain: how chronic ongoing activity in primary nociceptors can enhance evolutionary fitness after severe injury. *Philosophical Transactions of the Royal Society of London. Series B, Biological Sciences* 374: 20190277.

WBVM (Wyoming Board of Veterinary Medicine) (2018). Veterinary Medicine Practice Act, Chapter 30 Veterinarians. https://vetboard.wyo.gov/rules (accessed 19 February 2023).

Weir, M. (2019). How much airfare in the US costs today compared to 10 years ago. https://www.businessinsider.com/fight-prices-airfare-average-cost-usa-2019-11 (accessed 2019 10 December).

WFC (World Federation of Chiropractic) (2001). Definition of chiropractic. https://www.wfc.org/website/index.php?option=com_content&view=article&id=90&Itemid=110 (accessed 8 July 2020).

WFC (World Federation of Chiropractic) (2009). History of chiropractic. https://www.wfc.org/website/index.php?option=com_content&view=article&id=46&Itemid=109&lang=en (accessed 8 July 2020).

Woodley, K. (2018). Pet insurance for holistic and integrative practice. https://ivcjournal.com/pet-insurance-integrative-practices (accessed 11 August 2021).

Woolf, C. (2010). What is this thing called pain? *Journal of Clinical Investigation* 120 (11): 3742–3744.

Woolf, C. and Ma, Q. (2007). Nociceptors: noxious stimulus detectors. *Neuron* 55 (3): 353–364.

WSL (Washington State Legislature) (2023). Chapter 18.92 RCW Veterinary Medicine, Surgery, and Dentistry. https://app.leg.wa.gov/rcw/default.aspx?cite=18.92 (accessed 19 February 2023).

WVBVM (West Virginia Board of Veterinary Medicine) (2023). Series 4 Standards of Practice. https://www.wvbvm.org/Home/Laws/Rules-/Series-4-Standards-of-Practice (accessed 19 February 2023).

WVEB (Wisconsin Veterinary Examining Board) (2022). Chapter VE1 Veterinarians. https://docs.legis.wisconsin.gov/code/admin_code/ve/1.pdf (accessed 19 February 2023).

Yam, M.F., Loh, Y.C., Tan, C.S. et al. (2018). General pathways of pain sensation and the major neurotransmitters involved in pain regulation. *International Journal of Molecular Sciences* 19 (8): 2164.

Zhang, Z.-J., Wang, X.-M., and McAlonan, G.M. (2011). Neural acupuncture unit: a new concept for interpreting effects and mechanisms of acupuncture. *Evidence Based Complementary and Alternative Medicine* 2012: 429412.

Zhao, Z.-Q. (2008). Neural mechanism underlying acupuncture analgesia. *Progress in Neurobiology* 85 (4): 355–375.

Zhu, H. (2014). Acupoints initiate the healing process. *Medical Acupuncture* 26 (5): 264–270.

Zink, C. (2013). Locomotion and athletic performance. In: *Canine Sports Medicine and Rehabilitation* (ed. M.C. Zink and J.B. Van Dyke), 19–31. Oxford: Wiley-Blackwell.Nociception vs. Pain

11

Western Herbal Medicine

Introduction

Western herbal medicine (WHM) is a therapeutic modality using individual and combinations of plant materials, with minimal processing, to aid in the prevention and treatment of disease. Western herbs and herbal formulas are not classified as drugs and thus not regulated by the Food and Drug Administration (FDA). The lack of regulation highlights the importance of proper veterinarian training, as well as utilizing and recommending herbal products from trusted sources. WHM can be used to aid in the treatment of most veterinary conditions.

The introduction of WHM into veterinary practice can be beneficial for both the patient and the health of the practice. The successful incorporation and utilization of WHM does not end with the veterinarian's training.

Support staff training and client education are crucial. This chapter discusses the what, why, and how for effective integration of WHM within your practice.

The What

Definition

WHM is a medicinal system which utilizes individual and combinations of plant materials, with minimal processing, to help. Crude parts or extracts of the root, bark, and flower are used as individual herbs or part of a multiplant formulation (Niemeyer et al. 2013). The practice of WHM is also known as Western herbalism, botanical medicine, medical herbalism, and phytotherapy. In veterinary medicine, WHM is often referred to as veterinary herbal medicine (VHM). For the purposes of

Integrative Medicine in Veterinary Practice, First Edition. Lisa P. McFaddin.
© 2024 John Wiley & Sons, Inc. Published 2024 by John Wiley & Sons, Inc.
Companion website: www.wiley.com/go/mcfaddin/integrativemedicine

this chapter VHM and WHM are used interchangeably.

Human History

The first written record of medicinal plant usage is roughly 5000 years old (Petrovska 2012). From 1500 BCE the Ebers Papyrus contains a collection of 800 prescriptions comprising 700 plant species and drugs used for everyday therapy (Tucakov 1948). Homer referred to 63 medicinal plant species in *The Iliad* and *The Odyssey* in 800 BCE.

Botanical science was founded by Theophrastus (371–287 BCE), called the father of botany. In his books *De Causis Plantarium* (Plant Etiology) and *De Historia Plantarium* (Plant History), he described over 500 medicinal plants (Petrovska 2012).

WHM was popularized by the Greeks around 400 BCE. The concept of the Four Humors, a physical system believed to regulate human body functions, arose from Indian Ayurvedic medicine philosophies (Wynn and Fougère 2007d). The Father of Medicine, Hippocrates, promoted the humoral theory, focusing on medicinal plants, diet, and exercise as the keys to disease prevention and treatment. The humoral theory remained influential until the fifteenth century (Petrovska 2012).

During the Dark Ages Benedictine monks published on the use of herbal medicine. The monks were trained to translate Latin texts describing the humoral theories. The monks were also responsible for treating the sick due to a lack of trained physicians (Wynn and Fougère 2007d; Cabrera 2012).

WHM texts exploded in the sixteenth century with the invention of the printing press. The humoral theories were replaced with the belief that diseases affected humans chemically and drugs were needed to treat illness. Plants were still utilized but newer remedies, including opium and mercury, stole the spotlight. Chemical medicine evolved into alchemy, which concentrated on the chemical constituents of plants rather than the whole plant (Wynn and Fougère 2007d; Cabrera 2012).

During the Renaissance scientific experiments further divided the theoretical approaches of biomedicine and herbalism. America saw a resurgence in herbal medicine in the nineteenth century which declined following the release of the Flexner Report in 1910 (Stahnisch and Verhoef 2012). The Flexner Report, written by Abraham Flexner and commissioned by the Carnegie Foundation for the Advancement of Teaching, critically evaluated the current admission and graduation standards of medical schools, suggested improvements regarding the number, quality, and curriculum of medical schools, and disparaged the practice of almost all forms of complementary and alternative medicine (CAM) (Stahnisch and Verhoef 2012).

Since the 1960s, there has been renewed and persistent interest in WHM. WHM was and is seen to counteract the side effects of pharmaceutical drugs or as an alternative approach when traditional therapies are ineffective. The primary scientific approaches to WHM are phytotherapy and traditional herbalism. Phytotherapy is an evidence-based approach to the treatment of diseases using herbal remedies. Traditional herbalism is the application of different cultural medicinal systems, such as traditional Chinese medicine and Ayurvedic medicine (Wynn and Fougère 2007d).

Veterinary History

VHM was first documented in the Western hemisphere in a 12-volume text *On Agriculture*, in first-century Rome (Wynn and Fougère 2007d). The regular use of herbal remedies in veterinary medicine persisted through the twentieth century. As was seen with human medicine, the use of herbal remedies in veterinary medicine fell out of favor in the early 1900s. Again, following the human medicine trend, some veterinary textbooks mentioned herbal remedies in the 1960s, though most discussions focused on potential toxicological, not medicinal, properties. There was renewed interest in VHM, along with acupuncture and Chinese herbal medicine (CHM), in the 1970s (Wynn and Fougère 2007d).

The founding of the Veterinary Botanical Medicine Association (VBMA) in 2000 was a turning point in VHM. The VBMA's goal was and is to legitimize VHM by encouraging research and emphasizing the importance of training and education for all veterinarians interested in practicing herbal medicine.

Terminology

The world of WHM comes with its own vocabulary. A basic understanding of these terms is crucial, allowing effective communication amongst professionals and with clients. A summary of common terms is provided below.

Allopathic medicine (aka allopathy): The treatment of disease using pharmaceutical, surgical, or other modern therapies (Iftikhar 2019). The term is synonymous with traditional or mainstream medicine. This term originated as a central tenet within homeopathy, denoting all non-homeopathic treatments and carries with it negative connotations. Some practitioners discourage its use in professional literature.

Autonomic nervous system (ANS): Contains components of the central nervous system (CNS) and peripheral nervous system (PNS) which function to control involuntary activity, maintain homeostasis, and react to stress (Darby 2014). The ANS is divided into the sympathetic and parasympathetic nervous systems.

Ayurvedic medicine: One of the world's oldest medical systems developed in India. The practice utilizes herbs, diet,

massage, exercise, detoxification, and meditation to prevent and treat disease (NCCIH 2019).

Bioavailability: The amount or proportion of active drug or other constituent entering circulation after ingestion, injection, or absorption.

Botanical: An ingredient derived from a plant and used as an additive.

Chinese herbal medicine: CHM is one of the four branches within traditional Chinese veterinary medicine (TCVM): acupuncture, Chinese herbal medicine or therapy, Tui-na, and food therapy. CHM is a medicinal system which utilizes individual and combinations of herbs to diagnose, prevent, and treat disease.

Ethnoveterinary medicine (aka veterinary anthropology): The study of a community's knowledge base and skills pertaining to animal health care for companion animals and livestock (Matekaire and Bwakura 2004; Lans et al. 2007).

Heroic medicine (aka heroic depletion theory): A therapeutic system popular in the seventeenth to eighteenth centuries based on the belief that disease and illness developed as a result of humoral imbalance. Common treatments included bloodletting, purging (emesis induction), and diaphoresis (sweating) (Wynn and Fougère 2007e).

Humoral theory (aka humoralism): A medical theory, popularized by Hippocrates, focusing on the balance of four primary substances, called humors, within the body: yellow bile, black bile, phlegm, and blood. It was believed all diseases stemmed from an imbalance of one or more of the Four Humors. Humorism influenced medical theory and therapy from 400 bce through the fifteenth century (Wynn and Fougère 2007e).

Materia medica: Accumulated information pertaining to the therapeutic properties of a substance used for healing (Klein 2007). The materia medica is like an encyclopedia of herbal remedies composed of individual monographs.

Medical botany: The study of naturally occurring materials possessing medicinal properties (Klein 2007).

Monograph: A summary of compiled information outlining specific details about a particular herb or natural substance. The monograph generally includes the common name, scientific name, pseudonyms, distribution, similar species, scientific family, parts of the plant used, specific collection techniques, constituents or active medicinal compounds, clinical actions, history and traditional use, energetics, published research, indications, veterinary indications, contraindications, toxicology, adverse effects, drug interactions, preparation notes, dosage, combinations or multi-herb formulas, and references (Wynn and Fougère 2007e).

Pharmacodynamics: A branch of pharmacology focusing on the drug effects and mechanisms of actions (Chen 2013).

Pharmacokinetics: A branch of pharmacology focusing on the movement of drugs throughout the body (Chen 2013; Zhao et al. 2015).

Physiomedicalism: An herbal medicinal system based on the treatment of a patient's underlying condition. Resolution of the underlying condition would restore patient vitality, normalizing all body systems and functions, through the application of the following therapeutic ideals: detoxification; improving circulation; ANS balance; and tissue function restoration (Fougère 2007).

Phytopharmacology: The study of plants as medicine, specifically the active molecular components of plants possessing medicinal properties (Bone 2007).

Phytotherapy: The clinical application of plant-based extracts or medications in the prevention and treatment of disease (Ghosh 2016).

Phytotomy (aka plant anatomy): The study of the internal structures of plants (Klein 2007).

Taxonomy: A branch of biology centered on the scientific classification of related items (Klein 2007).

Traditional Chinese Medicine (TCM): A complex medical system, developed over thousands of years in China, used to prevent and treat disease. There are five branches within TCM: acupuncture, Chinese herbal medicine or therapy, Tui-na, Tai-Chi, and food therapy (Xie 2011a; NCCIH 2013). The study and application of TCM in animals is known as **traditional Chinese veterinary medicine (TCVM)**. Refer to Chapters 1–3 for further information.

Trophorestorative: Herbs with the ability to nurture, support, protect, and repair specific organs or tissues (Fougère 2007).

Vitalism: All living beings are born with a "vital force" which flows continuously through the body providing nourishment and sustaining life.

Zoopharmacognosy: The behavior of self-medication, through ingestion or topical application of plants, soil, or insects, by non-human animals. As an example, non-human primates, as well as domesticated companion and food animals, are known to ingest plants with antiparasitic or purgative properties to rid themselves of intestinal parasites (Engel 2007; Kapadia et al. 2014; Shurkin 2014).

Medical Botany

To utilize WHM safely and effectively, the veterinarian must know their botanical pharmacy inside out, including taxonomy, identification, anatomy, and chemistry (Klein 2007).

Plant and Fungi Taxonomy

All life is divided into three domains: Eukaryota, Archaea, and Bacteria (Figure 11.1). Plants and Fungi fall within the Eukaryota domain. The are five divisions within the plants (Plantae) and three within Fungi.

Eukaryota is divided into three Kingdoms: Plantae, Fungi, and Animalia (NRCS 2023). The science of hierarchical classification of plants is necessary to standardize the nomenclature of the herbs used in WHM (Bennett and Balick 2014). Common names are frequently used when practitioners and clients/patients discuss herbs. This practice can create confusion when a common name refers to two species. For example, two species of ginseng are commonly used, white ginseng or American ginseng (*Panax quinquefolius*) and red ginseng or Korean ginseng (*Panax ginseng*), each having their own characteristics and treatment effects. As another example, the common name salvia refers to dozens of plant species falling into three different families (Bennett and Balick 2014). The most common type of salvia used in veterinary WHM is *Salvia officinalis* L., also known as Sage (Wynn and Fougère 2007e).

Standardization eliminates confusion, ensuring the correct herb is used each time. This distinction is also vital in medicinal plant research which is used to legitimize and prove the therapeutic effectiveness of specific plants (Bennett and Balick 2014).

To avoid confusion and error, the following criteria should be followed when referencing medicinal plants and fungi (Klein 2007; Bennett and Balick 2014):

1) Provide common and scientific names.
2) The scientific name should include the complete (not abbreviated) genus and species name, as well as subspecies if applicable.
3) Indicate the part of the plant used: flower, stem, leaves, or root.

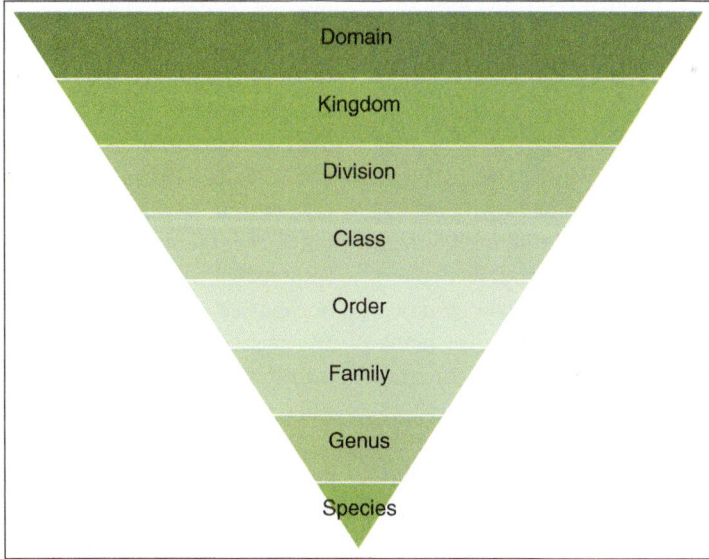

Figure 11.1 The hierarchical classification of taxonomy. The inverted pyramid illustrates the heightened specificity associated with each taxonomic classification. There is an inverse correlation between the category and the number of taxa within it. There are three domains: Eukaryota, Archaea, and Bacteria. Source: Lisa P. McFaddin.

The United States Department of Agriculture (USDA) Natural Resources Conservation Service (NRCS) has an amazing online search engine which provides detailed taxonomic nomenclature and hierarchy for all known plants called the Plants Database (https://plants.usda.gov/classification.html). This invaluable tool should be used to ensure all medicinal plants and fungi are referenced appropriately.

Plant and Fungi Identification

Experienced WHM practitioners should have the ability to correctly identify the morphology of live whole plants and raw, dried, and cut plant material. Identification methods typically involve visual, olfactory, and taste cues (Klein 2007). Herbal medicine manufacturers should also perform microscopic evaluation and chemical analyses (Klein 2007). Proper plant identification ensures the correct medicinal herb is selected and adulterated products are not used.

Plant and Fungi Anatomy

Knowledge of the internal structure of plants, particularly on a cellular level, is necessary to understand the chemical composition and physiologic effects exerted by medical plants (Klein 2007).

Plant and Fungi Chemistry

The therapeutic effects associated with medicinal plants and fungi are due to their chemical composition. There are primary and secondary chemical components. The primary components are essential for the survival of the plant or fungus, including carbohydrates, amino acids, proteins, and lipids (Yarnell 2007).

The secondary components are considered nonessential for plant or fungus survival but aid in maintaining overall health (Yarnell 2007). Secondary components prevent self-trauma from the by-products of photosynthesis (antioxidants), attract pollinators encouraging seed distribution (reproduction), prevent predation from insects and herbivores, as well as discourage nearby growth of other plants (self-defense), and improve cellular signals (Yarnell 2007). The secondary constituents are responsible for many of the plant or fungi's medicinal effects.

The categorization of the secondary components is complex and confusing. From a clinical perspective the most useful classification scheme utilizes biochemical metabolites. A metabolite is formed when a substance is broken down or structurally augmented. Examples of categories of botanical secondary metabolites (BSM) include alkaloids, phenolics, saponins, and terpenes (Klein 2007; Wink 2015; Kaushik et al. 2021). Further research continuously leads to the discovery of additional botanical metabolites and reorganization of their classifications.

Phytochemistry for Veterinarians

An in-depth discussion of phytochemistry is beyond the scope of this book and there are ample reference materials covering this information in detail. Let us examine phenolics more closely just to get a taste of the complexity of phytochemistry. Phenolics are likely the largest group of BSM, with more than 8000 phenolic compounds found in plants (Kumar and Pandey 2013). The chemical structure ranges from a single aromatic ring to complex polymers (Teoh 2015). Phenols are often responsible for the color, flavor, and taste of herbs used in drinks and food (Hussein and El-Anssary 2019). Phenolics can be divided into the subcategories of phenolic acids, tannins, coumarins, flavonoids, chromones and xanthones, quinones, stilbenes, curcuminoids, and lignans (Hussein and El-Anssary 2019; Kisiriko et al. 2021).

Many of the medicinal effects of phenolics are related to their ability to augment protein structure and function (including membrane proteins), modulate transcription factors, protect against oxidative stress (antioxidant and antiaging), protect against bacteria and fungi (antiseptic), reduce inflammation (anti-inflammatory), sedate, aid wound healing, function as a chemopreventative, protect the heart (cardioprotective), and protect skin from ultraviolet (UV) radiation exposure (photoprotective) (Teoh 2015; Wink 2015; Tungmunnithum et al. 2018; Kaushik et al. 2021). Alkyl phenols can be allergenic compounds and are hazardous to the eyes (potentially causing blindness) (van Wyk and Wink 2017).

Plants belonging to the Lamiaceae family, i.e. *Rosmarinus officinalis, Salvia officinalis, Thymus vulgaris, Origanum vulgare, Ocimum basilicum, Melissa officinalis, Mentha piperita, Origanum majorana, Satureja hortensis,* and *Hyssopus officinalis* are characterized by high levels of phenolic compounds . . . Among medicinal plants, those with the highest contents of phenolic compounds were the herbs oregano and thyme as well as the leaves of melissa and rosemary. Among spices, the highest TPC [total phenolic content] values were found in marjoram, sage, thyme, oregano and tarragon, and the latter belongs to the Asteraeae family (Ulewicz-Magulska and Wesolowski 2018).

Classification

The herbs used in WHM can be categorized by their botanical metabolites, traditional herb actions, target organ or tissue, and therapeutic goals.

Botanical Compounds

The compound or compounds responsible for the clinical activity of an herbal medicine is usually due to secondary metabolites, as discussed in the previous section. The clinical benefits of an herb or herbal formula may be predicted based on the compounds present but are also affected by the concentration of the active compounds and the type and presence of other compounds. This is one reason herbalists rely on traditional clinical activity and reported clinical benefits of an herb in the absence of controlled trials in cats and dogs.

Traditional Herbal Actions

The primary therapeutic effect exerted by a particular herb is also known as their traditional herbal action. Categorization by herbal actions is one of the simplest, yet effective, classification structures. Table 11.1 summarizes the most common traditional herbal actions.

Target Organ or Tissue

Some herbs have an affinity for a specific organ or tissue. These herbs can nurture, support, protect, and repair specific organs and tissues (Fougère 2007). Examples are provided in Table 11.2.

Therapeutic Action

Herbs can be organized by their therapeutic effects as reported anecdotally or in peer-reviewed literature. Examples are provided in Table 11.3.

Monographs

The materia medica is like an encyclopedia of herbal remedies and comprises individual monographs. Inclusion of an entire materia medica is beyond the scope of this book. The purpose of this section is to introduce the practitioner and hospital team to the concept of herbal monographs. Herbal monographs are often organized in a similar fashion from source to source. Table 11.4 lists the information contained within most herbal monographs. The order of the information may vary depending on the source. Table 11.5 provides an example herbal monograph for ginger root (*Zingiberis officinale rhizoma*). A list of excellent sources for herbal

Table 11.1 Common traditional herbal actions used to categorize herbs in veterinary WHM. A description of the category, examples of up to three therapeutic effects, and up to three herb examples are provided (Fougère 2007; Kolen 2013).

Adaptogens	Description	Normalize the body's response to stress; often tonics (give energy)
	Therapeutic effects	Chronic illness; support adrenal function; regulate the immune system
	Example herbs	*Avena sativa* (Oat); *Glycyrrhiza glabra* (Licorice); *Panax ginseng* (Asian Ginseng)
Alternatives	Description	Enhance body system functions by stimulating the metabolism; often work through detoxification, elimination, or immune modulation
	Therapeutic effects	Dermatologic conditions; gastrointestinal disorders; immune system conditions
	Example herbs	*Arctium lappa* (Greater Burdock); *Iris versicolor* (Blue Flag); *Urtica dioica* (Stinging Nettle)
Anthelmintic	Description	Goal is to kill parasites without harming the host; often given with a purgative
	Therapeutic effects	Kill and expel intestinal parasites
	Example herbs	*Allium sativum* (Garlic); *Artemesia* spp. (Mugwort); *Juglans nigra* (Eastern Black Walnut)
Antiemetics	Description	Stop vomiting and reduce nausea
	Therapeutic effects	Coat, protect, lubricate, and soothe the gastric mucosa; neutralize stomach pH; stimulate vomit centers locally and centrally (within the brain)
	Example herbs	*Cinnamomum cassia* (Chinese Cinnamon); *Mentha piperita* (Peppermint); *Zingiber officinale* (Ginger)
Aperients	Description	Mild laxative
	Therapeutic effects	Promote bowel movements
	Example herbs	*Articum lappa* (Greater Burdock); *Berberis vulgaris* (Barberry); *Plantago psyllium* (Psyllium)
Aromatics	Description	Contain strong aromas
	Therapeutic effects	Used for aromatherapy; support the digestive tract; support and clear the respiratory tract
	Example herbs	*Angelica archangelica* (Norwegian Angelica); *Elettaria cardamomum* (True Cardamon); *Salvia rosmariunus* (Rosemary)
Astringents	Description	Precipitate intracellular and extracellular protein; dry, draw, and shrink tissue creating a barrier; protect tissue from damage
	Therapeutic effects	Reduce pain; tone mucous membranes; reduce excess
	Example herbs	*Achillea millefolium* (Yarrow); *Camellia sinensis* (Tea); *Quercus alba* (White Oak)

Bitters	Description	Taste bitter; cooling; improve blood flow to the gastrointestinal tract
	Therapeutic effects	Liver disease; stimulate digestion; improve appetite
	Example herbs	*Artemisia absinthium* (Common Wormwood); *Humulus lupulus* (Hops); *Scutellaria* spp. (Skullcap)
Carminatives	Description	Encourage eructation and flatulence; primarily volatile compounds; cause mild gastrointestinal irritation and vasodilation; cause a mild warming sensation
	Therapeutic effects	Reduce gas pains; decrease colonic spasms (after an initial period of increased peristalsis)
	Example herbs	*Carum carvi* (Caraway); *Foeniculum vulgare* (Fennel); *Pimpinella anisum* (Anise)
Cholagogues	Description	Stimulate the release of bile from the liver; usually bitter; frequently combined with laxatives
	Therapeutic effects	Liver disease; liver dysfunction; gallbladder disease Contraindicated in cases of bile duct obstruction, icterus, septic cholecystitis, ileus, or hepatic neoplasia
	Example herbs	*Artemisia vulgaris* (Mugwort); *Chamomilla recutita* (German Chamomile); *Dioscorea villosa* (Wild Yam)
Choleretics	Description	Stimulate bile production within the liver; often function as a cholagogue
	Therapeutic effects	Liver disease; liver dysfunction; gallbladder disease Contraindicated in cases of bile duct obstruction, icterus, septic cholecystitis, ileus, or hepatic neoplasia
	Example herbs	*Berberis vulgaris* (Barberry); *Curcuma longa* (Turmeric); *Silybum marianum* (Milk Thistle)
Demulcents	Description	Mucilaginous or oily; lubricate, protect, and soothe mucous membranes; can be used as bulking agents
	Therapeutic effects	Disorders of the oral, pharyngeal, esophageal, and gastric mucosa
	Example herbs	*Althaea officinalis* root (Marsh Mallow Root); Honey; Malt extract
Diaphoretics	Description	Encourage sweating by raising body temperature and improving peripheral circulation
	Therapeutic effects	Fever
	Example herbs	*Achillea millefolium* (Yarrow); *Capsicum minimum* (Tabasco Pepper); *Eupatorium perfoliatum* (Common Boneset)
Diuretics	Description	Promote urine flow; increase renal blood flow and glomerular filtration rate; limit salt resorption; often administered as a tea
	Therapeutic effects	Urinary tract infections; water retention
	Example herbs	*Atractylodes macrocephala* (Bai Zhu); *Cynara scolymus* (Artichoke); *Juniperus communis* (Common Juniper)

(Continued)

Table 11.1 (Continued)

Eliminatives	Description	Promote or assist with elimination; patient should be strong
	Therapeutic effects	Diuretics; laxatives; expectorants; cholagogues
	Example herbs	*Cynara scolymus* (Artichoke); *Urtica dioica* (Stinging Nettle); *Withania somnifera* (Ashwagandha)
Emollients	Description	Similar function to demulcents; mucilaginous
	Therapeutic effects	Used topically to protect and soothe the skin
	Example herbs	*Aloe barbadensis* (Aloe Vera); *Althaea officinalis* (Marsh Mallow); *Stellaria media* (Chickweed)
Expectorant	Description	Remove mucus from the lungs; three main categories (stimulating, soothing, and tonics)
	Therapeutic effects	Reduce cough; soothe and lubricate the respiratory tract; encourage productive coughing
	Example herbs	*Angelica archangelica* (Norwegian Angelica); *Grindelia camporum* (Great Valley Gumweed); *Hyssopus officinalis* (Hyssop)
Laxatives	Description	Often contain anthraquinone glycosides and bitters; four groups (aperients, bulk laxatives, cathartics, and purgatives)
	Therapeutic effects	Constipation
	Example herbs	*Aloe barbadensis* (Aloe Vera); *Fumaria officinalis* (Common Fumitory); *Juglans cinerea* (Butternut)
Nervines	Description	Cause a beneficial effect on the nervous system; three groups (tonics, relaxants, and stimulants)
	Therapeutic effects	Chronic stress; depression/anxiety; reduce muscle spasms
	Example herbs	*Hypericum perforatum* (St. John's Wort); *Lavandula officinalis* (English Lavender); *Piper methysticum* (Kava)
Sialagogues	Description	Considered bitters; improve digestion and appetite by increasing saliva production; can increase gastric secretions; may stimulate gastric emptying; administer 5–15 minutes before eating or with food
	Therapeutic effects	Gastrointestinal disorders; inappetance; anorexia
	Example herbs	*Acmella oleracea* (Paracress); *Echinacea purpurea* (Purple Coneflower); *Zingiber officinalis* (Ginger)
Tonics	Description	Restore vital energy; increase tissue and organ tone; often used with adaptogens; classified by the target tissue or organ
	Therapeutic effects	Cardiovascular disease; gastrointestinal disease; immune system conditions
	Example herbs	*Hydrastis canadensis* (Goldenseal); *Panax quinquefolium* (American Ginseng); *Plantago lanceolata* (Common Dandelion)

Source: Lisa P. McFaddin.

Table 11.2 Examples of herbs with an affinity for a particular organ or tissue (Hoffmann 1989; Fougère 2007).

Target organ or tissue	Herb examples
Cardiovascular	*Crataegus oxycantha* (Hawthorn Berry); *Vaccinium myrtillus* (Billberry)
Connective tissue	*Centella asiatica* (Gotu Kola); *Equisetum arvense* (Horsetail)
Dermatologic	*Arctium lappa* (Greater Burdock); *Stellaria media* (Chickweed)
Endocrine	*Glycyrrhiza glabra* (Licorice); *Panax ginseng* (Asian Ginseng)
Gastrointestinal	*Glycyrrhiza glabra* (Licorice); *Filipendula ulmaria* (Meadowsweet)
Hepatic	*Silybum marianum* (Milk Thistle); *Taraxacum officinalis* (Dandelion Root)
Hypothalamic–pituitary–ovarian regulator	*Dioscorea villosa* (Wild Yam); *Glycyrrhiza glabra* (Licorice)
Immune stimulant	*Astragalus propinquus* (Astragalus); *Uncaria tomentosa* (Cat's Claw)
Lymphatic system	*Echinacea purpurea* (Echinacea); *Phytolacca americana* (Pokeweed Root)
Mucous membrane	*Hydrastis canadensis* (Goldenseal); *Solidago* spp. (Goldenrod)
Neurologic	*Avena sativa* (Oats); Turnera diffusa (Damiana)
Pancreas	*Gymnema sylvestre* (Gymnema); *Mahonia aquifolium* (Oregon Grape)
Renal	*Astragalus propinquus* (Astragalus); *Rehmannia glutinosa* (Rehmannia)
Respiratory	*Equisetum arvense* (Horsetail); *Verbascum thapsus* (Mullen)
Thyroid	*Fucus vesiculosus* (Bladderwrack); *Plectranthus barbatus* (Forskohlii)

Source: Lisa P. McFaddin.

Table 11.3 Examples of Western herbs organized by their therapeutic effects and traditional herbal actions (Fougère 2007; Wynn and Fougère 2007e; ABC 2023, 2013).

Anticancer	
Adaptogens	*Astragalus membranaceus* (Astragalus); *Panax ginseng* (Asian Ginseng); *Withania somnifera* (Ashwagandha)
Alteratives	*Articum lappa* (Burdock); *Mahonia aquifolium* (Oregon Grape); *Taraxacum officinale* (Dandelion Root)
Antioxidants	*Camella sinensis* (Green Tea); *Curcuma longa* (Turmeric); *Silybum marianum* (Milk Thistle)
Bladder cancer	*Allium sativum* (Garlic); *Piper methysticum* (Kava)
Fibrosarcoma	*Aloe vera* (Aloe); *Artemisia annua* (Wormwood)
Hematopoietic neoplasia	*Cordyceps sinensis* (Cordyceps); *Echinacea purpurea* (Echinacea); *Uncaria tomentosa* (Cat's Claw)
Immune modulators	*Astragalus membranaceus* (Astragalus); *Echinacea purpurea* (Echinacea); *Withania somnifera* (Ashwagandha)
Neurologic neoplasia	*Aloe vera* (Aloe); *Boswellia serrata* (Boswellia); *Cannabis sativa* (Cannabis)
Oral tumors	*Camellia sinensis* (Tea); *Curcuma longa* (Turmeric); *Ginkgo biloba* (Ginkgo)
Osteosarcoma	*Phytolacca americana* (Pokeweed); *Trifolium pratense* L. (Red Clover)

(Continued)

Table 11.3 (Continued)

Anticancer	
Pulmonary neoplasia	*Camella sinensis* (Green and Black Tea); *Linum usitatissimum* (Flaxseed); *Vitis vinifera* (Grape Seed)
Renal neoplasia	*Astragalus membranaceus* (Astragalus); *Ligustrum lucidum* (Conidium); *Viscum album* (Mistletoe)
Reproductive neoplasia	*Calendula officinalis* (Calendula); *Linum usitatissimum* (Flaxseed); *Silybum marianum* (Milk Thistle)
Cardiovascular	
ACE inhibitors	*Salvia miltiorrhiza* (Dan Shen); *Tribulus terrestris* (Tribulus)
Antiarrhythmics	*Convallaria majalis* (Lily of the Valley); *Coptis chinensis* (Coptis); *Mahonia aquifolium* (Oregon Grape)
Anticoagulants	*Allium sativum* (Garlic); *Salvia miltiorrhiza* (Dan Shen)
Cardiotonic and cardioprotective	*Astragalus membranaceus* (Astragalus); *Crataegus* spp. (Hawthorn); *Ginkgo biloba* (Ginkgo); *Slenicereus grandifloras* (Cactus)
Cardioactive	*Convallaria majalis* (Lily of the Valley); *Lycopus europaeus* (Bugleweed); *Slenicereus grandifloras* (Cactus)
Circulatory stimulants	*Angelica sinensis* (Dong Quai); *Capsicum annuum* (Cayenne); *Ginkgo biloba* (Ginkgo)
Diuretics	*Petroselinum crispum* (Parsley); *Taraxacum officinalis* (Dandelion)
Hypotensives	*Allium sativum* (Garlic); *Ginkgo biloba* (Ginkgo); *Valeriana officinalis* (Valerian)
Nervines	*Leonurus cardiac* (Motherwort); *Tilia platyphyllos* (Linden); *Valeriana officinalis* (Valerian)
Dermatologic	
Adaptogens	*Bupleurum falcatum* (Bupleurum); *Glycyrhiza glabra* (Licorice); *Withania somnifera* (Ashwagandha)
Alternatives	*Articum lappa* (Burdock Root); *Mahonia aquifolium* (Oregon Grape); *Viola tricolor* (Wild Pansy)
Antiallergy	*Albizia lebbeck* (Albizia); *Glycyrrhiza glabra* (Licorice); *Urtica dioica* folia (Nettle Leaf)
Anti-inflammatory	*Bupleurum falcatum* (Bupleurum); *Curcuma longa* (Tumeric); *Oenothera biennis* (Evening Primrose Oil)
Antioxidant	*Ginkgo biloba* (Ginkgo); *Ganoderma lucidum* (Reishi); *Zingiber officinale* (Ginger)
Antipruritics	*Camellia sinensis* (Tea); *Matricaria recutita* (Chamomile)
Immune-modulating	*Astragalus membranaceus* (Astragalus); *Hemidesmus indicus* (Hemidesmus)
Nervines	*Avena sativa* (Oats); *Hypericum perforatum* (St. John's Wort); *Scutellaria lateriflora* (Skullcap)
Endocrine	
Adrenal	*Cordyceps sinensis* (Cordyceps); *Panax ginseng* (Asian Ginseng); *Withania somnifera* (Ashwagandha)
Antidiabetic	*Curcuma longa* (Turmeric); *Panax ginseng* (Asian Ginseng); *Zingiber officinale* (Ginger)
Antihyperglycemic	*Gymnema sylvestre* (Gymnema); *Panax ginseng* (Asian Ginseng); *Trigonella foenum-graecum* (Fenugreek)

Hyperglycemic	*Camellia sinensis* (Tea); *Panax ginseng* (Asian Ginseng)
Thyroid-inhibiting	*Aloe vera* (Aloe); *Lycopus virginicus* (Bugleweed); *Melissa officinalis* (Lemon Balm)
Thyroid-stimulating	*Bacopa monniera* (Brahmi); *Fucus vesiculosus* (Bladderwrack); *Withania somnifera* (Ashwagandha)
Gastrointestinal	
Antacids and antiulcer	*Curcuma longa* (Turmeric); *Filipendula ulmaria* (Meadosweet); *Vaccinium myrtillus* (Bilberry)
Antiemetics	*Ballota nigra* (Black Horehound); *Panax ginseng* (Asian Ginseng); *Zingiber officinale* (Ginger)
Anthelmintics	*Allium sativum* (Garlic); *Artemsia* spp. (Wormwood); *Inula helenium* (Elecampane)
Anti-inflammatory	*Boswellia serrata* (Boswellia); *Petasites hybridus* (Butterbur); *Matricaria recutita* (Chamomile)
Antimicrobials	*Matricaria recutita* (Chamomile); *Thymus vulgaris* (Thyme)
Antiviral	*Potentilla erecta* (Tormentil Root); *Thuja occidentalis* (Thuja)
Bitters	*Berberis aquifolium* (Oregon Grape); *Dioscorea villosa* (Wild Yam); *Gentiana lutea* (Gentian)
Carminatives and spasmolytics	*Lavandula angustifolia* (Lavender); *Mentha piperita* (Peppermint); *Pimpinella anisum* (Aniseed Oil)
Cholagogues and choleretics	*Cynara scolymus* (Artichoke); *Matricaria recutita* (Chamomile); *Taraxacum officinale* (Dandelion)
Laxatives	*Aloe barbadensis* (Aloe); *Glycyrrhiza glabra* (Licorice); *Rheum officinale* (Rhubarb)
Hematologic and immune system	
Adaptogens	*Bacopa monnieri* (Bacopa); *Cordyceps sinensis* (Cordyceps); *Panax ginseng* (American ginseng)
Anticoagulant	*Allium sativum* (Garlic); *Curcuma longa* (Curcumin); *Salvia miltiorrhiza* (Dan Shen)
Antihyperlipidemics	*Commiphora mukui* (Gugulipid); *Cynara scolymus* (Artichoke); *Monascus purpureus* (Red Yeast Rice)
Blood tonics	*Rehmannia glutinosa* (Rehmannia); *Rhodiola rosacea* (Rhodiola); *Urtica dioica* (Nettles)
Hemostatics	*Equisetum arvense* (Horsetail); *Hamamelis virginiana* (Witch Hazel); *Urtica dioica* (Stinging Nettle)
Immune modulators	*Grifola frondosa* (Maitake); *Trametes versicolor* (Turkey Tail); *Tripterygium wilfordii* (Thunder God Vine)
Hepatic	
Hepatoprotective	*Schisandra chinensis* (Schisandra); *Silybum marianum* (Milk Thistle)
Musculoskeletal	
Alternatives	*Arctium lappa* (Greater Burdock); *Iris versicolor* (Blue Flag); *Phytolacca americana* (Pokeweed)
Analgesics	*Corydalis* spp. (Corydalis); *Hypericum perforatum* (St John's Wort); *Piscidea erythrina* (Jamaican Dogwood)

(Continued)

Table 11.3 (Continued)

Musculoskeletal	
Anti-inflammatory	*Harpagophytum procumbens* (Devils' Claw); *Salix alba* (Willow Bark); *Urtica dioica* (Stinging Nettle)
Antirheumatics	*Artemisia absinthium* (Wormwood); *Mahonia aquifolium* (Oregon Grape); *Urtica dioica* (Stinging Nettle)
Circulatory stimulants	*Capsicum annuum* (Capsicum); *Zanthoxylium americanum* (Prickly Ash); *Zingiber officinale* (Ginger)
Diuretic	*Achillea millefolium* (Yarrow); *Apium graveolens* (Celery); *Eupatorium perfoliatum* (Boneset)
Nervines	*Apium graveolens* (Celery); *Piscidia erythrina* (Jamaica Dogwood); *Valeriana officinale* (Valerian)
Spasmolytics	*Actaea racemosa* (Black Cohosh); *Valeriana officinalis* (Valerian); *Viburnum opulus* (Cramp Back)
Neurologic	
Antidepressants	*Bacopa monnieri* (Bacopa); *Lavandula* spp. (Lavender); *Hypericum perforatum* (St. John's Wort)
Anxiolytic	*Eschscholzia californica* (California Poppy); *Lavandula* spp. (Lavender); *Hypericum perforatum* (St. John's Wort)
Hypnotics	*Eschscholzia californica* (California Poppy); *Humulus lupulus* (Hops); *Piper methysticum* (Kava Kava)
Nervine	*Actaea racemosa* (Black Cohosh); *Humulus lupulus* (Hops); *Withania somnifera* (Ashwagandha)
Pain	
Adaptogens	*Panax ginseng* (Asian Ginseng); *Schisandra chinensis* (Schisandra); *Withania somnifera* (Ashwagandha)
Analgesics	*Corydalis* spp. (Corydalis); *Dioscorea viliosa* (Wild Yam); *Lavandula officinalis* (Lavender)
Anticonvulsants	*Gelsemium sempervirens* (Gelsemium); *Hypericum perforatum* (St. John's Wort); *Scutellaria laterifolia* (Skullcap)
Reproductive	
Anti-inflammatories	*Dioscorea villosa* (Wild Yam); *Paeonia lactiflora* (White Peony)
Emmenagogues	*Artemisia vulgaris* (Mugwort); *Mitchella repens* (Partridgeberry); *Ruta graveolens* (Rue)
Endocrine modulators	*Actaea racemosa* (Black Cohosh); *Foeniculum vulgare* (Fennel); *Salvia miltiorrhiza* (Dan Shen)
Galactagogues	*Foeniculum vulgare* (Fennel); *Galega officinalis* (Goat's Rue); *Vitex anguscastus* (Chaste Tree)
Nervine and antispasmodic	*Actaea racemosa* (Black Cohosh); *Viburnum prenifolium* (Black Haw)
Uterine astringents	*Alchemilla vulgaris* (Ladie's mantle); *Capsella bursa-pastoris* (Shepherd's Purse); *Geranium maculatum* (Cranesbill)
Uterine relaxants	*Caulophyllum thalictroides* (Blue Cohosh); *Viburnum opulus* (Cramp Bark)
Uterine tonics	*Angelica sinensis* (Dong Quai); *Chamaelirum luteum* (False Unicorn Root); *Rubus idaeus* (Raspberry)

Respiratory	
Anti-inflammatory and antiallergic	*Boswellia serrata* (Boswellia); *Perilla frutescens* (Perilla Seed); *Urtica dioica* (Stinging Nettle)
Antitussive	*Arctium lappa* (Burdock); *Glycyrrhiza glabra* (Licorice); *Prunus serotine* (Wild Cherry Bark)
Demulcent	*Althaea officinalis* (Marshmallow); *Plantago major* (English Plantain); *Ulmus fulva* (Slippery Elm)
Expectorant	*Lobella inflate* (Lobella); *Polygala senega* (Senega Snakeroot); *Sanguinaria canadensis* (Bloodroot)
Spasmolytic	*Ephedra sinica* (Ephedra); *Grindelia* spp. (Grindelia); *Thymus vulgaris* (Thyme)
Urinary tract	
Anti-inflammatory	*Piper methysticum* (Kava)
Antilithics	*Hydrangea arborescens* (Hydrangea); *Trigonella foenum-graecum* (Fenugreek); *Zea mays* (Corn Silk)
Antimicrobial	*Agathosma betulina* (Buchu); *Solidago viraurea* (Goldenrod); *Vaccinium macrocarpa* (Cranberry)
Bladder tonics	*Crataeva nurvala* (Crataeva)
Diuretics	*Apium graveolens* (Celery); *Petroselinum crispum* (Parsley); *Urtica dioica* (Stinging Nettle)
Renal protective	*Astragalus membranaceus* (Astragalus); *Cordyceps sinensis* (Cordyceps); *Oenothera biennis* (Evening Primrose)
Spasmolytics	*Cucurbita pepo* (Pumpkin Seed); *Viburnum opulus* (Cramp Bark)

ACE, angiotensin-converting enzyme. Source: Lisa P. McFaddin.

Table 11.4 The categories of information, with their descriptions, comprising most herbal monographs. The categories are listed in the most common order found within the monographs (Klein 2007; Wynn and Fougère 2007e).

Category	Description
Common name	The most common name as defined by the United States Department of Agriculture (USDA) Natural Resources Conservation Service (NRCS) Plant Database (https://plants.usda.gov/home) (NRCS 2023)
Botanical name	Scientific name, including genus and species, as defined by the USDA NRCS Plant Database (https://plants.usda.gov/home) (NRCS 2023)
Distribution	Helps identify locally available, invasive, and endangered plant species
Similar species	Used if multiple species within the same genus can be used
Other names	Often a plant has more than one common name
Family	Taxonomic classification as defined by the USDA NRCS Plant Database (https://plants.usda.gov/home) (NRCS 2023)
Parts used	Portions of the plant typically used in herbal formulations
Collection	Tips for harvesting plants
Selected constituents	Lists the most active secondary metabolites with therapeutic benefit found within the plant

(Continued)

Table 11.4 (Continued)

Category	Description
Clinical actions	Traditional therapeutic actions
Historical use	A brief lineage of the plant's medicinal use in human history
Energetics	Pertains the herb's taste properties and often references information pertaining to traditional Chinese medical applications
Research	Summarizes studies conducted using the herb
Indications	Traditional medical applications or conditions benefiting from use of the herb
Suggested veterinary indications	Traditional and integrative applications or conditions benefiting from use of the herb based on evidence-based medicine
Notes of interest	Miscellaneous pertinent information

Contraindications
Toxicology
Adverse effects
Drug interactions
	BSH safety grades:
	• **Class 1**: Herbs safely consumed when used appropriately
	• **Class 2**: Herbs with specific use restrictions:
	  - **2a** = External use only
	  - **2b** = Do not consume when pregnant
	  - **2c** = Do not consume when nursing
	  - **2d** = Other restrictions when noted
	• **Class 3**: Herbs to be used under expert supervision. Herbs often have the following labeling "To be used only under the supervision of an expert qualified in the appropriate use of this substance"
	• **Class 4**: Herbs with insufficient data available preventing classification
	
	BSH interaction classes:
	• **Class A**: Herbs with no clinically relevant interactions
	• **Class B**: Herbs with potential clinically relevant interactions
	• **Class C**: Herbs with known clinically relevant interactions
	(AHPA 2013)

Preparation notes	If specific preparation affects the herbal efficacy
Dosage	Small animal and human dosage suggestions
Combinations	This section may be included where specific combinations greatly benefit herbal efficacy
References	List of selected references used to compile the information found within the monograph

BSH, Botanical Safety Handbook. Source: Lisa P. McFaddin.

monographs can be found in the Veterinarians section. Additionally, the following websites are fantastic resources: American Botanical Council (http://www.cms.herbalgram.org), Herbal Medicines Compendium (http://www.hmc.usp.org/monographs/all), and Veterinary Botanical Medical Association (www.vbma.org).

Diagnoses

As with other modalities of veterinary integrative medicine (VIM), the patient's age, breed predilections, environment, lifestyle, diet, and concurrent illnesses are all taken into account when formulating a treatment plan.

Table 11.5 Herbal monograph for Ginger root (*Zingiberis officinale* rhizome).

Common name	Ginger root
Botanical name	*Zingiberis officinale* rhizome
Distribution	Native to Southeast Asia. Cultivated in almost all tropical and subtropical countries, especially China, India, Nigeria, Australia, Jamaica, and Haiti. China and India are the world's leading producers (ABC 2000)
Similar species	n/a
Other names	African Ginger, Common Ginger, Jamaica Ginger, Gan Jiang (dried rhizome), Sheng Jiang (fresh rhizome)
Family	Zingiberaceae
Parts used	Rhizome
Collection	Peeled, finger-long, fresh or dried rhizome, and its preparations (ABC 1990)
Selected constituents	"Ginger rhizome contains oleoresin (4.0–7.5%) composed of non-volatile pungent principles (phenols such as gingerols and their related dehydration products shogaols), non-pungent substances (fats and waxes), and volatile oils; volatile oil (1.0–3.3%), of which 30–70% are sesquiterpenes, mainly β-bisabolene, (−)-zingiberene, β-sesquiphellandrene, and (+)-ar-curcumene, and monoterpenes, mainly geranial and neral; carbohydrates, mainly starch (40–60%); proteins (9–10%); lipids (6–10%) composed of triglycerides, phosphatidic acid, lecithins, and free fatty acids; vitamins niacin and A; minerals; and amino acids (Bradley 1992; Bruneton 1995; Budavari 1996; Chrubasik et al. 2005; Leung and Foster 1996; Newall et al. 1996; Wichtl and Bisset 1994)." (ABC 2000) There are numerous phenolic (gingerols, shogaols, paradols, polyphenols, quercetin, zingerone, gingerenone-A, and 6-dehydrogingerdione) and terpene (β-bisabolene, α-curcumene, zingiberene, α-farnesene, and β-sesquiphellandrene) compounds in ginger (Schadich et al. 2016; Yeh et al. 2014; Mao et al. 2019)
Clinical actions	Carminative, antispasmodic, anti-inflammatory, antiplatelets, and diaphorectic (Wynn and Fougère 2007c)
Historical use	"Ginger has been used as a medicine since ancient times, recorded in early Sanskrit and Chinese texts and ancient Greek, Roman, and Arabic medical literature (Bone 1997). In Asian medical practices, dried ginger has been used as a drug to treat stomachache, diarrhea, and nausea for thousands of years. It is traditionally prepared in aqueous decoctions and infusions (Bruneton 1995; But 1997; Kapoor 1990; Leung and Foster 1996). In Africa, dried ginger is used much as it is in Asia (GHP 1992; Iwu 1990). Today, ginger is official in the national pharmacopeias of Austria, China, Egypt, Germany, Great Britain, Japan, and Switzerland (BP 1988; Bradley 1992; DAB 1997; JP 1993; Newall et al. 1996; ÖAB 1981–1983; Ph.Helv 1987; Tu 1992). Chinese pharmacopeia lists ginger for epigastric pain with cold feeling, vomiting and diarrhea accompanied by cold extremities and faint pulse, dyspnea, and cough with copious frothy expectoration (Tu 1992). The Ayurvedic Pharmacopeia specifically recommends ginger for flatulent intestinal colic (Karnick 1994)." (ABC 2000)
Energetics	Hot and dry (Wynn and Fougère 2007c)
Indications and research	*For the purposes of this monograph the indications have been combined with the supporting research.* The primary indications center around ginger's anti-emetic and anti-nausea (especially with pregnancy and chemotherapy) effects (Giacosa et al. 2015; Bodagh et al. 2018; Kim et al. 2022). Given the sheer volume of studies conducted on ginger meta-analyses and systematic reviews of pre-existing research are cited. Other cited indications include anti-inflammatory, antioxidant, antitumor, and antiulcer (ABC 1990; Wynn and Fougère 2007d; ABC 2000).

(Continued)

Table 11.5 (Continued)

Suggested veterinary indications	Anti-nausea, adjunct treatment for dirofilariasis, adjunct treatment for osteoarthritis, and improving circulation (especially non-ambulatory and geriatric patients) (Wynn and Fougère 2007c; Sharma et al. 1997; Merawin et al. 2010; Javdani et al. 2021)
Contraindications	Gallstones (ABC 1990, 2000)
Adverse effects and toxicology	None known. Fresh herb safety Class I and dried herb Class 2d (ABC 2000)
Drug interactions	None known (ABC 2000).
Preparation notes	"Chopped or comminuted rhizome and dry extracts for teas, other galenical preparations for internal use" (ABC 1990)
Dosage	Dried herb 15–200 mg/kg divided daily (Wynn and Fougère 2007c)
References	Included throughout the monograph

Source: Lisa P. McFaddin.

WHM Diagnosis for Veterinarians

WHM diagnoses are historically rooted in the concepts of the vital force, humoral theory, and physiomedicalism (Fougère 2007). **Vitalism** is based on the concept that all living beings are born with a "vital force," the energy coursing through their bodies (Fougère 2007). The vital force is crucial for survival and prosperity of the being, both physical and emotional. This concept is known as Qi in TCM. Refer to Chapters 1–3 for further information on TCM.

Humoral theory states the blood consists of Four Humors: Melancholic Humor (Black Bile), Phlegmatic Humor (Phlegm), Choleric Humor (Bile), and Sanguine Humor (Blood) (Fougère 2007). Homeostasis is achieved when all Four Humors are balanced, while disease results from an imbalance amongst the Four Humors.

Physiomedicalism is an herbal medicinal system based on the treatment of a patient's underlying condition. Resolution of the underlying condition would restore patient vitality, normalizing all body systems and functions, through the application of detoxification, improving circulation, ANS balance, and tissue function restoration (Fougère 2007).

WHM diagnoses are also based on the energetics of the patient (and disease) as well as the organ(s) affected. For example, is the patient weak (deficient) or excessive (often acute)? Is the patient hot or cold? What organ(s) is/are most affected? Answers to these questions guide herbal formula selection.

Figure 11.2 provides an example of a diagnostic algorithm for WHM based on viewing the disease condition from three perspectives: problem duration, energetics, and body system(s) effected. The length of the condition is divided into acute (excess) or chronic (deficiency). Energetics can refer to the presence of hot signs (think heat stroke), cold signs (think hypothyroid dog), moist signs (think infection), and dry signs (think old hyperthyroid cat). Conditions can contain multiple energies such as hot and moist or hot and dry. Finally, like traditional medicine, the affected organ(s) (body system) is determined to help focus where the herb needs to have the most beneficial effects.

Examples of the steps involved in modern physiomedicalism are outlined in Table 11.6. Keep in mind these concepts are complex and require advanced training to fully understand and utilize. The purpose of presenting this information here is to highlight the intricacies of WHM.

Regulation

The regulation of herbs and herbal formulas is discussed in detail in Chapter 3. A summary of the information is provided here.

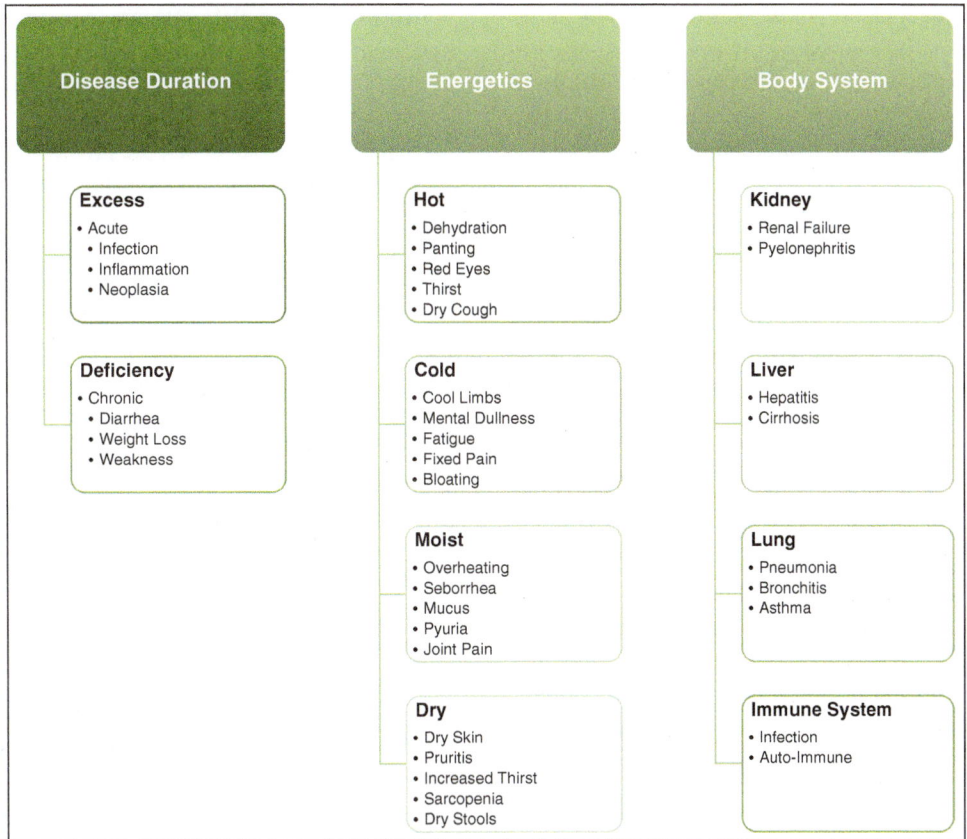

Figure 11.2 Example of diagnostic algorithms used is veterinary Western herbal medicine. Source: Lisa P. McFaddin.

Table 11.6 The steps comprising modern physiomedicalism.

Steps	Description	Example herbal categories
Physiologic enhancement	Utilizes diet, exercise, and environment to restore patient vitality	
	Primary focus = improve nutrition and detoxification	Bitters; cholagogues; hepatorestoratives; depuratives; laxatives
	Secondary focus = improve energy levels and the ability to cope with stress	Tonics; adaptogens
Physiologic compensation	Focuses therapy on correction of imbalances: overstimulation, deficiencies, and symptom relief	Anti-inflammatories; antispasmodics; antiviral anti-allergy; etc.
Treatment of underlying condition	Determine the underlying cause and treat accordingly. Causes can be divided into: predisposing, excitatory, and perpetuating	Dependent on the cause being treated
Patient specific	Ensure the herb choice is appropriate for the patient and their problems	Example = do not use warm herbs for hot patients

Source: Fougère (2007) with permission of Elsevier.

The regulation of herbs and herbal formulas is most influenced by their categorization and target consumer (human or animal). An herb or herbal formula may meet the definition of a drug, herbal drug, or dietary supplement.

Drugs

Drugs are defined as substances used to diagnose, cure, treat, or prevent disease in both humans and animals, as well as alter the body's functions or structure (FDA 2021c). The FDA does not develop or test products before approving them (FDA 2020, 2021b).

> "Manufacturers must … prove they are able to make the drug product according to federal quality standards … (and] FDA experts review the results of laboratory, animal, and human clinical testing done by manufacturers. If FDA grants an approval, it means the agency has determined that the benefits of the product outweigh the known risks for the intended use" (FDA 2020, 2021b).

Botanical Drugs

The FDA defines a botanical drug as a product "intended for use in the diagnosis, cure, mitigation, treatment or prevention of disease in humans." As of October 2022, there are two approved herbal drugs for human use.

Human Dietary Supplements

All herbs and herbal formulas marketed for human consumption are classified as dietary supplements. Dietary supplements are defined as substances which complement the diet and contain at least one of the following ingredients: a vitamin, a mineral, an herb, an amino acid, or a product which affects caloric intake (DSHEA 1994). Within the provisions established by The Dietary Supplement Health and Education Act (DSHEA) of 1994, an amendment to The United States Federal Food, Drug and Cosmetic Act (FDCA, Title 21) dietary supplements were classified as a separate regulatory category of food; in other words, dietary supplements are not considered food or drug.

Almost all dietary supplements are considered over the counter (OTC). FDA approval is not required to market or sell the products. The FDA is only responsible for ensuring the safety of supplements if there is gross risk of illness, inadequate evidence regarding product safety, or a supplement is adulterated (DSHEA 1994). The FDA does not regulate the development, manufacturing, or marketing of dietary supplements.

The FDA does specify what information pertaining to health claims can be made. Health claims assert a relationship between a particular substance and its ability to diagnose, treat, cure, or prevent disease. The FDA may approve health claims if there is enough scientific evidence supporting the correlation (FDA 2018).

In the December 2006 Draft Guidance, the FDA released a "Guidance for industry on complementary and alternative medicine (CAM) products and their regulation by the FDA" in response to an increasing number of CAM products and public confusion regarding the regulation of said products. Depending on how the herbal product is marketed and labeled it may be considered a dietary supplement, food, or drug. Dietary supplements receive very little to no FDA oversight. Food substances must meet the requirements defined by the Federal Food, Drug, and Cosmetic Act (FDCA, Title 21). If the herbal product is marketed or used to treat disease, then it is considered a "drug" and must meet the requirements defined by the FDCA (Title 21).

Animal Dietary Supplements

Animal supplements are considered food or food additives. According to the National Animal Supplement Council (NASC) there are over 400 unapproved substances marketed for use in animals (Grassie 2002).

The FDCA does not require pre-market FDA approval before new animal food is sold. The FDCA does require "that food for animals, like food for people, be safe to eat, produced under sanitary conditions, free of harmful substances, and truthfully labeled" (FDA 2021c).

The FDCA (Title 21) does require pre-market approval for animal food additives. Food additives are defined as "any substance that directly or indirectly becomes a component of a food or that affects a food's characteristics" (FDA 2021a,c). Substances generally recognized as safe (GRAS) are exempt from the pre-market approval requirements (FDA 2021a,c).

The FDA's Center for Veterinary Medicine (CVM) is responsible for regulating animal food products, including many botanicals. Failure of a food to meet the requirements outlined in the FDCA (Title 21) results in the food (or in this case the botanical) classified as adulterated or misbranded. The reality is a lot of botanicals used in veterinary medicine are considered unapproved food additives or unapproved animal drugs, and the FDA could take regulatory action (Burns 2017). Often the regulation of botanicals is low on the priority list for FDA regulators.

To summarize, an herb or herbal formula marketed as a food, containing ingredients with known and approved nutritional value, does not need CVM pre-market approval. An herb or herbal formula marketed as a food with unknown or unapproved ingredients requires CVM pre-market approval.

Production

The FDA does not approve manufacturing companies. "Owners and operators of domestic and foreign food, drug, and most device facilities must register their facilities with FDA, unless an exemption applies. FDA does have authority to inspect regulated facilities to verify that they comply with applicable good manufacturing practice regulations" (FDA 2017).

There appears to be room for error when it comes to manufacturing and bottling herbs. This highlights the importance of utilizing and recommending herbal products from trusted sources. Factors to consider when selecting a manufacturer include the existence of a seed to

seal guarantee, adherence to good manufacturing practices (GMP), existence of quality control measures, and potentially a seal of approval from a recognized third party (ConsumerLab, National Animal Supplement Council, or the United States Pharmacopeia). See Chapters 3 and 4 for further information on the production of botanicals.

Herbal Formulations

Several factors should be considered when dispensing an herb, including the use of an individual herb compared to a combination of herbs (formula), preparation, and dosing.

Individual Herb versus Formula

There are times when single herbs are chosen or added to pre-made formulas, but for the most part herbal formulas are preferred. Herbal formulas epitomize the saying "the sum is greater than the parts." While each herb has its own unique characteristics and beneficial properties, together herbal formulas can exact a greater effect on the patient.

Preparation

Western herbs are dispensed mostly in three forms: dried herbs (powdered), dried extract, and liquid extract. Powdered herbs are made from dried bulk herbs and can be administered as a loose powder or in capsules. Dried bulk herbs can be "concentrated by simmering in water removing the residue, and spraying the concentrated 'tea' in a vacuum chamber, resulting in powder or granules of remaining concentrated herbal constituents" (Wynn and Fougère 2007b). Liquid extracts are a concentrated liquid created by extracting bulk herbs in either boiling water or over a long period of time in alcohol, vinegar, or glycerin (Wynn and Fougère 2007b).

Dosage

Factors affecting herbal dosing include the formulation, route of administration, frequency of administration, bioavailability (i.e. how well it is absorbed by the body), patient signalment (age, breed, and sex), concurrent illnesses, concurrent medications, supplements, and herbs, clinical experience, and clinical studies (when available) (Wynn and Fougère 2007b). Ultimately the clinician is responsible for determining the appropriate dose for each patient.

Formulations for Veterinarians

The copious botanical metabolites found within each plant are responsible for the plethora of potential therapeutic actions. This complex chemical matrix results in nonlinear healing, meaning one plant can cause both local and systemic effects within the patient (Niemeyer et al. 2013).

Individual herbs are chosen based on the patient's needs and their chemical and therapeutic attributes. The creation, or selection, of herbal formulas is dependent on the patient, the chemical and therapeutic properties of the individual herbs, and the combined actions and interactions of the herbs when mixed together (Gonora 2015).

The American Herbalist Guild (2015) recommends herbal formulas be created to balance each individual herb's energetics and actions with the patient's temperament and problem. Herbs should be paired to modify and improve their individual actions (Gonora 2015). The science and practice of properly creating and balancing herbal formulas is an advanced technique, requiring additional training. To demonstrate the complexity, Table 11.7 provides several example strategies for creating herbal formulas.

Like pharmaceutical agents there is often a dose range. To avoid adverse effects patients are often started on a lower dose then slowly increased to the most effective dose for the patient. There are numerous herbal dosing strategies, most extrapolated from human dosing. The most common methods include drop dosing, manufacturer dosing, and proportionate dosing. Drop dosing is a low-dose method used for liquid preparations. One to two drops of herbal tincture are administered per two pounds of body weight, regardless of the extract concentration. This technique assumes that 1 ml equals 20–30 drops and tinctures are at least a 1 : 5 ratio of diluent to herb (Wynn and Fougère 2007b).

Each manufacturer has their own recommended dosing chart based on the herbal formula's concentration and patient weight.

Table 11.7 Example strategies used by Western herbal medicine practitioners when devising herbal formulas. The name or type of pairing strategy, its description, and an example herbal formula are provided.

Pairing strategy	Description	Example herbal formula
Circulatory stimulation	Improves the distribution and systemic effect of the herbs	Single herb (simples) + Ginger (*Zingiber officinale*)
Amplification	Two herbs with similar functions or actions	*Immunity support*: Astragalus (*Astragalus propinquus*) + Reishi (*Ganoderma lucidum*)
Steering	Using the action of one herb to heighten the action of another	*Liver tonic*: Agrimony (*Agrimonia eupatoria*) + Dandelion (*Taraxacum officinale*)
Balancing	The energetic properties of each balance one another	*Neutral thermal property*: Yellow Gentian (*Gentiana lutea*) + Ginger (*Zingiber officinale*)
Patient constitution	Use an herb to address the patient's condition	Golden seal (*Hydrastis Canadensis*) + Myrrh (*Commiphora myrrha*) are drying
		Adding a moistening herb, comfrey (*Symphytum* spp.), allows use of the formula in a dry patient

Source: adapted from Gonora (2015).

Different concentrations aside, some manufacturers provide more conservative dosing instructions than others. Finally, proportionate dosing is based on human dosing structure determined by the efficacy, toxicity, and clinical trials of herbal tinctures. Ultimately the dose is determined by the veterinarian on a case-by-case basis.

Safety

Safety concerns surrounding should focus on two concepts: adverse effects and herb–drug interactions.

Adverse Effects

Adverse effects (AEs), also known as side effects, are defined as any unwanted and harmful outcome caused by a drug or supplement. Like pharmaceuticals, a severity scale is often used when discussing AEs, mild to severe. Severe AEs can be considered a form of toxicity.

Given the sheer number of herbs and herbal formulas, the exact incidence of AEs is unknown. In a systematic review conducted by Di Lorenzo et al. (2015), 492 studies comprising a total of 66 botanical ingredients, of which 27 had no reported AEs. The two most cited plants were *Glycine max* (soybean) and *Glycyrrhiza glabra* (licorice). AEs of soybean were typically allergic reactions and hormone-like activity (phytoestrogens), while licorice caused low potassium (hypokalemia) and high blood pressure (hypertension) due to its glycyrrhetic acid content (Di Lorenzo et al. 2015). The authors drew the following conclusions:

"(1) Cases of adverse effects of botanicals are numerous, in term of citations by scientific literature or phytovigilance centers, but an assessment according to the WHO criteria indicates that the number of those with adequate evidence for a causal relationship is significantly less. (2) Given the long period of time considered and the number of plants included in the review, the occurrence of adverse effects of botanical ingredients is relatively low. (3) The number of severe clinical reactions is very limited, but some fatal cases have been described. (4) It is important to recognize that an underestimation is also possible, for the following reasons: (i) the consumer usually considers botanicals as safe products and does not report their use if they are admitted to hospital or emergency service; (ii) as they use PFS at their own discretion, consumers could avoid informing the family doctor, fearing a reprimand; (iii) data collected by poison centers are published only in a relatively few cases" (Di Lorenzo et al. 2015).

The 4Rs can be used to reduce the risk of AEs: right herb, right patient, right patient purpose, and right dose. The **right herb** refers to using trusted manufacturers and choosing the correct formulation of the herb. The **right patient** means the practitioner should ensure the use of botanicals is appropriate for the patient (consider their age, existing medical conditions, and concurrent medications, supplements, or herbs). The **right purpose** refers to the reason for using the herb(s), i.e. will this help or hinder this patient? The **right dose** is just that: does the recommended dose match the patient's needs? Sometimes a lower or even higher dosage is required. Additionally, the recommended treatment length should be considered.

Adverse Effects for Veterinarians

It is beyond the scope of this book to discuss every potential AE associated with all herbs and herbal formulas used in veterinary WHM. Table 11.8 provides examples of several herbs with known toxic potential, as well as methods to reduce the risk of toxicity.

There are additional studies highlighting the potential AEs associated with herbs in both people and animals. In a review of 50 systemtic reviews evaluating 50 different individual

Table 11.8 Examples of herbs with known toxic potential, descriptions of the clinical signs of toxicity, and methods to reduce the risk of toxicity (Poppenga 2007; Xie 2011b; Chen and Chen 2012; Marsden 2014).

Aconite (*Aconitum* spp.)	TCS	CV = arrythmias, angina, hypotension
		GI = nausea, vomiting, abdominal pain, diarrhea
	TR	Use only prepared herb; use lowest effective dose; do not use during pregnancy
Aloe (*Aloe vera*)	TCS	GI = (when ingested) irritant, nausea, intestinal cramping
		NS = numbness and weakness of the limbs, numbness of the face
	TR	Topical use primarily; use dried juice or resin if ingested
Aristolochia (*Aristolochia* spp.)	TCS	IS = carcinogenic, mutagenic
		RS = nephrotoxic
	TR	Use not recommended; can be found as a contaminant
Blue-green algae	TCS	HS = hepatoxic
		NS = neurotoxic
	TR	Use not recommended; *Spirulina* is a safe blue-green algae but can be contaminated with mercury
Cardiac glycosides	TCS	CV = arrhythmias
		GI = cramping, nausea
		NS = dizziness, weakness, muscle tremors, miosis
	TR	Use is generally not recommended; use only under direct veterinary supervision
	Examples	*Digitalis* spp., *Nerium oleander*, *Thevetia peruviana*, *Convallaria majalis*, *Taxus brevifolia*, *Strophanthus* spp., *Acokanthera* spp., and *Urginea maritma*
Chapparal (*Larrea tridentate*)	TCS	DS = contact dermatitis
		IS = carcinogenic
		HS = hepatotoxic
	TR	Use not recommended
Comfrey (*Symphytum* spp.)	TCS	HS = hepatoxocity
	TR	Ingestion is not recommended; can be used topically in people, but high risk of ingestion in animals
Ephedra (*Ephedra* spp.)	TCS	CV = hypertension, tachycardia
		GI = nausea, vomiting, abdominal pain
		NS = restlessness, irritability, excitement, hypersensitivity
	TR	Avoid use in pregnancy or weak or debilitated patients; use caution with patients with neurologic conditions; illegal to use in the United States
Garlic (*Allium sativum*)	TCS	DS = local irritation
		GI = vomiting, nausea, burning of the mouth, esophagus, and stomach
		IS = anemia
		NS = sweating, dizziness
	TR	Use under direct veterinary supervision; small amounts may be tolerated; avoid use in cats

Kava Kava (*Piper methysticum*)	TCS	HS = hepatotoxicity
	TR	Use under direct veterinary supervision; limit use to less than three months; potential herb–drug interactions
Pokeweed (*Phytolacca* spp.)	TCS	CV = hypotension
		GI = severe cramping, nausea, emesis, diarrhea
		NS = weakness, spasms, seizures
		RS = dyspnea
	TR	All parts of the plant are toxic; mature leaves and fruit are less toxic

Spp., species; TCS, clinical signs of toxicity; TR, toxicity reduction; CV, cardiovascular; GI, gastrointestinal; NS, neurologic; IS, immune system; RS, renal system; HS, hepatic system; DS, dermatologic system. Source: Lisa P. McFaddin.

herbal medicines, Posadzki et al. (2013) found that most of the systemtic reviews (62%, 31 of the 50) concluded the herbal medicines were safe; 30% (15 of 50) noted moderately severe AEs, and 8% (4 of 50) indicated the studied herbal medicine was not safe (Posadzki et al. 2013). The AEs ranged from mild to severe. Mild AEs included pain, allergic reaction, burning sensation, constipation, dermatitis, diarrhea, dizziness, drowsiness, dry mouth, fatigue, gastrointestinal update, headache, loss of appetite, muscle spasms, muscle weakness, nausea, rash, sleep disorders, and vomiting; severe AEs included acute psychosis, cerebral hemorrhage, death, coma, respiratory arrest, tachycardia, hallucinations, convulsions, rhabdomyolysis and renal failure, acute lung injury, hemorrhage, circulation failure, hepatitis, hyperkalemia, liver damage, nephrotoxicity, hyperkalemia, cirrhosis, liver failure, stroke, acute myocardial infarction, congestive heart failure, severe multiorgan hypoxic injury, carcinoma, gastrointestinal perforation, and seizures (Posadzki et al. 2013).

While the authors did evaluate 50 different herbal medicines, only a single systematic review was used for each herbal medicine. Herbal formulas with more than one herbal medicine were excluded. Additionally, the authors noted the quality of the methods in several studies was not optimal. The authors did conclude in general that the AEs of the studied herbal medicines were mild (Posadzki et al. 2013).

A five-year toxicological study in London, performed by Shaw et al. (1997), found that of the 1297 symptomatic enquires associated with both food supplements and traditional herbal remedies, 60% (785) experienced suspected or confirmed AEs. The overall public health risk was considered low, but several serious AE were associated with specific remedies, including a CHM for skin (liver disease), royal jelly and propolis (allergic reactions), and remedies from the Indian subcomtinent (heavy metal poisoning) (Shaw et al. 1997).

Haller et al. (2008) worked with the FDA Center for Food Safety and Nutrition (CFSAN) to conduct a one-year prospective surveillance study of dietary supplement-related poison control center calls in 2006. There were 275 dietary supplement-related calls, with 66% likely related to supplement use. Most of the AEs were considered minor. The toxic effects were most likely due to ingestion of caffeine- and yohimbe-containing products (Haller et al. 2008). Yobimbe (*Pausinystalia johimbe*) is an evergreen tree native to central and western Africa. The plant was traditionally used as an aphrodisiac and enhancer of sexual performance (NCCIH 2020). The primary compound believed responsible for its beneficial effects is yohimbine. There is a standardized prescription pharmaceutical form of yohimbine hydrochloride available in the United States. Yohimbe has been associated with heart attacks and seizures and is banned in many countries due to inaccurate labeling and potential toxicity (NCCIH 2020).

Herb–Drug Interactions

An herb–drug interaction (HDI) is any modification to the use, effect, efficacy, or mechanism of action of a prescription medication by an herbal substance, or vice versa (Pasi 2013). The modification may result in a beneficial, undesirable, or negative (harmful) effect. It is crucial the practitioner be aware of, and know how to research, potential HDIs. How the herbs and drug move through the body (pharmacokinetics) and function within the body (pharmacodynamics) explain how and why HDIs may occur. Table 11.9 provides examples of five potential HDIs. Table 3.26 in Chapter 3 lists additional HDI examples.

HDIs for Veterinarians

Pharmacokinetics is "the study of how the body interacts with administered substances for the entire duration of exposure" (Grogan and

Table 11.9 Examples of five potential herb–drug interactions (Xie 2011b; Fasinu et al. 2012; Chen 2013; Pasi 2013; Bhadra et al. 2015). Examples of individual herbs, their common use, drugs with which they may interact, and their mechanism(s) of action are provided.

Allium sativum (Garlic)	Common uses	Hyperlipidemia (high blood lipids), antimicrobial, anthelmintic, reduces blood clots, lower blood pressure
	Drug interaction candidates	Anticoagulants (warfarin), antiplatelet agents
	Mechanisms of action	Inhibits platelet aggregation, additive anticoagulant and antiplatelet effects, induces CYP and P-glycoprotein
Curcuma longa (Tumeric)	Common uses	Anti-inflammatory, antioxidant, support the immune system
	Drug interaction candidates	Aspirin
	Mechanisms of action	May potentiate antiplatelet activity
Ginkgo biloba (Ginkgo)	Common uses	Reduces behavioral disturbances (CCD, anxiety), retinal injuries, lung disease or injury, spinal cord injuries, clots
	Drug interaction candidates	Acetaminophen, aspirin
		Drugs reducing or affecting the seizure threshold (antiepileptic medications, oral flea and tick medications, antidepressants or anxiolytics)
	Mechanisms of action	Increased bleeding time due to antiplatelet activity
		Reduces seizure threshold
Hypericum perforatum (St. John's Wort)	Common uses	Mood stabilizer, reduces anxiety, reduces fear-based aggression
	Drug interaction candidates	Fluoxetine, sertraline, tramadol, trazodone
		Digoxin
		Clopidogrel
		Tacrolimus

	Mechanisms of action	Increases serotonin levels
		Induces P-glycoprotein reducing serum digoxin levels
		Induces CYP decreasing platelet clumping
		Induces CYP lowering blood levels
Vaccinium macrocarpon (Cranberry Fruit Extract)	Common uses	Supports the immune system, lowers blood sugar, reduces occurrence of UTI
	Drug interaction candidates	Any drug heavily metabolized by the liver (especially using CYP)
	Mechanisms of action	Inhibits CYP enzymes affecting drug metabolism and blood levels

CCD, canine cognitive dysfunction; CYP, cytochrome P450; UTI, urinary tract infections. Source: Lisa P. McFaddin.

Table 11.10 Examples of the mechanisms through which herbs can potentially affect the pharmacokinetics of medications including the absorption, metabolism, and excretion. Botanical examples and supporting literature (systematic reviews and clinical trials) are provided for each action.

Action	Herbal examples	Research
Absorption		
Decreased by soluble fiber such as those in tannins	*Cinnamomum* spp. (Cinnamon); *Punica granatum* (Pomegranate); *Rheum officinale* (Rheubarb)	Blumenthal (2000), Pasi (2013)
Decreased by insoluble fibers	*Plantago psyllium* (Psyllium)	
Metabolism		
Inhibition of cytochrome P450 which can increase serum drug concentrations	*Citrus paradisi* (Grapefruit); *Hydrastis canadensis* (Goldenseal); *Hypericum perforatum* (St. John's Wort)	Bailey and Dresser (2004), Wanwimolruk and Prachayasittikul (2014)
Elimination		
Altered renal elimination	*Glycyrrhiza glabra* (Licorice); *Juniperus communis* (Juniper); *Levisticum officinale* (Parsley)	Fasinu et al. (2012)

Source: Lisa P. McFaddin.

Preuss 2022). Pharmacodynamics is "the study of a drug's molecular, biochemical, and physiologic effects or actions" (Marino et al. 2023). Pharmacokinetics and pharmacodynamics help explain the mechanism of action behind HDIs. Specifically, pharmacokinetics describes how the HDI affects each substance's absorption, distribution, metabolism, and elimination throughout the body (Poppenga 2007; Chen and Chen 2012). Table 11.10 provides examples of the pharmacokinetics of several herbal substances.

Pharmacodynamics explains how the HDI can be synergistic, additive, or antagonistic through its effect on the organ systems, receptors, and enzymes (Pasi 2013). *Ginkgo biloba* (Ginkgo) should be administered with caution to patients on anticoagulants due to the potential negative synergistic effects. Ginkgo can alter platelet function, primarily through its flavonoid, ginkgolides, and ginkgolic acid content (Yagmur et al. 2005). Alternatively, *Zingiber officinale* (Ginger) can have positive synergistic effects with antiemetic drugs due to its ability to reduce nausea and vomiting, primarily through its zingerone and gingerol content (Lala et al. 2004).

Unfortunately, HDIs are still understudied due in large part to the sheer number of potential botanical–pharmaceutical combinations, underreporting of adverse effects, and lack of communication between the client/patient and clinician (human and veterinary). In one prospective study by Haller et al. (2008) of the 275 dietary supplement-related calls, six cases involved suspected HDIs including co-ingestion of yombine and buproprion (one case), yomhimbe and methamphetamine (three cases), nonsteroidal anti-inflammatories (NSAIDs) and fish oil (one case), and NSAIDs and ginkgo (one case).

The Why

Applications in Human Medicine

Analysis of the results from the 2015 National Consumer Survey on the Medication Experience and Pharmacists' Roles showed more than 33% of respondents use herbal supplements (Rashrash et al. 2017). Additionally, the study found people with chronic diseases, those having suffered a stroke, and those already taking OTC medications were more likely to take herbal supplements compared to the general population.

According to the Nutrition Business Journal, sales of herbal dietary supplements totaled over $11 billion in 2020, a 17.3% increase from 2019, and over $12 billion in 2021, a 9.7% increase (Smith et al. 2021a,b). The massive jump was due, in no small part, to the sales of immune health, stress relief, mood and energy support, and heart health supplements during the COVID-19 pandemic (Smith et al. 2021a).

The most common conditions for which herbal supplements are used include mental health (anxiety, depression, stress), immune health (especially for colds and flu), headache, pain, arthritis, dermatologic conditions, gastrointestinal conditions, reproductive conditions, and respiratory conditions (Wachtel-Galor and Benzie 2011; ATMS 2020). The National Institutes of Health (NIH) expresses concern regarding the lack of scientific evidence and potential for negative HDIs (NCCIH 2021a). The National Center for Complementary and Integrative Medicine (NCCIH) has a dedicated section of their website providing summary factsheets on a variety of herbs (https://nccih.nih.gov/health/herbsataglance.htm) (NCCIH 2021b).

Applications in Veterinary Medicine

In 2021, the global pet supplement market total almost $2 billion with an expected compounding annual growth rate of 5.9% from 2022 to 2030 (GVR 2021). The North American market accounted for the largest revenue share in 2021, 44.7% (GVR 2021). Botanical products are frequently grouped with pet supplements, making it difficult to tease out the revenue percentage dedicated specifically to herbal medicine.

Listing the most used botanicals is difficult as it is highly dependent on the practitioner (preference and level of experience) and patient condition. A study conducted by Romero et al. (2022) found the five most common herbs used by practitioners in Spain included *Cannabis sativa* (Cannabis), *Aloe vera* (Aloe), *Thymus vulgaris* (Thyme), *Artemisia annua* (Artemisia), and *Silybum marianum* (Milk Thistle). The top five botanicals listed by the online *Merck Veterinary Manual* include *Boswellia serrata* (Boswellia), *Curcuma longa* (Curcumin, Tumeric), *Zingiber officinale* (Ginger), *Harpagophytum procumbens* (Devil's Claw), and *Capiscum frutescens* (Cayenne or Capsaicin) (Merck Manual 2023). WHM practitioners also appear to frequently use herbs with one or more of the following secondary compounds: flavonoids, anthraquinones, coumarins, alkaloids, saponins, sterols and sterolins, tannins, and volatile oils (Fougère 2007, 2015).

Herbal medicine is commonly used to aid in the treatment of chronic infections, gastrointestinal disorders, geriatric health, immune-mediated conditions, musculoskeletal conditions, and cancer (Wynn and Fougère 2007a; Romero et al. 2022). Refer to Table 11.11 for specific disease conditions where veterinary WHM has been studied.

Veterinary Research

While several individual herbs and herbal formulas have been well studied, WHM as a whole modality is not. Due to the sheer number of herbs and herbal formulas it would be nearly impossible to study all veterinary herbs in detail.

Table 11.11 Examples of several studies demonstrating the efficacy of veterinary herbal medicine in the treatment of multiple diseases and conditions as of February 2023.

Condition	Species	Herb(s)	Research
Anxiety	Canine	*Magnolia officinalis* (Magnolia) and *Phellodendron amurense* (Phellodendron)	DePorter et al. (2012), Landsberg et al. (2017), and Stillo et al. (2021)
		Souroubea spp. and *Platanus* spp. (Sycamore)	Masic et al. (2021)
		Withania somnifera (Ashwagandha)	Kaur et al. (2022)
Cancer	AM	*Berberis vulgaris* (Barberry)	Xu et al. (2019)*
	Canine	*Coriolus versicolor* (Turkey Tail Mushroom)	Brown and Reetz (2012)
		Curcuma longa (Curcumin)	Withers et al. (2018)
		Multiple botanicals used in food	Levine et al. (2016)
	Canine Feline	*Artemisia annua* (Sweet Wormwood)	Saeed et al. (2019)
Cognitive function	Canine	*Ginkgo biloba* (Ginkgo)	Reichling et al. (2006) and Araujo et al. (2008)
Dermatology	Canine	Variety of botanicals used topically	Tresch et al. (2019)*
Environmental enrichment	Feline	*Actinidia polygama* (Silver Vine), *Lonicera tatarica* (Tatarian Honeysuckle), *Valeriana officinalis* (Valerian), *Nepeta cataria* (Catnip)	Bol et al. (2017)
GI health	Canine	*Curcuma longa* (Curcumin), *Salicornia europaea* (Glasswort), *Artemisia princeps* (Ganghwa Mugwort)	Park et al. (2019)
Hepatoprotective	Canine	Multi-ingredient supplement with *Silybum marianum* (Milk Thistle, Silymarin)	Giannetto et al. (2022)
Hepatotoxicity	Feline	*Silybum marianum* (Milk Thistle, Silymarin)	Avizeh et al. (2010)
Osteoarthritis	Canine	*Boswellia serrata* (Boswellia)	Reichling et al. (2004)
		Boswellia serrata (Boswellia) and *Curcuma longa* (Curcumin)	Caterino et al. (2021)
		Curcuma longa (Curcumin) and *Camellia sinensis* (Green Tea)	Comblain et al. (2017)
URI	Canine	*Echinacea purpurea* (Echinacea)	Reichling et al. (2003)
Viral infections	Canine	*Echinacea purpurea* (Echinacea)	Guan et al. (2018)

*, represent systematic reviews; AM, animal models; GI, gastrointestinal; URI, upper respiratory tract infection.
Source: Lisa P. McFaddin.

To provide a glimpse into the current research in VHM, presented below are the summaries of three studies. Additionally, Table 11.10 highlights several of the diseases and conditions, as well as the studies, for which WHM has shown a scientifically beneficial effect in veterinary medicine. This list is not all inclusive as new studies are continually published. There are also abundant case studies demonstrating the successful use of WHM in veterinary patients. Individual case studies were not included in the following table which focuses instead on clinical trials and several systematic reviews.

Not all studies have yielded positive results. A study by Griessmayr et al. (2008) investigated the effect of the use of an extract from *Grifola frondosa* (Maitake mushroom) as a single agent therapeutic in the treatment of canine lymphoma. While no AEs were noted with administration of Maitake PETfraction, neither were beneficial responses.

Although Brown and Reetz (2012) demonstrated that the polysaccharopeptide (PSP) from *Coriolus versicolor* delayed metastasis and improved survival time in splenectomized dogs with advanced splenic hemangiosarcoma, a study by Gedney et al. (2022) was unable to confirm the results, even when combined with a commonly used chemotherapeutic agent, doxorubicin.

A Randomized and Controlled Study of the Effect of *Echinacea purpurea* on Canine Parvovirus and Distemper Virus Antibody Levels in Dogs

Authors: Yucheng Guan, BS; Jiuzhi Chen, MS; Shanshan Zhou, MS; Cui Liu, PhD; Shining Guo, DVM, PhD; and Dayou Shi, DVM, PhD
Journal: *American Journal of Traditional Chinese Veterinary Medicine*
Date: 2018
Study design: Randomized controlled study
Sample size: 25 6–12-month-old poodles
Study hypothesis: The administration of one or more doses of *E. purpurea* to dogs vaccinated against canine parvovirus (CPV) and canine distemper virus (CDV) will increase serum antibody levels.
Materials and methods: All dogs received identical vaccination schedules: modified live canine adenovirus-2, CPV, and CDV combination vaccine at 8, 12, and 16 weeks of age. At the start of the experiment all dogs were vaccinated again on the dorsal thorax (T11–L1) and observed for three days for adverse reactions. Dogs were randomly divided into five groups of five dogs each: four treatment groups and one control group. The four treatment groups received oral preparations of *E. purpurea* (EP) at varying concentrations (0.1, 0.2, 0.4, and 0.8 g/kg)

with the food twice daily for 21 days followed by a seven-day observational period. CPV and CDV antibodies levels were checked on days 7, 14, 21, and 28 of the study. Data was analyzed using a one-way analysis of variance (ANOVA) and Duncan's new complex-difference test method.

Results

1) CPV antibody levels were higher in the treatment groups compared to the control groups at each measurement.
2) CPV antibodies were significantly higher at all four measurements in the group fed the highest concentration of EP compared to the control group.
3) The group fed the 0.4 g/kg EP dose has statistically significant higher CPV antibodies on days 14 and 28, while CPV antibodies were significantly higher on day 28.
4) Results for the CDV antibody levels were similar to the CPV findings, except the treatment group antibody levels decreased with each measured (while still remaining higher compared to the control group).

Study conclusions: The administration of *E. purpurea* following vaccination with a modified live combination CDV, CPV, and canine adenovirus type-2 vaccine improved CPV and CDV titers in a dose-dependent manner.

Study limitations

1) Small sample sizes within each group.
2) Study was not blinded.
3) Antibody levels were monitored for only 28 days.

5) Puppies received prior vaccination with the same vaccine which will affect antibody titers.

L.P.M. conclusions: The administration of *E. purpurea* following vaccination improved CPV and CDV antibody response suggesting the herb has immune-enhancing properties. Improved vaccination response would be especially helpful in at-risk puppies. Further studies should be conducted evaluating the effects with other vaccine antibody titers.

(Guan et al. 2018)

Dietary Support with Boswellia Resin in Canine Inflammatory Joint and Spinal Disease

Authors: J. Reichling, H. Schmökel, J. Fitzi, S. Bucher, and R. Saller
Journal: *Schweizer Archiv fur Tierheilkunde*
Date: 2004
Study design: Clinical trial
Study hypothesis: The dietary administration of Boswellia resin to dogs will reduce the clinical signs associated with osteoarthritis.
Sample size: 29 companion dogs (16 male and 13 female; age range 2–16 years)
Materials and methods: Patients with clinical and radiographic evidence of osteoarthritis were included in the study. The daily meal of all patients in the study was supplemented with a standardized Boswellia resin extract for six weeks. The extract was provided in blister packs containing 400 mg/10 kg of Boswellia resin. The patient's condition was evaluated by a clinician before treatment and at two, four, and six weeks of supplementation. Nine clinical signs were used as endpoint parameters for evaluation: permanent and intermittent lameness, local pain, stiff gait, reduced range of motion, crepitation, increased filling of the joint, thickening of the capsule, myoatrophy, excess weight and effects of external factors that aggravate lameness. Bowker's test was used for statistical analysis.

Results

1) Two weeks into supplementation 71% of the dogs showed overall improvement in clinical signs.
2) Statistically significant improvement in lameness was noted at weeks 2 and 6.
3) Statistically significant improvement in local pain was noted at weeks 2, 4, and 6.
4) Statistically significant improvement in gait stiffness was noted at week 6.

Study conclusions: Dietary supplementation with a Boswellia resin improves patient comfort through reduction of lameness, local pain, and gait stiffness.

Study limitations

1) No control group.
2) Patient age differences may have affected response to therapy.
3) Evaluation criteria was very subjective.
4) Client observations were not included in the study.

L.P.M. conclusions: Boswellia is a safe and effective supplement (herbal therapy) for the reduction of clinical signs associated with osteoarthritis in dogs.

(Reichling et al. 2004)

Reduction of Behavioral Disturbances in Elderly Dogs Supplemented with a Standardized Ginkgo Leaf Extract

Authors: J. Reichling, M. Frater-Schröder, K. Herzog, S. Bucher, and R. Saller
Journal: *Schweizer Archiv fur Tierheilkunde*
Date: 2006
Study design: Clinical trial
Study hypothesis: Once-daily supplementation with *G. biloba* in geriatric dogs will reduce behavioral disturbances.
Sample size: 42 senior dogs (19 females and 23 males; age 9–13 years old)
Materials and methods: Patients were diagnosed with behavioral changes secondary to age-related cognitive dysfunction based on six clinical signs. A scoring system was associated with the clinical signs to provide each patient with a "severity of geriatric condition."

- Score 1: disorientation
- Score 2: sleep and activity changes
- Score 3: house training
- Score 4: behavioral changes
- Score 5: general behavior
- Score 6: general physical condition

All patients were administered a daily dose of 40 mg/10 kg of tableted *G. biloba* leaf extract mixed in the food for eight weeks. Clinician evaluation was performed on days 1, 28, and 56. The last observation carried forward (LOCF) was used for statistical analysis.

Results

1) The "severity of geriatric condition" was significantly reduced after eight weeks of supplementation with *G. biloba*.
2) Improvement was seen within four weeks of supplementation.
3) 36% of dogs were symptom-free at the end of the study.
4) All scores (except house training) significantly improved during the clinical trial.

Study conclusions: *G. biloba* is a viable and safe alternative therapy for dogs with canine cognitive dysfunction.

Study limitations

1) No control group.
2) Patient age differences may have affected response to therapy.
3) Evaluation criteria were very subjective.
4) Client observations were not included in the study.

L.P.M. conclusions: *Ginkgo biloba* appears to be a safe and efficacious therapy for dogs experiencing clinical signs of canine cognitive dysfunction. Further studies are needed comparing these effects to control groups and other treatment groups (i.e. pharmaceutical drugs and other currently available supplements).

(Reichling et al. 2006)

The How

Team Members

This section reviews the potential return on investment (ROI), how to effectively train the entire team, how to promote, and how to integrate WHM.

Return on Investment

ROI can be determined by evaluating client interest, veterinarian demand, hospital costs, applicability of the service, revenue stream, appointment scheduling, and pricing.

Client Interest

Currently there are no studies or surveys documenting client interest and the popularity of veterinary WHM. Surveys and studies investigating client interest in animal supplements and CHM can be used to estimate client interest in WHM. Refer to Chapters 3 and 4 for more detailed information on these topics, respectively.

The bottom line is clients are very interested in supplements, CHM, and WHM, especially as an alternative to traditional pharmaceuticals. A survey, almost 20 years ago, of 254 owners with pets (cats and dogs) with cancer reported 76% were interested in VIM options for their pets (Lana et al. 2006). Given the growing interest in non-traditional options in human and veterinary medicine, this percentage has likely increased over time. Additionally, by evaluating trends in general interest herbal medicine, client interest in veterinary alternative or integrative medicine, and pet health insurance client interest in WHM can be inferred.

General Interest The NCCIH, a part of the NIH, annually interviews tens of thousands of Americans discussing current health and illness trends. The results of these studies are published as the National Health Interview Survey (NHIS). The NHIS evaluated complementary and alternative health topics in 2002, 2007, 2012, and 2017. The 2012 NHIS assessed the use of yoga, natural products, and chiropractic therapy.

The 2012 NHIS determined most people used natural products for the maintenance of general wellness and disease prevention, as opposed to disease treatment or management (NCCIH 2012). The study found that over 85% of participants used natural products for wellness, over 40% of participants used natural products to treat health problems, and over 65% of participants reported improved overall health because of using natural products (NCCIH 2012).

Wu et al. (2014) used the 2012 NHIS data to estimate 40.6 million adults in the United States used herbs and supplements. Interestingly there was a 1% decline in herb and supplement use compared to 2002 but use remained static compared to 2007 (Wu et al. 2014).

Client Opinion Table 11.12 summarizes the pet owner demographics and statistics mentioned in the My Lessons section of the

Table 11.12 Summary of the 2022 pet ownership and pet health insurance demographics in the United States discussed in the Introduction of the book (Burns 2018, 2022; MFAF 2018; APPA 2022; Nolen 2022; NAPHIA 2023).

- 83% of pets are owned by millennials (32%), generation X (24%), and baby boomers (27%)
- 69 million households owned dogs
- 45.3 million households owned cats
- Estimated over 81.1 million owned dogs
- Estimated over 60.7 million owned cats
- 68% of owners are interested in alternative treatment modalities for their pets
- 4.41 million pets have pet health insurance
- 82% of insurance pets are dogs

Source: Lisa P. McFaddin.

Introduction. Even if one-quarter of those owners are open to WHM, that is still 26.5 million potential patients.

Pet Health Insurance Many pet insurance plans include coverage for integrative therapies, especially acupuncture (Woodley 2018). The presence of this type of coverage re-emphasizes the mainstream incorporation of these treatment modalities, as well as reflecting client demand.

Veterinarian Demand

There is a definite need for small animal veterinarians in general, as well as integrative veterinarians. Refer to the Introduction and Chapter 1 for more specifics.

One way to examine the need in your specific area is to compare the number of general practitioners within a 5-, 10-, or 20-mile radius to the number of veterinarians advertising WHM. The search radius is dependent on your hospital's demographics. Most comparisons tend to follow the 5% trend, meaning no more than 5% of the surrounding hospitals are currently offering WHM. Ensuring your area is not saturated prevents the introduction of redundant service.

Hospital Costs

Let us start by reviewing all the potential costs associated with introducing and offering WHM: veterinarian training, staff training, supplies and equipment, staffing, facilities, and advertising. Tables 11.13 and 11.14 demonstrate the different potential start-up costs, primarily dependent on the hospital's contribution toward the veterinarian's training and prior utilization of regular all-staff meetings. For more information on potential hospital costs, refer to the Introduction of this book.

Veterinarian Training

Course There are three main organizations offering training programs in the United States. Two of the organizations offer online-only training, while the other offers on-site training only. The most basic introductory course, offered by the College of Integrative Veterinary Therapies (CIVT), has an estimated completion time of six to eight weeks, while the longest and most comprehensive course, also offered by CIVT, can take up to two years to complete. Most courses offer a problem-orientated approach, meaning veterinarians can usually start practicing herbal medicine, and generating revenue, while taking the course. Estimated cost reflects the average cost of all available courses. Additional information can be found in the Veterinarians section of this chapter (cost range, $765–8495; average cost, $3794).

Textbooks Textbooks may not be required for the courses but are highly recommended. The price range is based on a two to five book requirement (cost range, $250–1550; average cost, $600).

Travel Expenses The costs are based solely on attending the on-site course which consists of five modules each 3–3.5 days of training, estimated to four days including travel. Online-only training would eliminate the costs associated with travel and room and board.

Here is a breakdown of the costs if on-site training was chosen.

- *Airfare*: As of January 2023, the average roundtrip domestic flight was $412 (BLS 2023; Trcek 2023). The $412 value was used when calculating the cost of airfare for five roundtrip flights (total cost, $2060).
- *Lodging*: As of February 2023 the federal per diem rate for lodging on business trips is $98 per night (FederalPay.org 2023). The federal per diem rate was used for calculations, with four nights of lodging over five sessions (total cost, $1960).
- *Car rental*: As of January 2023, the average weekly car rental price is $551 (French and Kemmis 2023). Rideshare and cabbing are extremely popular, but the variability in travel distances makes calculating an average cost impractical. It is suspected this cost would be comparable, if not lower, than that of a rental car. The total was calculated using five-day car rentals for five sessions (total cost, $2755).
- *Meals*: The federal per diem rate for business trip meals from October 2022 through September 2023 is $59 a day (FederalPay.org 2023). Most training programs provide at least one meal, as well as snacks. Meal expenditure is estimated to be $40/day for a total of 25 days (total cost, $1000).
- *Time Off*: Veterinarian paid time-off (PTO) for on-site courses only factors in as an added expense if additional PTO is provided outside of their contractual annual PTO. Clinics offer an average of 4.1 paid continuing education (CE) days per year (AAHA 2019). Allowing the veterinarian to use CE days for the on-site courses would not "cost" the hospital anything additional. There is also no additional cost if the hospital requires the veterinarian use their PTO for the on-site training. Online training should not require additional PTO days, as the expectation is the veterinarian will complete the training on their own time.

Table 11.13 Potential hospital start-up costs for veterinary WHM as of February 2023.

Category	Sub-categories	Projected cost	
Veterinarian training	Course cost	$765–8495	Average $3749
	Textbooks	$250–1550	Average $600
	Travel expenses	$0–7775	
	Time-off	$0–6177	
Staff training	Variable	$230–1396	
Supplies	Herbs	$150–250	
	Measuring and dispensing instruments	$45	
Staffing	Variable	≥$0	
Facilities	Overhead	$2–5/minute per 30–60-minute appointment	
		$60–300 per patient	
Advertising	Variable	≤$420	

Source: Lisa P. McFaddin.

Table 11.14 Projected WHM start-up costs for six hospital scenarios, with varying hospital contributions toward veterinary certification and staff training as of February 2023. Examples 1–3 represent online-only training or on-site training with no hospital contribution toward travel and PTO, while examples 4–6 represent various contributions for on-site training. The cost of veterinarian training is based on the values presented in Table 11.13. Staff training costs assume a 1.5-hour-long all-staff meeting, using national averages for employee numbers: eight non-DVMs and two DVMs (AVMA 2019, 2023). The cost of office supplies and lunch as estimated based on 10 employees attending the meeting. The overhead is based on an average of $3.5/minute. Missed revenue is calculated using the 2022 national mean revenue per hour for companion animal practices ($567/hour) (AVMA 2023). Advertising includes printed materials, digital advertisement, and community engagement.

Category	Projected expenses	Ex. 1	Ex. 2	Ex. 3	Ex. 4	Ex. 5	Ex. 6
Veterinarian training	Average course cost	$3794	$3794	n/a	$3794	$3794	$3794
	Average textbooks	$600	n/a	n/a	$600	$600	$600
	Travel expenses	n/a	n/a	n/a	$7775	$7775	n/a
	Additional time-off	n/a	n/a	n/a	$6177	n/a	$6177
Staff training	Office supplies	$30	$30	$30	$30	$30	$30
	Lunch	$200	$200	$200	$200	$200	$200
	Overhead	$315	$315	$315	$315	n/a	n/a
	Missed DVM revenue	$851	$851	$851	$851	n/a	n/a
Supplies	Herbal pharmacy	$680	$680	$680	$680	$680	$680
	Measuring and dispensing	$30	$30	$30	$30	$30	$30
Advertising		$420	$420	$420	$420	$420	$420
Total		$6920	$6320	$2526	$20872	$13529	$11931
Total without supply costs		**$6210**	**$5610**	**$1816**	**$20162**	**$12819**	**$11221**

Source: Lisa P. McFaddin.

The clinic accrues an added expense if they agree to pay for the additional CE days. The median pay for a full-time veterinarian, calculated by the United States Bureau of Labor Statistics in 2022, was $100 370 or $48.26/hour (BLS 2022a). Each paid CE day was calculated as eight hours. The total cost provided represents a scenario in which a veterinarian selected the on-site only training, requiring at least 20 days for CE, and the clinic agrees to pay for an additional 16 days of PTO. The total does not include potential lost revenue due to the veterinarian's absence, nor does it include relief veterinarian expenses (total cost, $6177).

Staff Training Team training expenses are highly variable and dependent on the preexistence of staff meetings and use of a staff meeting for training (compared to self-study). Refer to the Introduction of the book for a breakdown of these variables (cost range, $230–1396).

Supplies The specific type and quantity of individual herbs and herbal formulas kept within the practice will be based on practitioner preference as well as the hospital's goal for inventory on-hand. Cost per patient is based on the premise that each patient will receive at least one full bottle of herbs per appointment. The hospital cost for each Chinese herbal formula depends on the formulation and bottle size. The hospital cost per bottle, jar, or bag can range from $5 to $60 each. The clinic should be prepared to carry at least 5–10 herbs to start with, likely one of each. For ease of calculations, the cost of each herb was estimated to be $30 (cost range, $150–250).

Potential materials necessary to mix and dispense herbs include graduated cylinders, funnels (PVDF, glass, and silicon), bottle brushes, prescription vials, glass dispensing bottles (various sizes, 2–8 ounces), measuring spoons, and a gram scale. Estimated cost for these materials was based on consultation with a senior technical representative for a major laboratory supply company in the United States (McFaddin 2023) (cost range, $200–500).

The supply cost is ultimately $0 appointment. The herbs are considered inventory, not supplies, as their cost is expected to be recouped when sold to the client. Typically, herbal formulas are sold for 2–2.25 times the purchase price plus a dispensing fee. The cost of the equipment is negligible when broken down per patient and is expected to be recouped.

Staffing Integrative appointments range from 30 to 60 minutes depending on the condition(s) being treated. Following the American Animal Hospital Association (AAHA) recommendations a veterinary assistant (VA) or licensed technician (LT) should always restrain patients for physical examinations and procedures. A VA/LT is usually required for 15–20 minutes. Support staff assistance is not required while discussing plans with the client. During this time the VA/LT are free to assist other team members.

If the VA/LT is only needed for the examination, there is no difference in staffing cost for a WHM appointment compared to a traditional appointment. If the VA/LT is required to stay in the exam room for the entire appointment the staff cost for the additional 15–45 minutes should be considered: $4.43–13.29 per patient. The provided expenses are based on a national average wage of $17.72 an hour for veterinary technologists and technicians as of September 2022 (BLS 2022b).

Facilities Facility expenses represent the costs needed to keep the doors open (aka overhead). Overhead includes rent or mortgage, utilities, administrative costs, and often employee costs divided by the minutes the practice is open (Stevenson 2016). The price per minute equals the amount of revenue needed just to break even. Overhead is extremely hospital specific, but the range tends to be $2–5/minute. The low end of the range in Table 11.13 represents the cost for a 30-minute appointment at a clinic with a $2/minute overhead, while the high end represents the cost for a 60-minute appointment at a clinic with a $5/minute overhead.

Designating a specific room, in a multi-exam room hospital, for integrative appointments minimizes the chances other associates will need the room for their appointments. However, there is then an added expense for designing the room and potential lost revenue if the room is not used regularly. The absence of a designated room theoretically reduces redecoration costs, but this can be disruptive for appointment flow if the treatment takes longer than the allotted time.

Advertising   There are numerous ways to advertise a new service. On average veterinary hospitals spend 0.7% of revenue on promotion and advertisement (AVMA 2019). Most of the advertising can be done with little to no additional expenditure. The Promotion section discusses advertising ideas in further detail. The national median gross revenue for companion animal practices was $1.2 million in 2022 (AVMA 2023). Advertising costs are calculated assuming no more than 5% of the current advertising budget would be used for the promotion of the new service (estimated maximal cost, $420).

Start-Up Costs   Table 11.13 summarizes projected start-up costs for WHM. Table 11.14 calculates potential start-up costs based on the type of course taken, degree of hospital contribution toward veterinarian, and staff training. Different scenarios are presented in which the hospital covers all, some, or none of the expenses.

Applicability
As stated earlier WHM is versatile and beneficial for numerous conditions and ailments. As the clinician becomes more comfortable and confident in their WHM skills, the variety of cases for which WHM is recommended increases.

Revenue Stream
A well-trained and effective WHM practitioner can generate a relatively "recession proof" revenue stream. When used appropriately herbs can be both safe and effective. Many veterinary patients suffer from chronic conditions making herbal medicine ideal for long-term use. Online pharmacies may not carry the most used veterinary herb brands. Veterinary herbal manufacturers and distributors frequently only sell through licensed practitioners and clinics. With each herb sold, either as a new prescription or refill, the income continues to build into the clinic over time.

Appointment Scheduling
There are four main factors to consider when planning WHM appointment protocols: appointment length; support staff availability; exam room availability; and follow-up appointment scheduling.

There are other issues to consider when scheduling WHM appointments. For example, will WHM appointments be scheduled separately from traditional Western appointments, or will the appointment length be increased?

The initial integrative appointment is often longer, 60 minutes, compared to follow-up appointments. Follow-up appointments are generally scheduled for 30–60 minutes depending on the patient and if additional treatments are performed.

Keep the appointment positive. You want the pet to enjoy the experience. A relaxed pet is more easily treated. Avoid ancillary procedures which may cause stress: nail trims, anal gland expression, sanitary trims, anything with the ears, etc. Additional information on appointment scheduling can be found in the Introduction of this book.

Pricing
An in-depth look into appointment pricing can be found in the Introduction of this book. Here we discuss two pricing methods: current market fees and hospital cost-based pricing.

Current Market Fees   There are no studies examining the average cost of veterinary WHM appointments. Current market fees may be estimated by examining acupuncture and CHM appointment pricing. A study of five

Table 11.15 Estimated hospital costs per patient for 30- and 60-minute western herbal medicine appointments as of February 2023. Start-up costs are taken from the totals in Table 11.13. Amortization is per patient and is based on the veterinarian seeing 952 integrative patients in two years. Overhead is calculated using $3.5/minute in a practice with two veterinarians. Multiple examples are provided with the variance determined by the total cost within each category. The total is rounded to the nearest whole number.

	Ex. 1	Ex. 2	Ex. 3	Ex. 4	Ex. 5	Ex. 6
30-minute appointments						
Table 11.14 totals	**$6210**	**$5610**	**$1816**	**$20162**	**$12819**	**$11221**
Amortization	$6.52	$5.89	$1.91	$21.18	$13.47	$11.79
Overhead	*$52.50*	*$52.50*	*$52.50*	*$52.50*	$52.50	$52.50
Total	**$59**	**$58**	**$54**	**$74**	**$66**	**$64**
60-minute appointments						
Table 11.14 totals	**$6210**	**$5610**	**$1816**	**$20162**	**$12819**	**$11221**
Amortization	$6.52	$5.89	$1.91	$21.18	$13.47	$11.79
Overhead	*$105*	*$105*	*$105*	*$105*	*$105*	*$105*
Total	**$112**	**$111**	**$107**	**$126**	**$118**	**$117**

Source: Lisa P. McFaddin.

general practices within Central Florida found the price of acupuncture appointments ranged from $45 to $150, with a mean of $95.80 (Marks and Shmalberg 2015). The average length of these appointments was 47 minutes. Assuming these clinics follow the average service fee increase of 3.9%, the mean price four years later would equate to $110.75 for a 50-minute session (Purdue University 2018).

Hospital Cost-Based Pricing Table 11.15 outlines the hospital cost per patient for 30- and 60-minute WHM appointments, respectively. The veterinarian training amortization per patient was calculated using the assumptions listed in Chapter 1. Supply assumptions were considered $0, as herbs are considered inventory, and their cost (plus nominal expenses for applicable vials, scales, etc.) is recouped when the product is sold.

The formula for determining service fees is quite simple: Service Fee = Hospital Cost + Profit. The big question becomes, how much profit? Table 11.16 illustrates the potential fee for integrative appointments based on hospital cost and variable markup percentages. It becomes readily apparent that the lower the hospital contribution, the higher the comparative profit.

Additional Considerations Many of my patients receive other treatments or diagnostics when they come in for their appointments. Frequently we adjust current medication regimens, run diagnostics (blood work, urinalysis, radiographs, etc.), discuss dietary and environmental modifications, and discuss nutrition and nutraceuticals. All of which increases revenue, average transaction charge (ATC), and DVM revenue per hour.

Offering integrative medicine also helps improve current client retention and drive new client acquisition. Marks and Shmalberg (2015) found 29% of new acupuncture and integrative patients returned for wellness and other services. Additionally, clients and surrounding veterinary practices are likely to refer patients once they see the benefit of WHM, especially in cases where traditional medicine was not effective. Improving client retention and new client referrals help drive revenue.

Table 11.16 Potential 30- and 60-minute integrative appointment prices using hospital costs from Table 11.15 at varying percentage markups as of February 2023.

		Ex. 1	Ex. 2	Ex. 3	Ex. 4	Ex. 5	Ex. 6
30-minute appointments							
Total hospital cost		**$59**	**$58**	**$54**	**$74**	**$66**	**$64**
Potential appointment price	40% Markup	$83	$81	$76	$104	$92	$90
	50% Markup	$89	$87	$81	$111	$99	$96
	60% Markup	$94	$93	$86	$118	$106	$102
	70% Markup	$100	$99	$92	$126	$112	$109
	80% Markup	$106	$104	$97	$133	$119	$115
	90% Markup	$112	$110	$103	$141	$125	$122
	100% Markup	$118	$116	$108	$148	$132	$128
60-minute appointments							
Total hospital cost		**$112**	**$111**	**$107**	**$126**	**$118**	**$117**
Potential appointment price	40% Markup	$157	$155	$150	$176	$165	$164
	50% Markup	$168	$167	$161	$189	$177	$176
	60% Markup	$179	$178	$171	$202	$189	$187
	70% Markup	$190	$189	$182	$214	$201	$199
	80% Markup	$202	$200	$193	$227	$212	$211
	90% Markup	$213	$211	$203	$239	$224	$222
	100% Markup	$224	$222	$214	$252	$236	$234

Source: Lisa P. McFaddin.

Team Training

The concept of phase training is used when introducing acupuncture to the hospital team. A multi-media approach is used to assist with the training program and is outlined in Table 11.17.

Practice Manager's Role in Training

To conquer this task the practice manager needs his or her own checklist which includes the following information:

- Schedule a date and time for the team training.
- Ensure all information pertaining to the new service is reviewed with the staff.
- Confirm all team members have completed the training.
- Certify all team members understand the information and can successfully educate clients.

Promotion

There are six common avenues of promotion for a VIM service: hospital website, social media, email blasts, mailers, in-hospital promotions, and client education.

Hospital Website

Advertise "Veterinary Western Herbal Medicine" or "Veterinary Herbal Medicine" in several locations on the website. On the made page insert "Now offering veterinary herbal medicine" with a link to success stories or client testimonials. Utilize the hospital website to advertise the VIM treatment under the "Services" section. Under Veterinarian Biograph include a description of the specialized training and professional initials. Create a VHM blog page discussing patient success stories.

Table 11.17 The breakdown of phase training steps and resources for the entire hospital team.

Phase 1: background information	
Team training guide	The handout walks the practice manager and/or veterinarian through Phase 1 of the training
	A downloadable and editable copy of the handout is located on the companion website
Training presentation	The video covers background information on the modality
	PowerPoints can be downloaded, edited, and personalized from the companion website.
	The document can be used as a PowerPoint or saved as an mp4 creating a personalized movie
Team training handout	The handout provides additional background information for the CSRs, VAs, and LTs to complement the knowledge gained from watching the training presentation
	A downloadable and editable copy of the handout is located on the companion website
Phase 2: knowledge proficiency	
Quiz	A short quiz to ensure all team members have a good understanding of the service being offered
	A downloadable and editable copy of the handout is located on the companion website
	A key is provided
Phase 3: expectations	
Training worksheets	A training checklist is provided for CSRs and VA/LTs with role-specific expectations and tasks for each staff member
	A recommended completion time is provided
	A downloadable and editable copy of the handout is located on the companion website
Phase 4: client education	
Client scripts	Bullet point information and scripted examples used when discussing the therapy with clients
	A downloadable and editable copy of the handout is located on the companion website
client education presentation	A short (5–7 minute) client educational video about the therapeutic modality
	PowerPoints can be downloaded, edited, and personalized from the companion website.
	The document can be used as a PowerPoint or saved as an mp4 creating a personalized movie
Client education handout	An informational handout about the therapeutic modality written specifically for clients
	A downloadable and editable copy of the handout is located on the companion website

CSR, customer service representative; VA, veterinary assistant; LT, licensed technician. Source: Lisa P. McFaddin.

Social Media

Utilize Facebook, Instagram, and/or Twitter to post facts, photographs, hashtags, and patient success stories. Include fun and intriguing facts about VHM. Clients love patient photos. Be sure to include ones with the herbal formulas they are taking. Create or utilize VHM specific hashtags.

Email Blasts

Send fun mass emails to your clients introducing VHM. Consider monthly case presentations illustrating how the service has benefited patients. Almost everyone has at least one email address these days. Customer service representatives should be amassing client emails at the same rate as phone numbers.

Mailers

Mailers can be expensive and are largely unnecessary in this digital age. Mailers can be used to announce the introduction of herbal medicine to existing clients. The mailer should include the name of the new service, a brief description of how VHM can help pet patients, the name of the doctor offering the service, a brief description of the training the doctor received, and one or more photographs of a pet taking VHM.

In-Hospital Promotions

Advertise VHM within the hospital using small promotions signs, informational signs, invoice teasers, and staff buttons. Small promotional signs can be placed in the waiting room and exam rooms. Include photos of pets and herbal formulas. Consider catchphrases such as "Got Herbs?" or "We got an herb for that!"

Informational signs should include a brief description of how VHM can help pet patients, photographs of pets with their formulas, the name of the doctor offering the service, and a brief description of the training the doctor received.

Invoice teasers should consist of short phrases reminding and enticing owners regarding a new service offered at the practice. Examples include "Now offering Veterinary Herbal Medicine", "Curious if herbal medicine can help your pet?", "Introducing Veterinary Herbal Medicine", and "Would your pet benefit from Veterinary Herbal Medicine?"

Buttons can be made for the staff to wear with kitchy phrases reminding owners, in a fun way, of the new VIM service. Examples include "Got Herbs" and "Want to learn more about Veterinary Herbal Medicine?".

Client Education

Education is crucial to understanding the purpose and importance of any given treatment, as well as answer client questions and any concerns that may arise. The client handouts and videos solidify pet owner knowledge base reducing concerns and conveying value.

Integration

The key components for proper integration include availability of the service to the right patients; appropriate patient scheduling; appropriate support staff scheduling; and STAFF buy-in (understanding the benefits of the offered service).

Veterinarians

There are several factors to consider when veterinarians prepare to incorporate a VIM in their clinical repertoire: state requirements and restrictions, return on investment, course availability, supplies and equipment, veterinary organizations, and continuing education.

State Requirements and Restrictions

Is WHM Considered the Practice of Veterinary Medicine?

Each state has its own veterinary provisions outlining what is and is not considered the practice of veterinary medicine. Currently no state specifically defines WHM as the practice of veterinary medicine. These rules can change, and careful review of your specific state requirements is recommended.

Does WHM Continuing Education Count toward Licensure Continuing Education Requirements?

Currently no states require specific CE hours for veterinarians offering WHM nor do they specifically reference WHM CE. Some states limit the use of integrative medicine CE hours toward the annual CE requirement for license renewal. Most states permit the use of integrative CE if the lectures or webinars are performed by an approved provider. Review your specific state's requirements for further details. Table 1.14 in Chapter 1 lists each state's CE requirements and provides links for their Board of Veterinary Medicine on the companion website.

Are Your Assets Covered?

Check with your liability insurance to determine if you are covered when practicing

WHM. Refer to the Introduction of this book for additional information.

Return on Investment

Specifics are discussed in the Team Members section of this chapter.

Course Availability

Formal training in VHM is not required but is highly recommended. Training and certification provide the foundations of understanding as to how WHM can best help your veterinary patients. Completion of formal training and certification also help legitimize the modality. Some veterinarians take courses offered by human herbalists. Depending on the instructors, these can provide high-quality information, but this is not recommended for technicians as it does require veterinary training to ascertain where the course information does and does not apply to animals.

As of 2023, there are no American Board of Veterinary Specialty (ABVS)-supported residencies in herbal medicine, although the American College of Veterinary Botanical Medicine (ACVBM) has been working for recognition by the ABVS.

Veterinarians who are on the fence about committing to a full training course are encouraged to attend introductory lectures first. Familiarizing yourself with the information is a great way to determine if pursuing this modality is right for you and your practice. State and national veterinary conferences generally offer at least a few lectures on various VIM topics. Online veterinary educational platforms offering introductory and advanced VIM lectures include the Veterinary Botanical Medical Association (VBMA), College of Integrative Veterinary Therapies (CIVT), International Veterinary Acupuncture Society (IVAS), International Herbal Symposium (HIS) Vet Track Classes, Veterinary Information Network (VIN), Vetfolio, DVM360 Flex, and Vet Girl on the Run.

Additionally, the annual conferences hosted by the AHVMA, VBMA, IVAS, and ACVBM consist solely of VIM topics, including

---

American College of Veterinary Botanical Medicine (ACVBM)

Vision Statement: "The [ACVBM] will provide a means to reach diplomate status through maintaining a standard base of post-graduate instruction and examination, offer educational opportunities designed to advance experience and proficiency, and enhance the integration of scientific, clinical, and traditional knowledge into veterinary medicine practice for the greater benefit of the health and well-being of animals."
Mission Statement: "The mission of the [ACVBM] is to increase the proficiency and competence of veterinarians in the use of medicinal plants, ultimately leading to diplomate status in the specialty of veterinary botanical medicine."

Objectives

1) "Establishing requirements for post-doctoral education and experience pre-requisite to certification in the specialty of veterinary botanical medicine.
2) Providing programs of required study including: Phytochemistry, Phytopharmacology, Pharmacognasy, Ethnopharmacology, Ethnoveterinary Medicine, Traditional and Cultural Uses of Herbal medicines, Traditional/Oriental Medicine & Western Medicine herbology.
3) Supporting scientific research in Phytochemistry, Phytopharmacology, Phytopharmacodynamics, and Toxicology.
4) Examining and certifying veterinarians as specialists in Botanical Veterinary Medicine."

Website: https://www.acvbm.org

WHM. Listed below are the currently available and recommended VHM courses, pricing as of February 2023.

College of Integrative Veterinary Therapies (CIVT)

- **Course name:** Essentials of Veterinary Western Herbal Medicine (WHM)
- **Prerequisites**: Veterinarians (with a license in good standing), veterinary students, veterinary technicians, or veterinary nurses
- **Description**
  - 12 hours American Association of Veterinary State Boards Registry of Approved Continuing Education (AAVSB RACE)-approved CE in veterinary WHM.
  - 10.75 hours of credits for the International Veterinary Acupuncture Society (IVAS).
  - Course objectives include:
    - Basic history of WHM, especially in veterinary medicine.
    - Applicability of WHM in global herbal medicine systems.
    - Introduction to phytomedicine, WHM terminology, classification of phytochemicals, understanding phytochemical functions, basic understanding of WHM applications in practice, and an introduction to HDIs.
    - Ability to prepare three basic herbal preparations.
    - Use of the top 10 herbs used in veterinary medicine.
  - Assessments include a multiple-choice open book test, short answer questions, and forum participation.
- **Online training**: Six online modules.
- **On-site training: Not appicable**
- **Completion time**: Six to eight weeks, self-paced.
- **Cost**: $765.00
  - Recorded lectures and tutorials.
  - Downloadable course materials and readings.
- **Contact information**
  - Address: 292 Lyons Rd., Russell Lea, 2046 NSW, Australia
  - Phone: (304) 930-5684
  - Website: www.civtedu.org
  - Email: admin1@civtedu.org

College of Integrative Veterinary Therapies (CIVT)

- **Course name**: Certification in Veterinary Western Herbal Medicine (WHM)
- **Prerequisites**: Veterinarians, with a license in good standing
- **Description**
  - 50 hours AAVSB RACE-approved CE.
  - Course objectives include:
    - History of WHM, especially in veterinary medicine.
    - Applicability of WHM in global herbal medicine systems.
    - Introduction to phytomedicine, WHM terminology, classification of phytochemicals, understanding phytochemical functions, basic understanding of WHM applications in practice, and an introduction to HDIs.
    - Ability to plan individualized prescriptions.
    - Manage an herbal dispensary.
    - Use of the top 40 herbs used in veterinary medicine.
  - Assessments include online quizzes, forum participation, case journals and case studies, and short answer questions and essays.
  - Students receive Certification in Veterinary Western Herbal Medicine (CVWHM) upon successful completion of the course.
- **Online training**: Four online modules, each lasting approximately three months.
- **On-site training**: Not applicable
- **Completion time**: 12 months, self-paced.
- **Cost**: $4230
  - Recorded lectures and tutorials.
  - Downloadable course materials and readings.
- **Contact information**
  - Address: 292 Lyons Rd., Russell Lea, 2046 NSW, Australia

– Phone: (304) 930-5684
– Website: www.civtedu.org
– Email: admin1@civtedu.org

College of Integrative Veterinary Therapies (CIVT)

- **Course name**: Advanced Certification in Veterinary Western Herbal Medicine (WHM)
- **Prerequisites**: Veterinarians, with a license in good standing, who have completed the CIVT Certification Veterinary Western Herbal Medicine course, completed a comparable course from a recognized herbal school, and can demonstrate proficiency in WHM.
- **Description**
  – 3 hours AAVSB RACE-approved CE.
  – Course focuses on
    o The Materia Medica especially the actions, indications, constituents, and contraindications of herbs.
    o At least 100 herbs.
    o Relationship of herbs with different body systems.
  – Assessments include online quizzes, forum participation, case journals and case studies, and short answer questions and essays.
  – Students receive Advanced Certification in Veterinary Western Herbal Medicine (ACVWHM) upon successful completion of the course.
- **Online training**: Four online modules, each lasting approximately three months.
- **On-site training**: Not applicable
- **Completion time**: 12 months, self-paced.
- **Cost**: $4230
  – Recorded lectures and tutorials.
  – Downloadable course materials and readings.
- **Contact information**
  – Address: 292 Lyons Rd., Russell Lea, 2046 NSW, Australia
  – Phone: (304) 930-5684
  – Website: www.civtedu.org
  – Email: admin1@civtedu.org

College of Integrative Veterinary Therapies (CIVT)

- **Course name**: Graduate Diploma of Veterinary Western Herbal Medicine (WHM)
- **Prerequisites**: Veterinarians (with a license in good standing), Licensed Veterinary Technicians or Nurses, or postgraduates with vocational practice.
- **Description**
  – 99 hours AAVSB RACE-approved CE.
  – Combine the information presented in the Certification and Advanced courses in WHM.
  – Assessments include online quizzes, forum participation, case journals and case studies, and short answer questions and essays.
  – Students receive Graduate Diploma Veterinary Western Herbal Medicine (GDVWHM) upon successful completion of the program.
- **Online training**: Seven online modules, total 1414 hours.
- **On-site training**: Not applicable
- **Completion time**: 24 months, self-paced.
- **Cost**: $8495
  – Recorded lectures and tutorials.
  – Downloadable course materials and readings.
- **Contact information**:
  – Address: 292 Lyons Rd., Russell Lea, 2046 NSW, Australia
  – Phone: (304) 930-5684
  – Website: www.civtedu.org
  – Email: admin1@civtedu.org

CuraCore

- **Course name**: Veterinary Botanical Medicine Consultant
- **Prerequisites**: Veterinarians (with a license in good standing), veterinary students, and veterinary technicians and nurses.
- **Description**
  – 110 hours AAVSB RACE-approved CE.
  – Course focuses on:
    o The mechanisms, indications, contraindications, and HDIs of herbs.

- o The potential legal and ethical concerns of botanical medicine.
- o The practical applications of herbal medicine within the veterinary practice.
- Each module contains videos, reading assignments, and homework.
- Students receive Veterinary Botanical Medicine Consultant (VBMC) certificate upon successful completion of the course.
- **Online training**: 16 modules, self-paced.
- **On-site training**: Not applicable
- **Completion time**: 12 months
- **Cost**: $1095
- **Contact information**:
  - Address: 4007 Automation Way, Fort Collins, CO 80525
  - Phone: (970) 818-0851
  - Website: www.curacore.org
  - Email: info@curacore.org

Purple Moon Herb Studies

- **Course name**: Veterinary Herbal Apprenticeship and Retreat
- **Prerequisites**: Veterinarian (with a license in good standing)
- **Description**
  - 64.5 hours AAVSB RACE-approved CE
  - 56 hour IVAS-approved CE.
  - A hands-on introductory, immersive, and comprehensive approach to herbal medicine.
    - o Covers the history of WHM, practice of formulation, prescribing, and phytopharmacology.
    - o Lectures center on Materia Medica organized primarily by Western organ systems.
    - o Laboratories will focus on making herbal products.
  - Assessments include:
    - o Producing two products and two new Materia Medicas for each successive module (based on topics covered in the previous module).
    - o Complete a pictorial and information herb walk of their home territory including 10 different herbs.

- o Optional self-care journaling and projects.
- **Online training**: Not applicable
- **On-site training**: Five modules, each with classes for 3–3.5 days.
- **Completion time**: Eight months
- **Cost**: $3950
- **Contact information**:
  - Class address: Lowood Educational Center, North Duck, North Carolina
  - Mail address: 1841 Bryant's Corner Road, Hartly, Delaware 19953
  - Phone: (302) 270-5095
  - Website: https://www.purplemoonherb-studies.com
  - Email: info@purplemoonherbstudies.com

Veterinary Botanical Medical Association (VBMA)

- **Course name**: VBMA Herbalist Certification
- **Prerequisites**: Veterinarians (license in good standing) or non-veterinary herbalists with prior herbal training
- **Description**
  - This is not a training course but an examination of competency in VHM.
  - The examination is held annually at the AHVMA.
  - A downloadable study guide is available on the VBMA website.
  - Successful completion requires:
    - o Passing the multiple-choice test with at least a 70%.
    - o Submission of three case reports (peer review is recommended).
    - o Donation of at least 10 questions for future examinations.
  - Veterinarians are certified by the VBMA as a Certified Veterinary Herbalist (CVH) upon successful completion of the test.
- **Cost**: $100
- **Contact information**
  - Address: 6410 Highway 92 * Acworth Georgia 30102
  - Phone: (302) 270-5095

– Website: https://www.vbma.org/index.html
– Email: office@vbma.org

Supplies

Inventory

Western herbal formulas can be purchased pre-blended or created by the practitioner in the hospital setting. Most WHM practitioners utilize both pre-made and hospital-made herbal formulas, depending on the formula and preparation needed for a particular patient. Like most pharmaceutical formulation decisions, there are pros and cons to using pre-blended formulas. The benefits include reduced inventory needs, reduced preparation time, and multiple preparations may be available. Potential negatives include the inability to change the herbal formula and multiple preparations may not be available.

When making your own herbal formulas the hospital must carry all the potential individual herbal components needed. For example, most granular herbs (individual and formulas) come as 100 g bottles of powder. If an herbal formula contains five herbs you would need 20 g of each herb to make a 100 g mixture with a 1 : 1 : 1 : 1 : 1 ratio. However, if you carried the pre-mixed formula you would only need one 100-g bottle.

If the mixture is a commonly used formula, it may be worth the expense of carrying all five individual herbs. If the formula is used infrequently, the remaining 80 g of each herb may expire before being used, resulting in lost inventory revenue.

Tinctures are also recommended given their long shelf-life and ease of mixing. The specific herbs and herbal formulas a veterinary herbalist elects to carry are based on their training and level of experience. Figure 11.3 pictures the inventory of a veterinarian practicing WHM. Table 11.18 lists several commonly used suppliers of veterinary herbal products.

Preparation Time

It takes longer to measure and mix hospital-created herbal formulas compared to the time needed to place a prescription label on a bottle of pre-packaged herbs. The overhead cost

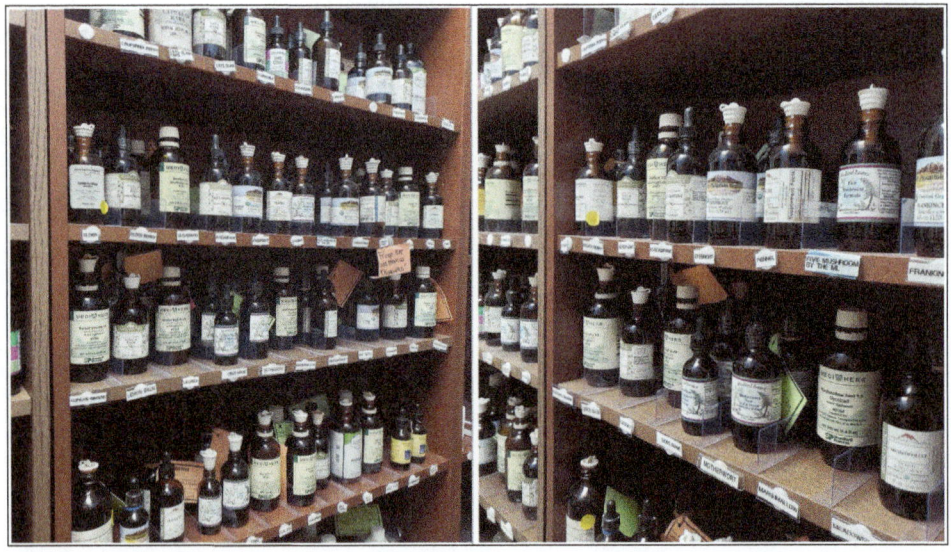

Figure 11.3 Examples of the inventory in the herbal pharmacy of a veterinarian practicing Western herbal medicine. Source: Lisa P. McFaddin.

Table 11.18 Several commonly used suppliers and brands of veterinary herbs and herbal formulas as of February 2023.

Supplier	Brands	Available formulation
Animal Essentials 1518 W Knudsen Dr #102, Phoenix, AZ 85027 (888) 551-0416 www.animalessentials.com info@animalessentials.com	Animal essentials	Most are tinctures or liquid; extracts; some are granular powder or capsules
A Time to Heal 140 Webster Road, Shelburne, VT 05482 (802) 497-2375 www.atimetohealherbs.com admin@atimetohealherbs.com	Natural path	Most are granular powder; several liquid extracts
Buck Mountain Botanicals HC 30 Miles City, MT 59031 (406) 332-1185 www.buckmountainbotanicals.net buckmountainherbs@hotmail.com	Buck mountain	Most are tinctures or liquid; extracts; some are granular powder
Herbalist and Alchemist 51 South Wandling Ave, Washington, NH 07882 (908) 689-9020 http://www.herbalist-alchemist.com	Herbalist and alchemist	Human Western herbal medicine company, offer a variety of single herbal extracts
Veterinarian's Apawthecary 1518 W Knudsen Dr. #102, Phoenix, AZ 85027 (888) 551-0416 www.vetpawthecary.com apawlab@montana.com	Veterinarian's Apawthecary	Mostly tinctures; some granular powders

Source: Lisa P. McFaddin.

required for the physician, or trained support staff, and time needed to measure and mix individual herbs must be considered.

Available Preparations

Some pre-blended formulas come as granular powders, liquid extracts, or capsules. This variety may improve owner and patient compliance with respect to ease of administration.

Specialized Formulations

Pre-made herbal formulas cannot be easily altered, especially when manufactured as liquid extract. Some patients may require specific formulas that can only be achieved if made in the hospital. Having a well-stocked herbal pharmacy allows for the creation of herbal formulas not routinely mass produced. Customized formulas usually take advanced formal training to perfect, which is why commercial formulas may be helpful for beginners.

Storage

Hospital remodeling and/or redecorating is generally not required. Additional storage space is required for the herbal bottles in the pharmacy or a separate area of the hospital.

Veterinary Organizations

A description of the most common veterinary organizations with a special interest in VIM and WHM are provided below. Table 11.19

Table 11.19 Veterinary associations and organizations with a special interest in veterinary integrative medicine and herbal medicine) as of February 2023.

Organization	Contact information	Membership dues
American College of Veterinary Botanical Medicine (ACVBM)	cyndvm@gmail.com	None
American Holistic Veterinary Medical Association (AHVMA)	PO Box 630, Abingdon, MD 21009 (410) 569-0795 office@ahvma.org	$300/year
College of Integrative Veterinary Therapies (CIVT)	PO Box 352, Yeppoon, 4703 QLD, Australia (303) 800-5460 membership@civtedu.org	$185/year
Veterinary Botanical Medicine Association (VBMA)	6410 Highway 92, Acworth, GA 30102 office@vbma.org	$85/year

Source: Lisa P. McFaddin.

summarizes the organizations' names, contact information, and membership dues.

American College of Veterinary Botanical Medicine (ACVBM)
- **Description**: Founded in 2014 to establish requirements for post-doctoral education and certification in veterinary botanical medicine. The goal was to create a diplomate status for the specialty of veterinary botanical medicine. Patrons can become supporting members through donations or apply to become members of the organizing committee. No required annual CE to maintain membership.
- **Membership benefits**: The ACVBM offers an annual CE conference.

American Holistic Veterinary Medical Association (AHVMA)
- **Description**: The AHVMA was founded in 1982 at the Western States Veterinary Conference with the goal of advancing integrative medicine through the education of integrative and non-integrative veterinarians, the introduction of integrative medicine to veterinary students, the promotion of research, and representation in the AVMA House of Delegates. There is no annual CE requirement to maintain membership.
- **Membership benefits**
  - Free subscription to the *AHVMA Journal*, a peer-reviewed journal.
  - Online resources for client education.
  - Searchable member directory.
  - Discounted vaccination titers through Kansas State University (KSU) Diagnostic Lab.
  - Free access to the Natural Medicines Database, an online resource for supplements, natural medicines, and integrative therapies.
  - Reduced cost for the AHVMA annual conference.

College of Integrative Veterinary Therapies (CIVT)
- **Description**: An online organization open to all licensed animal health providers interested in integrative medicine. There are two membership options: full membership for veterinarians and associate membership for registered animal health professionals. CIVT strives to promote all aspects of evidence-based integrative medicine through online education and discussion forums. CIVT

provides financial support to veterinary students interested in studying integrative medicine. CIVT also helps fund integrative medicine research. There is no annual CE requirement to maintain membership.

- **Membership benefits**
  - Access to the online electronic library.
  - Access to the electronic *Journal of Integrative Veterinary Therapies.*
  - Three free CE webinars annually.
  - 20% discount on all webinars.
  - Discounts on specific CIVT courses.
  - Searchable member directory.
  - Access to the Natural Medicines Databases and the American Botanical Council Library.

Veterinary Botanical Medicine Association (VBMA)

- **Description**: Founded by Susan Wynn, DVM, CVA, CVCH, AHG in 2002. The VBMA comprises veterinarians and herbalists interested in promoting the responsible application of herbal therapies for animals. No required annual CE to maintain membership.
- **Membership benefits**
  - VBMA members receive daily email discussion threads detailing real-life case questions and expert practical advice.
  - Weekly and monthly emails are also shared highlighting herbs commonly used in veterinary medicine.
  - Free subscription to the biannual online *Journal of Veterinary Botanical Medicine.*
  - Access to Herbal Wiki, an online herbal materia medica.
  - Access to additional educational articles, websites, and videos.
  - Discounted cost for telemedicine conferences and webinars.
  - Searchable member directory.
  - The VBMA offers an annual conference and multiple webinars.

Reference Books

The following is a recommended list of TCVM and VHM books as of February 2023. A summary of each book is provided.

A Clinical Guide to Blending Liquid Herbs: Herbal Formulations for the Individual Patient
- Author: Kerry Bone
- Summary: Clinical guide and reference book for the use of liquid herbal remedies in people. The book contains 125 monographs.

American College of Veterinary Botanical Medicine (ACVBM) Annual Conference Proceedings
- Authors: Various
- Summary: Contains the lecture notes from the conference as well as key presentations from 2015 to 2019. There are audio recordings available for the 2020–2022 conferences (https://www.acvbm.org/bookstore.html).

The Complete Herbal Handbook for the Dog and Cat
- Author: Juliette de Baïracli Levy
- Summary: An introduction into the applications of integrative pet care and herbal therapy for owners.

Dr. Pitcairn's Complete Guide to Natural Health for Dogs and Cats
- Authors: Richard Pitcairn, DVM, PhD and Susan Pitcairn
- Summary: An introduction into the applications of integrative pet care for owners.

The Fungal Pharmacy: The Complete Guide to Medicinal Mushrooms and Lichens of North America
- Author: Robert Rogers, RH (AHG)
- Summary: Comprehensive summary of more than 300 species of North American medicinal mushrooms and lichens, including physical characteristics and medicinal properties.

Herbal Vade Mecum: 800 Herbs, Spices, Essential Oils, Liquids, etc. Constituents, Properties, Uses, and Caution
- Author: Gazmend Skenderi
- Summary: A quick reference guide for the general public with information and practical applications for herbs and essential oils, including 657 abbreviated monographs.

The Identification of Medicinal Plants: A Handbook of the Morphology of Botanicals in Commerce

- Author: Wendy Applequist
- Summary: A comprehensive handbook published by the American Botanical Council designed to review the basic plant structure, identification tips, and botanical nomenclature for over 150 species of medicinal botanicals.

Integrating Complementary Medicine into Veterinary Practice

- Authors: Robert S. Goldstein, VMD, Paula Jo Broadfoot, DVM, Richard E. Plamquist, DVM, Karen Johnstons, DVM, Jiu Jia Wen, DVM, Barbara Fougère, BSc, BVMs (Hons), BHSc (comp Med), MODT, MHSc (Herb Med), CVA (IVAs), CVBM, CVCP, and Margo Roman, DVM
- Summary: A comprehensive review of multiple integrative therapies including: Chinese herbal medicine, acupuncture, homotoxicology, nanopharmacology, homotoxicology, and therapeutic nutrition. The book aims to educate veterinary practitioners on the validity, effectiveness, and incorporation of each modality within daily practice.

Manual of Natural Veterinary Medicine: Science and Tradition

- Authors: Susan G. Wynn, DVM, DACVN and Steve Marsden, DVM, ND, MSOM, Lac, Dipl.CH., RH(AHG)
- Summary: A quick reference book discussing the integrative therapy options for numerous diseases in veterinary medicine. The book is organized by Western conditions. For each category the potential TCVM diagnoses and treatment options are then discussed in succinct detail. A must-have for all integrative veterinarians.

Phytotherapy in Veterinary Medicine: Place of Medicinal Plants in the Treatment of Canine Diseases

- Authors: Aïmen Abbassi and Hela Gana
- Summary: An introduction into the science of VHM. Provides a reference for veterinarians and owners.

Principles and Practice of Phytotherapy: Modern Herbal Medicine

- Authors: Kerry Bone and Simon Mills
- Summary: An introduction to the theories and applications of Western herbal medicine for the human practitioner. The book contains 50 evidence-based monographs.

Veterinary Herbal Medicine

- Authors: Susan Wynn, DVM, DACVN and Barbara Fougère, BSc, BVMS (Hons), MODT, BHSc (Comp Med), CVA (IVAS), CVCP, CV Herb Med, MHSc (Herb Med)
- Summary: Comprehensive reference book on veterinary WHM. The book is divided into five sections covering the history of WHM, controversies surrounding WHM, materia medica, clinical uses within veterinary medicine, and appendices. This book is a must-have for all veterinarians practicing western herbal medicine.

Veterinary Herbal Pharmacopoeia

- Author: Sun-Chong Wang
- Summary: Covers herbal recipes for various disease conditions in dogs and cats. The book is meant as a reference for both owners and veterinarians.

Promotion

Information regarding the hospital's promotion of WHM can be found in the Team Members section.

Integration

Key components for proper integration include availability, scheduling, and staff buy-in. Availability means offering the service to the right patient. Scheduling refers to appropriate patient and support staff scheduling. Staff buy-in ensures all team members understand the benefits of the offered service.

Conclusion

Veterinary WHM is a well-studied and increasingly popular therapeutic modality.

The effects and benefits are numerous for veterinary patients. This chapter and companion website describe in detail how veterinary WHM can be successfully introduced into daily practice, as well as provide practical tools for implementation.

Acknowledgment

I would like to thank Dr. Susan G. Wynn for reviewing the first draft of this chapter for content. Susan G. Wynn, DVM, DACVN is certified in acupuncture (IVAS 1997), Chinese herbal medicine (Chi Institute 2001), and accepted as a peer-reviewed professional member of the American Herbalists Guild (2002). She is a former president of the American Holistic Veterinary Medical Association and the American Academy of Veterinary Acupuncture, founder of the Veterinary Botanical Medical Association and has served on the boards of directors for the American Academy of Veterinary Nutrition and the Georgia Veterinary Medical Association. Dr. Wynn also founded Pets Are Loving Support (PALS), an Atlanta-based support organization for pet owners living with chronic illnesses, and she headed the charitable arm of the GVMA, rebranding it as VetHeart while leading a new development campaign. She has consulted with a variety of pet food and supplement companies, and is now the Senior Director of Scientific Affairs with Instinct Pet Food. She also serves as a consultant for the Veterinary Information Network (VIN), speaks locally and internationally on nutrition and holistic veterinary medicine, is an adjunct faculty member with Auburn University's College of Veterinary Medicine, and has authored four professional textbooks including *Veterinary Herbal Medicine* (2007), *Manual of Natural Veterinary Medicine: Science and Tradition* (2003), *Emerging Therapies: Herbal and Natural Medicine for Small Animals*, and the seminal *Complementary and Alternative Veterinary Medicine: Principles and Practice* (1998).

References

AAHA (American Animal Hospital Association) (2019). *Compensation and Benefits*, 9e. Denver, CO: AAHA Press.

ABC (American Botanical Council) (1990). Ginger root. http://cms.herbalgram.org/herbstream/library/CommissionE/#param.wapp?sw_page=@@@@ceHome%3Fufgp%3DMonographs/Monograph0181.html (accessed 30 April 2023).

ABC (American Botanical Council) (2000). Ginger root. http://cms.herbalgram.org/herbstream/library/HerbalMedicine/#param.wapp?sw_page=@@@@@expEView%3Fufgp%3DGingerroot.html (accessed 30 April 2023).

ABC (American Botanical Council) (2013). The ABC Clinical Guide to Herbs. http://cms.herbalgram.org/herbstream/library/ABCguide (accessed 30 April 2023).

ABC (American Botanical Council) (2023). HerbMedPro. http://cms.herbalgram.org/herbstream/library/HerbMedPro (accessed 30 April 2023).

AHPA (American Herbl Products Association) (2013). *Botanical Safety Handbook*, 2e. Baton Rouge, FL: CRC Press.

APPA (American Pet Products Association) (2022). Pet industry market size and ownership statistics. https://www.americanpetproducts.org/press_industrytrends.asp (accessed 23 February 2023).

Araujo, J., Landsberg, G., Milgram, N., and Miolo, A. (2008). Improvement of short-term memory performance in aged beagles by a nutraceutical supplement containing phosphatidylserine, Ginkgo biloba, vitamin E, and pyridoxine. *Canadian Veterinary Journal* 49 (4): 379–385.

ATMS (Australian Traditional-Medicine Society) (2020). Western Herbal Medicine. www.atms.com.au/modalities/western-herbal-medicine (accessed 8 June 2020).

Avizeh, R., Najafrzadeh, H., Razijalali, M., and Shirali, S. (2010). Evaluation of prophylactic and therapeutic effects of silymarin and N-acetylcysteine in acetaminophen-induced hepatotoxicity in cats. *Journal of Veterinary Pharmacology and Therapeutics* 33 (1): 95–99.

AVMA (American Veterinary Medical Association) (2019). Economic state of the veterinary profession. https://www.avma.org/news/press-release/AVMA-2019-Economic-State-of-the-Veterinary-Profession-Report-now-available (accessed 26 July 2021).

AVMA (American Veterinary Medical Association) (2023). *2023 AVMA Report on the Economic State of the Veterinary Profession.* Schaumburg, IL: AVMA.

Bailey, D.G. and Dresser, G.K. (2004). Interactions between grapefruit juice and cardiovascular drugs. *American Journal of Cardiovascular Drugs* 4 (5): 281–297.

Bennett, B. and Balick, M. (2014). Does the name really matter? The importance of botanical nomenclature and plant taxonomy in biomedical research. *Journal of Ethnopharmacology* 152 (3): 387–392.

Bhadra, R., Ravakhah, K., and Ghosh, R.K. (2015). Herb–drug interaction: the importance of communicating with primary care physicians. *Australasian Medical Journal* 8 (10): 315–319.

BLS (Bureau of Labor Statistics) (2022a). Occupational outlook handbook: veterinarians 2022 median pay. https://www.bls.gov/ooh/healthcare/veterinarians.htm (accessed 18 February 2023).

BLS (Bureau of Labor Statistics) (2022b). Occupational outlook handbooks: veterinary technologists and technicians median pay 2020. https://www.bls.gov/ooh/healthcare/veterinary-technologists-and-technicians.htm (accessed 18 February 2023).

BLS (Bureau of Labor Statistics) (2023). News Release: Consumer Price Index January 2023. https://www.bls.gov/news.release/pdf/cpi.pdf (accessed 18 February 2023).

Blumenthal, M. (2000). Interactions between herbs and conventional drugs: introductory considerations. *HerbalGram* 49: 52–63.

Bodagh, M.N., Maleki, I., and Hekmatdoost, A. (2018). Ginger in gastrointestinal disorders: a systematic review of clinical trials. *Food Science and Nutrition* 7 (1): 96–108.

Bol, S., Caspers, J., Buckingham, L. et al. (2017). Responsiveness of cats (Felidae) to silver vine (*Actinidia polygama*), Tatarian honeysuckle (*Lonicera tatarica*), valerian (*Valeriana officinalis*) and catnip (*Nepeta cataria*). *BMC Veterinary Research* 13 (1): 70.

Bone, K. (1997). Ginger. *British Journal of Phytotherapy* 4 (3): 110–120.

Bone, K. (2007). Evaluating, designing, and accessing herbal medicine research. In: *Veterinary Herbal Medicine* (ed. S.G. Wynn and B. Fougere), 87–97. St. Louis, MO: Mosby Elsevier.

BP (1988). *British Pharmacopoeia*. London: Her Majesty's Stationery Office.

Bradley, P. (1992). *British Herbal Compendium*. Bournemouth: British Herbal Medicine Association.

Brown, D. and Reetz, J. (2012). Single agent polysaccharopeptide delays metastases and improves survival in naturally occurring hemangiosarcoma. *Evidence-Based Complementary and Alternative Medicine* 2012: 384301.

Bruneton, J. (1995). *Pharmacognosy, Phytochemistry, Medicinal Plants*. Paris: Lavoisier Publishing.

Budavari, S. (1996). *The Merck Index: An Encyclopedia of Chemicals, Drugs, and Biologicals*, 12e. Whitehouse Station, NJ: Merck & Co, Inc.

Burns, K. (2017). Assessing pet supplements. https://www.avma.org/javma-news/2017-01-15/assessing-pet-supplements (accessed 4 February 2021).

Burns, K. (2018). Pet ownership stable, veterinary care variable. https://www.avma.org/javma-news/2019-01-15/pet-ownership-stable-veterinary-care-variable (accessed 11 August 2021).

Burns, K. (2022). New report takes a deep dive into pet ownership. https://www.avma.org/news/new-report-takes-deep-dive-pet-ownership (accessed 6 November 2022).

But, P. (1997). *International Collation of Traditional and Folk Medicine*. Singapore: World Scientific.

Cabrera, C. (2012). The history of western herbal medicine. http://www.chanchalcabrera.com/history-of-western-herbal-medicine (accessed 2 May 2020).

Caterino, C., Aragosa, F., Della Valle, G. et al. (2021). Clinical efficacy of Curcuvet and Boswellic acid combined with conventional nutraceutical product: an aid to canine osteoarthritis. *PLoS One* 16 (5): e0252279.

Chen, J. (2013). *Concurrent Use of Herbal Medicines and Pharmaceuticals: Pharmacodynamics Interactions*. College of Integrative Veterinary Therapies.

Chen, J.K. and Chen, T.T. (2012). *Chinese Medical Herbology and Pharmacology*. City of Industry, CA: Art of Medicine Press, Inc.

Chrubasik, S., Pittler, M.H., and Roufogalis, B.D. (2005). *Zingiberis rhizoma*: a comprehensive review on the ginger effect and efficacy profiles. *Phytomedicine* 12 (9): 684–701.

Comblain, F., Barthélémy, N., Lefèbvre, M. et al. (2017). A randomized, double-blind, prospective, placebo-controlled study of the efficacy of a diet supplemented with curcuminoids extract, hydrolyzed collagen and green tea extract in owner's dogs with osteoarthritis. *BMC Veterinary Research* 13: 395.

DAB (1997). *Deutscher Apotheker Verlag*. Stuttgart: Deutsches Arzneibuch.

Darby, S.A. (2014). Neuroanatomy of the autonomic nervous system. In: *Clinical Anatomy of the Spine, Spinal Cord, and ANS*, 3e (ed. G.D. Cramer and S.A. Darby), 413–507. St. Louis, MO: Elsevier.

DePorter, T.L., Landsberg, G.M., Araujo, J.A. et al. (2012). Harmonease Chewable tablets reduces noise-induced fear and anxiety in a laboratory canine thunderstorm simulation: a blinded and placebo-controlled study. *Journal of Veterinary Behavior* 7 (4): 225–232.

Di Lorenzo, C., Ceschi, A., Kupferschmidt, H. et al. (2015). Adverse effects of plant food supplements and botanical preparations: a systematic review with critical evaluation of causality. *British Journal of Clinical Pharmacology* 79: 578–592.

DSHEA (1994). Dietary Supplement Health and Education Act (DSHEA) of 1994 Public Law 103-417. https://ods.od.nih.gov/About/DSHEA_Wording.aspx#sec3 (accessed 2 February 2021).

Engel, C. (2007). Zoopharmacognosy. In: *Veterinary Herbal Medicine* (ed. S.G. Wynn and B. Fougere), 7–15. St. Louis, MO: Mosby Elsevier.

Fasinu, P.S., Bouic, P.J., and Rosenkranz, B. (2012). An overview of the evidence and mechanisms of herb–drug interactions. *Frontiers in Pharmacology* 3: 69.

FDA (Food and Drug Administration) (2017). Is it really FDA Approved? https://www.fda.gov/consumers/consumer-updates/it-really-fda-approved (accessed 4 February 2021).

FDA (Food and Drug Administration) (2018). Label Claims for Conventional Foods and Dietary Supplements. https://www.fda.gov/food/food-labeling-nutrition/label-claims-conventional-foods-and-dietary-supplements (accessed 3 February 2021).

FDA (Food and Drug Administration) (2020). The Ins and Outs of Extra-Label Drug Use in Animals: A Resource for Veterinarians. https://www.fda.gov/animal-veterinary/resources-you/ins-and-outs-extra-label-drug-use-animals-resource-veterinarians (accessed 2 February 2021).

FDA (Food and Drug Administration) (2021a). Animal Food & Feeds: Product Regulation. https://www.fda.gov/animal-veterinary/animal-food-feeds/product-regulation (accessed 20 February 2021).

FDA (Food and Drug Administration) (2021b). Animal Medicinal Drug Use Clarificaiton Act of 1994 (AMDUCA). https://www.fda.gov/animal-veterinary/guidance-regulations/

animal-medicinal-drug-use-clarification-act-1994-amduca (accessed 24 January 2022).

FDA (Food and Drug Administration) (2021c). CFR – Code of Federal Regulations Title 21. https://www.accessdata.fda.gov/scripts/cdrh/cfdocs/cfcfr/CFRSearch.cfm?CFRPart= 211&showFR=1 (accessed 16 December 2021).

FederalPay.org (2023). FY 2023 Federal Per Diem Rates October 2022–September 2023. https://www.federalpay.org/perdiem/2023 (accessed 18 February 2023).

Fougère, B. (2007). Approaches in veterinary herbal medicine prescribing. In: *Veterinary Herbal Medicine* (ed. S.G. Wynn and B. Fougere), 275–290. St. Louis, MO: Mosby Elsevier.

Fougère, B. (2015). *How Do Herbs Work? An Introduction to Herbal Modes of Action and Use*. Veterinary Information Network.

French, S. and Kemmis, S. (2023). Rental Car Pricing Statistics:2023. https://www.nerdwallet.com/article/travel/car-rental-pricing-statistics#:~:text=The%20average%20weekly%20rental%20price,in%20advance%2C%20it%20was%20%24513 (accessed 18 February 2023).

Gedney, A., Salah, P., Mahoney, J.A. et al. (2022). Evaluation of the anti-tumour activity of Coriolus versicolor polysaccharopeptide (I'm-Yunity) alone or in combination with doxorubicin for canine splenic hemangiosarcoma. *Veterinary Comparative Oncology* 20: 688–696.

Ghosh, D. (2016). Seed to patient in clinically proven natural medicines. In: *Nutraceuticals: Efficacy, Safety, and Toxicity* (ed. R. Gupta), 925–931. San Diego, CA: Elsevier.

GHP (1992). *Ghana Herbal Pharmacopoeia*. Accra: Policy Research and Strategic Planning Institute (PORSPI).

Giacosa, A., Morazzoni, P., Bombardelli, E. et al. (2015). Can nausea and vomiting be treated with ginger extract? *European Review for Medical and Pharmacological Sciences* 19 (7): 1291–1296.

Giannetto, C., Arfuso, F., Giudice, E. et al. (2022). Antioxidant and hepatoprotective effect of a nutritional supplement with silymarin phytosome, choline chloride, l-cystine, artichoke, and vitamin E in dogs. *Antioxidants* 11 (12): 2339.

Gonora, L. (2015). The action formula. https://www.americanherbalistsguild.com/sites/default/files/the_action_formula_-_ganora_-_ahg_2015_1.pdf (accessed 1 November 2021).

Grassie, L. (2002). Update on Animal Dietary Supplements. https://www.nasc.cc/historical-summary (accessed 4 February 2021).

Griessmayr, P., Gauthier, M., Barber, L., and Cotter, S. (2008). Mushroom-derived Maitake PETfraction as a single agent for the treatment of lymphoma in dogs. *Journal of Veterinary Internal Medicine* 21 (6): 1409–1412.

Grogan, S. and Preuss, C.V. (2022). Pharmacokinetics. Treasure Island, FL: StatPearls. https://www.ncbi.nlm.nih.gov/books/NBK557744 (accessed 6 May 2023).

Guan, Y., Chen, J., Zhou, S. et al. (2018). A randomized and controlled study of the effect of Echinacea Purpurea on canine parvovirus and distemper virus antibody levels in dogs. *American Journal of Traditional Chinese Veterinary Medicine* 13 (2): 13–18.

GVR (Grand View Research) (2021). Pet supplements market size, share & trends analysis repert by bet type (dogs, cats), by form (pills, chewables, powders), by application, by distribution channel (online, offline), by region, and segment forcasts, 2022–2030. https://www.grandviewresearch.com/industry-analysis/pet-supplements-market (accessed 10 May 2023).

Haller, C.A., Kearney, T., Bent, S. et al. (2008). Dietary supplement adverse events: report of a one-year poison center surveillance project. *Journal of Medical Toxicology* 4: 84–92.

Hoffmann, D. (1989). *The Herbal Handbook: A User's Guide to Medical Herbalism*. Rochester, VT: Healing Arts Press.

Hussein, R. and El-Anssary, A. (2019). Plants secondary metabolites: the key drivers of the pharmacological actions of medicinal plants. In: *Herbal Medicine*. IntechOpen: Online https://www.intechopen.com/chapters/61866.

Iftikhar, N. (2019). What is allopathic medicine? https://www.healthline.com/health/allopathic-medicine (accessed 2 November 2021).

Iwu, M. (1990). *Handbook of African Medicinal Plants*. Boca Raton, FL: CRC Press.

Javdani, M., Aali, A., Mohebi, A. et al. (2021). Oral administration of ginger rhizome powder and postoperative inflammation indices in ovariohysterectomized dogs. *Iranian Journal of Veterinary Surgery* 16 (2): 91–99.

JP (1993). *Japanese Pharmacopoeia*. Tokyo: Government of Japan Ministry of Health and Welfare—Yakuji Nippo, Ltd.

Kapadia, M., Zhao, H., Ma, D. et al. (2014). Zoopharmacognosy in diseased laboratory mice: conflicting evidence. *PLoS One* 9 (6): e100684.

Kapoor, L. (1990). *Handbook of Ayurvedic Medicinal Plants*. Boca Raton, FL: CRC Press.

Karnick, C. (1994). *Pharmacopoeial Standards of Herbal Plants*. Delhi: Sri Satguru Publications.

Kaur, J., Seshadri, S., Golla, K.H., and Sampara, P. (2022). Efficacy and safety of standardized Ashwagandha (*Withania somnifera*) root extract on reducing stress and anxiety in domestic dogs: a randomized controlled trial. *Journal of Veterinary Behavior* 51: 8–15.

Kaushik, B., Sharma, J., Kumar, P. et al. (2021). Phytochemical properties and pharmacological role of plants: secondary metabolites. *Biosciences and Biotechnology Research in Asia* 18 (1): 23–35.

Kim, S.-D., Kwag, E.-B., Yang, M.-X., and Yoo, H.-S. (2022). Efficacy and safety of ginger on the side effects of chemotherapy in breast cancer patients: systematic review and meta-analysis. *International Journal of Molecular Science* 23 (19): 11267.

Kisiriko, M., Anastasiadi, M., Terry, L.A. et al. (2021). Phenolics from medicinal and aromatic plants: characterisation and potential as biostimulants and bioprotectants. *Molecules* 26 (21): 6343.

Klein, R. (2007). Medical botany. In: *Veterinary Herbal Medicine* (ed. S.G. Wynn and B. Fougere), 139–158. St. Louis, MO: Mosby Elsevier.

Kolen, R. (2013). Guide to basic herbal actions. https://blog.mountainroseherbs.com/understanding-herbal-actions (accessed 11 November 2020).

Kumar, S. and Pandey, A. (2013). Chemistry and biological activities of flavonoids: an overview. *Scientific World Journal* 2013: 162750.

Lala, L., D'Mello, P., and Naik, S. (2004). Pharmacokinetic and pharmacodynamic studies on interaction of "Trikatu" with diclofenac sodium. *Journal of Ethnopharmacology* 91 (2–3): 277–280.

Lana, S., Kogan, L.R., Crump, K.A. et al. (2006). The use of complementary and alternative therapies in dogs and cats with cancer. *Journal of the American Animal Hospital Association* 42 (2): 361–365.

Landsberg, G., Huggins, S., Fish, J., and Milgram, N.W. (2017). The effects of a nutritional supplement (Solliquin) in reducing fear and anxiety in a laboratory model of thunder-induced fear and anxiety. *Proceedings of the 11th International Veterinary Behaviour Meeting* (14–16 September 2017), Samorin, Slovakia. https://doi.org/10.1079/9781786394583.0094

Lans, C., Khan, T., Curran, M., and McCorkle, C. (2007). Ethnoveterinary medicine: potential solutions for large-scale problems? In: *Veterinary Herbal Medicine* (ed. S.G. Wynn and B. Fougere), 17–32. St. Louis, MO: Mosby Elsevier.

Leung, A. and Foster, S. (1996). *Encyclopedia of Common Natural Ingredients Used in Food, Drugs, and Cosmetics*, 2e. New York: Wiley-Interscience.

Levine, C.B., Bayle, J., Biourge, V., and Wakshlag, J.J. (2016). Effects and synergy of feed ingredients on canine neoplastic cell proliferation. *BMC Research* 12: 159.

Mao, Q.-Q., Xu, X.Y., Cao, S.Y. et al. (2019). Bioactive compounds and bioactivities of ginger (*Zingiber officinale* Roscoe). *Foods* 8 (6): 185.

Marino, M., Jamal, Z. and Zito, P.M. (2023). Pharmacodynamics. Treasure Island, FL: StatPearls. https://www.ncbi.nlm.nih.gov/books/NBK507791 (accessed 6 May 2023).

Marks, D. and Shmalberg, J. (2015). Profitability and financial benefits of acupuncture in small animal private practice. *American Journal of Traditional Chinese Veterinary Medicine* 10 (1): 43–48.

Marsden, S. (2014). *Essential Guide to Chinese Herbal Formulas: Bridging Science and Tradition in Integrative Veterinary Therapies*. College of Integrative Veterinary Therapies.

Masic, A., Landsberg, G., Milgram, B. et al. (2021). Efficacy of Souroubea-platanus dietary supplement containing triterpenes in beagle dogs using a thunderstorm noise-induced model of fear and anxiety. *Molecules* 26 (7): 2049.

Matekaire, T. and Bwakura, T. (2004). Ethnoveterinary medicine: a potential alternative to orthodox animal health delivery in Zimbabwe. *International Journal of Applied Research in Veterinary Medicine* 2 (4): 269–273.

McFaddin III, J.G. (2023). Current cost of common measuring and dispensing materials. A discussion with a Senior Technical Representative for Avantor. Interview, 14 May 2023.

Merawin, L., Arifah, A.K., Sani, R.A. et al. (2010). Screening of microfilaricidal effects of plant extracts against *Dirofilaria immitis*. *Research in Veterinary Science* 88 (1): 142–147.

Merck Manual (2023). Common Botanical Products in Veterinary Medicine. https://www.merckvetmanual.com/multimedia/table/common-botanical-products-in-veterinary-medicine (accessed 13 May 2023).

MFAF (Michelson Found Animals Foundation) (2018). Furred lines: Pet trends. https://www.prnewswire.com/news-releases/furred-lines-pet-trends-2019-300741947.html (accessed 26 July 2021).

NAPHIA (North American Pet Health Insurance Association) (2023). Industry Data. https://naphia.org/industry-data/#my-menu (accessed 18 February 2023).

NCCIH (National Center for Complementry and Integrated Health) (2012). Wellness-Related Use of Common Complementary Health Approaches Among Adults: United States, 2012. https://www.nccih.nih.gov/research/wellness-related-use-of-common-complementary-health-approaches-among-adults-united-states-2012 (accessed 3 January 2021).

NCCIH (National Center for Complementry and Integrated Health) (2013). Traditional Chinese medicine: what you need to know. https://www.nccih.nih.gov/health/traditional-chinese-medicine-what-you-need-to-know (accessed 2 November 2021).

NCCIH (National Center for Complementry and Integrated Health) (2019). Ayurvedic medicine in depth. https://www.nccih.nih.gov/health/ayurvedic-medicine-in-depth (accessed 2 November 2021).

NCCIH (National Center for Complementry and Integrated Health) (2020). Yohimbe. https://www.nccih.nih.gov/health/yohimbe#:~:text=Yohimbe%20has%20been%20associated%20with,or%20banned%20in%20many%20countries (accessed 3 May 2023).

NCCIH (National Center for Complementry and Integrated Health) (2021a). Herb–Drug Interactions. https://www.nccih.nih.gov/health/providers/digest/herb-drug-interactions (accessed 10 May 2023).

NCCIH (National Center for Complementry and Integrated Health) (2021b). Herbs at a Glance. https://www.nccih.nih.gov/health/herbsataglance (accessed 17 Decenber 2021).

Newall, C., Anderson, L., and Phillipson, J. (1996). *Herbal Medicines: A Guide for Health-Care Professionals*. London: The Pharmaceutical Press.

Niemeyer, K., Bell, I., and Koithan, M. (2013). Traditional knowledge of Western herbal medicine and complex systems science. *Journal of Herbal Medicine* 3 (3): 112–119.

Nolen, R.S. (2022). Pet ownership rate stabilizes as spending increases. https://www.avma.org/news/pet-ownership-rate-stabilizes-spending-increases (accessed 22 February 2023).

NRCS (Natural Resources Conservation Service) (2023). US Department of Agriculture (USDA) NRCS. https://www.nrcs.usda.gov (accessed 29 April 2023).

ÖAB (1981–1983). *Österreichisches Arzneibuch*. Wien: Verlag der Österreichischen Staatsdruckerei.

Park, D., Kothari, D., Niu, K.M. et al. (2019). Effect of fermented medicinal plants as dietary additives on food preference and fecal microbial quality in dogs. *Animals* 9 (9): 690.

Pasi, A.K. (2013). Herb–drug interaction: an overview. *International Journal of Pharmaceutical Sciences and Research* 4 (10): 3770–3774.

Petrovska, B.B. (2012). Historical review of medicinal plants' usage. *Pharmacognosy Review* 6 (11): 1–5.

Ph.Helv (1987). *Pharmacopoeia Helvetica*. Bern: Office Central Fédréal des Imprimés et du Matériel.

Poppenga, R. (2007). Herbal medicine: potential for intoxication and interactions with conventional drugs. In: *Veterinary Herbal Medicine* (ed. S.G. Wynn and B. Fougere), 183–207. St. Louis, MO: Mosby Elsevier.

Posadzki, P., Watson, L.K., and Ernst, E. (2013). Adverse effects of herbal medicines: an overview of systematic reviews. *Clinical Medicine Journal* 13 (1): 7–12.

Purdue University (2018). Veterinary price index mid-year 2018 yodate. http://nationwidedvm.com/wp-content/uploads/2018/07/NWP-VPI0708182.pdf (accessed 12 December 2020).

Rashrash, M., Schommer, J., and Brown, L. (2017). Prevalence and predictors of herbal medicine use among adults in the United States. *Journal of Patient Experience* 4 (3): 108–113.

Reichling, J., Fitzi, J., Fürst-Jucker, J. et al. (2003). Echinacea powder: treatment for canine chronic and seasonal upper respiratory tract infections. *Schweizer Archiv für Tierheilkunde* 145 (5): 223–231.

Reichling, J., Schmökel, H., Fitzi, J. et al. (2004). Dietary support with Boswellia resin in canine inflammatory joint and spinal disease. *Schweizer Archiv für Tierheilkunde* 146 (2): 71–79.

Reichling, J., Frater-Schröder, M., Herzog, K. et al. (2006). Reduction of behavioural disturbances in elderly dogs supplemented with a standardised Ginkgo leaf extract. *Schweizer Archiv für Tierheilkunde* 148 (5): 257–263.

Romero, B., Susperregui, J., Sahagún, A.M. et al. (2022). Use of medicinal plants by veterinary practitioners in Spain: a cross-sectional survey. *Frontiers in Veterinary Science* 9: 1060738.

Saeed, M., Breuer, E., Hegazy, M.-E., and Efferth, T. (2019). Retrospective study of small pet tumors treated with Artemisia annua and iron. *International Journal of Oncology* 56: 123–138.

Schadich, E., Hlaváč, J., Volná, T. et al. (2016). Effects of ginger phenylpropanoids and quercetin on Nrf2-ARE pathway in human BJ fibroblasts and HaCaT keratinocytes. *BioMed Research International* 2016: 2173275.

Sharma, S.V.K., Gupta, S.K., Seth, S.D., and Gupta, Y.K. (1997). Antiemetic efficacy of ginger (*Zingiber officinale*) against cisplatin-induced emesis in dogs. *Journal of Ethnopharmacology* 57 (2): 93–96.

Shaw, D., Leon, C., Kolev, S., and Murray, V. (1997). Traditional remedies and food supplements. A 5-year toxicological study (1991–1995). *Drug Safety Journal* 17 (5): 342–356.

Shurkin, J. (2014). News feature: animals that self-medicate. *Proceedings of the National Academy of Sciences of the United States of America* 111 (49): 17339–17341.

Smith, T., Eckl, V., and Reynolds, C.M. (2021a). Herbal supplement sales in US increase by record-breaking 17.3% in 2020. *HerbalGram* 131: 52–65.

Smith, T., Resetar, H., and Morton, C. (2021b). US Sales of herbal supplements increase by 9.7% in 2021. *HerbalGram* 19 (11): https://www.herbalgram.org/resources/herbalegram/volumes/volume-19/issue-11-november/news-and-features-1/2021-herb-market-report/.

Stahnisch, F.W. and Verhoef, M. (2012). The Flexner report of 1910 and its impact on complementary and alternative medicine and psychiatry in North America in the 20th century. *Evidence- Based Complementary and Alternative Medicine* 2012: 647896.

Stevenson, P. (2016). How to set practice service fees. https://cliniciansbrief.com/article/how-set-practice-service-fees (accessed 10 June 2020).

Stillo, T., Norgard, R.J., Stefanovski, D. et al. (2021). The effects of Solliquin administration on the activity and fecal cortisol production of shelter dogs. *Journal of Veterinary Behavior* 45: 10–15.

Teoh, E.S. (2015). *Medicinal Orchids of Asia* (ed. 73), 59. Nature Public Health Emergency Collection.

Trcek, L.(2023). This is How Much Flight Prices Increase in 2023 (+FAQs). https://www.travelinglifestyle.net/this-is-how-much-flight-prices-increase-in-2023 (accessed 18 February 2023).

Tresch, M., Mevissen, M., Ayrle, H. et al. (2019). Medicinal plants as therapeutic options for topical treatment in canine dermatology? A systematic review. *BMC Veterinary Research* 15: 174.

Tu, G. (1992). *Pharmacopoeia of the People's Republic of China (English Edition 1992).* Beijing: Guangdo Science and Technology Press.

Tucakov, J. (1948). *Pharmacognosy*, 8–21. Belgrade: Academic Books.

Tungmunnithum, D.A.T., Pholboon, A., and Yangsabai, A. (2018). Flavonoids and other phenolic compounds from medicinal plants for pharmaceutical and medical aspects: an overview. *Medicines* 5 (3): 93.

Ulewicz-Magulska, B. and Wesolowski, M. (2018). Total phenolic contents and antioxidant potential of herbs used for medical and culinary purposes. *Plant Foods for Human Nutrition* 74 (1): 61–67.

Wachtel-Galor, S. and Benzie, I.F. (2011). An introduction to its history, usage, regulations, current trends, and research needs. In: *Herbal Medicine: Biomolecular and Clinical Aspects*, 2e (ed. I.F.F. Benzie and S. Wachtel-Galor). Boca Raton, FL: CRC Press/Taylor & Francis.

Wanwimolruk, S. and Prachayasittikul, V. (2014). Cytochrome P450 enzyme mediated herbal drug interactions (part 1). *Experimental and Clinical Sciences Journal* 13: 347–391.

Wichtl, M. and Bisset, N. (1994). *Herbal Drugs and Phytopharmaceuticals*. Stuttgart: Medpharm Scientific Publishers.

Wink, M. (2015). Modes of action of herbal medicines and plant secondary metabolites. *Medicines* 2 (3): 251–286.

Withers, S., York, D., Johnson, E. et al. (2018). In vitro and in vivo activity of liposome-encapsulated curcumin for naturally occurring canine cancers. *Veterinary and Comparative Oncology* 16 (4): 571–579.

Woodley, K. (2018). Pet insurance for holistic and integrative practice. https://ivcjournal.com/pet-insurance-integrative-practices (accessed 11 August 2021).

Wu, C.-H., Wang, C.C., Tsai, M.T. et al. (2014). Trend and pattern of herb and supplement use in the United States: results from the 2002, 2007, and 2012 National Health Interview Surveys. *Evidence-Based Complementary and Alternative Medicine* 2014: 872320.

van Wyk, B.-E. and Wink, M. (2017). *Medicinal Plants of the World*. Pretoria: Briza Publications.

Wynn, S. and Fougère, B. (2007a). Clinical practice: getting started. In: *Veterinary Herbal Medicine* (ed. S.G. Wynn and B. Fougere), 453–458. St. Louis, MO: Mosby Elsevier.

Wynn, S. and Fougère, B. (2007b). Herb manufacture, pharmacy, and dosing.

In: *Veterinary Herbal Medicine* (ed. S.G. Wynn and B. Fougere), 221–236. St. Louis, MO: Mosby Elsevier.

Wynn, S. and Fougère, B. (2007c). Materia medica. In: *Veterinary Herbal Medicine* (ed. S.G. Wynn and B. Fougère), 459–672. St. Louis, MO: Mosby Elsevier.

Wynn, S. and Fougère, B. (2007d). The roots of veterinary biomedicine. In: *Veterinary Herbal Medicine* (ed. S.G. Wynn and B. Fougere), 33–49. St. Louis, MO: Mosby Elsevier.

Wynn, S. and Fougère, B. (2007e). *Veterinary Herbal Medicine*. St. Louis, MO: Mosby Elsevier.

Xie, H. (2011a). Chronicle of Chinese history and traditional Chinese veterinary medicine. In: *Xie's Chinese Veterinary Herbology* (ed. H. Xie and V. Preast), 558–591. Ames, IA: Wiley-Blackwell.

Xie, H. (2011b). Toxicity of Chinese veterinary herbal medicines. *American Journal of Traditional Chinese Veterinary Medicine* 6 (2): 45–53.

Xu, J., Long, Y., Ni, L. et al. (2019). Anticancer effect of berberine based on experimental animal models of various cancers: a systematic review and meta-analysis. *BMC Cancer* 19: 589.

Yagmur, E., Piatkowski, A., Gröger, A. et al. (2005). Bleeding complication under Gingko biloba medication. *American Journal of Hematology* 79 (4): 343–344.

Yarnell, E. (2007). Plant chemistry in veterinary medicine: medicinal consituents and their mechanisms of action. In: *Veterinary Herbal Medicine* (ed. S.G. Wynn and B. Fougere), 159–182. St. Louis, MO: Mosby Elsevier.

Yeh, H.-y., Chuang, C.H., Chen, H.C. et al. (2014). Bioactive components analysis of two various gingers (*Zingiber officinale* Roscoe) and antioxidant effect of ginger extracts. *LWT Food Science and Technology* 55 (1): 329–334.

Zhao, J., Geng, T., Wang, Q. et al. (2015). Pharmacokinetics of Ginkgolide B after oral administration of three different Ginkgolide B formulations in beagle dogs. *Molecules* 20 (11): 20031–20041.

12

Multimodal Approach

Introduction

Veterinary integrative medicine (VIM) is a form of multimodal medicine. This chapter explores this concept further, providing examples of how VIM functions as a multimodal approach and how multiple VIM therapies can be used to treat one patient. Six case studies are provided as real-life examples of the practicality and applicability of VIM in everyday practice.

The What

Word Origin

Multimodal is a portmanteau of the words "multiple" and "modes."

Definition

The National Cancer Institute (NCI), a subsidiary of the National Institutes of Health (NIH), defines multimodality treatment as "therapy that combines more than one method of treatment" (NCI 2023).

Traditional Medicine History

The term "multimodal approach" or "multimodal medicine" appears the most when referencing the management of pain and cancer, in both human and veterinary medicine. Veterinarians practice multimodal medicine all the time. Multiple treatment factors are considered and treated with each patient, including diet, environment, systemic, and topical. Refer to Figure 12.1 for examples of how multimodal medicine can be used in traditional veterinary medicine.

Integrative Medicine History

VIM is a blended practice in which traditional (aka Western) and non-traditional (aka Eastern, Holistic, and Alternative) diagnostics

Integrative Medicine in Veterinary Practice, First Edition. Lisa P. McFaddin.
© 2024 John Wiley & Sons, Inc. Published 2024 by John Wiley & Sons, Inc.
Companion website: www.wiley.com/go/mcfaddin/integrativemedicine

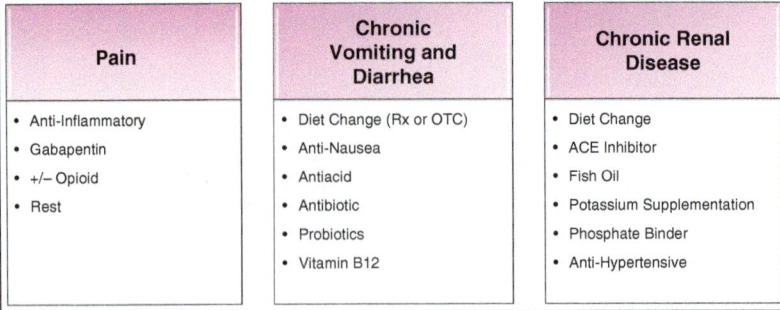

Figure 12.1 An algorithmic representation of the multimodal traditional approach to three common problems seen in veterinary medicine. Potential treatments are provided for each problem. Diagnostics are not included but presumed to have been completed prior to instituting therapy. The list of potential treatments is not all encompassing. TVM, traditional veterinary medicine; Rx, prescription; OTC, over the counter; ACE, angiotensin-converting enzyme. Source: Lisa P. McFaddin.

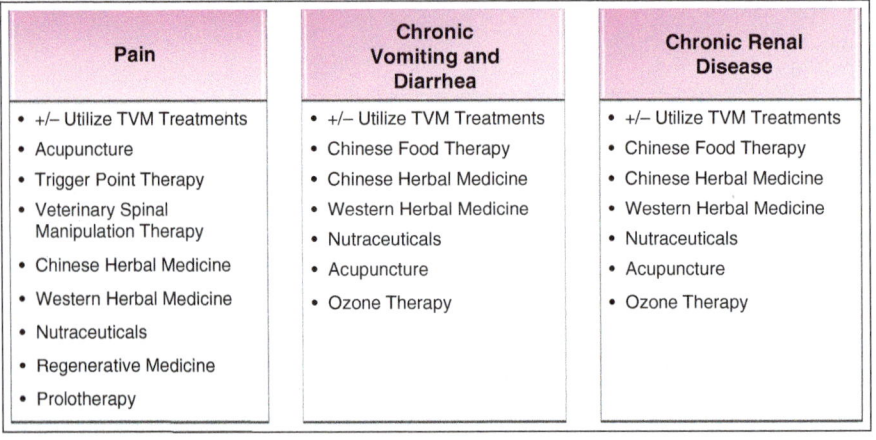

Figure 12.2 An algorithmic representation of the multimodal integrative approach to same three problems presented in Figure 12.1. Potential integrative treatments are provided for each problem. Diagnostics are not included but presumed to have been completed prior to instituting therapy. The list of potential treatments is not all encompassing. VIM, veterinary integrative medicine; Source: Lisa P. McFaddin.

and treatments are used to provide the best possible veterinary care to patients. Integrative medicine is the best of both worlds. By its own definition, VIM is inherently a multimodal approach to medicine. Not only does the incorporation of traditional and non-traditional medicine qualify as multimodal, but practitioners also frequently combine multiple VIM modalities. Figure 12.2 provides examples of how multiple modalities within VIM can be combined (refer to the Case Studies sections for further examples).

Terminology

Refer to Appendix C for a recap of the terminology referenced in Chapters 1–11.

VIM Key Takeaways

This section summarizes key information for each modality covered in Chapters 1–11.

Chapter 1: Acupuncture

- Acupuncture has been used in veterinary medicine for almost 3000 years.

- Acupuncture is the insertion of a needle, or other object, into the skin or stimulation of a specific area of the body causing a beneficial response.
- Acupuncture points, acupoints, are most commonly located on 14 major channels or meridians covering the entire body.
- Acupoints have high concentrations of free nerve endings, small blood vessels, and lymphatic channels.
- Stimulation of acupoints can cause local and systemic effects.
- There are multiple types of acupuncture
  - Acupressure: application of fingers and hands to specific acupoints or regions with multiple points.
  - Aquapuncture: injection of sterile fluid (usually vitamin B12) into acupuncture points.
  - Dry needle: insertion of small sterile, single-use, needles into acupoints. This is the most common form.
  - Electroacupuncture: electric current is applied to pre-placed acupuncture needles using small leads.
  - Hemoacupuncture: intentional bloodletting (small amounts) from specific areas of the body.
  - Moxibustion: burning an herb (Moxa) over acupoints with or without attachment of the herb to the needle.
  - Pneumoacupuncture: injection of air into specific acupoints or larger areas of subcutaneous tissue. Generally used in large animals.
  - Laser acupuncture: low-power cold laser used to stimulate acupoints.
- Acupuncture is used most to help with the management of pain (acute and chronic), anxiety, gastrointestinal disorders, immune system support and disorders, musculoskeletal disorders, neurologic disorders, reproductive disorders, and respiratory dysfunction.
- Acupuncture is considered very safe with few cautions, contraindications, and potential adverse effects.

Cautions
  - Extra caution should be used when placing needles around the eye.
  - Shorter needles should be used at specific points over the chest.
  - Fewer needles should be used in severely debilitated and geriatric patients.
  - Avoid certain points around the lower back and abdomen during pregnancy.
  - Avoid electroacupuncture on animals with seizures and pacemakers.
- **Contraindications**
  - Do not needle through skin infections.
  - Do not needle through open wounds.
  - Do not needle through tumors.
  - Avoid moxibustion in the summer.
  - Avoid hemoacupuncture in weak or geriatric patients.
  - Do not needle CV-8.
- **Adverse effects**
  - Bleeding
  - Bruising
  - Local irritation
  - Bent needle
  - Difficult to remove needle
  - Needle ingestions

Chapter 2: Chinese Food Therapy
- Chinese food therapy (CFT) is one of the four branches within traditional Chinese veterinary medicine (TCVM): acupuncture, Chinese herbal medicine or therapy, Tui-na, and food therapy
- CFT is a medicinal system utilizing food and herbs to prevent and treat diseases and disharmonies diagnosed using TCVM principles.
- The safe and effective use of CFT can only be accomplished once a TCVM diagnosis has been obtained.
- The TCVM exam is different from the typical Western exam taking into account a more detailed history and physical components.
- The primary components of TCVM theory include:

- **Yin and Yang Theory**: Philosophical view dividing all things into two halves which oppose, complement, control, create, and transform into each other.
- **Five Element Theory**: Philosophical view categorizing everything in the natural world five categories: Wood, Fire, Earth, Metal, and Water. Animal personalities are also based on their primary element type.
- **Eight Principle Theory**: A diagnostic system containing three paired categories each of which is define by their Yin or Yang properties.
  - ○ Yin and Yang Theory
  - ○ Cold and Heat Patterns: Reflect the thermal nature of a disease condition and can be subdivided by their location within the body.
  - ○ Deficiency and Excess Patterns: Reflect the body's ability to resist disease, Zheng Qi. There are four categories of Deficiency Patterns: Qi, Blood, Yin and Yang.
- **Five Treasures**: Categorization of life essence into five substances: Qi (energy), Shen (spirit), Jing (essence), Blood, and Body Fluid.
- **Zang-Fu Physiology**: Classification of the 12 organ systems as either solid structures used for storage (Zang) or hollow tube-like structures used to transmit and excrete (Fu).
  - ○ Zang Organs: Lung, Spleen, Heart, Pericardium, Liver, and Kidney.
  - ○ Fu Organs: Large Intestine, Stomach, Small Intestine, Triple Heater, Gallbladder, and Urinary Bladder.
- **Bian Zheng**: Utilization of one or more of the eight diagnostic systems for pattern differentiation.
- CFT uses multiple classification structures applied to all food items simultaneously:
  - **The Five Tastes**: Sour, Bitter, Sweet, Pungent, and Salty
  - **The Five Energies**: Cold, Cool, Neutral, Warm, and Hot

- **The Eight Principles**: Yin, Yang, Interior, Exterior, Deficiency, Excess, Cold and Heat
- **Zang-Fu Organ(s) Affinity**: The Zang-Fu organ(s) most directly affected by the food item.
- **TCVM Therapeutic Actions**: Tonify (Qi, Blood, Yin, Yang, Zang-Fu Organ), Clear (Wind, Heat, Cold), Drain (Damp), Warm, Dissolve (Phlegm), etc.
- CFT is used in one or more of the following situations:
  - Guide commercial diet selection
  - Supplement commercial diets
  - Recreate an herbal formula
  - Temporary therapeutic diet
  - Maintenance diet
- Maintenance diets must be appropriate for the age and health status of the patient.
- A well-balanced diet is critical for patient health. Inclusion of vitamins, supplements, and consultation with a board-certified veterinary nutritionist may be warranted.
- CFT is not well studied in human or veterinary medicine. The overall effects of food on general well-being and disease prevention/management are well studied in both medical fields.
- CFT is commonly used in veterinary medicine to aid in the treatment of cancer, cardiovascular disease, chronic inflammation, dermatologic disorders, endocrine dysfunction, gastrointestinal disorders, general health maintenance, geriatric patients, kidney disorders, and liver diseases.

Chapter 3: Chinese Herbal Medicine

- Chinese herbal medicine (CHM) is one of the four branches within TCVM: acupuncture, Chinese herbal medicine or therapy, Tui-na, and food therapy.
- CHM is a medicinal system which utilizes individual and combinations of herbs to diagnose, prevent, and treat disease.
- The safe and effective use of CHM can only be accomplished once a TCVM diagnosis has been obtained.

- The TCVM exam is different from the typical Western exam taking into account a more detailed history and physical components.
- The primary components of TCVM theory include:
  - **Yin and Yang Theory**: Philosophical view dividing all things into two halves which oppose, complement, control, create, and transform into each other.
  - **Five Element Theory**: Philosophical view categorizing everything in the natural world five categories: Wood, Fire, Earth, Metal, and Water. Animal personalities are also based on their primary element type.
  - **Five Treasures**: Categorization of life essence into five substances: Qi (energy), Shen (spirit), Jing (essence), Blood, and Body Fluid.
  - **Zang-Fu Physiology**: Classification of the 12 organ systems as either solid structures used for storage (Zang) or hollow tube-like structures used to transmit and excrete (Fu).
    - Zang Organs: Lung, Spleen, Heart, Pericardium, Liver, and Kidney.
    - Fu Organs: Large Intestine, Stomach, Small Intestine, Triple Heater, Gallbladder, and Urinary Bladder.
  - **Bian Zheng**: Utilization of one or more of the eight diagnostic systems for pattern differentiation.
  - **Treatment Strategies**: Chinese herbs and herbal formulas are used to treat the TCVM diagnosis: Clear Heat, Drain Damp, Reduce Excess, Tonify Deficiency, etc.
- The organization of both individual Chinese herbs and Chinese herbal formulas is complex and typically characterized by:
  - TCVM effects
  - Taste
  - Thermal properties
  - Direction
  - Zang-Fu channel and organ affinity
  - Source
  - Adverse effects
  - Pharmacologic effects.

- Chinese herbs and herbal formulas marketed for animals are technically classified as animal food or food additives. The Food and Drug Administration (FDA) does not require pre-market approval before new animal food is sold. The FDA does require pre-market approval for animal food additives unless it is generally recognized as safe (GRAS).
- The FDA's Center for Veterinary Medicine (CVM) is responsible for regulating animal food, including herbs and herbal formulas. Failure to meet the CVM requirements results in the adulterated or misbranded herbs and the FDA could take regulatory action. Typically, veterinary botanicals are low on the priority list for the FDA regulators.
- According to the National Animal Supplement Council (NASC) there are over 400 unapproved substances marketed for use in animals (Grassie 2002).
- When selecting an herbal company ensure the following criteria are met:
  - Seed to seal guarantee.
  - Meet or exceed good manufacturing practices (GMP).
  - Excellent quality control measures.
- Adverse effects are uncommon and if noted generally resolve within 24 hours.
- Most herb–drug interactions are positive, i.e. herbs can be used to negate the negative side effects of many pharmaceuticals.
- When dispensing CHM the practitioner must consider the best herb or herbal formula, best preparation method, and best dosing instructions.
- CHM can be used to aid in the treatment of almost all veterinary conditions.

Chapter 4: Nutraceuticals

- Veterinary Nutraceuticals (VN) (aka animal health supplement) are products isolated or derived from a food source(s) used to support normal biological processes within animals. VN are not drugs and cannot treat, diagnose, prevent, or cure disease.

- Dietary supplement (aka food supplement) are substances which complement the diet and contain at least one of the following ingredients: a vitamin, a mineral, an herb, an amino acid, or a product which affects caloric intake (FDA 2018).
- Drug is a substance used to diagnose, cure, treat, or prevent disease in both humans and animals, as well as alter the body's functions or structure (Law Revision Counsel US Code 2018).
- Regulation information: refer to Chapter 3.
- Factors to consider when selecting a VN manufacturer:
  - The company can trace its source materials.
  - The company follows GMP.
  - The company can provide their quality control measures.
  - The products are accurately labeled.
  - The products have a seal of approval from an outside regulatory agency.
- Adverse effects are relatively uncommon and generally mild. To avoid side effects follow the 4Rs when prescribing a VN: right supplement, right patient, right purpose, and right dose. If adverse effects are noted, they should be report to the veterinarian and manufacturer.
- VN–drug interactions (VNDI) are possible which is why it is critical to record everything a pet is taking to avoid interactions.
- VN are classified in the chapter as vitamins, minerals, microbiome therapy, joint supplements, amino acids, antioxidants and free radical scavengers, and botanicals (Burns 2017).
- There are potential cautions, contraindications, and adverse effects associated with each supplement.

Chapter 5: Ozone Therapy

- Veterinary ozone therapy (VOT) is the introduction of medical-grade ozone gas into or onto the body with the intent to treat or cure a specific disease condition.
- Ozone is administered (alone or in solution) intravenously, subcutaneously, rectally, or topically, but never through inhalation.

- VOT has been practiced for roughly 50 years, with increasing use over the last 20 years.
- Ozone, an inorganic molecule, is a colorless to pale blue explosive gas with a characteristic odor comprising three oxygen atoms, O_3.
- A medical-grade ozone generator, or ozonator, is a device used to create ozone from oxygen gas using either an electrical discharge (corona), UV light, plasma, or electrolysis.
- The following variables must be considered when performing VOT:
  - *Concentration*: Ozone is divided into low, medium, and high concentrations.
  - *Formulation*: Ozone is typically administered as a gas, percolated in a liquid, or mixed in an oil.
  - *Volume*: Typically measured in milliliters (ml).
  - *Route of administration*: Ozone can be administered systemically (through injection or insufflation) or locally (bagging or topically with gas, percolated liquid, or oil).
  - *Frequency*: Ozone can be administered daily, multiple times a week, weekly, every other week, or as needed.
  - *Patient factors*: Including age, health status, and disease condition addressed.
- Ozone has antimicrobial, immune-stimulating, analgesic, anti-inflammatory, and anti-hypoxic effects.
- Ozone gas is toxic to the lungs and extrapulmonary organs if inhaled directly.
- Ozone is considered safe, with few adverse effects, when administered using the appropriate formulation, correct dose, and length of exposure.
- VOT is most used for the treatment of chronic inflammatory and infectious conditions.

Chapter 6: Photobiomodulation

- Photobiomodulation (PBM) is a portmanteau of the words "photo" (meaning light) and "biomodulation" (meaning modifying or changing a biological or biochemical process).
- PBM therapy (PBMT) is also known as low-level laser or light therapy or cold laser therapy.

- PBMT is the use of light (most commonly red or near-infrared) to stimulate, heal, regenerate, and protect damaged tissue.
- **Laser basics**
  - Laser is an acronym for light amplification by stimulated emission of radiation.
  - A laser is a device which can convert light or electrical energy into a focused and high energy beam.
  - The light is monochromatic (one color), contains a single light frequency (coherent), and does not spread out very far over long distances.
  - The most common lasers used in PBMT are in the red or near-infrared spectrum.
  - Lasers are classified based on their potential risk to the user (aka hazard potential), with Class IIIb and Class IV being the most used in veterinary PBMT.
- **LED basics**
  - Light-emitting diodes (LEDs) are very small light bulbs without filaments, which do not produce heat.
  - The light is not monochromic and is non-coherent.
  - The most common LEDs used in veterinary PBM are in the red or near-infrared spectrum.
- **Parameters**
  - Wavelength: Distance between the peaks of a wave, usually measured in nanometers (nm). Determines the depth of tissue penetration, with longer wavelengths penetrating deeper. Normally fall between 600 and 1000 nm (red and near-infrared spectrum).
  - Power: Rate at which energy is delivered, expressed in watts (W) or milliwatts (mW). Determines the treatment length. 1 watt equals 1 joule (J) per second, i.e. $1 W = 1 J/s$. Lower watt lasers (Class III, <500 mW) are best suited for superficial tissues, and higher watt lasers (Class IV, >500 mW) are typically used for conditions affecting deeper tissues.
  - Dose: Laser's energy measured in joules (J). Expressed as the amount of energy delivered over a surface area (J/cm^2). Range is dependent on the condition being treated, typically between 2 and $10 J/cm^2$.
  - Treatment interval: Length of time between treatments and varies by condition (days to weeks).
- **Techniques**
  - Point-to-point: The desired treatment area is divided into a specific number of points, and the probe is held in place for a set period of time (seconds) depending on the treatment length.
  - Non-point-to-Point: Require continuous movement throughout the treatment period; gridding or surrounding.
  - Probe: Must always be kept perpendicular (90° angle) to the target tissue to reduce reflection and scatter.
  - Treatment area: Should include target tissue and surrounding healthy/non-affected tissue.
- **Mechanisms of action**
  - Particles of light (photons) hitting the surface of the skin, and other tissue layers, can either be reflected, transmitted, scattered, or absorbed.
  - Only absorbed photons produce a therapeutic effect.
  - The interaction of light with damaged or diseased tissue causes changes at the molecular, cellular, and tissue level (Cheng et al. 2021).
  - Light photons interact with chromophores (contribute to the color of a substance) which cause changes at the molecular, cellular, and tissue levels.
  - There are four major biological or therapeutic effects: pain reduction (analgesia), anti-inflammatory, immune modulation, and an increase in tissue healing and regeneration.
- **Safety**
  - OSHA requires all veterinary hospitals with a medical laser institute a laser safety program.
  - A hospital must have a designated Laser Safety Officer (LSO).

– A hospital must designate specific areas for laser storage and use.
– Safety signs must be used when the laser is in use and where the laser is stored.
– All persons in a room with a working laser must wear protective eyewear.
– Protective laser goggles are made to block specific wavelengths and are not universal.
– The patient's eyes should be protected from indirect and direct ocular exposure.
– PBMT is a very safe and effective therapy, and the only true contraindication is ocular exposure.
- PBMT is most used in veterinary medicine to aid in the treatment of skin wounds and infections, musculoskeletal injuries, osteoarthritis, neurologic injuries, postoperative pain and healing, and other sources of pain.

Chapter 7: Prolotherapy

- Other names for prolotherapy are nonsurgical ligament and tendon reconstruction and regenerative joint Injection.
- Prolotherapy is the injection of a small volume of a sterile irritant into a painful joint, tendon, or ligament. The irritating solution induces a local inflammatory response, stimulating the body's natural healing ability, stabilizing the weakened tissues, and reducing pain.
- The most common substance used is dextrose, diluted with sterile saline.
- Refer to Terminology section for common terms, and their definitions, used when discussing prolotherapy
- Mechanism of action is complex and not fully understood.
  – The injection of a substance into a tendon, ligament or joint causes a controlled injury or insult which incites a predictable inflammatory and healing response by the body.
  – The result is improved stability, strength, and reduction of pain.
  – Pain relief is achieved by improving stability within the joint, tendon, or ligament.

- Prolotherapy incites the body's natural phases of wound healing: hemostasis, inflammatory phase, proliferative phase, and remodeling phase.
- Prolotherapy is used to aid in the treatment of a variety of musculoskeletal and neurologic conditions.
- Prolotherapy should be used with caution in senior pets and immunocompromised patients.
- Prolotherapy should be avoided in cases of cancer (affecting local muscle, connective tissue, and bone), acute non-reduced luxations or dislocations, septic arthritis, post-traumatic arthritis, acute tendonitis, acute bursitis, and allergies to the injectable solution.
- Potential adverse effects of prolotherapy include infection at the injection site, pain, stiffness, bruising or bleeding, transient nerve damage, and potentially therapy failure.

Chapter 8: Veterinary Regenerative Medicine

- Veterinary regenerative medicine (VRM) is defined as the injection of a substance derived from animal cells or tissues into a joint, tendon, or ligament with the intent of reducing pain and inflammation by promoting the body's natural healing abilities.
- VRM is frequently used as an adjunct to surgery or as part of a multimodal approach to rehabilitation.
- The two primary biologicals used in regenerative medicine are platelet-rich plasma and stem cells.
- Refer to Terminology section for common terms, and their definitions, used when discussing prolotherapy
- The Food and Drug Administration (FDA) classifies platelet-rich plasma (PRP) and stem cells as drugs. Use of animal-based cell products must follow FDA guidelines.
- There is a lack of standardization in the processing of both PRP and stem cells.
- Samples (both PRP and stem cells) should be validated prior to administration.

- PRP samples are typically obtained, processed, and administered within the veterinary hospital using commercially available PRP kits.
- Stem cell samples are typically send to an outside laboratory for processing causing a delay between the time of sample collection and sample administration.

- PRP and stem cells can be injected within or around joints, tendons, ligaments, and muscles.
- There are four phases of wound healing: hemostasis, inflammation, proliferation, and remodeling.
- Following injection both PRP and stem cells reduce pain and inflammation, as well as encouraging tissue healing, through direct and indirect effects on the tissue itself. The result is improved stability, strength, and reduction of pain.
- Regenerative medicine is a newer science without strict regulation and protocols. Validation of sample preparation, storage, and application, along with continued scientific research, is critical to the advancement of this therapy.
- VRM is used primarily to aid in the treatment of musculoskeletal injuries but other applications are gaining popularity.
- VRM should be used with caution in immunocompromised individuals.
- VRM is contraindicated in patients with cancers affecting local muscle, connective tissue, and bone, acute non-reduced luxations or dislocations, septic arthritis, post-traumatic arthritis, acute tendonitis, acute bursitis, bleeding disorders, and clotting disorders.
- Potential adverse effects include infection, pain, stiffness, bruising, bleeding, transient nerve damage, and therapy failure.

Chapter 9: Trigger Point Therapy

- A trigger point (TrP) (aka myofascial trigger point) is a hyperirritable palpable nodule or taut band within the skeletal muscle or associated fascia (Finando 2005).

- Direct manipulation of the nodule or band will elicit a disproportionately painful response locally and often distantly (referred pain) (Finando 2005).
- A TrP leads to three primary issues: muscle dysfunction (a hard nodule within the muscle); pain; and motor dysfunction (reduced range of motion and weakness).
- Characteristics of TrP in veterinary patients:
  - A tight band or nodule within the muscle which causes marked pain upon palpation.
  - Visible or palpable contraction of the muscle during TrP palpation (local twitch response, LTR).
  - Weakness of the affected muscle, without atrophy.
  - Reduced range of motion of the associated joint.
  - Jump sign seen after palpation of a TrP.
- The most common conditions causing TrP formation include trauma, overuse, neurologic, orthopedic, hormone disorders, overweight/obesity, and viscero-somatic pain.
- TrP are diagnosed using either flap or pincher palpation.
- Trigger point therapy (TrPT) refers to a group of treatment modalities used to reduce the pain associated with, and ideally resolve, myofascial trigger points.
- TrPT techniques include physical therapy (massage, stretching, ischemic compression technique, taping, and neuromuscular techniques); therapeutic ultrasound; photobiomodulation (cold laser); thermal techniques (hot and cold packs); dry needling; and trigger point injection.
- Trigger point pressure release (TPPR) is the most common manual technique used in the management of TrP in people and animals.
  - Digital compression is applied to the palpable TrP until relaxation of the taut band is appreciated.
  - Blood flow to the TrP is initially decreased then returns restoring circulation, improving muscle fiber relaxation, reducing inflammation, and promoting healing.

- Dry needling (DN) is the placement of a thin solid acupuncture needle through the skin directly into a TrP.
  - Veterinary patients are often sedated for DN.
  - Placement of the needle punctures the skin causing counter-irritation within the epidermis, dermis, subcutaneous tissues, and muscle leading to microtrauma (Clemmons 2007).
  - This tissue disruption directly affects local nerves, muscle fibers, blood vessels, and immune cells improving blood flow, immune response, and relaxation of tissues and muscles (Dommerholt 2011).
  - Signals carried by the nerve cells spread from the point of impact to the spinal cord and eventually the brain, propagating the beneficial effects throughout the body (Chiu et al. 2001).
- Trigger point injections (TrPI) involve the injection of a small amount of a sterile solution into a TrP.
  - The most used solutions include local anesthetics (lidocaine or bupivacaine, with or without sodium bicarbonate), corticosteroids, sterile saline, or dextrose (Tantanatip et al. 2021; Hammi et al. 2022).
  - The exact mechanism(s) of TrPI is unknown.
  - The injection of a sterile liquid into or near a TrP has similar effects to that of DN (Hammi et al. 2022).
  - TrPIs also improve the movement of myofascial tissues helping to normalize muscle function and reduce pain (Tantanatip et al. 2021).
  - TrPIs incite a predictable response by the body: controlled inflammation followed by healing (Osborn 2018).
- TPPR is contraindicated in patients with fractures, bone infections (osteomyelitis), muscle or bone cancer, and active bleeding (especially internally).
  - Caution is required when treating patients with cancer or immune-mediated diseases.

- Pain and bruising are the most likely adverse effects (Wall 2010, 2019).
- The contraindications, cautions, and adverse effects of invasive techniques (DN and TrPIs) are like those seen with TPPR.
  - Invasive TrPTs are also contraindicated in areas with skin infections and patients with a high anesthetic or sedation risk, if required (Wall 2010, 2019).
  - Pain, bruising, bleeding, hematoma formation, and an adverse reaction to the sedation/anesthetic are the most likely adverse effects (Wall 2010, 2019).

Chapter 10: Veterinary Spinal Manipulation Therapy

- VSMT was first utilized by Dr. Sharon Willoughby, a veterinarian, and Doctor of Chiropractic (DC), in the 1980s. With the help of Tom Offen DC, the pair adapted chiropractic techniques to animals.
- VSMT (aka veterinary chiropractic and animal chiropractic) is an integrative medical system rooted in the diagnosis and treatment of hypomobile joints, especially those within the spinal column, which cause local and systemic dysfunction of nerves, muscles, and organs. Improvement in joint mobility, generally through manual therapy, allows the body's innate forces to heal itself, achieving homeostasis.
- A strong foundation in veterinary anatomy, physiology, and neurology are required to understand and apply VSMT.
- A VSMT exam consists of a general physical exam, comprehensive neurologic examination and orthopedic examination.
- Common VSMT techniques include:
  - **Manual adjustments or manipulation**: The application of unidirectional high-velocity low-amplitude thrust to specific motion segment. Commonly performed on the entire spine and appendicular skeleton.
  - **Traction**: Gentle sustained pressure is used to separate joint surfaces for

15–30 seconds, then pressure is slowly released. Typically performed on the neck, elbows, wrists (carpi), and tail.

- **Mobilization**: The joint is passively moved through its range of motion multiple times loosening areas and breaking up adhesions. Performed on the digits (thoracic and pelvic), metacarpals/metatarsals, wrist (carpus), accessory carpal bone, ankles (hocks), and tail (coccygeal) vertebrae.
- **Stretch and hold**: Muscle, connective tissue, and fascia relaxation is achieved through sustained elongation, approximately 90–120 seconds, of the affected muscles. Most often performed on the shoulder and hip flexors.

- VSMT may help with the management of pain, lameness, paresis (weakness), behavioral changes, sporting dog injuries, incontinence, TMJ issues, and as an adjunct to postoperative orthopedic rehabilitation.
- VSMT should be used with caution in patients with hypermobile joints, spondylosis deformans, cancer, seizures, immune-mediated diseases, and poor patient compliance (very aggressive or scared pets).
- VSMT should be avoided in cases severe acute pain, fracture (spine or limb), vertebral abnormalities (hemivertebrae, block vertebrae)*, intervertebral disk protrusion*, bone infection (osteomyelitis), bone cancer, splenic cancer, active bleeding (especially internally), fever, and immediately postoperative. (*Refer to the affected motion units.)
- Patients may experience muscle stiffness or pain or loose bowel movements within the first 24 hours following VSMT.

Chapter 11: Western Herbal Medicine

- Western herbal medicine (WHM) is a medicinal system which utilizes individual and combinations of plant materials, with minimal processing, to prevent and treat disease.
  - Crude parts or extracts of the root, bark, and flower are used as individual herbs or

part of a multi-plant formulation (Niemeyer et al. 2013).
  - The practice of WHM is also known as Western herbalism, botanical medicine, medical herbalism, and phytotherapy.
  - In veterinary medicine, WHM is often referred to as veterinary herbal medicine (VHM).
- To utilize WHM safely and effectively, the veterinarian must know their botanical pharmacy inside out, including taxonomy, identification, anatomy, and chemistry (Klein 2007).
- The therapeutic effects associated with medicinal plants and fungi are due to their chemical composition.
  - The primary components are essential for the survival of the plant or fungus including carbohydrates, amino acids, proteins, and lipids (Yarnell 2007).
  - The secondary components are considered nonessential for plant or fungus survival but aid in maintaining overall health by preventing self-trauma from the by-products of photosynthesis (antioxidants), attracting pollinators and encouraging seed distribution (reproduction), preventing predation from insects and herbivores, as well as discouraging nearby growth of other plants (self-defense), and improving cellular signals (Yarnell 2007).
  - The secondary constituents are responsible for many of the plant or fungi's medicinal effects.
  - Examples of categories of botanical secondary metabolites (BSM) include alkaloids, phenolics, saponins, and terpenes (Klein 2007; Wink 2015; Kaushik et al. 2021).
- Herbs can be categorized by their botanical metabolites, traditional herb actions, target organ or tissue, and therapeutic goals.
- The materia medica is like an encyclopedia of herbal remedies comprising individual monographs.

- There are multiple WHM diagnostic categories, and the one(s) used are dependent on the practitioner's training and level of experience.
- To develop a treatment plan, the practitioners must consider multiple factors including the patient's age, breed predilections, environmental factors, lifestyle, diet, and concurrent illness.
- Herbs used in veterinary WHM are either classified as animal dietary supplements (considered food) or food additives.
  - Pre-market FDA approval is not required before selling new animal foods, but the food must "be safe to eat, produced under sanitary conditions, free of harmful substances, and truthfully labeled" (FDA 2021a).
  - Pre-market approval is required for animal food additives.
- The FDA does not approve manufacturing companies. "Owners and operators of domestic and foreign food, drug, and most device facilities must register their facilities with FDA, unless an exemption applies. FDA does have authority to inspect regulated facilities to verify that they comply with applicable good manufacturing practice regulations" (FDA 2017).
- Due to the overall lack of regulation, it is crucial the veterinary herbalist knows how to choose reputable and safe products including critically evaluating the companies used to source, manufacture, bottle, and store herbal products.
- Herbs can be dispensed as individual herbs, in-clinic combined formula, or a pre-made formula.
- Herbs are primarily dispensed as dried herbs (powdered), dried extract, or liquid extract.
- Factors affecting herbal dosing include the formulation, route of administration, frequency of administration, bioavailability (i.e. how well it is absorbed by the body), patient signalment (age, breed, and sex), concurrent illnesses, concurrent medications, supplements, and herbs, clinical experience, and clinical studies (when available) (Wynn and Fougère 2007).

- WHM can be used to aid in the treatment of a large number of veterinary conditions. Adverse effects (AEs), also known as side effects, are defined as any unwanted and harmful outcome caused by a drug or supplement.
  - The type and severity of potential AEs is dependent on the herb or herbs administered.
  - Ensuring the right herb is used for the right patient at the right dose and for the right purpose should reduce the risk of AEs.
- A herb–drug interaction (HDI) is any modification to the use, effect, efficacy, or mechanism of action of a prescription medication by an herbal substance, or vice versa (Pasi 2013).

  - The modification may result in a beneficial, undesirable, or negative (harmful) effect. It is crucial the practitioner be aware of, and know how to research, potential HDIs.

The Why

Figures 12.3–12.5 summarize the conditions for which each modality has shown beneficial effects. The VIM therapies are divided into three groups: manual therapies, injectable therapies, and oral therapies. Manual therapies include acupuncture, photobiomodulation, trigger point therapy, and veterinary spinal manipulation. Injectable therapies include ozone, prolotherapy, and regenerative medicine. Oral therapies include Chinese herbal medicine, Western herbal medicine, nutraceuticals, and Chinese food therapy.

The How

Frequently a multimodal approach incorporates all therapies equally. But almost as often one of the therapies is primary while the other modalities serve as adjuncts, aiding in improvement or resolution of the clinical signs. In this section several case studies are provided showcasing one

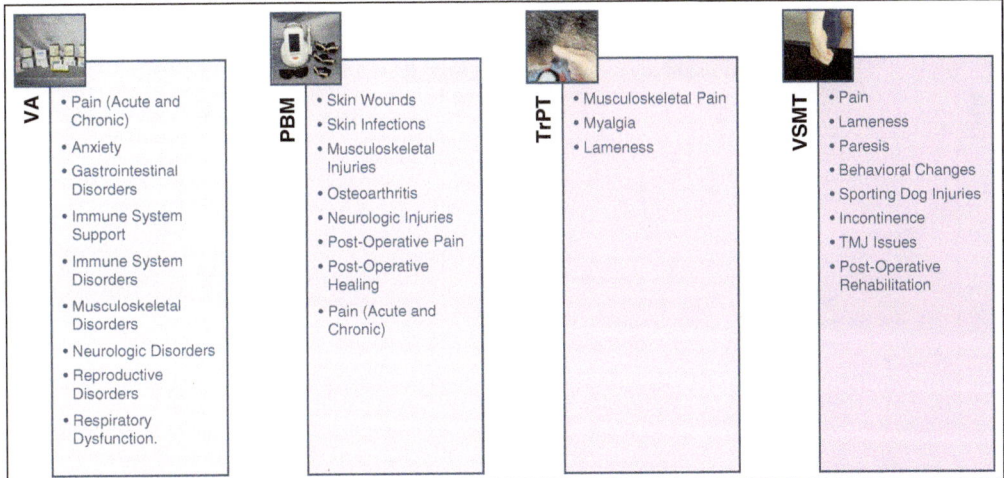

Figure 12.3 A list of many conditions for which the incorporation of veterinary acupuncture (VA), photobiomodulation (PBM), trigger point therapy (TrPT), and veterinary spinal manipulation therapy (VSMT) has shown beneficial therapeutic effects. This is not an exhaustive list. Refer to each modality's chapter for further information. TMJ, temporomandibular joint. Source: Lisa P. McFaddin.

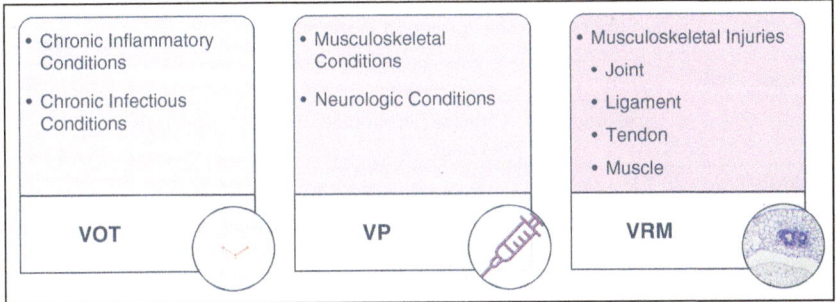

Figure 12.4 A list of many of the conditions for which the incorporation of veterinary ozone therapy (VOT), veterinary prolotherapy (VP), and veterinary regenerative medicine (VRM) has shown beneficial therapeutic effects. This is not an exhaustive list. Refer to each modality's chapter for further information. Source: Lisa P. McFaddin.

modality while referencing the concurrent use of other modalities. Table 12.1 summarizes the primary and secondary modalities used in each case study.

Case studies are a valuable means through which clinical experience can be relayed in a clear and succinct format (Morresey 2019). Outlines the reasons for which case studies are written in his editorial "How to write a clinical case report":

1) To describe a novel disease.
2) To present a new diagnosis for a previously known disease.
3) To define a new treatment for a previously known disease.
4) To impart knowledge, either new or reinforcing previous dogma, in veterinary medicine.
5) To be used as a foundation upon which clinical research will be based (aka case rounds).

The case studies in this book function to demonstrate new ways to approach previously known conditions and impart new knowledge to the veterinary field supporting the use of VIM.

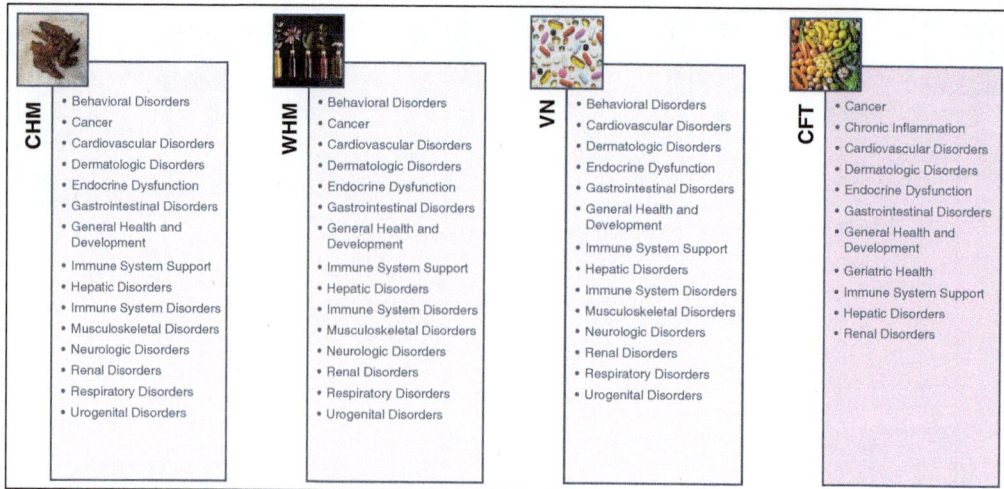

CHM	WHM	VN	CFT
• Behavioral Disorders	• Behavioral Disorders	• Behavioral Disorders	• Cancer
• Cancer	• Cancer	• Cardiovascular Disorders	• Chronic Inflammation
• Cardiovascular Disorders	• Cardiovascular Disorders	• Dermatologic Disorders	• Cardiovascular Disorders
• Dermatologic Disorders	• Dermatologic Disorders	• Endocrine Dysfunction	• Dermatologic Disorders
• Endocrine Dysfunction	• Endocrine Dysfunction	• Gastrointestinal Disorders	• Endocrine Dysfunction
• Gastrointestinal Disorders	• Gastrointestinal Disorders	• General Health and Development	• Gastrointestinal Disorders
• General Health and Development	• General Health and Development	• Immune System Support	• General Health and Development
• Immune System Support	• Immune System Support	• Hepatic Disorders	• Geriatric Health
• Hepatic Disorders	• Hepatic Disorders	• Immune System Disorders	• Immune System Support
• Immune System Disorders	• Immune System Disorders	• Musculoskeletal Disorders	• Hepatic Disorders
• Musculoskeletal Disorders	• Musculoskeletal Disorders	• Neurologic Disorders	• Renal Disorders
• Neurologic Disorders	• Neurologic Disorders	• Renal Disorders	
• Renal Disorders	• Renal Disorders	• Respiratory Disorders	
• Respiratory Disorders	• Respiratory Disorders	• Urogenital Disorders	
• Urogenital Disorders	• Urogenital Disorders		

Figure 12.5 A list of many of the conditions for which the incorporation of Chinese herbal medicine (CHM), Western herbal medicine (WHM), veterinary nutraceuticals (VN), and Chinese food therapy (CFT) has shown beneficial therapeutic effects. This is not an exhaustive list. Refer to each modality's chapter for further information. Source: Lisa P. McFaddin.

Table 12.1 Summary of the primary and secondary veterinary integrative modalities used in the case studies provided in this chapter.

Case Study 1	Primary	Acupuncture
	Secondary	Chinese herbal medicine, nutraceuticals, massage
Case Study 2	Primary	Chinese food therapy
	Secondary	Chinese herbal medicine, nutraceuticals
Case Study 3	Primary	Chinese herbal medicine
	Secondary	Nutraceuticals
Case Study 4	Primary	Photobiomodulation
	Secondary	Rehabilitation
Case Study 5	Primary	Trigger point therapy
	Secondary	Rehabilitation, massage, photobiomodulation
Case Study 6	Primary	Veterinary spinal manipulation therapy
	Secondary	Acupuncture, Chinese herbal medicine, nutraceuticals, massage, trigger point therapy

Source: Lisa P. McFaddin.

Case Study 1 Focus on Acupuncture

Title: Dry needle acupuncture and aquapuncture treatment for C6 radiculoneuritis in a dog
Author: Lisa P. McFaddin, DVM, GDCVHM, CVSMT, CVA, FCoAC

Summary: A historically paraplegic dog with an acute onset of neck pain secondary to C6 radiculoneuritis was successfully managed using traditional pharmaceuticals, acupuncture, and aquapuncture. The patient's pain level greatly improved after the first session. Despite the cessation of opioid pain medication and steroid tapering, the patient remained pain-free with successive acupuncture treatments.

Introduction: Cervical radiculoneuritis is defined as inflammation of a nerve root within the cervical vertebrae generally caused by compression of the nerve as it leaves the spinal cord. Common causes in veterinary medicine include trauma, intervertebral disk disease, immune-mediated inflammation, infections, and neoplasia (Chrisman 2011). Traditional treatment involves strict rest, anti-inflammatories in the form of nonsteroidals or steroids, nerve pain medication (gabapentin, amantadine), muscle relaxants (methocarbamol), and opioid pain medication (tramadol, codeine, hydromorphone).

The successful use and effectiveness of acupuncture as a stand-alone or adjunct treatment for cervical spinal cord disease is well documented in both human and veterinary medicine (Gülanber 2008; Hayashi et al. 2007; Joaquim et al. 2010; Chien 2011; Liu et al. 2015; Silva et al. 2017; Rovnard et al. 2018; Zuo et al. 2019). Acupuncture, in its most elemental form, is the insertion of a needle, or other object, into the skin on a specific area of the body which causes a beneficial response. Aquapuncture is the injection of a sterile liquid, usually vitamin B12, into an acupuncture point (acupoint).

The mechanism through which acupuncture exerts its effects, especially with respect to the reduction of pain and inflammation, is complex and not fully understood. Anatomically acupoints comprise free nerve endings, small vessels (arteries and veins), and lymphatics (this includes immune cells and channels carrying immune cells). Placement of the acupuncture needle punctures the skin causing counter-irritation within the epidermis, dermis and subcutaneous tissues, leading to microtrauma (Clemmons 2007). This tissue disruption directly affects local nerves, blood vessels, and immune cells improving blood flow, immune response, and relaxation of tissues and muscles. Signals carried by the nerve cells spread from the point of impact to the spinal cord and eventually the brain, propagating the beneficial analgesic effects of acupuncture throughout the body (Chiu et al. 2001).

The addition of acupuncture to the treatment regimen for cervical nerve pain is safe, effective, and can reduce the need for Western pharmaceuticals. The following case demonstrates the effective incorporation of acupuncture and aquapuncture in the treatment of a dog with cervical radiculoneuritis. An in-depth evaluation and explanation of the use of traditional chinese veterinary medicine (TCVM) examinations and diagnoses are beyond the scope of this case study. The TCVM examination results and diagnoses are provided for the sake of completeness, but their significance is not discussed.

Case Presentation: Winston is a seven-year-old male neutered beagle with a history of complete pelvic limb paralysis and spinal walking secondary to a Type III disk herniation at T13–L1 in 2013. He was receiving regular acupuncture and spinal manipulation therapy, approximately every three months, to improve mobility of his thoracic limbs. His last maintenance integrative therapy session was on 15 March 2019.

One month later, 13 April 2019, Winston became acutely painful with right thoracic limb lameness after a digging episode in the front yard. The owner started methocarbamol, rest, and hot/cold compresses at home. On 15 April 2019 Winston was taken to his regular

(Continued)

Case Study 1   (Continued)

veterinarian who diagnosed neck pain and prescribed carprofen.

The owner consulted with a neurologist on 20 April 2019 due to minimal improvement in his pain level. The neurologic exam revealed paraplegia with spinal walking, lowered head-carriage, and ambulatory thoracic limbs without paresis. There was absent pelvic limb placement with hyperreflexia and mass reflexes. Limb placement and reflexes were normal in the thoracic limbs. The cutaneous trunci was absent caudal to T10. There was reduced cervical range of motion, especially on dorsal flexion. Discomfort was noted in the caudal cervical region and on shoulder palpation. All diagnostics were declined at the time. Differential diagnoses included intervertebral disk disease, inflammatory response, and neoplasia. Medications prescribed included, gabapentin (100 mg, one to two capsules orally every 8–12 hours), codeine (30 mg, half to one tablet orally every 8–12 hours), diazepam (5 mg, one tablet orally every 8–12 hours), prednisolone (5 mg tapering dose starting at 1.5 tablets every 12 hours after a 48-hour washout period), omeprazole (20 mg, one tablet orally once daily 20 minutes before meals for seven days), and trazodone (25 mg, one tablet orally in the evening).

Further diagnostics were performed with the neurologist on 1 May 2019 after minimal improvement in neck pain. Toxoplasma and Neospora were negative. Baseline blood work was unremarkable. Magnetic resonance imaging (MRI) and analysis of the cerebrospinal fluid (CSF) were consistent with C6 radiculo-neuritis. The steroid taper was lengthened in an effort to reduce inflammation.

Winston presented for acupuncture on 9 May 2019. The owner noted little improvement in the pain level as well as increasing restlessness. Winston's clinical condition improved with each recheck and acupuncture

appointment over the next two months. The pertinent patient history, abnormal physical exam findings associated with the thoracic limbs and cervical region, acupoints utilized, and recommendations for each recheck examination are described.

9 May 2019

- Client observations: Initial presentation for acupuncture. Little improvement in the pain level with increased restlessness.
- Abnormal exam findings: Hypertrophied shoulder muscles bilaterally with occasional muscle spasm. Tight brachiocephalicus, omotransversarius, caudal cervical muscles, and trapezius muscles bilaterally. Restricted cervical range of motion.
- TCVM exam findings:
  - *Shen*: Quiet, Nervous, and Sad
  - *Personality*: Metal
  - *Hot/Cold*: Mild heat noted at the pole (back of the head near the neck) and caudal cervical region.
  - *Tongue*: Pink with slight purple hue.
  - *Pulse*: Superficial, wiry, and taut.
  - *Active acupoints*: An Shen, GB-20, BL-13, BL-20, LI-11, BL-60
- TCVM diagnosis: Qi Stagnation, Blood Deficiency, Shen Disturbance
- Dry needle (25 minutes): GV-20, GB-20, An Shen, JJJ C3/C5/C6, A-Shi Mid-brachiocephalicus bilaterally, BL-13, BL-20, LI-11, and KID-3 to BL-60
- Aquapuncture: Vitamin B12 with 0.1 ml at each acupoint = GV-20, GB-20, and An Shen.
- Recommendations: Continue exercise restriction. Taper off the codeine. Stop the trazodone. Continue exercise restriction. Recheck two weeks based on owner availability.

24 May 2019

- Client observations: Patient has been anxious and stir-crazy because of the exercise restriction. No obvious pain. Developed diarrhea over the last week.

- Abnormal exam findings: Persistent shoulder muscle hypertrophy. Reduced muscle tension associated with the brachiocephalicus, omotransversarius, caudal cervical muscles, and trapezius muscles. Improved cervical range of motion.
- TCVM exam findings: No change except tongue now had a faint purple hue.
- TCVM diagnosis: Qi Stagnation, Blood Stagnation, Blood Deficiency, Spleen Qi Deficiency, Shen Disturbance
- Dry needle (25 minutes): GB-20, An Shen, JJJ C3 and C6, BL-14, BL-20, BL-23, BL-26, Bai Hui, GV-4, Left SP-9, KID-3 to BL-60, LIV-3
- Aquapuncture: Vitamin B12 with 0.1 ml at each acupoint = GV-20, GB-20, An Shen, GV-14.
- Recommendations: Continue exercise restriction. Start a Chinese herbal formula for anxiety. Recheck four weeks based on owner availability.

21 June 2019

- Client observations: Moderate improvement in the patient's level of anxiety. No observed pain and continued improvement in the thoracic limb mobility. Neurologist recheck on 1 June confirmed resolution of spinal pain and inflammation. Diarrhea resolved. Patient was started on Clavamox™ after the regular veterinarian diagnosed a urinary tract infection (UTI) one week earlier.
- Abnormal exam findings: Persistent shoulder muscle hypertrophy. Greatly improved muscle tension associated with the brachiocephalicus, omotransversarius, caudal cervical muscles, and trapezius muscles. Good cervical range of motion.
- TCVM exam findings: No change.
- TCVM Diagnosis: Bladder Damp Heat, Qi and Blood Stagnation, Blood Deficiency, Spleen Qi Deficiency, Improved Shen Disturbance

- Dry needle (25 minutes): GB-20, An Shen, JJJ C3 and C6, LI-11, LI-4, BL-14, BL-20, BL-23, BL-26, Bai Hui, Jian Jiao, GB-34, ST-36, and KID-3 to BL-60
- Aquapuncture: Vitamin B12 with 0.1 ml at each acupoint = GB-20, An Shen, GV-14, and A-shi shoulder joint.
- Recommendations: Slowly reintroduce normal activity level. Continue Clavamox and prednisolone taper as directed. Continue Chinese herbal formula for anxiety. Recheck two weeks based on owner availability.

5 July 2019

- Client observations: No recurrence of anxiety. No neck or shoulder pain. Still undergoing treatment for UTI.
- Abnormal exam findings: No change.
- TCVM exam findings: No change.
- TCVM diagnosis: Qi Stagnation, Blood Stagnation, Blood Deficiency, Spleen Qi Deficiency, Damp Resolving
- Dry needle (25 minutes): GB-20, An Shen, JJJ C3/C5/C7, LI-11, GV-14, BL-12, BL-15, BL-23, GV-4, Bai Hui, BL-60 to KID-3
- Aquapuncture: Not performed.
- Recommendations: Continue reintroduction of normal activity level. Reinstitute spinal manipulation going forward. Continue all medications, supplements, and herbs as directed. Recheck four weeks for maintenance therapy.

After 5 July 2019 Winston's treatments were gradually lengthened to monthly appointments with continued tapering and eventual cessation of the prednisone therapy. His cervical and shoulder mobility and muscle tension remain stable with monthly to bimonthly acupuncture sessions, with added spinal manipulation and manual therapy.

The acupuncture points utilized during the treatments are shown in Figure 12.6 and described in Table 12.2.

(Continued)

Case Study 1   (Continued)

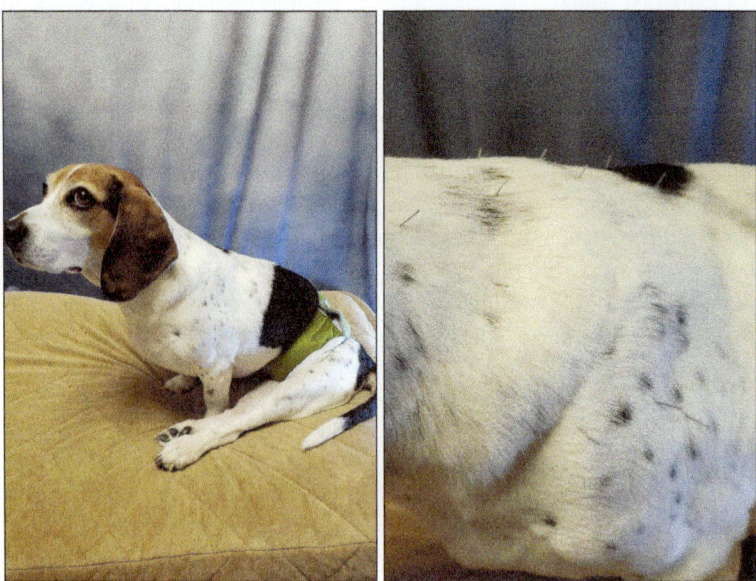

Figure 12.6   Photographs taken during Winston's dry needle acupuncture session. The needles used were very small Korean hand needles, most often used for cats and small dogs. Winston was very sensitive and responded better when smaller needles were used. Typically, for a dog of Winston's size, approximately 30 lbs (13.5 kg), the 34g 0.5–1 inch acupuncture needles would be used. Source: Lisa P. McFaddin.

Discussion: Unlike most Western pharmaceuticals, acupuncture side effects are very uncommon. Acupuncture is not only very safe but generally well tolerated by veterinary patients (Xie and Ortiz-Umpierre 2006). The most common, though still infrequent, issue is bleeding or bruising following needle removal. Comparatively the most common side effects of chronic steroid therapy include increased thirst, increased urination, increased hunger, mood changes, hepatopathy, cardiovascular effects, insulin resistance, weight gain, iatrogenic hyperadrenocorticism, and dermatologic changes.

The local, regional, and systemic effects generated by acupuncture are dependent on several variables: the acupuncture points selected, the method of stimulation, and the length of stimulation (Karavis 1997). Needle placement through the skin causes counter-irritation within the epidermis, dermis, and subcutaneous tissues, leading to microtrauma. This stimulation causes a combination of three potential, and often simultaneously occurring, reactions at the acupoint: neuronal reactions, biophysical reactions, and biochemical reactions (Zhu 2014). Each of these reactions contributes to the analgesic effects of acupuncture.

The neuronal effects occur primarily through stimulation of afferent pain signals transmitted by thin slow unmyelinated C fibers (Group IV fibers) and thin faster myelinated Adelta (Aδ) fibers, while afferent mechanical signals are primarily transmitted through Aδ fibers (Zhu 2014).

Signal transmission through these afferent sensory nerves enters the spinal cord via the dorsal horn where nociceptive information is blocked through the stimulation of local interneurons and higher brain centers via the spinothalamic tract (Mittleman and Gaynor 2000;

Table 12.2 The anatomic locations, traditional Chinese veterinary medicine (TCVM) information, and indications of the acupoints used during Winston's dry needle and aquapuncture sessions. Details regarding the acupoint locations and indications were taken from Xie and Preast (2007c) and Ferguson (2007).

LI-4	Location	Dorsal paw at the midpoint between the third and fourth metacarpal bones	
	TCVM information	Master point for the face and mouth	
	Treatment indications	Head	Nasal congestion, nasal discharge, epistaxis, dental pain, pharyngitis, facial paralysis
		Immune system	Fever, immune support (especially skin disease)
		Other	General pain
LI-10	Location	Craniolateral proximal antebrachium below the elbow in the facial groove between the extensor carpi radialis and common digital extensor	
	TCVM information	Thoracic limb "Three Mile Point"; used for Qi Deficiency, Wind-heat	
	Treatment indications	Immune system	General support
		Head	Dental pain and inflammation
		Gastrointestinal	Abdominal pain, diarrhea
		Thoracic limb	Pain, weakness, paralysis, generalized weakness
ST-36	Location	Long linear point in the craniolateral tibia in the cranial tibialis muscle	
	TCVM information	Pelvic limb "Three Mile Point"; master point for the gastrointestinal tract and abdomen; used for Qi Deficiency	
	Treatment indications	Pelvic limb	Knee pain, generalized weakness
		Gastrointestinal	Nausea, vomiting, abdominal pain, constipation, diarrhea
SP-10	Location	Medial thigh proximal to the stifle in the fascia cranial to the sartorius. "One kneecap up and over"	
	TCVM information	"Sea of Blood"; used for blood deficiency, blood heat, and blood stagnation	
	Treatment indications	Immune system	Fever
		Pelvic limb	Weakness or paralysis
BL-12	Location	Within the paraspinal muscles running along either side of the dorsal spinous processes caudal to the second thoracic vertebrae	
	TCVM information	Used for Wind-cold and Wind-heat	
	Treatment indications	Respiratory	Nasal congestion, cough
		Immune system	Fever
		Dermatologic	Pruritis
		Pain	Cervical, thoracic

(Continued)

Case Study 1: Table 12.2 (Continued)

BL-13	Location	Within the paraspinal muscles running along either side of the dorsal spinous processes caudal to the third thoracic vertebrae	
	TCVM information	Association point for the lung; used for Yin Deficiency, Wind-heat, and Wind-cold	
	Treatment indications	Respiratory	Cough, dyspnea, pneumonia, bronchitis, nasal congestion
BL-14	Location	Within the paraspinal muscles running along either side of the dorsal spinous processes caudal to the fourth thoracic vertebrae	
	TCVM information	Association point for the pericardium; used for Shen disturbances	
	Treatment indications	Mentation	Anxiety
		Gastrointestinal	Vomiting
		Respiratory	Coughing, thoracic pain
BL-15	Location	Within the paraspinal muscles running along either side of the dorsal spinous processes caudal to the fifth thoracic vertebrae	
	TCVM information	Association point for the heart; use for Shen disturbance	
	Treatment indications	Cardiovascular	Chest pain, arrhythmias, heart disease
		Neurology	Epilepsy, cognitive disorders
BL-20	Location	Within the paraspinal muscles running along either side of the dorsal spinous processes caudal to the twelfth thoracic vertebrae	
	TCVM information	Association point for the Spleen; used for Spleen Deficiency and Damp	
	Treatment indications	Gastrointestinal	Digestive disorders, pancreatitis, vomiting, diarrhea
		Hematologic	Anemia, edema
		Hepatic	Liver disease (especially jaundice)
		Neurologic	Thoracolumbar intervertebral disk disease
BL-23	Location	Within the paraspinal muscles running along either side of the dorsal spinous processes caudal to the second lumbar vertebrae	
	TCVM information	Association point for the kidney; used for kidney Yin deficiency and kidney Qi deficiency	
	Treatment indications	Urogenital	Kidney disease, urinary incontinence
		Pelvic limb	Hip arthritis
		Neurologic	Thoracolumbar intervertebral disk disease, pelvic limb weakness
		Other	Hearing loss, edema
BL-26	Location	Within the paraspinal muscles running along either side of the dorsal spinous processes caudal to the sixth lumbar vertebrae	
	TCVM information	Used for kidney Yang deficiency and kidney Qi deficiency	
	Treatment indications	Urogenital	Urinary incontinence
		Gastrointestinal	Diarrhea, abdominal pain
		Neurologic	Lumbosacral pain

BL-60	Location	In the fleshy skin on the lateral hock proximal to the angle of the hock (opposite KID-3)	
	TCVM information	"Aspirin Point"	
	Treatment indications	Neurologic	Intervertebral disk disease; cervical and thoracolumbar pain; epilepsy
		Cardiovascular	Epistaxis, hypertension
		Pain	Generalized
KID-3	Location	In the fleshy skin on the medial hock proximal to the angle of the hock (opposite BL-60)	
	Treatment indications	Urogenital	Kidney disease, difficulty urinating
		Endocrine	Diabetes mellitus
		Respiratory	Pharyngitis, dyspnea
		Head	Dental pain, otitis, hearing loss
		Neurologic	Thoracolumbar intervertebral disk disease
LIV-3	Location	PELVIC LIMB = On the dorsal paw between the second and third metatarsal bones proximal to the metatarsophalangeal joint	
	TCVM information	Used for liver Qi stagnation	
	Treatment indications	Hepatic	Liver and gallbladder disease
		Pelvic limb	Weakness, paralysis, pain
GB-20	Location	At the pole on either side of the occipital protuberance	
	TCVM information	Used for Wind (external and internal)	
	Treatment indications	Neurologic	Cervical pain, intervertebral disk disease, epilepsy
		Head	Epistaxis, nasal discharge, nasal congestion
GB-34	Location	In the lateral stifle/distal femur caudal to the lateral epicondyle cranial to the biceps femoris tendon	
	TCVM information	Influential point for tendon and ligament; used for stomach Qi Stagnation and liver Qi Stagnation	
	Treatment indications	Cardiovascular	Hypertension
		Gastrointestinal	Vomiting
		Hepatic	Liver and gallbladder disease
		Musculoskeletal	Tendon and ligament disorders
		Pelvic limbs	Lameness, weakness, paralysis, pain
GV-14	Location	On dorsal midline cranial to the dorsal spinous process of the first thoracic vertebrae	
	TCVM information	Used for Heat and Yin deficiency	
	Treatment indications	Immune system	Fever, immune support
		Respiratory	Cough, dyspnea
		Neurologic	Cervical pain, intervertebral disk disease, epilepsy
		Dermatologic	Skin inflammation

(Continued)

Case Study 1: Table 12.2 (Continued)

GV-20	Location	On dorsal midline on top of the head, using the tips of the pinna as a perpendicular guide	
	TCVM information	"Sedation Point"; used for Shen disturbances	
	Treatment indications	Mentation	Anxiety, sleep disturbance
		Gastrointestinal	Anal prolapse
An Shen	Location	Caudal aspect of the head behind the base of the ear (near the bend of the vertical and horizontal canals)	
	TCVM information	Used for Shen disturbance and Internal Wind	
	Treatment indications	Mentation	Anxiety
		Neurologic	Epilepsy, facial paralysis
		Head	Epistaxis, nasal discharge, nasal congestion, facial swelling, otitis, hearing problems
Jian Jiao	Location	On the lateral pelvis in the depression ventral to the iliac spine	
	Treatment indications	Musculoskeletal	Hip arthritis, hip pain, hip dysplasia, pelvic limb lameness, pelvic limb weakness, pelvic limb paralysis
Jing-Jia-Ji	Location	Two rows of acupoints above and below the lateral spinous processes of each cervical vertebrae. Acupoints associated with C3, C5, and C6 used	
	Treatment indications	Neurologic	Cervical pain, cervical intervertebral disk disease, cervical vertebral instability (Wobbler's)
A-shi	Location	Active region of skin or muscle not associated with a specific meridian or acupoint. Many trigger points (focal areas of hyperirritable skeletal muscle) are considered A-shi points	
	Treatment indications	Musculoskeletal	Muscle spasms, pain relief
Bai Hui	Location	On dorsal midline between the seventh lumbar vertebrae and sacrum	
	TCVM information	Used for Yang Deficiency	
	Treatment indications	Neurologic	Pelvic limb paresis, pelvic limb paralysis, lumbosacral pain, lumbosacral intervertebral disk disease
		Musculoskeletal	Hip arthritis
		Gastrointestinal	Abdominal pain, diarrhea

Source: Lisa P. McFaddin.

Clemmons 2007). Additionally, there are several connections in the midbrain, especially the periaqueductal gray matter (PAG) and rostral ventral medulla (RVM), which regulate the response and integration of painful stimuli, in part through the release of endogenous opioids and cannabinoids (Yam et al. 2018).

The PAG helps regulate the response to nociceptive input integrating information from the higher brain centers, including the cortex, and the dorsal horn of the spinal cord. The RVM downregulates excitatory information from the dorsal horn of the spinal cord. Both the PAG and RVM express a variety of neurotransmitters (endogenous opioids and cannabinoids, 5-hydroxytryptamine or 5-HT, and norepinephrine or NE) that are heavily involved in the regulation and recognition of pain (Yam et al. 2018). The importance of endogenous opioids in perpetuating the effects of acupuncture is emphasized by the fact that administration of drugs known to inhibit opioid biosynthesis (cycloheximide) or block opioid action (naloxone) reduce the analgesic effects of acupuncture (Mittleman and Gaynor 2000).

The primary effect of the biophysical reactions is the stimulation of local mechanoreceptors, especially muscle spindle cells (MSCs) and Golgi tendon organs (GTOs) within the skin, muscle, and tendons. Activation of MSC and GTO inhibit pain (Purves et al. 2012).

Needle stimulation causes the release of a whole host of neural and nonneuronal bioactive factors (Zhu 2014). These biochemical substances contribute to the local and systemic beneficial effects of acupuncture primarily through regulation of blood and lymphatic flow, as well as stimulation of afferent signals to the central nervous system (Clemmons 2007). Opioid peptides, β-endorphins, enkephalins, dynorphins, serotonin, NE and GABA (γ-aminobutyric acid)

are also released and produced within the central nervous system as a direct result of acupuncture, particularly electroacupuncture (Zhao 2008). The primary function of these biochemical modulators and neurotransmitters is the central inhibition of pain.

The incorporation of acupuncture and aquapuncture in this case not only improved the patient's pain level but also allowed reintroduction of his normal activity level, facilitating the successful taper of traditional medications, especially prednisolone. This case also illustrated the flexibility of acupuncture therapy with respect to client lifestyle. Not all clients can confirm to a rigid recheck schedule. In an ideal setting Winston would have rechecked weekly for four to five treatments, with a gradual lengthening of the treatment frequency. Despite the scheduling conflicts Winston still appeared to benefit greatly from the treatments.

As stated in the introduction the focus of this case study is to highlight the beneficial effect of acupuncture and aquapuncture as an adjunct treatment for cervical pain. As such the TCVM examination findings, diagnoses, and Chinese herbal formula used for Winston are beyond the scope of this report and not discussed. One other issue to address is the lack of electroacupuncture (EAP) in this case. EAP can be extremely effective in reducing neurologic pain and speeding recovery (Hayashi et al. 2007). Unfortunately, Winston historically did not tolerate EAP which is why the modality was not utilized.

Conclusion: The application of acupuncture and aquapuncture, along with traditional medications, successfully improved neck pain secondary to C6 radiculoneuritis in a dog. The report demonstrates the applications and efficacy of integrative therapy in the management of a common neurologic condition.

Case Study 2   Focus on Chinese Food Therapy

Title: Management of canine atopic dermatitis using traditional chinese veterinary medicine food and herbal therapy

Author: Lisa P. McFaddin, DVM, GDCVHM, CVSMT, CVMRT, FCoAC, CVA

Summary: Whole food therapy is crucial to animal well-being. Without a proper diet the body cannot maintain homeostasis and disease ensues. The correction of a home-made diet combined with Chinese herbal therapy led to the resolution of Damp Heat and Spleen Deficiency in a dog, as well as improvement in chronic skin issues due to atopic dermatitis. This case also highlights the importance of reassessment in proper patient management. Diseases are not static and therapeutic adjustments are necessary as the conditions evolve.

Introduction: Atopic dermatitis (AD) is a common and frustrating condition affecting many canine and feline patients. Atopy is characterized by a genetic predisposition to excessive inflammatory responses, frequently associated with the overproduction of immunoglobulin (Ig)E against environmental allergens resulting in excessive pruritus (Gedon and Mueller 2018). Traditional management is often lifelong and focused on hypoallergenic diets, immunosuppressive pharmaceuticals, allergen-targeted therapy, monoclonal antibody injections, and topical therapy (Gedon and Mueller 2018).

Diet is crucial in the management of canine AD. First, a six to eight week trial of a hypoallergenic diet can aid in the diagnosis of true AD versus food allergies (Kawarai et al. 2010). Second, proper nutritional management of dogs with AD can improve the skin barrier on a cellular level reducing its susceptibility to environmental allergens (van Beeck et al. 2015; Witzel-Rollins et al. 2019). Third, the manipulation of the intestinal microbiome through diet and probiotics reduces intestinal permeability, improves the local immune system (gut-associated lymphoid tissue or GALT), improves the neuroendocrine system, and reduces the hyperreactivity of systemic IgE and mast cells (Craig 2016).

Hypoallergenic diets, in veterinary medicine, focus on feeding either a novel protein/carbohydrate source or a hydrolyzed protein diet. These diets are most often prescription products sold as canned and dry varieties. Prescription dog foods are expensive when compared to most non-prescription options. Palatability can also be an issue.

There is often a negative stigma associated with home-made diets in veterinary medicine. Concerns involve inadequate macronutrients and micronutrients, as well as recent fears regarding the exact nature of dilated cardiomyopathy and grain-free diets. A nutritionally sound whole-food home-cooked diet can offer a safe and effective alternative for clients with atopic dogs.

The negative effects associated with chronic immunosuppressive medications (including increased thirst, increased urination, increased hunger, increased panting, elevated liver enzymes, risk of diabetes mellitus, and risk of pancreatitis), as well as the required chronic laboratory monitoring, is often daunting to owners. Clients must balance these risks with the frustration associated with a chronically itchy, uncomfortable, and often smelly canine companion. The use of nutraceuticals and Chinese herbal therapy can provide a safe and effective alternative to traditional pharmaceuticals.

The purpose of this case report is to illustrate the effective management of a dog with known AD through the modification of a home-cooked diet, nutraceuticals, and Chinese herbal therapy.

Case Presentation: Patient A, an eight-year-old male neutered Shih Tzu Mix, presented for an initial integrative medicine consultation on 22 November 2014 to discuss chronic skin issues. Previous medical history included a migrating foreign body, one episode of pancreatitis, and chronic recurrent skin issues secondary to atopic dermatitis.

The migrating foreign body was surgically removed from the caudal aspect of the left rear leg in August 2014. Patient A then underwent a six-week course of Clavamox based on culture and sensitivity results.

The episode of pancreatitis occurred five years earlier after which the owner elected to home-cook a majority of Patient A's meals. Historically, Patient A only ate once daily even when offered food multiple times a day. The past six to eight weeks Patient A refused to eat any kibble. His diet consisted of rice, pumpkin, peas and turkey. He was eating approximately 400 kcal/day.

The recurrent skin lesions predominantly involved crusting and red scaly lesions around his face and paws, and copious serous to mucopurulent ocular discharge. The allergies occurred throughout the year but would flare up when the seasons changed.

The owner described Patient A as very friendly with people but not other dogs. He would run and hide if he became too excited. The owner reported no preference for hot or cold. His energy level was good. He chronically dreamed for the past few years. The owner noted he had lost the fur along his lumbar spine while on the antibiotics. The fur was slow to regrow and the texture became coarser once fully regrown.

Current medications and supplements include monthly Heartgard Plus, monthly topical Vectra for fleas and ticks, Standard Process Dermal Support daily, and Standard Process Immune Support daily. He received his rabies vaccine one week prior to presentation. Repeat blood work performed the day of the integrative examination was within normal limits.

The client observations, abnormal Western and TCVM examination findings, Western and TCVM diagnoses, TCVM treatment goals, dietary recommendations, nutraceutical and herb recommendations for initial examination and all recheck exams are outlined below.

22 November 2014

- Client observations: Appetite is off, refusing to eat kibble. Historically only eats once daily. Recurrent crusting, red and scaly skin lesions. Seasonal and non-seasonal allergies.
- Western examination findings: Left semimembranous and semitendinous muscle atrophy. Slightly enlarged and firm left popliteal lymph node. Minimal redness and inflammation of the pelvic limb interdigital skin. Dry skin with fine powdery dandruff. Patch of coarse fur along dorsum.
- TCVM examination findings: Good Shen, Earth personality, light pink tongue, and pulse was deep, deficient, slightly wiry, and weaker on the left compared to the right.
- Western diagnoses: Mild recurrent skin infections, reactive left popliteal lymph node, muscle atrophy left rear limb, chronic recurrent allergies and possible atopy
- Historical foreign body left rear leg, and historical pancreatitis.
- TCVM diagnoses: Blood Deficiency, Spleen Deficiency, Tendency toward Damp Accumulation, and Wind–Damp Invasion.
  - **Blood deficiency**: Light pink tongue, deficient wiry pulse weaker on the left (yin and blood), historical mild to moderate itch, recurrent low-grade skin rashes, recurrent paw infections, current mild redness associated with paws, cool paws and ear tips, dry coat, fine powdery dandruff, fur took a while to regrow and change in texture when it regrew, frequent dreaming, fear aggression with other dogs, historical kibble diet.
  - **Spleen deficiency**: Historic kibble diet, poor appetite (eats once daily and no interest at other times), historical damp accumulation (ear infections, skin infections, pancreatitis), and active BL 20 and ST 36.

(Continued)

Case Study 2   (Continued)

- **Tendency toward Damp Accumulation**: Historical ear infections and skin infections, historic pancreatitis, pronounced inflammation and infection of the left rear limb secondary to foreign body (wind heat invasion), historic kibble diet, and active BL 20.
- **Wind-Damp Invasions** – Initially generalized lymphadenopathy followed by only enlargement of the left popliteal lymph node (as if the problem was moving), Swollen infected left rear limb, Active LI 11, and historical chronic recurrent skin infections.
- TCVM treatment goals: Tonify Blood, Support the Spleen, and Clear Wind-Damp.
- Diet: Continue a home-made diet at 400 kcal/day. Add in beef liver (cooked or freeze-dried).
- Supplement and herbs: Stop the Standard Process Dermal and Immune Support™. Start Standard Process Whole Body Support™, Rx Biotics™, Nordic Naturals Omega 3 Pet™, Rx Vitamins Canine Minerals™, and Si Wu Xiao Feng Yin.

19 January 2015

- Client observations: Feeding previous diet plus 2 tsp of cooked beef liver and one to two beef liver treats daily. Stools were a little soft. Less licking but no change in scratching. Nail beds appeared inflamed and crust. The left eye was red.
- Western examination findings: Periocular dermatitis medial to left eye. Thickened nail beds with brown waxy discharge between the cuticle and nail. Remainder of the exam was unchanged.
- TCVM examination findings: Red-pink tongue; pulse deep, deficient and thin.
- Western diagnoses: pododermatitis, periocular dermatitis left eye, and historical diagnoses remained unchanged.

- TCVM diagnoses: Damp Heat, Blood Deficiency, and Spleen Qi Deficiency.
  - **Damp Heat**: Periocular dermatitis, thickened nail beds with waxy discharge, ulcerated nail beds, and red tongue.
  - **Blood Deficiency**: Dry skin with small dandruff flakes, and thin and weak pulse.
  - **Spleen Qi Deficiency**: Soft stool and thin and deficient pulses.
- TCVM treatment goals: Drain Damp, Clear Heat, Support the Spleen, and Tonify Blood.
- Diet: Added Stella and Chewy's Lamb Dehydrated Meal. Current diet cut in half.
- Supplement and herbs: Add in Si Miao San with Dang Gui. All other supplements and herbs continued.

16 March 2015

- Client observations: Gained 0.5 lbs which was unusual for him. Eye was improved. Licking less. One digit remained alopecic. Enlarging cystic growth on back. Normal stools. Loved the lamb patties.
- Western examination findings: Fifth digit on the right front paw was alopecic with thickened hyperkeratosis and dried skin with crusts. Fourth digit on the right front paw had a 2-mm round, firm, raised white dermal lesion. Enlarged epidermal inclusion cyst on the right hip. Slight discoloration of the nail beds. Enlarged left popliteal and right prescapular lymph nodes. Skin was less dry without dandruff.
- TCVM examination findings: Tongue was red-pink; pulse was thin and weak.
- Western diagnoses: Pododermatitis, epidermal inclusion cyst, and historical diagnoses remained unchanged.
- TCVM diagnoses: Damp Heat, Blood Deficiency, and Spleen Qi Deficiency.
  - **Damp Heat**: Thickened hyperkeratotic and crusting digit, round raised dermal lesion, epidermal cyst, enlarged right

prescapular lymph node, red-pink tongue, and weight gain.

- **Blood Deficiency**: Dry coat and Thin pulse.
- **Spleen Qi Deficiency**: Historic kibble diet, previous diarrhea, as well as propensity for Damp indicate a generally deficient Spleen, and Thin and deficient pulse.
- TCVM treatment goals: Drain Damp, Clear Heat, Support the Spleen, and Tonify Blood.
- Diet: Stop the lamb, rice, and chicken. Calorie content reduced to 300–350 kcal/day. Ratio of 33% carbohydrates, protein, and vegetables/fruit. New diet: turkey, peas, broccoli, applesauce, and beef liver.
- Supplement and herbs: Si Wu Xiao Feng Yin was discontinued. All other supplements and herbs continued.

15 May 2015

- Client observations: Resolved itching, licking, and growth on the fourth right front digit. Persistent flaking right front fifth digit. Scratching and rubbing right ear since grooming. Normal stool.
- Western examination findings: Mild pinnal erythema on the right ear without discharge or inflammation. Fifth digit right front paw alopecic with regrowing fur. Persistent but smaller epidermal inclusion cyst.
- TCVM examination findings: Red-pink tongue; pulse mid-range and thin.
- Western diagnoses: No change
- TCVM Diagnoses: Damp Heat, Blood Deficiency, and Spleen Qi Deficiency.
  - **Damp Heat**: Hyperkeratosis and crusting of the digit, epidermal inclusion cyst, nail discoloration and crusting, enlarged lymph nodes, and red-pink tongue.
  - **Blood Deficiency**: Mildly dry skin and pulses thin and mildly deficient.
  - **Spleen Qi Deficiency**: Historic kibble diet, previous diarrhea, as well as propensity for Damp indicate a generally

deficient Spleen, and Thin and deficient pulse.
- TCVM treatment goals: Drain Damp, Clear Heat, Support the Spleen, and Tonify Blood.
- Diet: No change.
- Supplements and herbs: No change.

3 July 2015

- Client observations: No scratching or itching. Clear eyes, skin, and ears. Odor from the right ear.
- Western examination findings: Mild pinnal erythema on the right ear with discharge and yeasty odor. Fur fully regrown on the right front fifth digit. Slightly smaller right prescapular lymph node.
- TCVM examination findings: Faint red hue associated with the tongue. Pulse was mid-range, deficient and thin, weaker on the right compared to the left.
- Western diagnoses: Yeast otitis externa right ear. No other changes to historical diagnoses.
- TCVM diagnoses: Mild Damp Heat, Blood Deficiency, and Spleen Qi Deficiency
  - **Damp Heat**: Yeast otitis externa AD, minimal crusting of digit, slight red hue associated with the tongue, and enlarged left popliteal lymph node.
  - **Blood Deficiency** – Slightly deficient pulses and left weaker than right.
  - **Spleen Qi Deficiency** – Historic kibble diet, previous diarrhea, as well as propensity for damp indicate a generally deficient Spleen, and Deficient pulse.
- TCVM treatment goals: Drain Damp, Clear Heat, Support the Spleen, and Tonify Blood.
- Diet: No change.
- Supplements and herbs: Started Zymox with Hydrocortisone Ear Medication. No other changes to supplements or herbs.

Patient A's Standard Process supplements were transitioned to a single product, Whole Body Support, in an effort to reduce the number of supplements he received on a daily

(Continued)

Case Study 2   (Continued)

basis and provide a more generalized whole-food micronutrient approach. Probiotics, Rx Biotics, were started to support the gut and overall immune system. Fish oil, Nordic Naturals Omega 3 Pet, was started to support the skin, immune system, and function as a blood tonic. Finally, a calcium and mineral supplement, Canine Minerals, was added to prevent nutritional deficiencies secondary to the home-made diet. The following is a list of the names, ingredients, and dosages of the supplements Patient A was taking.

Canine Dermal Support

- Ingredients: Bovine liver, L-glutamine, *Silybum marianum*, bovine kidney, defatted wheat germ, alfalfa juice, *Emblica officinalis*, carrot (root), fat-soluble extract (from alfalfa [whole plant], sunflower [seed], carrot (root), *Tillandsia usneoides*, buckwheat [leaf and seed], and pea [vine]), bovine and ovine spleen, bovine adrenal PMG™ extract, *Strombus gigas*, calcium lactate, bovine liver fat extract, blackcurrant juice, *Carthamus tinctorius*, bovine liver PMG extract, nutritional yeast, mushroom, porcine jejunum, porcine stomach, betaine hydrochloride, bovine parotid PMG extract, para-aminobenzoate, beet leaf juice, beet root, oat flour, porcine brain, bovine adrenal Cytosol™ extract, purified bovine bile salts, bone meal, *Taraxacum officinale*, and inositol.
- Dose: ¼ tsp twice daily
- Manufacturer: Standard Process

Canine Immune Support

- Ingredients: Bovine liver, nutritional yeast, bovine and ovine spleen, rice bran, bovine spleen PMG extract, bovine thymus PMG extract, carrot, bovine kidney, bovine thymus Cytosol extract, buckwheat leaf juice and seed, bovine pancreas Cytosol extract, pea vine juice, *Eleutherococcus senticosus*, porcine duodenum, blackcurrant juice, porcine jejunum, bovine adrenal Cytosol

extract, veal bone PMG extract, oat flour, calcium lactate, purified bovine bile salts, defatted wheat germ, mushroom, Spanish black radish, ribonucleic acid, bovine adrenal PMG extract, *Tillandsia usneoides*, *Withania somnifera*, zinc rice chelate, kelp, and blackcurrant seed oil.
- Dose: ¼ tsp twice daily
- Manufacturer: Standard Process

Canine Whole Body Support

- Ingredients: Defatted wheat germ, bovine liver, pea vine juice, nutritional yeast, carrot, rice bran, bovine and ovine spleen, alfalfa juice, *Silybum marianum*, beet root, porcine stomach, oat flour, bovine heart PMG extract, *Tillandsia usneoides*, L-carnitine, Brussels sprouts, bovine orchic Cytosol extract, kidney bean extract, kelp, bovine liver PMG extract, bone meal, bovine trachea, bovine kidney PMG extract, mushroom, bovine kidney, inositol, choline bitartrate, thiamine hydrochloride, bovine adrenal Cytosol extract, celery, bentonite, veal bone PMG extract, bovine liver fat extract, calcium lactate, manganese glycerophosphate, carbamide, bovine adrenal PMG extract, bovine hypothalamus Cytosol extract, bovine thymus PMG extract, bovine pituitary PMG extract, zinc liver chelate, copper liver chelate, iron liver chelate, soybean lecithin, bovine hypothalamus PMG extract, bovine thymus Cytosol extract, bovine thyroid PMG extract, para-aminobenzoate, porcine brain, and ascorbic acid.
- Ingredients: ¼ tsp twice daily
- Manufacturer: Standard Process

Omega 3 Pet

- Ingredients: Wild anchovy and sardine oil (EPA per serving = 150 mg; DHA per serving = 90 mg).
- Dose: One Soft Gel Daily
- Manufacturer: Nordic Naturals

Rx Biotics

- Ingredients: DDS-1 ProbioPlus Probiotic Blend (*Lactobacillus acidophilus, Bifidobacterium bifidum, Bifidobacterium longum, Bifidobacterium lactis*), fructooligosaccharides, and Larch Arabinogalactan.
- Dose: ⅛ tsp daily
- Manufacturer: Rx Vitamins

Canine Minerals

- Ingredients: (per ½ tsp) Calcium 500 mg, Magnesium 322 mg, Iron 0.77 mg, Strontium

0.27 mg, Sodium 0.20 mg, Manganese 0.08 mg, Phosphorus 0.07 mg, Potassium 0.04 µg, Chromium 6 µg.
- Dose: ⅓ tsp daily
- Manufacturer: Rx Vitamins

Patient A's initial diet change focused on adding in beef liver to tonify blood and support the liver. The owner was instructed to use either cooked beef liver (1–2 tbsp) or freeze-dried beef liver treats (four to six pieces) at least three times a week. Tables 12.3–12.6 list the dietary ingredients,

Table 12.3 Summary of the individual ingredients, amount fed, and calorie content of the home-made diet fed on 22 November 2014 through 19 January 2015 (Pitchford 2002; Xie 2015; Wynn 2010).

Food	Amount	Kcal
Cooked white rice	3 tbsp/day	60
Cooked lean ground turkey	⅓ cup/day	176
Plain canned pumpkin	⅓ cup/day	28
Cooked peas	⅓ cup/day	45
Beef liver	4–6 pieces/day	50
Calcium/phosphorus ratio, 0.18:1 Amount of canine minerals added: ½ tsp Corrected calcium/phosphorus ratio, 1.2:1		**Total = 359**

Source: Lisa P. McFaddin.

Table 12.4 Summary of the individual ingredients, amount fed, and calorie content of the home-made diet fed 20 January 2014 through 16 March 2015 (Pitchford 2002; Xie 2015; Wynn 2010).

Food	Amount	Kcal
Cooked white rice	2 tbsp/day	40
Cooked lean ground turkey	⅙ cup/day	88
Plain canned pumpkin	⅙ cup/day	14
Cooked peas	⅙ cup/day	23
Beed liver	4–6 pieces/day	50
Freeze-dried lamb patty	Two patties	160
Calcium/phosphorus ratio, 0.18:1 Amount of canine minerals added, ½ tsp Corrected calcium/phosphorus ratio, 1.2:1		**Total = 375**

Source: Lisa P. McFaddin.

(Continued)

Case Study 2   (Continued)

Table 12.5   Summary of the individual ingredients, amount fed, and calorie content of the home-made diet fed 17 March 2015 through 15 May 2015 (Pitchford 2002; Xie 2015; Wynn 2010).

Food	Amount	Kcal
Cooked lean ground turkey	⅓ cup/day	176
Cooked peas	⅓ cup/day	45
Beed liver	4–6 pieces/day	50
Cooked broccoli	½ cup/day	27
Applesauce plain	½ cup/day	60
Calcium/phosphorus ratio, 0.17:1 Amount of canine minerals added, ½ tsp Corrected calcium/phosphorus ratio, 1.2:1		**Total = 358**

Source: Lisa P. McFaddin.

Table 12.6   Summary of the individual ingredients, amount fed, and calorie content of the home-made diet fed 16 May 2015 until patient was lost to follow-up (Pitchford 2002; Xie 2015; Wynn 2010).

Food	Amount	Kcal
Cooked peas	⅓ cup/day	45
Plain canned pumpkin	⅓ cup/day	28
Cooked broccoli	½ cup/day	27
Cooked chicken breast (no skin)	⅓ cup/day	100
Canned kidney beans	¼ cup/day	53
Calcium/phosphorus ratio, 0.3:1 Amount of canine minerals added, ⅓ to ½ tsp Corrected calcium/phosphorus ratio, 1.2:1 to 1.5:1		**Total = 253**

Source: Lisa P. McFaddin.

quantity fed, and caloric content of the home-made diets. Table 12.7 describes the TCVM properties of the dietary ingredients.

19 January 2015

Stella and Chewy's Freeze-dried Lamb was added to see if the addition of a novel protein would positively affect the gut and skin. Stella and Chewy's Dandy Lamb Freeze Dried Patties contain multiple ingredients, but lamb is the sole source of protein.

- Ingredients: Lamb, lamb spleen, lamb liver, lamb bone, lamb heart, lamb kidney, pumpkin seed, potassium chloride, organic cranberries, organic spinach, organic broccoli, organic beets, sodium phosphate monobasic, organic carrots, organic squash, organic apples, organic blueberries, choline chloride, dried

Table 12.7 The TCVM properties of the ingredients used in the diets from 22 November 2014 through 16 May 2015 (Marsden 2015a-c; Pitchford 2002; Marsden 2015a-c; Xie 2015).

Apples	Properties	Sweet, sour, cool
	Channels entered	Spleen, stomach
	TCVM function	Produces body fluids and reinforces the spleen
	Indications	Debility, indigestion, and loss of appetite
Beef liver	Properties	Sweet, neutral
	Channels entered	Liver
	TCVM function	Nourish the blood; reinforces the liver
	Indications	Blood deficiency and liver blood deficiency
Cooked broccoli	Properties	Sweet, cool
	Channels entered	Liver
	TCVM function	Yin tonic and blood tonic
	Indications	Yin deficiency and blood deficiency
Chicken breast	Properties	Sweet, warm
	Channels entered	Spleen, liver
	TCVM function	Strengthens spleen and stomach; nourishes liver and kidney; Qi energy tonic; increases Jing essence; and improves condition of the bone marrow
	Indications	Spleen Qi deficiency; Qi deficiency; weakness; emaciation; edema; frequent urination; and chronic illness
Kidney beans	Properties	Sweet, cooling
	Channels entered	Heart, stomach
	TCVM function	Diuretic; increases Yin fluids; drains damp; and blood tonic
	Indications	Blood deficiency; Damp; and Yin deficiency with dryness
Lamb	Properties	Sweet, hot
	Channels entered	Spleen, kidney
	TCVM function	Warm the middle burner; enrich Qi and blood; and tonify Yang
	Indications	Cold intolerance; weakness in the lower back; profuse clear urine; abdominal pain; cold limbs; and fatigue
Peas	Properties	Sweet, neutral
	Channels entered	Spleen, stomach
	TCVM function	Strengthens the spleen; relieves edema; and produces body fluids
	Indications	Dry throat; thirst; and spleen deficiency
Pumpkin	Properties	Sweet, warm
	Channels entered	Spleen, stomach
	TCVM function	Reinforce the middle burner; replenish Qi; dissolve phlegm; promote discharge of pus; expel roundworms; and dries dampness in the GI tract
	Indications	Weak spleen, spleen Qi deficiency, coughing up thick sputum, GI parasites, malnutrition, chronic IBD, and diabetes (stimulates β-cell insulin release)

(Continued)

Case Study 2: Table 12.7   (Continued)

Turkey	Properties	Sweet, cool
	Channels entered	Kidney, liver, heart
	TCVM function	Yin tonic
	Indications	Yin deficiency
White Rice	Properties	Sweet, warm or neutral
	Channels entered	Spleen, stomach
	TCVM function	Nourish the spleen; harmonize the stomach; relieve thirst; and Yin Tonic but Dampening
	Indications	Vomiting; anorexia; thirst and dry mouth; and stomach Yin impairment and heat

Source: Lisa P. McFaddin.

Pediococcus acidilactici fermentation product, dried *Lactobacillus acidophilus* fermentation product, dried *Bifidobacterium longum* fermentation product, taurine, tocopherols (preservative), zinc proteinate, zinc sulfate, iron sulfate, iron proteinate, vitamin E supplement, niacin, copper sulfate, copper proteinate, manganese sulfate, sodium selenite, manganese proteinate, thiamin mononitrate, pyridoxine hydrochloride, vitamin D3 supplement, folic acid, calcium iodate, vitamin B12 supplement

- https://www.stellaandchewys.com/dog-food/freeze-dried-raw-dinners/patties/dandy-lamb

16 March 2015

The Si Wu Xiao Feng Yin was discontinued. The owner was instructed to stop the lamb, pumpkin, chicken, and rice at this time. The goal of the diet change was to eliminate warm/hot foods and focus more on cooling or neutral foods which support the spleen and tonify the blood (Marsden 2015a-c). Grains were eliminated from the diet at this time to prevent further inflammation and determine if grains may be contributing to the recurrent skin problems. His daily caloric requirement was recalculated, based on his current weight, to 300–350 kcal/day. The diet comprised 33% carbohydrates, 33% protein, and 33% vegetables/fruit. The specific dietary ingredients are provided in Table 12.4.

15 May 2015

There was mild improvement with the continuation of the herbs and diet modification. Changes made to the diet are provided in Table 12.4. The supplements and Chinese herbal formulas remained the same.

3 July 2015

Patient A's condition was greatly improved at the fourth recheck appointment. The diet change improved the Damp Heat. Approximately three weeks after the last recheck appointment the owner sent an email stating Patient A's ear and skin were completely clear and he was not itching or scratching. The owner noted his aggression toward other dogs had worsened. The owner was instructed to increase the beef liver to daily administration and add a part of a hard-boiled egg to the food daily. An email update two weeks later indicated Patient A's mood had improved.

TCVM Discussion: The Spleen during the process of digestion extracts the clear (pure) from the impure (turbid). Only the turbid descends to the small intestine. The clear substance, called Gu Qi (Food Essence), ascends to the Lung, combining with Qing Qi (Universal Clean Air) to form Zong Qi (Pectoral

Qi) (Xie and Preast 2007b). Gu Qi also forms Ying Qi (Nutrient Blood) which circulates in the blood vessels and transforms into Blood (Xie and Preast 2007b).

The Spleen also extracts fluids from the food. The clear fluid ascends to the Heart where Blood is made under the influence of the Kidney. Any unusable or pathologic fluid, called Damp, extracted by the Spleen is stored in the body (Marsden 2015a-c). The accumulation of Damp causes many diseases commonly seen in veterinary medicine (Marsden 2015a-c). The less nutrient dense and more processed the diet, the more unusable fluid (Damp) is made. Damp accumulation likely contributed to the recurrent ear infections and skin infections in Patient A's history.

If the diet is poor then Gu Qi and clear fluid are poor and Blood is not made resulting in Blood Deficiency (Marsden 2015a-c). Damp accumulation also impedes Qi flow. Qi propels Blood, and lack of Qi worsens Blood Deficiency. If the body is deficient in Blood then blood flow to the periphery is weakened leading to cool paws and ear tips (Xie and Preast 2007a).

Lack of Blood supply to the limbs leads to drying of tissues causing the low-grade itch, dry skin, mild redness, recurrent low-grade skin infections, and fine powdery dandruff (Xie and Preast 2007a). This leaves the skin vulnerable to external Wind invasions causing recurrent low-grade infections. The historical lymphadenopathy and swelling of the left rear limb was likely the result of a Wind Heat Invasion.

The light pink tongue supported Blood Deficiency as poor blood flow to the tongue would dampen the color (Xie and Preast 2007a). The pulse was deficient and weaker on the left supporting Blood or Yin Deficiency. Chronic Blood Deficiency can lead to Qi deficiency because Blood governs Qi. Additionally Qi propels Blood, so deficient Qi can cause a wiry pulse (Marsden 2015a-c).

Blood Deficiency will also affect the Heart causing Shen disturbances, often demonstrated as frequent dreaming and dog aggression (Xie and Preast 2007a). Lack of blood frequently causes Liver Blood Deficiency because the Liver stores Blood. Liver Blood Deficiency frequently causes Liver Qi Stagnation because Blood governs Qi, and the Liver regulates the smooth flow of Qi. Both pathologies can cause Liver Qi Stagnation which contributes to dreaming and aggressive tendencies (Xie and Preast 2007a).

Initial Appointment: On initial presentation Patient A's signs were most consistent with Blood Deficiency and Spleen Deficiency. Based on his response Si Wu Xiao Fang Yin was not the best initial formula and should have been discontinued sooner. The herbal formula did help reduce the itch but allowed the development of Damp Heat symptoms which indicated both Blood Deficiency and Spleen Deficiency with Secondary Damp needed to be addressed first.

Dang Gui Shao Yao San may have been a better herbal formula with which to begin. This formula belongs to the category of Tonify and Move Blood with the secondary categories Draining Damp and Tonifying the Spleen (Chen et al. 2012). TCM indications for which this formula works best include Damp, Blood Stasis, Blood Deficiency, Spleen Qi Deficiency, and Elements of Liver Blood Deficiency (Chen et al. 2012; Marsden 2014a). Patients' tongues are often pale, lavender and moist or swollen. The pulses are thin, wiry, or slippery. The formula includes Dang Gui (Angelica), Bai Shao (White Peony), Chuan Xiong (Ligusticum), Bai Zhu (White Atractylodes), Fu Ling (Poria), and Ze Xie (Alisma) (Chen et al. 2012; Marsden 2014a).

19 January 2015

Based on the TCVM diagnoses the treatment goals were to Tonify Blood and Support the Spleen. Si Wu Xiao Feng Yin (Four Materials Eliminate Wind Combination, Natural Path)

(Continued)

Case Study 2 (Continued)

was chosen because it is a very useful formula for skin disease due to Blood Deficiency, as well as Blood Deficiency leading to external Wind invasions (Marsden 2014c). Given the historical Wind Damp Heat invasion, the objective was to tonify the Blood and prevent further Wind invasions and eliminate any potentially lingering subclinical Wind from the skin and collaterals. Si Wu Xiao Feng Yin belongs to the category of formulas that Expels Wind and Releases Wind from the Skin and Collaterals (Chen et al. 2012; Marsden 2014c). TCVM indications for the formula include Liver Blood Deficiency, Blood Deficiency, and Wind Heat Invasions (Chen

et al. 2012; Marsden 2014c). The formula improves blood synthesis and peripheral circulation and increases immune surveillance. The tongues of patients benefiting from this formula are pale purple or lavender (Chen et al. 2012; Marsden 2014c). The pulse is generally thin, choppy, and/or wiry. Si Wu Xiao Feng Yin was started at ⅛ tsp daily and slowly increased to ¼ tsp daily over three to five days. The herbs were given once daily because they were mixed with the food and Patient A would only eat once a day. Table 12.8 provides additional information about the individual herbs comprising Si Wu Xiao Feng Yin.

Table 12.8 The Chinese herbs comprising the Chinese herbal formula Si Wu Xiao Feng Yin. The herbal properties, channels entered, and TCVM functions of each herb within the formula (Chen et al. 2012; Marsden 2014c).

Bai Xian Pi	English name	Dictamnus root
	Properties	Bitter, cold
	Channels entered	Spleen, stomach
	Functions	Expels wind heat pathogens; clears heat, eliminates toxins, and alleviates itching; and clears damp-heat
Bo He Ye	English name	Peppermint
	Properties	Acrid, cool
	Channels entered	Lung, liver
	Functions	Expels wind heat pathogens; clears eyes, head, and throat; vents rashes; and disperses liver Qi
Chai Hu	English name	Bupleurum root
	Properties	Bitter, slightly cold
	Channels entered	Liver, gallbladder
	Functions	Helps mobilize liver Qi stagnating secondary to liver blood deficiency; expels wind heat pathogens; immune stimulant; resolves Shao Yang disorders and lowers fever; raises Yang Qi in cases of Middle Jiao deficiency; guides formula to the Triple Burner; and prevents Qi and blood stasis
Chi Shao	English name	Red Peony root
	Properties	Bitter, slightly cold
	Channels entered	Liver
	Functions	Relieves itch; cools blood; clears heat and cools blood; invigorates blood, removes stagnation and swelling; and clears liver fire

Chuan Xiong	English name	Ligusticum (Szechuan) root
	Properties	Acrid, warm
	Channels entered	Liver, gallbladder, pericardium
	Functions	Activates Qi and blood circulation and dispels wind and relieves pain
Da Zao	English name	Jujube
	Properties	Sweet, warm
	Channels entered	Spleen, stomach
	Functions	Tonifies blood; tonifies spleen and stomach. benefits Qi; calms Shen; and harmonizes other herbs
Dang Gui	English name	Angelica
	Properties	Sweet, acrid, warm
	Channels entered	Heart, liver, spleen
	Functions	Nourish blood and relieves pain; tonifies blood; moistens intestines and unblocks bowels; stops cough and treats dyspnea; and prevents Qi and blood stasis
Du Huo	English name	Angelica root
	Properties	Acrid, bitter
	Channels entered	Kidney, bladder
	Functions	Dispel wind, cold, and dampness; relieves pain; and releases the exterior
Jing Jie	English name	Schizonepeta
	Properties	Acrid, slightly warm
	Channels entered	Lung, liver
	Functions	Expels wind heat pathogen; relieves the exterior and dispels winds; alleviates itching and rashes; and stops bleeding
Sheng Di Huan	English name	Rehmannia root
	Properties	Sweet, cold
	Channels entered	Heart, liver, kidney
	Functions	Clears heat and cools blood; nourishes Yin and increases fluids; clears heart fire; and stops bleeding
Chan Tui	English name	Cicada molting
	Properties	Sweet, cold
	Channels entered	Liver, lung
	Functions	Disperses wind cold; relieves sore throat and produces sound; relieves itching and promotes eruption; Improves vision; and extinguishes wind and relieves spasms

Source: Lisa P. McFaddin.

(Continued)

Case Study 2   (Continued)

Based on the TCM diagnoses the goal was to Drain Damp, Clear Heat, Support the Spleen, and Tonify Blood. The Si Wu Xiao Feng Yin was continued to help with Blood Deficiency and because the itch was improved. Si Miao San with Dang Gui was added to Drain Damp and Clear Heat while Supporting the Spleen, Tonifying the Spleen Qi, and Tonifying the Blood (Marsden 2014b; Chen et al. 2012). Si Miao San belongs to the category of formulas that Expels Damp, Clears Heat, Tonifies, and Moves. TCVM indications for the formula include Dampness Accumulation, Damp Heat, Blood Stasis, Spleen Qi Deficiency, and Yang Ming Pathogens, especially in the Large Intestine and Stomach (Marsden 2014b; Chen et al. 2012). Patients' tongues are often swollen, damp, pink to red or purple-red. The pulses are slippery and wiry; however, if the Spleen is really deficient the pulses may be weaker. Dang Gui belongs to the Blood Tonifying category (Chen et al. 2012). Table 12.9 provides additional information about the individual herbs comprising Si Miao San with Dang Gui.

The Si Wu Xiao Fang Yin should have been discontinued and only Si Miao San started. At that time it was more important to Drain Damp, Clear Heat, and Support the Spleen and Spleen Qi than Tonify Blood. It is always better to clear the excess before trying to tonify deficiencies.

The diet should have been changed sooner. The original home-made diet contained warm foods (White Rice), Yin Tonics (Turkey, White Rice), and was overall too Dampening (especially with the addition of White Rice) (Pitchford 2002; Xie 2015; Marsden 2015a-c). The addition of Lamb further increased the heat associated with the diet.

16 March 2015

Si Wu Xiao Feng Yin was discontinued due to the persistent Damp Heat signs. Si Miao San + Dang Gui was continued to Drain Damp, Clear Heat, Support the Spleen, and Tonify the Blood. If Patient A had been on Si Miao San only at this time, Dang Gui would not have been added because the biggest problem was the Damp Heat due to a deficient Spleen. However, the owner already had the herbal combination and it was continued. The diet change at the second recheck appointment was geared toward further Clearing of Heat, Supporting the Spleen, and Tonifying the Blood. Ideally the diet should have focused more on Clearing Heat, Draining Damp, and Supporting the Spleen. Tonifying the Blood is important but Dang Gui could have been added once the Damp Heat was cleared.

15 May 2015

At this point many of the Damp Heat signs had improved, and the decision was made to focus on the diet. The ingredients were chosen, in part, based on Patient A's finicky tendencies. The goal of the diet was to Drain Damp (Pumpkin, Kidney Beans), Support the Spleen (Chicken, Peas, Pumpkin), and Tonify Blood (Kidney Beans, Broccoli). The diet's overall thermal property was neutral. All of the foods were sweet helping to Tonify and support the Spleen.

3 July 2015

The cause for the aggression was assumed to be persistent Blood Deficiency and development of Liver Blood Deficiency. Both beef liver and whole eggs function as blood tonics and

Table 12.9 The Chinese herbs comprising the Chinese herbal formula Si Miao San+Dang Gui. The herbal properties, channels entered, and TCVM functions of each herb within the formula are listed (Chen et al. 2012; Marsden 2014b).

Cang Zhu	English name	Atractylodes rhizome
	Properties	Acrid, bitter, warm
	Channels entered	Spleen, stomach, liver
	Functions	Tonifies spleen; dispels damp and wind; induces diaphoresis and releases the exterior; dries dampness in the Lower Jiao; and improves vision and night blindness
Huai Niu Xi	English name	Achryanthes root
	Properties	Bitter, sour, neutral
	Channels entered	Liver, kidney
	Functions	Relaxes sinews of lower back and moves blood. moves blood; helps formula with acutely inflamed, subacute, and chronic inflammatory conditions; astringent effect on fluid loss helping to relieve aching of lower back, lower limbs, and knees caused by dehydrating influence of longstanding damp heat accumulation; and counteracts the drying effects of the other three herbs making herb safe for long-term use
Yi Yi Ren	English name	Coix seed
	Properties	Sweet, tasteless, slightly cold
	Channels entered	Spleen, stomach, lung
	Functions	Leaches damp and clears heat from lower burner while providing mild support to the spleen; supports the effects of the two marvels by draining damp
Huang Bai	English name	Phellodendron bark
	Properties	Bitter, cold
	Channels entered	Kidney, bladder
	Functions	Dried damp and clears heat from lower burner; strong cooling action; and focuses on lower burner but strong enough for systemic effect
Dang Gui	English name	Angelica
	Properties	Sweet, acrid, warm
	Channels entered	Heart, liver, spleen
	Functions	Nourish blood and relieves pain; tonifies blood; moistens intestines and unblocks bowels; stops cough and treats dyspnea; and prevents Qi and blood stasis

Source: Lisa P. McFaddin.

(Continued)

Case Study 2 (Continued)

contain higher levels of tryptophan which is a precursor to serotonin and can improve mood (Pitchford 2002; Xie 2015; Marsden 2015a-c).

Western Discussion: An in-depth discussion of the pharmacologic effects of each nutraceutical is beyond the scope of this report. A brief overview of the pharmacologic benefits of the two Chinese herbal formulas and key dietary ingredients will be discussed.

Si Wu Xiao Feng Yin is effective through improving cutaneous blood flow (Dang Gui) and reducing inflammation (Bai Shao Yao and Chai Hu) (Marsden 2014c). With improved blood flow comes white blood cells, antibodies, and immune complexes which help deal with inflammation and allergens (Marsden 2014c).

Si Miao San is a potent anti-inflammatory. Phellodendron (Huang Bai) inhibits the production of inflammatory cytokines and nitric

oxide, acts as an antioxidant, inhibits gene expression of tumor necrosis factor (TNF)-α, and enhances the effectivity of antimicrobials (Marsden 2014b). Coix (Yi Yi Ren) decreases nitric oxide synthesis and superoxide production (Marsden 2014b).

The nutritional and therapeutic properties associated with the ingredients comprising Patient A's home-cooked diet are outlined Table 12.10.

Conclusion: The incorporation of a TCVM-based home-cooked diet, Chinese herbal formulas, and nutraceuticals successfully improved and managed a dog with chronic skin and ear issues due to atopic dermatitis. The report demonstrates the useful nature of integrative medicine in the management of common and chronic dermatologic disorders in canine patients.

Table 12.10 The nutritional properties and therapeutic benefits of each ingredient within Grissom's home-cooked diet.

Applesauce	Nutritional properties	*High fiber*	4 g per medium-sized apple
		Vitamins	A, B1, B2, B6, C, E, K
		Minerals	Copper, manganese, potassium
		Antioxidants	Catechin, cholorgenic acid, phloridzin, polyphenols, quercetin
	Therapeutic benefits		Improves cognitive function; reduces risk of stroke; lowers levels of low-density lipoprotein cholesterol; helps manage blood pressure; lowers risk of developing type 2 diabetes; and may lower the risk of lung, breast, and colorectal cancer development (Brazier 2019; Jennings 2018)
Beef liver	Nutritional properties	*High protein*	22 g per 3 ounces
		Vitamins	A, B2, B9, B12, D, E, K
		Minerals	Choline, copper, iron, zinc
		Bioactive compounds	Creatine, conjugated linoleic acid, glutathione, taurine
	Therapeutic benefits		Improves immune system health; improves retinal health (Enviromedica 2018; Rowles 2017)

Broccoli	Nutritional properties	*High fiber*	2.4 g per 1 cup
		Vitamins	A, B9, C, K
		Minerals	Calcium, phosphorus, potassium, selenium, zinc
		Antioxidants	Kaempferol, lutein, sulforaphane, zeaxanthin
	Therapeutic benefits	Improves blood sugar levels; protects against osteoporosis; improves small intestinal and colonic health; lowers levels of low-density lipoprotein cholesterol; has cardioprotective and neuroprotective effects; may reduce systemic inflammation; and may lower the risk of developing breast, prostate, gastric, colorectal, renal, and bladder cancer (Hill 2018; Ware 2018)	
Chicken breast	Nutritional properties	*High protein*	26 g per 3 ounces
		Vitamins	B3, B6
		Minerals	Phosphorus, selenium
		Antioxidants	Creatine, conjugated linoleic acid, glutathione, and taurine
	Therapeutic benefits	Low glycemic index; maintains muscle mass (Frey 2020)	
Kidney beans	Nutritional properties	*High fiber*	6.4 g per 3.5 ounces
		High protein	8.7 g per 3.5 ounces
		Vitamins	Folate, K1
		Minerals	Copper, iron, potassium, manganese, molybdenum
		Bioactive compounds	Anthocyanins, isoflavones, phytohemagglutinin, phytic acid, and starch blockers
	Therapeutic benefits	Low glycemic index, helping control blood sugar levels; may prevent colorectal cancer (Arnarson 2019a)	
Lamb	Nutritional properties	*High protein*	25.6 g per 3.5 ounces
		Vitamins	B3, B12
		Minerals	Iron, phosphorus, selenium, and zinc
		Antioxidants	Creatine, conjugated linoleic acid, glutathione, taurine
	Therapeutic benefits	Maintains muscle tone; lowers glycemic index helping regular blood sugar (Arnarson 2019b)	

(Continued)

Case Study 2: Table 12.10   (Continued)

Peas	Nutritional properties	*High fiber*	4 g per ½ cup
		Moderate protein	4 g per ½ cup
		Vitamins	A, folate, K
		Minerals	Iron, phosphorus, manganese, thiamine
	Therapeutic benefits	Low glycemic index, helping control blood sugar; helps control blood pressure; and may lower the risk of developing prostate cancer (Alliott 2017; Elliott 2017)	
Pumpkin	Nutritional properties	*High fiber*	3 g per 1 cup
		Vitamins	A, B2, C, E
		Minerals	Copper, iron, manganese, potassium
		Antioxidants	α-Carotene, β-carotene, β-cryptoxanthin, lutein, and zeaxanthin
	Therapeutic benefits	Systemic antioxidant and anti-inflammatory effects; promotes systemic immunity; improves retinal health; lowers levels of low-density lipoprotein cholesterol; regulates blood pressure; controls blood sugar levels; and may lower the risk of colon and prostate cancer (Raman 2018a; Ware 2019)	
Turkey	Nutritional properties	*High protein*	22 g per 4 ounces
		Vitamins	B3, B6, B12
		Minerals	Choline, magnesium, phosphorus, potassium, selenium, sodium, zinc
		Bioactive compounds	Creatine, conjugated linoleic acid, glutathione, taurine
	Therapeutic benefits	High B vitamin content improves cardiovascular function; low glycemic index helps regulate blood sugar; and vitamin B6 has cardioprotective and neuroprotective effects (Tourney 2011; O'Brien 2019)	
White rice	Nutritional properties	*Low fiber*	0.9 g per 2.5 ounces
		Vitamins	B3, B6, folate
		Minerals	Copper, iron, magnesium, manganese, phosphorus, selenium, thiamine, zinc
	Therapeutic benefits	Improves fecal consistency and output in dogs (Raman 2018b; Teixeira et al. 2019)	

Source: Lisa P. McFaddin.

Case Study 3   Focus on Chinese Herbal Medicine

Title: The use of Xiao Yao San in the management of generalized anxiety in a dog

Author: Lisa P. McFaddin, DVM, GDCVHM, CVSMT, CVMRT, FCoAC, CVA

Summary: An eight-year old female spayed Labrador mix presented for an integrative consultation and alternative treatment options for recurrent paw licking and anxiety. Her symptoms included chronic low-grade pruritus, licking, and redness of the paws as well as generalized anxiety. Treatment with the Chinese herbal formula Xiao Yao San resolved the pododermatitis, improved the anxiety, and allowed reduction of the fluoxetine dosage.

Introduction: The fifth edition of the Diagnostic and Statistical Manual of Mental Disorders (DSM-5) defines human generalized anxiety disorder (GAD) as excessive worrying about a variety of events or activities which persists for more than six months (Kupper and Regeir 2013). Common clinical signs include restlessness, fatigue, difficulty concentrating, irritability, muscle tension, and sleep disturbances (Kupper and Regeir 2013). The DSM-5 separates the diagnosis of GAD and obsessive-compulsive disorder (OCD) but considers them comorbidities.

Canine anxiety is defined as the anticipation of danger without a specific threat or cause (Horowitz 2006). Anxiety is believed to develop because of genetic proclivities, improper or incomplete socialization as a puppy, disruptive household or life changes, and trauma (Horowitz 2006). There are multiple manifestations of canine anxiety including, but not limited to, generalized anxiety, separation anxiety, thunderstorm or firework phobias, and obsessive-compulsive behaviors (Horowitz 2006). Unlike human medicine, veterinary medicine does classify OCD behaviors as a form of generalized anxiety. Common canine obsessive-compulsive behaviors include shadow and light chasing, spinning, tail chasing, lick granulomas, self-mutilation, fly biting, pica, fence running, flank sucking, and excessive surface licking (Frank 2016).

Lick granulomas, self-mutilation, excessive self-licking, and flank sucking also fall into a category of conditions known as behavioral dermatoses. Behavioral dermatoses are divided into psychophysiological disorders, primary behavioral disorders, secondary behavioral disorders, and cutaneous sensory disorders (Vigra 2003). Each category of the dermatoses can cause similar clinical signs and more than one disease process can be present at a time.

Western treatment recommendations for most forms of canine anxiety include behavior and environmental modification, as well as pharmacological intervention (Horowitz 2006).

The Chinese herbal formula Xiao Yao San (Wandering Ease Combination; Bupleurum and Dang Gui Formula) is frequently used to treat depression and anxiety in people. Zhang et al. (2011) discussed numerous studies investigating the use of Xiao Yao San for depression and anxiety. The paper concluded the herbal formula was helpful in treating depression and anxiety with fewer side effects compared to traditional antidepressants and anxiolytics. Zhang et al. (2011) later suggested the use of Xiao Yao San with an antidepressant, such as fluoxetine, may have a faster beneficial effect compared to treating with an antidepressant alone. This case study highlights the efficacy of using Xiao Yao San in canine patients with generalized anxiety and obsessive-compulsive disorders causing bodily harm.

Case Presentation: Patient B, an eight-year-old female spayed 73 lb (33 kg) Labrador mix, presented with a two-day exacerbation of excessive paw chewing. She was adopted at one year of age. Since adoption she had a history of recurrent itching, scratching, yeast otitis externa, and pododermatitis (paw

(Continued)

Case Study 3 (Continued)

infections). The paw infections were attributed to obsessive chewing and licking which worsened when she was alone. She had a history of generalized anxiety, hiding, and hyperactivity. She was very friendly to the owner's daughter but standoffish with the son. She was not destructive when anxious. She dreamed frequently. She was diagnosed with hypothyroidism and started on levothyroxine 0.7 mg twice daily in 2009. Records from the diagnosis were not available. She was started on fluoxetine 40 mg once daily in 2010 to treat the signs of generalized anxiety. The owner noted modest improvement in her anxiety level with medication. She was started on hydroxyzine 50 mg twice daily, Catalystz™ (a fish oil supplement with a rice bran base), and Dermal Support (a dietary supplement made by Standard Process) in 2012 to treat the recurrent dermatitis. The owner noted minimal improvement in the pruritis with treatment. Her current diet was a dry kibble, Natural Balance™.

On Western physical examination she was very anxious, hiding under the bench and shivering. Both ears had mild waxy debris. There was a small amount of erythema associated with the palmar and plantar aspects of the third and fourth digits on all four paws. There were no active lesions. The skin and hair coat were dry with fine powdery dandruff.

On TCVM examination she had a Water personality (generally characterized by dogs who are timid, hiding, often fear aggressive or submissive). The paws and ear tips were cool to the touch. The tongue was red with a slight purple hue. The pulses were deep, thin, and slightly wiry bilaterally. Active acupuncture points were not evaluated.

Impression cytology of the digits was unremarkable. Baseline blood work, Michigan State University therapeutic thyroid panel, and urinalysis were declined by the owner. The traditional Western medicine diagnoses included mild pododermatitis, historical generalized anxiety, and historical hypothyroidism. The pododermatitis was considered secondary to obsessive compulsive paw licking, likely a symptom of the generalized anxiety. The TCVM diagnosis was Liver Blood Deficiency.

Treatment options discussed with the owner included dietary changes, adjustment of the supplements, acupuncture, topical anti-itch medication for the paws, and the Chinese herbal formula Xiao Yao San (XYS). They approved starting the herbal formula, declining all other recommendations. At the owner's request all other medications and supplements were continued. XYS was dispensed as a tablet made by Kan Herb called Happy Wanderer™. The dose was one tablet (550 mg) by mouth every 12 hours for three days then increased to two tablets (1100 mg) every 12 hours.

Four weeks after starting the Xiao Yao San the owner reported a 70% improvement in the paw licking but no change in the anxiety. The Xiao Yao San dose was increased to three tablets (1650 mg) twice daily. The hydroxyzine was discontinued at this time, but all other supplements and medications were continued. Six weeks later, 10 weeks after starting XYS, the owner reported resolution of the paw licking and a 30–40% improvement in the anxiety. Four months later, 6.5 months after starting XYS, the owner reported further improvement in the anxiety, and the fluoxetine dose was reduced to 30 mg once daily. Four weeks later, 7.5 months after starting XYS, the owner reported continued improvement in her anxiety level, and the fluoxetine was reduced to 20 mg once daily. Six weeks later, nine months after starting XYS, the owner reported continued improvement but declined further dose reduction of the fluoxetine. The Xiao Yao San, levothyroxine, Catalyst™, and Dermal Support were continued long term.

TCVM Discussion: The historical findings of Patient B that supported Liver Blood Deficiency included anxiety, fearfulness, chronic low-grade dermatitis, hypothyroidism, and frequent dreaming (Xie and Preast 2007a-d; Xie and Preast 2007a,d). Western and TCVM examination findings consistent with Liver Blood Deficiency included anxiety, mild dermatitis, dry skin, fine powdery dandruff, cool paws and ears, purple hue to the tongue, and deficient, thin, wiry pulses. The history of yeast otitis and repeat pododermatitis suggested a propensity for Dampness accumulation. No Damp signs were noted on presentation.

Blood Deficiency can result from a variety of causes including a weakened Spleen, poor diet, and Dampness accumulation. The Spleen is considered responsible in Chinese medicine for transforming and transporting food, to generate Ying Qi (plasma), along with Jing or Essence, which make up the cellular components of Blood. If the diet is poor then Essence and Ying Qi are not formed and Blood is not made resulting in Blood Deficiency. Damp accumulation also impedes Qi flow. Qi propels Blood, and lack of Qi worsens Blood Deficiency. Lack of Blood flow to the limbs causes the tissues to dry leading to dry skin, dandruff, and low-grade itch. Blood Deficiency also affects the Shen because blood flow to the Heart is lessened. This contributes to anxiety, fearfulness, and frequent dreaming. Any condition in which Blood is deficient will cause Liver Blood Deficiency. The Liver is responsible for the storage of Blood and its volume in circulation. Blood Deficiency reduces the amount of Blood supplied to and stored by the Liver, resulting in this failure of peripheral circulation being commonly termed "Liver Blood deficiency" (Marsden 2015a-c; Wynn and Marsden 2003).

Liver Blood Deficiency can theoretically lead to a reduction in circulating thyroid hormone levels and slowing of the metabolic rate which then reduces peripheral circulation (Marsden 2015a-c; Wynn and Marsden

2003). This so-called adaptive hypothyroidism can result in reduction of total T4 levels with normal TSH levels (Wynn and Marsden 2003). The means by which Patient B was diagnosed with hypothyroidism was not known. It is possible she suffered from adaptive hypothyroidism and not autoimmune primary hypothyroidism.

The primary TCVM treatment goal was to tonify Liver Blood. Xiao Yao San belongs to the category of herbal formulas that Regulates and Harmonizes the Liver and Spleen, Disperses Liver Qi, Relieves Stagnation, Tonifies Spleen Qi, and Nourishes Blood (Marsden 2014d). TCVM indications for its use include Liver Blood Deficiency, Blood Deficiency, Disharmonies between the Liver and Spleen, Spleen Deficiency, and Liver Qi Stagnation (Marsden 2014d). The tongue is often pale, lavender, and occasionally swollen. The pulses are usually thin, soft, tense, weak, or taut.

Xiao Yao San should be avoided in Damp conditions. Administration of Xiao Yao San in patients with preexisting cholestasis may cause liver enzyme elevations (Marsden 2014d). The formula should be avoided during pregnancy and lactation (Marsden 2014d).

Xiao Yao San is composed of eight individual herbs: Chai Hu, Dang Gui, Bai Shao Yao, Bo He, Bai Zhu, Fu Ling, Gan Cao, and Sheng Jiang. Table 12.11 summarizes the properties and functions of each herb within the formula; while Figure 12.7 depicts the dried version of each ingredient. Figure 12.8 shows the powdered version of the herbal formula used.

Western Discussion: The recurrent paw licking was likely due to an obsessive-compulsive behavior (primary behavioral disorder) but the presence of neuropathic itch (psychophysiologic disorder) cannot be ruled out. Neuropathic itch is defined as pruritus resulting from damage to the central or peripheral sensory neurons resulting in cutaneous pruritogenic stimulation (Rossmeisl 2016). Regardless of

(Continued)

Case Study 3   (Continued)

Table 12.11   The individual herbs comprising the Chinese herbal formula Xiao Yao San. The pinyin, common name, herbal properties, channels entered, and TCVM functions for each herb within the formula are described (Chen and Chen 2012; Marsden 2014d).

Pin Yin	Common name	Properties	Channels	Function
Chai Hu	Bupleurum	Bitter Slightly cold	Liver Gallbladder	Moves stagnant Liver Qi. Moves Qi
Dang Gui	Angelica	Sweet Acrid Warm	Heart Liver Spleen	Moves and tonifies Liver Blood and Yin. Blood tonic
Bai Shao Yao	White Peony	Bitter Sour Cool	Liver Spleen	Nourishes, moves, and tonifies Liver Blood and Yin. Nourishes Liver to calm Liver Yang and Liver Wind. Softens the Liver and relieves pain
Bo He	Mint	Acrid Cool	Lung Liver	Expels wind heat pathogens. Clears eyes, head, and throat. Disperses Liver Qi. Clears heat that has accumulated in the Liver channel from longstanding stasis
Bai Zhu	White Atractylodes	Bitter Sweet Warm	Spleen Stomach	Drains and dries Damp from the Spleen and Stomach while supporting Spleen and Lung Qi formation
Fu Ling	Poria	Sweet Bland Neutral	Heart Lung Spleen Kidney	Drains Damp and reduces swelling. Promotes urination for difficult urination and scant urination due to damp-heat. Tonifies Spleen Qi. Calms Shen
Gan Cao	Licorice root	Sweet Neutral	Spleen Stomach Lung Heart	Qi Tonifying. Harmonizes the formula. Tonifies Stomach Qi
Sheng Jiang	Fresh ginger	Acrid Slightly warm	Lung Spleen Stomach	Warms the middle energizer to stop vomiting. Leaches and dries dampness. Harmonizes the middle jiao. Dispels water and reduces edema. Releases the exterior and induces perspiration. Warms the Lung and stops coughing. Eliminates toxins

Source: Lisa P. McFaddin.

the inciting cause Patient B likely developed sensitivity in her paws over time. Recurrent microtrauma to the skin from licking could lead to inflammation and continual stimulation of C-fibers increasing their sensitivity and perpetuating the itch–lick cycle (Rossmeisl 2016).

Medical management of Patient B's anxiety was instituted but there was no record of behavior or environmental changes. Fluoxetine is a selective serotonin reuptake inhibitor used to treat depression, anxiety, and anti-compulsive behaviors in canines and felines. While there is an FDA-approved

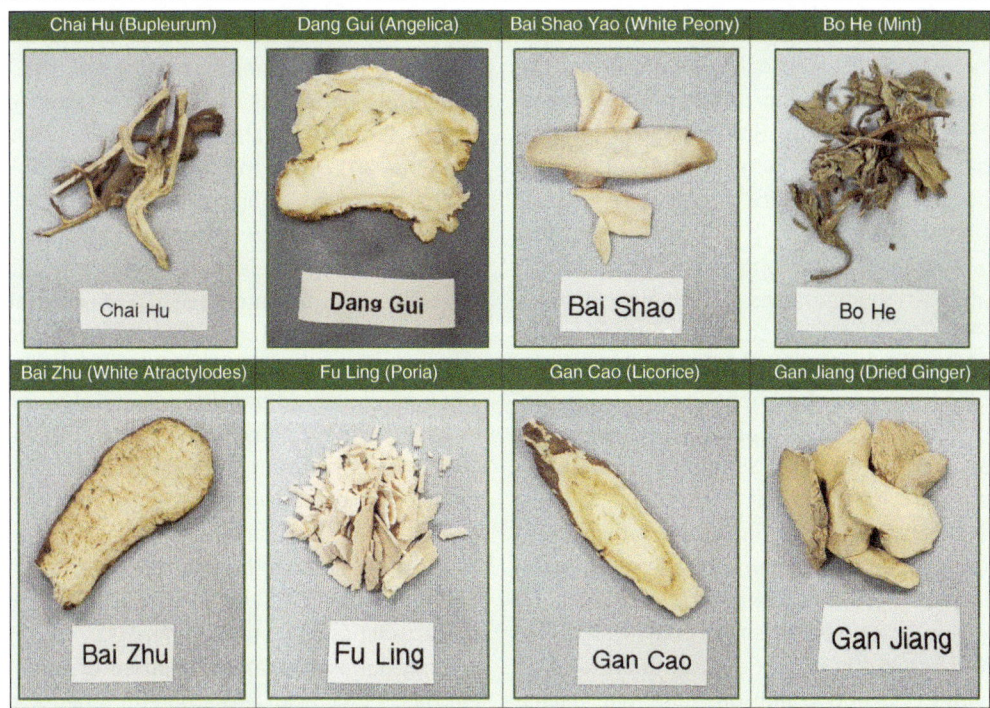

Figure 12.7 The individual herbs comprising Xiao Yao San. A sample ground, instead of dried, Angelica (Dang Gui) is provided. A sample of dried ginger (Gan Jiang), not fresh ginger (Sheng Jiang) is pictured. Source: Lisa P. McFaddin.

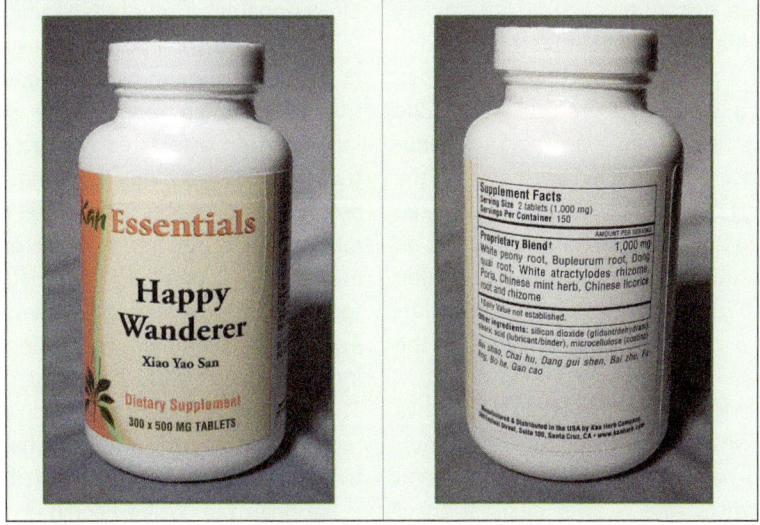

Figure 12.8 The Kan Essentials tablet preparation of Happy Wanderer (Xiao Yao San). Source: Lisa P. McFaddin.

(Continued)

Case Study 3 (Continued)

canine product, Reconcile, Patient B was taking the generic version. Adverse effects associated with fluoxetine include lethargy, gastrointestinal effects, anxiety, irritability, insomnia/hyperactivity, anorexia, or panting (Plumb 2015).

Xiao Yao San is a commonly used herbal formula in humans and companion animals. Beneficial Western medical properties associated with its use include improved hepatic blood flow, increased hepatic nitric oxide production, limited neutrophil activity, free radical scavenging (through superoxide dismutase), analgesia, inhibition of fibrosis and collagen synthesis, changes to insulin sensitivity, relief from depression and anxiety, and mood stabilization (Marsden 2014d; Yin et al. 2012).

The exact mechanism through which Xiao Yao San exerts its anxiolytic and antidepressant is unknown. Multiple potential mechanisms have been studied. Marsden (2014a–d) suggests the formula's ability to alter cortical blood flow likely contributes to its beneficial effects. This notion is supported by Karim et al.'s (2017) study which demonstrated adults with a history of generalized anxiety disorder exhibited increased cerebral blood flow to multiple areas of the brain when experiencing periods of severe worry. Zhu et al. (2014) determined Xiao Yao San modulated β-Arrestin 2-mediated pathways in the hippocampus. Yin et al. (2012) demonstrated Xiao Yao San had a dose-dependent effect on glial cell proliferation and neuroprotection against oxidative stress as well as stimulating certain 5-HT (serotonin) receptors in the cerebrum.

Xiao Yao San, as a whole, works to improve circulation while at the same time each individual herb has its own unique and useful pharmacological role. A brief description of each component of the formula is provided to better understand the pharmacologic effects of Xiao Yao San.

Chai Hu (Bupleurum) is composed of triterpenoids, essential oils, carbohydrates, flavone, saponins, coumarin, and organic acids (Chen and Chen 2012). The formula has been shown to be analgesic, antipyretic, sedative, anti-inflammatory, hepatoprotective, cholagogic, antihyperlipidemic, immunostimulant, and antibacterial (Chen and Chen 2012). Lee et al. (2012) determined bupleurum reduced depression and anxiety-like symptoms in rats when administered prior to a stressful event. Li et al. (2013) suggested the antidepressant effects of bupleurum were due to the neuronal cytoprotective properties of its saponins. Based on the pharamacologic properties and recent studies bupleurum contributes heavily to the anxiolytic and antidepressant characteristics of Xiao Yao San.

Dang Gui (Angelica) is composed of essential oils, ferulic acid, and scopletin (Chen and Chen 2012). Known pharmacologic effects include modulation of uterine smooth muscle tone, improved blood circulation, antiplatelet and immunostimulant activity, reduction in bronchospasm, hepatoprotection, antibacterial effects, analgesia, relief of inflammation and a reduction in insomnia (Chen et al. 2012). Lee et al. (2016) determined the topical application of Angelica reduced the pruritus and inflammation associated with atopic dermatitis. The exact mechanism was not determined but beneficial effects were noted on mast cell numbers and the level of serum IgE (Lee et al. 2016). Hsiao et al. (2012) determined the topical application of an ethanol extract of Angelica improved wound healing by promoting human epithelial fibroblast proliferation. The addition of Angelica to Xiao Yao San likely reduced Patient B's pruritus and helped resolve the mild paw inflammation and dermatitis.

Bai Shao Yao (White Peony) is composed of paeoniflorin, albiflorin, oxypaoniflorin, benzoyl-paeoniflorin, paeonin, and hydroxypaeoniflorin (Chen and Chen 2012). Studied pharmacologic properties include CNS suppression, inhibition of smooth muscle contraction in the gut and uterus. The formula has antibacterial, antipyretic, anti-inflammatory, antiplatelet, and vasodilatory effects as well (Chen and Chen 2012). Additionally, Wang et al. (2013) demonstrated an oral preparation of white peony could relieve the pain associated with radiation-induced esophagitis. The anti-inflammatory and analgesic properties of white peony likely contributed to the resolution of Patient B's pododermatitis.

Bo He (Mint) is composed of essential oils, lipophilic flavones, and coumarins (Chen and Chen 2012). Known pharmacologic effects include improved local blood circulation with topical application and antipyretic, diaphoretic, and anti-inflammatory properties (Chen and Chen 2012). Cash et al. (2016) determined oral preparations of peppermint oil reduced symptoms of irritable bowel syndrome in susceptible patients through a viscero-somatic effect. The addition of Mint to Xiao Yao San likely contributed to the resolution of inflammation and itch associated with the pododermatitis.

Bai Zhu (White Atractylodes) is composed of atractylol, atractylon, junipercamphor, atractylolide, hydroxyactyldide, sesquiterpenelon, β-eudesmol,hinesol,8-β-ethoxyatractylenolide, palmitic acid, anhydroatractyolide, fructose, and synanthrin (Chen and Chen 2012). Studied pharmacologic effects include adaptogenic, immunostimulant, antiplatelet, diuretic, antidiabetic, and antineoplastic influences along with resolution of constipation and diarrhea (Chen and Chen 2012). Chen et al. (2016) demonstrated White Atractylodes reduced inflammation and pain through the inhibition of nitric oxidase, prostaglandins, and cyclooxygenase. Inclusion of White Atractylodes in Xiao Yao San likely contributes to its anti-inflammatory and analgesic properties.

The chemical composition of Fu Ling (Poria) includes pachymose, pachyman, pachymaran, tumulosic acid, and poriaic acid ABC (Chen and Chen 2012). The studied pharmacological effects include diuretic, antineoplastic, sedative, and antibacterial properties (Chen and Chen 2012). Hu et al. (2014) determined Poria had neuroprotective effects against oxidative stress experimentally induced in the hippocampus of rats. Inclusion of Poria in Xiao Yao San expectedly contributes to the neuronal, antioxidant, and anti-inflammatory effects of the formula.

Gan Cao (Licorice) contains triterpenoids and flavonoids (Chen and Chen 2012). Studied pharmacologic effects include mineralocorticoid and glucocorticoid action and anti-inflammatory, antiarrhythmic, and immunologic effects. Use results in inhibition of gastric acid as well as antitoxin, hepatoprotective, antitussive, expectorant, analgesic, antibiotic, and antihyperlipidemic influences (Chen and Chen 2012). Ofir et al. (2003) suggested the phytoestrogens in Licorice inhibit serotonin reuptake. Fan et al. (2012) demonstrated the flavonoids in Licorice have neuroprotective effects in conditions of chronic stress. The addition of Licorice in Xiao Yao San likely has a direct effect on the level of anxiety and depression.

The chemical composition of Sheng Jiang (Ginger) includes essential oils, geraniol, geranial, β-bisabolene, α-terpineol, β-sesquiphellandrene, arcurcumene, nerodiol, sesquiphellandrol, gingerol, methylgingerol, and gingerdiones (Chen et al. 2012). Pharmacologic effects include gastrointestinal protective effects, increased heart and respiratory rates, increased blood pressure, and antibiotic influences (Chen and Chen 2012). Yi et al. (2009) reported the combination of Magnolia Bark and Ginger Rhizome had synergistic antidepressant actions by affecting serotonin and norepinephrine activities. It is reasonable to speculate that Ginger combined with Bupleurum, Poria, and Licorice has similar effects on neurotransmitters associated with depression and anxiety.

Conclusion: Anxiety and OCD-type behaviors are common conditions seen in canine companions. Side effects associated with traditional anxiolytic and antidepressant

(Continued)

Case Study 3 (Continued)

medications can be cumbersome for patients and owners. Additionally, paw licking is a common complaint noted by owners. In this case the cause of the recurrent paw licking and mild pododermatitis were linked to an OCD-type behavior and possible neurogenic itch. Xiao Yao San was shown to be effective in the resolution of mild pododermatitis, obsessive paw licking, and anxiety when the underlying cause was Liver Blood Deficiency.

Case Study 4 Focus on Photobiomodulation

Title: Management of acral lick dermatitis in a dog with resultant hip osteoarthritis

Author: Kirsty Oliver, VN, DipAVN (surgical), RVT, CCRP, CVPP, VTS (physical rehabilitation)

Summary: This case illustrates the successful use of photobiomodulation therapy (PBMT) in the treatment of an adult dog with a chronic lick granuloma and hip osteoarthritis (OA). In this patient, there was significant change in chronic self-mutilation, weight-bearing, hip range of motion and comfort after the third treatment. Symptoms resolved after the tenth treatment and the continuation of maintenance treatments allowed the cessation of steroid use.

Introduction: Acral lick dermatitis (ALD) lesions (aka acral lick granulomas or ALG) typically present as red, swollen, and irritated areas made worse by repetitive self-trauma which causes the formation of a thickened plaque, called a granuloma (George et al. 2001). Many ALGs are associated with stress, anxiety, boredom, or compulsiveness (Luescher 2000). ALD can also be caused by referred pain from another body part, caused by neuralgia or peripheral neuropathy (Rosychuk 2011). Frequently found in distal limbs, care should be taken to rule out pain or discomfort from joints proximal to the lesion.

Case Presentation: Patient C was a 10-year-old female spayed Labrador retriever with a more than nine-year history of aALG, chronic licking, and pyoderma. Previous biopsies, radiographs, and baseline blood work was unremarkable. Previous treatments included judicious use of antibiotics and steroids.

Treatment protocol: A Class IV laser was used. The first three sessions used a peripheral treatment setting with 808 nm and 905 nm, 242 Hz, 75 W, for 95 seconds at 38.5 J. The secondary treatment involved 808 nm and 905 nm, 465 Hz, at 75 W, for 3 minutes 25 seconds at 150 J to both the left tarsus and coxofemoral joint. Treatment frequency was three times the first week, twice the second week, then weekly.

Treatment summary: The ALD showed obvious visual improvement after the third treatment, between the second and seventh days. The owners began noticing reduced licking during this time as well. Figure 12.9 shows photographs of the tarsus before six of the treatments. The tarsus and licking continued to improve with each treatment. Over 16 weeks after the final treatment the owners reported no recurrence of the licking or ALD.

Discussion: Light is essential to almost all life forms. Plants draw energy directly from solar radiation by photosynthesis. Light regulates the biological rhythms of many living beings. Science has proven that certain light emissions are able to effectively transfer energy to animal cells and tissue.

Not all light emissions are of the same quality, nor do they have the same therapeutic effect. The extent of therapeutic effect depends on the coherence of the emission used, wavelength, and the way in which the energy is supplied over time (form of the impulse used).

There are two distinct types of laser treatments in veterinary medicine: laser surgery

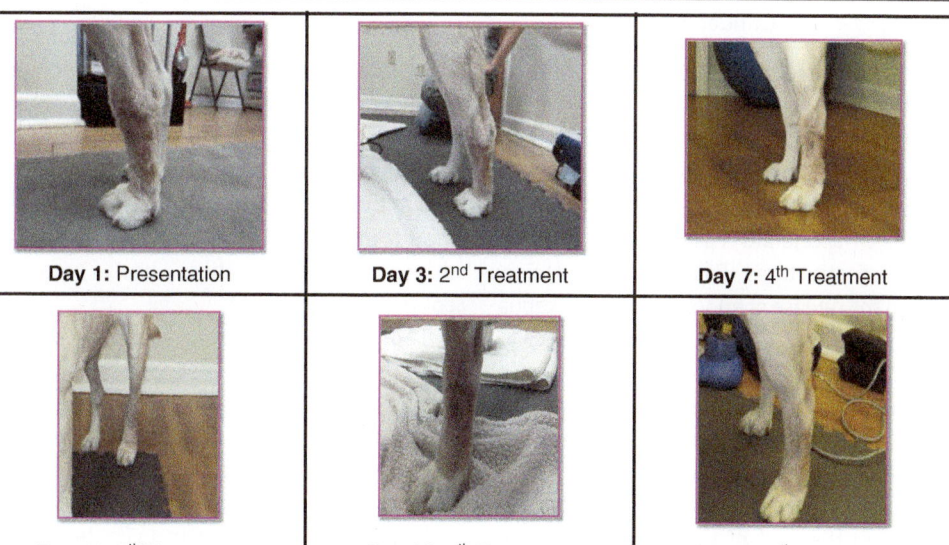

Day 1: Presentation	**Day 3:** 2nd Treatment	**Day 7:** 4th Treatment
Day 11: 5th Treatment	**Day 14:** 6th Treatment	**Day 21:** 7th Treatment

Figure 12.9 Photographs of the tarsus of a 10-year-old female spayed Labrador retriever with ALD receiving PBMT. Photographs were taken on the day of presentation, day 3 (before the second PBMT), day 7 (before the fourth PBMT), day 11 (before the fifth PBMT), day 14 (before the sixth PBMT), and day 21 (before the seventh PBMT). Source: Kirsty Oliver.

and laser therapy. Laser surgery is used to cut, cauterize, and coagulate tissue. Laser therapy uses low-dose photons to stimulate healing and reduce pain.

Energy is generated by activating electrons into an excited state. When these electrons drop from this excited state to their ground state, photons are emitted. Some of the photons stimulate the emission of other photons, amplifying the stimulated emission leading to a chain reaction. These emitted photons resonate between the mirrored ends in the laser chamber. Momentum builds until a highly concentrated beam of light passes through a partially transmissive mirror at one end of the laser chamber.

Lasers are classified by their output power and potential risks. Class I are found in supermarket scanners, Class II are found laser pointers, Class IIIA are visible light therapy lasers, and Class IIIB are non-visible light, therapy lasers with a power output of up to 500 mW and wavelength ranging from 300 nm up to infrared (FDA 2021b). Class IV

are non-visible light, therapy lasers with a power output of greater than 500 mW which may cause thermal skin effects and eye damage (FDA 2021b).

There are many different veterinary laser products, each with different characteristics. The most important qualities to consider are energy, time, wavelength, frequency, power, emission, and fluency (dose). Energy, measures in joules, is a property of objects that can be transformed to another object or converted into different forms but cannot be created or destroyed (Kittel and Kroemer 1980). Time is defined as the duration of the treatment or irradiance.

Wavelength is measured in nanometers (nm) (Gould 1959). Photon wavelength determines the effect. Smaller wavelengths penetrate tissue with greater ability. Laser affects tissue because the photons delivered to the cell and tissue triggers biologic change and reactions (Gould 1959), Photons are absorbed by cytochromes within the cell mitochondria and cell membrane

(Continued)

Case Study 4 (Continued)

causing increased oxygen production and the formation of a proton gradient across the cell and mitochondrial membranes. This leads to ATP and DNA production, stimulating cellular metabolism and growth. Laser photons can potentially accelerate tissue repair and cell growth of structures. Pain relief is attained through the release of endorphins and enkephalins (Anders et al. 2015). As photons enter cellular matter it may be scattered, reflected, or absorbed by different tissue types and density (Jacques 2013). This intensity of light decreases with the depth of tissue penetration.

Frequency is the number of impulses emitted during the unit of time (Siegman 1986), i.e. the number of light waves passing a fixed point in a specific time interval, measured in hertz (Hz) (Siegman 1986; Silfvast 1996). For 1 Hz, one light wave passes a fixed point in 1 second. Therefore, a machine producing 500 Hz creates 500 light waves per second.

Power is expressed in watts (W), where 1 watt is equal to 1 J/s and is the expression of energy over time. A common misconception is that power is equal to the total amount of energy emitted. One milliwatt is equal to 0.001 W. The emission mode can be either continuous, pulsed, or a combination (Paschotta 2016).

As no two patients are alike, neither is the dosing of laser therapy. Individual patient characteristics and the target tissue result in individual responses to therapy due to tissue thickness, body type, hair color and length.

The most common indications for laser therapy in veterinary medicine include pain reduction, reduction of inflammation and edema, improvement of local blood circulation, repair of wounds and ulcers, arthritis, and before- and/or after surgery.

Recent improvements in laser technology have resulted in a change of nomenclature. Today the preferred term is "photobiomodulation," recognized by 15 international participants at a joint meeting of NAALT (North American Association of Photobiomodulation Therapy) and WALT (World Association for Photobiomodulation Therapy) in 2014 as being "the most descriptive of science that involves complex mechanisms, some of which are stimulatory and some that are inhibitory" (Anders et al. 2015).

Case Study 5 Focus on Trigger Point Therapy

Title: Release of myofascial trigger points by dry needling to reduce pain in an adult canine with chronic intervertebral disk disease and hip osteoarthritis

Authors: Krysta E. Bailey, DVM, CCRP, DACVSMT, Jennifer A. Barnhard, BS, MS, and Matthew W. Brunke, DVM, CCRP, CVPP, CVA, CCMT, DACVSMR

Summary: A seven-year-old Cocker Spaniel with chronic intervertebral disk disease (IVDD) and hip osteoarthritis (OA) was found to have diffuse myofascial trigger points (MTrPs), postural changes, and pain. Dry needling (DN) is one modality used to promote myofascial release. Pain was measured using the Colorado State University (CSU) pain scale; no increase in pain was observed throughout treatment. An overall reduction in the pain score was observed.

MTrP DN therapy was incorporated using sterile, 30g, 1-inch stainless steel monofilament needles. Each needle was inserted into the center of the tight band of tissue, and then the needle was hand spun clockwise or counter-clockwise until a local twitch response (LTR) was elicited. Each needle was then left in place for another three to five minutes; the treatment was repeated if needed.

Within eight DN sessions over the course of four weeks resolution of the initially noted MTrPs was observed. DN was used in addition to several other therapeutic modalities and after four weeks of rehabilitation the patient's CSU pain score was 0. The use of DN is not contraindicated with the other modalities used in this case.

There should be further investigation in the canine species to explore the distinct benefits of DN, develop detailed treatment protocols and explore the relationship between patients with MTrPs, chronic IVDD, and hip OA.

Introduction: Intramuscular manual stimulation using monofilament needles to release MTrP pain, otherwise known as trigger point DN, has been taught through continuing education certification programs to physiotherapists and human doctors in the United States since the 1980s (FSBPT 2017). DN was initially integrated into manual techniques for treatment of canine lameness in 1991 (Janssens 1991; Wolfe et al. 1992). Further research is needed regarding the efficacy of DN and the etiology of the trigger points being treated. Natalie Lenton, director of the Canine Massage Therapy Centre Ltd. (CMTC), which is externally accredited with LANTRA, pioneered the Lenton Method™ for treatment of musculoskeletal problems and chronic pain management in canines. As part of the world's first double-blind clinical trials on MTrP release with Winchester University and Sparsholt University Centre, the Lenton Method™ is not specifically looking at DN, but serves as a research platform for the basis of the benefits of MTrP release in canines. Resolving MTrPs "can address, resolve, and support chronic ongoing pain with great success and is key to pain management" (Lenton 2018).

Healthy muscles are pliable and non-reactive to normal palpation. MTrPs are

"hyperirritable bands of focal point tension whereby the fibers in the muscles have stayed in a contracted state due to the restrictive binding of the fascia that surround them. This produces ischemia, nerve irritation, tenderness, muscular fatigue, reduced range of motion (ROM), and referred pain. Commonly the patient will experience hyperalgesia upon compression of the nodule. Muscles holding multiple MTrPs can suffer from restriction fatigue and mimic symptoms of other diseases such as arthritis" (Lenton 2018).

This is often seen by a patient adopting an abnormal posture or gait. Methods such as DN aim to resolve the MTrPs and thus reduce pain through improving an animal's range of motion and willingness to remain active (Hong and Simons 1998).

MTrPs exist in both active and latent forms; the acute form can cause pain at rest or in motion. Both forms can lead to shortening, weakness and stiffness of the affected muscle. This may initiate referred tenderness and autonomic phenomena in the pain reference zone. MTrPs are activated either directly or indirectly. Direct activation occurs via microtrauma such as acute overload, overwork fatigue, chilling, or gross trauma of the affected muscle. Indirect activation of MTrPs may occur as a result of nearby MTrPs, visceral disease, arthritic joints, or emotional distress (Frank 2007).

DN is not an injection, rather it is the specific placement of monofilament needles to resolve MTrPs. The advantage of trigger point DN is that the confirmed production of one or more LTRs can cause an immediate reduction in local sensitivity or pain (Wall 2014).

(Continued)

Case Study 5   (Continued)

A DN technique used to resolve MTrPs in canines is as follows:

1) Insert sterile, 30g, 1-inch stainless steel, monofilament needles into the center of a tight band of tissue, approximately 1–2 cm deep.
2) Hand spin each needle clockwise or counter-clockwise until an LTR is elicited.
3) Leave each needle in place for an additional three to five minutes.
4) Repeat treatment as needed to help resolve MTrPs.

This case study depicts the use of trigger point DN as a part of a multimodal pain management approach for a canine patient with IVDD and hip OA. Both IVDD and hip OA, which are common comorbidities in adult canines, result in patients with increased MTrPs, muscular tension, decreased ROM, and lowered motivation to be active (Coates 2000; Dycus et al. 2017). The CSU Pain Scale is used for objective evaluation of the patient's progress.

Case Presentation: A seven-year-old intact male Cocker Spaniel presented to the rehabilitation service for further evaluation as a transfer from the emergency (ER) service. Two years prior he was diagnosed with a myelopathy between the third thoracic and third lumbar vertebrae and a right-sided hemilaminectomy between the 13th thoracic and first lumbar vertebrae was performed. The patient recovered ambulatory ability after formal rehabilitation therapy, no chronic medications were used. There were no known comorbidities.

On presentation to the ER service, the patient had acute-onset moderate kyphosis, mildly delayed left and right pelvic limb placing and hopping proprioceptive deficits, a cutaneous trunci reflex that terminated at L4, and spinal hyperesthesia in the cranial lumbar spine. Baseline blood work (complete blood count, chemistries, and electrolytes) and urinalysis were all within normal limits. With a CSU pain score of 3/4, he was started on a constant rate infusion of fentanyl, lidocaine, and ketamine; and given a 0.2 mg/kg dose of meloxicam subcutaneously.

On presentation to the rehab service, the patient had a body condition score (BCS) of 6/9, a CSU pain score of 1/4, and was moderately kyphotic. Mild placing and hopping proprioceptive deficits were noted in the pelvic limbs only. Bilateral hindlimb atrophy and decreased muscle tone was observed. Orthopedic abnormalities included symmetrically reduced coxofemoral extension bilaterally (130°, normal 155–160°), with crepitus. Moderate diffuse MTrPs were appreciated bilaterally in the quadriceps, sartorius, latissimus dorsi, longissimus dorsi, teres minor, and middle gluteal muscles. A review of the survey radiographs showed no vertebral abnormalities, but bilateral moderate coxofemoral osteoarthritic changes were present.

At the initial rehab evaluation, the working diagnosis was an acute IVDD episode, with chronic coxofemoral OA, and secondary diffuse MTrPs. The patient was discharged with a plan for medical management, home exercise, and formal rehabilitation.

As a part of formal rehabilitation, a multimodal approach was adopted including massage therapy, trigger point DN, and photobiomodulation.

MTrP therapy was incorporated using sterile, 30g, 1-inch, stainless steel monofilament needles. Each needle was inserted into the center of the tight band of tissue, and then the needle was hand spun clockwise or counter-clockwise until an LTR was elicited. The needle was then left in place for another three to five minutes.

The formal rehabilitation sessions occurred twice a week for six weeks. DN was repeated at each session and by the end of the fourth week no MTrPs were appreciated, and the patient's CSU pain score was 0/4. The patient continued in formal rehabilitation for additional strengthening, and by the fifth week had a normal posture (no kyphosis). In the sixth week, the patient was reevaluated and still had a BCS of 6/9, but he continued to have a pain score of 0/4. Muscle circumference remained unchanged. The patient was subsequently transferred to a maintenance rehabilitation program for further work on conditioning and weight loss. Table 12.12 outlines the history, patient evaluation, and treatment plan at each visit.

Discussion: The theory of treatment in this case was to resolve muscular tension that was limiting the patient's ROM. The addition of DN as a part of a multimodal approach was feasible, caused no harm, and played a role in the overall reduced pain score. The patient presented with multiple MTrPs that were resolved after eight sessions of DN over four weeks.

Although few studies highlight the best treatment methods for managing canine patients with chronic hip osteoarthritis (OA) or IVDD, a multimodal approach is often described with goals of improving function, reducing pain, improving ROM, and building muscle mass (Frank 1999; Dycus et al. 2017). DN was used as a part of this program; while the benefits are not completely understood, there were no reported complications from treatment. Prior literature supports the safety of DN, with the risk of major adverse reactions with DN by physiotherapists to be less than 0.04% (Kalichman and Vulfsons 2010; Cashman et al. 2014).

At presentation the patient displayed crepitant coxofemoral joints with reduced extension. In 2019, an assessment of kinetic and kinematic function in dogs with hip OA compared to healthy dogs showed a major difference in hip extension and acceleration (Souza et al. 2019). Over the six-week course of biweekly formal rehabilitation sessions, this patient showed a 20° improvement of hip extension. Another study using gait analysis would be needed to determine if improvement in acceleration was achieved.

While this rehabilitation timeline will not fit every patient, it is notable that while DN may release MTrPs in one session, if ROM and posture are still abnormal, new formation or reformation of MTrPs may occur and need to be released in another DN session (Hsieh et al. 2007). Evaluation of MTrPs at each session is recommended for optimal results. As described in the Lenton Method™, multiple MTrPs can cause muscle restriction fatigue, which results in abnormal posture or gait (Lenton 2018). After this patient's MTrPs were resolved in week 4, there was improved muscle function leading to a greater willingness to be active. The combination of controlled low-impact activity allowed the patient to regain his normal posture at week 5. The physical exam at each rehabilitation session addressed the current MTrPs, the DN therapy resolved the MTrPs, and the ongoing formal rehabilitation including massage therapy and photobiomodulation supported the patient in a holistic manner.

The research behind the effect of MTrPs on canine performance is limited; however, in other species such as horses, rats, rabbits, and humans more specific documentation exists. An equine cross-sectional study in 2017 demonstrated that aversive behavior to the girth and altered performance were associated with the presence of MTrPs. The MTrPs interfered with muscle lengthening, strength, and pain. MTrPs inhibited muscle performance and motor control (Bowen et al. 2017).

The patient's rehabilitation plan was adjusted weekly. Pain medication was decreased and then ultimately stopped by week 5. The patient's CSU pain score was 0/4 and remained as such after the MTrPs were resolved. At this point, the patient's rehabilitation plan was adjusted to focus on building muscle mass.

(Continued)

Case Study 5   (Continued)

Table 12.12   The history, patient evaluation, and therapeutic plan at each visit.

Initial rehabilitation therapy assessment		
History	One day post ER transfer for acute-onset postural changes, worsening bilateral hindlimb proprioception, and lumbar hyperesthesia. CSU pain score 3/4. Radiographs revealed bilateral moderate coxofemoral OA changes	
Patient evaluation	Gait and stance	Ambulatory with mild proprioceptive pelvic limb ataxia, moderate kyphosis
	MSK	Moderate diffuse MTrPs bilateral quadriceps, sartorius, latissimus dorsi, longissimus dorsi, teres minor, and middle gluteal muscles
	Pain score	CSU pain score 1/4
	Physical exam	Mild delay in bilateral pelvic limb placing and hopping proprioceptive testing, cutaneous trunci reflex that terminated at L4. Spinal hyperesthesia was present in the cranial lumbar spine
	Objective measurements	Muscle mass: LF 18 cm, RF 18 cm, LH 26 cm, RH 26 cm *Relevant goniometry*: Left hip: flexion 45°, extension 130° Right hip: flexion 45°, extension 130° (Normal: flexion 48–52°, extension 160–164°)
Plan	Medical management	Meloxicam 0.1 mg/kg PO for 3 weeks Gabapentin 100 mg PO BID for 30 days
	Home exercises	Adjusted walks to short interval high frequency. Basic initial home exercises including passive ROM, weight shifting, paw stimulation, and assisted sit to stands
	Formal rehabilitation	Outpatient 1 hour twice weekly sessions for 12 weeks
	At-home care	Activity restricted
First and second week of twice weekly rehabilitation therapy (1 hour)		
Patient evaluation	Gait and posture	Ambulatory with mild proprioceptive pelvic limb ataxia, moderate kyphosis
	MSK	Moderate diffuse MTrPs cervicothoracic, longissimus dorsi, quadriceps, sartorius, and iliopsoas muscles
	Pain score	CSU pain score 1/4
	Physical exam	Reduced extension of the coxofemoral joints bilaterally
Manual therapy and AROM	Manual therapy	Effleurage and petrissage massage techniques, followed by passive stretching of affected areas
	Dry needling	Monofilament needles inserted into MTrPs and hand spun until an LTR is noted. Treatment time: 3–5 minutes
	Photobiomodulation	Photobiomodulation Class IV: 8–10 J/cm² to the thoracolumbar spine and each hip joint twice a week

Third and fourth week of 2 × weekly rehabilitation therapy (1 hour)		
Patient evaluation, manual therapy and AROM	Gait and posture	Mild kyphosis
	Physical exam	Reduced extension bilateral coxofemoral joints
	Pain score	CSU pain score 1/4
	Medical management	No medications starting week 4
	MSK	Moderate cervicothoracic, longissimus dorsi, quadriceps, sartorius and iliopsoas muscle tension
	Manual	Effleurage and petrissage massage techniques, passive stretching
	Dry needling	Monofilament needles inserted into MTrPs and hand spun until an LTR is noted. Treatment time: 3–5 minutes
	Photobiomodulation	Photobiomodulation Class IV: 8–10 J/cm^2 to the thoracolumbar spine and each hip joint twice a week
Fifth and sixth week of 2 × weekly rehabilitation therapy (1 hour)		
Patient evaluation	Gait and posture	Normal spinal posture
	MSK	Resolution of all previously noted trigger points
	Pain score	CSU pain score 0/4
	Physical exam	Normal proprioception × 4, reduced extension bilateral coxofemoral joints
	Dry needling	Not performed since not indicated/improved
	AROM	UWTM acclimation water at level of the greater trochanter. Speed 0.7–1.0 mph. Time 10 minutes
	Photobiomodulation	Photobiomodulation Class IV: 8–10 J/cm^2 to the thoracolumbar spine and each hip joint once a week
Final recheck		
History	Doing great at home, the owner has noted improved comfort and mobility. No concerns Current medications: none	
Patient evaluation	Gait and posture	Ambulatory, normal posture
	Physical exam	Normal proprioception × 4
	Pain scale	CSU pain score 0/4
	Objective measurements	Muscle mass: LF 18 cm, RF 18 cm, LH 26 cm, RH 26 cm Target for hindlimbs: 27–28 cm *Relevant goniometry*: Left hip: flexion 45°, extension 150° (firm) Right hip: flexion 45°, extension 150° (firm)
Plan	Formal rehabilitation	Patient graduated from previous formal rehabilitation Maintenance rehabilitation for continued weight loss and muscle strengthening

OA, osteoarthritis; MTrP, myofascial trigger point; CSU, Colorado State University; LF, left forelimb; RF, right forelimb; LH, left hindlimb; RH, right hindlimb; PO, per os (orally); BID, twice daily; ROM, range of motion; AROM, active range of motion; UWTM, underwater treadmill; J/cm^2, joules per centimeter squared. Source: Krysta E. Bailey.

(Continued)

Case Study 5   (Continued)

Limitations included limited data, and short-term follow-up. Access and incorporation of force plate analysis would expand the objective measurements for patient outcome. Further research is needed as to how much of a role the DN had in the patient's recovery.

New methods of treatment are being formulated daily to treat pain more effectively in veterinary medicine. Less invasive methods that target disease-related issues will be paramount in providing better outcomes for patients with chronic disease. Further investigation is needed to explore the role of MTrP therapy and DN components of a multimodal rehabilitation approach.

Conclusion: This case study depicts the use of trigger point DN as a part of a multimodal approach to managing a canine patient with IVDD and hip OA. This case study is not intended to be prescriptive or imply that it is the only option for managing these cases. Practitioners interested in DN are encouraged to check if they are within jurisdiction to perform DN techniques and then view continuing education resources on how to become certified in these techniques.

Case Study 6   Focus on Veterinary Spinal Manipulation

Title: Management of postoperative forelimb lameness in a dog with bilateral elbow dysplasia

Author: Lisa P. McFaddin, DVM, GDCVHM, CVSMT, CVMRT, FCoAC, CVA

Summary: This case illustrates the successful use of veterinary spinal manipulation therapy (VSMT) in the postoperative management of a young dog with elbow dysplasia. The patient's gait, pain level, attitude, and energy level improved within the first six sessions despite the cessation of a nonsteroidal anti-inflammatory drug (NSAID).

Introduction: Elbow dysplasia (ED) is an umbrella term for multiple developmental pathologies within the joint, including ununited anconeal process (UAP), fragmented medial coronoid process (FCP), osteochondrosis (OC) or osteochondrosis dissecans (OCD), and elbow joint incongruity (Hazelwinkle 2015). ED is believed to result from the asynchronous growth of the radius and ulna secondary to genetic, heritable, and nutritional factors (Canapp and Kirby 2013). The complete pathogenesis of ED is not fully understood.

ED appears to affect purebred and large or giant breed dogs more often than mixed breed and smaller dogs. ED has a 17% prevalence rate in United States Labrador Retrievers, both American and English varieties (O'Neill et al. 2020). Epidemiological studies of ED are primarily limited to patients treated at tertiary facilities or those undergoing disease screening programs (O'Neill et al. 2020). This population bias may skew our understanding of the overall impact of ED on the general dog population.

Most dogs with ED present with thoracic limb lameness prior to two years of age (Beale 2016). The most common physical examination findings include persistent or intermittent forelimb lameness, elbow joint effusion, reduced elbow joint range of motion, and joint pain (Beale 2016). Radiographs may aid in the diagnosis, but definitive diagnosis often requires computed tomography (CT) and/or arthroscopy.

Ultimately treatment recommendations are dependent on the pathologies affecting each dysplastic elbow. In general surgical correction coupled with rehabilitation and lifelong prevention and management of elbow osteoarthritis are recommended (Canapp and Kirby 2013; Beale 2016).

Though not always considered or recommended, VSMT is an invaluable management tool for canine patients with ED, especially when incorporated postoperatively. Changes in a dog's gait due to pain or lameness affect the entire musculoskeletal system causing compensatory changes within the spine and other limbs (Bliss 2013). This case study shows how the addition of VSMT to the postoperative treatment regimen for ED is safe, effective, and can reduce the need for Western pharmaceuticals.

Case Presentation: Otter, a nine-month-old male intact Labrador Retriever, presented on 6 April 2019 for an initial integrative appointment as a referral from a local rehabilitation service. Otter started limping on the left front limb November 2018. He was referred to a local surgical and sports medicine center by his primary veterinarian. In December 2018 bilateral elbow arthroscopy revealed a left OC lesion, left fragmented medial coronoid process, mild to moderate left elbow incongruity, and mild incongruity of the right elbow. The left OC lesion and medial coronoid process were removed arthroscopically via a subtotal coronoidectomy, and an abrasion arthroplasty was performed. The patient was started on Adequan®, Dasuquin Advanced®, Welactin®, Denamarin®, probiotics, carprofen, gabapentin, and trazodone as needed. Rehabilitation, at home and in clinic, was started two weeks following surgery. Dry needle acupuncture was started one month after surgery.

After three months of rehabilitation there was some improvement in elbow mobility with mild left forelimb muscle atrophy. Persistent left forelimb lameness and a generalized lack of endurance were noted by the rehabilitation practitioners and the owner. Otter was extremely limited in his ability to stand for more than 90 seconds without sitting. Walks were limited to seven minute intervals with a two minute rest period. While off-leash Otter preferred to lay down, with short intermittent bursts of attempting to play with the other dogs in the house. Chiropractic therapy was recommended to improve posture, gait, and endurance.

The only abnormalities noted on his initial examination involved the musculoskeletal system. VSMT and dry needle acupuncture were performed at the initial and subsequent integrative appointments. Due to the owner's long commute, recheck examinations and VSMT treatments were recommended monthly. Between treatments Otter received weekly rehabilitation sessions and every other week dry needle acupuncture from veterinarians closer to the owner. Table 12.13 describes the owner's observations, physical examination findings and VSMT treatments performed during the first six appointments. Figure 12.10 demonstrates some of the VSMT techniques performed. Acupuncture information was not included as the focus of the case study is on spinal manipulation, and acupuncture was not a new treatment variable.

After the third session Otter graduated from physical therapy. After six treatments the owner reported Otter's adjustments provided relief for four to eight weeks. The length of pain-free time was dependent on Otter's activity level. Otter lives in a multi-dog household, and he has a propensity for mischief when playing. The owner was instructed to return every four to eight weeks for VSMT depending on his energy level, stamina, and signs of lameness.

Discussion: Pathologic changes in the anatomy, physiology, and biomechanics of the spine negatively affect the nervous system. VSMT is used to correct these irregularities, restoring neurologic and musculoskeletal function. The mechanisms of action can be broken down into neurophysiologic and biomechanical effects. Figure 12.11 summarizes

(Continued)

Case Study 6 (Continued)

Table 12.13 Owner's observations, musculoskeletal abnormalities (MSA), and VSMT adjustments for each visit. The Colorado State University Veterinary Medical Center Acute Pain Scale was used for pain assessment.

	6 April 2019 = initial visit	27 April 2019 = first recheck
History	Poor stamina and endurance, limited ability to stand, left forelimb lameness	Tired for 24 hours after adjustment. Improved energy level and stamina for 2 weeks
Pain score	2/4 = moderate pain	2/4 = moderate pain
Lameness	Grade 2/5 left forelimb	Grade 1/5 left forelimb
Gait and stance	Wide-based pelvic limbs	Slightly wide-based pelvic limbs
Thoracic limbs	Reduced shoulder joint extension bilaterally Reduced left elbow joint flexion Reduced internal rotation right shoulder joint	Reduced shoulder joint extension bilaterally Reduced left elbow joint flexion Reduced internal rotation right shoulder joint
Pelvic limbs	Reduced hip joint extension bilaterally	Reduced extension right hip joint
Occiput	LS	RS
Cervical vertebrae	3 BR, 5 BR, 7 BR	3 BR, 5 BR, 7 BR
Thoracic vertebrae	6 P, 9 P, 10th rib PS, 12 PR	6 P, 9 P, 12 PR
Lumbar vertebrae	2 PR, 4 PR, Sacral Apex PR	2 PR, 4 PR, Sacral Apex R
Pelvis	R&L PI Ilium, R&L Logan Basic	R&L PI Ilium, R&L Logan Basic
Thoracic limbs	L externally rotated humerus, R MP scapula	L externally rotated humerus, R MP scapula, lateral radius left and right, caudal ulnas bilaterally
Mobilization	Digits, ACB, MC, hip joints	Digits, ACB, MC, hip joints
Traction	Cervical, carpal, elbow	Cervical, carpal, elbow, tail
	17 May 2019 = second recheck	**5 July 2019 = third recheck**
History	No lethargy following treatment. Improved stamina and energy level persisted for 2 weeks. Stopped carprofen	Still limps daily. Improved energy level and stamina lasting 4 weeks
Pain score	1/4 = mild pain	1/4 = mild pain
Lameness	Grade 1/5 left forelimb	Grade 1/5 left forelimb
Gait and stance	Slightly wide-based pelvic limbs	Slightly wide-based pelvic limbs
Thoracic limbs	Reduced shoulder joint extension bilaterally Reduced internal rotation right shoulder joint	Reduced shoulder joint extension bilaterally Reduced internal rotation right shoulder joint
Pelvic limbs	Reduced extension right hip joint	Stands with stifles turned outward and hocks turned inward causing slight tarsal valgus bilaterally
Occiput	Atlas RS, 3 BR, 6 BR	LS

Cervical vertebrae	4P, 8A, 12 PR, Sternum L	Atlas RP, 7 BR
Thoracic vertebrae	2 PR, 4 PR, Sacral Apex R	6P, 9P, 12 PL, right first rib S, Sternum L
Lumbar vertebrae	R&L PI Ilium, R&L Logan basic	2 PL, 4 PR, Sacral Apex L
Pelvis	R MP scapula	R&L PI Ilium, R&L Logan basic
Thoracic limbs	Digits, ACB, MC, hips	R internally rotated humerus
Mobilization	Cervical, carpal, elbow, tail	Digits, ACB, MC, hips
Traction	1/4 = mild pain	Cervical, carpal, elbow, tail
	2 August 2019 = fourth recheck	**5 September 2019 = fifth recheck**
History	Was doing really well until he ran off and fought with a wild animal (unknown type). Has been off in the rear since then	Did really well after last treatment until owner went out of town. Suspects he injured himself while owner was away. Limping more on left forelimb now
Pain score	0/4 = no pain	0/4 = no pain
Lameness	Grade 0/5 left forelimb	Grade 1/5 left forelimb
Gait and stance	Slightly wide-based pelvic limbs	Slightly wide-based pelvic limbs Off-loading onto the right front and right rear Standing with pelvic limbs tucked underneath
Thoracic limbs	Reduced shoulder joint extension bilaterally (left worse than right)	Left elbow joint heat with mild effusion and reduced flexion Reduced left shoulder joint extension
Pelvic limbs	Stands with stifles turned outward and hocks turned inward causing slight tarsal valgus bilaterally	Slight tarsal valgus bilaterally
Occiput	RS	RS
Cervical vertebrae	R Atlas S, 3 BR, 7 BR	R Atlas P, 3 BL, 6 BR
Thoracic vertebrae	4 P, 6 P, 9 P, 12 PL, first ribs S bilaterally	4 P, 6 P, 9 A, 12 PL, first ribs S bilaterally
Lumbar vertebrae	2 PL, 4 PR, Sacral Apex R	2 PL, 4 PR, Sacral Apex L
Pelvis	R&L PI Ilium, R&L Logan basic	R&L PI Ilium, R&L Logan basic
Thoracic limbs	Lateral radii bilaterally, caudal ulnas bilaterally	L internally rotated humerus, lateral radii bilaterally, caudal ulnas bilaterally
Mobilization	Digits, ACB, MC, hips	Digits, ACB, MC, hips
Traction	Cervical, carpal, elbow, tail	Cervical, carpal, elbow, tail
	11 October 2019 = sixth recheck	
History	Patient is much more mobile and comfortable. If he runs around too much he will stop, drop, and roll to the right instead of turning to the right	
Pain score	Grade 0/5 left forelimb	
Lameness	Slightly wide-based pelvic limbs Lays down with left carpus flexed	
Gait and stance	Reduced extension shoulder joints bilaterally (left > right)	
Thoracic limbs	Reduced extension right hip joint Slight tarsal valgus bilaterally	

(Continued)

Case Study 6: Table 12.13   (Continued)

Pelvic limbs	3 BR, 7 BR
Occiput	4 P, 6 P, 9 P, 12 PL, first ribs S bilaterally
Cervical vertebrae	2 PL, 4 PR, Sacral Apex P
Thoracic vertebrae	L PI Ilium, R&L Logan Basic
Lumbar vertebrae	L internally rotated humerus, lateral radii bilaterally, caudal ulnas bilaterally
Pelvis	Digits, ACB, MC, hips
Thoracic limbs	Cervical, carpal, elbow, tail
Mobilization	Grade 0/5 left forelimb
Traction	Cervical, carpal, elbow, tail

A, anterior; ACB, accessory carpal bone; B, body; I, inferior; L, left; M, medial; MC, metacarpals; P, posterior; R, right; S, superior. Source: Lisa P. McFaddin.

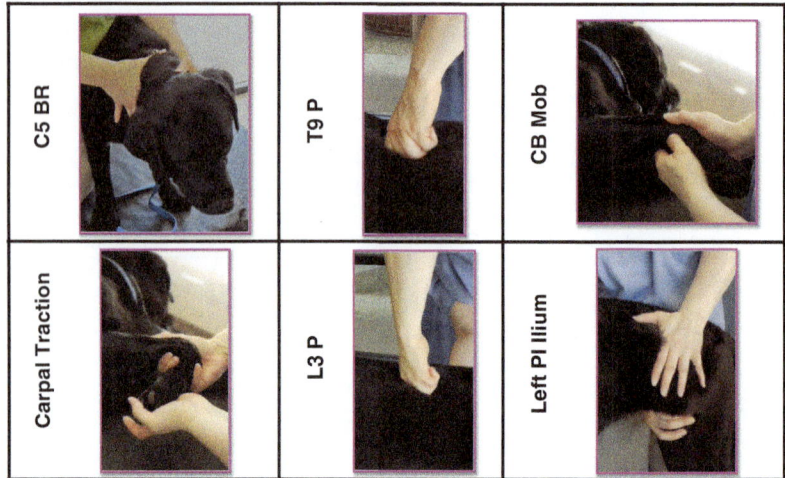

Figure 12.10 Photographs of spinal manipulation, mobilization, and traction techniques used on a canine. *C5 BR*: adjustment of a fifth cervical vertebrae body right. The lateral aspect of the practitioner's right index finger makes contact with the skin and soft tissues covering the lamina pedicle junction of the fifth cervical vertebrae. The left hand is used to stabilize and maintain joint tension on the left side of the neck. The angle of adjustment is lateral to medial, posterior to anterior, and inferior to superior (Rivera 2015). *T9 P*: adjustment of a ninth thoracic vertebrae posterior. The practitioner's thumb and bent index finger make contact with the skin and soft tissue covering the dorsal spinous process of the ninth thoracic vertebrae. The opposite hand is used to stabilize the underside of the thorax. The angle of adjustment is posterior to anterior and inferior to superior (Rivera 2015). *ACB Mob*: Mobilization of the accessory carpal bone (ACB). One hand is used to stabilize the superior portion of the carpus. The other hand is used to grasp the skin and soft tissue surrounding the ACB. Gentle steady pressure is used to mobilize the ACB 360° clockwise and counterclockwise (Rivera 2015). *Carpal traction*: two fingers are placed behind the carpal joint, while the other hand is used to gently flex the carpal joint around the stabilizing fingers. Traction is held for 15–30 seconds then slowly released (Rivera 2015). *L3 P*: adjustment of a third lumbar vertebrae posterior. The practitioner's thumb and bent index finger make contact with the skin and soft tissue covering the dorsal spinous process of the third lumbar vertebrae. The opposite hand is used to stabilize the underside of the abdomen. The angle of adjustment is posterior to anterior (Rivera 2015). *Left PI Ilium*: adjustment of a left dorsal caudal tubersacral (posterior inferior ilium). The practitioner's thenar prominence (heel of the hand) makes contact with the skin and soft tissue covering the wing of the left ilium. The other hand supports the thigh of the leg being adjusted. The adjustment angle is posterior to anterior, medial to lateral, and inferior to superior (Rivera 2015). Source: Lisa P. McFaddin.

the neurophysiologic and biochemical mechanisms involved in VSMT.

Spinal manipulation directly affects the structures comprising the intervertebral foramen, intervertebral disk (IVD), zygapophyseal joints, muscles and connective tissue around the spine, blood flow, and nervous input and output (Cramer and Darby 2005). High-velocity, low-amplitude (HVLA) therapy of these components causes movement within the joints, breakdown of adhesions, improved blood flow, and improved nervous system function (Cramer 2015; Rivera 2015). The end result is muscle relaxation, improved joint mobility, and pain reduction.

VSMT directly affects all structures within the portion of the spine (motion segment) being adjusted, including the zygapophyseal joints (Z-joint), intervertebral foramen, IVD, paraspinal muscles, connective tissue, vascular supply, and neural structures (Cramer 2015). Stimulation of these structures through spinal manipulation causes a host of biomechanical changes, including movement of the meniscus within the Z-joint, disruption of adhesions, stimulation of mechanoreceptors

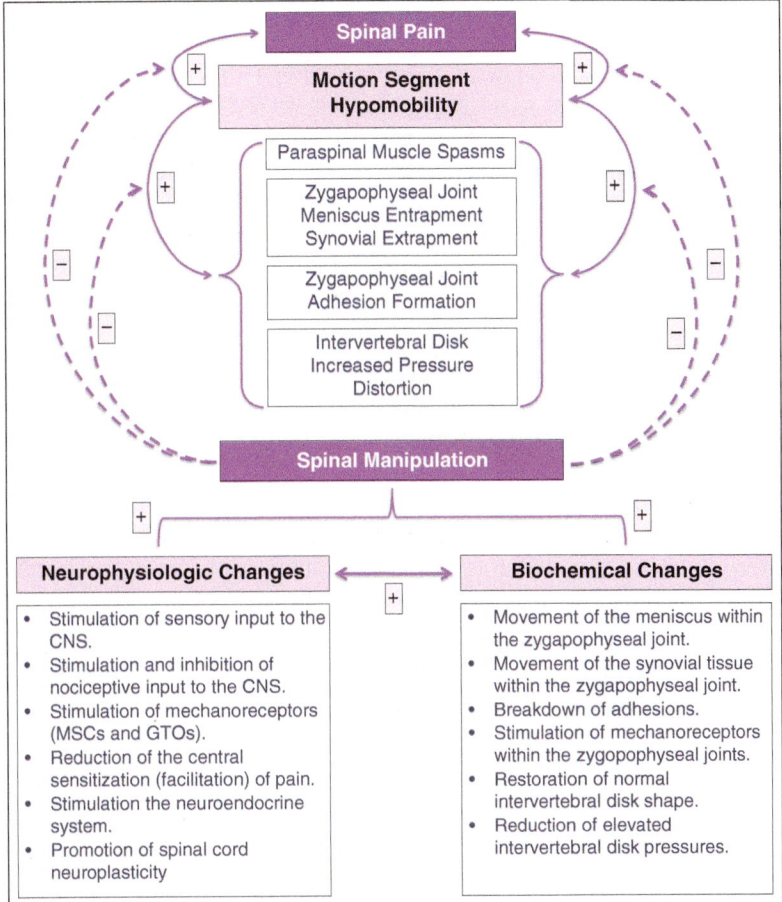

Figure 12.11 The primary causes of motion segment hypomobility, neurophysiologic and biochemical mechanisms involved in spinal manipulation, and the effects of both on pain (Mootz 2005; Pickar et al. 2007; Cramer 2015). (+) indicates promotion; (−) signifies inhibition. Source: Lisa P. McFaddin.

(Continued)

Case Study 6   (Continued)

within the Z-joints, and restoration of normal IVD shape and pressure (Panzer 2005; Cramer 2015).

Unlike most Western pharmaceuticals, VSMT side effects are uncommon. VSMT is not only very safe but generally well tolerated. Patients may experience mild soreness within the first 24 hours following the adjustment (Rivera 2015).

Conclusion: The incorporation of VSMT in this case not only improved the patient's pain level but also allowed reintroduction of his normal activity level, facilitating the successful cessation of the NSAID (carprofen). This case also illustrates the flexibility of VSMT therapy with respect to client lifestyle. Not all clients can confirm to a rigid recheck schedule. In an ideal setting Otter would have initially received treatments every two weeks with a gradual lengthening of the treatment frequency. Despite the scheduling conflicts Otter still benefited greatly from the treatments.

Conclusion

VIM offers effective alternatives and adjuncts treatments to traditional medical therapies. Growing client and veterinarian interest, combined with increasing scientific research, is encouraging the evolution of VIM. Inclusion of VIM within veterinary practices offers a profitable addition to the practitioners' arsenal improving patient care. This chapter provides real-life examples of how easily VIM modalities can be incorporated into day-to-day practice management.

Throughout the book the plethora of VIM training opportunities are listed. In fact, most VIM education is postdoctoral with little to no consensus on the information taught. There is a definite need for appropriate integration of the material within veterinary schools.

Memon et al. (2021) conducted a survey of 49 veterinary schools accredited by the Association of American Veterinary Medical Colleges; of the 88% who responded (43 schools), 30% (13 schools) offered formal courses in VIM. Approximately 77% (33 schools) briefly covered certain aspects of VIM within the curriculum. Roughly 74% (32 schools) offered clinical VIM services. The most common VIM topics were rehabilitation and acupuncture (Memon et al. 2016). (I would argue that while rehabilitation contains elements of VIM within it, the practice as a whole should not fall under the umbrella of VIM.)

In an article by Memon et al. (2016), the authors discuss the need for VIM courses within veterinary schools stating "IVM [Integrative veterinary medicine] by definition requires constant refinement and should be guided by available scientific evidence. Consumer demand has accelerated the incorporation of many CAVM [complementary and alternative veterinary medicine] modalities into conventional practice. Consequently, students should receive adequate exposure to the principles, theories, and current knowledge supporting or refuting such techniques."

The authors go on to say "Such a course should be evidence-based, unbiased, and unaffiliated with any particular CAVM advocacy or training group. Each institution should ensure compliance and consistency with their college's educational standards by performing periodic evaluation of integrative medicine courses" (Memon et al. 2016).

Introducing veterinary students to VIM will open their minds to alternative therapeutic options and improve client communication. Clients are actively seeking alternative treatments for their pets. An uninformed veterinarian can shut down dialogue and negatively affect the veterinarian–client–patient bond. It is impossible to learn everything there is to know about the various VIM modalities in veterinary school, but inclusion of the material within the curriculum can spur interested persons to pursue further education.

References

Alliott, B. (2017). Why green peas are healthy and nutritious. https://www.healthline.com/nutrition/green-peas-are-healthy (accessed 2 April 2020).

Anders, J., Lanzadame, R., and Arany, P. (2015). Low-level light/laser therapy versus photobiomodulation therapy. *Photomedicine and Laser Surgery* 33 (4): 183–184.

Arnarson, A. (2019a). Kidney beans 101: nutrition facts and health benefits. https://www.healthline.com/nutrition/foods/kidney-beans (accessed 2 April 2020).

Arnarson, A. (2019b). Lamb 101: nutrition facts and health effects. https://www.healthline.com/nutrition/foods/lamb (accessed 2 April 2020).

Beale, B. (2016). Current treatment of elbow dysplasia in the juvenile and adult dog. Wild West Veterinary Conference, 10–12 October 2016, Reno-Tahoe. https://www.vin.com/members/cms/project/defaultadv1.aspx?pid=20006&catId=&id=8282539&said=&meta=&authorid=&preview=

van Beeck, F.L., Watson, A., Bos, M. et al. (2015). The effect of long-term feeding of skin barrier-fortified diets on the owner-assessed incidence of atopic dermatitis symptoms in Labrador retrievers. *Journal of Nutritional Science* 4: e5.

Bliss, S. (2013). Musculoskeletal structure and physiology. In: *Canine Sports Medicine and Rehabilitation* (ed. M.C. Zink and J.B. Van Dyke), 32–59. Oxford: Wiley-Blackwell.

Bowen, A., Goff, L., and McGowan, C. (2017). Investigation of myofascial trigger points in equine pectoral muscles and girth-aversion behavior. *Journal of Equine Veterinary Science* 48: 154–160.e1.

Brazier, Y. (2019). What to know about apples. https://www.medicalnewstoday.com/articles/267290 (accessed 2 December 2020).

Burns, K. (2017). Assessing pet supplements. https://www.avma.org/javma-news/2017-01-15/assessing-pet-supplements (accessed 4 February 2021).

Canapp, S. and Kirby, K. (2013). Disorders of the canine forelimb: veterinary diagnosis and treatment. In: *Canine Sports Medicine and Rehabilitation* (ed. M.C. Zink and J.B. Van Dyke), 223–249. Oxford: Wiley-Blackwell.

Cash, B., Epstein, M., and Shah, S. (2016). A novel delivery system of peppermint oil is an effective therapy for irritable bowel syndrome symptoms. *Digestive Diseases and Sciences* 61: 560–571.

Cashman, G., Mortenson, W., and Gilbart, M. (2014). Myofascial treatment for patients with acetabular labral tears: a single-subject research design study. *Journal of Orthopaedic and Sports Physical Therapy* 44 (8): 604–614.

Chen, J.K. and Chen, T.T. (2012). *Chinese Medical Herbology and Pharmacology*. City of Industry, CA: Art of Medicine Press, Inc.

Chen, J.K., Chen, T.T., Beebe, S., and Salewski, M. (2012). *Chinese Herbal Formulas for Veterinarians*. City of Industry, CA: Art of Medicine Press, Inc.

Chen, L.-G., Jan, Y.-S., Tsai, P.-W. et al. (2016). Anti-inflammatory and antinociceptive constituents of *Atractylodes japonica* Koidzumi. *Journal of Agricultural Food Chemistry* 64 (11): 2254–2262.

Cheng, K., Martin, L.F., Slepian, M.J. et al. (2021). Mechanisms and pathways of pain photobiomodulation: a narrative review. *Journal of Pain* 22 (7): 763–777.

Chien, C.H. (2011). Canine intervertebral disk disease treated with aquapuncture and Chinese herbal and western medicine. In: *Traditional Chinese Veterinary Medicine for Neurological Disease* (ed. H. Xie and C. Chrisman), 311. Reddick, FL: Jing Tang Publishing.

Chiu, J.-H., Cheng, H.C., Tai, C.H. et al. (2001). Electroacupuncture-induced neural activation detected by use of manganese-enhanced functional magnetic resonance imaging in rabbits. *American Journal of Veterinary Research* 62 (2): 178–184.

Chrisman, C.L. (2011). Spinal cord disorders. In: *Traditional Chinese Veterinary Medicine for Neurological Diseases* (ed. H. Xie and C. Chrisman), 225–330. Reddick, FL: Jing Tang Publishing.

Clemmons, R.M. (2007). Functional neuroanatomical physiology of acupuncture. In: *Xie's Veterinary Acupuncture* (ed. H. Xie and V. Preast), 341–347. Ames, IA: Blackwell Publishing.

Coates, J.R. (2000). Intervertebral disk disease. *Veterinary Clinics of North America: Small Animal Practice* 30 (1): 77–110.

Craig, J.M. (2016). Atopic dermatitis and the intestinal microbiota in humans and dogs. *Veterinary Medicine and Science* 2 (2): 95–105.

Cramer, G. (2015). *The Clinical Anatomy of Spinal Manipulative Therapy*. Sturtevant, WI: Healing Oasis Wellness Center.

Cramer, G. and Darby, S. (2005). Anatomy related to spinal subluxation. In: *Foundations of Chiropractic Subluxation*, 2e (ed. M.I. Gatterman), 30–46. St. Louis, MO: Elsevier Mosby.

Dommerholt, J. (2011). Dry needling: peripheral and central considerations. *Journal of Manual and Manipulative Therapy* 19 (4): 223–227.

Dycus, D., Levine, D., and Marcellin-Little, D. (2017). Physical rehabilitation for the management of canine hip dysplasia. *Veterinary Clinics of North America Small Animal Practice* 47 (4): 823–850.

Elliott, B. (2017). Why green peas are healthy and nutritious. https://www.healthline.com/nutrition/green-peas-are-healthy (accessed 2 April 2020).

Enviromedica (2018). Beef liver: nature's perfect food. https://www.enviromedica.com/learn/beef-liver-natures-perfect-food (accessed 2 April 2020).

Fan, Z.-Z., Zhao, W.-H., Guo, J. et al. (2012). Antidepressant activities of flavonoids from Glycyrrhiza uralensis and its neurogenesis protective effect in rats. *Yao Xue Xue Bao* 47 (12): 1612–1617.

FDA (Food and Drug Administration) (2017). Is it really FDA Approved? https://www.fda.gov/consumers/consumer-updates/it-really-fda-approved (accessed 4 February 2021).

FDA (Food and Drug Administration) (2018). Label Claims for Conventional Foods and Dietary Supplements. https://www.fda.gov/food/food-labeling-nutrition/label-claims-conventional-foods-and-dietary-supplements (accessed 3 February 2021).

FDA (Food and Drug Administration) (2021a). CFR - Code of Federal Regulations Title 21. https://www.accessdata.fda.gov/scripts/cdrh/cfdocs/cfcfr/CFRSearch.cfm?CFRPart=211&showFR=1 (accessed 16 December 2021).

FDA (Food and Drug Administration) (2021b). Laser Products and Instruments. https://www.fda.gov/radiation-emitting-products/home-business-and-entertainment-products/laser-products-and-instruments (accessed 22 January 2023).

Ferguson, B. (2007). Techniques of veterinary acupuncture and moxibustion. In: *Xie's Veterinary Acupuncture* (ed. H. Xie and V. Preast), 329–339. Ames, IA: Blackwell Publishing.

Finando, D.S.F. (2005). *Trigger Point Therapy for Myofascial Pain*. Rochester, VT: Healing Arts Press.

Frank, E. (1999). Myofascial trigger point diagnostic criteria in the dog. *Journal of Musculoskeletal Pain* 7 (1–2): 231–237.

Frank, E. (2007). Clinical applications of myofascial trigger point therapy. *World Small Animal Veterinary Association World Congress Proceedings*. https://www.vin.com/apputil/content/defaultadv1.aspx?id=3860821&pid=11242

Frank, D. (2016). Obsessive-compulsive disorders: do they really exist? 62nd Convention of the Canadian Veterinary Medical Association. https://www.vin.com/members/cms/project/defaultadv1.aspx?pi

d=11313&catId=&id=4737167&said=&meta
=&authorid=&preview=

Frey, M. (2020). Chicken breast nutrition facts
and health benefits. https://www.verywellfit.
com/how-many-calories-in-chicken-
breast-3495665 (accessed 2 April 2020).

FSBPT (Federation of State Boards of Physical
Therapy) (2017). Resource Paper Regarding
Dry Needling, 7th edn. Alexandria, VA:
FSBPT. https://www.fsbpt.org/Portals/0/
documents/news-events/Vol_20_No_01.pdf

Gedon, N.K.Y. and Mueller, R.S. (2018). Atopic
dermatitis in cats and dogs: a difficult disease
for animals and owners. *Clinical and
Translational Allergy* 8: 41.

George, H.M., Kirk, R.W., Miller, W.H., and
Griffin, C.E. (2001). *Muller & Kirk's Small
Animal Dermatology*, 1058. Philadelphia:
Saunders.

Gould, G. (1959). *The LASER: Light Amplification by Stimulated Emission of Radiation*.
Ann Arbor, MI: University of Michigan.

Grassie, L. (2002). Update on Animal Dietary
Supplements. https://www.nasc.cc/historical-
summary (accessed 4 February 2021).

Gülanber, E.G. (2008). The clinical effectiveness
and application of veterinary acupuncture.
*American Journal of Traditional Chinese
Veterinary Medicine* 3 (1): 9–22.

Hammi, C., Schroeder, J., and Yeung, B. (2022).
Trigger Point Injection. Treasure Island, FL:
StatPearls. https://www.ncbi.nlm.nih.gov/
books/NBK542196 (accessed 26 March
2023).

Hayashi, A., Matera, J.M., Soares da Silva,
T. et al. (2007). Electro-acupuncture and
Chinese herbs for treatment of cervical
intervertebral disk disease in a dog. *Journal of
Veterinary Science* 8 (1): 95–98.

Hazelwinkle, H. (2015). Introduction, clinical
investigation and force plate of patients with
elbow dysplasia. Veterinary Investigation
Network. https://www.vin.com/apputil/
content/defaultadv1.aspx?id=7259255&pi
d=14365&print=1

Hill, A. (2018). Top 14 health benefits of
broccoli. https://www.healthline.com/
nutrition/benefits-of-broccoli (accessed 2
April 2020).

Hong, C. and Simons, D. (1998).
Pathophysiologic and electrophysiologic
mechanisms of myofascial trigger points.
*Archives of Physical Medicine and
Rehabilitation* 79 (7): 863–872.

Horowitz, D. (2006). Canine anxieties and
phobias. *Western Veterinary Conference* (19–23
February) Las Vegas, NV. https://www.vin.
com/members/cms/project/defaultadv1.aspx?
pid=11208&catId=&id=3855008&said=&met
a=&authorid=&preview=

Hsiao, C.-Y., Hung, C.-Y., Tsai, T.-H., and Chak,
K.-F. (2012). A study of the wound healing
mechanism of a traditional Chinese medicine,
Angelica sinensis, using a proteomic approach.
*Evidence-Based Complementary and
Alternative Medicine* 2012: 467531.

Hsieh, Y.-L., Kao, M.-J., Kuan, T.-S. et al. (2007).
Dry needling to a key myofascial trigger point
may reduce the irritability of satellite MTrPs.
*American Journal of Physical Medicine and
Rehabilitation* 86 (5): 397–403.

Hu, S., Peng, R., Wang, C. et al. (2014).
Neuroprotective effects of dietary supplement
Kang-fu-ling against high-power microwave
through antioxidant action. *Food and
Function* 5 (9): 2243–2251.

Jacques, S.L. (2013). Optical properties of
biological tissues: a review. *Physics in Medicine
and Biology* 58 (11): R37–R61.

Janssens, L.A.A. (1991). Trigger points in 48 dogs
with myofascial pain syndromes. *Veterinary
Surgery* 20 (4): 274–278.

Jennings, K.-A. (2018). 10 impressive health
benefits of apples. https://www.healthline
.com/nutrition/10-health-benefits-of-apples
(accessed 2 December 2020).

Joaquim, J., Luna, S.P.L., Brondani, J.T. et al.
(2010). Comparison of decompressive surgery,
electroacupuncture, and decompressive
surgery followed by electroacupuncture for
the treatment of dogs with intervertebral disk
disease with long-standing severe neurologic
deficits. *Journal of the American Veterinary
Medical Association* 236 (11): 1225–1229.

Kalichman, L. and Vulfsons, S. (2010). Dry needling in the management of musculoskeletal pain. *Journal of the American Board of Family Medicine* 23 (5): 640–646.

Karavis, M. (1997). The neurophysiology of acupuncture: a viewpoint. *Acupuncture in Medicine* 15 (1): 33–42.

Karim, H., Tudorascu, D.L., Butters, M.A. et al. (2017). In the grip of worry: cerebral blood flow changes during worry induction and reappraisal in late-life generalized anxiety disorder. *Translational Psychiatry* 7: e1204.

Kaushik, B., Sharma, J., Yadav, K. et al. (2021). Phytochemical properties and pharmacological role of plants: secondary metabolites. *Biosciences Biotechnology Research Asia* 18 (1): 23–35.

Kawarai, S., Ishihara, J., Masuda, K. et al. (2010). Clinical efficacy of a novel elimination diet composed of a mixture of amino acids and potatoes in dogs with non-seasonal pruritic dermatitis. *Journal of Veterinary Medical Science* 72 (11): 1413–1421.

Kittel, C. and Kroemer, H. (1980). *The Scattering of Light*. New York: Academic Press.

Klein, R. (2007). Medical botany. In: *Veterinary Herbal Medicine* (ed. S.G. Wynn and B. Fougere), 139–158. St. Louis, MO: Mosby Elsevier.

Kupper, D. and Regeir, D. (2013). Generalized anxiety disorder. In: *Diagnostic and Statistical Manual of Mental Disorders*, 5e (ed. D.C. Washington), 222–226. American Psychiatric Association.

Lee, B., Yun, H.-Y., Shim, I. et al. (2012). Bupleurum falcatum prevents depression and anxiety-like behaviors in rats exposed to repeated restraint stress. *Clinical Microbiology and Biomedical Sciences* 22 (3): 422–430.

Lee, J., Choi, Y.Y., Kim, M.H. et al. (2016). Topical application of *Angelica sinensis* improves pruritus and skin inflammation in mice with atopic dermatitis-like symptoms. *Journal of Medicinal Food* 19 (1): 98–105.

Lenton, N. (2018). Clinical trials of the Canine Massage Guild's Lenton Method. https://www.k9-massage.co.uk/canine-massage/ clinical-trials-canine-massage-guilds-lenton-method (accessed 2020).

Li, Z.-Y., Guo, Z., Liu, Y.-M. et al. (2013). Neuroprotective effects of total saikosaponins of *Bupleurum yinchowense* on corticosterone-induced apoptosis in PC12 cells. *Journal of Ethnopharmacology* 148 (3): 794–803.

Liu, C.M., Chang, F.C., and Lin, C.T. (2015). Retrospective study of the clinical effects of acupuncture on cervical neurological diseases in dogs. *Journal of Veterinary Science* 17 (3): 337–345.

Luescher, A. (2000). Compulsive Behavior in Companion Animals. https://www.ivis.org/ library/recent-advances-companion-animal-behavior-problems/compulsive-behavior-companion-animals (accessed 2021).

Marsden, S. (2014a). Dang Gui Shao Yao San (Angelica and Peony Combination). In: *Essential Guide to Chinese Herbal Formulas: Bridging Sicence and Tradition in Integrative Veterinary Medicine*, 80–83. College of Integrative Veterinary Therapies.

Marsden, S. (2014b). Si Miao san (Four Marvels Combination). In: *Essential Guide to Chinese Herbal Formulas: Bridging Science and Tradition in Integrative Veterinary Medicine*, 128–134. College of Integrative Veterinary Therapies.

Marsden, S. (2014c). Si Wu Xiao Feng Yin. In: *Essential Guide to Chinese Herbal Formulas: Bridging Science and Tradition in Integrative Veterinary Medicine*, 135–137. College of Integrative Veterinary Therapies.

Marsden, S. (2014d). Xiao Yao san (Rambling Ease Powder, Easy Wanderer). In: *Eassential Guide to Chinese Herbal Formulas: Bridging Science and Tradition in Integrative Veterinary Medicine*, 155–157. College of Integrative Veterinary Therapies.

Marsden, S. (2015a). *Chinese Herbal Treatment of Gastrointestinal Disorders*, 249–265. College of Integrative Medicine.

Marsden, S. (2015b). *Chinese Herbal Treatment of some Small Animal Endocrine Disorders*, 125–138. College of Integrative Veterinary Medicine.

Marsden, S. (2015c). *Lecture Notes and Videos: Nutritional Strategies in Chinese Herbal Medicine - Building on the Success of Herbs with Diet Change*, 135–137. College of Integrative Therapies.

Memon, M., Shmalberg, J., Adair, H.S. et al. (2016). Integrative veterinary medical education and consensus guidelines for an integrative medicine curriculum within veterinary colleges. *Open Veterinary Journal* 6 (1): 44–56.

Memon, M.A., Shmalberg, J.W., and Xie, H. (2021). Survey of integrative veterinary medicine training in AVMA-accredited veterinary colleges. *Journal of Veterinary Medical Education* 48 (3): 289–294.

Mittleman, E. and Gaynor, J. (2000). A brief overview of the analgesic and immunologic effects of acupuncture in domestic animals. *Journal of the American Veterinary Medical Association* 217 (8): 1201–1205.

Mootz, R. (2005). Theoretic models of subluxation. In: *Foundations of Chiropractic: Subluxation*, 2e (ed. M.I. Gatterman), 227–244. St. Louis, MO: Elsevier Mosby.

Morresey, P. (2019). Editorial: How to write a clinical case report. *Equine Veterinary Education* https://doi.org/10.1111/eve.13026.

NCI (National Cancer Institute) (2023). NCI Dictionary of Cancer Terms. https://www.cancer.gov/publications/dictionaries/cancer-terms/def/multimodality-treatment (accessed 12 March 2023).

Niemeyer, K., Bell, I.R., and Koithan, M. (2013). Traditional knowledge of Western herbal medicine and complex systems science. *Journal of Herbal Medicine* 3 (3): 112–119.

O'Brien, S. (2019). All you need to know about turkey meat. https://www.healthline.com/nutrition/turkey (accessed 2 April 2020).

Ofir, R., Tamir, S., Khatib, S., and Vaya, J. (2003). Inhibition of serotonin re-uptake by licorice constituents. *Journal of Molecular Neuroscience* 20 (2): 135–140.

O'Neill, D., Brodbelt, D.C., Hodge, R. et al. (2020). Epidemiology and clinical management of elbow joint disease in dogs under primary veterinary in the UK. *Canine Medicine and Genetics* 7: 1.

Osborn, J. (2018). Prolotherapy in practice. https://ivcjournal.com/prolotherapy-practice (accessed 5 May 2023).

Panzer, D. (2005). Facet subluxation syndrome. In: *Foundations of Chiropractic Subluxation*, 2e (ed. M.I. Gatterman), 509–521. St. Louis, MO: Elsevier Mosby.

Paschotta, R. (2016). Modes of laser operation. https://www.rp-photonics.com/modes_of_laser_operation.html (accessed 10 December 2020).

Pasi, A.K. (2013). Herb–drug interaction: an overview. *International Journal of Pharmaceutical Sciences and Research* 4 (10): 3770–3774.

Pickar, J.G., Sung, P.S., Kang, Y.-M., and Ge, W. (2007). Response of lumbar paraspinal muscles spindles is greater to spinal manipulative loading compared with slower loading under length control. *Spine Journal* 7 (5): 583–595.

Pitchford, P. (2002). *Healing with Whole Foods*. Berkeley, CA: North Atlantic Books.

Plumb, D. (2015). Fluoxetine HCl. In: *Plumb's Veterinary Drug Handbook*, 8e. Oxford: Wiley-Blackwell.

Purves, D., Augustine, G., FitzPatrick, D. et al. (2012). The somatic sensory system: touch and proprioception. In: *Neuroscience*, 5e, 189–208. Sunderland, MA: Sinauer Associates.

Raman, R. (2018a). 9 impressive health benefits of pumpkin. https://www.healthline.com/nutrition/pumpkin (accessed 2 April 2020).

Raman, R. (2018b). Is white rice health or bad for you? https://www.healthline.com/nutrition/is-white-rice-bad-for-you (accessed 2 April 2020).

Rivera, P. (2015). *Introduction to Veterinary Spinal Manipulation: Lecture and Notes*. Sturtevant, WI: Healing Oasis Wellness Center.

Rossmeisl, J. (2016). Intersections of neuropathic pain and itch. Veterinary Information Network.

Rosychuk, R. (2011). Canine lick granuloma. *Proceedings of the 36th World Congress of the World Small Animal Veterinary Association.* https://www.ivis.org/library/wsava/wsava-annual-congress-korea-2011/canine-lick-granuloma

Rovnard, P., Frank, L., Xie, H., and Fowler, M. (2018). Acupuncture for small animal neurologic disorders. *Veterinary Clinics of North America Small Animal Practice* 48 (1): 201–219.

Rowles, A. (2017). Why liver is a nutrient-dense superfood. https://www.healthline.com/nutrition/why-liver-is-a-superfood (accessed 2 April 2020).

Siegman, A.E. (1986). *Lasers.* Melville, New York: University Science Books.

Silfvast, W. (1996). *Laser Fundamentals.* Cambridge: Cambridge University Press.

Silva, N.E., Luna, S.P.L., Joaquim, J.G.F. et al. (2017). Effect of acupuncture on pain and quality of life in canine neurological and musculoskeletal diseases. *Canadian Veterinary Journal* 58: 941–951.

Souza, A., Escobar, A.S.A., Germano, B. et al. (2019). Kinetic and kinematic analysis of dogs suffering from hip osteoarthritis and healthy dogs across different physical activities. *Veterinary and Comparative Orthopaedic Traumatology* 32 (2): 104–111.

Tantanatip, A., Patisumpitawong, W., and Lee, S. (2021). Comparison of the effects of physiologic saline interfascial and lidocaine trigger point injections in treatment of myofascial pain syndrome: a double-blind randomized controlled trial. *Archives of Rehabilitation Research and Clinical Translation* 3 (2): 100119.

Teixeira, L., Pinto, C.F.D., de Mello Kessler, A., and Trevizan, L. (2019). Effect of partial substitution of rice with sorghum and inclusion of hydrolyzable tannins on digestibility and postprandial glycemia in adult dogs. *PLoS One* 14 (5): e0208869.

Tourney, A. (2011). Gound turkey nutrition information. https://www.livestrong.com/article/343597-ground-turkey-nutrition-information (accessed 2 April 2020).

Vigra, V. (2003). Acral lick dermatitis, psychogenic alopecia, and hyperesthesia. *Western Veterinary Conference* (16–19 February), Las Vegas, NV. https://www.vin.com/members/cms/project/defaultadv1.aspx?pid=11155&catId=&id=3846700&said=&meta=&authorid=&preview=

Wall, R. (2010). Myofascial pain in dogs. https://www.dvm360.com/view/myofascial-pain-dogs-proceedings (accessed 22 September 2020).

Wall, R. (2014). Introduction to myofascial trigger points in dogs. *Top Companion Animal Medicine* 29 (2): 43–48.

Wall, R. (2019). Myofascial pain and dysfunction: trigger points (part 1 and 2). *Pacific Veterinary Conference* (21–23 June), Long Beach, CA. https://www.vin.com/members/cms/project/defaultadv1.aspx?pid=23140&catId=&id=9111958&said=&meta=&authorid=&preview=

Wang, Z., Shen, L., Li, X. et al. (2013). Pain-relieving effect of a compound isolated from white peony root oral liquid on acute radiation-induced esophagitis. *Molecular Medicine Reports* 7 (6): 1950–1954.

Ware, M. (2018). Is turkey good for you? https://www.medicalnewstoday.com/articles/285736 (accessed 2 April 2020).

Ware, M. (2019). What are the heatlh benefits of pumpkins? https://www.medicalnewstoday.com/articles/279610 (accessed 2 April 2020).

Wink, M. (2015). Modes of action of herbal medicines and plant secondary metabolites. *Medicine* 2 (3): 251–286.

Witzel-Rollins, A., Murphy, M., Becvarova, I. et al. (2019). Non-controlled, open-label clinical trial to assess the effectiveness of a dietetic food on pruritus and dermatologic scoring in atopic dogs. *BMC Veterinary Research* 15 (1): 220.

Wolfe, F., Simons, D.G., Fricton, J. et al. (1992). The fibromyalgia and myofascial pain syndromes: a preliminary study of tender points and trigger points in persons with fibromyalgia, myofascial pain syndrome and no disease. *Journal of Rheumatology* 19 (6): 944–951.

Wynn, S. (2010). Clinical aspects of energy metabolism. https://www.vin.com/members/cms/project/defaultadv1.aspx?pid=373&id=4561229&f5=1

Wynn, S. and Fougère, B. (2007). Herb manufacture, pharmacy, and dosing. In: *Veterinary Herbal Medicine* (ed. S.G. Wynn and B. Fougere), 221–236. St. Louis, MO: Mosby Elsevier.

Wynn, S. and Marsden, S. (2003). Therapies for digestive disorders. In: *Manual of Natural Veterinary Medicine*, 157–216. St. Louis, MO: Mosby, Inc.

Xie, H. (2015). *DrXie's Lecture Notes*, 1–176. Reddick, FL: Jing Tang Publishing.

Xie, H. and Ortiz-Umpierre, C. (2006). What acupuncture can and cannot treat. *Journal of the American Animal Hospital Association* 42: 244–248.

Xie, H. and Preast, V. (2007a). Diagnostic systems and pattern differentiation. In: *Traditional Chinese Veterinary Medicine: Fundamental Principles*, 249–303. Reddick, FL: Chi Institute.

Xie, H. and Preast, V. (2007b). Qi, Shen, Jing, blood, and body fluid. In: *Traditional Chinese Veterinary Medicine: Fundamental Principles*, 69–100. Reddick, FL: Chi Institute.

Xie, H. and Preast, V. (2007c). *Xie's Veterinary Acupuncture*. Ames, IA: Blackwell Publishing.

Xie, H. and Preast, V. (2007d). Zang-Fu Physiology. In: *Traditional Chinese Veterinary Medicine: Fundamental Principles*, 105–114. Reddick, FL, Chi Institute.

Yam, M.F., Loh, Y.C., Tan, C.S. et al. (2018). General pathways of pain sensation and the major neurotransmitters involved in pain regulation. *International Journal of Molecular Sciences* 19 (8): 1–23.

Yarnell, E. (2007). Plant chemistry in veterinary medicine: medicinal consituents and their mechanisms of action. In: *Veterinary Herbal Medicine* (ed. S.G. Wynn and B. Fougère), 159–182. St. Louis, MO: Mosby Elsevier.

Yi, L.-T., Xu, Q., Li, Y.-C. et al. (2009). Antidepressant-like synergism of extracts from magnolia bark and ginger rhizome alone and in combination in mice. *Progress in Neuro-Psychopharmacology and Biological Psychiatry* 33 (4): 616–624.

Yin, S.-H., Wang, C.-C., Cheng, T.-J. et al. (2012). Room-temperature super-extraction system (RTSES) optimizes the anxiolytic and antidepressant like behavioral effects of traditional Xiao Yao san in mice. *Chinese Medicine* 7 (1): 24.

Zhang, Y., Han, M., Liu, Z. et al. (2011). Chinese herbal formula Xiao Yao san for treatment of depression: a systematic review of randomized controlled trials. *Evidence-Based Complementary and Alternative Medicine* 2012: 931636.

Zhao, Z.-Q. (2008). Neural mechanism underlying acupuncture analgesia. *Progress in Neurobiology* 85 (4): 355–375.

Zhu, H. (2014). Acupoints initiate the healing process. *Medical Acupuncture* 26 (5): 264–270.

Zhu, X., Xia, O., Han, W. et al. (2014). Xiao Yao san improves depressive-like behavior in rats through modulation of β-Arrestin 2-mediated pathways in hippocampus. *Evidence-Based Complementary and Alternative Medicine* 2014: 902516.

Zuo, G., Gao, T.-C., Xue, B.-H. et al. (2019). Assessment of the efficacy of acupuncture and chiropractic on treating cervical spondylosis radiculopathy: a systematic review and met-analysis. *Medicine* 98 (48): e17974.

Appendixes

CHAPTER MENU

Appendix A: Terminology

Absorption coefficient: Measure of the degree of electromagnetic radiation absorbed as the light passes through a substance (Patil and Dhami 2008).

AAFCO (Association of American Feed Control Officials): Members are individuals from various governmental agencies throughout North America responsible for the regulation of animal feed. The United States Food and Drug Administration (FDA) is a member. The individual members have the ability to regulate animal feed requirements within their jurisdiction, but AAFCO as a whole is not a regulatory body.

Action potential (aka nerve spike or nerve impulse): Electrical signals generated by neurons which travel along their axons (Purves et al. 2012a).

Acupoint: Also known as an acupuncture point. Anatomically acupoints comprise free nerve endings, small vessels (arteries and veins), and lymphatics (this includes immune cells and channels carrying immune cells) (Clemmons 2007). Most are found along the 14 major meridians, and each channel has its own specific number of points. There are additional acupoints, classical points, found elsewhere on the body.

Acupressure: The application of fingers and hands to specific acupoints or regions of multiple acupoints.

Acupuncture: The insertion of a sterile needle, or other object, into the skin on a specific area of the body causing a beneficial response.

Adjustment: The application of any chiropractic technique on a specific motion segment or anatomic region resulting in the improvement, and ideally restoration, of neurologic and physiologic function to that area (Cooperstein and Gleberzon 2004; Gatterman 2005).

Adulterated food: "Food packaged or held under unsanitary conditions, food or ingredients that are filthy or decomposed, and food that contains any poisonous or deleterious substance, or other contaminant" (FDA 2021a).

Afferent: Signals or nerve cells (neurons) sending information toward the central nervous system (CNS).

Alcohols: An organic compound containing one or more hydroxyl (oxygen–hydrogen) groups bound to a carbon atom (Vitz et al. 2022).

Aldehyde: An organic compound containing a carbon double bonded to an oxygen atom (carbonyl group), single bonded with a hydrogen atom, and single bonded with another atom or groups of atoms (March and Brown 2020).

Allodynia: A form of neuropathic pain in which nonpainful stimuli cause pain.

Allogeneic transplant: Cells or tissue obtained from a donor are transplanted into a different patient.

Allopathic medicine (aka allopathy): The treatment of disease using pharmaceutical, surgical, or other modern therapies (Iftikhar 2019). The term is synonymous with traditional or mainstream medicine. This term originated as a central tenet within homeopathy, denoting all non-homeopathic treatments and carries with it negative connotations. Some practitioners discourage its use in professional literature.

Amino acids: Organic nitrogen-containing compounds. Of the hundreds of identified, 20 are used to make up almost every protein found in plants and animals.

Analgesia: The inability to feel pain. An analgesic is a substance or drug which reduces or relieves pain.

Anterior (aka ventral): Closer to the front of the body.

Antigens: A foreign substance or toxin causing an immune response (and often antibody production) in the body.

Antioxidants: Synthetic or natural substances which prevent or delay cell damage. Antioxidants are considered a type of free radical scavenger.

Apoptosis: Cell death.

Aquapuncture: The injection of sterile fluid into acupuncture points.

Arthritis (aka osteoarthritis): Degeneration of the cartilage (smooth covering) within a joint. Over time, physical changes occur to the underlying bone (CDC 2020).

Articular cartilage (aka hyaline cartilage): The translucent, blue-hued cartilage covering the joint end of bones, comprising synovial joints. The tissue serves to reduce concussive forces and friction within the joint (Pasquini et al. 2003). Cartilage thickness is dependent on the joint location and function.

Atmosphere: Layers of gas surrounding the Earth maintained in place by gravity.

Atom: Smallest unit of ordinary matter of a chemical element (Trefil et al. 2022). Atoms contain a nucleus (comprising one or more positive protons and several neutral neutrons) and one or more negatively charged electrons.

Autohemotherapy: Removal, infusion with ozone, and re-injection of patient's own blood in an aseptic technique.

Autonomic nervous system (ANS): Contains components of the CNS and peripheral nervous system (PNS) which function to control involuntary activity, maintain homeostasis, and react to stress (Darby 2014). The ANS is divided into the sympathetic and parasympathetic nervous systems.

Autologous transplant: Cells or tissue obtained from and transplanted into the same patient.

Ayurvedic medicine: One of the world's oldest medical systems developed in India. The practice utilizes herbs, diet, massage, exercise, detoxification, and meditation to prevent and treat disease (NCCIH 2019).

Bian Zheng: The utilization of one or more of the diagnostic systems to discern a traditional Chinese veterinary medicine (TCVM) diagnosis or pattern. The diagnostic systems include Five Element Theory, Yin–Yang Theory, Interior vs. Exterior Patterns, Cold vs. Hot Patterns, Deficiency vs. Excess Patterns, Five Treasures, and Zang-Fu Physiology (Xie and Preast 2007a).

Bioavailability: The amount or proportion of active drug or other constituent entering circulation after ingestion, injection, or absorption.

Biomechanics: The study of the structure, function, and mechanical motion of biological systems.

Biophysics: A field of study using physics to better understand biological systems from cells to entire organisms, including the human body (Biophysical Society 2023).

Bioregulatory medicine: The use of non-pharmaceutical agents to stimulate the body's natural healing abilities (Reinders and Haghighat 2019).

Body fluid: Fluid found within the body including tears, nasal discharge, sweat, urine, saliva, digestive juices, and joint fluid (Xie and Preast 2007d).

Botanical: An ingredient derived from a plant and used as an additive.

Bursa: A fluid-filled sac located between bone and other tissues (muscles, tendons, ligaments, and skin) which reduces friction during movement (Pasquini, et al. 2003).

Bursitis: Inflammation of the small fluid-filled cushions, called bursa, found between bone and other tissues, such as muscles, tendons, ligaments, and skin (MedlinePlus 2016).

Carbonyl group: An organic compound composed of a carbon atom double bonded to an oxygen atom (LibreTexts 2022b).

Carboxyl group: An organic compound composed of a carbon atom double bonded to an oxygen atom and single bonded to a hydroxyl group (OH) (Helmenstine 2020).

Carboxylic acid: An organic compound with acidic properties (aka organic acid) containing a carboxyl group attached to another atom or chain of molecules (Helmenstine 2020).

Caudal: Located farther from the head.

Cell-mediated immunity: Part of the adaptive immune response not reliant on the production of antibodies. Cell-mediated immunity takes longer to respond, occurs within tissues, and is primarily driven by T cells, divided into helper T cells (which function to activate other immune cells) and killer or cytotoxic T cells (which directly kill cells containing the pathogen).

Central nervous system: Brain and spinal cord.

Chiropractic (aka spinal manipulation): An integrative medical system rooted in the diagnosis and treatment of hypomobile joints, especially those within the spinal column, which cause local and systemic dysfunction of nerves, muscles, and organs. Improvement in joint mobility, generally through manual therapy, allows the body's innate forces to heal itself, achieving homeostasis (WFC 2001; Cooperstein and Gleberzon 2004; Rivera 2015).

Chromophore: An atom or group of atoms contributing to the color of a compound (Patil and Dhami 2008).

Also described as the portion of a molecule responsible for its color.

Coherence: Waves of radiation have a fixed phase and frequency (Heiskanen and Hamblin 2018).

Collagen: The most abundant protein in the body found within all types of connective tissue, including skin, cartilage, tendon, ligaments, and bone (Bliss 2013).

Concentric muscle contraction: A type of isotonic (normal) contraction in which muscle tension increases as the muscle shortens (Padulo et al. 2013).

Conductivity: How well a specific material conducts electricity (Heiskanen and Hamblin 2018).

Contralateral: Opposite side.

Corona discharge: An electrical discharge caused by the exposure of a fluid or gas (air) surrounding a conductor carrying a high voltage (ME 2022).

Covalent bond: A chemical bond involving the sharing of an electrons, forming electron pairs, between atoms (Ouellette and Rawn 2014).

Cranial: Located closer to the head.

Damp: Used to describe environments and disease conditions. One of the six evils or conditions in TCVM. Represents conditions with excessive moisture, infection, heaviness, and often pain (Xie and Preast 2007b).

Deficiency pattern: A condition in which the patient is lacking, often due to overwork, blood loss, or chronic illness. A patient can be deficient in one or more of the following: Qi, Blood, Yin, and Yang. Patients are often dry, thin, weak, lethargic, and have a pale tongue and weak pulse (Xie and Preast 2007a).

Dextrose (aka D-glucose): A natural sugar, or more specifically a D-isomer of glucose (Hauser et al. 2016).

Dietary ingredient: "A vitamin, mineral, herb or other botanical, amino acid, dietary substance for use by man to supplement the diet by increasing the total dietary intake or a concentrate, metabolite, constituent, extract, or combinations of the preceding substances" (FDA 2021b).

Dietary supplement (aka food supplement): Substances which complement the diet and contain at least one of the following ingredients: a vitamin, a mineral, an herb, an amino acid, or a product which affects caloric intake (FDA 2021c).

Diode: A semiconductor device with two terminals which allows electrons and energy to only flow in one direction (Heiskanen and Hamblin 2018).

Dipolar: An electrically neutral compound or molecule which carries both a positive and negative charge.

Dismutation (aka disproportionation): A reaction in which a chemical undergoes oxidation and reduction (redox reaction). Ozone dismutation refers to the breakdown of two ozone molecules (O_3) into three oxygen molecules (O_2).

Distal: Away from the body.

Dorsal: Closer to the back of the body.

Double bond: A covalent bond in which two electron pairs are shared between two atoms (Ouellette and Rawn 2014).

Drain: To remove from an area. Typically applied to Damp conditions.

Drug: A substance used to diagnose, cure, treat, or prevent disease in both humans and animals, as well as alter the body's functions or structure (FDA 2021b).

Eccentric muscle contraction: A type of isotonic (normal) contraction in which muscle elongates under tension (Padulo et al. 2013).

Efferent: Signals or nerve cells (neurons) sending information away from the CNS.

Eight Principle theory: A diagnostic system dividing the natural world into two categories (Yin or Yang) and three pairs (Interior vs. Exterior; Cold vs. Heat; and Deficiency vs. Excess) (Xie and Preast 2007a).

Elastin: A highly elastic protein found in connective tissue, tendons, ligaments, joint capsules, and cartilage (Frantz et al. 2010).

Electroacupuncture: An electric current is applied to pre-placed acupuncture needles using small leads. The frequency and intensity of the current is controlled by the electroacupuncture unit. Electric stimulation mimics and exceeds repeat manual manipulation of the acupuncture needle (Shmalberg et al. 2014).

Electromagnetic spectrum: All types of electromagnetic energy (NASA 2013).

Endogenous: Originating within an organism or body or something caused by internal factors.

Enthesis: The fibrocartilaginous junction where tendon attaches to bone (Tresoldi et al. 2013).

Ethnoveterinary medicine (aka veterinary anthropology): The study of a community's knowledge base and skills pertaining to animal health care for companion animals and livestock (Matekaire and Bwakura 2004; Lans et al. 2007).

Excess pattern: A condition in which the patient has too much of something. The condition is most often due to an exogenous (outside) pathogen (Wind, Cold, Dampness, Summer Heat, Dryness, and Fire) or secondary to another issue (overeating, blood stagnation, phlegm) (Xie and Preast 2007a,b). Patients often breathe rapidly and are excitable and have a fever, distended abdomen, red tongue with a coating, and surging pulse (Xie and Preast 2007a,b).

Exogenous: Originating outside an organism or body or something caused by outside (external) factors.

Exogenous pathogens: Also known as the 6 Exogenous Xie Qi or 6 Excessive Qi or 6 Evils. There are six weather changes which normally do not cause disease, but under the right circumstances (i.e. extreme weather changes and/or preexisting disease) can invade the body causing illness: Wind, Cold, Summer-Heat, Damp, Dryness, and Fire (Xie and Preast 2007b).

Exterior patterns: Issues, typically chronic in nature, associated with organ systems (Xie and Preast 2007a).

Extracellular matrix (ECM): A three-dimensional network of large non-cellular molecules, including collagen, elastin, and proteoglycans, outside of the cells found within all tissues and organs (Frantz et al. 2010). The ECM functions as a physical framework for cells and is intimately involved in numerous biochemical and biomechanical processes crucial for tissue health and growth (Frantz, et al. 2010).

Facilitation: Increased nerve cell (neuronal) stimulation causing hyperactive responses.

Fascia: A band of connective tissue composed primarily of collagen, covering and separating muscles, tendons, ligaments, joint capsules, blood vessels, nerves, and internal organs (Evans and Lahunta 2013). The terms "deep fascia" or "myofascia" are used when referring to the connective tissue surrounding individual muscle groups.

Fibrocartilage: A tough and strong avascular connective tissue found at the insertion sites of ligaments and tendons, as well as intervertebral disks (Benjamin and Evans 1990).

Five Element theory: Everything in the natural world can be broken down into five elements (Wood, Fire, Earth, Metal, and Water) which promote, restrain, and regulate each other maintaining order (Xie and Preast 2007c).

Five Energies: Food can be divided by thermal properties into cold, cool, neutral, warm, and hot (Xie 2015).

Five Tastes: Food can be divided by taste into sour, bitter, sweet, pungent, and salty (Xie 2015).

Five Treasures: The organization of life into five substances: Qi, Shen, Jing, Blood, and Body Fluid (Xie and Preast 2007d).

Fluence: Energy delivered per unit area, measured in joules per square centimeter (J/cm^2) (JEDEC 2023).

Food additive: Substances added to food with the direct or indirect result of becoming part of the food or altering the properties of the food itself (FDA 2021b).

Free radicals: Unstable molecules naturally created during cell metabolism or formed due to toxins, radiation, or pollutant. Free radicals accumulate within tissues and call cell damage.

Free radical scavengers: Substances which stabilize or neutralize free radicals to prevent harmful chain reactions and resultant cell damage.

Frequency: The rate at which something (in this case waves) passes during a specific period of time (JEDEC 2023). Frequency and wavelengths are inversely proportional. Waves with shorter wavelengths have a higher frequency, while waves with lower frequencies have longer wavelengths.

Fu organs: Yang organs located within the interior of the body. These organs are hollow or tube-like and function to transport or excrete. Examples include the large intestine, stomach, small intestine, triple heater, gallbladder, and urinary bladder (Xie and Preast 2007g).

Functional foods: Foods that have additional health benefits beyond basic nutritional requirements. This is a contentious term, as most foods have a function or purpose.

Glycolysis: The enzymatic breakdown of glucose releasing energy and pyruvic acid.

Heroic medicine (aka heroic depletion theory): A therapeutic system popular in the seventeenth to eighteenth centuries based on the belief that disease and illness developed as a result of humoral imbalance. Common treatments included bloodletting, purging (emesis induction), and diaphoresis (sweating) (Wynn and Fougère 2007a).

Hertz (Hz): A unit of frequency equal to one cycle per second (JEDEC 2023).

Hydrocarbon: An organic compound exclusively composed of hydrogen and carbon atoms.

Hyperalgesia: A form of neuropathic pain in which there is an abnormally increased sensitivity to pain.

Humoral immunity: Part of the adaptive immune response driven by B cells, involving the production of antigen-specific antibodies by effector B cells (plasma cells). Humoral immunity provides the immune system with a memory of the antigen through the production of memory B cells, allowing quick neutralization of the antigen if seen in the future.

Humoral theory (aka humoralism): A medical theory, popularized by Hippocrates, focusing on the balance of four primary substances, called humors, within the body: yellow bile, black bile, phlegm and blood. It was believed all diseases stemmed from an imbalance of one or more of the four humors. Humorism influenced medical theory and therapy from 400 BCE through the fifteenth century (Wynn and Fougère 2007a).

Hypoxia: Low levels of oxygen within tissues.

Inferior (aka caudal): Located farther from the head.

Ipsilateral: Same side.

In vitro (Latin for "within the glass"): Studies performed outside of a living being. Most commonly microorganisms, tissue cultures, and cells are studied in petri dishes and/or test tubes.

In vivo (Latin for "in glass"): Studies performed within living organisms, not tissue extracts or cells.

Insufflation: Blowing a substance (gas, liquid, or powder) into a body cavity.

Interior patterns: Issues, often acute in nature, affecting the inside of the body (Xie and Preast 2007a,b).

Interneurons: Nerve cells transmitting information from one neuron to another within the brain or spinal cord (Purves et al. 2012a).

Intervertebral disk: A fibrocartilaginous joint located between the vertebral bodies helping hold the vertebrae together, and also functioning as a shock absorber for the spine (Cramer and Darby 2005).

Intervertebral foramen: The hole (or foramen) between two vertebrae through which the spinal nerve exits (Evans and Lahunta 2013).

Ipsilateral: Same side.

Irradiance: The flux of radiant energy per unit area, or the power divided by the area (W/cm^2) (de Freitas and Hamblin 2016). Often referred to as power density, but this is technically incorrect (Chung et al. 2012).

Isometric muscle contraction: There is no change in muscle

length as tension (aka contraction) increases (Padulo et al. 2013).

Isotonic muscle contraction: There is change in muscle length as tension (aka contraction) increases (Padulo et al. 2013).

Jing: Also known as Essence. There are two forms of Jing: Prenatal and Postnatal Jing. You are born with Prenatal Jing, also known as Kidney Jing or Congenital Jing (Xie and Preast 2007d). Postnatal Jing (aka Zang-Fu Jing or Acquired Jing) is acquired through the ingestion of food and stored in each Zang-Fu organ (Xie and Preast 2007d).

Jing Luo: A system of interconnected channels covering the outer surface of the body. The channels function as a conduit through which Qi (energy) and Blood circulate throughout the entire body (Xie and Preast 2007e).

Joint (aka articulations): Area where two or more bones meet covered by a fibrous, elastic, cartilaginous, or combination of connective tissue types (Evans and Lahunta 2013).

Joint capsule: Tissue covering a joint that comprises two layers: an outer fibrous layer and an inner synovial membrane (Pasquini et al. 2003).

Joint cavity: The space within a synovial joint containing synovial fluid (Pasquini et al. 2003).

Jump sign: A behavioral response involving an involuntary movement or jerk of the head or limb, and often vocalization, after digital palpation of a trigger point (Al-Shenqiti and Oldham 2005). The reaction represents a disproportionate pain response when pressure is applied to a trigger point (Al-Shenqiti and Oldham 2005).

Joule (J): A measure of energy. More specifically, the Système International (SI) unit of work (energy) created by the force of 1 newton acting through a distance of 1 meter (Britannica 2020). With respect to light, each photon contains a certain amount of energy measured in joules. Joules and photons have a proportional relationship: the more photons, the higher the joules (or energy) (JEDEC 2023).

Ketone: An organic compound containing a carbon atom covalently bonded to an oxygen atom (carbonyl group), while also bonded to two other carbon-containing molecules (Brown 2022).

Laser: An acronym for *l*ight *a*mplification by *s*timulated *e*mission of *r*adiation. A narrow beam of single-frequency light emitted by a device which utilizes light, electrical energy, or electromagnetic energy as its source (NASA 2021).

Lateral: Farther away from the median plane or midline of the body or organ.

LED (light-emitting diode): A semiconductor diode which produces light when a current flows through it (Edwards 2005).

Ligament: Bands of fibrous connective tissue connecting bone to bone. Intracapsular ligaments are located within a joint, while extracapsular ligaments are found outside of the joint or function as part of the joint capsule (Pasquini et al. 2003).

Ligament laxity: A ligament which is too loose to properly stabilize the joint and prevent misalignment during movement.

Local twitch response: Mechanical stimulation of the trigger point, most commonly needling, results in a visible or palpable contraction of the muscle and skin. This is most often observed when needling the trigger point (Perreault et al. 2017).

Lymphocytes: A type of white blood cell involved in the immune system, formed in the bone marrow, and found in blood and lymph tissue. T cells, B cells, and natural killer cells are types of lymphocytes.

Lysis: Rupture of a cell.

Luxation: Dislocation of a joint.

Macrophage: A type of white blood cell involved in the immune system, found within almost all tissues, which directly engulfs (ingests) and destroys (digests) pathogens.

Manipulation: Movement of a joint through passive range of motion to the paraphysiologic space without exceeding the joint's anatomical barrier (Gatterman 2005).

Materia medica: Accumulated information pertaining to the therapeutic properties of a substance used for healing (Wynn and Fougère 2007b; Klein 2007). The materia medica is like an encyclopedia of herbal remedies comprising individual monographs.

Medial: Closer to the median plane or midline of the body or organ.

Medical botany: The study of naturally occurring materials possessing medicinal properties (Klein 2007).

Meridians: A set of 12 paired and two unpaired pathways or channels on the outer surface of the body through which blood and energy (Qi) flow to the main organ systems (Zang-Fu organs), joints, muscles, bone, and brain (Xie and Preast 2007e).

Meridian clock: Also known as the traditional Chinese medicine (TCM) circadian clock. Qi flows through the 12 Zang-Fu organ channels in a specific order: lung → large intestine → stomach → spleen → heart → small intestine → bladder → kidney → pericardium → triple burner → gallbladder → liver. There is a two-hour period during which the passage of Qi through each meridian and corresponding organ is greatest (Xie and Preast 2007e).

Microbiome: A group of microorganisms, their genes, and surrounding environmental conditions in a defined area (Marchesi and Ravel 2015).

Microbiota: A group of microorganisms in a defined environment (Marchesi and Ravel 2015). Most often used to describe the bacteria within the gastrointestinal tract.

Mineral: An inorganic substance required in various quantities by the body for normal growth, nutrition, and development.

Molecule: Smallest part of a substance that maintains the physical and chemical properties of the substance, consisting of two or more atoms (LibreTexts 2022a).

Mobilization: Movement of a joint through normal range of motion to passive range of motion (Gatterman 2005).

Monochromatic: Containing one color.

Monograph : A summary of compiled information outlining specific details about a particular herb or natural substance. The monograph generally includes the common name, scientific name, pseudonyms, distribution, similar species, scientific family, parts of the plant used, specific collection techniques, constituents or active medicinal compounds, clinical actions, history and traditional use, energetics, published research, indications, veterinary indications, contraindications, toxicology, adverse effects, drug interactions, preparation notes, dosage, combinations or multi-herb formulas, and references (Wynn and Fougère 2007b).

Motion unit (spinal) (aka motion segment): The smallest unit of motion within the spine consisting of two articular facets and a disk (Rivera 2015).

Motor neurons: Nerve cells transmitting information from the brain and spinal cord to muscles and some glands (Purves et al. 2012b).

Myalgia: Muscle pain.

Myofascia (aka deep fascia): The connective tissue sheath surrounding and passing between muscles. The myofascia is particularly thick in the limbs. For some muscles the myofascia takes the place of a tendon (aponeurosis) attaching to the outside of the bone (periosteum) at the origin or insertion of the muscle (Evans and Lahunta 2013).

Myofascial pain: Pain associated with one or multiple muscles and surrounding fascia.

Myofascial pain syndrome (MPS): A chronic condition in people affecting a specific area or areas of muscle and the surrounding fascia (Akamatsu et al. 2015; Shah et al. 2015). Associated clinical signs include the presence of one or more trigger point(s), regional pain, with or without referred pain, increased tension, and reduced flexibility (Akamatsu et al. 2015; Shah et al. 2015). MPS is classified as a separate disorder from fibromyalgia, tendonitis and bursitis.

Myopathology: Abnormal muscle function.

Neuron (aka nerve cell): A cell capable of electrical excitability which sends signals to other cells over long distances (Purves et al. 2012a).

Neuropathic pain: Pathologic pain caused by damage or injury to nerves responsible for transferring information from the body (PNS) to the spinal cord or brain (CNS).

Neuropathology: Abnormal nervous system function.

Neuroplasticity: Ability of the nervous system to reorganize and create new synaptic connections within the CNS (Jackman and Regehr 2017; Maltese et al. 2019). Typically used to describe the brain's ability to learn and heal following injury, but the concept can also be applied to the spinal cord (Maltese et al. 2019).

Neurotransmitters: A chemical released at the end of a neuron whose release is triggered by an action potential (Nolte 2009). Neurotransmitters serve to stimulate other cells (nerve, muscle) or structures.

Nociception: Detection and communication of noxious stimuli by the nervous system.

Nociceptors (aka free nerve endings): Sensory nerves stimulated by damaging or noxious stimuli which send information to the CNS where the information is interpreted as pain (Purves et al. 2012c).

Nociceptive pain: Physiologic pain caused by damage to the body and is typically well localized and temporary.

Noxious stimulus: A signal which is damaging or threatening to normal tissue.

Orthobiologics: The use of biological materials to treat musculoskeletal injuries.

Oxidation: The loss of electrons and increase in charge (becomes more positive) (Wiley 2002).

Oxidizing agent (aka oxidant or oxidizer): A substance that removes or accepts electrons from a reducing agent during a redox reaction (Wiley 2002).

Oxygen: An element with the atomic symbol O. Oxygen gas is colorless, odorless, tasteless, and noncombustible (but does promote the burning of combustible materials) (PubChem 2022a).

Ozone: An inorganic molecule composed of three oxygen atoms, O_3, which create a colorless to pale blue volatile gas with a distinct odor (PubChem 2022b).

Ozonide: A chemical compound formed by the reaction of ozone with another compound (Hassan et al. 2020).

Ozone generator (aka ozonator): A device designed to create ozone from either room air or pure oxygen gas using primarily an electrical discharge (corona) or ultraviolet (UV) light.

Ozonolysis (aka Criegee mechanism): The process by which ozone interacts with and breaks apart (cleaves) the double bonds in hydrocarbons (OCP 2022).

Pain: The sensation and emotional experience associated with tissue damage (perceived or actual).

Parasympathetic nervous system ("rest and digest"): Sends signals from the brain and spinal cord to the internal organs ensuring normal day-to-day function.

Pathoanatomy: Abnormal organ and tissue function.

Pathobiochemistry: Abnormal biochemical processes or reactions.

Pathogen: A broad term referring to an organism (bacteria, fungus, virus, or other microorganism) or agent (cancer, chemical, organic or inorganic material) which causes disease.

Pathophysiology: Abnormal physiologic function.

Percolating: Filtering of a liquid or gas slowly through a porous substance, such as a filter or surface.

Periosteum: The fibrous tissue covering the non-articulating surfaces of a bone. The periosteum nourishes and repairs bone and functions as the attachment site for tendons and ligaments (Pasquini et al. 2003).

Peripheral nervous system: Cranial nerves and spinal nerves.

Phagocytosis: Ingestion (engulfing) of a large particle by a cell using its plasma membrane, creating an internal compartment within the cell.

Pharmacodynamics: A branch of pharmacology focusing on the effects and mechanisms of actions of drugs (Chen 2013)

Pharmacokinetics: A branch of pharmacology focusing on the movement of drugs throughout the body (Chen 2013; Zhao et al. 2015).

Phlegm: An abnormal form of Body Fluid which can accumulate within the body (Xie and Preast 2007a). Often any "strange" condition or illness is due to phlegm.

Photoacceptor: A pigment that uses light (photons) as the first step in a photochemical reaction (Sineshchekov 1995).

Photobiomodulation (aka low-level laser or light therapy or cold laser therapy): The use of light (most commonly red or near-infrared) to stimulate, heal, regenerate, and protect damaged tissue (Hamblin 2017).

Photobiophysics: A branch of biophysics studying how light interacts with biological systems (Reusch 2013).

Photochemical reaction: A chemical reaction induced by the absorption of light energy (Reusch 2013).

Photochemistry: A branch of chemistry studying the chemical effects of light (Reusch 2013).

Photon: A particle of electromagnetic radiation with zero mass at rest, which carries energy proportional to the radiation frequency (Reusch 2013). For example, short wavelengths have high frequencies and high-energy photons.

Physiomedicalism: An herbal medicinal system based on the treatment of a patient's underlying condition. Resolution of the underlying condition would restore patient vitality, normalizing all body systems and functions, through the application of the following therapeutic ideals: detoxification; improving circulation; ANS balance; and tissue function restoration (Fougère 2007).

Phytopharmacology: The study of plants as medicine, specifically the active molecular components of plants possessing medicinal properties (Bone 2007).

Phytotherapy: The clinical application of plant-based extracts or medications in the prevention and treatment of disease (Ghosh 2016).

Phytotomy (aka plant anatomy): The study of the internal structures of plants (Klein 2007).

Platelet-rich plasma (PRP): Blood that has been processed, generally spun down using a centrifuge, to separate and concentrate the platelets from the blood. PRP has a higher concentration of platelets than that found in whole blood (Reinders and Haghighat 2019).

Platelet-rich therapy: The injection of PRP into damaged and painful areas of the musculoskeletal system with the goal of stimulating the body's natural healing ability, stabilizing the weakened tissues, and reducing pain (Reinders and Haghighat 2019).

Posterior (aka dorsal): Closer to the back of the body.

Power: Rate of energy delivery measured in watts (W): $1\,W = 1\,J/s$ (Patil and Dhami 2008).

Prolotherapy (aka nonsurgical ligament and tendon reconstruction and regenerative joint injection): The injection of a small volume of a sterile irritant into a painful joint, tendon, or ligament with the goal of stimulating the body's natural healing ability, stabilizing the weakened tissues, and reducing pain (Hauser et al. 2016; AOAPRM 2020).

Prolozone: The injection of ozone or a combination of ozone plus an irritant or pharmaceutical into a joint, tendon, or ligament for the purposes of relieving pain and improving dysfunction (Shallenberger 2011).

Proprioception: Perception or awareness of the body and limb positions in space (Purves et al. 2012d).

Proteoglycans: Glycosylated proteins present in all connective tissues which form hydrogel matrices allowing tissues to withstand intense compressive forces (Frantz et al. 2010).

Proximal: Closer to the body.

Qi: Energy. There are eight primary forms of Qi: Yuan Qi, Zong Qi, Gu Qi, Ying Qi, Wei Qi, Zang-Fu Qi, Jing Luo Qi, and Zheng Qi (Xie and Preast 2007d).

Radiation: Energy which travels and spreads out through space (NASA 2013).

Reactive oxygen species (ROS): Highly reactive and unstable molecules containing oxygen which react with other molecules in a cell; examples include singlet oxygen, peroxides, superoxides, and hydroxyl radicals (Shields et al. 2021).

Reducing agent (aka reductant): A substance that donates electrons to an oxidizing agent during a redox reaction (Wiley 2002).

Reduction: The gaining of electrons and subsequent decrease in charge (becomes more negative) (Wiley 2002).

Referred pain: Pain perceived in a site distant from the painful stimulus or origin of the pain (Physiopedia 2016). Referred pain maps have been created for human trigger points and visceral pain.

Regenerative medicine: The use of biological materials, including stem cells and PRP, to treat disease and injury through the restoration of the body's natural healing abilities (Barrett 2016).

Repetitive motion disorder (RMD): A category of muscular conditions caused by repeated motions performed during routine work or daily activities (NINDS 2019).

Rheological properties: The ability of a material to change shape, distort, or change its flow.

Sclerotherapy: The injection of an irritating solution into a vein or lymphatics causing transient swelling of the area, followed by collapse of the abnormal vein or lymph vessel. Most commonly used to treat varicose veins (aka chronic venous insufficiency), hemorrhoids, and malformed lymph vessels in people (Villines 2017).

Semiconductor: A solid substance comprising an insulator and a metal which has conductivity (Heiskanen and Hamblin 2018).

Sensory neurons: Nerve cells which respond to stimuli (touch, sound, light, and temperature changes) and send information to the spinal cord or brain (Purves et al. 2012d).

Shen: Also known as the Spirit or Affect. An outward expression of an individual's mental state (Xie and Preast 2007d).

Single bond: A covalent bond in which one electron pair is shared between two atoms (Ouellette and Rawn 2014).

Spinal cord: A long column of nervous tissue, housed within the spinal canal of the vertebrae, extending from the level of the foramen magnum to the lumbosacral region (Pasquini et al. 2003).

Spinal manipulation: The use of manual therapy, most often a high-velocity low-amplitude thrust, to restore normal pain-free range of motion to a joint or motion unit (Gatterman 2005).

Sprain: Injury to one or more ligaments. Ligaments are either stretched or torn (NIAMSD 2015).

Stem cells: Cells which can self-renew and develop into specific cells. Self-renewal involves the unlimited production of daughter cells identical to the original cell (Biehl and Russell 2009).

Stem cell therapy: The injection of prepared stem cells into the body with the goal of stimulating the body's natural healing ability.

Strain: Injury to a muscle or tendon because of stretching or tearing of the tissue (NIAMSD 2015).

Stratosphere: Second layer of the atmosphere, 6–30 miles above the Earth's surface.

Stratospheric ozone: Layer of ozone located within the stratosphere, responsible for absorbing much of the harmful ultraviolet (UV) radiation from the sun (EPA 2022). Considered the "good ozone."

Stretch and hold: The application of a sustained stretch to a tight muscle with the intent of passively inducing muscle relaxation.

Subluxation: A joint with reduced mobility (i.e. hypomobility), restriction, fixation, or joint dysfunction (Gatterman 2005; Mai-Roecker and Roecker 2018).

Superior (aka cranial): Closer to the head.

Sympathetic nervous system ("fight or flight"): Sends signals from the brain and spinal cord to the internal organs in times of stress.

Synovial fluid: The thick gelatinous liquid produced by the synovial membrane used to lubricate and nourish a synovial joint (Pasquini et al. 2003).

Taxonomy: A branch of biology centered on the scientific classification of related items (Klein 2007).

Traditional Chinese medicine (TCM): A complex medical system, developed over thousands of years in China, used to prevent and treat disease. There are five branches within TCM: acupuncture, Chinese herbal medicine or therapy, Tui-na, Tai-Chi, and food therapy (Xie 2011; NCCIH 2013). The study and application of TCM in animals is known as **traditional Chinese veterinary medicine (TCVM)**.

TCVM: Traditional Chinese veterinary medicine is a Chinese medicine system used to treat animals n comprises four branches: acupuncture, Chinese herbal medicine or therapy, Tui-na, and food therapy.

TCVM therapeutic actions: A beneficial effect associated with a specific TCVM therapy.

Thrust: The use of a specific contact point to deliver a deliberate, controlled, and unidirectional force to a particular motion segment (Gatterman 2005; Rivera 2015).

Tissue penetration: How deep (or how many tissue layers) a beam of light can penetrate.

Tendon: Fibrous connective tissue attaching muscle to bone (Pasquini et al. 2003).

Tendonitis: Inflammation of a tendon.

Tonify: To increase energy (Qi), blood flow, Yin, Yang, or organ function in an area. A substance which tonifies is often referred to as a "tonic."

Trigger point (TrP) (aka myofascial trigger point): A hyperirritable palpable nodule or taut band within the skeletal muscle or associated fascia (Finando 2005). Direct manipulation of the nodule or band will elicit a disproportionately painful response locally and often distantly (referred pain) (Finando 2005).

Trigger point therapy (TrPT): TrPT refers to a group of treatment modalities used to reduce and/or resolve the pain associated with myofascial trigger points. Therapeutic techniques include physical therapy (massage, stretching, ischemic compression technique, taping, and neuromuscular techniques), therapeutic ultrasound, photobiomodulation, thermal techniques (hot and cold packs), dry needling, and trigger point injection (Physiopedia 2016).

Trophorestorative: Herbs with the ability to nurture, support, protect, and repair specific organs or tissues (Fougère 2007).

Troposphere: First layer of the atmosphere starting at the Earth's surface and extending upward for 6–7 miles.

Tropospheric ozone: Ozone found within the troposphere which contributes to air pollution. Considered the "bad ozone" (EPA 2022).

Ultraviolet (UV) light or radiation: A form of invisible light energy (aka electromagnetic radiation) with a wavelength shorter than that of visible light (10–400 nm) but longer than that of X-rays (FDA 2020). Sunlight is the primary source of UV radiation. There are three main forms of UV radiation, in order of decreasing wavelengths: UVA, UVB, and UVC. The stratospheric ozone layer filters the amount and type of UV radiation reaching the Earth's surface, absorbing all UVC and some UVB radiation (FDA 2020). UV radiation reaching the Earth's surface can penetrate different layers of the skin depending on their wavelength, with UVA (longest wavelength) penetrating to the middle skin layer (dermis) and UVB (shorter wavelength) penetrating the outer skin layer (dermis) (EPA 2022).

Vertebral subluxation complex (VSC): A model explaining the cascade of events resulting from and contributing to spinal segment hypomobility. The VSC comprises nine components which function individually and synergistically following the restriction of vertebral segments: kinesiology, neuropathology, myopathology, vascular pathology, connective tissue pathology, inflammatory response, pathoanatomy, pathophysiology, and pathobiochemistry (Seaman and Faye 2005).

Veterinary nutraceutical (aka animal health supplement): A product isolated or derived from a food source used to support normal biological processes within animals. They are not drugs so they cannot treat, diagnose, prevent, or cure disease.

Veterinary regenerative medicine: The injection of a substance derived from animal cells or tissues into a joint, tendon, or ligament with the intent of reducing pain and inflammation and promoting the body's natural healing abilities.

Visible light: A specific range of electromagnetic radiation, typically between 380 and 700 nm, visible to the human eye (Nagaraja 2021).

Vitalism: All living beings are born with a "vital force" which flows continuously through the body providing nourishment and sustaining life.

Vitamin: Organic compounds which cannot be synthesized by the body and are required in small doses for normal growth, nutrition, and development (Hand et al. 2010).

Wavelength: Distance between the peaks of a wave, usually measured in nanometers or nm (Patil and Dhami 2008).

Wind: Used to describe environments and disease conditions. One of the six evils or conditions in TCVM. Often considered the primary cause of disease. Wind can invade the body from the outside world (exogenous wind) or originate within the body (internal wind) (Xie and Preast 2007b). The presence of Wind often allows other pathogens or conditions to develop concurrently.

Yang: Half of the Yin–Yang division. The descriptor can be applied to all manner of items both animate and inanimate. Characteristics considered Yang include day, brightness, summer, hot, fast, male, healthy, strength, birth, top or back, Qi, pungent or bitter, and Fu organs (Xie and Preast 2007f).

Yin: Half of the Yin–Yang division. The descriptor can be applied to all manner of items both animate and inanimate. Characteristics considered Yin include night, darkness, winter, cold, slow, female, illness, weakness, death, bottom or belly, blood, salty and sweet, and Zang organs (Xie and Preast 2007f).

Yin–Yang Theory: Divides all things into two halves which oppose, complement, control, create, and transform into each other (Xie and Preast 2007f).

Z-joints (aka zygapophyseal joints): Joint between two articular facets.

Zang-Fu physiology: The classification of the 12 organs as either Zang or Fu.

Zang organs: Yin organs located within the interior of the body, are solid in structure, and whose primary function is manufacturing and storage: lung, spleen, heart, pericardium, liver, and kidney (Xie and Preast 2007g).

Zoopharmacognosy: The behavior of self-medication, through ingestion or topical application of plants, soil, or insects, by non-human animals. As an example, non-human primates, as well as domesticated companion and food animals, are known to ingest

plants with antiparasitic or purgative properties to rid themselves of intestinal parasites (Engel 2007; Kapadia et al. 2014; Shurkin 2014).

Appendix B: Veterinary Organizations

American Academy of Veterinary Acupuncture (AAVA)

- **Description**: The AAVA was founded in 1998 and is affiliated with international veterinary acupuncture society (IVAS). The goals of the AAVA are to promote the education, understanding, and professional development of veterinarians practicing veterinary acupuncture, TCVM, and other Eastern medicine practices. There is no annual CE requirement to maintain membership.
- **Membership benefits**
  - Free subscription to the *American Journal of Traditional Chinese Veterinary Medicine*, a peer-reviewed journal.
  - Searchable member directory.
  - Help advance integrative medicine through the AAVA's seat on the AVMA House of Delegates.
  - Access to the career center with open positions and potential candidates.
  - Option to advance the veterinarian's acupuncture development through completion of the Fellows of American Academy of Veterinary Acupuncturists (FAAVA) certification process.
  - The AAVA hosts an annual CE.

American College of Veterinary Botanical Medicine (ACVBM)

- **Description**: Founded in 2016 as a means to establish requirements for post-doctoral education and certification in veterinary botanical medicine. The ultimate goal is to create a diplomate status for the specialty of veterinary botanical medicine. Patrons can become supporting members through donations or apply to become members of the organizing committee. No required annual continuing education (CE) to maintain membership.

- **Membership benefits**: The ACVBM offers an annual CE conference.

American Holistic Veterinary Medical Association (AHVMA)

- **Description**: The AHVMA was founded in 1982 at the Western States Veterinary Conference with the goal of advancing integrative medicine through the education of integrative and non-integrative veterinarians, the introduction of integrative medicine to veterinary students, the promotion of research, and representation in the AVMA House of Delegates. There is no annual CE requirement to maintain membership.
- **Membership benefits**
  - Free subscription to the *AHVMA Journal*, a peer-reviewed journal.
  - Online resources for client education.
  - Searchable member directory.
  - Discounted vaccination titers through Kansas State University (KSU) Diagnostic Lab.
  - Free access to the Natural Medicines Database, an online resource for supplements, natural medicines, and integrative therapies.
  - Reduced cost for the AHVMA annual conference.

American Veterinary Chiropractic Association (AVCA)

- **Description**
  - A non-governmental organization which aims to develop standards of care for animal chiropractic in North America.
  - AVCA has created a certification program and awards time-limited credentials to interested individuals meeting their criteria.
  - AVCA created a voluntary, non-licensure, membership which issues certificates of competency to veterinarians and chiropractors meeting the standards outlined in

the following section. Recertification is required to maintain the credentials.

- **Requirements**
  - Complete a postgraduate animal chiropractic program approved by the Education Committee of the AVCA.
  - Pass the AVCA exit examination.
  - Pass the AVCA written and practical examinations.
  - Hold a veterinary or chiropractic license in good standing.
  - Initial certification is granted for three years.
  - Recertification requires a minimum of 30 hours of AVCA approved continuing education every three years and pass the written and practice examinations.
- **Membership benefits**
  - Access to current articles and clinical information.
  - Network with other members through the "Community of Practice" forum.
  - Name is listed on the "Find a Certified Doctor" directory.
  - Information about upcoming CE seminars and conventions, including the annual meeting.
  - Discounted prices on logo apparel and conferences.

College of Integrative Veterinary Therapies (CIVT)

- **Description**: An online organization open to all licensed animal health providers interested in integrative medicine. There are two membership options: full membership for veterinarians and associate membership for registered animal health professionals. CIVT strives to promote all aspects of evidence-based integrative medicine through online education and discussion forums. CIVT provides financial support to veterinary students interested in studying integrative medicine. CIVT also helps fund integrative medicine research. There is no annual CE requirement to maintain membership.

- **Membership benefits**
  - Access to the online electronic library.
  - Access to the electronic *Journal of Integrative Veterinary Therapies*.
  - Three free CE webinars annually.
  - 20% discount on all webinars.
  - Discounts on specific CIVT courses.
  - Searchable member directory.
  - Access to the Natural Medicines Databases and the American Botanical Council Library.

International Veterinary Academy of Pain Management (IVAPM)

- **Description**: Originally known as the Companion Animal Pain Management Consortium, then the Academy of Pain Management Interest Group, and finally IVAPM. Founded in 2001 to provide pain management education and certification programs. The organization's goal is to provide acute and chronic pain relief for veterinary patients. Both traditional and alternative therapies are embraced, including acupuncture and rehabilitation and physical therapy.
- **Membership benefits**
  - Members can become Certified Veterinary Pain Practitioners (CVPP).
  - Access to member's only Facebook group offering case consultations and questions.
  - Reduced subscription rate for IVAPM's journal *Veterinary Anesthesia and Analgesia*.
  - Reduced registration fee for the International Veterinary Emergency and Critical Care (IVECCS) conference.
  - Reduced registration for all IVAPM continuing education events (online and onsite).
  - Complementary World Small Animal Veterinary Association (WSAVA) membership.

International Veterinary Acupuncture Society (IVS)

- **Description**: IVAS was founded in 1974 to promote and educate veterinarians and non-veterinarians on the subject of veterinary acupuncture. IVAS held the first veterinary acupuncture course in 1974 in Cincinnati, Ohio. Current membership numbers are over 1800 veterinarians. IVAS helps promote, educate, and set the global standards for veterinary acupuncture. Certified Veterinary Acupuncturists (CVA) are required to have 10 hours of acupuncture CE every two years.
- **Membership benefits**
  - Searchable member directory.
  - Access to IVAS member-only publications: *The Point* published quarterly and *The Flashpoint* published monthly.
  - Discounted IVAS events and seminars.
  - Online access to IVAS Congress Proceedings.
  - Free digital subscription to *American Journal of Traditional Chinese Veterinary Medicine*, a peer-reviewed journal.
  - Access to the in-print and online IVAS classifieds.
  - Access to online forums with other IVAS members.
  - Access to veterinary acupuncture templates for in-hospital promotion.
  - Access to veterinary acupuncture educational materials.
  - IVAS has multiple CE events annually.

International Veterinary Chiropractic Association (IVCA)

- **Description**
  - An international nonprofit organization promoting veterinary chiropractic.
  - IVCA created a voluntary, non-licensure, membership which issues certificates of competency to veterinarians and chiropractors meeting the standards outlined in the following section. Recertification is required to maintain the credentials.
- **Requirements**
  - Hold a veterinary or chiropractic license in good standing.
  - Complete an IVCA approved course.
  - Pass the IVCA certification examination.
  - Complete the IVCA requirements.

– Annual membership fee.
– Recertification is required every three years.
- **Membership benefits**
  – Source of patient referrals.
  – Case consultation with other IVCA members.
  – Free client education and promotional information.
  – Access to worldwide CE courses and seminars.
  – Access to research funding.

World Association of Traditional Chinese Veterinary Medicine (WATCVM)
- **Description**: The WATCVM promotes the education, research, and practice of TCVM throughout the world. The WATCVM provides financial support to veterinary students interested in studying TCVM as well as establishing student organizations within veterinary schools. The WATCVM funds TCVM research programs. There is no annual CE requirement to maintain membership.
- **Membership benefits**
  – Access to online case discussion forums.
  – Free subscription to the *American Journal of Traditional Chinese Veterinary Medicine*, a peer-reviewed journal.
  – Access to the quarterly online TCVM newsletter.
  – Access to the online TCVM library.
  – Discounted TCVM conferences.
  – Access to the online classified ads.
  – Assistance with scientific writing as well as research design of grant proposals.
  – Dual membership in WATCVM and American Association of Traditional Chinese Veterinary Medicine (AATCVM).
  – The WATCVM and AATCVM offer an annual International Conference on TCVM.

Veterinary Botanical Medicine Association (VBMA)
- **Description**: Founded by Susan Wynn, DVM, CVA, CVCH, AHG in 2002. The VBMA comprises veterinarians and herbalists interested in promoting the responsible application of herbal therapies for animals. No required annual CE to maintain membership.
- **Membership benefits**
  – VBMA members receive daily email discussion threads detailing real-life case questions and expert practical advice.
  – Weekly and monthly emails are also shared highlighting herbs commonly used in veterinary medicine.
  – Free subscription to the biannual online *Journal of Veterinary Botanical Medicine*.
  – Access to Herbal Wiki, an online herbal materia medica.
  – Access to additional educational articles, websites, and videos.
  – Discounted cost for telemedicine conferences and webinars.
  – Searchable member directory.
  – The VBMA offers an annual conference and multiple webinars.

Appendix C: Reference Materials

A Clinical Guide to Blending Liquid Herbs: Herbal Formulations for the Individual Patient
- Author: Kerry Bone
- Summary: Clinical guide and reference book for the use of liquid herbal remedies in people. The book contains 125 monographs.

American College of Veterinary Botanical Medicine Annual Conference Proceedings
- Authors: Various
- Summary: Contains the lecture notes from the conference as well as key presentations from 2015 to 2019. There are audio recordings available for the 2020–2022 conferences (https://www.acvbm.org/bookstore.html).

Acu-Cat: A Guide to Feline Acupressure
- Authors: Nancy Zidonis and Amy Snow
- Summary: An introduction to TCVM theory, the location of feline acupuncture points (acupoints), practical tips for performing acupressure, and suggested acupressure acupoints by disease condition. This book can be

utilized by veterinarians, non-veterinarians working in the animal health field, and owners.

Acu-Dog: A Guide to Canine Acupressure
- Authors: Amy Snow and Nancy Zidonis
- Summary: A introduction to TCVM theory, the location of canine acupoints, practical tips for performing acupressure, and suggested acupressure acupoints by disease condition. This book can be utilized by veterinarians, non-veterinarians working in the animal health field, and owners.

Acupuncture for Dogs and Cats: A Pocket Atlas
- Author: Christina Matern, DVM
- Summary: A quick reference pocket guide introducing the basic concepts of TCVM and veterinary acupuncture. A brief outline of the location, indication, systemic effect, and technique for each canine acupoint is discussed.

Anatomy of Domestic Animals: Systemic and Regional Approach
- Authors: Chris Pasquini, DVM, MS, Tom Spurgeon, PhD, and Susan Pasquini, DVM
- Summary: Most veterinarians already own a copy from vet school. This in-depth, thorough, and entertaining anatomy book provides tons of information on the anatomy of most domestic animals.

Application of Traditional Chinese Veterinary Medicine in Exotic Animals
- Authors: Zhiqiang Yang and Huisheng Xie, DVM, MS, PhD
- Summary: Proceedings from the 13th Annual International TCVM Conference discussing the introduction and implementation of TCVM therapies for exotic animals.

Applied Veterinary Clinical Nutrition
- Authors: Andrea Fascetti, VMD, PhD, DACVIM, DACVN and Sean Delaney, DVM, MS, DACVN
- Summary: Meant to be a quicker reference for the busy practitioner allowing the practical application of canine and feline nutrition

during daily practice. The book provides an overview of nutrition basics, pet food options, and dietary supplement information.

Bone Broth for Dogs and Cats: Supercharged Nutrition for Allergies, Stiffness, Skin Problems, Intestinal Issues, Inflammation, and the Immune System
- Author: Judy McFarlen, DVM
- Summary: An in-depth discussion of the beneficial effects of bone broth, as well as practical recipes.

Canine and Feline Nutrition: A Resource for Companion Animal Professionals
- Authors: Linda P. Case, MS, Leighann Daristotle, DVM, PhD, Michael G. Hayek, PhD, and Melody Foess Rassch, DVM
- Summary: A point-of-reference guide for animal professionals regarding companion animal nutrition, as well as practical approaches to interpreting and understanding nutritional myths, pet food safety, pet food ingredient lists, pet food formulations, and dietary supplementation.

Canine Ergonomics: The Science of Working Dogs
- Author: William S. Helton
- Summary: A comprehensive review of the physiology, cognition, and ergonomics of working dogs. There is also a discussion on training service dogs.

Canine Lameness
- Author: Felix Duerr, DVM
- Summary: An in-depth reference book covering the diagnosis and treatment of musculoskeletal diseases in dogs. There is a companion website with videos of examination techniques and lameness conditions.

Canine Nutrigenomics: The New Science of Feeding Your Dog for Optimum Health
- Authors: Jean Dodds, DVM and Diana Laverdure
- Summary: An in-depth discussion into the study of how nutrition affects gene expression in canines.

Canine Rehabilitation and Physical Therapy
- Authors: Darryl Mills, DVM, DACVS, DACVSMT, CCRP, and David Levine, PhD, PT
- Summary: A comprehensive reference book covering canine rehabilitation protocols for a variety of conditions, printable medical record forms, canine exercises, therapeutic modality options available, physical examination specifics, and a companion website. A must-have for veterinarians interested in manual therapy, orthopedics, and rehabilitation.

Canine Sports Medicine and Rehabilitation
- Authors: M. Christine Zink, DVM, PhD, DACVP, DACVSMR and Janet D. Van Dyke, DVM, DACVSMR
- Summary: A comprehensive reference book discussing common canine musculoskeletal conditions and ailments, with particular interest in the canine athlete. The book covers gait analysis and physiology, various therapeutic approaches (including nutrition, rehabilitation, manual therapy, acupuncture, chiropractic, therapeutic exercise, aquatic therapy, conditioning and retraining, and assistive devices), and specific diagnoses and treatment recommendations for disorders of the forelimbs and pelvic limbs. A must-have for veterinarians interested in manual therapy, orthopedics, and rehabilitation.

Chinese Herbal Formulas for Veterinarians
- Authors: John Chen, PhD, Pharm D, OMD, Lac, Tina Chen, MS, Lac, Signe Beebe, DVM, and Michael Salewski, DVM
- Summary: Monograms of Chinese herbal formulas used in veterinary medicine organized by their TCVM category. Each monogram discusses the nomenclature, formula composition, dosage, Chinese therapeutic actions, clinical manifestations, veterinary clinical applications, veterinary modifications, cautions and contraindications, pharmacological effects, human clinical studies and research, toxicology, suggested acupuncture therapies, and often additional author comments.

Chinese Medical Herbology and Pharmacology
- Authors: John Chen, PhD, Pharm D, OMD, Lac and Tina Chen, MS, Lac
- Summary: Monograms of Chinese herbs organized by their TCM category. Each monogram discusses the nomenclature, Chinese therapeutic actions, dosages, cautions and contraindications, chemical composition, pharmacological effects, clinical studies and research, herb–drug interactions, toxicology, and often additional author comments.

Chinese Veterinary Herbal Handbook: 216 Most Commonly Used Veterinary Herbal Formulas
- Authors: Huisheng Xie, DVM, MS, PhD, Lauren Frank, DVM, CVA, Vanessa Preast, DVM, CVA, and Lisa Trevisanello, DVM, CVA
- Summary: The third edition is an earlier version of the *Clinical Manual of Veterinary Herbal Medicine* functioning as a faster reference guide. Focuses on formulas carried by Jing Tang Herbal.

Clinical Application of Different TCM Schools and Thoughts in Veterinary Practice
- Authors: Huisheng Xie, DVM, MS, PhD and Aituan Ma, DVM, PhD, MS
- Summary: Proceedings from the 18th Annual International TCVM Conference discussing the different TCVM schools and theories and TCVM therapy for infectious and inflammatory diseases, behavioral disorders, and other conditions.

Clinical Manual of Chinese Veterinary Herbal Medicine: 178 Commonly Used Veterinary Herbal Formulas
- Authora: Huisheng Xie, DVM, MS, PhD and Aituan Ma, DVM, PhD, MS
- Summary: A quick reference book covering the safe use of Chinese herbal medicine in veterinary patients with an emphasis on practical information on commonly used Chinese herbal formulas as well as formula selection using TCVM and Western diagnoses. Scientific studies focusing on the referenced herbal formulas are provided.

Focuses on formulas carried by Jing Tang Herbal.

Clinician's Guide to Canine Acupuncture
- Authors: Curtis Wells Dewey, DVM, MS, DACVIM (Neurology), DACVS, and Huisheng Xie, DVM, MS, PhD
- Summary: An in-depth discussion of canine acupuncture focusing on the anatomic location of acupoints. A summary of the Western and Eastern indications for each acupoint is provided.

Clinical Nutrition: Veterinary Clinics of North America Small Animal Practice
- Authors: Dottie Laflamme, DVM, PhD, DACVN and Debra Zoran, DVM, PhD, DACVIM
- Summary: A condensed summary covering the foundation of small animal nutrition, its practical applications to everyday life, and the nutritional management of common canine and feline diseases.

The Complete Herbal Handbook for the Dog and Cat
- Author: Juliette de Baïracli Levy
- Summary: An introduction into the applications of integrative pet care and herbal therapy for owners.

Dogs in Motion
- Authors: Martin S Fischer and Karin E Lije
- Summary: An in-depth look into the anatomy of canine locomotion across 32 different breeds. There is a companion DVD with over 400 movies, X-rays, and 3D animations.

Dr. Becker's Real Food for Health Dogs and Cats: Simple Homemade Food
- Authors: Beth Taylor and Karen Becker, DVM
- Summary: An introduction to the theory and applications of raw food diets for dogs and cats, as well as multiple raw food diet recipes.

Dr. Pitcairn's Complete Guide to Natural Health for Dogs and Cats
- Authors: Richard Pitcairn, DVM, PhD and Susan Pitcairn
- Summary: An introduction into the applications of integrative pet care for owners.

Essential Guide to Chinese Herbal Formulas: Bridging Science and Tradition in Integrative Veterinary Medicine
- Author: Steve Marsden, DVM, ND, MSOM, Lac, Dipl.CH., RH(AHG)
- Summary: A quick reference book covering the safe use of Chinese herbal medicine in veterinary patients with an emphasis on practical information on commonly used Chinese herbal formulas as well as formula selection using TCVM and Western diagnoses. Focuses on formulas carried by A Time to Heal Herbs.

Essentials of Western Veterinary Acupuncture
- Authors: Samantha Lindley, BVSc, MRCVS and Mike Cummings, DVM
- Summary: A discussion of the history, mechanisms of action, safety, and practical uses of veterinary acupuncture from a Western medicine perspective.

Feeding Dogs: The Science Behind the Dry Versus Raw Debate
- Author: Conor Brady, BSC Hons, PhD
- Summary: A scientific review of the current commercial dog food, including its major pitfalls, and suggested canine diets going forward.

Foundations of Chiropractic: Subluxation
- Author: Meridel Gatterman, MA, DC, MED
- Summary: Evidence-based approach to the theories of joint dysfunction, common clinical syndromes, and practical application of chiropractic therapy in people.

Four Paws Five Directions: A Guide to Chinese Medicine for Cats and Dogs
- Author: Cheryl Schwartz, DVM
- Summary: An introduction to TCVM in veterinary medicine focusing on TCVM theory and acupuncture. Additional therapies are briefly covered: food therapy, herbal supplements, nutritional supplements, environmental modifications. The disease processes are organized by body system and the Five Element Theory.

Frontiers in Stem Cell and Regenerative Medicine Research
- Editors: Atta-ur-Rahman, FRS and Shazia Anjum
- Summary: A review of the use of stem cell therapy through retrodifferentiation, mesodermal regeneration, hematopoiesis, and mesenchymal stem cells.

The Fungal Pharmacy: The Complete Guide to Medicinal Mushrooms and Lichens of North America
- Author: Robert Rogers, RH (AHG)
- Summary: Comprehensive summary of more than 300 species of North American medicinal mushrooms and lichens, including physical characteristics and medicinal properties.

Healing with Whole Foods: Asian Traditions and Modern Nutrition
- Author: Paul Pitchford
- Summary: An in-depth look into the applications of Chinese food therapy with TCM descriptions of common food items and a multitude of recipes for various human diseases.

Herbal Vade Mecum: 800 Herbs, Spices, Essential Oils, Liquids, etc. Constituents, Properties, Uses, and Caution
- Author: Gazmend Skenderi
- Summary: A quick reference guide for the general public with information and practical applications for herbs and essential oils, including 657 abbreviated monographs.

Home-Prepared Dog and Cat Diets
- Author: Patricia Schenck
- Summary: An introduction for owners into the basics of companion animal nutrition, the effect of diet on specific disease conditions, and home-cooked recipes.

The Human Brain: An Introduction to its Functional Anatomy
- Author: John Nolte
- Summary: A comprehensive look into the anatomy and functional neurology of the brain. While geared toward the study of the human brain the information is applicable to veterinary patients.

The Identification of Medicinal Plants: A Handbook of the Morphology of Botanicals in Commerce
- Author: Wendy Applequist
- Summary: A comprehensive handbook published by the American Botanical Council designed to review the basic plant structure, identification tips, and botanical nomenclature for over 150 species of medicinal botanicals.

Integrating Complementary Medicine into Veterinary Practice
- Authors: Robert S. Goldstein, VMD, Paula Jo Broadfoot, DVM, Richard E. Plamquist, DVM, Karen Johnstons, DVM, Jiu Jia Wen, DVM, Barbara Fougère, BSc, BVMs (Hons), BHSc (comp Med), MODT, MHSc (Herb Med), CVA (IVAs), CVBM, CVCP, and Margo Roman, DVM
- Summary: A comprehensive review of multiple integrative therapies including Chinese herbal medicine, acupuncture, homotoxicology, nanopharmacology, homotoxicology, and therapeutic nutrition. The book aims to educate veterinary practitioners on the validity, effectiveness, and incorporation of each modality within daily practice.

Integrative and Traditional Chinese Veterinary Medicine Food Therapy Small Animal and Equine
- Authors: Margaret Fowler, DVM and Huisheng Xie, DVM, MS, PhD
- Summary: A thorough explanation of Western and Eastern nutritional science with a TCVM foundation. Food therapy for specific disease conditions, based on TCVM pattern differentiation and traditional diagnoses, are discussed. The book includes information on specific dietary ingredients, as well as 300 AAFCO compliant homemade small animal recipes and recipes for equine top-dressings.

Interactive Medical Acupuncture Anatomy
- Author: Narda G. Robinson, DO, DVM, MS, FAAMA
- Summary: A combination book and CD set providing detailed anatomic locations for human acupoints.

Kan Essentials Chinese Herbal Formula Guide
- Author: Steve Marsden, DVM, ND, MSOM, Lac, Dipl.CH., RH(AHG)
- Summary: Product booklet discussing the clinical uses and dosing for the Kan Essentials herbal formulas.

Laser Therapy in Veterinary Medicine: Photobiomodulation
- Authors: Ronald J. Riegel, DVM and Hohn C. Godbold, Jr., DVM
- Summary: An in-depth review of the science behind photobiomodulation as well as a practical reference for the clinical applications of laser therapy in veterinary medicine.

Manual of Natural Veterinary Medicine: Science and Tradition
- Authors: Susan G. Wynn, DVM and Steve Marsden, DVM, ND, MSOM, Lac, Dipl. CH., RH(AHG)
- Summary: A quick reference book discussing the integrative therapy options for numerous diseases in veterinary medicine. The book is organized by Western conditions. For each category the potential TCVM diagnoses and treatment options are then discussed in succinct detail. A must-have for all integrative veterinarians.

Mesenchymal Stem Cell in Veterinary Services
- Editors: Mudasir Bashir Gugjoo, PhD and Amar Pal
- Summary: Discusses the production, properties, clinical applications, and mechanisms of action for mesenchymal stem cells in regenerative medicine.

Miller's Anatomy of the Dog
- Authors: Howard Evans, PhD and Alexander de Lahunta, DVM, PhD

- Summary: Most veterinarians already own a copy from vet school. This is a comprehensive guide to the canine anatomy.

Myofascial Pain and Dysfunction: The Trigger Point Manual Volumes 1 and 2
- Authors: David Simons, MD, Janet Travell MD, and Lois Simons PT
- Summary: A comprehensive look into the etiology, diagnosis, and treatment of human trigger points.

Natural Path Herb Company Guide to Chinese Veterinary Herbal Medicine for Small Animals
- Author: Steve Marsden, DVM, ND, MSOM, Lac, Dipl.CH., RH(AHG)
- Summary: Product booklet discussing the clinical uses and dosing for the Natural Path herbal formulas. Natural Path produces a few formulas classified as Western herbal medicine.

Nutraceuticals in Veterinary Medicine
- Authors: Ramesh Gupta, Ajay Srivastava, and Rajiv Lall
- Summary: An in-depth look into veterinary nutraceuticals evaluating common ingredients, classifications, applications, utilization, safety and toxicity data, recent trends in research and product development, and regulation.

Nutrient Requirements of Dogs and Cats
- Author: National Research Council
- Summary: A detailed description of the nutrient requirements for dogs and cats based on age and lifestyle, as well as nutrient metabolism and diseases related to nutritional deficiencies.

Pain, Lameness, Neurological and Endocrine Disorders
- Authors: Huisheng Xie, DVM, MS, PhD and Aituan Ma, DVM, PhD, MS
- Summary: Proceedings from the 20th Annual International TCVM Conference discussing the use of TCVM for the treatment of pain, lameness, neurologic disorders, endocrine disorders, infertility, and other conditions.

Phytotherapy in Veterinary Medicine: Place of Medicinal Plants in the Treatment of Canine Diseases

- Authors: Aïmen Abbassi and Hela Gana
- Summary: An introduction into the science of veterinary herbal medicine. Provides a reference for veterinarians and owners.

Practical Guide to Traditional Chinese Veterinary Medicine: Emergencies and Five Element Syndromes

- Authors: Huisheng Xie, DVM, MS, PhD, Lindsey Wedemeyer, MA, VetMB, MRCVS, and Cheryl L Chrisman, DVM, MS, EdS, DACVIM (Neurology)
- Summary: The first of a four-volume series discussing the practical use of TCVM in veterinary medicine. The book breaks down the TCVM pattern diagnosis and treatment options (acupuncture, Chinese herbal formulas, Tui-na, food therapy, and environmental changes) for common small animal emergencies. The book is organized using the Five Element Theory of disease as it relates to emergent disorders.

Practical Guide to Traditional Chinese Veterinary Medicine: Exotic, Zoo, and Farm Animals

- Authors: Huisheng Xie, DVM, MS, PhD and Harvey E Ramirez
- Summary: The final part of a four-volume series discussing the practical use of TCVM in veterinary medicine. The book breaks down the TCVM pattern diagnosis and treatment options (acupuncture, Chinese herbal formulas, Tui-na, food therapy, and environmental changes) for exotic, zoo, and farm animals.

Practical Guide to Traditional Chinese Veterinary Medicine: Small Animal Practice

- Authors: Huisheng Xie, DVM, MS, PhD, Lindsey Wedemeyer, MA, VetMB, MRCVS, Cheryl L Chrisman, DVM, MS, EdS, DACVIM (Neurology), and Lisa Trevisanellow, DrMEDVET

- Summary: The second of a four-volume series discussing the practical use of TCVM in veterinary medicine. The book breaks down the TCVM pattern diagnosis and treatment options (acupuncture, Chinese herbal formulas, Tui-na, food therapy, and environmental changes) for common small animal diseases. The book is organized by the Western medical diagnoses and then further divided into the possible TCVM diagnoses for each disease process.

Principles and Practice of Phytotherapy: Modern Herbal Medicine

- Authors: Kerry Bone and Simon Mills
- Summary: An introduction to the theories and applications of Western herbal medicine for the human practitioner. The book contains 50 evidence-based monographs.

Raw and Natural Nutrition for Dogs: The Definitive Guide to Homemade Diets

- Author: Lew Olson, PhD
- Summary: A reference guide for owners providing an introduction to canine nutrition, the benefits of a raw food diet, and practical raw food recipes.

Real Food for Dogs and Cats: A Practice Guide to Feedings Your Pet a Balanced, Natural Diet

- Author: Clare Middle, DVM
- Summary: A quick reference for pet owners regarding how to properly balance natural diets.

Safety of Dietary Supplements for Horses, Dogs, and Cats

- Authors: National Research Council
- Summary: An in-depth discussion centered on the safety and efficacy of dietary supplements as well as current laws and regulations.

See Spot Live Longer

- Authors: Steve Brown and Beth Taylor
- Summary: An introductory guide for pet owners to the complexity of canine nutritional science. The book includes background educational information, as well as

practical tips for augmenting and designing companion canine diets.

Small Animal Clinical Nutrition, **5th Edition**
- Authors: Michael Hand DVM, PhD, Craig Thatcher, DVM, MS, PhD, Rebecca Remillard PhD, DVM, Philip Roudebush, DCM, and Bruce Novotny, DVM
- Summary: The gold-standard for small animal nutritional information covering dogs, cats, birds, reptiles, and small mammals with over 125 contributing authors. The book discusses the fundamental principles of small animal nutrition, commercial and home-made pet foods, nutritional management of canine and feline diseases, and dietary husbandry information for many exotic species. There are now digital excerpts of the 6th edition available through Clinician's Brief.

Spark in the Machine: How the Science of Acupuncture Explains the Mysteries of Western Medicine
- Author: Daniel Keown
- Summary: A discussion of how Western medicine can be used to validate Chinese medicine theories.

Stem Cells in Veterinary Science
- Authors: Ratan Kumar Choudhary, PhD, MS and Shant Choudhary, PhD
- Summary: An overview of the use of stem cell therapy in veterinary medicine focusing on the mechanisms of action, preclinical evidence, safety, and therapeutic efficacy. The book covers a variety of stem cell types and practical applications.

Therapeutic Applications of Mesenchymal Stem Cells in Veterinary Medicine
- Author: Mudasir Bashir Gugjoo, PhD
- Summary: An in-depth review of the application of mesenchymal stem cells in veterinary regenerative and reproductive medicine. The book discusses applications for the musculoskeletal, nervous, gastrointestinal, cardiovascular, urogenital, respiratory, and integumentary systems.

Traditional Chinese Veterinary Medicine Approach to Gastrointestinal and Hepatobiliary Diseases
- Authors: Liting Cao DVM, PhD and Huisheng Xie DVM, PhD
- Summary: Proceedings from the 22nd Annual International TCVM Conference discussing the use of TCVM for the treatment of gastrointestinal and hepatobiliary diseases.

Traditional Chinese Veterinary Medicine Approach to Veterinary Dermatological and Immune-mediated Diseases
- Authors: Aituan Ma, DVM, PhD, MS, Cui Liu, DVM, PhD, Chang Yu, DVM, MS, and Huisheng Xie, DVM, MS, PhD
- Summary: Proceedings from the 21st Annual International TCVM Conference discussing the use of TCVM for the treatment of dermatologic and immune-mediated diseases.

Traditional Chinese Veterinary Medicine Empirical Technique to Scientific Validation
- Authors: Zhiqiang Yang and Huisheng Xie, DVM, MS, PhD
- Summary: Proceedings from the 1st Annual International TCVM Conference discussing the scientific study of TCVM including, basic scientific research, small animal specific studies, exotic animal specific studies, large animal specific studies, and pediatric and geriatric medicine.

Traditional Chinese Veterinary Medicine for the Diagnosis and Treatment of Kidney and Water Element Disorders
- Authors: Aituan Ma, DVM, PhD, MS and Huisheng Xie, DVM, MS, PhD
- Summary: Proceedings from the 23rd Annual International TCVM Conference discussing the use of TCVM for the treatment of kidney and water element disorders.

Traditional Chinese Veterinary Medicine for Geriatric Medicine and Palliative Care
- Authors: Huisheng Xie, DVM, MS, PhD and Aituan Ma, DVM, PhD, MS
- Summary: Proceedings from the 19th Annual International TCVM Conference

discussing the use of TCVM for geriatric medicine and palliative care.

Traditional Chinese Veterinary Medicine for Neurologic Diseases
- Authors: Huisheng Xie, DVM, MS, PhD, Cheryl L Chrisman, DVM, MS, EdS, DACVIM (Neurology), and Lisa Trevisanellow, DrMEDVET
- Summary: Proceedings from the 13th Annual International TCVM Conference discussing the use of TCVM for a variety of neurologic conditions.

Traditional Chinese Veterinary Medicine from Dragon Legend to Modern Practice
- Authors: Xiuhuii Zhong, Aituan Ma, DVM, PhD, MS, Lisa Trevisanellow, DrMEDVET, and Qingbo Wang
- Summary: Proceedings of the 14th Annual International TCVM Conference discussing the use of TCVM for the treatment of liver, gastrointestinal, equine specific, and exotic animal specific diseases. A variety of other topics are also covered, including the longitudinal muscle system, PRP in aquapuncture, and the adverse effects of Chinese herbal medicine and acupuncture.

Traditional Chinese Veterinary Medicine Fundamental Principles
- Authors: Huisheng Xie, DVM, MS, PhD and Vanessa Preast, DVM, CVA
- Summary: The quintessential introduction to TCVM theory with self-study quizzes, case examples, and practical application of TCVM therapies for small animal and equine patients.

Traditional Chinese Veterinary Medicine for Pain, Lameness, Neurological, and Endocrine Disorders
- Authors: Huisheng Xie, DVM, MS, PhD and Aituan Ma, DVM, PhD, MS
- Summary: Proceedings from the 20th Annual International TCVM Conference discussing the use of TCVM for the treatment of pain, lameness, neurologic disorders, endocrine disorders, infertility, and other conditions.

Trigger Point Dry Needling: An Evidence and Clinical-Based Approach
- Authors: Jan Dommerholt, PT, DPT, MPS and Cesar Fernandez de las Penas, PT, PhD Dr. SciMed
- Summary: The neurophysiology of trigger points and dry needling in people. Contains detailed descriptions and images of dry needling techniques.

Trigger Point Therapy for Myofascial Pain: The Practice of Informed Touch
- Authors: Donna Finando, Lac, LMT and Steven Finando, PhD, Lac
- Summary: Human reference book for the evaluation, common locations, and treatment of trigger-points. The book is organized by muscle grouping.

Unlocking the Canine Ancestral Diet: Healthier Dog Food the ABC Way
- Author: Steve Brown
- Summary: A practical reference for dog owners on how to augment their dog's current diet to improve overall health. Recipes for complete dog foods are also included.

The Ultimate Pet Health Guide: Breakthrough Nutrition and Integrative Care for Dogs and Cats
- Author: Gary Richter, MS, DVM
- Summary: A practical reference for pet owners discussing integrative medicine and non-traditional (aka kibble) food options.

Veterinary Acupuncture
- Author: Allen M. Schoen, DVM, MS
- Summary: A detailed discussion of the history, anatomy, neurophysiologic mechanisms of action, scientific research, techniques, and practical application of veterinary acupuncture for small and large animals.

Veterinary Clinics of North America Small Animal Practice
- Published July 2023, Volume 53, issue 4, pp. 757–774. DOI: 10.1016/j.cvsm.2023.02.008.
- Chapter title: Veterinary Spinal Manipulative Therapy or Animal Chiropractic in Veterinary Rehabilitation.

- Summary: "Veterinary rehabilitation is a multimodal diagnostic and treatment approach that is recommended and provided to patients daily. One therapeutic modality that may be beneficial (diagnostically and therapeutically) is veterinary spinal manipulative therapy or animal chiropractic (AC). AC is a receptor-based health-care modality being provided more frequently in veterinary practices. All clinicians should strive to understand the mode of action, indications, contraindications, how it affects the patient from the neuro-anatomical and biomechanical point of view, and most importantly, when not to provide the requested modality, as further diagnostics may be indicated" (LoGiudice and Rivera 2023).

Veterinary Herbal Medicine
- Authors: Susan Wynn, DVM, DACVN and Barbara Fougère, BSc, BVMS (Hons), MODT, BHSc (Comp Med), CVA (IVAS), CVCP, CV Herb Med, MHSc (Herb Med)
- Summary: Comprehensive reference book on veterinary Western herbal medicine. The book is divided into five sections covering the history of Western herbal medicine, controversies surrounding Western herbal medicine, materia medica, clinical uses within veterinary medicine, and appendices. This book is a must-have for all veterinarians practicing Western herbal medicine.

Veterinary Herbal Pharmacopeia
- Author: Sun-Chong Wang
- Summary: Covers herbal recipes for various disease conditions in dogs and cats. The book is meant as a reference for both owners and veterinarians.

Veterinary Laser Therapy in Small Animal Practice
- Authors: Maria Suárez Rendondo, DVM, PhD, CVA and Bryan J. Stephens, PhD
- Summary: Practical guide to laser therapy for the clinician discussing the fundamentals of light therapy and clinical applications. Case studies are included to demonstrate how laser therapy can be incorporated into everyday practice.

Xie's Chinese Veterinary Herbology
- Authors: Huisheng Xie, DVM, MS, PhD and Vanessa Preast, DVM, CVA
- Summary: A practical guide covering the theory and application of veterinary Chinese herbal medicine. The book is organized into three sections: herbal materia medica, herbal formulas, and clinical applications.

Yin and Yang Nutrition for Dogs: Maximizing Health with Whole Foods, Not Drugs
- Author: Judy Morgan, DVM
- Summary: Quick reference for pet owners discussing based concepts in Chinese veterinary medicine and dog food recipes.

Your Guide to Health with Foods and Herbs: Using the Wisdom of TCM
- Authors: Zhang Yifang and Yao Yingzhi
- Summary: A quick-reference guide introducing the application of TCM to common foods and herbs.

References

Akamatsu, F., Ayres, B.R., Saleh, S.O. et al. (2015). Trigger points: an anatomical substratum. *BioMed Research International* 2015: 623287.

Al-Shenqiti, A. and Oldham, J. (2005). Test–retest reliability of myofascial trigger point detection in patients with rotator cuff tendonitis. *Clinical Rehabilitation* 19 (5): 482–487.

AOAPRM (American Osteopathic Association of Prolotherapy Regenerative Medicine) (2020). What is prolotherapy. https://prolotherapy college.org/ (accessed 29 October 2020).

Barrett, J. (2016). A set of grand challenges for veterinary regenerative medicine. *Frontiers in Veterinary Science* 3: 20.

Benjamin, M. and Evans, E. (1990). Fibro cartilage. *Journal of Anatomy* 171: 1–15.

Biehl, J. and Russell, B. (2009). Introduction to stem cell therapy. *Journal of Cardiovascular Nursing* 24 (2): 98–103.

Biophysical Society (2023). What is biophysics? https://www.biophysics.org/what-is-biophysics (accessed 5 February 2023).

Bliss, S. (2013). Musculoskeletal structure and physiology. In: *Canine Sports Medicine and Rehabilitation* (ed. M.C. Zink and J.B. van Dyke), 32–59. Oxford: Wiley-Blackwell.

Bone, K. (2007). Evaluating, designing, and accessing herbal medicine research. In: *Veterinary Herbal Medicine* (ed. S.G. Wynn and B. Fougère), 87–97. St. Louis: Mosby Elsevier.

Britannica (2020). Joule. https://www.britannica.com/science/joule (accessed 7 January 2023).

Brown, W. (2022). Ketone Chemical Compound. https://www.britannica.com/science/ketone (accessed 29 September 2022).

CDC (Centers for Disease Control and Prevention) (2020). Arthritis: Osteoarthritis. http://www.cdc.gov/arthritis/basics/osteoarthritis.htm (accessed August 2020).

Chen, J. (2013). *Concurrent Use of Herbal Medicines and Pharmaceuticals: Pharmacodynamics Interactions*. College of Integrative Veterinary Therapies.

Chung, H., Dai, T., Sharma, S.K. et al. (2012). The nuts and bolts of low-level laser (light) therapy. *Annals of Biomedical Engineering* 40 (2): 516–533.

Clemmons, R.M. (2007). Functional neuroanatomical physiology of acupuncture. In: *Xie's Veterinary Acupuncture* (ed. H. Xie and V. Preast), 341–347. Ames, IA: Blackwell Publishing.

Cooperstein, R. and Gleberzon, B. (2004). *Technique Systems in Chiropractic*. Philadelphia: Elsevier Science.

Cramer, G. and Darby, S. (2005). Anatomy related to spinal subluxation. In: *Foundations of Chiropractic Subluxation*, 2e (ed. M.I. Gatterman), 30–46. Elsevier Mosby: St. Louis, MO.

Darby, S.A. (2014). Neuroanatomy of the autonomic nervous system. In: *Clinical Anatomy of the Spine, Spinal Cord, and ANS*, 3e, 413–507. St. Louis, MO: Elsevier.

Edwards, K.D. (2005). Light emitting diodes. https://web.archive.org/web/20190214175634/http://faculty.sites.uci.edu/chem1l/files/2013/11/RDGLED.pdf (accessed 10 January 2023).

Engel, C. (2007). Zoopharmacognosy. In: *Veterinary Herbal Medicine* (ed. S.G. Wynn and B. Fougère), 7–15. St. Louis, MO: Mosby Elsevier.

EPA (Environmental Protection Agency) (2022). Ozone pollution and your patients' health. https://www.epa.gov/ozone-pollution-and-your-patients-health/what-ozone (accessed 13 September 2022).

Evans, H. and de Lahunta, A. (ed.) (2013). *Miller's Anatomy of the Dog*, 4e. St. Louis, MO: Elsevier.

FDA (Food and Drug Administration) (2020). Ultraviolet (UV) radiation. https://www.fda.gov/radiation-emitting-products/tanning/ultraviolet-uv-radiation (accessed 17 September 2022).

FDA (Food and Drug Administration) (2021a). Animal food and feeds: product regulation. https://www.fda.gov/animal-veterinary/animal-food-feeds/product-regulation (accessed 20 February 2021).

FDA (Food and Drug Administration) (2021b). CFR: Code of Federal Regulations Title 21. https://www.accessdata.fda.gov/scripts/cdrh/cfdocs/cfcfr/CFRSearch.cfm?CFRPart=211&showFR=1 (accessed 16 December 2021).

FDA (Food and Drug Administration) (2021c). Facts about the Current Good Manufacturing Practices (CGMPs). http://www.fda.gov/Drugs/DevelopmentApprovalProcess/Manufacturing/ucm169105.htm (accessed 17 December 2021).

Finando, D.S.F. (2005). *Trigger Point Therapy for Myofascial Pain*. Rochester, VT: Healing Arts Press.

Fougère, B. (2007). Approaches in veterinary herbal medicine prescribing. In: *Veterinary Herbal Medicine* (ed. S.G. Wynn and B. Fougère), 275–290. St. Louis, MO: Mosby Elsevier.

Frantz, C., Stewart, K., and Weaver, V. (2010). The extracellular matrix at a glance. *Journal of Cell Science* 123: 4195–4200.

de Freitas, L. and Hamblin, M. (2016). Proposed mechanisms of photobiomodulation or low-level light therapy. *IEEE Journal of Selected Topics in Quantum Electronics* 22 (3): 7000417.

Gatterman, M. (2005). What's in a word? In: *Foundations of Chiropractic Subluxation* (ed. M.I. Gatterman), 5–18. Elsevier Mosby: St. Louis, MO.

Ghosh, D. (2016). Seed to patient in clinically proven natural medicines. In: *Nutraceuticals: Efficacy, Safety, and Toxicity* (ed. R.C. Gupta). London: Academic Press.

Hamblin, M. (2017). Mechanisms and applications of the anti-inflammatory effects of photobiomodulation. *AIMS Biophysics* 4 (3): 337–361.

Hand, M., Thatcher, C.D., Remillard, R.L. et al. (2010). *Small Animal Clinical Nutrition*, 5e. Topeka, KS: Mark Morris Institute.

Hassan, Z., Stahlberger, M., Rosenbaum, N., and Bräse, S. (2020). Criegee intermediates beyond ozonolysis: synthetic and mechanistic insights. *Angewandte Chemie International Edition* 60 (28): 15138–15152.

Hauser, R., Lackner, J., Steilen-Matias, D., and Harris, D. (2016). A systematic review of dextrose prolotherapy for chronic musculoskeletal pain. *Clinical Medicine Insights. Arthritis and Musculoskeletal Disorders* 9: 139–159.

Heiskanen, V. and Hamblin, M. (2018). Photobiomodulation: lasers and light emitting diodes? *Photochehmical and Photobiological Sciences* 17 (8): 1003–1017.

Helmenstine, A.M. (2020). Definition of carboxyl group in chemistry. https://www.thoughtco. com/definition-of-carboxyl-group-and-examples-604879 (accessed 29 September 2022).

Iftikhar, N. (2019). What is allopathic medicine? https://www.healthline.com/health/allopathic-medicine (accessed 2 November 2021).

Jackman, S. and Regehr, W. (2017). The mechanisms and functions of synaptic facilitation. *Neuron* 94 (3): 447–464.

JEDEC (2023). Dictionary: JESD88. https://www.jedec.org/standards-documents/dictionary (accessed 7 January 2023).

Kapadia, M., Zhao, H., Ma, D. et al. (2014). Zoopharmacognosy in diseased laboratory mice: conflicting evidence. *PLoS One* 9 (6): e100684.

Klein, R. (2007). Medical botany. In: *Veterinary Herbal Medicine* (ed. S.G. Wynn and B. Fougère), 139–158. St. Louis, MO: Mosby Elsevier.

Lans, C., Khan, T., Curran, M., and McCorkle, C. (2007). Ethnoveterinary medicine: potential solutions for large-scale problems? In: *Veterinary Herbal Medicine* (ed. S.G. Wynn and B. Fougère), 17–32. St. Louis, MO: Mosby Elsevier.

LibreTexts (2022a). 3.3: Molecules and Chemical Nomenclature. https://chem.libretexts.org/Bookshelves/Introductory_Chemistry/Beginning_Chemistry_(Ball)/03%3A_Atoms_Molecules_and_Ions/3.03%3A_Molecules_and_Chemical_Nomenclature (accessed 29 September 2022).

LibreTexts (2022b). The Carbonyl Group. https://chem.libretexts.org/Bookshelves/Organic_Chemistry/Supplemental_Modules_(Organic_Chemistry)/Aldehydes_and_Ketones/Properties_of_Aldehydes_and_Ketones/The_Carbonyl_Group#:~:text=A%20carbonyl%20group%20is%20a,contributing%20to%20smell%20and%20taste (accessed 29 September 2022).

LoGiudice, R. and Rivera, P.L. (2023). Veterinary spinal manipulative therapy or animal chiropractic in veterinary rehabilitation.

Veterinary Clinics of North America. Small Animal Practice 53 (4): 757–774.

Mai-Roecker, H. and Roecker, C. (2018). Improving interprofessional communication. https://www.acatoday.org/News-Publications/ACA-News-Archive/ArtMID/5721/ArticleID/347 (accessed 8 July 2020).

Maltese, P., Michelini, S., Baronio, M., and Bertelli, M. (2019). Molecular foundations of chiropractic therapy. *Acta Biomedica* 90 (10-S): 93–102.

March, J. and Brown, W. (2020). Aldehyde. https://www.britannica.com/science/aldehyde (accessed 29 September 2022).

Marchesi, J. and Ravel, J. (2015). The vocabulary of microbiome research: a proposal. *Microbiome* 3: 31.

Matekaire, T. and Bwakura, T. (2004). Ethnoveterinary medicine: a potential alternative to orthodox animal health delivery in Zimbabwe. *International Journal of Applied Research in Veterinary Medicine* 2 (4): 269–273.

ME (Michigan Engineering) (2022). Ozonators. https://encyclopedia.che.engin.umich.edu/ozonators (accessed 17 September 2022).

MedlinePlus (2016). Bursitis. https://medlineplus.gov/bursitis.html (accessed 1 May 2020).

Nagaraja, M. (2021). Visible light. https://science.nasa.gov/ems/09_visiblelight (accessed 10 January 2023).

NASA (National Aeronautics and Space Administration) (2013). The Electromagnetic Spectrum. https://imagine.gsfc.nasa.gov/science/toolbox/emspectrum1.html (accessed 8 April 2021).

NASA (National Aeronautics and Space Administration) (2021). What is a laser? https://spaceplace.nasa.gov/laser/en (accessed 10 January 2023).

NCCIH (National Center for Complementary and Integrative Health) (2013). Traditional Chinese medicine: what you need to know. https://www.nccih.nih.gov/health/traditional-chinese-medicine-what-you-need-to-know (accessed 2 November 2021).

NCCIH (National Center for Complementary and Integrative Health) (2019). Ayurvedic medicine in depth. https://www.nccih.nih.gov/health/ayurvedic-medicine-in-depth (accessed 2 November 2021).

NIAMSD (National Institute of Arthritis and Musculoskeletal and Skin Diseases) (2015). Sprains and strains. http://niams.nih.gov/health-topics/sprains-and-strains (accessed 3 May 2020).

NINDS (National Institute of Neurological Disorders and Stroke) (2019). Repetitive motion disorders. https://www.ninds.nih.gov/health-information/disorders/repetitive-motion-disorders#:~:text=Definition,%2C%20tenosynovitis%2C%20and%20trigger%20finger (accessed 2 May 2020).

Nolte, J. (2009). Synaptic transmission between neurons. In: *The Human Brain*, 6e, 177–200. Philadelphia, PA: Mosby Elsevier.

OCP (Organic Chemistry Portal) (2022). Ozonolysis. https://www.organic-chemistry.org/namedreactions/ozonolysis-criegee-mechanism.shtm (accessed 29 September 2022).

Ouellette, R. and Rawn, J.D. (2014). Structure and bonding in organic compounds. In: *Organic Chemistry: Structure, Mechanism, and Synthesis* (ed. R. Ouellette and J.D. Rawn), 1–39. San Diego, CA: Elsevier.

Padulo, J., Laffaye, G., Chamari, K., and Concu, A. (2013). Concentric and eccentric: muscle contraction or exercise? *Sports Health: A Multidisciplinary Approach* 5 (4): 306.

Pasquini, C., Spurgeon, T., and Pasquini, S. (2003). *Anatomy of Domestic Animals: Systemic and Regional Approach*, 10e. Pilot Point, TX: Sudz Publishing.

Patil, U. and Dhami, L. (2008). Overview of lasers. *Indian Journal of Plastic Surgery* 41 (Suppl): S101–S113.

Perreault, T., Dunning, J., and Butts, R. (2017). The local twitch response during trigger point dry needling: is it necessary for successful outcomes? *Journal of Bodywork and Movement Therapies* 21 (4): 940–947.

Physiopedia (2016). Trigger points. https://www.
physio-pedia.com/Trigger_Points?utm_
source=physiopedia&utm_
medium=search&utm_campaign=ongoing_
internal (accessed 20 September 2020).

PubChem (2022a). Oxygen. https://pubchem.
ncbi.nlm.nih.gov/compound/977 (accessed
17 September 2022).

PubChem (2022b). Ozone. https://pubchem.
ncbi.nlm.nih.gov/compound/24823 (accessed
5 September 2022).

Purves, D., Augustine, G., FitzPatrick, D. et al.
(2012a). Electrical signals of nerve cells. In:
Neuroscience, 5e, 25–40. Sunderland, MA:
Sinauer Associates.

Purves, D., Augustine, G., FitzPatrick, D. et al.
(2012b). Lower motor neuron circuits and
motor control. In: *Neuroscience*, 5e, 343–374.
Sunderland, MA: Sinauer Associates.

Purves, D., Augustine, G., FitzPatrick, D. et al.
(2012c). Pain. In: *Neuroscience*, 5e, 209–227.
Sunderland, MA: Sinauer Associates.

Purves, D., Augustine, G., FitzPatrick, D. et al.
(2012d). The somatic sensory system: touch
and proprioception. In: *Neuroscience*, 5e,
189–227. Sunderland, MA: Sinauer Associates.

Reinders, M. and Haghighat, S. (2019). Modified
platelet rich plasma (PRP) for cruciate
ligament injuries in dogs. https://ivcjournal.
com/prp-cruciate-ligament-injuries (accessed
5 May 2020).

Reusch, W. (2013). Photochemistry. https://
www2.chemistry.msu.edu/faculty/reusch/
VirtTxtJml/photchem.htm (accessed
10 January 2023).

Rivera, P. (2015). *Introduction to Veterinary
Spinal Manipulation: Lecture and Notes,
Modules 1–5*. Sturtevant, WI: Healing Oasis
Wellness Center.

Seaman, D. and Faye, L.J. (2005). The vertebral
subluxation complex. In: *Foundations in
Chiropractic Subluxation*, 2e (ed.
M.I. Gatterman), 195–226. St. Louis, MO:
Elsevier Mosby.

Shah, J., Thaker, N., Heimur, J. et al. (2015).
Myofascial trigger points then and now: a

historical and scientific perspective. *Physical
Medicine and Rehabilitation* 7 (7): 746–761.

Shallenberger, F. (2011). Prolozone™:
regenerating joints and eliminating pain.
Journal of Prolotherapy 3 (2): 630–638.

Shields, H., Traa, A., and Raamsdonk, K.V.
(2021). Beneficial and detrimental effects of
reactive oxygen species on lifespan: a
comprehensive review of comparative and
experimental studies. *Frontiers in Cell and
Developmental Biology* 9: 628157.

Shmalberg, J., Burgess, J., and Davies, W.
(2014). A randomized controlled blinded
clinical trial of electro-acupuncture
administered one month after cranial cruciate
ligament repair in dogs. *American Journal
of Traditional Chinese Veterinary Medicine*
9 (2): 43–51.

Shurkin, J. (2014). News feature: animals that
self-medicate. *Proceedings of the National
Academy of Sciences of the United States of
America* 111 (49): 17339–17341.

Sineshchekov, V. (1995). Photobiophysics and
photobiochemistry of the heterogeneous
phytochrome system. *Biochimica et Biophysica
Acta Bioenergetics* 1228 (2–3): 125–164.

Trefil, J., Bertsch, G., and McGrayne, S.B. (2022).
Atom. https://www.britannica.com/science/
atom (accessed 29 September 2022).

Tresoldi, I., Oliva, F., Benvenuto, M. et al. (2013).
Tendon's ultrastructure. *Muscles, Ligaments
and Tendons Journal* 3 (1): 2–6.

Villines, Z. (2017). What is sclerotherapy?
https://www.medicalnewstoday.com/
articles/320282 (accessed 2 May 2020).

Vitz, E., Moore, J.W., Shorb, J., et al. (2022). 8.14:
Alcohols. https://chem.libretexts.org/
Bookshelves/General_Chemistry/Book%3A_
ChemPRIME_(Moore_et_al.)/08%3A_
Properties_of_Organic_Compounds/8.14%3A_
Alcohols (accessed 29 September 2022).

WFC (World Federation of Chiropractic) (2001).
Definition of chiropractic. https://www.wfc.
org/website/index.php?option=com_content
&view=article&id=90&Itemid=110 (accessed
8 July 2020).

Wiley (2002). Redox reactions. https://www.wiley.com/college/boyer/0470003790/reviews/redox/redox.htm (accessed 26 September 2022).

Wynn, S. and Fougère, B. (2007a). The roots of veterinary biomedicine. In: *Veterinary Herbal Medicine* (ed. S.G. Wynn and B. Fougère), 33–49. St. Louis, MO: Mosby Elsevier.

Wynn, S. and Fougère, B. (2007b). *Veterinary Herbal Medicine*. St. Louis, MO: Mosby Elsevier.

Xie, H. (2011). Chronicle of Chinese history and traditional Chinese veterinary medicine. In: *Xie's Chinese Veterinary Herbology*, 558–591. Ames, IA: Wiley-Blackwell.

Xie, H. (2015). *Dr. Xie's Lecture Notes*, 1–176. Reddick, FL: Jing Tang Publishing.

Xie, H. and Preast, V. (2007a). Diagnostic systems and pattern differentiation. In: *Traditional Chinese Veterinary Medicine: Fundamental Principles*, 249–303. Reddick, FL: Chi Institute Press.

Xie, H. and Preast, V. (2007b). Etiology and pathology. In: *Traditional Chinese Veterinary Medicine: Fundamental Principles*, 249–303. Reddick, FL: Chi Institute Press.

Xie, H. and Preast, V. (2007c). Five element theory. In: *Traditional Chinese Veterinary Medicine: Fundamental Principles*, 27–62. Reddick, FL: Chi Institute Press.

Xie, H. and Preast, V. (2007d). Qi, Shen, Jing, blood, and body fluid. In: *Traditional Chinese Veterinary Medicine: Fundamental Principles*, 69–100. Reddick, FL: Chi Institute Press.

Xie, H. and Preast, V. (2007e). The meridians. In: *Traditional Chinese Veterinary Medicine: Fundamental Principles*, 149–204. Reddick, FL: Chi Institute Press.

Xie, H. and Preast, V. (2007f). Yin and Yang. In: *Traditional Chinese Veterinary Medicine: Fundamental Principles*, 1–24. Reddick, FL: Chi Institute Press.

Xie, H. and Preast, V. (2007g). Zang-Fu Physiology. In: *Traditional Chinese Veterinary Medicine: Fundamental Principles*, 105–114. Reddick, FL: Chi Institute Press.

Zhao, J., Geng, T., Wang, Q. et al. (2015). Pharmacokinetics of Ginkgolide B after oral administration of three different Ginkgolide B formulations in beagle dogs. *Molecules* 20 (11): 20031–20041.

Index

Page numbers in italics indicate *figures* and bold indicate **tables**.

Integrative Medicine in Veterinary Practice, First Edition. Lisa P. McFaddin.
© 2024 John Wiley & Sons, Inc. Published 2024 by John Wiley & Sons, Inc.
Companion website: www.wiley.com/go/mcfaddin/integrativemedicine